Chaos in Medicine: Source Readings

Dedication

To our parents
Ruth and Joseph Sataloff
and
Jean and Paul Hawkshaw

Chaos in Medicine: Source Readings

Robert T. Sataloff, MD, DMA
Professor
Department of Otolaryngology—Head and Neck Surgery
Thomas Jefferson University
Chairman, Department of Otolaryngology—Head and Neck Surgery
Graduate Hospital
Adjunct Professor
Department of Otorhinolaryngology—Head and Neck Surgery
The University of Pennsylvania
Adjunct Professor of Otolaryngology
Department of Otolaryngology—Head and Neck Surgery
Georgetown University
Chairman, Board of Directors
The Voice Foundation
Chairman, American Institute for Voice and Ear Research
Faculty, Academy of Vocal Arts
Faculty, The Curtis Institute of Music
Philadelphia, Pennsylvania

Mary Hawkshaw, RN, BSN, CORLN
Otolaryngologic Nurse-Researcher
Executive Director
American Institute for Voice and Ear Research
Philadelphia, Pennsylvania

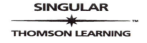
SINGULAR
THOMSON LEARNING

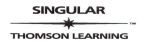

Chaos in Medicine: Source Readings

Robert T. Sataloff, MD, DMA
Mary Hawkshaw, RN, BSN, CORLN

Health Care Publishing Director: William Brottmiller
Acquisitions Editor: Candice Janco
Development Editor: Kristin Banach
Executive Marketing Manager: Dawn F. Gerrain
Channel Manager: Tara Carter

Project Editor: Patricia Gillivan
Production Editor: James Zayicek
Art/Design Coordinator: Timothy J. Conners .
Marketing Manager: Kathryn Bamberger

Printed in the United States
1 2 3 4 5 XXX 05 04 02 01 00

For more information contact Singular Publishing Group,
401 West "A" Street,
Suite 325
San Diego, CA 92101.

Or find us on the World Wide Web at
http://www.singpub.com

For permission to use material from this text or product,
contact us by
Tel (800) 730-2214
Tax (800) 730-2215
www.thomsonrights.com

Library of Congress Cataloging-in-Publication Data
Chaos in medicine : source readings / [edited by] Robert T. Sataloff, Mary Hawkshaw.
   p.   cm.
  Includes bibliographical references and index.
  ISBN 1-56593-953-0 (hardcover : alk. paper)
  1. Chaotic behavior in systems. 2. Medicine—Mathematical models. 3. Fractals. I. Sataloff, Robert Thayer. II. Hawkshaw, Mary.
  [DNLM: 1. Nonlinear Dynamics—Collected Works. 2. Fractals—Collected Works. Q 172.5.C45 C4605 2001]
R852.C445 2001
610'.1'514742—dc21

00-029135

NOTICE TO THE READER

Contents

Preface

This book is one of a series of collections of Source Readings scheduled for publication by Singular Publishing Group, Inc., San Diego, California. This ambitious publishing project was designed to make important, classic articles on chaos theory and its applications in the numerous fields of medicine readily available for interested readers. For many subjects, selection of articles required the mature perspective of experienced clinicians and scientists. Only such experts are able to digest centuries of literature and select germinal articles that have influenced the field. In the area of chaos theory and its biological applications, the task was easier. This remarkable science is new, and biological application is just being explored. Nevertheless, important articles have already been written by farsighted scientists and they appear in diverse sources and are often difficult to find. This book was prepared in order to make many of the existing articles pertaining to biological applications of nonlinear dynamic theory easily available to researchers and clinicians in diverse specialities. The editors hope that this text will not only prove interesting, but will also facilitate research by making it easier for biomedical researchers to find out what clinical practice and research has already been reported, what works and what does not. This should inspire new approaches and prevent repetition of mistakes that have already been made.

We believe that the new understanding of biological systems and how they function has been made possible through application of chaos theory and is of critical importance to future advances in medical science. Many of the articles included in this text have already made important contributions in clinical care. We are confident that many more insights and advances are forth-coming. We hope that this collection of articles makes such new discoveries and applications a little easier, and perhaps makes them arrive a little bit faster than they might have otherwise.

The editors are most indebted to several colleagues who facilitated the completion of this book. We express our thanks and appreciation to our colleague Rajeev Bhatia for his ideas, consultation, and collaboration in our first writings on this subject. We are also indebted to Helen Caputo for her expert preparation of the manuscript. We express appreciation to B. B. Mandelbrot who pioneered chaos theory, to James Gleick whose classic book originally developed our interest in chaos and to the many other colleagues who have shared our fascination with nonlinear dynamic theory and enhanced our involvement in the field. We express a special thanks to Dr. Sadanand Singh for his willingness to publish this series of Source Readings in general, and this book in particular. His willingness to publish works of academic importance has added much to the literature and exemplifies the highest traditions of publishing.

Robert Thayer Sataloff, MD, DMA   **Mary Hawkshaw,** RN, BSN, CORLN

Introduction

M. Hawkshaw and R.T. Sataloff

As we begin a new century, despite all the research and technical achievements in science (particularly medicine), there remain large gaps in our understanding of how the human body works. Scientists are still searching for explanations for "erratic" and unpredictable behavior by attempting to create adequate models of instability.

Chaos or nonlinear dynamics is a young science that is shedding light on an apparent inner order to seemingly random phenomena. Chaos is a nonlinear, predictable order of actions or events that lacks periodic repetition. This relatively new field is fascinating to those who seek better understanding of constantly fluctuating systems in medicine such as the heart's electrical system and the human voice in medicine, as well as the weather, and even the stock market!

Nonlinear dynamic theory provides a means of describing the complex interactions of mathematical, physical and biological systems that exhibit nonlinear characteristics. The distinct and complementary mathematical concepts of fractals and chaos are central to nonlinear dynamics theory. Gleick[1] has provided a particularly good introduction to chaos theory and fractal dimensions which is commercially available. Other excellent nontechnical introductions are also available.[2-12]

The articles by Denton, et al, Herzel, et al, Baken and others included in this book provide useful introductions to nonlinear dynamic theory, and additional references. Denton's article also contains a working glossary of terms, as well as a review of five important aspects of nonlinear dynamics: phase plane plots, poincare sections, return maps, fractal dimension, and spectral analysis. Familiarity with and comprehension of the terminology and basic concepts underlying this science are critical groundwork for anyone interested in further readings and study.

In medicine, chaos and nonlinear dynamics have been used to investigate complex problems plaguing cardiology, neurology, epidemiology, endocrinology, immunology, gerentology, voice and other disciplines.

Fractals, and particularly fractal dimensions appear useful for quantifying nonlinearities in biological systems. To understand the application of nonlinear dynamics, one must first understand that fractals are a spectral concept. For review, lines, rectangles, triangles, and cubes are **regular** structures. Fractals are **irregular** but they possess an underlying pattern or regularity to their irregularity. Simply, fractals are data sets that remain similar at all scales. Many authors have suggested that fractal dimensions may serve as a useful clinical index by helping to describe and quantify pathologic changes even at the cellular level that have previously been presumed aberrant and random. Clinical applications are already being used in cardiology, neurology, and other fields, as illustrated in articles appearing in this text. We believe that the potential for clinical applications is limitless.

BIBLIOGRAPHY

1. Gleick, J. *Chaos: Making a new science.* Viking Penguin Inc., NY, 1987.
2. Gulick, D. *Encounters with Chaos.* McGraw-Hill, Inc., NY, 1992.
3. Mandelbrot, B.B. *Fractals: Form, chance and dimension.* Freeman Press, NY, NY, 1977.
4. Stewart, I. *Does God play dice? The mathematics of chaos.* Basil Blackwell, Limited, NY, NY, 1989.
5. Barnsley, M.P. *Fractals everywhere.* Academic Press. San Diego, CA.: 1988.
6. Briggs, J. *Fractals. The patterns of chaos, discovering a new aesthetic of art, science and nature.* Touchstone. Simon and Schuster, NY: 1992.
7. Farmer, J.D. *Dimension, fractal measures and chaotic dynamics in evolution of order and chaos.* Editor: H. Haken; Springer-Verlag, NY, 1982.
8. Ferris, T. *The University and Eye. Making sense of the new science.* Chronicle Books, CA; 1992.
9. Hawkin, S. *A brief history of time. From the big bang to black holes.* Bantam Books. USA; 1988.
10. Peitgen, H.O. Richter, P.H. *The beauty of fractals.* Springer-Verlag, NY; 1986.
11. Stauffer, D., Stanley, H.E. *From Newton to Mandelbrot. The primer in theoretic physics.* Springer-Verlag, NY; 1990.
12. Stewart, I. *Does God play with dice? The mathematics of chaos.* Basal-Blackwell Limited, NY; 1989.

Application of Chaos Theory in Biomedical Research: An Overview

R.T. Sataloff, M. Hawkshaw, R. Bhatia

Inspired by the successful early application of nonlinear dynamics theory to the electrophysiology of the heart and frustrated by the failure of conventional statistical or stochastic approaches to compute the inherent morphological or temporal nonlinearities present in biological systems, biomedical researchers have turned to fractals (particularly the use of the fractal dimension) as a method of quantifying these inherent nonlinearities. A broad overview of the use of fractals in biomedical research can be found in the June 1992 issue of the IEEE Engineering in Medicine and Biology.[1,2]

Both morphological and temporal nonlinear complexity in biological systems have been quantified successfully with the use of fractals. It is noteworthy that there is a wide variety of methods employed to calculate fractal dimension.[2] Researchers seeking to quantify morphological (geometric) nonlinearities in biological systems have typically computed the fractal dimension using the box-counting algorithm for digitized data.[3] Temporal nonlinearities have been successfully quantified in biological systems by computing fractal dimension using the D algorithm developed by Grassberger and Procaccia for discrete time data samples.[4] Examples of the use of fractals in quantifying the morphological and temporal nonlinear complexity in biological systems are growing in number and importance.

As previously stated, modern chaos theory has wide application to various biological phenomena with fractal analysis now being used as a measurement of complexity. It is being applied by scientists, researchers, and physicians as we continue to study changes in man, from fetal life through senescence. Review of the literature yields many biological applications of chaos theory. Fractal analysis appears useful in understanding and quantifying structure, function, and even texture of various body systems that have previously been difficult or impossible to study adequately. It seems particularly important at the cellular level where scientists examine structure, ion exchange, protein sequences and their dynamics, DNA, genetics, fluidity and transport, and diffusion kinetics. Scientists and physicians continue to pursue the explanations for currently unexplainable events, for example, sudden death due to ventricular fibrillation. Current investigations of chaotic dynamics and fractal architectures in the human body are shedding light on such occurrences, challenging long-held principles of medicine, and revealing possible methods of predicting disease.

GENERAL AND MOLECULAR BIOMEDICAL RESEARCH

Some of the most interesting and early research into the applications of chaos theory has taken place in the study of human biology and medicine. Biology and medicine have many poorly understood problems such as lethal cardiac arrhythmias and epileptic seizures. Chaotic systems, such as the heart's electrical system and the nervous system, can now be quantified by calculating the correlation dimension of a sample of data which the systems generate.

The point correlation dimension in biologic calculations is advantageous in that it does not presume a stationary state. This enables researchers to track the transient nonstationary events that occur routinely in constantly variable biologic systems. Skinner et al[5] found that dimensional measurements appeared far more sensitive and accurate in evaluating stochastic events as compared to the standard deviation and power spectrum measures employed traditionally. They also suggest that deterministic measurements are far more accurate in quantifying time-series measurements. Sadanna and Madagula[6] also employed fractal analysis in their investigations of the time-dependent binding rate coefficients on external diffusion limited kinetics. They found the fractal approach was conducive to analyzing reactions in a low dimensional environment. Their analyses suggest a frame-work for estimation of the effects of external diffusion limitations and variable absorption rate coefficients on the attachment of antigen-antibody in first-order systems.

The application of fractal analysis in the interpretation of the diminution curves occurring in the estimation of membrane transport has also been investigated. Bassingthwaighte et al[7] believe that the fractal approach removes bias in the estimation of permeability-surface area products for capillary and cell membranes, thus reducing random error. They developed a rather novel approach to describing heterogeneity of regional blood flows, by fractals, in space and time. They suggest that when estimating regional flows, cutting of the organ's tissues into finer segments reveals broader heterogeneity. Their research focused on fractal analysis of the structures in biology, and it is hoped that their methodology will allow for useful comparison of data between laboratories. Solovyev[8] based his research on the graphical representation of sequences which suggest a global view of sequence features. He believes that the graphical images of sequences are readily compared both visually and by computer models. His work suggests new patterns of recognition for the classifying of particular genome functional regions. He also suggests that his graphic model can be used in the investigation of both DNA and protein genetics.

Researchers Li, Li, and Zhao[9] present a practical method for characterizing confirmation of protein chains, which are neither strictly random fabrication of co-polymers nor regularly recurrent. They do, however, have statistical self-similarities, and thus can be characterized by fractal dimension. The authors suggest that fractal dimensions will be useful in the interpretation of thermodynamic properties, reaction kinetics, and catalysis of protein molecules, especially enzymes. They also propose applications of fractal dimensions may be quite helpful in the study of the allosteric enzymes. Researchers EL-Jaick and Wajnberg[10] have also focused their efforts on the application of fractal analysis to the study of protein dynamics. They put forth a model, based on fractal concepts, for analysis of the photolysis of nitrosyl hemoglobin. In their previous research, they have shown that the kinetic curve of photolysis of nitrosyl hemoglobin, obtained by electron paramagnetic resonance at low temperatures, is fitted equally well by a biphasic exponential and a distribution of activation energies. Their research shows that photodissociation experiments may be interpreted by use of a fractal model. The fractal dimension is sensitive to the quaternary conformation of the protein. It is their hope that the fractal model will serve as a framework for further study of protein dynamics. Liebovitch and Sullivan[11] have proposed a model of ion channel kinetics based on the fractal model. In their fractal model, closed and open states are represented as a continuum of many conformational states. Their model shows value in their description of the open and closed time, and the voltage dependence of channel gating.

Smith et al[12] have focused their research efforts also at the cellular level with greater concentration on structure. They studied the morphologic shapes of the borders of central nervous system neurons grown as a monolayer in cell culture. Their findings showed that cells with simple, uncomplicated structure had a small fractal dimension and cells with a complex structure have large fractal dimension. They remind us that fractal dimension alone does not completely describe the cell's morphology; but in combination with other measures it may serve as an adjunct in the measurement of more complex cell structure.

Further review of the literature reveals an emergence in the study of chaos and complexity and the application of fractal analysis in almost all the disciplines of human anatomy, biology and physiology. Much of the research focuses on cellular identification and tissue classification. For example, MacAulay and Palcic[13] have applied the technique of fractal dimension in the evaluation of the nuclear features of stained cells of the human uterine cervix.

Along with physiologists, physicians have also begun to quantify the possibilities of chaotic dynamics and fractal architectures in the human body. Glenny et al[14] have focused their energies on the application of various fractal measurements of correlation in spatial properties and temporal fluctuations, by comparing the regional heterogeneities of pulmonary and myocardial blood flows. Goldberger et al[15] suggest that chaos in bodily functions signals health, and periodic behavior can forewarn disease. They strongly suggest continued investigation of how developmental processes lead to construction of fractal architectures, and how the dynamic processes in the body generate apparent chaos.

CARDIOLOGY

Janse[17] in his article "Is there chaos in cardiology?" reviews modern chaos theory and its wide application to various biological phenomena, in particular the electrophysiologic system of the heart. He believes that chaos theory might be extremely useful in the study of ventricular fibrillation and its predictors. He suggests that if ventricular fibrillation is found to be chaotic, that would suggest there might be a single mechanism at work in potentially lethal arrhythmias. He believes a great deal can be expected from further studies applying chaos theory to cardiac rhythms and hopefully, more insight will be gained into the early identification of individuals at high risk for sudden cardiac death. His research also shows that chaotic behavior can be induced in cardiac tissue. Although he is enthusiastic about applying modern chaos theory to cardiology, he cautions us not to forget our knowledge of "old fashioned electrophysiology".

Denton et al[17] in their article "Fascinating Rhythm", have written an excellent primer and introduction to the application of chaos theory in the science of cardiology. They provide a generally good review of chaos;

what it is; what causes it; and how to detect it. These authors reviewed the five tools of modern linear dynamics including phase plane plots, return maps, Poincare sections, fractal dimensions and spectral analysis. They detail the way in which nonlinear systems can become chaotic and they apply these findings to cardiac arrhythmias. Their article also provides a very useful glossary of terms.

Rambihar[18] reminds us that the laws of nonlinear dynamics describe an essential and inherent unpredictability in systems. She too believes that chaos and complexity offer a model for understanding the variety, variability and unpredictability seen in cardiology. She suggests that a greater understanding of the role of chaos and chance in clinical medicine leads us to believe that we may have a variable degree of impact on individual systems and outcome.

Stein and Kligfield[19] too, have focused their research effort the understanding of cardiac arrhythmia and sudden death. They suggest that the distribution of an individual's premature ventricular contractions over time is best represented by a particular kind of fractal known as the fractal dust. This enables one to measure dimension for purposes of quantification of uniformity or non-uniformity of an individual's ectopic heart beats. In their study group of patients with congestive heart failure, dimension was found to have prognostic significance. Berenfeld et al[20] have also focused their research on the heart's conduction system. They remind us that the Purkinje fibers (part of the heart's electrical system) share structures common to a tree with repeatedly bifurcating branches that decrease in length with each generation. Assuming that this bifurcating and decreasing process is the same at each generation, the heart's conduction system is a fractal tree. They developed a model of a heart's ventricles which reflects the QRS complex exhibiting a form of an inverse power law that was predicted by the fractal depolarization hypothesis. They then studied the frequency spectrum of the QRS complex and reported that its high frequency enhancement increased as generations were added to the conduction system. The results of their research showed that the slope of the inverse power law might be a useful index of spectral reserve, adding to the list of useful physiologic parameters.

Vasomotion, or the fluctuation in blood vessel diameter, seems amenable to fractal analysis, as well. The nature of these fluctuations at first appear to be random, but have readily observable periodicities. It is the apparent randomness that had made the application of amplitude and frequency measurements currently in use, difficult. Yamashiro et al[21] questioned whether this apparent randomness is actually the result of a low-dimensional nonlinear system. They applied fractal analysis to vasomotion data, and their findings suggest that a model is needed with at least two coupled relaxation oscillators for more accurate explanation.

Herzel, who has written some of the germinal articles in nonlinear dynamics theory related to voice, has also provided important observations in research on the heart, respiration and baroreflex.[22] Herzel observed that the interaction of heartbeat, respiration and carotid sinus nerve stimulation may induce complicated trains of heart beat intervals under normal circumstances. Also, respiratory and cardiac rhythms are not entrained, although slight interactions occur, such as sinus arrhythmia. However, under abnormal circumstances such as extremely rapid respiration (which approaches heart rate), entrainments on bifurcations and presumably chaotic cardiac rhythms are observed. Herzel describes characteristic sequences or heart beat intervals that display bifurcations. It appears that respiration and cardiac rate interactions can be classified in terms of entrainment zones and bifurcations, which may give useful insights into the dynamics of the system. Elegantly, Herzel also identified the attractor in this system, finding it topologically equivalent to an electrocardiographic time series. In related research, Warzel et al[23] studied the dependence of heart period on carotid sinus nerve stimulation at different positions of the cardiac and respiratory cycles, and looked at influences, such as the effect of alcohol on the heart's rate and rhythm. Doublings were identified, and nonlinear dynamic theory provided the best method of data analysis. In follow up research, Seidel et al[24] studied phase dependencies of the human baroreflex. In this research, the authors credit the influence of respiratory and sinus node phase on the effects of baroreceptor stimulation, measured indirectly from electrocardiographic changes of heart period. This research, built upon their previous work on a nonlinear model, depicts the short-term dynamics of the baroreceptor control loop.[25] Their research indicated that the phase response period which depends upon both respiratory and sinus node phase can be represented as the product of two independent factors. They also found that the measured phase response curve of the sinus node is the integration of its response during the length of the stimulus cycle. This research evolved from prior work in nonlinear dynamics and moves toward more physiologically representative baroreceptor loop modelling.

Review of the cardiology literature also shows that fractal analysis of fetal heart rate variability, arterial pressure oscillations, and echocardiographic images is ongoing.[26-28]

NEUROLOGY

Most of the research in neurology has been focused on interpretation of electroencephalogram EEG signals and in research of the complicated soma-dendritic borders of the cerebral cortex neurons. Fractal analysis has been applied to EEG data since the mid-1980s.

Bullmore, et al. proposed a method of fractal analysis that offers significant operational advantages over previously published techniques, and they illustrate the application of this method to the quantification of ictal EEG changes.[29] They suggest that further development of their methodology will lead to advanced definition of initial ictal changes in the EEG and synaptic visualization of long periods of EEG data. Mandelbrot[30] reported that the pyramidal neurons in the mammalian cerebral cortex can be described by fractal dimension, which provides quantitative objective measurements of the soma-dendritic borders. Porter, et al. studied the fractal dimensions of the cell's border and reported measurements via camera lucida reconstructions of cat and monkey neurons in the motor cortex sending axons into the pyramidal tract.[31] They found statistically significant differences among the fractal dimensions of several different neuronal types which may be relevant, given the nature of their physiologic function.

VASCULAR SYSTEM

The fractal branching model has been applied to the study of the pulmonary vasculature, renal and retinal circulation, along with the cardiac system. Cross, et al. set out to determine whether the renal arterial system was a fractal structure.[32] The renal arterial tree is a branching structure in which the small peripheral branches have a similar appearance to the larger divisions. Thus, it is considered subjectively self-similar. These researchers successfully employed fractal geometry to describe the renal arterial tree, and they assessed the utility of fractal dimension as a measurement of normality in the kidney. The method appears useful, and they believe their methodology can be applied to vascular "trees" elsewhere in the body.

Wang and Wang[33] have focused their research on the practicality of applying fractal analysis in the interpretation of doppler ultrasound signals. They found that the fractal dimension curve of doppler signals corresponds with the maximum frequency curve of those signals. As we know, doppler signals are time domain signals whose horizonal coordinates and vertical coordinates have different dimensions. Wang and Wang's method normalizes time and amplitude of a signal wave form. This enabled them to utilize the method of calculating the fractal dimensions of graphs that are used to analyze the fractal dimensions of time domain signals.

OPHTHALMOLOGY

It is generally believed that the higher the fractal dimension, the more complex the pattern. Morigawa, Tauchi, and Fukuda demonstrated in their research that the ganglion cells of the rat's retina, which exhibit dendric branching, in fact have fractal structures.[34] They examined how fractal dimension varies in cells undergoing developmental changes. Also using animal models, Smith and Behar[35] studied glial cell maturity and compared it to the growth of fractal dimension. They found that fractal dimension did correlate, and increased in value as the glial cells matured. They also examined self-similarity by determining the fractal dimension of cells over a range of magnifications. Their research showed that fractal dimension remained constant over a tenfold range in optical magnification. They suggest that fractal dimension analysis along with traditional histologic and immunologic assays will augment cellular assessment.

Studying oligodendrocytes or Type II astrocytes from neonatal rat optic nerves, they confirmed that fractal dimension correlated with perceived complexity and increased as glial cells matured. Thus fractal dimension appears to be a useful and consistent descriptor for quantifying complexity in this system.[36]

Wingate et al[37] in studying the retinal ganglion cells of the ferret employed fractal measurements in the characterization and classification of cells, and also found chaos theory appropriate and useful.

PULMONARY

Pulmonary research has focused primarily on the fractal dimension of the lung's arterial system. It has been shown that the fractal dimension of the pulmonary arteries of normal control lungs was higher than that of those with pulmonary arterial hypertension.[38] These researchers also found that the fractal dimension of the pulmonary arteries of hypoxic and hyperoxic lungs was not significantly different. They suggest that the fractal character of the pulmonary arteries may be related to the mechanism of their tree-like formation. The major airways are developed by approximately the sixteenth week of gestation from dichotomous branching of the diverticulum. The self-similar branching of the pulmonary arteries may result from a self-similar pattern of morphogenesis.

Witten and his team of researchers[39] performed fractal and morphometric analysis of lung structures in beagle puppies after causing canine adenovirus II-induced bronchiolitis. They found that fractal analysis gave additional information about the changes in lung function after a viral illness and compared it to standard morphometric techniques. Using fractal analysis, they attempted to determine whether the canine adenovirus II-induced bronchiolitis altered the puppies' lung growth. They also compared the sensitivity of fractal analysis to standard morphometric techniques. Using fractal analysis, they attempted to determine whether the canine adenovirus II-induced bronchiolitis altered the puppies' lung growth. They also compared the sensitivity of fractal analysis to standard morphometrics used in the assessment of lung function after a viral infection. Fractal analysis showed an increased fractal dimension D_1 of the alveolar perimeter length in the CAV2 group associated with increased growth that was similar to the percentage of V_1 and ISA, where V_1 is lung volume by water displacement and ISA is internal surface area. This information suggests that the single viral infection in the puppies accelerated their lung growth and increased the complexity of the alveolar surface.

RADIOLOGY

Some very interesting research has taken place in the field of radiology. Texture analysis of medical radiographs has been a subject of interest for many years. Visible texture represents the summation of the attenuation from numerous thin plates of bone. Lynch and colleagues[40] have utilized fractal signature in the analysis of texture in macroradiographs of osteoarthritic knees. By variation of the fractal dimension with resolution, the fractal signature indicates how images deviate from fractal surfaces. They further developed the texture analysis method by using the fractal signature that withstood changes in image acquisition and digitization. Their findings indicate that peaks in the fractal signature (heightened position) matched the visual assessment of the degree of the arthritic changes seen in the knee.

Retinal blood flow has also been evaluated through the interpretations of retinal angiograms. Landini et al[41] measured the fractal dimension of the retinal vasculature, isolating venous and arterial trees in the review of twenty-three routine, fluorescein angiograms of normal retinas. The estimated fractal dimension showed no significant difference between isolated venous and arterial trees, which is not supported by previous reports. They found fractal analysis to be an easy method for evaluating the images of the branching structures of the retina. Moreover, they proposed that diseases which alter the distribution of the retinal vasculature, such as proliferative retinopathies, would also change their fractal dimensions.

Grant and Lunsden[42] attempted to quantify perfusion by interpretation of computerized tomography (CT) images. They reviewed CT images of the canine renal cortex to determine whether the heterogenous pixel intensity patterns were amenable to fractal analysis and whether fractal analysis could be used as a method of quantification. They concluded that fractal dimension was a sound means for examining the invivo organization of the kidney's vascular perfusion by quantifying pixel heterogeneity in CT images.

Priebe and his colleagues[43] have applied fractal analysis to the interpretation of mammographic images of breast tissue. They developed a pattern recognition technique which used features derived from the fractal nature of the image. In comparing the medical images of malignant vs. non-malignant breast tissue, their results indicate that discrimination based on the fractal analysis represents a viable approach to using computers to assist in diagnosis.

DENTISTRY

Oshida and his research team[44] have used fractal dimension analysis in the study of surface texture of metallic materials commonly used in dentistry. These authors studied the effect of recycling aluminum oxide particles on the surface texture of metallic materials. Each week, the aluminum powder was sampled and analyzed for weight fraction and contaminants. The surface texture of sand blasted standard samples was also characterized by fractal dimension analysis. Results indicated that little change was seen in particle size despite an increase in fractal dimension.

VOICE

The application of chaos theory to voice analysis has already proven exciting and tantalizing. Voice research has been plagued by the existence of numerous, apparently random, unpredictable aspects of phonation. These have defied measurements and study. Chaos has helped address these problems. As Baken points out, it is important to remember that the existence of a noninteger fractal dimension by itself is not an indicator that the nonlinearity exhibited by a biological system can be characterized as being chaotic.[45] Baken reminds us that the following criteria must be satisfied before the behavior of a nonlinear system can be classified as being chaotic:

1. The behavior of the system is the product of a deterministic nonlinear system. There must exist some nonlinear rule(s) that govern the behavior of the system.
2. Despite the determinism of the generating system, the output of the system must nonetheless be unpredictable.
3. The behavior of the system must be sensitive to initial conditions.

From an implementation perspective, for a system to be considered chaotic, it must have not only a noninteger fractal dimension but more importantly its behavior must be describable by the presence of strange attractors as generated by phase plane plots, return maps or it must show evidence of bifurcations.

Baken further reports that several researchers working independently have yielded evidence of the chaotic nature of voice production.[46] Bifurcation behavior has been observed in mathematical models of phonatory function, normal infant cry, and the abnormal phonation of adults with demonstrable laryngeal disorders. Awrejcewicz has shown that an important class of laryngeal models is chaotic, producing bifurcations.[47] Wong and Ito have demonstrated that a hybrid of Ishizaka-Flanagan and Titze models is also chaotic and produces outputs that mimic important characteristics of the voices of pathological larynges.[48] In addition, evidence of bifurcations observed in infant's cries have been reported by Mende and Herzel.[49] A few early works are worthy of particular attention.

In "Evidence of Chaos in Vocal Fold Vibration,"[50] Titze, Baken and Herzel describe the need in voice science for a method of summarizing all the dynamic properties of the vocal folds. Predictable physical phenomena are easily described by classical modeling methods. Unpredictable/unstable phenomena have proven highly refractory to such descriptions. Years of research have shown that vocal fold motion exhibits orderliness and underlying unity. These authors review the essential properties of chaotic systems, starting with a review of Poincare's seminal papers in topology which date back to 1891 and the early work of Mandelbrot in the late 1960s. They bring us up to date in the development of the science of nonlinear dynamics and fractal geometry. Their research efforts have certified the applicability of nonlinear dynamics to understanding vocal function.

In "Analysis of Vocal Disorders of Methods from Nonlinear Dynamics," Herzel, Berry, Titze and Saleh present simple techniques that will aid all voice researchers in identification of the nonlinear dynamics of voice signals.[51] Within the context of chaos theory, these authors attempt to clarify and standardize some of the terms that have been used in the literature to describe abnormal voice. It appears as if much of the terminology used to describe vocal "roughness" can be unified using nonlinear dynamics. They also suggest directions for future research. This practical article provides a first step in the transition between more complex chaos theory, and clinical application. It is incumbent upon the leaders in the field of chaos theory to provide such practical simplification. Only in this way will these new concepts be applied. Moreover, only such application and analysis of the resultant clinical data will clarify the true importance and utility of chaos theory in voice care.

This research has obvious applications for our understanding of control of phonation. Considering the speed at which phonatory events occur, the maximal speed of any given system has obvious implications for its ability to control specific phonatory functions. In addition, it is clinically important to note the nature of neural communication systems. They are obviously involved in respiration and phonation. Because of their speed, the activities which they control must be slow, relative to phonatory events such as high frequency vibratory margin vibration, but they are probably important. One may hypothesize that anything that

further slows, conduction might have a disportionate effect in a system which is also relatively slow in comparison with other body systems. This may help explain some of the disportionately great voice effects seen in patients who seem to have relatively minor pulmonary, thoracic or abdominal disease or injury, particularly those which alter rib cage and related functions.

Herzel, in "Bifurcations and Chaos in Voice Signals,"[52] examines speech production through speech synthesis and recognition. In this article, he reviews bifurcation and chaotic behavior that are apparent in voice signals. He also reviews the basic physiologic mechanism of speech production including the bifurcations seen in the newborn infant's cry and during voicing. He believes there is convincing evidence of voice bifurcations and low dimensional attractors in the voice signal. He also believes that fractal analysis will aid in diagnosis of voice disorders and vocal fold pathology.

In "Bifurcations in an Asymmetric Vocal Fold Model," Steinecke and Herzel reaffirm that normal voice contains periodic signals, and pathologic voice sounds contain many signal irregularities.[53] Acoustical analysis has shown voice to be a highly nonlinear, dynamic system. All existing models of vocal fold vibration exhibit chaos and bifurcations at different parameter values. These authors discuss a left to right asymmetry in a two mass model. They have shown through bifurcation analysis that the system is relatively stable against small deviations from normal parameters. However, sufficiently large right to left tension imbalances induce bifurcations to subharmonic regimes, toroidal oscillations and chaos. Bifurcations are located in parameter planes such as vocal fold stiffness and subglottal pressure.

In our opinion, these observations are consistent with clinical observations that the phonatory system can compensate for small, or even substantial, variations from normal. Since variations and initial conditions of this magnitude might be expected to cause greater effect in a predominantly chaotic system, this model helps clarify the combined effect of chaotic and periodic phenomena within the phonatory system. Intuitively, it also may help explain why minor changes in vocal fold condition are tolerated much more poorly by patients who have vocal fold injury. One might infer that, when such an injury impairs the periodic function of normal vocal fold vibration by inducing structural asymmetries, then the chaotic activity becomes more dominant; and any change in initial condition or phase plane thereafter results in a greater effect on phonatory output. In addition one might often cause about as much asymmetry as the system can handle, and even a little more (due to swelling from voice abuse, for example) will be enough to provoke pronounced chaotic behavior.

The property of nonlinearity, seen in nearly all biological systems, suggests the possibility of complex behavior and thus, the need for special control strategies for satisfactory function or performance. Fletcher points out that, in the vocal system, nonlinearity is observed in the multidimensional vocal fold vibrations and in the aerodynamics of flow through the vocal fold opening.[54] It is encountered in the interaction between these two quantities, as well. Considering the physical features of the vocal system that lead to complex behavior, Fletcher suggests that some strategies of control need to be employed to produce desired sound. Linear methods are insufficient to describe phonatory systems, but chaos theory shows promise in doing so, and concomitantly in allowing us to understand subtle complexities. Such precise descriptions and understandings are invaluable to the clinician. They allow us to analyze system function, pinpoint areas of failure in vocal behavior, articulate therapeutic strategies for the restoration of normal phonatory behavior when possible, and assess post-treatment success by comparing quantitated data.

Herzel states that voice instabilities/abnormalities include *hoarseness* which still remains the overall description for deviation from normal voice, and breathiness which is turbulent noise.[55] (NOTE: The editors (RTS and MH) disagree with Herzel's definitions of these terms, particularly the assertion that "hoarseness" may be used to describe abnormal voice in general.) Herzel has found that roughness especially can be analyzed using the framework of bifurcation theory and chaos. He believes that convincing evidence exists that a rough voice is intimately related to nonlinear dynamics such as period doubling. The goal of his research has been an attempt to achieve quantitative agreement between observations and computer simulation, developing methods for quantification of irregularities commonly seen in vocal fold dysfunction such as hoarseness, paralysis and masses. He employs two parameter bifurcation diagrams, mode concept, excised larynx studies and high speed digital imaging. This work is particularly important and interesting. It provides the clinician with the opportunity to understand the importance of asymmetries, the nature of their interference with phonatory function, and perhaps to quantify the degree of symmetry required for clinically satisfactory phonatory functions. When asymmetries are present at the vocal fold level, bifurcations and subharmonics are seen in areas of instability. There is also a relationship between the degree of asymmetry and subglottal pressure. Recognition of these phenomena provides the clinician with not only a new set of behaviors which are helpful for diagnostic purposes, but also a new set of measures to allow pretreatment/posttreatment comparisons for assessment of therapeutic efficacy.

Herzel's work has great potential clinical applications. If it can be demonstrated that selected pathological conditions result in chaotic phonatory events, then it should be possible to predict and explain their be-

havior more accurately, assess the degree of pathology (perhaps by comparing chaotic and periodic events in a voice sample) and model and/or simulate voice pathology. Although all previous attempts at computer diagnosis have failed, it would certainly be interesting to look at nonlinear dynamic phenomenon associated with certain types of pathology to determine whether they are consistent from case to case. Chaos theory provides another window for voice recognition and quantification and as such has great potential value in the clinical voice laboratory.

It is known that normal voice sound contains periodic signals. Steinecke and Herzel point out that pathologic voice sounds contain many signals irregularities.[56] Acoustical analysis has shown voice to be a highly nonlinear, dynamic system. Many models simulating vocal fold vibration exist.[57,58] All models exhibit chaos and bifurcations at different parameter values. These authors discuss a left to right asymmetry in a two mass model. They have shown that through bifurcation analysis, the analyzed system is relatively stable against small deviations from normal parameters. These observations are consistent with clinical observations that the phonatory system can compensate for small, or even substantial, variations from normal. The editors (RTS and MJH) believe this work is particularly important.

Voice irregularities are related to the intrinsic nonlinearities in vocal fold vibrations. Herzel et al. used narrow band spectrograms to analyze bifurcations and chaos in voice signals.[59] They have found that the human voice source exhibits several essential nonlinearities that include:

1. Nonlinear stress-strain characteristics of vocal fold tissue
2. Highly nonlinear relation between pressure and glottal area
3. Collision of the vocal folds
4. Vortices and jet instabilities

In simulations utilizing the two mass model, these researchers have shown that the various bifurcations appear to be due to the synchronization of the right and left vocal fold for over-critical asymmetry. The resulting instabilities are similar to those seen in patients with vocal fold paralysis.

From our clinical perspective, assuming that the nonlinearities are important in vocal function, and in the distinct and desirable acoustic output of the vocal mechanism in some situations, this research provides particularly interesting insights for the clinician. It shows that not only are chaotic activities present and potentially measurable, but also that they are intimately related to vocal fold synchronization and symmetry. It is essential for the physician to understand exactly what degree of symmetry is necessary to maintain such effects, and what aspects of vocal fold motion are critical. Such considerations are key in designing vocal fold therapy, especially surgery; and measurement of nonlinear functions restored following treatment may prove a valuable measure of the success of each intervention.

Sato et al point out that artificial voice sources differ from the human voice source in that human speech involves small wave forms and spectral fluctuations.[60] It has been shown that recurrent neural networks with arbitrary feedback are highly nonlinear dynamic systems. These researchers hypothesize that if recurrent networks could learn the voice source waveforms, including their chaotic aspects, and if they could reproduce them under some control, a recurrent net driven synthesizer could yield synthetic speech that would be much more natural. They tested their idea on computer simulation utilizing APOLONN, the recurrent network they chose. APOLONN was trained to generate voice source waveforms and to produce fluctuations of frequency and amplitude amongst 32 pitches.

CONCLUSION

It is clear that chaos theory and fractal analysis have been employed successfully in characterizing nonlinear behavior of biological systems. The articles that constitute the remainder of this book, and the references contained within those articles, constitute much of the original biomedical research utilizing nonlinear dynamic theory.

BIBLIOGRAPHY

1. Goldberger, A.L. *Fractal mechanisms in the electrophysiology of the heart.* IEEE Engineering in Medicine and Biology, 1992; 47–52.
2. Schepers, H.E., van Beek, J.H.G.M., Bassinghwaighte, J.B. *Four methods to estimate the fractal dimension from Self-Affine Signals.* IEEE Engineering in Medicine and Biology, 1992; 57–64.
3. Liebovitch, L.S., Toth, T.A. *A fast algorithm to determine fraction dimensions by box counting.* Physics Letter A, 1989; 141:386–390.
4. Grassberger, P, Procaccia, I. *Measuring the strangeness of strange attractors.* Physica 9D, 1983; 9:183–208.
5. Skinner, J.E., Molnar, M., Vybiral, P., Mitra, M. *Application of Chaos theory to biology and medicine.* Integrative Physiologic and Behavioral Science, Jan/Mar 1992; 27(1):39–53.
6. Sadanna, A., Madagula, A. *A fractal analysis of external diffusion limited first-order kinetics for the binding of antigen by immobilized antibody.* Biosensors and bioelectronics, 1994; 9:45–55.
7. Bassingthwaighte, J., King, R., Sambrook, J.E., van Steenwyk, B. *Fractal analysis of blood-tissue exchange kinetics.* Advances in Experimental Medicine and Biology, (ed) Mochizuki, Honig, Koyama, Goldstick, Bruely 1988; pp. 222:15–23.
8. Solovyev, V.D. *Fractal graphical representation and analysis of DNA and protein sequences.* Biosystems, 1993; 30:137–160.
9. Li, H., Li, Y., Zhao, H. *Fractal analysis of protein chain conformation.* International Journal of Biological Macromolecules, 1990; 12:6–8.
10. EL-Jaick, L.J., Wajnberg, E. *Fractal analysis of photolysis of nitrosyl haemoglobin at low temperatures.* International Journal of Biological Macromolecules, 1993; 15:119–123.
11. Liebovitch, L.S., Sullivan, J.M. *Fractal analysis of a voltage-dependent potassium channel from cultured mouse hippocampal neurons.* Biophysical Journal, 1987; 52:979–988.
12. Smith, T.G., Marks, W.B., Lange, G.D., Sheriff, W.H., Neale, E.A. *A fractal analysis of cell images.* Journal of Neuroscience Methods, 1989; 27:173–180.
13. MacAulay, C., Palcic, B. *Fractal texture features based on optical density of surface area used in imaging analysis of cervical cells.* Analytical and Quantitative Cytology and Histology, 1990; 12(6):394–398.
14. Glenny, R.W., Robertson, H.T., Yamashiro, S., Bassingthwaighte, J.B. *Applications of fractal analysis to physiology.* Journal of Applied Physiology, 1991; 70:2351–2367.
15. Goldberger, A., Rigney, D., West, B. *Chaos and Fractals in Human Physiology.* Scientific American, 1990; 43–49.
16. Janse, MJ. *Is there Chaos in cardiology?* British Heart Journal, 1992; 67(1):3–4.
17. Denton, T.A., Diamond, G.A., Helfant, R.H., Khan, S., Karagueuzian, H. *Fascinating rhythm: A primer on chaos theory and its application to cardiology.* American Heart Journal, 1990; 120(6)(part 1):1419–1439.
18. Rambihar, V. *Jurassic heart: from the heart to the edge of chaos.* Canadian Journal of Cardiology, Nov 1993; 9(9):787–788.
19. Stein, K., Kligfield, P. *Application of fractal geometry to the analysis of ventricular premature contractions.* Journal of Electrocardiology, 1990; 23(Supp):82–84.
20. Berenfeld, O., Sadeh, D., Abboud, S. *Modeling of the heart's ventricular conduction system using fractal geometry: spectral analysis of the QRS complex.* Annals of Biomedical Engineering, 1993; 21:125–134.
21. Yamashiro, S.M., Slaaf, D.W., Reneman, R.S., Tangelder, G.J., Bassingthwaighte, J.B. *Fractal analysis of vasomotion.* Annals New York Academy of Sciences, 1990; 591:410–416.
22. Herzel, H., Seidel, H., Warzel, H. *Heart Rate, Respiration, and Baroreflex: Entrainment, Bifurcations, and Chaos.* Wiss. Zeitschrift der Humboldt-Universitat zu Berlin, R. Medizin, 1992; 41(4):51–57.
23. Warzel, H., Seidel, H., Herzel, H. *Heart Rate, Respiration, and Baroreflex: Motivation and Experiments.* Wiss. Zeitschrift der Humboldt-Universitat zu Berlin, R. Medizine, 1992; 41(4):59–61.
24. Seidel, H., Herzel, H., Eckberg, D.L. *Phase dependencies of the human baroreflex.* Department of Physics, Technical University, Berlin, Germany, May 17, 1995 (submitted for publication.)
25. Seidel, H., Herzel, H. *Modeling heart rate variability due to respiration and baroreflex.* In E. Mosekilde and O.G. Mouritsen (eds.) Modeling the Dynamics of Biological Systems, Springer-Verlag, 1995, pp 205–229.
26. Griffith, T.M., Edwards, D.H., *Fractal analysis of role of smooth muscle Ca^{2+} fluxes in genesis of chaotic arterial pressure oscillations.* American Journal of Physiology, 1994; 226 (Heart Circ Physiol, 35): H1801–H1811.
27. Gough, N.A.J. *Fractal analysis of fetal heart rate variability.* Physiological Measurement, 1993; 14:309–315.
28. Verhoeven, J.T.M., Thijssen, J.M. *Potential fractal analysis for lesion detection in echographic images.* Ultrasonic Imaging, 1993; 15:304–323.
29. Bullmore, E., Brammer, M., Alarcon, G., Binnie, C. *A new technique for fractal analysis applied to human, intracerebrally recorded, ictal electroencephalographic signals.* Neuroscience Letters, 1992; 146:227–230.
30. Mandelbrot, B.B. *Fractal geometry of nature.* WH Freeman, NY, NY, 1982.
31. Porter, R., Ghosh, S., Lange, D.G., Smith, T.G. *A fractal analysis of pyramidal neurons in mammalian motor cortex.* Neuroscience Letters, 1991; 130(1);112–116.
32. Cross, S.S., Start, R.C., Silcocks, P.D., Bull, A.D., Cotton, D.W.K., Underwood, J.C. *Quantitation of the renal arterial tree by fractal analysis.* Journal of Pathology, 1993; 170:479–484.

33. Wang, Y.Y., Wang, W.Q. *Fractal concept and its analysis method of doppler ultrasound signals.* Ultrasound in Medicine and Biology, 1993; 19(8):661–666.

34. Morigiwa, K., Tauchi, M., Fukuda, Y. *Fractal analysis of ganglion cell dendritic branching patterns of the rat and cat retinae.* Neuroscience Research, 1989; Supp. 10:S131–S140

35. Smith, T.G., Behar, T.N. *Comparative fractal analysis of cultured glia derived from optic nerve and brain demonstrate different rates of morphological differentiation.* Brain Research, 1994; 634:181–190.

36. Smith, T.G., Behar, T.N., Lange, G.D., Marks, W.D., Sheriff, W.H. *The fractal analysis of cultured rat optic nerve glial growth and differentiation.* Neuroscience, 1991; 41(1):159–166.

37. Wingate, R., Fitzgibbon, T., Thompson, I.D. *Lucifer yellow, retrograde tracers, and fractal analysis characterise adult ferret retina ganglion cells.* Journal of Comparative Neurology, 1992; 323(4):449–474.

38. Boxt, L.M., Katz, J., Liebovitch, L.S., Jones, R., Esser, P.D., Reid, L. *Fractal analysis of pulmonary arteries: the fractal dimension is lower in pulmonary hypertension.* Journal of Thoracic Imaging, 1994; 9(1):8–13.

39. Witten, M.L., McKee, J.L., Lantz, R.C., Hays, A.M., Quan, S.S., Sobonya, R.E., Lemen, R.J. *Fractal and morphometric analysis of lung structures after canine adenovirus-induced bronchiolitis in beagle puppies.* Pediatric Pulmonary, 1993; 16:62–68.

40. Lynch, J.A., Hawkes, D.J., Buckland-Wright, J.C. *Analysis of texture in macroradiographs of osteoarthritic knees using the fractal signature.* Physics in Medicine and Biology, 1991; 36(6):709–722.

41. Landini, G., Misson, G.P., Murray, P.I. *Fractal analysis of the normal human retinal fluorescein angiogram.* Current Eye Research, 1993; 12(1):23–27.

42. Grant, P.E., Lumsden, C.J. *Fractal analysis of renal cortical perfusion.* Investigation Radiology, Jan 1994; 29:16–23.

43. Priebe, C.E., Solka, J.L., Lorey, R.A., Rogers, G.W., Poston, W.L., Kallergi, M., Qian, W., Clarke, L.P., Clark, R.A. *The application of fractal analysis to mammographic tissue classification.* Cancer letters, 1994; 77:183–189.

44. Oshida, Y., Munoz, C., Winkler, M.M., Hashem, A., Itoh, M. *Fractal dimension analysis of aluminum oxide particle for sandblasting dental use.* Biomedical Materials in Engineering, 1993; 3(3): 117–126.

45. Baken, R.J. *Epilogue: Into a chaotic future.* In Rubin, J.S., Sataloff, R.T., Korovin, G.S., Gould, W.J. (eds): *Diagnosis and Treatment of Voice Disorders.* Igaku-Shoin, NY, 1995, pp 502–509.

46. Baken, R.J. *Irregularity of vocal period and amplitude: a first approach to the fractal analysis of voice.* Journal of Voice, 1990; 4:185–197.

47. Awrejcewicz, J. *Bifurcation portrait of the human vocal cord oscillations.* Journal of Sound and Vibration, 1990; 136:151–156.

48. Wong, D., Ito, M.R., Cox, N.B., Titze, I.R. *Observation of perturbations in a lumped-element model of the vocal folds with application to some pathological cases.* Journal of the Acoustical Society of America, 1991, 89:383–391.

49. Mende, W., Herzel, H., Wermke, K. *Bifurcations and chaos in newborn infant cries.* Physical Letter A,1990; 145:418–424.

50. Titze, I.R., Baken, R.J. Herzel, H. *Evidence of chaos in vocal fold vibration.* In Titze IR (ed): *Vocal Fold Physiology: Frontiers in Basic Science,* San Diego CA, Singular Press, 1993, p 143.

51. Herzel, H., Berry, D.A., Titze, I.R., Saleh, M. *Analysis of vocal disorders with methods from nonlinear dynamics.* Journal of Speech and Hearing Research. 1994; 37:1008–1019.

52. Herzel, M. *Bifurcations and chaos in voice signals.* Applied Mechanics Review, 1993; 46:399–413.

53. Steinecke, I., Herzel, H. *Bifurcations in an asymmetric vocal-fold model.* Acoustical Society of America, 1995; 97:1–11.

54. Fletcher, N. *The human voice: a highly nonlinear dynamic system.* In Davis P, Fletcher N (eds): *Controlling Chaos and Complexity.* Singular Publications, San Diego, CA, in press.

55. Herzel, H. *Possible mechanisms of vocal instabilities.* In Davis P, Fletcher N (eds): *Controlling Chaos and Complexity.* Singular Publications, San Diego, CA. 1997.

56. Steinecke, I. *Bifurcations in an asymmetric vocal fold model.* Journal of Acoustical Society of America, 1995; 97:1–11.

57. Ishizaka, K., Flanagan, J.L. *Synthesis of voiced sounds from a two-mass model of the vocal cords.* Bell Systems Technical Journal, 1972; 51:1233–1268.

58. Titze, I., Talkin, D.T. *A theoretical study of the effects of various laryngeal configurations on the acoustics of phonation.* Journal of Acoustical Society of America, 1979; 66:60–74.

59. Herzel, H., Berry, D., Titze, I.R., Steinecke, I. *Nonlinear dynamics of the voice: signal analysis and biomechanical modeling.* In Davis P, Fletcher N (eds): *Controlling Chaos and Complexity.* Singular Publications, San Diego, CA.

60. Sato, M., Joe, K., Hirahara, T. *APOLONN brings us to the real world: learning nonlinear dynamics and fluctuations in nature.* ATR Aud and Vis-Perc Res Lab, 1990; 1:I-581-I-586.

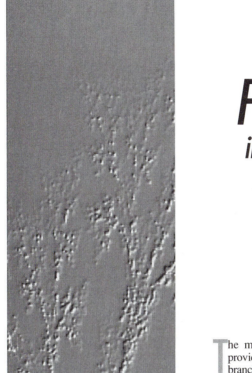

Fractal Mechanisms
in the Electrophysiology of the Heart

Ary L. Goldberger
Cardiovascular Division
Beth Israel Hospital
Harvard Medical School

The mathematical concept of fractals provides insights into complex anatomic branching structures that lack a characteristic (single) length scale, and certain complex physiologic processes, such as heart rate regulation, that lack a single time scale. Heart rate control is perturbed by alterations in neuro-autonomic function in a number of important clinical syndromes, including sudden cardiac death, congestive failure, cocaine intoxication, fetal distress, space sickness and physiologic aging. These conditions are associated with a loss of the normal fractal complexity of interbeat interval dynamics. Such changes, which may not be detectable using conventional statistics, can be quantified using new methods derived from "chaos theory."

What Is a Fractal?

The term fractal, coined by the mathematician B. Mandelbrot [1], is currently used in three related contexts: geometric, temporal (dynamical), and statistical. In the most general terms, fractals are defined by a property called self-similarity [1-3]. Fractal objects are composed of subunits that resemble the larger scale shape. These subunits in turn are composed of yet smaller units that also look similar to the larger ones, and so on. Fractals, therefore, do not have a single length scale, but rather have structure on multiple scales of length (Fig. 1).

The term fractal also relates to the fact that these irregular structures may have a noninteger (fractional) dimension. For example, the branching tracheo-bronchial tree, a fractal-like structure, has a dimension between 2 and 3, since it converts a volume of gas in the trachea (D = 3) into something approaching a surface area (D = 2) in the alveoli.

The notion of self-similarity has also been extended into temporal and statistical domains. A temporal fractal

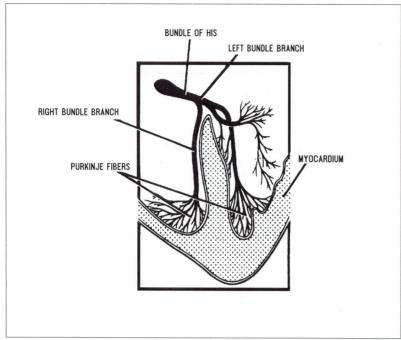

1. The self-similar branchings of the His-Purkinje system constitute a fractal-like network.

is a process that does not have a characteristic scale of time, analogous to a fractal structure that lacks a characteristic scale of length. Instead, fractal processes have self-similar fluctuations on multiple scales of time. This property is reflected by a type of broadband frequency spectrum, i.e., one having multiple frequencies. The concept of temporal fractals is closely related to that of "chaos." Finally, the fractal concept has been applied in a statistical context. One example is the irregular structure of the mammalian lung, where there is a self-similar distribution of

scale sizes across multiple generations of branchings [4, 5].

The Heart's Fractal-like Anatomy

A number of cardiac structures have a self-similar or fractal-like appearance [6-8]. Examples of this nonlinear architecture include the coronary arterial and venous trees, the chordae tendineae, certain muscle bundles, and the His-Purkinje network (Fig.1). The latter provides an efficient way of distributing the depolarization stimulus to the ventricles. Recently, there has been interest in model-

ing the electrogenesis of the QRS complex using a fractal-like conduction system, as well as for studying alterations in the frequency content of the normal QRS due to changes in His-Purkinje geometry or in myocardial conduction [6, 9, 10]. Abboud and colleagues [8, 9] have shown that slow conduction in myocardial cells activated by such a fractal network can lead to "late potentials" or to selective attenuation of higher frequency content of the QRS, simulating changes seen in ischemic coronary syndromes.

Controversy surrounding the fractal hypothesis of QRS electrogenesis centers on two questions [11-12]:

1. Is the His-Purkinje system really a fractal?
2. Does its macroscopic structure actually relate in any way to the frequency content of the QRS complex?

Idealized (computer-generated) fractals have infinite scales of length and literally have no smallest scale. Physiologic fractals are obviously bounded at both the upper and lower ends. However, the definition of a fractal does not require infinite scales of length [3]. Furthermore, it is also apparent that physiological fractals are not identical on different scales of magnification. However, structures such has the tracheo-bronchial tree and the His-Purkinje system do maintain a similarity of dichotomous branching for which the term "fractal-like" is mathematically appropriate [1-8]. Interconnections between branches of the His-Purkinje system, which makes the system more than a simple branching structure, also do not undermine the fractal-like nature of the geometry.

Spectral analysis of normal QRS complexes reveals a broadband frequency

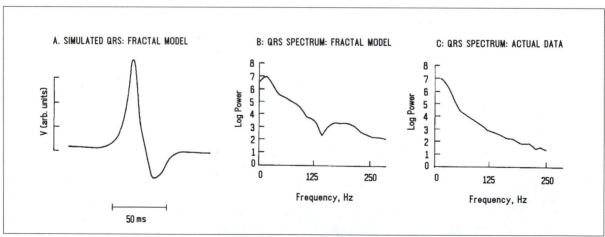

2. Activation of a three-dimensional network of myocardial "cells" by a self-similar conduction system (see Fig. 1) in a computer model generates realistic QRS complexes (left panel), with a broadband frequency spectrum (middle panel) comparable to that obtained from actual ECG data in healthy men (right panel). Computer model QRS and spectrum are from [9] and [10]; clinical data from [6].

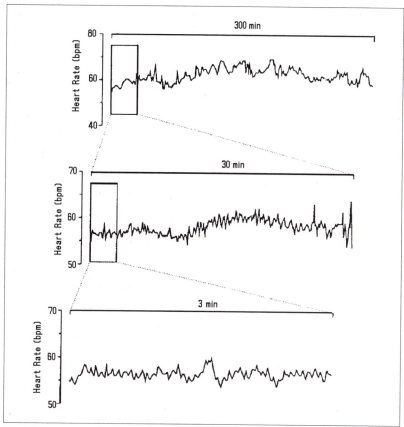

3. Normal sinus rhythm time series. Heart rate in healthy subjects, even at rest, is not strictly regular but fluctuates in a complex way (bpm, beats/min). Furthermore, there are self-similar fluctuations on multiple different orders of temporal magnitude, a fractal feature of healthy variability. (Adapted from [8].)

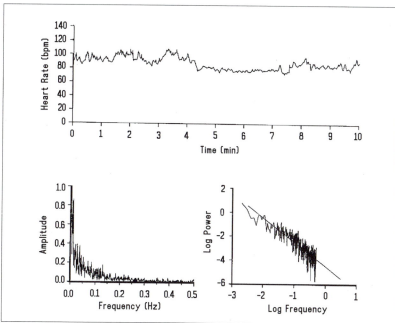

4. Normal sinus rhythm heart rate time series (top panel) from a 61 year old woman reveals erratic fluctuations. The frequency spectrum (lower left panel) is broadband, with a 1/f-like (inverse power-law) distribution, evident when the spectral data are replotted on double log axes (lower right panel).

spectrum (Fig. 2). While most of the frequency content of the QRS is comprised of frequencies below 20-30 Hz, there is a small but important contribution of higher frequencies, which go up to several hundred Hz. Furthermore, spectral analysis has indicated an inverse power-law distribution to the frequency components of the normal QRS. That is, a graph of log QRS frequency versus log power makes a good fit to a straight-line plot with a negative slope [6, 7].

A theoretical argument has been made that this broadband spectrum with its inverse power-law distribution is consistent with depolarization of the myocardium via an irregular, self-similar branching network [5]. Therefore, according to this fractal theory, the frequency content of the QRS complex is importantly related to the macroscopic structure of the His-Purkinje system, and not exclusively to the microscopic nature of the Purkinje-myocardial cell interactions and local wavefront propagation. Support for this counterintuitive notion has come from computer modeling studies in which a self-similar branching network has been used to depolarize a 3-dimensional network of cells [9, 10]. Such experiments reveal that with nine or ten generations of conduction system branchings, one can generate QRS complexes that are essentially indistinguishable from those seen clinically. Furthermore, the simulated QRS complexes have a broadband frequency spectrum comparable to that observed physiologically (Fig.2). Such models also confirm that changes in the geometry of the branching conduction system may alter the frequency content of the QRS complexes, independent of any changes in myocardial conduction. This macroscopic fractal model of QRS electrogenesis, based on myocardial activation via an irregular conduction network, is not inconsistent with microscopic observations on the nature of the Purkinje-subendocardial muscle cell interface [13].

The Healthy Heartbeat is a Temporal Fractal

As noted, the fractal concept can be extended from geometry to dynamics. In this latter context, one can describe certain complex processes that do not have a characteristic scale of time. The regulation of the heart rate may be one such fractal process [6-8]. This notion has proven controversial, in part because it runs counter to the conventional dictum that the normal heartbeat is highly regular ("regular sinus rhythm"). Palpation of the pulse and observation of the electrocardiogram in a healthy individual gives the appearance of metronomic regularity. However, actual measurements of interbeat interval fluctuations reveal quite a different impression (Fig. 3).

Normal subjects, even those at rest, show a high degree of heart rate variability, which is not subjectively perceptible. Furthermore, these fluctuations are not simply those associated with respiration. In fact, spectral analysis of heart rate data from healthy subjects shows a broadband spectrum with a so-called 1/f-like distribution (Fig. 4). Note that the term 1/f-like is synonymous with the inverse power-law type of scaling defined above.

Another controversial aspect of the concept of the fractal heartbeat relates to its mechanism. The interbeat interval fluctuations of the healthy heart may be due, in part, to intrinsic variability of autonomic control ("chaos") [8]. This hypothesis apparently conflicts with the theory of homeostasis enunciated by Walter B. Cannon [14] and others, which states that apparently erratic fluctuations of variables such as heart rate are due primarily to external influences, and that the normal condition of the cardiovascular system, and of other physiologic systems, is that of a steady state. A number of lines of evidence support the countervailing theory that deterministic chaos, not homeostasis, is the "wisdom of the body" [15]. The broadband spectrum of the healthy heartbeat is consistent with, but not diagnostic of, deterministic chaos. Additional tests for chaos include the measurement of a finite correlation dimension and of a positive Lyapunov exponent. Measurement of these nonlinear metrics from biologic data sets is fraught with potential problems, which have been discussed in detail elsewhere [16]. However, preliminary attempts to perform such measurements from heart rate data have been consistent with the hypothesis that these fluctuations do in fact represent deterministic chaos [17-19]. Finally, phase space portraits (delay maps) of interbeat interval time series are also consistent with those of so-called strange (chaotic) attractors (Fig. 5).

The mechanism for such physiologic chaos of the heartbeat, if it exists, is not certain. However, it is clear that heart rate fluctuations are primarily due to autonomic nervous system control and, therefore, any chaos of the heartbeat must reflect chaos in nervous system dynamics. There is evidence for this kind of deterministic chaos even in the nervous systems of more simple organisms [19].

Chaos and Disease

A corollary of the classical notion of homeostasis relating health to constancy is that disease and other perturbations are likely to cause a loss of regularity. The chaos hypothesis advanced above predicts just the opposite, namely, a variety of disease states that alter autonomic function may lead to a loss of physiologic complexity and, therefore, to greater, not less regularity [8]. Support for this notion comes from the comparison of heart rate time series from patients with a variety of different clinical syndromes, including those at high risk of sudden death and those with heart failure, whose sinus rhythm dynamics are typically *less* complex than those seen normally (Fig. 6) [20]. Similar changes are found in experimental animals with severe cocaine toxicity [21]. The term "complexity" is used here to include the fractal type of variability described above. It should be emphasized that quantifying losses of this type of nonlinear complexity cannot be accomplished by use of traditional statistics such as variance. An illustration of this principle comes from comparing two signals, one a large amplitude sine wave and the other a lower amplitude, highly erratic signal. Clearly, the sine wave is less complex despite its greater variance. This observation is of more than theoretical import, since there has been a flurry of interest in recent years in the analysis of heart rate variability using conventional statistics.

Aging is also associated with a loss of physiologic complexity [22, 23]. We have recently observed a reduction in both the *approximate dimension* and *approximate*

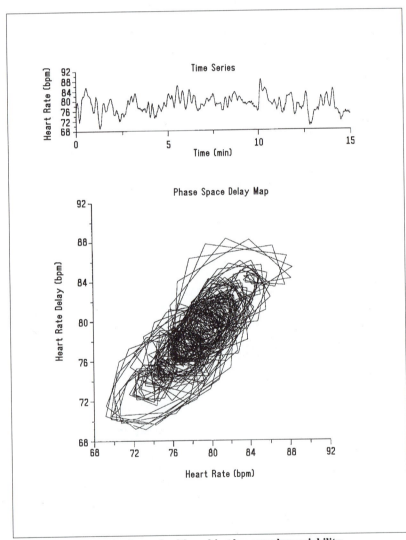

5. Heart rate time series from a healthy subject has complex variability. Two-dimensional phase space plot reveals a complex trajectory suggestive of a so-called strange attractor. Delay map plots heart rate in beats per minute (bpm) at a given time against the heart rate after a fixed delay (in this case, 4 seconds), and then tracks the evolution of this heart rate vector after an arbitrary time (also 4 seconds in this case). Data in this example and Fig. 6 were filtered with singular value decomposition.

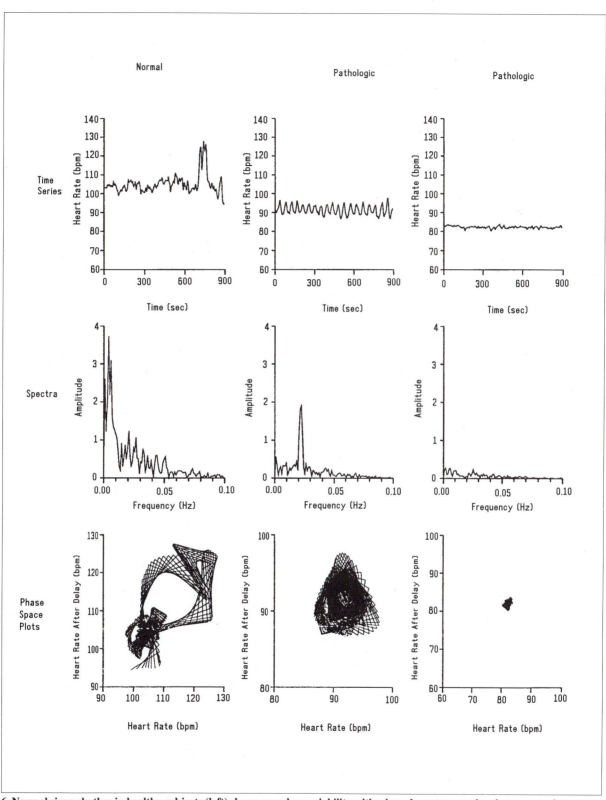

6. Normal sinus rhythm in healthy subjects (left) shows complex variability with a broad spectrum and a phase space plot consistent with a strange (chaotic) attractor. Patients with heart disease may show altered dynamics, sometimes with oscillatory sinus rhythm heart rate dynamics (middle) or an overall loss of sinus variability (right). With the oscillatory pattern, the spectrum shows a sharp peak, and the phase space plot shows a more periodic attractor, with trajectories rotating about a central hub. With the flat pattern, the spectrum shows an overall loss of power, and the phase space plot is more reminiscent of a fixed-point attractor. (Adapted from [8].)

entropy of heart rate and blood pressure signals in healthy, old versus young subjects, despite an increased blood pressure variance in the older subjects [24]. Loss of cardiovascular complexity also appears to be an important feature of a number of other pathologic conditions, including fetal distress and space sickness [7, 8, 15, 25]. Therefore, the loss of physiologic complexity may provide a new prognostic and diagnostic indicator that may greatly expand the accuracy and utility of physiologic monitoring systems.

Conclusions

This brief review has attempted to highlight key aspects of the application of fractals to clinical cardiac physiology, and to discuss some of the more controversial aspects of this theory. The fractal concept has been applied at two specific levels of cardiac function: 1) ventricular depolarization and 2) heart rate regulation. In the first case, that of ventricular depolarization, we have attempted to relate the self-similar and irregular branching structure of the His-Purkinje system to the dynamics of ventricular activation and to the resultant frequency spectrum of the QRS complex. Computer modeling studies have supported the counterintuitive notion that the macroscopic geometry of the conduction system may play a more important role than previously acknowledged in the genesis of the frequency content of the QRS complex under both normal and pathologic conditions.

In the second instance, that of heart rate variability, we have suggested that complex fluctuations in healthy heart rate may be due in part to deterministic chaos in the neuroautonomic control system. Furthermore, perturbations of this control system, such as those seen in heart failure and in sudden cardiac death syndromes, may lead to a loss of complexity of heart rate dynamics. These anomalies may be detectable with new nonlinear metrics based on calculations of dimension, entropy and Lyapunov exponents.

Acknowledgment

This work was supported in part by The National Heart, Lung and Blood Institute, the National Aeronautics and Space Administration, the National Institute on Drug Abuse, and by grants from Colin Electronics, Ltd., and the G. Harold and Leila Y. Mathers Charitable Foundation. This article is the author's updated, revised version of chapter 13 in *Cardiac Electrophysiology, Circulation and Transport*, edited by S. Sideman, R. Beyar, and A. Kleber, Norwell, MA, Kluwer Academic Publishers, 1991.

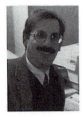
Ary Goldberger was born in New York City in 1949. He currently resides in Newton Centre, MA. He received the A.B., Summa Cum Laude, from Harvard College in 1970, and the M.D. from Yale Medical School in 1974. He did his medical internship and residency at Yale New Haven Hospital (1974-77) and then moved to San Diego on a cardiology fellowship at UCSD (1977-79). He remained on the faculty until 1985. Currently, he is Associate Professor of Medicine at Harvard Medical School, and Clinical Director of the Electrocardiography and Arrhythmia Laboratories at Beth Israel Hospital in Boston.

Dr. Goldberger and his colleagues were among the first to apply concepts from nonlinear dynamics, chaos theory and fractals to sudden cardiac death and bedside cardiology. Dr. Goldberger is the author of more than 90 scientific papers and two textbooks on electrocardiography. In 1988, he was the recipient of the S. Robert Stone Award for excellence in teaching at Harvard Medical School and Beth Israel Hospital. Address for correspondence: Beth Israel Hospital, 330 Brookline Ave. Boston, MA 02215.

References

1. **Mandelbrot BB:** *The Fractal Geometry of Nature.* New York, Freeman, 1982.

2. **Feder J:** *Fractals.* New York, Plenum, 1988.

3. **Stauffer D, Stanley HE:** *From Newton to Mandelbrot. A Primer in Theoretical Physics.* New York, Springer-Verlag, 1990.

4. **West BJ, Bhargava V, Goldberger AL:** Beyond similitude: renormalization in the bronchial tree. *J Appl Physiol* 1986; 60:1089-1097.

5. **Nelson TR, West BJ, Goldberger AL:** The fractal lung: universal and species-related scaling patterns. *Experientia* 1990:46:251-254.

6. **Goldberger AL, Bhargava V, West BJ, Mandell AL:** On a mechanism of cardiac electrical stability: the fractal hypothesis. *Biophys J* 1985; 48:525-528.

7. **Goldberger AL, West BJ:** Fractals in physiology and medicine. *Yale J Biol Med* 1987; 60:421-435.

8. **Goldberger AL, Rigney DR, West BJ:** Chaos and fractals in human physiology. *Sci Am* 1990; 262:42-49.

9. **Berenfeld O:** Simulation of the ventricular depolarization process using a three dimensional heart model with a self-similar conduction system. Master's Thesis, Tel Aviv University, 1989.

10. **Abboud S, Berenfeld O, Sadeh D:** Simulation of high-resolution QRS complex using a ventricular model with a fractal conduction system. Effects of ischemia on high-frequency QRS potentials. *Circ Res* 1991; 68:1751-1760.

11. **Lewis PJ, Guevara MR:** A $1/f^a$ power law spectrum of the QRS complex does not imply fractal activation of the ventricles (letter). *Biophys J.* 1991; 60:1297-1300.

12. **Goldberger AL:** Comments on the $1/f^a$ power spectrum of the QRS complex revisited (letter). *Biophys J.* 1991; 60:1301-1302.

13. **Rawling DA, Joyner RW:** Characteristics of junctional regions between Purkinje and ventricular muscle cells of canine ventricular subendocardium. *Circ Res* 1987; 60:580-585.

14. **Cannon WB:** Organization for physiological homeostasis. *Physiol Rev* 1929; 9:399-431.

15. **Goldberger AL:** Is the normal heartbeat chaotic or homeostatic? *News Physiol Sci* 1991; 6:87-91.

16. **Goldberger AL, Rigney DR:** Nonlinear dynamics at the bedside. In Glass L, Hunter P, McCulloch A, eds. *Theory of Heart.* New York/Berlin, Springer-Verlag, 1990.

17. **Destexhe A, Babloyantz A:** Is the normal heart a periodic oscillator? *Biol Cybern* 1988; 58:203-11.

18. **Mayer-Kress G, Yates FE, Benton L, Keidel M, Tirsch W, et al:** Dimensional analysis of nonlinear oscillations in brain, heart and muscle. *Math Biosci* 1988; 90:155-182.

19. **Skinner JE, Carpeggiani C, Landisman CE, Fulton KW:** The chaotic correlation dimension of the heartbeat is reduced in conscious pigs by myocardial ischemia. *Circ Res* 1991; 68:966-976.

20. **Mpitsos GJ, Burton MR Jr, Creech HC, Soinila SO:** Evidence for chaos in spike trains of neurons that generate rhythmic motor patterns. *Brain Res Bull* 1988; 21:529-538.

21. **Goldberger AL, Rigney DR, Mietus J, Antman EM, Greenwald S:** Nonlinear dynamics in sudden cardiac death syndrome: heartrate oscillations and bifurcations. *Experientia* 1988; 44:-983-987.

22. **Stambler BS, Morgan JP, Mietus J, Moody GB, Goldberger AL:** Cocaine alters heart rate dynamics in conscious ferrets. *Yale J Biol Med* 1991; 64:143-153.

23. **Lipsitz LA, Mietus J, Moody GB, Goldberger AL:** Spectral characteristics of heart rate variability before and during postural tilt: relations to aging and risk of syncope. *Circulation* 1990; 81:1803-1810.

24. **Kaplan D, Furman MI, Pincus S, Ryan SM, Lipsitz LA, Goldberger A:** Aging and the complexity of cardiovascular dynamics. *Biophys J* 1991; 59:945-949.

25. **Goldberger AL:** Nonlinear dynamics, fractals, cardiac physiology and sudden death. In: Temporal Disorder in Human Oscillatory Systems; Rensing L, an der Heiden U, Mackey MC, eds. New York/Berlin, Springer-Verlag, 1987, pp 118-125.

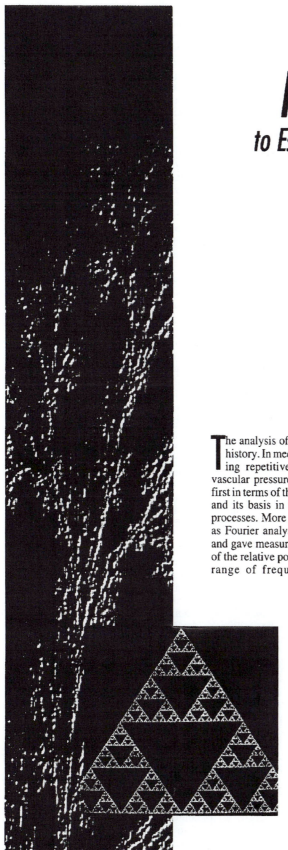

Four Methods
to Estimate the Fractal Dimension from Self-Affine Signals

Hans E. Schepers
Max Planck Institute

Johannes H.G.M. van Beek
Physiology Laboratory
The Free University, Amsterdam

James B. Bassingthwaighte
Center for Bioengineering
University of Washington

The analysis of a time series has a deep history. In medicine, waveforms showing repetitive patterns (ECG, EEG, vascular pressure pulses) were analyzed first in terms of the specifics of the pattern and its basis in the underlying physical processes. More general techniques such as Fourier analysis were also applicable and gave measures of the periodicity and of the relative power contributions over a range of frequencies. Such analyses showed that the periodicities were not exact. Exact periodicity of cardiovascular events is an abnormal phenomenon [1], presumably because biological control systems are multidimensional, low-gain, and remarkably redundant. They balance well without any set-points. Nonlinearity in biological control systems is evident and leads, in a natural way, to their examination as low-dimension, chaotic dynamical systems [2], wherein there is a fractal attractor. Such systems operate within bounds and without apparent predictability.

Demonstrating the fractal or chaotic nature of a signal is valuable, for it provokes the development of new ways for discovering how the system works. It is in this spirit that we undertake to examine time series using one-dimensional approaches. Fractal systems (in time or space) have neighbor-to-neighbor correlation at all levels of scale. In spatial statistics, the variance of a local measure depends on the resolution of the measurement [3]. For instance, the variance of regional blood flow in the heart increases as the resolution of measurement is increased. In an experiment where the heart is divided into many sections for the measurement of the concentration of a flow-proportional marker (e.g., radioactive microspheres) in each of the sections [4], the relation between the resolution mass of observed tissue element, m, and the variance (Var) of regional blood flows is well described by a power law function:

$$Var(m) = Var(m_o)(\frac{m}{m_o})^{2H-2} \quad (1)$$

where H is the Hurst coefficient, H = 2-D, and D is the fractal dimension lying between 1.0 and 2.0. The spatial distribution is considered to have fractal properties because it shows statistical self-similarity. Voss [5] showed that in a fractal system all of the moments of the distribution have the same power law slope. In our early analyses [6], we examined the relationship between the measure of variation (the coefficient of variation) and the resolution of the measurement. This was a simple one-dimensional spatial analysis which we label as RD analysis, where RD is the relative dispersion, i.e., the standard deviation divided by the mean.

The dependence of the variance of a variable on the resolution was also found by the same fractal analysis of a time series [6], for example, the velocity of blood cells passing through a small artery as a function of time. If a signal, y(t), is divided into intervals of length, Δt, and the mean is calculated for each interval, one can also calculate the variance of these means; there will be a lower variance when the interval length is increased. The relationship between the variance and the sample time may fit a power law, and if so, the fractal dimension of the time series can be calculated by the same RD analysis as was used for a spatial measure.

In this article, we shall examine four methods for analyzing a one-dimensional time signal, y(t). The first of these is our RD analysis. The others are correlation analysis, rescaled range analysis, and

Relative dispersion, correlation, rescaled range, and Fourier analyses all yield the fractal dimension, D

power spectral analysis. All methods yield the fractal dimension, D.

When neighboring elements in a time series or a spatial distribution are positively correlated, the measured variance will drop less rapidly as the resolution is decreased. Based on this phenoenon, Bassingthwaighte and Beyer [7] reinvented the expression for the autocorrelogram (originally provided by Mandelbrot and van Ness [8]) from the relationship for covariances among neighboring units fulfilling Eq. 1. The one parameter of this function is the fractal dimension, and it can be estimated directly from an autocorrelogram (correlation analysis).

Another statistical measure from which the fractal dimension can be calculated is Hurst's rescaled range analysis [9, 10] for analyzing flows in rivers. The "range" is of the integral of deviations from the mean over an interval, and it is normalized by dividing by the standard deviation of the differences from the mean. Mandelbrot and Wallis published a series of papers was published on this analysis [11, 12, 13, 14, 15], showing that Hurst's method could be used to estimate the fractal dimension from a fractional Brownian noise. They modified the method by using the differences from a trend line, rather than differences from the mean.

The signals analyzed here are examples

of fractional Brownian noises; they are characterized by a specific power spectrum of the form $S(f) \sim f^{-\beta}$, where f is frequency. Thus Fourier analysis [5, 16] is the fourth procedure used to estimate the fractal dimension. The 1/f noise, as it is frequently called, is common in nature, although the physical reason is not well understood. Recently, Bak et al. [18] proposed a general model for systems with a very high number of degrees of freedom, called 'self-organized criticality,' which accounts for both the occurrence of 1/f noise and fractals. Fractional Brownian noises and spatial fractals are, respectively, the temporal and the spatial fingerprints of a system that has evolved towards a critical state.

Do these four procedures to estimate the fractal dimension provide the same answer? Are they equally accurate? To find out, we generated signals with a known fractal dimension (D = 1.1 - 1.9), then used the four methods to estimate its value. The first problem is how to distinguish between the effects from the different signal generating algorithms, and the estimation methods. However, the estimation methods also perform better on long signals. The production of a truly fractal signal is itself a non-trivial exercise and may be as difficult as producing real random noise. So we must worry about the adequacy of the generating algorithms as well as the analysis algorithms. Some estimation procedures may require a very long signal, whereas others provide good results at shorter signal length. These four methods, however, are not exhaustive. The article by Fortin et al. in this issue [17] describes the use of a maximum likelihood estimator, another useful method.

The significance of D is that it describes, very compactly, the relation between the variance of the signal, and the time scale. No assumptions on the underlying system from which the signal was observed are made, and it is therefore a purely statistical tool. The fractal dimension estimated by these techniques from a time series is between one and two, i.e., for a one dimension function y(t), the fractal D lies between the Euclidean dimension E (= 1) and E + 1. (This is not at all the same fractal dimension that one attempts to derive from an embedding or correlation analysis [2], where one seeks a measure related to the order of the set of underlying differential equations.) For our analysis, 1 < D < 2; values of D near 1 indicate high correlation or "memory" over time. (This can be seen, for example, in the nearest neighbor correlation coefficient $r_1 = 2^{3 - 2D} - 1$.) For random signals, D = 1.5 (Table 1).

We will test methods for estimating the fractal dimension of self-affine and self

Table I
D and H for Fractal Times Series

Correlation	D	H = 2 - D
Positive	1 < D < 1.5	1 > H > 0.5
Random	1.5	0.5
Negative	1.5 < D < 2	0.5 > H > 0

similar curves. Self-affine curves repeat themselves only when the different axes are magnified by different factors, whereas self-similar curves use the same factor for each axis. Both a time series and a spatial distribution of local blood flows are classed as self affine, because the variable has units different from that of the axes [5]. Therefore, the standard methods of calculating the fractal dimension for spatial, self-similar fractal patterns (box-, divider- and similarity dimension) [19], require modification for the analysis of self-affine signals. The four methods described below can be used on either self-similar or self-affine signals.

Generating a Fractal Signal

To generate a signal with a known fractal dimension, two algorithms were used which generate a fractional Brownian motion, fBm, with a parameter, H, that defines the fractal dimension of the signal. The well known ordinary Brownian motion, such as a random walk of diffusing particles, is a fractional Brownian motion with H = 0.5. The successive differences between points of an fBm are called a fractional Brownian noise, fBn. Because determining H or D from fBm is difficult [8, 16], the fBn is needed to estimate fractal dimension. White noise is the uncorrelated form of fBn, being the increments or successive steps from the normal Brownian motion. Fractional Brownian noise signals with positive autocorrelation have H > 0.5, whereas fBn signals with negative correlations have H < 0.5. The fBn is always a stationary signal, and while fBm is stationary over long times, its short term behavior appears non-stationary. Since "short" and "long" are relative, and the signal has statistically self-similar behavior, the overall stationarity may not be demonstrable. Mandelbrot and Wallis [11-15] presented a simple definition of the fBn's with spectral theory: white noise and all its repeated integrals and derivatives have a spectral density of the form $1/f^{2}\beta$, where f is the frequency; and β is an integer. Fractional Brownian noises are defined as having a spectral density of the same form, with β a non-integer fraction, hence the name fractional (Brownian) noise, $\beta = 2H - 1$. The fractal dimension relates to H as D = E + 1 - H, where E is the Euclidian dimension [5].

The spectral synthesis method (SSM) generates the signal by computing the backtransform of a Fourier spectrum of known form: the squared amplitude must be a power law function of the frequency. The method is described in some detail by Voss [5]. Saupe [20], in the same volume, gives a pseudocode outline of the program, which requires only a few lines. The phases are usually randomly drawn from

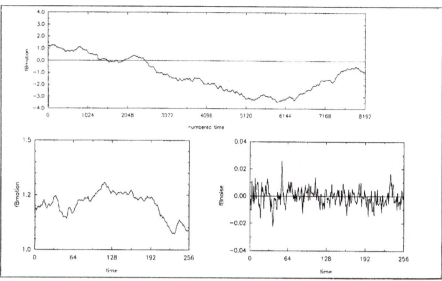

1. Fractional Brownian motion of H = 0.75, N = 8192, created by the Spectral Synthesis method (a). Magnification of the first part of (a), N = 256 (b). The corresponding fractional Brownian noise (c).

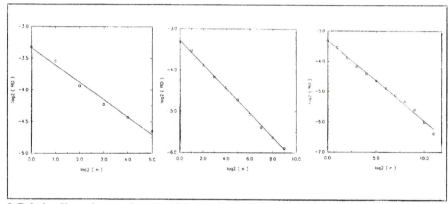

2. Relative dispersion as a function of the number of data points averaged. The signals analyzed are fractional Brownian noises with H = 0.75, consisting of 512 (left), 8192 (middle) and 32768 (right) points (SSM algorithm). Estimated H = 0.726, 0.726, and 0.733, respectively.

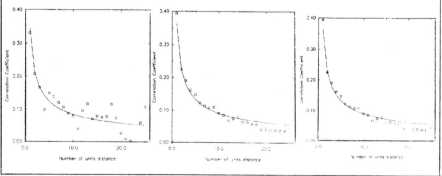

3. Estimation of H in Eq. 6 (autocorrelation analysis). The signals analyzed are the same as in Fig. 2 using the SSM algorithm, N = 512 (left), 8192 (middle) and 32768 (right). Estimated H: 0.716, 0.743, and 0.717, respectively.

a uniform distribution. An alternative method is presented by Osbourne and Provenzale [21]. The derivative of a fractal signal has the exponent of the power law function of the Fourier spectrum reduced by two, as compared to the original signal. Thus, an fBn can also be directly computed from the power spectrum. Fractional Brownian noises with H near 1.0 are smooth, while those with H near 0.5 are rough. For other examples see Fortin, et al. [17]. Figure 1 shows an example of both an fBm and its derivative, fBn, with H = 0.75.

The successive random addition (SRA) algorithm of Saupe [20] generates an fBm as follows: a random displacement is added to the middle and to the ends of a straight line. Each half of the line is replaced by the connecting line between the new points. Each of the daughter line segments is then treated as in the first step, but with random displacements of lower variance, depending on the parameter H:

$$Var_i = \sigma_o^2 \frac{1-2^{2h-2}}{2^{2h}} \quad (2)$$

where σ_o^2 is the variance in the first step, and the index, i, denotes the number of steps. In order to get the fractional Brownian noise that is required for all the estimation procedures, the differences of successive points in the fBm are taken.

The Estimation Procedures
Relative Dispersion Analysis

In spatial statistics, the relative dispersion (RD) analysis compares the variance of a variable as the measurement resolution increases [22]. The RD equals the standard deviation divided by the mean.

Relative dispersion analysis is well suited for long signals

In time series analysis, one starts by measuring, at the highest level of resolution, the variance of the signal over its whole time course. The next step is to average the signal over pairs of consecutive values, find the variance, and repeat for longer strings of values of y(t$_i$). String length increasing geometrically, grouping by 2, 4, 8, etc., is efficient because pairs of averages are combined for a next iteration. When the signal is uncorrelated (white noise), with H = 0.5, one expects that the standard deviation, when two consecutive values are averaged, is reduced by a factor of $1/2^{0.5}$, or when n consecutive values are averaged, by $1/n^{0.5}$. The mean remains the same. Now one will find that with a correlated fBn, and H not equal to 0.5, the SD will be proportional to n^{H-1}, n being the bin size or the time resolution interval. By calculating the RD (RD = SD/mean) for different bin sizes, n, and fitting the exponent of the power law function:

$$RD = RD_o \left(\frac{n}{n_o}\right)^{H-1} \quad (3)$$

where RD_o is the RD for some reference bin size n_o, the fractal dimension (via H) is easily computed. The whole of the data set is used for each calculation of RD(n) at each level of resolution or number of pieces, n.

The exponent can best be estimated after a log-log transformation (Fig. 2):

$$log(RD) = log(RD_o) + (H-1)log(n/n_o) \quad (4)$$

As can be seen from Fig. 2, the fit is a little improved when a longer signal is used. The RD analysis yields essentially the same results when only the first three or four points in the graph (i.e., the smallest bin sizes, 2, 4, 8 and 16) are used. With very large bin sizes, the number of bins is of course small and the measure of variance is less accurate. This relationship is an important advantage of the RD analysis, because especially in spatial statistics, signals may not be very long due to limited resolution and domain size.

Correlation Analysis

Van Beek et al.[23] derived an equation for the correlation between measurements in adjacent units from the assumption that RD diminishes by a factor of 2^{H-1} when two pieces (values in the time series) are lumped together, or are averaged (the bin size is doubled):

$$r_1 = 2^{2H-1} - 1 \quad (5)$$

The correlations between neighboring pieces are independent of the piece size, which is the reciprocal (approximately) of the number of units into which a domain has been divided. Bassingthwaighte and Beyer [7] extended the formula to the autocorrelation coefficients between pieces which are separated by n - 1 intervening pieces:

$$r_n = \frac{(n+1)^{2H}}{2} - \frac{n+1}{2} - \sum_{i=1}^{n-1}(n-i+1)r_i \quad (6)$$

From this, they derived an expression r_n, that is not recursive, for all n > 0, integer or non-integer:

$$r_n = \frac{1}{2}\{ |n-1|^{2H} -2|n|^{2H} + |n+1|^{2H}\} \quad (7)$$

In doing so, they rediscovered the relationship described by Mandelbrot and van Ness [8], and Mandelbrot [24], and used by others since. For example, Burrough [25, 26] used it for soil characterization, and Lundahl et al.[16] show its meaning and merit with respect to fractional Brownian motion. The relationship for H > 0.5 for large n goes asymptotically to a power law relationship [27]:

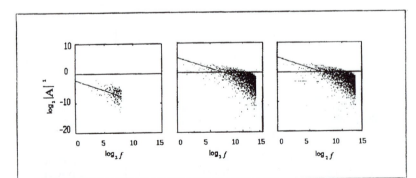

4. Power in fBn as a function of frequency. Estimation of H in Eq. 9 $|A|^2\alpha^{-b}$ using spectral analysis. The signals are the same as those analyzed for Fig. 2 using SSM algorithm, N = 512 (left), 8192 (middle) and 32768 (right). True H = 0.75. Estimated H = 0.802, 0.741, and 0.756 respectively.

$$\frac{r_n}{r_{n-1}} = \left(\frac{n}{n-1}\right)^{2H-2} \qquad (8)$$

The slope is the same as that of Eq. 1, and the meanings now coalesce: when the variances are fractal, there is a defined degree of correlation and an extended correlation. This simple expression is quite good for $n \geq 3$, and so H can be simply determined from the plot of $\log r_n$ versus $\log n$.

We obtained a nonlinear fit of Eq. 7 to the data with the procedure GGOPT [28] from the National Simulation Resource, Center for Bioengineering, University of Washington, Seattle. The correlograms for the longer signals are much smoother than for the shorter ones. This can be seen in Fig. 3, where three plots are compared. With N = 512 (left panel), the correlation curve is noisy, whereas for N = 8192, the noise is smaller, but the distant correlations are erroneously low. The error has almost disappeared with N = 32768.

The long time span over which correlation persists is very remarkable. The autocorrelogram tends very slowly to zero. For high H (= 0.5 to 1), the correlations are positive and extend longer. Mandelbrot and Wallis [11 - 15] called this a long-term persistence. When the signal is a straight line, there is no decrease in the correlogram and H = 1. For H < 0.5 the correlations are negative, which is termed anti-persistence. Examples of correlation versus separation are shown by Fortin, et al. [17].

For the estimation of H from the autocorrelogram, it is important that not too many correlation coefficients be used in the estimation procedure. With long separations, even minuscule degrees of random noise or measurement error will cause the estimate to be biased towards H = 0.5 as shown by Lundahl et al.[16].

A further test of the self-affine nature of the signal using the autocorrelation function follows the style of the RD analysis. It is particularly useful for distinguishing a single fractal process from a multifractal. A true fractal will follow Eq. 7 for any chosen sample size. Therefore, the test is to group successive samples, take the mean of the groups, and repeat the calculation of r_n. Repeat this for groups of a few different sizes, e.g., of two, four, etc. points of the original signal. If different group sizes all give the same estimate of H, it is strong evidence of a fractal signal that is stationary over long times, given the context that the signal set is a finite sampling of an infinite and stationary signal.

Fourier analysis

The power spectrum (the square of the amplitude from the Fourier transform) of a pure fractional Brownian motion is known to be described by a power law function [5]:

$$|A|^2 \approx \frac{1}{f^\beta} \qquad (9)$$

where |A| is the magnitude of the spectral density at frequency f, with an exponent equal to $\beta = 2H + 1$. In general, fractal signals always have such a very broad spectrum. When the derivative is taken

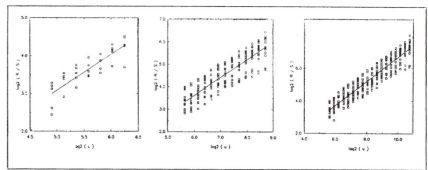

5. Estimation of H in Eq. 14 (R/S analysis). The signals analyzed are the same as in Figure 2 using SSM algorithm, N = 512 (left), 8192 (middle) and 32768 (right). Estimated H =

0

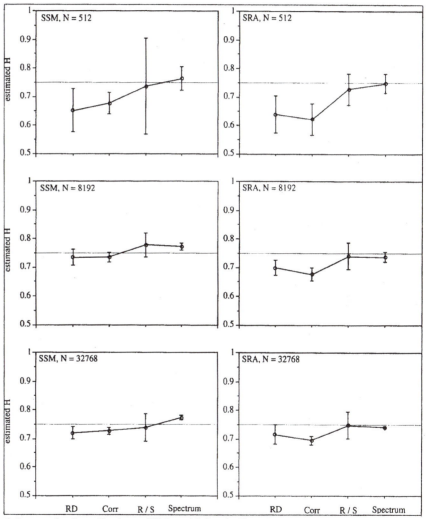

6. Averaged values of estimated H from 10 signals. Error bars denote ± one standard deviation. The preset value of H is 0.75, indicated by the horizontal line on each panel. The panel headings indicate the synthesis method (SSM or SRA) and the numbers of points, N. The abbreviations on the abscissa are RD = relative dispersion analysis; Cor = autocorrelation analysis; R/S = rescaled range analysis; Spectrum = Fourier analysis.

from a fractal signal, β is reduced by two. Thus, for fractional Brownian noise, fBn, β is expected to be:

$$\beta = 2H - 1 \qquad (10)$$

Here again, a straight line is fitted from a log-log plot, and H is calculated from the slope β, as in the examples in Fig. 4. The influence for longer signals in the Fourier analysis is not clear from the individual plots, but the estimates are quite accurate even for shorter signals.

Rescaled Range Analysis

Edwin Hurst [9, 10] a hydrology engineer, had a statistical problem when designing the Aswan dam on the Nile River. He wanted to know how high the dam should be to contain all incoming river water and provide a constant outflow. When the inflow of the dam is a stationary random variable, the water level of the lake is the integral of the differences of the inflow and the constant outflow. He took data on the annual flow in the Nile and other rivers, and computed the range, R(u), defined as the maximum value minus the minimum value of the integral of the differences of the annual flow from the mean flow, divided by the standard deviation of the yearly inflow for different time spans ("time lag" u), averaged at different starting times, t_0. He found that a power law relation between the quotient of the range $R(t_0, u)$ and the standard deviation, S(u), of the inflow and the time span u described the data very well:

$$\frac{R(u)}{S(u)} \approx u^H \qquad (11)$$

where R/S is called the rescaled range. The longer time a dam should be able to hold all inflow, the higher it must be.

Mandelbrot and Wallis used Hurst's rescaled range analysis as an estimation procedure to estimate the fractal dimension of a signal [8, 11, 12, 13, 14, 15]. The quantity $R(t_0, u)/S(t_0, u)$ is calculated for subsets of the data over intervals of time lag u, starting from each of many starting points, t_0 separated by some interval, $\Delta t > u$, so that there are no overlapping subsets. The range is:

$$R(t_0, u) = MAX\{X(t_0, u)\} - \\ MIN\{X(t_0, u)\} \qquad (12)$$

where:

$$X(t_0, u) = \int_{t_0}^{t_0+u} [B(s) - <B(s)>] \, ds \qquad (13)$$

and <B(s)> denotes the mean value of the fBn over the interval B(t_0, t_0+u). The standard deviation S(t_0, u) is the standard deviation of B(t) over the same interval. For a data set of N evenly spaced observations, there are N/(u/Δt) estimates of R/S obtainable from non-overlapping intervals of length u. We abbreviate R(t_0, u)/S(t_0, u) to R(u)/S(u), which is a function of t_0 and u, and plot the individual calculations for each interval length, u, in Fig. 5, giving the "pox plot" [11]. A straight line is fitted in the log-log plot:

$$log[R(u)/S(u)] = c + H \, log(u) \qquad (14)$$

The individual points for a given u in Fig. 5 are calculated independently of each other, since there is no overlap between subsets. Using the GGOPT optimizer or a maximum likelihood estimator as used by Fortin et al. [17] gives a minimally biased estimate of H, which is better than fitting the means of R/S at each u.

The estimations from the R/S analysis depend on the way the subsets from the signal are taken to calculate the rescaled range. With longer signals, larger lags can be used, along with more points per lag.

Correlation and rescaled range analyses yield biased results under many circumstances

Also, the length of the shortest lag can be increased, which improves the fit further, as reported by Mandelbrot and Wallis [11-15].

Results
In Fig. 6, the results are summarized for estimates obtained with the four methods for ten signals generated by the spectral synthesis method (SSM) and the successive random addition method (SRA) for H = 0.75. Several conclusions can be drawn from this Figure. Except from the R/S analysis and the Fourier analysis, the estimates of H tend to be too low. Some of the deviation may be blamed on the synthesis algorithm. For instance, deviations from the preset value of H = 0.75 with signals generated by the SSM algorithm are smaller than the deviations with the SRA algorithm (Figs 6a, 6b).

In general, estimates from the Fourier analysis come closest to the correct value of H = 0.75, and have a small standard deviation. The estimates from the RD and correlation analyses are low. The correlation estimates may be biased towards 0.5 because correlation coefficients over too

---

Table 2

Estimates of H from y(t), ten trials each; actual H = 0.75

Synthesis Algorithm	Analysis Method	Estimates of H at different N (± SD)		
		N = 512	N = 8192	N = 32768
SSM	RD	0.652 (0.076)	0.735 (0.028)	0.7043 (0.027)
	Cor	0.678 (0.036)	0.736 (0.018)	0.724 (0.007)
	R/S	0.736 (0.169)	0.778 (0.042)	0.738 (0.032)
	Spectrum	0.764 (0.042)	0.773 (0.013)	0.770 (0.008)
SRA	RD	0.639 (0.065)	0.698 (0.027)	0.716 (0.033)
	Cor	0.622 (0.057)	0.676 (0.023)	0.696 (0.015)
	R/S	0.727 (0.054)	0.740 (0.046)	0.748 (0.047)
	Spectrum	0.748 (0.033)	0.738 (0.018)	0.742 (0.003)

large distances are taken into account. The mean of the estimations from the rescaled range analysis is fairly good, but the standard deviation is very large. The estimates from Fig. 6 are listed in Table 2.

The estimates of H obtained via these procedures are presented in Fig. 7 for signals with true values of H from 0.1 to 0.9. The Fourier analysis yields the best results (right lower panel). It is apparent that the correlation analysis yields estimates biased towards H = 0.5. The correlation estimates for high values of H are clearly improved when a longer signal is analyzed.

Estimates of the R/S analysis tend to be too high, but with a large standard deviation (Fig. 7, right upper panel). The RD analysis yields excellent results with 8192 points. Even with only 512 points, at H = 0.1 and 0.3, the RD analysis provides almost correct values, underestimating at higher H.

An important difference between the correlation structure of signals generated by the SRA and SSM algorithm is shown in Fig. 8. The first 25 correlation coefficients of 10 signals for each algorithm are plotted along with Eq. 7 with H = 0.75. The SRA algorithm appears to produce a more nearly randomly structured signal, as the estimates tend toward 0.5 and therefore fall mostly below the expected correlation for H = 0.75 (Fig. 8a). The values for the correlations are too low, and the scatter is large. The SSM produced signals whose autocorrelograms are only a little below the model function equation, Eq. 7 (Fig. 8b).

Discussion

A major problem of the work described above involves the question: "What is being tested, the estimation procedures by the signal generating algorithm, or the signal generating algorithm by the estimation procedures?" When a signal generating algorithm produces a signal with a different fractal dimension from the dimension corresponding to the parameter H, it cannot be expected that the estimation procedures will be unbiased with respect to the preset parameter value. But because the estimations were done on the same signals, it is still possible to determine which of the methods comes closest to the preset value, and the variances of the estimation procedures can be compared.

The variance of estimates from the R/S analysis is much larger than those of the other estimation procedures. This occurs because in the R/S analysis, the signal must be divided into several subintervals, which can be done in many ways. The results for the R/S analysis clearly depend on the number of subintervals (the number of points in Fig. 5 at each lag), the mini-

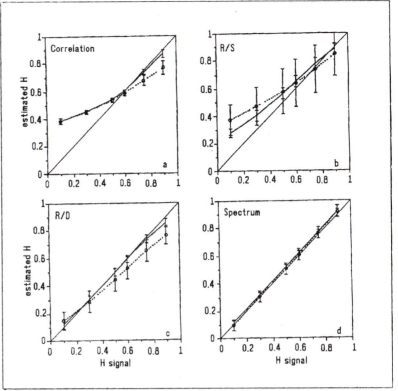

7. Comparison of estimates of H from short (N = 512, dotted lines) and long (N = 8192, solid lines) signals from the different estimation procedures. The error bars denote standard deviations of estimates of H from ten signals at each H. Signals were generated by the SSM algorithm. Correlation analysis (a); R/S analysis (b); RD analysis (c); spectral analysis (d).

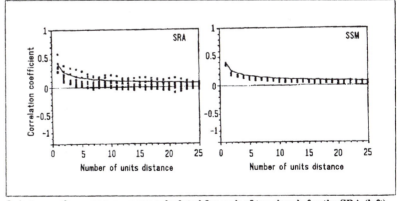

8. Autocorrelograms r_n versus n calculated for each of ten signals for the SRA (left) and the SSM (right) algorithms, both for N = 8192, H = 0.75. The lines represent the expected correlation function with H = 0.75.

mum and maximum lags. It is not clear how important the number of subintervals is. Mandelbrot and Wallis noted that the smallest lags (under 30) can't be expected to be on the line, and should not be included in the procedure. In this article, we chose not to use overlapping subintervals, so that no extra dependence between these subintervals occurs. Hurst reported that the estimates from the R/S analysis might

be biased towards 0.72, in agreement with our finding at short signal lengths. However, at long signal lengths the bias seemed to be toward H = 0.8. It is not clear why this would occur. Further work needs to be done, especially on the influence of picking the particular subintervals from the main signal. As can be seen with the correlation analysis for signals of length 512, 8192 and 32768, in Fig. 3, the SSM algorithm produces a better correlation structure for longer signals. From Fig. 6, it can be seen that the same applies to the SRA algorithm, because the estimations also become progressively better; compare Figs. 6b, 6d, and 6f.

In the estimation of H from the correlogram, the estimates of r are biased towards zero when n is large. Figure 9 shows the estimations of H as a function of lags included in the correlogram for the fit of the correlation function, Eq. 6. The signal was generated with the SSM algorithm with an H = 0.9. The bias towards 0.5 becomes progressively more apparent when more distant correlation coefficients are included. With n large, the calculation of r_n is also rendered less accurate, simply because there are fewer pairs of values to correlate at large distances. These difficulties are exacerbated when H is closer to 0.5, and lessened when H is > 0.8.

In the range of H between 0 and 0.5, all estimations except for the Fourier analysis and RD analysis with long signals are not

Spectral analysis yields the least biased results, and the lowest variance in estimates of D

very good. The reason is that the data points from which the Fourier analysis estimates the fractal dimension are independent of each other. With the correlogram this is not the case. The correlations are negative for the first few lags, but very quickly become scattered around zero When too many correlation coefficients are included in the estimation procedure, a biased estimate towards H = 0.5 is obtained. The estimation from only the first autocorrelation coefficient is not good, either. The first autocorrelation coefficient as a function of H is described by Eq. 5 [23]. Why a first autocorrelation coefficient of less than -0.5 is not possible for a fractal signal is not well understood.

Of all the methods discussed, the Fourier method is generally best. However, the variance (or SD) of the estimate is still larger than that given by the maximum likelihood methods (MLE) in Lundahl et al. [16] and Fortin et al. [17]. For example, with the Fourier method and N = 512 points, the SD is 0.033. Use of the MLE yeilds an SD =

0.01. The major liability of the MLE is its extensive computation time.

The procedure to calculate the fractal dimension of the strange attractor of the underlying dynamical system [2] is not discussed here. The fractal dimension of the strange attractor is conceptually different: it gives a measure of the minimal order of a system, the order N of N-dimensional phase space in which the time signal and its derivatives (or the order of the set of differential equations defining the system) can be mapped, plus the degree to which the signal fills the space. Although one would think that a little noise would encourage overestimating the dimension, in the situation where the system is relatively stable, the noise actually has the effect of revealing the dimensionality of the attractor more fully [29]. A main drawback of the analysis in [2] is that it requires a very large (long) time series in order to converge on the estimate of the dimension.

Conclusion

The fractal dimension provides a measure of the heterogeneity of the system and takes the correlation structure into account: D ≠ 1.5 implies that we are not dealing with a random distribution, but that there is correlation between adjacent regions. We compared four numerical methods to estimate the fractal dimension. Correlation analysis and rescaled range analysis yield seriously biased results under many circumstances. Relative dispersion analysis is well suited for long signals. Spectral analysis gives the least biased results, and also has lowest variance in the estimates of the fractal dimension. The same methods can be used for the one-dimensional analysis of spatial signals, as Hurst et al. [10] did for the analysis of thicknesses of tree growth rings, and mud layers. For the analysis of two- and three-dimensional signals, the methods can be extended to account for anisotropy, making the analysis more complicated but adhering to the same basic theory.

James Bassingthwaighte, born 1929, MD (Toronto), Ph.D. (Minnesota) is Professor of Bioengineering at the University of Washington, Seattle. His research is centered on cardiac blood flow and metabolism and the kinetics of exchange of substrates and ions. Address for correspondence: Center for Bioengineering WD 12, Seattle, WA 98195

Johannes H.G.M. van Beek, born 1952, B.S. (University of Utrecht, The Netherlands), Ph.D. (University of Leiden), is Assistant Professor at the Laboratory.

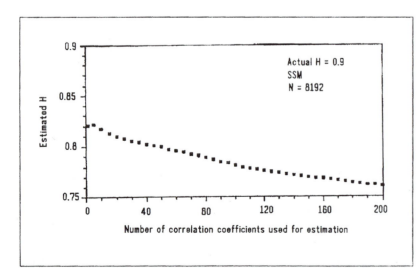

9. The effect of the number of correlation coefficients that are included in the estimation for H from a signal generated by the SSM algorithm, with N = 8129 and H = 0.9.

Volume 141, number 8,9 PHYSICS LETTERS A 20 November 1989

A FAST ALGORITHM TO DETERMINE FRACTAL DIMENSIONS BY BOX COUNTING

Larry S. LIEBOVITCH and Tibor TOTH

Department of Ophthalmology, Columbia University, 630 West 168th Street, New York, NY 10032, USA

Received 28 June 1989; revised manuscript received 14 September 1989; accepted for publication 21 September 1989
Communicated by D.D. Holm

A new algorithm is used to determine fractal dimensions by box counting for dynamic and iterated function systems. This method is fast, accurate, and less dependent on data specific curve fitting criteria than the correlation dimension.

The fractal dimension of a set in a metric space such as a geometric object or the phase space trajectory of a dynamical system can be computed from several different measures including: the first three generalized dimensions [1], the capacity [2–4], the information dimension [5], and the correlation dimension [6]; the Liapunov exponents [7,8]; and the singular value decomposition [9]. These methods are reviewed in refs. [10–12].

Recently, one of the most used measures has been the spatial correlation dimension computed from the algorithm of Grassberger and Procaccia [6]. The correlation dimension d_C is defined by

$$d_C = d \log C(r)/d \log r \qquad (1)$$

for small $r > 0$, where $C(r)$, the correlation integral, is given by

$$C(r) = \lim_{N \to \infty} \frac{1}{N^2} \sum_{j=1}^{N} \sum_{i=j+1}^{N} \theta(r - \|R_i - R_j\|). \qquad (2)$$

Here N is the number of points, θ is the Heaviside function, and the norm is the Euclidean one. In practise, however, the slope of $\log C(r)$ versus $\log r$, and thus d_C, determined from experimental data is not often a constant, but varies as a function of r [9,13,14]. One of the reasons this happens is that the correlation sum from points near the edge of the set is underestimated. Since there is no general procedure to choose the best estimate of d_C, the criteria to determine the fit of $\log C(r)$ versus $\log r$ depend on the details of each data set analyzed. Moreover, these computations can be time consuming. To compute all pairs of distances increases as N^2. This time can be reduced to order $N \log N$ by organizing the points into boxes [15]. Sometimes, only a small number, typically a few per cent, of "reference" points are chosen as R_i, which decreases the computational time at the expense of increasing the uncertainty in d_C [16].

An alternative measure of the dimension is the capacity [2,4,10,12,17]

$$d_B = \lim_{\epsilon \to 0} \log N_B(\epsilon)/\log(1/\epsilon). \qquad (3)$$

This is called "box-counting" because one counts the minimal number of boxes, $N_B(\epsilon)$, that cover the set, for boxes of size ϵ. Useful algorithms to implement this were described by Grassberger [3], Hunt and Sullivan [18], Giorgilli et al. [19], and Theiler [15]. Barnsley [4] provides a number of examples demonstrating the utility of box counting to determine the fractal dimension in the plane. However, this method has not been widely used because it required: (1) too large a number of datapoints and (2) too much computer memory and computation time. We will show how these limitations can be overcome. Moreover, our method does not require the curve fitting decisions dependent on the details of each data set required by the use of the correlation dimension.

Greenside et al. [20] found that taking the limit in eq. (3), that is, using very small box sizes, required an impractically large number of datapoints. However, this criterion is more restrictive than nec-

Volume 141, number 8,9   PHYSICS LETTERS A   20 November 1989

essary. The fractal dimension describes how many new pieces of a set are resolved as the resolution scale is decreased [21]. Since a fractal is self-similar, this means that the fractal dimension can be evaluated by comparing properties between any two scales, namely,

$$d_B \approx d \log N_B(\epsilon) / d \log(1/\epsilon). \tag{4}$$

In practice, the correlation dimension is also evaluated using this fact by fitting $\log C(r)$ versus $\log r$ over an intermediate range of r values and excluding the regimes near $r \to 0$ and near $r \to r_{max}$ where the accuracy of the determination of $C(r)$ is affected by the finite size of the data set. We will show below that the fractal dimension can be determined accurately from eq. (4), and present an efficient algorithm that requires only approximately $N d_e$ memory locations where d_e is the embedding dimension and executes in time of order $N \log N$.

This box counting method to determine the fractal dimension is particularly useful when the dimension is low. For example it is very efficient for the analysis of two-dimensional images such as the sets illustrated by Barnsley [4]. However, since it requires approximately 10^d data points, where d is the dimension of the attractor, it is less useful when the dimension is high. Note that other methods of determining the dimension may also be subject to a similar limitation, for example, Wolf et al. [7] note that their method, using Liapunov exponents, also requires 10^d or more data points.

To compute d_B, we need to count the number of boxes in a minimal cover that contain at least one element of the set. This is then carried out for a sequence of decreasing box sizes. Our algorithm does this by using an efficient hashing to code all the points within one box with the same number and then to count the number of distinct values.

Each of the N points of a set embedded in d_e dimensions can be represented by a vector with coordinates $\{X_i; i=1, d_e\}$. The values of X_i are normalized to cover the range $(0, 2^k - 1)$. The set is covered by a grid of d_e dimensional cubes of edge size 2^m, $0 \le m \le k$, called boxes. For each coordinate we form $Y_i = (X_i \text{ AND } M)$ where AND is the binary conjunction of the corresponding bits in X_i and M, and M is a binary number with 1's in the first $k-m$

places and 0's the remainder. Then for each $n=1, ..., N$ we construct $Z_n = Y_1 + Y_2 + Y_3... + Y_{d_e}$, where the operation "+" indicates concatenation (for example, "10"+"01"="1001"). All the points within the same box of size 2^m will have coordinates that have identical binary digits in the first $k-m$ places. Thus, distinct Z_n correspond to points in distinct boxes. We count the number of distinct Z_n efficiently by ordering them using a quicksort or heapsort [22] to order all N strings Z_n, and then walk down the list once to count the number of times the values change. The procedure is then repeated for different boxes of edge size 2^m, where $m=k, k-1, ..., 0$.

We performed the above procedure in a BASIC program by means of the concatenation of alphanumeric variables (strings) to form Z_n, and a quicksort algorithm [23]. Note that the memory required is determined by the number of data points and not the number of boxes in the grid. The data points were two-byte integers, so that the total memory required was approximately $2 N d_e$ bytes, where N is the number of data points and d_e the embedding dimension. The computational time for this box counting algorithm depends mostly on the time required by the sort which is approximately $N \log N$. The computational time increases slowly with d_e, the details of which depend on the hardware used.

The limited resolution due to the finite number N of the data points is reached when ϵ is small enough so that all the points lie in distinct boxes, that is, when $N_B(\epsilon) = N$. At this value of ϵ the function $N_B(\epsilon)$ is saturated. Values of $N_B(\epsilon)$ near saturation should be disregarded when the slope of $\log N_B(\epsilon)$ versus $\log(1/\epsilon)$ is calculated. To be enough below this point, only values of $N_B(\epsilon) \le N/5$ were taken into account. Moreover, since the largest box sizes have such poor resolution, we also ignore $N_B(\epsilon)$ for $m=k, k-1$. We then use a least squares fit to determine d_B as the slope of $\log N_B(\epsilon)$ versus $\log(1/\epsilon)$. Note, we always use the same procedure of fitting $N_B(\epsilon)$ versus $\log(1/\epsilon)$ from $m=k-2$ to $N_B(\epsilon) \le N/5$. Thus, we always have a fixed procedure to determine this fit. This is a significant improvement over the evaluation of the correlation dimension, where the fit of $\log C(r)$ versus $\log r$ depends on the details of the particular data set analyzed that determine the range of r over which d_C is evaluated. However, if the data consisted of a union

Volume 141, number 8,9 PHYSICS LETTERS A 20 November 1989

of subsets of different dimensions, our procedure would lump them together.

To compare their accuracy and computational times, we computed the correlation dimension d_C by the Grassberger–Procaccia algorithm and the capacity dimension d_B by our new algorithm for two types of attractors. The first type was an example of a deterministic dynamic system. We used the Hénon map [24]:

$$x_{i+1} = 1 + y_i - 1.4x_i^2, \quad y_{i+1} = 0.3x_i. \tag{5}$$

The fractal dimension for this map is known from estimates based on Liapunov numbers [25], capacity dimension [3,19,25] and correlation dimension [6]. However, the fractal dimension cannot be determined analytically for this, or many other, deterministic dynamic systems. Thus, to test the accuracy of these methods we also applied them to analyze a second type of set where the fractal dimension can be evaluated analytically. Such fractals were constructed using the Collage theorem [4]. They were generated from a set of affine transformations applied in random order. The transformations are such that the union of their images approximates the fractal desired. For example, the middle third Cantor set which has fractal dimension $\log 2/\log 3 \approx 0.631$ was formed by consecutive applications of the following set of affine transformations,

$$x_{i+1} = x_i/3, \quad x_{i+1} = 2/3 + x_i/3, \tag{6}$$

applied with equal probability to the result of the previous transformation. To produce a modified Sierpinski triangle map with fractal dimension $\log 3/\log 2 \approx 1.58$ the set of three transformations ($k=1$, 2, 3)

$$x_{i+1} = y_i/2 + a_k, \quad y_{i+1} = x_i/2 + b_k, \tag{7}$$

where $a_1 = a_2 = b_1 = 1$ and $a_3 = b_2 = b_3 = 125$, were applied with equal probability. The Hénon and modified Sierpinski attractors are shown in fig. 1.

The Hénon map and the iterated function systems were used to compute N values of $\{x_i\}$ for $N = 1000$ and 10000. In analyzing experimental data, typically the time series of only one of the variables is known. The attractor can then be reconstructed, in an embedding space of dimension d_e, from points whose coordinates are values of the time series separated by a constant lag time [26,27]. For the test cases here,

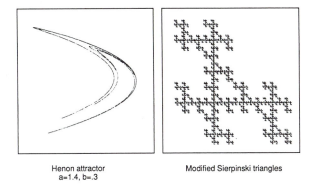

Henon attractor
a=1.4, b=.3

Modified Sierpinski triangles

Fig. 1. Plot of $\{x_i, y_i\}$ for the Hénon attractor of eq. (5) and the iterated function system representing the modified Sierpinski triangle map described by eq. (7).

the correlation length is one iteration, and thus the points $(x_i, x_{i+1}, x_{i+2}, ..., x_{i+d_e-1})$ for $i=1$ to $N - d_e + 1$ were used to reconstruct the trajectories. Embedding dimensions from $d_e = 3$ to $d_e = 11$ were used. The correlation function $C(r)$ versus r and the number of boxes of size ϵ occupied by at least one point of the trajectory $N_B(\epsilon)$ were then computed. The dimensions were determined as the least squares estimates of

$$d_C = \frac{d \log C(r)}{d \log r} \quad \text{and} \quad d_B = \frac{d \log N_B(\epsilon)}{d \log(1/\epsilon)}.$$

These results are shown in fig. 2 for the Hénon map and in fig. 3 for the modified Sierpinski triangle map. Note that d_B is a function of $1/\epsilon$, but that its average over different scales, always using the same fixed range from $m = k - 2$ to $N_B(\epsilon) = N/5$, yields an accurate estimate of the fractal dimension. The estimates of the dimensions are given in table 1 when the embedding dimension $d_e = 3$ and the number of points $N = 1000$ and 10000. All computations were done using an Apple Macintosh II and compiled Microsoft® QuickBASIC.

We have described a simple, fast, and accurate box counting method to determine the fractal dimension. This method has a fixed rule to fit the experimental data. This is an advantage over the correlation dimension where the range of r chosen to evaluate the dimension will vary with each particular data set. This box counting method is particularly well suited for low dimensional systems, such

Volume 141, number 8,9   PHYSICS LETTERS A   20 November 1989

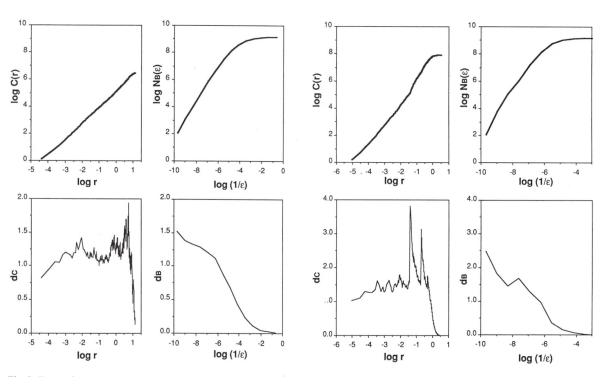

Fig. 2. Shown for the Hénon map with $d_e = 3$ and $N = 10000$ are the correlation function $C(r)$, and the number of boxes $N_B(\epsilon)$, of size ϵ occupied by the set. Below, are the correlation dimension $d_C = \mathrm{d} \log C(r) / \mathrm{d} \log r$ and the capacity dimension $d_B = \mathrm{d} \log N_B(\epsilon) / \mathrm{d} \log(1/\epsilon)$.

Fig. 3. Shown for the iterated function system representing the modified Sierpinski triangle map with $d_e = 3$ and $N = 10000$ are the correlation function $C(r)$, and the number of boxes $N_B(\epsilon)$, of size ϵ occupied by the set. Below, are the correlation dimension $d_C = \mathrm{d} \log C(r) / \mathrm{d} \log r$ and the capacity dimension $d_B = \mathrm{d} \log N_B(\epsilon) / \mathrm{d} \log(1/\epsilon)$.

as the analysis of two-dimensional images.

Note added. Daniel Kaplan has suggested to us a revision of our algorithm that considerably reduces

the execution time by using binary operations. If the high to low ordering of the bits in Z_n is the cyclic ordering of the bits in the coordinates Y_i, then the Z_n

Table 1
The results displayed correspond to embedding dimension 3. The Grassberger–Procaccia algorithm was used with reference points being 1% of the total amount of data points. The errors stated are those of the least-squares fit, which underestimate the systematic errors in both methods.

	Exact fractal dimension	Correlation dimension by Grassberger–Procaccia algorithm (computational time in minutes)		Capacity dimension by new box counting algorithm (computational time in minutes)	
		$N = 1000$	$N = 10000$	$N = 1000$	$N = 10000$
Hénon attractor	1.26	1.15 ± 0.01 (2)	1.21 ± 0.002 (420)	1.32 ± 0.02 (2)	1.27 ± 0.02 (19)
modified Sierpinski	1.58	1.50 ± 0.03 (2)	1.53 ± 0.01 (580)	1.62 ± 0.001 (2)	1.63 ± 0.04 (17)
middle third Cantor set	0.631	0.611 ± 0.012 (2)	0.630 ± 0.003 (570)	0.701 ± 0.015 (2)	0.639 ± 0.007 (16)

Volume 141, number 8,9   PHYSICS LETTERS A   20 November 1989

need to be sorted only once for all box sizes. Then for each box size, the box size dependent masking is performed, and the list of Z_n searched for distinct numbers.

This work was done during the tenure of an established investigatorship of the American Heart Association for L.S.L. This work was also supported by grants from the Whitaker Foundation and the National Institutes of Health, EY6234.

References

[1] H.G.E. Hentschel and I. Procaccia, Physica D 8 (1983) 435.

[2] A.N. Kolmogorov, Dokl. Akad. Nauk SSSR 119 (1958) 861.

[3] P. Grassberger, Phys. Lett. A 97 (1983) 224.

[4] M. Barnsley, Fractals everywhere (Academic Press, New York, 1988).

[5] A.N. Kolmogorov, Dokl. Akad. Nauk SSSR 124 (1959) 754.

[6] P. Grassberger and I. Procaccia, Phys. Rev. Lett. 50 (1983) 346.

[7] A. Wolf, J.B. Swift, H.L. Swinney and J.A. Vastano, Physica D 16 (1985) 295.

[8] J.P. Eckmann, S.O. Kamphorst, D. Ruelle and S. Ciliberto, Phys. Rev. A 34 (1986) 4971.

[9] A.M. Albano, J. Muench, C. Schwartz, A.I. Mees and P.E. Rapp, Phys. Rev. A 38 (1988) 3017.

[10] G. Mayer-Kress, ed., Dimensions and entropies in chaotic systems (Springer, Berlin, 1986).

[11] H.G. Schuster, Deterministic chaos (VCH, 1988).

[12] N. Gershenfeld, in: Directions in chaos, Vol. 2, ed. Hao Bai-Lin (World Scientific, Singapore, 1988).

[13] D.T. Kaplan, Dynamics of cardiac electrical instability, Ph.D. thesis Div. Appl. Sci. Harvard Univ. (1989).

[14] F. Caserta, H.E. Stanley, W.D. Eldred, G. Daccord, R.E. Hausman and J. Nittmann, Can we measure the shape of a neuron, preprint.

[15] J. Theiler, Phys. Rev. A 36 (1987) 4456.

[16] J. Holzfuss and G. Mayer-Kress, in: Dimensions and entropies in chaotic systems, ed. G. Mayer-Kress (Springer, Berlin, 1986) p. 114.

[17] P. Grassberger and I. Procaccia, Physica D 9 (1983) 189.

[18] F. Hunt and F. Sullivan, in: Dimensions and entropies in chaotic systems, ed. G. Mayer-Kress (Springer, Berlin, 1986) p. 74.

[19] A. Giorgilli, D. Casati, L. Sironi and L. Galgani, Phys. Lett. A 115 (1986) 202.

[20] H.S. Greenside, A. Wolf, J. Swift and T. Pignataro, Phys. Rev. A 25 (1982) 3453.

[21] B.B. Mandelbrot, The fractal geometry of nature (Freeman, San Francisco, 1983).

[22] W.H. Press, B.P. Flannery, S.A. Teukolsky and W.T. Vetterline, Numerical recipes (Cambridge Univ. Press, Cambridge, 1986).

[23] R. Dayton, Microsoft BASIC (Reston Publishing Co., Inc., Reston, VA, 1985) p. 83.

[24] J.M.T. Thompson and H.B. Stewart, Nonlinear dynamics and chaos (Wiley, New York, 1988).

[25] D.A. Russel, J.D. Hanson and E. Ott, Phys. Rev. Lett. 45 (1980) 1175.

[26] N.H. Packard, J.P. Crutchfield, J.D. Farmer and R.S. Shaw, Phys. Rev. Lett. 45 (1980) 712.

[27] F. Takens, Detecting strange attractors in turbulence, in: Dynamical systems and turbulence, eds. D.A. Rand and L.-S. Young (Springer, Berlin, 1980) p. 336.

Physica 9D (1983) 189–208
North-Holland Publishing Company

MEASURING THE STRANGENESS OF STRANGE ATTRACTORS

Peter GRASSBERGER† and Itamar PROCACCIA
Department of Chemical Physics, Weizmann Institute of Science, Rehovot 76100, Israel

Received 16 November 1982
Revised 26 May 1983

We study the correlation exponent v introduced recently as a characteristic measure of strange attractors which allows one to distinguish between deterministic chaos and random noise. The exponent v is closely related to the fractal dimension and the information dimension, but its computation is considerably easier. Its usefulness in characterizing experimental data which stem from very high dimensional systems is stressed. Algorithms for extracting v from the time series of a single variable are proposed. The relations between the various measures of strange attractors and between them and the Lyapunov exponents are discussed. It is shown that the conjecture of Kaplan and Yorke for the dimension gives an upper bound for v. Various examples of finite and infinite dimensional systems are treated, both numerically and analytically.

1. Introduction

It is already an accepted notion that many nonlinear dissipative dynamical systems do not approach stationary or periodic states asymptotically. Instead, with appropriate values of their parameters, they tend towards strange attractors on which the motion is chaotic, i.e. not (multiply) periodic and unpredictable over long times, being extremely sensitive on the initial conditions [1–4].

A natural question is by which observables this situation is most efficiently characterized. Even more basically, when observing a seemingly strange behaviour, one would like to have clear-cut procedures which could exclude that the attractor is indeed multiply periodic, or that the irregularities are e.g. caused by external noise [5].

The first possibility can be ruled out by making a Fourier analysis, but for the second one has to turn to some other measures. These measures should be sensitive to the *local* structure, in order to distinguish the blurred tori of a noisy (multi-) periodic motion from the strictly deterministic

† Permanent address: Department of Physics, University of Wuppertal, W. Germany.

motion on a fractal. Also, they should be able to distinguish between different strange attractors.

In this paper we shall propose such a measure. Before doing so we shall discuss however the existing approaches to the subject.

In a system with F degrees of freedom, an attractor is a subset of F-dimensional phase space towards which almost all sufficiently close trajectories get "attracted" asymptotically. Since volume is contracted in dissipative flows, the volume of an attractor is always zero, but this leaves still room for extremely complex structures.

Typically, a strange attractor arises when the flow does not contract a volume element in *all* directions, but stretches it in some. In order to remain confined to a bounded domain, the volume element gets folded at the same time, so that it has after some time a multisheeted structure. A closer study shows that it finally becomes (locally) Cantor-set like in some directions, and is accordingly a fractal in the sense of Mandelbrot [6].

Ever since the notion of strange attractors has been introduced, it has been clear that the Lyapunov exponents [7, 8] might be employed in studying them. Consider an infinitesimally small F-dimensional ball in phase space. During its evolution it will become distorted, but being infinitesimal, it will remain an ellipsoid. Denote the principal axes of this ellipsoid by $\epsilon_i(t)$ $(i = 1, \ldots, F)$. The Lyapunov exponents λ_i are then determined by

$$\epsilon_i(t) \approx \epsilon_i(0)\, e^{\lambda_i t}. \tag{1.1}$$

The sum of the λ_i, describing the contraction of volume, has of course to be negative. But since a strange attractor results from a stretching and folding process, it requires at least one of the λ_i to be positive. Inversely, a positive Lyapunov exponent implies sensitive dependence on initial conditions and therefore chaotic behaviour.

One drawback of the λ_i's is that they are not easily measured in experimental situations. Another limitation is that while they describe the *stretching* needed to generate a strange attractor, they don't say much about the *folding*.

That these two are at least partially independent is best seen by looking at a horshoe-like map† embedded in 3-dimensional space (fig. 1). Assume that each step of the evolution consists of (i) stretching in the x-direction by a factor of 2, (ii) squeezing in the y- and z-direction by different factors $\mu_z < \mu_y < \tfrac{1}{2}$, and (iii) folding in the (x, y) plane (fig. 1a) or in the (x, z) plane (fig. 1b). From fig. 1 one realizes already that the attractor will in both cases be a Cantorian set of lines, being more "plane-filling" in the first case than in the second case. Indeed, using the results of Section 7, one finds easily that the fractal dimensions are $D_a = 1 + \ln 2/|\ln \mu_y|$ and $D_b = 1 + \ln 2/|\ln \mu_z|$, respectively.

It is this fractal (or Hausdorff–Besikovich) dimension which has until now attracted most attention [9–14] as a measure of the local structure of fractal attractors. In order to define it [5], one first covers the attractor by F-dimensional hypercubes of side length l and considers the limit $l \to 0$. If the

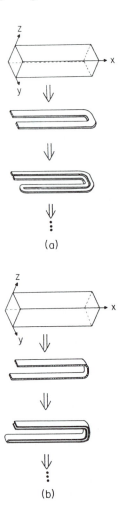

Fig. 1. Shape of an originally rectangular volume element after two iterations, each consisting of stretching, squeezing and folding. In fig. 1a (1b), the folding is in the $y(z)$-direction, which is the direction of lesser (stronger) squeezing.

minimal number of cubes needed for the covering grows like

$$M(l) \underset{l \to 0}{\simeq} l^{-D}, \tag{1.2}$$

the exponent D is called the Hansdorff dimension of the attractor [5].

Being a purely geometric measure, D is independent of the frequency with which a typical trajectory visits the various parts of the attractor.

---

† Notice that this is not a Smale's horseshoe. We also neglect in the following the bent parts of the horseshoe, in comparison to the parallel parts (i.e. we assume $L_x \gg L_y$, L_z; see fig. 1).

Even if these frequencies are very inequal, developing maybe even singularities somewhere, all parts contribute to D equally. It has been documented [12, 14] that the calculation of D is exceedingly hard and in fact impractical for higher dimensional systems.

Another measure which has been considered and which is sensitive to the frequency of visiting, is the information entropy of the attractor. By "information entropy" here we understand the information gained by an observer who measures the actual state $X(t)$ of the system with accuracy l, and who knows all properties of the system but not the initial condition $X(0)$. This is very similar to the entropy in statistical mechanics if we relate $X(t)$ to the microstate ($F \approx 10^{23}$), and the "system" to the macrostate. It is *not* the Kolmogorov entropy which is essentially the sum of all positive Lyapunov exponents.

Using the above partition of phase space into cells with length l, the information entropy can be written as

$$S(l) = - \sum_{i=1}^{M(l)} p_i \ln p_i, \qquad (1.3)$$

where p_i is the probability for $X(t)$ to fall into the ith cell. For all attractors studied so far, $S(l)$ increases logarithmically with $1/l$ as $l \to 0$, and we shall accordingly make the ansatz

$$S(l) \simeq S_0 - \sigma \ln l. \qquad (1.4)$$

The constant σ will be called, following ref. 8, the information dimension. It is always a lower bound to the Hausdorff dimension, and in most cases they are almost the same within numerical errors.

The measure on which we shall concentrate mostly in this paper, has been recently introduced by the present authors [15]. It is obtained from the correlations between random points on the attractor. Consider the set $\{X_i, i = 1 \cdots N\}$ of points on the attractor, obtained e.g. from a time series, i.e. $X_i \equiv X(t + i\tau)$ with a fixed time increment τ between successive measurements. Due to the exponential divergence of trajectories, most pairs (X_i, X_j) with $i \neq j$ will be *dynamically* uncorrelated pairs of essentially random points. The points lie however on the attractor. Therefore they will be spatially correlated. We measure this spatial correlation with the correlation integral $C(l)$, defined according to

$$C(l) = \lim_{N \to \infty} \frac{1}{N^2} \times \{\text{number of pairs } (i,j) \text{ whose}$$

$$\text{distance } |X_i - X_j| \text{ is less than } l\}. \qquad (1.5)$$

The correlation integral is related to the standard correlation function

$$c(r) = \lim_{N \to \infty} \frac{1}{N^2} \sum_{\substack{i,j=1 \\ i \neq j}}^{N} \delta^F(X_i - X_j - r) \qquad (1.6)$$

by

$$C(l) = \int_0^l \mathrm{d}^F r \, c(r). \qquad (1.7)$$

One of the central aims of this paper is to establish that for small l's $C(l)$ grows like a power

$$C(l) \sim l^\nu, \qquad (1.8)$$

and that this "correlation exponent" can be taken as a most useful measure of the local structure of a strange attractor. It seems that ν is more relevant, in this respect, than D. In any case, its calculation yields also an estimate of σ and D, since we shall argue that in general one has

$$\nu \leqslant \sigma \leqslant D. \qquad (1.9)$$

We found that the inequalities are rather tight in most cases, but not in all. Given an experimental signal, if one finds eq. (1.8) with $\nu < F$, one knows that the signal stems from deterministic chaos rather than random noise, since random noise will always result in $C(l) \sim l^F$. Explicit algorithms will be proposed below.

One of the main advantages of v is that it can easily be measured, at least more easily than either σ or D. This is particularly true for cases where the fractal dimension is large ($\gtrsim 3$) and a covering by small cells becomes virtually impossible. We thus expect that the measure v will be used in experimental situations, where typically high dimensional systems exist.

In theoretical cases, when the evolution law is known analytically, the easiest quantities to evaluate are the Lyapunov exponents. General formulae expressing D in terms of the λ_i have been proposed by Mori [9] and by Kaplan and Yorke [10]. If they were correct, they would obviously be very useful. They have been verified in simple cases [11, 14]. But Mori's formula was shown to be wrong in one case by Farmer [8], and the above example shown in fig. 1 shows that also the Kaplan–Yorke formula

$$D = D_{KY} \equiv j + \frac{\lambda_1 + \lambda_2 + \cdots + \lambda_j}{|\lambda_{j+1}|} \qquad (1.10)$$

does not hold even in all those cases where $v = \sigma = D$. Here, the exponents are ordered in descending order $\lambda_1 \geq \lambda_2 \geq \cdots \geq \lambda_F$, and j is the largest integer for which $\lambda_1 + \lambda_1 + \ldots + \lambda_j \geq 0$.

In section 7 we shall take up this question again. We shall show that the counterexample in fig. 1b is not generic. We shall however claim that eq. (1.10) cannot generally be expected to be correct, and that in fact D_{KY} is an upper bound, if $v = \sigma = D$.

In the next section, we shall present numerical results for several simple models, for which the fractal dimensions are known from the literature. This will serve to illustrate the scaling law (1.8), and to verify the inequality $v \leq D$. This inequality and its stronger version, eq. (1.9), will be derived in section 3. The case of one-dimensional maps at infinite bifurcation (Feigenbaum [16]) points is special in that there the information dimension σ and the exponent v can be calculated exactly, with the result $v \neq \sigma \neq D$. It is treated in section 4. Section 5 is dedicated to an important modification

which allows to extract v from a time series of one single variable, instead of from the series $\{X_i\}$. This is of course most important for infinite-dimensional systems, but it is also very useful in low-dimensional cases where it diminishes systematic errors. Among others, we shall apply this method in section 6 to the Mackey–Glass [17] delay equation studied in great detail in ref. 8.

In section 7 we discuss the relation of v to the Lyapunov exponents, and establish the result

$$v \leqslant D_{KY} . \qquad (1.11)$$

A summary and a discussion of the actual method of treating experimental signals is offered in section 8.

2. Case studies of low-dimensional systems

In this section we shall establish that $C(l)$ can be very well represented by a power law l^v, by exhibiting numerical results for a number of low dimensional systems. These results are summarized in table I. In section 5 we shall show that this is the case also in high (and infinite) dimensional systems. Details of the numerical algorithms are discussed in appendix A.

2.1. One-dimensional maps

The simplest cases of chaotic system are represented by maps of some interval into itself, as e.g. the logistic map [2]

$$x_{n+1} = ax_n(1 - x_n) . \qquad (2.1)$$

We shall study this map both at the point of onset of chaos via period doubling bifurcations, i.e. when $a = a_\infty = 3.5699456\ldots$ and for the case $a = 4.0$. In fig. 2 we show the result for the first case. It is well known [2, 16] that for this map the attractor* is

---

* Note that the term "attractor" would not be universally accepted here due to the fact that in any neighbourhood there exist trajectories which do not tend towards it asymptotically.

P. Grassberger and I. Procaccia / Measuring the strangeness of strange attractors   193

Table I

	v	No. of iterations, time increment τ	D	σ
Hénon map $a = 1.4$, $b = 0.3$	$1.21 \pm 0.01^{d)}$ $1.25 \pm 0.02^{e)}$	15000	1.26 (ref. 11)	-
Kaplan–Yorke map $\alpha = 0.2$	1.42 ± 0.02	15000	1.431(ref. 11)	-
Logistic eq., $b = 3.5699456\cdots$	0.500 ± 0.005 $0.4926 < v < 0.5024^{f)}$	25000	0.538(ref. 13)	0.5170976
Lorenz eq.$^{a)}$	2.05 ± 0.01	15000; $\tau = 0.25$	2.06 ± 0.01	-
Rabinovich–$^{b)}$ Fabrikant eq.	2.19 ± 0.01	15000; $\tau = 0.25$	-	-
Zaslavskii map$^{c)}$	(≈ 1.5)	25000	1.39(ref. 11)	-

$^{a)}$Parameters as in refs. 7 and 11.
$^{b)}$Parameters as in section 3 of ref. 20.
$^{c)}$Parameters as in ref. 11.
$^{d)}$From eqs. (1.5) and (1.8).
$^{e)}$From single variable time series, with $f = 3$.
$^{f)}$Exact analytic bound.

Cantor-like with a fractal dimension satisfying the exact bound [13] $0.5376 < D < 0.5386$. In section 4 we shall prove exactly that $\sigma = 0.517097\ldots$, and that $0.4926 < v < 0.5024$ while from Fig. 2 we find $v = 0.500 \pm 0.005$. For very small distances, the data for $C(l)$ deviate from a power law, but that was to be expected: the behaviour at $a = a_{\infty}$ is not yet chaotic, and therefore the values x_n are strongly

correlated. We verified that indeed the powerlaw holds down to smaller values of l if we increase N or use only values x_i, x_{i+p}, x_{i+2p}, x_{i+2p}, ... with p being a large odd number.

The same map can be used also to introduce the important issue of corrections to scaling. These are found for the parameter value $a = 4$. It is well known that in this the attractor* consists of the interval $[0, 1]$, and that the invariant probability density is equal to

$$p(x) \equiv \lim_{N \to \infty} \frac{1}{N} \sum_{i=1}^{N} \delta(x_i - x) \qquad (2.2)$$

$$= \frac{1}{\pi} [x(1-x)]^{-1/2}. \qquad (2.3)$$

From this, one finds easily

$$v = \sigma = D = 1. \qquad (2.4)$$

Notice, however, that while the scaling laws (1.2) and (1.4) are exact, the scaling law (1.8) for $C(l)$

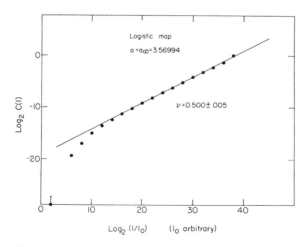

Fig. 2. Correlation integral for the logistic map (2.1) at the infinite bifurcation point $a = a_{\infty} = 3.699\ldots$ The starting point was $x_0 = \frac{1}{2}$, the number of points was $N = 30.000$.

*Again, the term is questionable, as no point outside the interval [0, 1] gets attracted towards it. We shall ignore this irrelevant point, which could be avoided by using $a = 4 - \epsilon$.

194   *P. Grassberger and I. Procaccia / Measuring the strangeness of strange attractors*

requires logarithmic corrections, due to the singular behaviour of $p(x)$:

$$C(l) = \int_0^1 \int dx\, dy p(x)p(y)\theta(|x-y|-l)$$

$$\simeq_{l\to 0} \frac{4}{\pi^2} l \ln 1/l. \qquad (2.5)$$

Thus, a numerical calculation of v is expected to converge very slowly. This problem and a remedy for it are discussed further in section 5.

2.2. Maps of the plane

Here we examined the Hénon [18] map

$$x_{n+1} = y_n + 1 - ax_n^2,$$
$$y_{n+1} = bx_n, \qquad (2.6)$$

with $a = 1.4$ and $b = 0.3$, the Kaplan–Yorke [10] map

$$x_{n+1} = 2x_n \quad (\text{mod } 1),$$
$$y_{n+1} = \alpha y_n + \cos 4\pi x_n, \qquad (2.7)$$

with $\alpha = 0.2$, and the Zaslavskii [19] map

$$x_{n+1} = [x_n + v(1 + \mu y_n) + \epsilon v\mu \cos 2\pi x_n] \quad (\text{mod } 1),$$
$$y_{n+1} = e^{-\Gamma}(y_n + \epsilon \cos 2\pi x_n), \qquad (2.8)$$

with the parameters

$$\mu = \frac{1 - e^{-\Gamma}}{\Gamma} \qquad (2.9)$$

and $\Gamma = 3.0$, $v = 400/3$, and $\epsilon = 0.3$ taken from ref. 11.

Figs. 3–5 exhibit the results for the correlation integrals. In the first two cases, we find excellent agreement with a power law; while for the Kaplan–Yorke map we find $v = 1.42 \pm .02$ in agreement with the published [11] value of D, a fit to the Hénon map yields $v_{eff} = 1.21$, smaller than

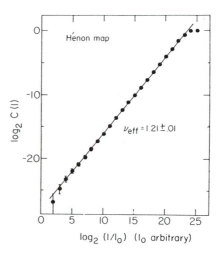

Fig. 3. Correlation integral for the Hénon map (2.6) with $a = 1.4$, $b = 0.03$ and $N = 15.000$.

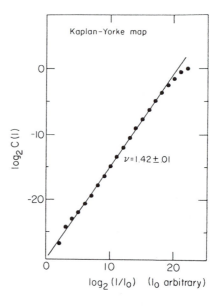

Fig. 4. Same as fig. 3, but for Kaplan–Yorke map (2.7) with $\alpha = 0.2$.

the value [11] $D = 1.261 \pm 0.003$. We shall argue in sectin 5 that actually the value of v for the Hénon map is underestimated here, and that instead $v = 1.25 \pm 0.02 \approx D$.

The case of the Zaslavskii map is exceptional as it was the only system for which we did not find

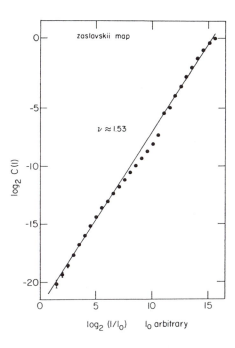

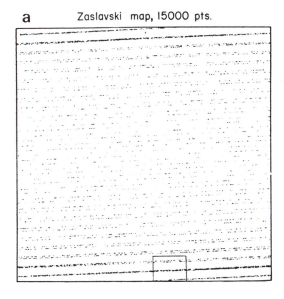

a Zaslavski map, 15000 pts.

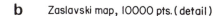

b Zaslavski map, 10000 pts. (detail)

Fig. 5. Correlation integral for Zaslavskii map (eqs. (2.8), (2.9)); $N = 25.000$, parameters as in the text. For faster scaling, the y-coordinate was blown up by a factor of 25, rendering the attractor square-like at low resolution (see fig. 6; without this, the attractor would have looked effectively 1-dimensional for $l \gtrsim l_{max}/25$).

Fig. 6. Attractor of the Zaslavskii map. a) entire attractor (15.000 points plotted; y-scale blown up by factor 25); b) Blown up view of part indicated in part a (10.000 points plotted).

clear-cut power behaviour. Also, an (admittedly poor) fit would yield $v \approx 1.5$, in clear violation of the bound $v < D$. The reasons why our method has to fail for this map – with the parameters as quoted above – becomes clear when looking at fig. 6. Call l_0 the outer length scale. From fig. 6a one sees that the attractor looks 2-dimensional for $l \gtrsim l_0 \times 2^{-5}$ and $\approx$ 1-dimensional for $l_0 \times 2^{-5} \gtrsim l \gtrsim l_0 \times 2^{-9}$. From fig. 6b one sees that it looks $\approx$ 2-dimensional again down to $\approx l_0 \times 2^{-14}$, scaling behaviour setting in only at about that scale (which is beyond our resolution). It seems to us that the box-counting algorithm of ref. 11 in which D is evaluated, should confront the same problem†.

2.3. *Differential equations*

We have studied the Lorenz [1] model

$$\dot{x} = \sigma(y - x),$$
$$\dot{y} = -y - xz + Rx, \qquad (2.10)$$
$$\dot{z} = xy - bz,$$

† Note added: Dr. Russel kindly provided us with the original data of $M(\epsilon)$ versus ϵ. From these, it seems that indeed a similar phenomenon occurs and that accordingly a value $D \approx 1.5$ cannot be excluded.

with $R = 28$, $\sigma = 10$, and $b = 8/3$, and the Rabinovich–Fabrikant [20] equations

$$\dot{x} = y(z - 1 + x^2) + \gamma x ,$$
$$\dot{y} = x(3z + 1 - x^2) + \gamma y , \qquad (2.11)$$
$$\dot{z} = -2z(\alpha + xy) ,$$

with $\gamma = 0.87$ and $\alpha = 1.1$.

As seen in fig. 7 we get adequate power laws for $C(l)$, and in the case of the Lorenz model, where D is known [11], we obtain $\nu \simeq D$.

Further examples will be studied in section 6, in the context of higher dimensional systems.

It should be stressed that the algorithm used to calculate ν converged quite rapidly. Although each entry in table I and figs. 2–7 were based on ≈ 15.000–25.000 points each, reasonable results (i.e. results for ν within $\pm 5\%$) were obtained in most cases already with only a few thousand

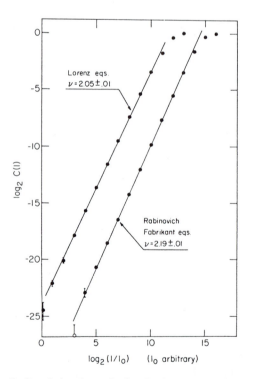

Fig. 7. Correlation integrals for the Lorenz equations (eq. (2.10); dots) and for the Rabinovich–Fabrikant equation (eq. (2.11); open circles). In both cases, $N = 15.000$ and $\tau = 0.25$.

points. This should be contrasted with the difficulties associated with estimating D in box-counting algorithms [11, 14].

Summarizing this section, we can say that except for the logistic map at $a = a_\infty$ ("Feigenbaum attractor") we found in all cases that $\nu \approx D$ within the limits of accuracy. We now turn to a theoretical analysis of the relations between ν, σ and D.

3. Relations between ν, σ and D

In this section we shall establish the inequalities (1.9). We shall do this in 3 steps.

a) The easiest inequality to prove is $\sigma \leqslant D$. Consider a covering of the attractor by hypercubes ("cells") of edge length l, and a time series $\{X_k; k = 1, \ldots, N\}$. The probabilities p_i for an arbitrary X_k to fall into cell i are simply

$$p_i = \lim_{N \to \infty} \frac{1}{N} \mu_i . \qquad (3.1)$$

where μ_i is the number of points X_k which fall into cell i.

If the coverage of the attractor is uniform, one has,

$$p_i = \frac{1}{M(l)} , \qquad (3.2)$$

where $M(l)$ is the number of cells needed to cover the attractor, and one finds from eqs. (1.3) and (1.2)

$$S(l) = S^{(0)}(l) = \ln M(l) = \text{const} - D \ln l . \qquad (3.3)$$

In the general case, one uses the convexity of $x \ln x$ in the usual way to prove that $S(l) \leqslant S^{(0)}(l)$. Invoking the ansatz $S(l) = \text{const} - \sigma \ln l$, we find $\sigma \leqslant D$.

b) Instead of showing immediately $\nu \leqslant \sigma$, let us proceed slowly and show first that $\nu \leqslant D$.

From the definition of $C(l)$, we get up to a factor

P. Grassberger and I. Procaccia / Measuring the strangeness of strange attractors 197

of order unity

$$C(l) \simeq \lim_{N \to \infty} \frac{1}{N^2} \sum_{i=1}^{M(l)} \mu_i^2 = \sum_{i=1}^{M(l)} p_i^2 . \qquad (3.4)$$

Here, we have replaced the number of pairs with distance $< l$ by the number of pairs which fall into the same cell of length l. The error committed should be independent on l, and thus should not affect the estimation of v. Using the Schwartz inequality we get

$$C(l) = M(l)\langle p_i^2 \rangle \geqslant M(l)\langle p_i \rangle^2 = \frac{1}{M(l)} \sim l^D . \quad (3.5)$$

In this equation square brackets denote average over all cells. Comparing eqs. (3.5) and (1.8) we find immediately $v \leqslant D$.

c) In order to derive $v \leqslant \sigma$, consider two nested coverings with cubes of lengths l and $2l$. The numbers of cubes that contain a piece of the attractor are then related by

$$M(l) = 2^D M(2l) . \qquad (3.6)$$

Denote by p_i the probability to fall in cube i of the finer coverage, and by P_j the probability to fall in cube j of the coarser. Define $\omega_i (i = 1, \ldots M(l))$ by

$$p_i = \omega_i P_j \quad (i \in j) . \qquad (3.7)$$

Evidently we have

$$P_j = \sum_{i \in j} p_i, \quad \sum_{i \in j} \omega_i = 1 . \qquad (3.8)$$

We can then write the correlation integral as

$$C(l) \simeq \sum_{i=1}^{M(l)} p_i^2 = \sum_{j=1}^{M(2l)} P_j^2 \sum_{i \in j} \omega_i^2 . \qquad (3.9)$$

Consider now the ratio

$$\frac{C(l)}{C(2l)} = \frac{\sum_j P_j^2 \sum_{i \in j} \omega_i^2}{\sum_j P_j^2} , \qquad (3.10)$$

and compare it to the entropy difference

$$S(2l) - S(l) = \sum_{i=1}^{M(l)} p_i \ln p_i - \sum_{j=1}^{M(2l)} P_j \ln P_j$$
$$= \sum_{j=1}^{M(2l)} P_j \sum_{i \in j} \omega_i \ln \omega_i . \qquad (3.11)$$

In order to estimate eq. (3.10) in terms of eq. (3.11), we have to introduce a new assumption. We assume that the ω_i's are distributed independently of the P_j. This means essentially that locally the attractor looks the same in regions where it is rather dense (P_j large) as in regions where P_j is small. Although we cannot further justify this assumption, it seems to us very natural. It leads immediately to

$$\frac{C(l)}{C(2l)} = \frac{\langle \omega^2 \rangle}{\langle \omega \rangle} = 2^D \langle \omega^2 \rangle , \qquad (3.12)$$

and to

$$S(2l) - S(l) = 2^D \langle \omega \ln \omega \rangle . \qquad (3.13)$$

Define now a normalized variable W by

$$W = \frac{\omega}{\langle \omega \rangle} = 2^D \omega . \qquad (3.14)$$

Using the inequality [21]

$$\langle W^2 \rangle > \exp \langle W \ln W \rangle , \qquad (3.15)$$

we establish

$$\frac{C(l)}{C(2l)} \geqslant \exp[S(2l) - S(l)] \qquad (3.16)$$

and thus

$$v \leqslant \sigma . \qquad (3.17)$$

Remarks. From the proofs it is clear that if the attractor is uniformly covered, one has equalities

$$v = \sigma = D . \qquad (3.18)$$

It is an interesting question how non-uniform the coverage must be in order to break them. With the exception of the Feigenbaum map (logistic map with $a = a_\infty$), which is however not generic, all examples of the last section were compatible with eq. (3.18).

In cases where $v \neq D$, we claim that indeed v is the more relevant observable. In these cases, the neighbourhoods of certain points have higher "seniority" in the sense that they are visited more often than others. The fractal dimension is ignorant of seniority, being a purely geometric concept. But both the correlation integral and the entropy dimension weight regions according to their seniority.

Eqs. (1.9) and (3.18) have been used previously in the context of fully developed homogeneous turbulence [22]. The connection

$$c(l) \propto l^{D-F}, \quad l \in R^f$$

following from $v = D$ has been used previously also in percolation theory [23] and in a model for dendritic growth [24].

4. Information entropy and v of the Feigenbaum attractor

In this section we shall compute exactly the information dimension and v of one-dimensional maps

$$x_{n+1} = F(x_n) \tag{4.1}$$

at the onset of chaos. The method follows closely the one of ref. 13.

It is well known that such maps – provided they have a unique quadratic maximum – have universal scaling features, studied in most detail by Feigenbaum [16]. This behaviour is most easily described by observing that the iterations

$$F^{(2^n)}(x) = \underbrace{F(F(\ldots F(x)\ldots))}_{2^n \text{ times}} \tag{4.2}$$

tend after a suitable rescaling towards a universal function

$$g(x) = \lim_{n \to \infty} \frac{1}{F^{(2^n)}(0)} F^{(2^n)}(x F^{(2^n)}(0)). \tag{4.3}$$

This "Feigenbaum function" $g(x)$ satisfies the exact scaling relation

$$g(g(x)) = -\frac{1}{\alpha} g(\alpha x), \tag{4.4}$$

with $\alpha = 2.50290\ldots$, and the normalization condition $g(0) = 1$. We have here assumed that the maximum of $F(x)$ is at $x = 0$, which can always be achieved by a change of variables. In order to obtain the information dimension of the logistic map at $a = a_\infty = 3.5699345\ldots$, it is thus sufficient to compute σ for the Feigenbaum map.

The "attractor" (see the reservations in section 2) of $g(x)$ consists of the sequence $\{\xi_n, n = 0, 1, 2, \ldots\}$ with

$$\xi_0 = 0 \tag{4.5}$$

and

$$\xi_{n+1} = g(\xi_n). \tag{4.6}$$

The first few ξ_k's are shown in fig. 8. There, it is also indicated how they build up the Cantorian structure of the attractor: the points ξ_1, ξ_2, $\xi_3, \ldots, \xi_{2^k+1}$ form the end-points of 2^k intervals, and the following ξ_k's fall all into these intervals. Furthermore, any sequence $\{\xi_n, \xi_{n+1} \ldots \xi_{n+2^k-1}\}$ of 2^k successive points visits each of these intervals exactly once. Thus, the a priori probabilities $p_i(i = 1, \ldots, 2^k)$ for an arbitrary x_n to fall into the ith interval are all equal to $p_i = 2^{-k}$.

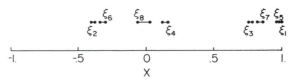

Fig. 8. First 16 points $\xi_1, \ldots, \xi_{16}$ of the attractor of the Feigenbaum equation describing the onset of chaos in 1-dimensional systems.

P. Grassberger and I. Procaccia / Measuring the strangeness of strange attractors   199

By the grouping axiom, we can first write the information entropy as

$$S(l) = \tfrac{1}{2}[S_{[2,4]}(l) + S_{[3,1]}(l)] + \ln 2 , \qquad (4.7)$$

where we denote by $S_{[i,j]}$ the information needed to specify the point on the interval $[\xi_i, \xi_j]$, and where we have used the fact that an arbitrary x_n has equal probability to be on $[\xi_2, \xi_4]$ or on $[\xi_3, \xi_1]$. From eq. (4.4) we find, however, that

$$\xi_{2.} = -\frac{1}{\alpha} \xi_n . \qquad (4.8)$$

Thus, the interval $[\xi_2, \xi_4]$ is a down-scaled image of the whole attractor, and we have

$$S_{[2,4]}(l) = S(\alpha l) \approx S(l) - \sigma \ln \alpha , \qquad (4.9)$$

where we have used the scaling ansatz (1.4).

In order to estimate $S_{[3,1]}(l)$, we decompose the interval $[3, 1]$ into the 2^{k-1} subintervals discussed above, defined by the ξ_n with odd n's:

$$S_{[3,1]}(l) = (k-1)\ln 2 + 2^{-k+1} \sum_{i=1}^{2^{k-1}} S_i(l) .$$

Again, we have applied the grouping axiom, using that $p_i = 2^{-k}$. The $S_i(l)$ are the informations needed to pin down x_n provided one knows that it falls into the ith subinterval. Since each subinterval maps onto one on the left-hand piece $[\xi_2, \xi_4]$, each $S_i(l)$ is equal to the information $\tilde{S}_i(|g_i'|l)$ needed to pin x_{n+1} on the corresponding interval on the left-hand side. Here, g_i' is some average derivative of $g(x)$ in the ith subinterval. Using that $\tilde{S}_i(|g_i'|l) \simeq \tilde{S}_i(l) - \sigma \ln|g_i'|$, we obtain

$$S_{[3,1]}(l) = (k-1)\ln 2 + 2^{-k+1} \sum_{i=1}^{2^{k-1}} \tilde{S}_i(l)$$

$$- \sigma \sum_{i=1}^{2^{k-1}} \ln|g_i'|$$

$$= S_{[2,4]}(l) - \sigma \sum_{i=1}^{2^{k-1}} \ln|g_i'| . \qquad (4.10)$$

Inserting this and eq. (4.9) into eq. (4.7), we find

after a few manipulations and after taking the limit $k \to \infty$

$$\sigma = \lim_{k \to \infty} \frac{\ln 2}{\ln \alpha + \dfrac{1}{2^{k+1}} \displaystyle\sum_{i=1}^{2^k} |g'(\xi_{2i-1})|} . \qquad (4.11)$$

The limit converges very quickly, leading (for $k > 7$) to

$$\sigma = 0.5170976 . \qquad (4.12)$$

The calculation of the correlation exponent, or rather of the exponent of the Renyi entropy (see eq. (3.4))

$$R(l) = \sum_{i=1}^{M(l)} p_i^2 \qquad (4.13)$$

follows even more closely the one in ref. 13.

As in that paper, we obtain a nested set of bounds. The first (and least stringent) is obtained by writing

$$R(l) = \tfrac{1}{4}\{R_{[2,4]}(l) + R_{[3,1]}(l)\} \qquad (4.14)$$

and using $R_{[2,4]}(l) = R(\alpha.l)$ and $R_{[3,1]}(l) = R(\alpha g'l)$ with

$$|g'(\xi_3)| < g' < |g'(\xi_1)| . \qquad (4.15)$$

Assuming $R(l) \sim l^\nu$, we obtain

$$1 + |g'(\xi_3)|^\nu < \frac{4}{\alpha^\nu} < 1 + |g'(\xi_1)|^\nu , \qquad (4.16)$$

leading to $0.4857 < \nu < 0.5235$.

For the next more stringent bounds, we write further

$$R_{[3,1]}(l) = \tfrac{1}{4}\{R_{[3,7]}(l) + R_{[5,1]}(l)\} , \qquad (4.17)$$

with

$$R_{[3,7]}(l) + R(\alpha^2 g^{(1)}.l), \quad |g'(\xi_3)| < g^{(1)} < |g'(\xi_7)|$$
$$(4.18)$$

and

$$R_{[5,1]}(l) + R_{[3,1]}(\alpha g^{(2)}l), \quad |g'(\xi_5)| < g^{(2)} < |g'(\xi_1)| .$$
(4.19)

Some algebra leads then to

$$|g'(\xi_5)|^\nu + \frac{\alpha^\nu}{4 - \alpha^\nu} |g'(\xi_3)|^\nu < \frac{4}{\alpha^\nu}$$

$$< |g'(\xi_1)|^\nu + \frac{\alpha^\nu}{4 - \alpha^\nu} |g'(\xi_7)|^\nu ,$$
(4.20)

with the result

$$0.4926 < \nu < 0.5024 ,$$
(4.21)

in agreement with the numerical value $\nu = 0.500 \pm 0.005$.

5. Using a single-variable time series

Very often one does not have access to a time series $\{X_n\}$ of F-dimensional vectors. Instead one follows only one or at most a few components of X_n. This is particularly relevant for real (as opposed to computer) experiments where the number of degrees of freedom often is very high if not infinite. Such systems nevertheless can have low-dimensional attractors. It would be very desirable to have a reliable method which allows a characterization of this attractor from a single-variable time series. $\{x_i, i = 1, \ldots, N; x_i \in R\}$.

The essential idea [25, 26] consists in constructing d-dimensional vectors

$$\xi_i = (x_i, x_{i+1}, \ldots, x_{i+d-1})$$
(5.1)

and using ξ-space instead of X-space. The correlation integral would e.g. be

$$C(l) = \lim_{N \to \infty} \frac{1}{N^2} \sum_{i,j=1}^{N} \theta(l - |\xi_i - \xi_j|) .$$
(5.2)

More generally, one can use

$$\xi_i = (x(t_i), x(t_i + \tau) \ldots x(t_i + (d-1)\tau)),$$
(5.3)

with τ some fixed interval. The magnitude of τ should not be chosen too small since otherwise $x_i \approx x_{i+\tau} \approx x_{i+2\tau} \approx \cdots$ so that the attractor in ξ-space would be stretched along the diagonal and thus difficult to disentangle. On the other hand, τ should not be chosen too large since distant values in the time series are not strongly correlated (due to the exponential divergence of trajectories and unavoidable small errors).

A similar compromise must be chosen for the dimension d. Clearly, d must be larger than the Hausdorff dimension D of the attractor (otherwise, $C(l) \sim l^d$). If the attractor is Cantorian in more than one dimension, this might however not be sufficient. Also, it might be that, when looked at in d dimension, the density

$$p(\xi) = \lim_{N \to \infty} \frac{1}{N} \sum_{i=1}^{N} \delta(\xi_i - \xi)$$
(5.4)

develops singularities which are absent in more than d dimensions (such singularities occur e.g. when one projects a sphere with constant density, $p(\xi) = p\delta(x^2 + y^2 + z^2 - R^2)$, onto the $x-y$ plane: the new density $\tilde{p}(x, y)$ is infinite at $x^2 + y^2 = R^2$).

On the other hand, one cannot make d too large without getting lost in experimental errors and lack of statistics.

In the next section, we shall study an infinite-dimensional system from this point of view. In the remainder of the present section, we shall apply these considerations to the logistic map with $a = 4$, and to the Hénon map.

In the logistic map, we have seen that there are logarithmic corrections to the power law $C(l) \sim l^\nu$. They result precisely from singularities of $p(x)$, at $x = 0$ and $x = 1$. While embedding the attractor in a higher dimensional space does not completely remove these singularities, it substantially reduces their influence. The reason is that embedding in higher dimensional space always results in stretching the attractor. However, the portions which are most strongly stretched are those which are most densely populated at the lower dimension. For example in the logistic map with $a = 4$ the "attractor" is the interval [0, 1] in $1d$ but is the parabola in $2d$. The parabola has highest slopes at the end points, exhibiting the stronger stretching associated with regions of singular distributions at a lower dimension. A similar effect appears when going·from $d = 2$ to $d = 3$. We thus expect that the importance of the singularities in the distribution would be reduced in higher dimensions.

In order to check this, we have calculated for the logistic map at $a = 4$ the original correlation integral and the modified integral obtained by embedding in a 2- and 3-dimensional space. The results are shown in fig. 9. We observe indeed the expected decrease of systematic error when increasing d, accompanied by an increase of the statistical error.

Analogous results for the Hénon map are shown in fig. 10. There, we used as time series the series $\{x_n, x_{n+2}, x_{n+4}, \dots\}$. While the 2-dimensional correlation integral gives an effective ν in agreement with the result of section 2, the 3-dimensional embedding gives a larger values $\nu = 1.25 \pm 0.02$ which agrees with the value of D found in refs. 11 and 14.

No such effects were observed in the Lorenz model, where both the originally defined $C(l)$ and

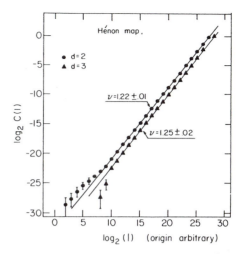

Fig. 10. Modified correlation integrals for the Hénon map (2.6). The time series consisted of coordinates x_n, x_{n+2}, $x_{n+4} \dots$, and $\xi = (x_n, x_{n+2}, \dots, x_{n+2(d-1)})$ for each d. For $d = 2$, we took $N = 30.000$; for $d = 3$, we took $N = 20.000$.

the modified correlation integral using only a single coordinate time series gave values of ν which agreed with D [15].

The conclusion drawn from these examples is that it is often useful to represent the attractor in a higher dimensional space than absolutely necessary, in order to reduce systematic errors. These errors result from a strongly non-uniform coverage of the attractor, provided this non-uniformity is not so strong as to make $\nu \neq D$.

6. Infinite-dimensional systems: an example

An extremely convenient way of generating very high dimensional systems is to consider delay differential equations of the type

$$\frac{dx(t)}{dt} = F(x(t), x(t - \tau)), \qquad (6.1)$$

where τ is a given time delay. Such a delay equation is in fact infinite dimensional, as is most easily seen from the initial conditions necessary to solve eq. (6.1): they consist of the function $x(t)$ over a whole interval of length τ.

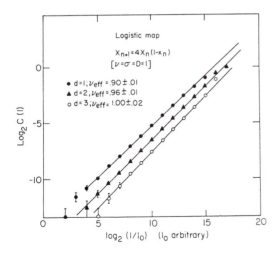

Fig. 9. Modified correlation integrals for the logistic map (2.1) with $a = 4$. The distance l between 2 points ξ_n and ξ_m on the attractor is defined as $l^2 = (\xi_n - \xi_m)^2 = (x_n - x_m)^2 + \dots + (x_{n+d-1} - x_{m+d-1})^2$. For each value of d, we took $N = 15.000$.

Following ref. 8, we shall study a particular example, introduced by Mackey and Glass [17] as a model for regeneration of blood cells in patients with leukemia. It is

$$\dot{x}(t) = \frac{ax(t-\tau)}{1 + [x(t-\tau)]^{10}} - bx(t). \qquad (6.2)$$

As in ref. 8, we shall keep $a = 0.2$ and $b = 0.1$ fixed, and study the dependence on the delay time τ.

For the numerical investigation, eq. (6.2) is turned into an n-dimensional set of difference equations, with $n = 600$–1200. Details are described in the appendix. The time series was always chosen as $\{x(t), x(t+\tau), x(t+2\tau), \dots\}$ except for some runs with $\tau = 100$, where we took points at times $t, t+\tau/2, t+2\tau/2, \dots$.

The results for the correlation integral are shown in figs. 11–14. Estimated values of ν are given in table II, together with values of D obtained in ref. 8 by applying the defining eq. (1.2) to a Poincaré return map. Also shown in table II are the

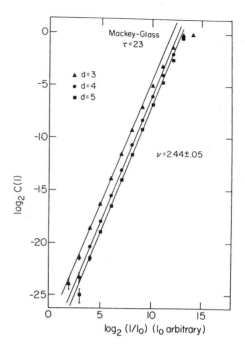

Fig. 12. Same as fig. 11, but for $\tau = 23$.

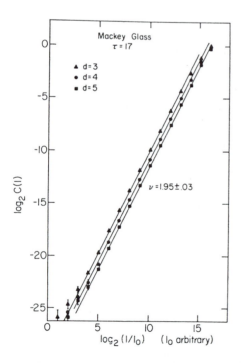

Fig. 11. Modified correlation integrals for the Mackey–Glass delay equation (6.2), with delay $\tau = 17$. The time series consisted of $\{X(t + i\tau); i = 1, \dots, 25.000\}$.

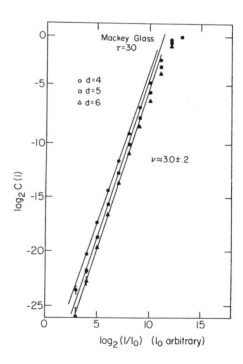

Fig. 13. Same as fig. 11, but for $\tau = 30$.

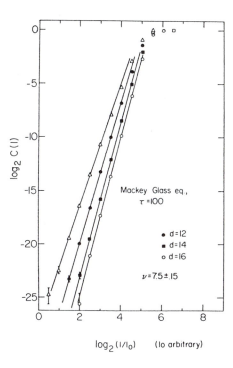

Fig. 14. Same as fig. 11, but for $\tau = 100$. For $d = 16$, the time series consisted of points $\{X(t + i\tau/2); i = 1, \ldots, 25.000\}$.

Kaplan–Yorke dimension D_{KY} (see eq. (1.10)) which will in the next section be shown to be an upper bound to v, and the number of positive Lyapunov exponents, both taken from ref. 8. It is obvious that this latter number, called D_{LB}, is a lower bound to D. If the density of trajectories on the attractor is not too non-uniform, we expect that D_{LB} yields also a lower bound to v.

From table II we see that indeed in all cases

$$D_{LB} \leqslant v \leqslant D \leqslant D_{KY}, \qquad (6.3)$$

except for $\tau = 17$ where v is slightly less than D_{LB}. However, for those small values of τ for which box-counting according to the definition of D had been feasible, our values of v are considerably smaller than the values of D found in ref. 8, while the values of D were fairly close to D_{KY}.

In all cases, the linearity of the plot of $\log C(l)$ versus $\log l$ improved substantially when increasing d above its minimal required value. For increasing values of d, the effective exponent at first also

Table II
Estimates of the correlation exponent v for the Mackey–Glass equation (6.2) with $a = 0.2$, $b = 0.1$. Values for D_{LB}, D and D_{KY} are from ref. 8. For $\tau = 100$ the value of v saturated at $d = 16$

τ	D_{LB}	v	D	D_{KY}
17.0	2	1.95 ± 0.03 ($d = 3$) 1.35 ± 0.03 ($d = 4$) 1.95 ± 0.03 ($d = 5$)	2.13 ± 0.03	2.10 ± 0.02
23.0	2	2.38 ± 0.15 ($d = 3$) 2.43 ± 0.05 ($d = 4$) 2.44 ± 0.05 ($d = 5$) 2.42 ± 0.1 ($d = 6$)	2.76 ± 0.06	2.92 ± 0.03
30.0	3	2.87 ± 0.3 ($d = 4$) 3.0 ± 0.2 ($d = 5$) 3.0 ± 0.2 ($d = 6$) 2.8 ± 0.3 ($d = 7$)	> 2.94	3.58 ± 0.04
100.0	6	5.8 ± 0.3 ($d = 10$) 6.6 ± 0.2 ($d = 12$) 7.2 ± 0.2 ($d = 14$) 7.5 ± 0.15 ($d = 16$)	-	≈ 10.0

increases, but settles at a value which we assume to be the true value of v. We must stress that we have no *proof* that the values of v obtained with the highest chosen d represent the "true" exponent. We feel however that they surely represent reasonable estimates even for attractors with dimensions as high as ≈ 7.

In real experiments, where Lyapunov exponents are not available and thus D_{LB} and D_{KY} not easily obtained, our method seems the only one which could distinguish such an attractor from a system where the stochasticity is due to random noise. In that case, one would expect $C(l) \sim l^d$ as the trajectory is space-filling, in clear distinction from what we observe.

7. Relation to Lyapunov exponents and the Kaplan–Yorke conjecture

As we already mentioned in the introduction, the Lyapunov exponents are related to the evolution of the shape of an infinitesimal F-dimensional ball in phase space: being infinitesimal, it depends only on the linearized part of the flow, and thus becomes an ellipsoid with exponentially shrinking or growing axes. Denoting the principal axes by $\epsilon_i(t)$, the Lyapunov exponents are given by

$$\lambda_i = \lim_{t \to \infty} \lim_{\epsilon_i(0) \to 0} \frac{1}{t} \ln \frac{\epsilon_i(t)}{\epsilon_i(0)}. \tag{7.1}$$

Directions associated with positive Lyapunov exponents are called "unstable", those associated with negative exponents are called "stable".

Originally [10], Kaplan and Yorke had conjectured that D_{KY} is equal to D. In a recent preprint [27], they claim that D_{KY} is generically equal to a "probabilistic dimension", which seems to be the same as σ.

This latter claim has been partially supported in ref. 28, where essentially D_{KY} is proven to be an upper bound to the probabilistic dimension.

As shown by the counter example mentioned in the introduction, there are (possibly exceptional)

cases where this bound is not saturated. In this section, we shall elucidate this question by giving a heuristic proof for the inequality $v \leqslant D$. From this, we see necessary conditions for the Kaplan–Yorke conjecture to hold, and which do not seem to be met generally.

Consider two infinitesimally close-by trajectories $X(t)$ and $X'(t) = X(t) + \Delta(t)$, where the latter could indeed be $X'(t) = X(t + T)$, which for sufficiently large T is essentially independent of $X(t)$. We assume that $\Delta_i(t)$ increase exponentially, without any fluctuations, as

$$\Delta_i(t) = \Delta_i(0)\, e^{\lambda_i t}, \tag{7.2}$$

where the components are along the principal axes discussed above. This is of course a strong assumption which would imply, in particular, that $v = \sigma = D$. Corrections to it will be treated in a forthcoming paper, but our main conclusion will remain unchanged. Conservation of the number of trajectories implies that the correlation function increases like

$$c(\Delta(t)) = \left| \frac{\partial(\Delta(0))}{\partial(\Delta(t))} \right| c(\Delta(0)) = e^{-t\Sigma_{i=1}^{F} \lambda_i} c(\Delta(0)). \tag{7.3}$$

To proceed further, we need a scaling assumption which generalizes the scaling ansatz

$$c(|\Delta|) \sim |\Delta|^{v-F}. \tag{7.4}$$

Observing that the attractor is locally a topological product of an R^n with Cantor sets, and that the relevant axes are the principal axes, we associate with each axis an exponent v_i, $0 < v_i < 1$, and make the ansatz

$$c(\Delta) \approx \prod_{i=1}^{F} c_i(\Delta_i), \tag{7.5}$$

with

$$c_i(x) \propto \begin{cases} x^{v_i - 1}, & \text{if} \quad 0 < v_i \leqslant 1, \\ \delta(x), & \text{if} \quad v_i = 0. \end{cases} \tag{7.6}$$

If $v_i = 0$, this means that the motion along this axis dies asymptotically (example: directions normal to a limit cycle). Directions with $v_i = 1$ are the unstable directions, with the continuous density. Directions with $0 < v_i < 1$, finally, are either Cantorian or, in exceptional cases, directions along which the distribution is continuous but singular at $\Delta_i = 0$. Notice that $v_i > 1$ is impossible.

Substituting eq. (7.5) into (7.3), we find

$$\prod_i (\Delta_i(0)^{v_i - 1} e^{t\lambda_i(v_i - 1)}) = e^{-t\Sigma_i\lambda_i} \prod_i \Delta_i(0)^{v_i - 1}, \qquad (7.7)$$

or

$$\sum_{i=1}^{F} \lambda_i v_i = 0. \qquad (7.8)$$

In addition we have, from eqs. (7.5) and (7.4),

$$\sum_{i=1}^{F} v_i = v, \qquad (7.9)$$

and

$$0 \leqslant v_i \leqslant 1. \qquad (7.10)$$

It is now easy to find the maximum of v subject to the constraints (7.8)–(7.10). It is obtained when

$$v_i = \begin{cases} 1, & \text{for } i \leqslant j, \\ 0, & \text{for } i \geqslant j + 2, \end{cases} \qquad (7.11a)$$

and

$$v_{j+1} = \frac{1}{|\lambda_{j+1}|} \sum_{i < j} \lambda_i. \qquad (7.11b)$$

Here, we have used that $\lambda_1 \geqslant \lambda_2 \geqslant \dots$, and that $\Sigma_j \lambda_i < 0$. Expressed in words, the distribution (7.11) means that the attractor is the most extended along the most unstable directions. Inserting it into eq. (7.9), we obtain

$$v \leqslant j + \frac{\sum_{i \leqslant j} \lambda_i}{|\lambda_{j+1}|} \equiv D_{\mathrm{KY}}. \qquad (7.12)$$

as we had claimed.

From the derivation it is clear that the Kaplan–Yorke conjectures $\sigma = D_{\mathrm{KY}}$ or $D = D_{\mathrm{KY}}$ cannot be expected to hold when *either the attractor is Cantorian in more than one dimension, or if the folding occurs in a direction which is not the minimally contracting one.* The latter was indeed the case for example b in fig. 1. But example b of fig. 1 is not generic, the generic case being the one where the folding is in a plane which encloses an arbitrary angle ϕ with the z-axis (see fig. 15). It is easy to convince oneself that $D = D_{\mathrm{KY}}$ whenever $\phi \neq 0$, i.e. nearly always. A still more general case is obtained if we fold in each $(2n)$th iteration in a plane characterized by ϕ_1, and each $(2n + 1)$st iteration in a different plane. Again, it seems that $D = D_{\mathrm{KY}}$ is generic.

The examples might suggest that indeed $D = D_{\mathrm{KY}}$ in all those generic cases in which $v = D$, but we consider it as not very likely in high-dimensional cases. For invertible two-dimensional maps, the above conditions are of course satisfied, and thus $\sigma = D_{\mathrm{KY}}$ if $v = \sigma = D$ (see ref. 29).

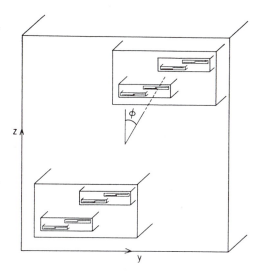

Fig. 15. Cross section through a rectangular volume element and its first 4 iterations under a map which stretches in x-direction, contracts in y- and z-directions (factors $\frac{1}{2}$ and $\frac{1}{4}$, respectively), and folds back under an angle ϕ with respect to the z-direction.

8. Conclusions

The theoretical arguments of section 3 and 6 of this paper have shown (though not with mathematical rigour) that the correlation exponent v introduced in this paper is closely related to other quantities measuring the local structure of strange attractors.

The numerical results presented in section 2, 5 and 7 have yielded proof that v can indeed be calculated with reasonable efforts. While all results presented in this paper were based on time series of 10.000–30.000 points, reasonable estimates of v can already be obtained with series of a few thousand points, in most cases. Surely, for higher dimensional attractors one needs longer time series. However, rather than taking longer time series, we found it in general more important to embed the attractor in higher dimensional spaces, and to choose this embedding dimension judiciously. Compared to box-counting algorithms used previously by other authors, our method has two advantages: First, our storage requirements are drastically reduced. Secondly, in a box-counting algorithm one should iterate until *all* non-empty boxes of a given size l have been visited. This is clearly impractical, in particular if l is very small. Thus, one has systematic errors even if the number of iterations N is excessively large. In our method, there is no such problem. In particular, the finiteness of N induces no systematic errors beyond the corrections to the scaling law $C(l) \sim l^v$.

We found that in most cases v was very close to the Hausdorff dimensions D and to the information dimension σ, with two notable exceptions. One was the Feigenbaum map, corresponding to the onset of chaos in 1 dimension. In that case, we were able to compute σ exactly in an analytic way, with the result $\sigma \neq D$, supporting the numerical evidence for $v < \sigma$.

The other exception was the Mackey–Glass delay equation, where we found numerically $v < D$. The information dimension has not been calculated directly in this case. Accepting the claim made in ref. 8 that the Kaplan–Yorke formula

(1.10) predicts correctly σ, we would have $v < \sigma = D = D_{KY}$. This seems somewhat surprising, since we argued in section 7 that a rather direct connection (as an inequality $v \leqslant D_{KY}$) exists between v and D_{KY}, while a connection between σ and D_{KY} seems less evident to us.

The main conclusion of this paper, as far as experiments are concerned, is that one can distinguish deterministic chaos from random noise. By analyzing the signal as explained in section 5, and embedding the attractor in an increasingly high dimensional space, one finds whether $C(l)$ scales like l^v or l^d. With a random noise the slope of $\log C(l)$ vs. $\log l$ will increase indefinitely as d is increased. For a signal that comes from a strange attractor the slope will reach a value of v and will then become d independent.

An issue of experimental importance is the effect of random noise *on top* of the deterministic chaos. The treatment of this question is beyond the scope of this paper and is treated elsewhere [30]. Here we just remark that when there is an external noise of a given mean square magnitude, a plot of $\log C(l)$ vs. $\log l$ has two regions. For length scales above those on which the random component blurs the fractal structure, $C(l)$ continues to scale like l^v. On length scales below those that are affected by the random jitter of the trajectory, $C(l)$ scales like l^d. The analysis of experimental signals along these lines can therefore yield simultaneously a characterization of the strange attractor *and* and estimate of the size of the random component. For more details see ref. 30.

It is thus our hope that the correlation exponent will indeed be measured in experiments whose dynamics is governed by strange attractors.

Acknowledgements

This work has been supported in part by the Israel Comission for Basic Research. P.G. thanks the Minerva Foundation for financial support. We thanks Drs. H.G.E. Hentschel and R.M. Mazo for a number of useful discussions.

Appendix A

All numerical calculations were performed in double precision arithmetic on an IBM 370/165 at the Weizmann Institute.

The integrations of the Lorenz and Rabinovich–Fabrikant equations were done using a standard Merson–Runge–Kutta subroutine of the NAG library.

In order to integrate the Mackey–Glass delay equation we approximated it by a N-dimensional set of difference equations by introducing a time step

$$\Delta t = \tau/n, \tag{A.1}$$

with n being some large integer, and writing

$$x(t + \Delta t) \approx x(t) + \frac{\Delta t}{2}(\dot{x}(t) + \dot{x}(t + \Delta t)). \tag{A.2}$$

Notice that this, being the optimal second-order approximation, is a very efficient algorithm – provided we can compute $\dot{x}(t + \Delta t)$. In the present case we can, due to the special form

$$\dot{x}(t) = f(x(t - \tau)) - bx(t). \tag{A.3}$$

Inserting this in eq. (A.2) and rearranging terms, we arrive at

$$x(t + \Delta t) = \frac{2 - b\Delta t}{2 + b\Delta t}x(t) + \frac{\Delta t}{2 + b\Delta t}$$
$$\times \{f(x(t - \tau)) + f(x(t - \tau + \Delta t))\}. \tag{A.4}$$

In all runs shown in this paper, we used $n = 600$ (corresponding to $0.03 \lesssim \Delta t \lesssim 0.15$), except for the runs with $\tau = 100$, where we used $n = 1200$ and with $n = 600$, finding no appreciable differences.

We also performed control runs with a fourth-order approximation instead of eq. (A.2). The correlation integral was unchanged within statistical errors, and the stability of the solutions did not seem to improve much. This could result from the very large higher derivatives of x, resulting from the tenth power in eq. (6.2).

In order to ensure that all x_i are on the attractor, the first 100–200 iterations were discarded.

Generating the time series $\{X_i\}_{i=1}^N$ was indeed the less time-consuming part of our computation, the more important part consisting of calculating the $N(N-1)/2 \gtrsim 10^8$ pairs of distances $r_{ij} = |X_i - X_j|$ and summing them up to get the correlation integral.

In particular, we found that an efficient algorithm for the latter was instrumental in applying the method advocated in this paper.

Such a fast algorithm was found using the fact that floating-point numbers are stored in a computer in the form

$$r = \pm \text{ mantissa} \cdot \text{base}^{+\exp}. \tag{A.5}$$

with base $= 16$ in our case $1/\text{base} < \text{mantissa} < 1$, and exp being an integer. If one can extract the exponent, one can bin the r_{ij}'s in bins of widths increasing geometrically. By extracting the exponent of an arbitrary power r^p of r, one can furthermore choose the width of this binning arbitrarily. Access to the exponent is made very easy and fast by using the shifting and masking operations available e.g. in extended IBM and in CDC Fortran. After having computed the numbers N_K of pairs (i, j) in the interval $2^{k-1} < r_{ij} < 2^k$, the correlation integrals are obtained by

$$c(r = 2^k) = \frac{1}{N^2} \sum_{k'=-\infty}^{k} N_{k'}. \tag{A.6}$$

We found this method to be nearly an order of magnitude faster than computing e.g. the logarithmics of r_{ij} directly, and binning by taking their integer parts. A typical run with 20.000 points took – depending on the model studied – between 15 and 30 minutes CPU time.

References

[1] E.N. Lorenz, J. Atmos. Sci. 20 (1963) 130.
[2] R.M. May, Nature 261 (1976) 459.
[3] D. Ruelle and F. Takens, Commun. Math. Phys. 20 (1971) 167.

[4] E. Ott, Rev. Mod. Phys. 53 (1981) 655.

[5] J. Guckenheimer, Nature 298 (1982) 358.

[6] B. Mandelbrot, *Fractals – Form, Chance and Dimension* (Freeman, San Francisco, 1977).

[7] V.I. Oseledec, Trans. Moscow Math. Soc. 19 (1968) 197. D. Ruelle, Proc. N.Y. Acad. Sci. 357 (1980) 1 (R.H.G. Helleman, ed.).

[8] J.D. Farmer, Physica 4D (1982) 366.

[9] H. Mori, Progr. Theor. Phys. 63 (1980) 1044.

[10] J.L. Kaplan and J.A. Yorke, in: Functional Differential Equations and Approximations of Fixed Points, H.-O. Peitgen and H.-O. Walther, eds. Lecture Notes in Math. 730 (Springer, Berlin, 1979) p. 204.

[11] D.A. Russel, J.D. Hanson and E. Ott, Phys. Rev. Lett. 45 (1980) 1175.

[12] H. Froehling, J.P. Crutchfield, D. Farmer, N.H. Packard and R. Shaw, Physica 3D (1981) 605.

[13] P. Grassberger, J. Stat. Phys. 26 (1981) 173.

[14] H.S. Greenside, A. Wolf, J. Swift and T. Pignataro, Phys. Rev. A25 (1982) 3453.

[15] P. Grassberger and I. Procaccia, Phys. Rev. Lett. 50 (1983) 346. Related discussions can be found in a preprint by F. Takens "Invariants Related to Dimensions and Entropy".

[16] M. Feigenbaum, J. Stat. Phys. 19 (1978) 25; 21 (1979) 669.

[17] M.C. Mackey and L. Glass, Science 197 (1977) 287.

[18] M. Hénon, Commun. Math. Phys. 50 (1976) 69.

[19] G.M. Zaslavskii, Phys. Lett. 69A (1978) 145.

[20] M.I. Rabinovich and A.L. Fabrikant, Sov. Phys. JETP 50 (1979) 311. (Zh. Exp. Theor. Fiz. 77 (1979) 617).

[21] W. Feller, An Introduction to Probability Theory and its Applications, vol. 2, 2nd ed. (Wiley, New York, 1971) p. 155.

[22] B.B. Mandelbrot, in: *Turbulence and the Navier–Stokes Equations*, R. Teman, ed., Lecture Notes in Math. 565 (Springer, Berlin, 1975). H.G.E. Hentschel and I. Procaccia, Phys. Rev. A., in press.

[23] D. Stauffer, Phys. Rep. 54C (1979) 1.

[24] T.A. Witten, Jr., and L.M. Sander, Phys. Rev. Lett. 47 (1981) 1400.

[25] N.H. Packard, J.P. Crutchfield, J.D. Farmer and R.S. Shaw, Phys. Rev. Lett. 45 (1980) 712.

[26] F. Takens, in: Proc. Warwick Symp. 1980, D. Rand and B.S. Young, eds, Lectures Notes in Math. 898 (Springer, Berlin, 1981).

[27] P. Frederickson, J.L. Kaplan, E.D. Yorke and J.A. Yorke, "The Lyapunov Dimension of Strange Attractors" (revised), to appear in J. Diff. Eq.

[28] F. Ledrappier, Commun. Math. Phys. 81 (1981) 229.

[29] L.S. Young, "Dimension, Entropy, and Lyapunov Exponents" preprint.

[30] A. Ben-Mizrachi, I. Procaccia and P. Grassberger, Phys. Rev. A, submitted.

Application of Chaos Theory to Biology and Medicine

JAMES E. SKINNER,
MARK MOLNAR,
TOMAS VYBIRAL,
and
MIRNA MITRA
Baylor College of Medicine

Abstract—The application of "chaos theory" to the physical and chemical sciences has resolved some long-standing problems, such as how to calculate a turbulent event in fluid dynamics or how to quantify the pathway of a molecule during Brownian motion. Biology and medicine also have unresolved problems, such as how to predict the occurrence of lethal arrhythmias or epileptic seizures. The quantification of a chaotic system, such as the nervous system, can occur by calculating the correlation dimension (D2) of a sample of the data that the system generates. For biological systems, the point correlation dimension (PD2) has an advantage in that it does not presume stationarity of the data, as the D2 algorithm must, and thus can track the transient non-stationarities that occur when the systems changes state. Such non-stationarities arise during normal functioning (e.g., during an event-related potential) or in pathology (e.g., in epilepsy or cardiac arrhythmogenesis). When stochastic analyses, such as the standard deviation or power spectrum, are performed on the same data they often have a reduced sensitivity and specifity compared to the dimensional measures. For example, a reduced standard deviation of heartbeat intervals can predict increased mortality in a group of cardiac subjects, each of which has a reduced standard deviation, but it cannot specify which individuals will or will not manifest lethal arrhythmogenesis; in contrast, the PD2 of the very same data can specify which patients will manifest sudden death. The explanation for the greater sensitivity and specificity of the dimensional measures is that they are *deterministic*, and thus are more *accurate* in quantifying the time-series. This accuracy appears to be significant in detecting pathology in biological systems, and thus the use of deterministic measures may lead to breakthroughs in the diagnosis and treatment of some medical disorders.

Key Words—correlation dimension, event-related potentials, sudden cardiac death, heart-attack, epilepsy

THE APPLICATION OF "chaos theory" to the physical and chemical sciences has resolved some long-standing problems, such as how to calculate a turbulent event in fluid dynamics or how to quantify the pathway of a molecule during Brownian motion (Gleick, 1987). Because biology and medicine have unresolved problems, such as how to predict the occurrence of

Address for correspondence: James E. Skinner, Mail Station F603, Baylor College of Medicine, 1 Baylor Plaza, Houston, TX 77030.

Integrative Physiological and Behavioral Science, January–March, 1992, Vol. 27, No. 1, 39-53.

lethal arrhythmias or epilepsy, it may be appropriate to consider the application of chaos theory to these areas, as well.

The quantification of a chaotic system, such as the nervous system, can occur by calculating the correlation dimension (D2) of a sample of the data that the system generates (Takens, 1981, 1985; Theiler, 1988). The dimension is the number of independent variables or degrees of freedom necessary for explaining the system's *total* behavior or dynamics (Babloyantz, 1990). The algorithm of Grassberger and Procaccia (1983) has been used extensively to calculate the D2 of both biological and physical systems. Application of this mathematical tool to biological systems can determine whether the seemingly random behaviors of the intrinsic electrochemical processes are stochastic or are governed by the rules of deterministic chaos (Schuster, 1988; Graf & Elbert, 1990). The breakthrough for biology is that what was thought to be higher-dimensional noise in many of the systems turns out to be low-dimensional chaos (Basar, 1990; Mayer-Kress et al., 1988). This means that these systems are not as complex as we had previously thought and therefore may be understood in relatively simple terms.

The algorithm found to be the most accurate in estimating dimension from limited data is the "Point Correlation Dimension" (PD2). This algorithm does not presume stationarity of the data, as the D2 algorithm of Grassberger and Procaccia must (Skinner, Carpegianni, Landisman, & Fulton, 1991a). Rather the PD2 tracks the transient non-stationarities that occur when the generator changes state, as often happens in biological systems (e.g., during behavioral arousal, epileptic seizure, or heart attack).

Biological data show transient dimensional changes during normal functioning, as during an event-related potential (Molnar & Skinner, in press), or in pathology, as in epilepsy (Babloyantz & Destexhe, 1986) or cardiac arrhythmogenesis (Skinner et al., 1991a; Skinner, Pratt, & Vybiral, in press). When the more common analyses are performed on these very same data epochs (e.g., the standard deviation, power spectrum, etc.) they are unable to make such discriminations; they, unlike the PD2, cannot indicate which electrocorticography leads are within an epileptic focus or which specific patients will manifest lethal arrhythmogenesis.

The explanation for why the dimensional indices are superior in their sensitivity and specifity for underlying pathology compared to the more common measures, is that they sense changes in the signals that are *deterministic*, not *stochastic*. The deterministic measures are inherently *more accurate* and therefore *more sensitive* (see Mayer-Kress et al., 1988). This greater sensitivity appears to be significant in detecting pathology in biological systems, and thus may lead to breakthroughs in the diagnosis and treatment of some recalcitrant medical disorders.

The Correlation Dimension: The D2 and PD2 Algorithms

To determine a system's dimension its state space has to be constructed. The coordinates of this space are the degrees of freedom of the analyzed system. It is possible to construct the state space from a single time series (such as the EEG), the structure of which is interpreted as involving a condensed image of the whole system generating the analyzed signal (Packard, Crutchfield, Farmer, & Shaw, 1980; Takens, 1981; Takens, 1985). These time series can be continuously different or aperiodic. Haken (1983) suggested that the dimensionality measures represent a "pattern" that exists in the minimum phase space in which the time series is plotted (i.e., embedded). Thus the dimensional measures are sensitive in identifying these "patterns" that can exist in aperiodic signals.

The correlation dimension (D2) of a time-series is defined as $C(r, n) = r^{D2}$ where $C(r, n)$ is the cumulative number of all rank-ordered vector-differences within a range (r) and n is the number of vector-differences. Vector-differences are made as follows. A reference vector (nref) is made that begins at a specific point in the data and takes a specified number (m) of sequential time-steps in the data stream that are of a fixed length (Tau); each value encountered in the time-steps is used as one coordinate of the m-dimensional vector. A different vector is then made by moving to a new starting point, for example to the next point in the time-series, and then using the same number of Tau-steps. Then another vector is made by starting at the third point in the series, and so on for all of the points in the data series. *All possible* vector-differences for every possible nref made with a given embedding dimension (i.e., number of Tau-steps, m) are then rank-ordered and a log C(r, n) versus log r plot is made. The slope of the linear region in this plot is then measured; this linear region reflects the range of r over which the model $C(r, n) = r^{D2}$, or $D2 = \log C(r, n)/\log r$, is valid. The value of m is incremented and the corresponding slope noted, thus yielding slope and m pairs. The values of m are selected to span the size of the expected D2 value (that is, m ranges from 1 to 2D2 + 1). The number of embedding dimensions is relevant up to the point where its increment is no longer associated with an increase in slope (i.e., it converges). D2 then is the slope of the linear region at the convergent values of m.

Mathematical stationarity is presumed in the above application, a presumption which is rarely tenable for biological data, as the generator is constantly changing. The "pointwise" scaling dimension was suggested by Farmer, Ott, and Yorke (1983) to estimate the D2 of biological data because it does *not* presume stationarity. This is so, because nref remains fixed for each D2 estimate: the difference-vectors made with respect to this *single* nref still span and probe the entire data-epoch, but they alone are the basis for the log-log plot and the consequent slope and m pairs. As nref is chosen sequentially for each digitized point in the time-series, dimension thus is estimated as a function of time. Because each nref has a new coordinate in each of its m-dimensional nref vectors, the series of estimates are independent of each other.

The "point-D2" estimate of the correlation dimension (PD2) was initially developed by Skinner et al. (1990a; 1991a). It was found to reduce the variance of the estimates compared to the "pointwise" D2 method. The point-D2 does *not* use all possible vector-differences, like the Grassberger and Procaccia algorithm, nor all vector-differences with respect to a fixed nref, like the Farmer, Ott, and Yorke algorithm; rather it rejects those nref vector-differences for which linear scaling and smooth convergence cannot be found. Accepting every data-point as an nref means erroneously including those vectors for which the relationship $C(r, n) = r^{D2}$ does not hold. In other words, the dimension cannot be estimated at some nrefs because the data points, being finite, are not distributed on the m-dimensional "strange-attractor" in a manner suitable for estimating the correlation dimension starting at that particular nref. The model for the point-D2 is $C(r, n, nref^*) = r^{D2}$, where nref* passes two criteria: (a) linear scaling in the log C(r, n, nref) versus log r plots and (b) convergence of slope versus m. The Point-D2 algorithm is available free of charge from Neurotech Laboratories, Inc., P.O. Box 9797, The Woodlands, TX 77387–6797.

The value of Tau is irrelevant if the number of points in the time-series is infinite, a condition which is never approached for biological data. A conventional way of determining the Tau to use is to calculate the first zero crossing of the autocorrelation function of the data time-series (i.e., approximately one quarter cycle of the dominant frequency). One should be cautious about new Tau requirements when non-stationarities arise in finite data; the autocorrelation function and Tau selection should be evaluated for each subepoch.

Figure 1A shows that the PD2 values are not related to either amplitude or frequency shifts in the time series being analyzed. Thus the information obtained by the deterministic PD2 measure is fundamentally different from that of stochastic measures, such as the power spectrum or standard deviation. Figure 1B illustrates the precision of the PD2 algorithm for estimating the D2

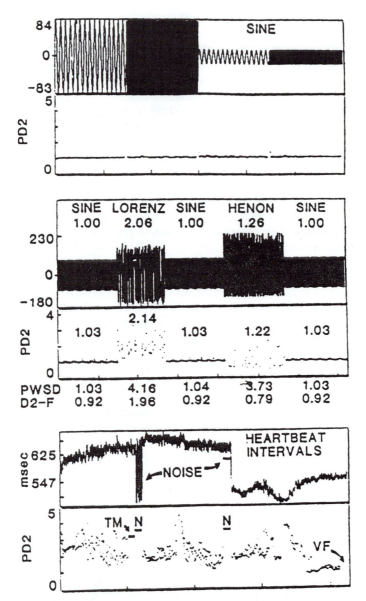

Fig. 1.   The "point correlation-dimension" (PD2) is not sensitive to changes in frequency or amplitude (upper panel), is more accurate than other methods (middle panel), and rejects bursts of high-dimensional noise in the data (lower panel). *Upper*: both a 10 points/Hz and a 100 points/Hz sine wave recorded by our data acquisition system are shown; each mark on the x-axis of each panel represents 1,000 data-points. *Middle*: 1,500 point Lorenz and Henon time series are embedded in a sine wave (the Lorenz equations used dp/dt =.001 and every 12th point was selected for the data analyzed); Tau = 1 was used to analyze the linked 7,200-point data set containing the non-stationary subepochs; the mean PD2 for each subepoch is shown above each series; the pointwise scaling dimension (PWSD) was also calculated for the 7,200 points and the subepoch means corresponding to the PD2 subepoch means are shown at the bottom; the Grassberger-Procaccia algorithm (D2-F) was used to analyze the individual 1,500 point subepochs (it is not valid to use the D2 algorithm for finite data when non-stationarities are within the epoch analyzed). *Lower*: An R-R interval from a human subject who

of several linked time-series, each of which was generated by a mathematical function for which the dimension is different and is known: the sine (D2 = 1.00), the Lorenz (D2 = 2.06), and the Henon (D2 = 1.26) functions (Mandelbrot, 1983). The "sampling rate" of each series was made so that a Tau = 1 could be used (the Henon series naturally has a Tau = 1). Note that the accuracy of the PD2 (subepoch mean) for each of these finite data samples is superior to that of the classical D2 algorithms (D2-F; i.e., the D2 assessed on finite data; Grassberger & Procaccia, 1983; Takens, 1981) or that of the "pointwise" scaling dimension (PWSD; Farmer, Ott, & Yorke, 1983). Figure 1C shows that the PD2 algorithm can sense and reject bursts of noise; continuous noise of as little as 1% of the amplitude of the signal, however, it can cause errors in calculation (Skinner et al., 1991).

Comparison of the D2 and PD2 algorithms when used on biological data also suggests that the PD2 has some advantages. When using the Grassberger and Procaccia D2-algorithm on event-related EEG data obtained during a cognitive experiment, Rapp et al. (1989) found it necessary to relax the criteria for *linearity* and *convergence*. By necessity they also had to presume stationarity within the 1-s epochs. These data samples were the smallest that could be used and still obtain sufficient data for the calculation. They found, as will be presented in more detail in the next section, a dimensional decrease in the epochs in which the target stimulus was present compared to that in which the control stimulus was present. In contrast, the PD2 algorithm was used on the same kind of data (Molnar & Skinner, in press) and the results confirmed the findings by Rapp et al. (1989) (i.e., a dimensional decrease), but the PD2 algorithm did *not* require relaxing either the linearity or convergence standards. Furthermore, it enabled the study of event-related dimensional shifts in *smaller* EEG epochs (i.e., "points" of Tau × m interval). The significance here is that these intervals were small enough so that the PD2 could be related to the brief event-related potentials that are presumed to represent cognitive processes.

Thus we conclude that the use of the PD2 algorithm to assess biological data is: (a) *appropriate*, as it meets all data requirements (i.e., it does not require data stationarity and thus can analyze small subepochs or "points"), (b) *accurate*, even in its estimate of D2 using relatively *small* epochs of data, and (c) *timely*, as recent dimensional assessment has been proposed to reveal deterministic processes that may underlie poorly understood phenomena, such as cognition and sudden cardiac death.

Low-Dimensional Chaos in the Brain

Event-related potentials (ERPs) are physiological correlates of cognitive processes in the brain. The experimental circumstances necessary to elicit the ERPs are well known (Donchin, Karis, Boshore, Coles, & Gratton, 1986), as most of the studies in the field are *correlational*. That is, the experimenter tries to find relationships between ERP components and experimental conditions, like that of "task relevance" and "stimulus probability" as in the case of the P3 component (Donchin, Ritter, & McCallum, 1978). To be able to know what physiological processes the ERP components may represent, the neural mechanisms underlying the *causes* or the *electrogeneses* of these potentials must be known (Karmos, Molnar, & Csepe, 1986; Molnar, Karmas, Csepe, & Winkler, 1988; Vaughan & Arezzo, 1988; Wood et al., 1984); furthermore new methods capable

FIG. 1 (*continued*)   manifested lethal ventricular fibrillation (VF) while wearing a Holter-monitor; white noise bursts of varying amplitude were inserted in the time-series; in the lower part of the panel the corresponding noise epochs are marked (N); note that for the large and small amplitude noise, all PD2 estimates were rejected; for the large amplitude noise the points in the preceding interval (TM), of duration Tau x m, were also rejected.

of accounting for the enormous *complexity* of the system causing the potentials must be developed (Albano et al., 1986; Babloyantz, 1985; Freeman & Skarda, 1985; Mayer-Kress et al., 1988; Rapp et al., 1990; Schuster, 1988).

Application of dimensional measures to the EEG have shown D2-reduction during epileptic seizures (Babloyantz & Destexhe, 1986; Skinner, Molnar, & Harper, in press) and sleep (Babloyantz, 1985; Babloyantz, 1986; Roschke & Basar, 1990; Skinner, Molnar, & Harper, in press). Little is known, however, about how cognitive processes influence the observed value of D2. According to Elbert and Rockstroch (1987) and Rapp et al. (1989), any "cognitive effort" should increase the value of D2. Our laboratory (Skinner et al., 1990b; 1991b) found in a simple model system (the olfactory bulb) that indeed a "novel" stimulus caused the D2s of the surface potentials (500 msec epochs) to increase from a baseline control level. The increase became spatially uniform, as all the D2s calculated for each electrode in an 8 × 8 array showed the same values. The same stimulus did *not* evoke an increase in D2 when it was familiar.

Figure 2 shows a replication of this spatial effect in the bulb using the PD2 algorithm (Mitra & Skinner, in press). During the quiescent control condition the spatial array of 64 simultaneously recorded electrodes shows that the EEG at each location has its own unique PD2 value; an area in the anteroventral quadrant seems to have smaller resting PD2s. During the 1.3 secs after the inspiration of the novel odor, each of the PD2s in the array increased, with those in the anteroventral quadrant increasing the most. What was apparent in all five of the rabbits studied is that the PD2s approach the *same* increased value; the bulb suddenly begins to manifest a homogeneous dynamical pattern while the novel odor is being evaluated by the rabbit.

D2-changes in epochs of the EEG that overlap the 500 ms interval of the human ERPs have been analyzed by Rapp et al. (1989, 1990). They reported *lower* dimensional values for the 1-sec epochs following an attended target stimulus compared to that which occurred when the stimulus was ignored. Their D2 method, however, could only analyze epochs greater than 1 sec, an interval during which stationarity had to be presumed; this interval is not suitable for tracking dimensional changes in sufficiently small intervals to enable correlation with ERP components.

Using the PD2 method, however, associations between human ERPs and their PD2s can be sought. Figure 3 shows averaged auditory ERPs and the corresponding averaged PD2s that occur during an auditory "odd-ball" task. The data were recorded when the subjects were instructed to ignore all stimuli (CONTROL), or when required to respond to the low-frequency tone, a target stimulus that was presented with a probability of occurrence of 10% (TARGET 10%). The ERP components are designated conventionally by their polarity (N, P) and order of occurrence. The peak latencies of these components are shown in milliseconds by the numbers. The background auditory stimuli (small arrows at left in both upper and lower panels) elicited the large N1 and P2 components and in the case of the target stimuli (large arrow at right in lower panel) these were followed by the N2 and P3 waves. The P1 component was small in all cases as usual. Compared to the background stimulus (Figure 3, upper left arrow) the ignored control tone (upper right arrow), which occurred less frequently, evoked a small second negative wave (N317).

Accompanying the ERPs, the PD2s related to the attended target stimulus were found to decrease instantly from baseline and peak at around 240 to 260 msec. This event-related decrease in dimension terminated at about the same time as the P3 component. The magnitude of the peak dimensional decrease was *not* significantly correlated with the amplitude of the P3, a finding which suggests independence of the generator processes of these two cortical events; however, the event-related PD2-decrease never occurred without the appearance of the P3 wave.

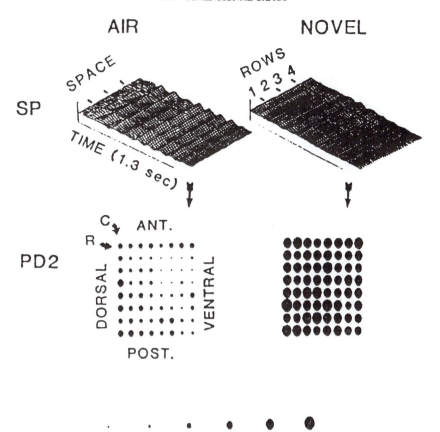

FIG. 2. Event-related potentials and their corresponding PD2 values recorded by an 8 × 8 electrode array on the surface of the olfactory bulb of the conscious rabbit. SP = surface potentials; PD2 = mean values during a 1.3-sec epoch after inspiration of air or a weak novel odor; R = row; C = column; scale at bottom ranges from 4.6 to 6.4 dimensions.

When the same physical stimulus had no significance for the subject (i.e., the subject was instructed to ignore the tones) it did not evoke PD2-changes. In contrast, the ERPs to the ignored lower tone manifested a second negative component (Figure 3, N317); this occurred because the lower tone was less-frequent and the potential corresponds to what is called the "mismatch negativity" (Naatanen, 1987). The presence of the small peak at N317 demonstrates that an ERP component can occur independently of any PD2 shift.

Since reducing Tau increased the PD2 onset slightly, and since in all cases the PD2 latency *is prior to* the N1 wave (which occurs around 100 msec after the stimulus), it is apparent that the initial event-related PD2 response approximates that of the small-amplitude ERP components that occur prior to P1; in the somatosensory system these early components are in the 30 to 90 ms range (Desmedt & Tomberg, 1989) and in the auditory system they are 20 to 70 ms in range (Cacace, Satya-Murti, & Wolpaw, 1990).

It has been interpreted that since the early ERPs occur at about the time of arrival of the afferent sensory signal in the cortex, there is no possibility for *feedback* to alter them (Desmedt & Tomberg, 1989). Thus their regulation by the stimulus contingencies of the task (e.g., "target" vs. "nontarget") suggests that they represent a sensory process of template-

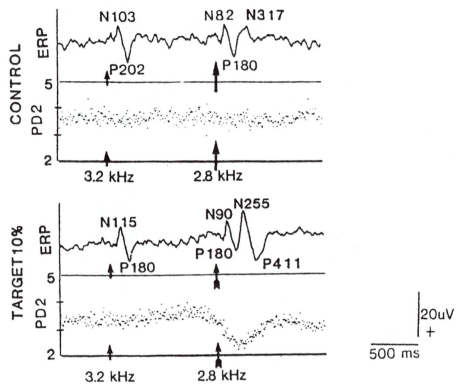

FIG. 3. Grand means of auditory event-related potentials (ERPs) and corresponding point correlation dimensions (PD2s) values recorded from 11 subjects in an auditory "odd-ball" experiment in which the subject had to identify the low-frequency target stimulus, which was presented during 10% of the trials. *Upper:* control experiment with 3.2 kHz background and 2.8 kHz control stimuli; the subject was told to ignore all auditory stimuli and to read a book (CONTROL, n = 340). *Lower:* "odd-ball" experiment with 3.2 kHz background and 2.8 kHz target stimuli; the subject was told to detect the low tones and count their total number; targets were presented at 10% probability (TARGET 10%, n = 340). The numbers represent the negative (N) and positive (P) peak latencies after the onset of the ignored or target stimulus. The PD2 values are displayed between 2 and 5 dimensions.

matching due to a "selective set" that exists in the thalamo-cortical projections (Desmedt & Tomberg, 1989). The neurophysiological mechanism for this sensory gating has been shown in animals to be carried out by the thalamic reticular system which is under the joint control of the mesencephalic reticular activating system and the frontal cortex (Skinner & Yingling, 1977).

The significance of the dimensional *decrease* when the signal is a "target stimulus" is not yet understood. One might consider that the dimensional decrease means the opposite of a dimensional increase. That is, a dimensional increase, evoked by either a "novel stimulus" (Skinner et al., 1990b) or "cognitive effort" (Rapp et al., 1989), suggests that the system has become more complex; its opposite simply means that the system has become *less* complex. But why fewer degrees of freedom or less complexity would be necessary to process the same signal when it has meaning compared to or when it is ignored, as in the present data, or why greater degrees of freedom or more complexity would be necessary to process the signal when it is unfamiliar and/or requires effort is simply not yet apparent. The "selective set," as carried out by the thalamic gating mechanism, suggests limited information flow into the cerebral cortex, and thus could reasonably be associated with a lowered dimension; but why the dimension remains high during the immediately preceeding control condition is not understood. Finding answers to these questions may lead to considerable insight into the mechanism underlying the cognitive processes.

Alternatively, the significance of the dimensional decrease in response to an expected target stimulus is more related to a change in the EEG *pattern* than to a reduction in the complexity of the generator. During the "odd-ball" task the decrease is sometimes a whole degree of freedom, a finding which could suggest that the system is reducing its complexity by eliminating a discrete variable. More often, however, the change is small and a fraction of an integer; in this case, perhaps, the simplest explanation is that the *pattern* of the generator dynamics has changed. It is not evident, for example, that the time-series generated by the Lorenz function, which has 2.06 degrees of freedom, is more or less complex than that of the Henon function, which has 1.26 degrees of freedom, or that either of these is more complex than the modulated sine wave seen in Figure 1A, which has 1.00 degrees of freedom. No subepoch within any one of these data-series is the same as another (i.e., they are all aperiodic time-series), yet each is fundamentally the *same in its pattern*. That is, each subepoch has a "strange attractor" that is invariant for the aperiodic data-stream. Changes in PD2 simply show that the attractor has changed.

The significance of the spatial effect showing dimensional homogeneity, as seen in the olfactory bulb (Figure 2), is also unclear, but its explanation may prove enlightening. For example, in these bulbar experiments it is seen that a novel odor rapidly causes all of the EEGs recorded by a 64-electrode surface-array to suddenly manifest *the same* dimension. As the odor is known to produce point-activation in the tissue initially (Wilson & Leon, 1988), it would appear that the information has become amplified *spatially* at the time the homogenous dimensionality occurs. It is interesting that this homogeneous dimensionality is only seen with dimensional increases.

Other spatial control mechanisms have been described for the processing of sensory information. It has been proposed that there is a dynamic spatial linkage between similar orientation-columns in the visual cortex of the adult cat. According to Gray and Singer (1989) and Gray, Konig, Engel, and Singer (1989) *precise* synchronization of activity occurs between neurons in widely separated columns with the *same* orientation, a linkage which suggests some type of dynamic "glue" that binds stimulus features to form an "object." The control of spatial patterns of activity through chaotic dynamics could be related to a fundamental mechanism by which object-recognition occurs.

The main question is, how does this spatial control mechanism work in a highly interconnected system like the olfactory bulb or visual cortex? Recently Ditto, Rauseo, and Spano (1991) showed that the application of a small pattern of displacements in an elastic (i.e., interconnected) mechanical system manifesting chaotic motion had the effect of controlling large amplitude displacements throughout the system. This controlling effect was predicted mathematically by Ott, Grebogi, and Yorke (1990) and is recognized as an instance of "initial conditions sensitivity," a mathematical property of all chaotic systems. What is significant here is that this property, which is usually observed in the *temporal domain*, may also exist in the *spatial domain*. For example, in a chaotic system being analyzed by the correlation dimension, it does not matter whether it is time or space that is used for the Tau-steps (Babloyantz, 1988). By analogy with the physical control experiment above, this means that a small signal exerted in a neural chaotic system may control the dynamics in either space or time, or both—i.e., just as it appears to happen neurophysiologically in the olfactory bulb during the processing of a "novel" stimulus.

In conclusion the cerebral data show a small event-related dimensional *increase* to an attended "novel" stimulus, and a *decrease* to a previously set "target" stimulus. The dimensional changes, which represent alterations in deterministic patterns in the EEG, appear to be independent of the ERPs, which represent stochastic means distributed in time. The dimensional data from the brain have a lot of *potential* for interpretation because of what we know about chaos in physical systems. We do not yet understand, however, what a dimensional change in a given direction means in a neural system or whether or not spatial amplification occurs in an interconnected neuropile as it does in an interconnected physical system. It would, therefore, be premature to speculate beyond our simple interpretation that the neural process has reduced complexity when it is analyzing a "target" stimulus and increased complexity when it is analyzing a "novel" stimulus. Finding out why this is the case, however, is a challenge that may eventually lead to a more complete (and we hope, simple) understanding of the complex biological system that underlies cognition.

The PD2 of the EEG, in addition to serving an explanatory purpose, may be used as a neural *discriminator*, as it is sensitive to evoked changes in the underlying dynamics of the system. That is, the PD2 may discriminate transient alterations in dynamics that can be associated with neural pathologies. A better illustration of the sensitivity of the PD2 and its potential use in detecting pathology can be seen in its application to the cardiovascular system.

Low-Dimensional Chaos in the Heart

Sudden cardiac death is predominantly due to ventricular fibrillation (VF) and it accounts for over 500, 000 yearly fatalities in the United States alone (Rapaport, 1988). A low ventricular ejection-fraction or a high degree of premature ventricular complexes observed in a 24-hour electrocardiogram are non-invasive indicators of risk (Multicenter Postinfarction Research Group, 1983). Although their sensitivity is statistically significant, their predictive power for a given individual (i.e., specificity) is not very good, nor do they suggest when the lethal event might occur (Pratt et al., 1987).

Based upon recent insight into the involvement of the autonomic nervous system and higher cortical centers in animal models of sudden cardiac death (Gillis et al, 1976; Parker, Michael, Hartley, Skinner, & Entman 1990; Skinner, Lie, & Entman, 1975; Skinner & Reed, 1981; Verrier & Lown, 1981), the relationship of the neurocardiac reflexes to cardiac vulnerability to VF is being closely examined (Billman, Schwartz, & Stone, 1982; Hull et al., 1990). In patients with a myocardial infarction, the standard deviation of spontaneously varying interbeat intervals (i.e., R-R intervals) and the sensitivity of these intervals to forced changes in blood pressure have both been shown to be prospective predictors of mortality (Bigger et al., 1988; Bigger et al., 1989; Kleiger, Miller, Bigger, & Moss, 1987; Kleiger, Miller, Krone, & Bigger, 1990; Martin et al., 1987; Myers et al, 1986; Rich et al., 1988). Power-spectrum analysis of heartbeat intervals suggests an increase in sympathetic- as well as a decrease in parasympathetic-reflexes in the vulnerable individuals (Bigger et al., 1989; Lombardi et al., 1987; Mayer-Kress et al., 1988).

It has been proposed that fluctuations in R-R intervals manifest deterministic chaos (Babloyantz 1988; Chialvo & Jalife, 1987; Goldberger, Rigney, Mietus, Antman, &

Greenwald, 1987; Guevara, Glass, & Shrier, 1981; Mayer-Kress et al., 1988; Skinner et al., 1991a); consequently the use of stochastic predictors, such as above, may be *inappropriate* for accurately describing the dynamics of the heartbeat pattern. In pursuit of this proposal, our laboratory studied neurocardiac reflex behavior in the conscious pig during experimental myocardial infarction, and we were able to demonstrate that low-dimensional chaos, as measured by the PD2-algorithm, predicts imminent VF (Skinner et al., 1991a). That is, after occlusion of the left anterior descending coronary artery, the mean PD2s of the R-R intervals dropped from 2.50 ± 0.81SD dimensions to 1.07 ± 0.18SD many minutes before VF occurred. Occlusions which did not result in VF did not produce such low-dimensional shifts in heartbeat behavior. Changes in the standard deviation of these same R-R intervals was not found to be a statistically significant predictor of VF.

We have demonstrated similar reductions in the PD2s of the heartbeats in electrocardiograms from ambulatory cardiac patients who manifested VF while being monitored (Skinner et al., in press). We found PD2 reductions below 1.2 in 21 of 21 subjects with pre-existing coronary heart disease who experienced VF while wearing a Holter-monitor. In 23 of 27 controls, who had severe arrhythmias but no history of VF, the PD2s did not drop to such low levels. Figure 4 shows in one of these VF-subjects that the low-dimensional excursions (POINT-D2) occurred repeatedly throughout the 12-hr period before VF. These excursions were independent of changes in mean heart rate and occurred without alteration of the QRS complex (ECG).

What is perhaps even more significant here is that the stochastic measure of the R-R data (i.e., the standard deviation) was *unable* to make a statistically significant discrimination between the VF-subjects and their controls (Skinner et al., in press). The controls had

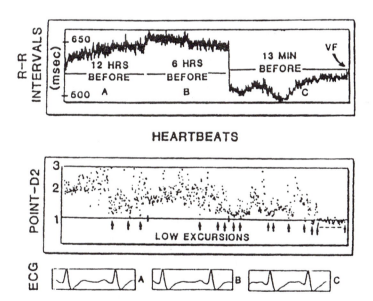

FIG. 4. R-R intervals and their corresponding PD2 values for a human subject who experienced lethal ventricular fibrillation (VF) at the far right of the figure. Three 13-min epochs were recorded at the time the Holter-monitor was attached (A), just before VF (C) and midway between them (B), and the PD2s of the linked epochs were calculated. Note the low-dimensional excursions below 1.2 dimensions during all three epochs.

reductions in left ventricular ejection-fraction and 24-hr ectopy profiles equivalent to those of the VF-subjects. Therefore, the heartbeat "pattern" recognized by the PD2 approaching 1.0 was detecting something pathological about the dynamics leading to VF, not simply detecting pathology caused by ischemic injury. Even without knowing the significance of the 1.0 value, these above data illustrate the use of the dimensional measure as a superior discrinimator over the stochastic measure.

As far a theory is concerned, it has been suggested that VF is produced by rotor waves that arise in the myocardium when the conditions of excitability become favorable (Winfree, 1987). Apparently the PD2 of the R-R intervals approaching 1.0 describes this deleterious condition (Skinner, Goldberger, Mayer-Kress, & Ideker, 1990a). It is the antecedent condition, not VF itself, that exhibits the significant pathology, and this pathology is dynamical, not anatomical. Pursuit of what the significance of the 1.0 value means to the dynamics could lead to an important theoretical insight into the mechanism underlying lethal arrhythmogenesis.

Conclusions

The *deterministic* analyses (i.e., D2 and PD2) of the EEG and ECG (i.e., R-R intervals) appear to be more sensitive to changes in the biological generators during normal functioning and abnormal pathology than the more common stochastic analyses. The further use of these measures of low-dimensional chaos as simple discriminators may lead to breakthroughs in the diagnosis and treatment of recalcitrant medical disorders. The theoretical implications of the data are also important and they may eventually lead to an understanding of why the biological systems normally change their dynamics and thus why the pathologies manifest their deleterious states at the times they do.

Note

Grant Support: National Institutes of Health HL31164 and NS27745

References

Albano, A.M., Abraham, N.B., Guzman de, G.C., Tarropja, M.F.H., Bandy, D.K., Gioggia, R.S., Rapp, P.E., Zimmerman, I.D., Greenbaun, N.N., & Bashore, T.R. (1986). Lasers and brains: Complex systems with low-dimensional attractors. In G. Mayer-Kress (Ed.), *Dimensions and entropies in chaotic systems* (pp. 231-240). Berlin: Springer.

Babloyantz, A. (1985). Strange attractors in the dynamics of brain activity. In H. Haken (Ed.), *Complex systems—Operational approaches in neurobiology, physics, and computers* (pp. 116-122). Berlin: Springer.

Babloyantz, A. (1986). Evidence of chaotic dynamics of brain activity during the sleep cycle. In G. Mayer-Kress (Ed.), *Dimensions and entropies in chaotic systems* (pp. 241-245). Berlin: Springer.

Babloyantz, A., & Destexhe, A. (1986). Low-dimensional chaos in an instance of epilepsy. *Proceedings of the National Academy of Sciences*, USA, 83, 3513-3517.

Babloyantz, A. (1988). Is the normal heart a periodic oscillator? *Biological Cybernetics, 58*, 203-211.

Babloyantz, A. (1990). Chaotic dynamics in brain activity. In E. Basar, (Ed.), *Chaos in brain function* (pp. 42-48.). Berlin: Springer.

Basar, E. (1990). *Chaos in brain function*. New York: Springer-Verlag.

Bigger, J.T., Kleiger, R.E., Fleiss, J.L., Rolnitzky, L.M., Steinman, R.C., & Miller, J.P. (1988). Multicenter post-infarction research group: Components of heart rate variability measured during healing of acute myocardial infarction. *American Journal of Cardiology, 61*, 208-215.

Bigger, J.T. Jr., La Rovere, M.T., Steinman, R.C., Fleiss, J.L., Rottman, J.N., Rolnitzky, L.M., & Schwartz, P.J. (1989). Comparison of baroreflex sensitivity and heart period variability after myocardial infarction. *Journal of the American College of Cardiology, 14,* 1511-1518.

Billman G.E., Schwartz P.J., & Stone H.L. (1982). Baroreceptor reflex control of heart rate: A predictor of sudden cardiac death. *Circulation, 66,* 874-880.

Cacace, A.T., Satya-Murti, S., & Wolpaw, J.R. (1990). Human middle-latency auditory evoked potentials: Vertex and temporal components. *Electroencephalography and Clinical Neurophysiology, 77,* 6-18.

Chialvo D.R., & Jalife J. (1987). Non-linear dynamics of cardiac excitation and impulse propagation. *Nature, 330,* 749-752.

Desmedt, J.E., & Tomberg, C. (1989). Mapping early somatosensory evoked potentials in selective attention: Critical evaluation of control conditions used for titrating by difference the cognitive P30, P40, P100 and N140. *Electroencephalography and Clinical Neurophysiology, 74,* 321-346.

Ditto, W.L., Rauseo, S.N., & Spano, M.L. (1990). Experimental control of chaos. *Physical Review Letters, 65,* 3211-3214.

Donchin, E., Karis, D., Bashore, T.R., Coles, M.G.H., & Gratton, G. Cognitive psychophysiology and human information processing (1986). In M.G.H. Coles, E. Donchin, & S. Porges (Eds.), *Psychophysiology: Systems, processes and applications.* (pp. 244-267). New York: Guildford Press.

Donchin, E., Ritter, W., & McCallum, W.C. (1978). Cognitive psychophysiology: The endogenous components of the ERP. In E. Callaway, P. Tueting, & S.H. Koslow, (Eds.), *Event-related potentials in man.* (pp. 349-412). New York: Academic Press.

Elbert, T., & Rockstroh, B. (1987). Threshold regulation—A key to the understanding of the combined dynamics of EEG and event-related potentials. *Journal of Psychophysiology, 4,* 317-333.

Farmer, J.D., Ott, E., & Yorke, J.A. (1983). Dimension of chaotic attractors. *Physica 7D,* 153-180.

Freeman, W., & Skarda, C.A. (1985). Spatial EEG-patterns, non-linear dynamics and perception: The neo-Sherringtonian view. *Brain Research Reviews, 10,* 147-175.

Gillis, R.A., Corr, P.B., Pace, D.G., Evans, D.E., DiMicco, J., & Pearle, D.L. (1976). Role of the nervous system in experimentally induced arrhythmias. *Cardiology, 61,* 37-49.

Gleick, J. (1987) *Chaos: Making a new science.* New York: Penguin.

Goldberger, A.L., Rigney, D.R., Mietus, J., Antman, E.M., & Greenwald, S. (1988). Nonlinear dynamics in sudden cardiac death syndrome: Heartrate oscillations and bifurcations. *Experientia, 44,* 983-987.

Graf, K.E., & Elbert, T. (1990). Dimensional analysis of the waking EEG. In E. Basar (Ed.), *Chaos in brain function.* (pp. 135-152). Berlin: Springer.

Grassberger, P., & Procaccia, I. (1983). Measuring the strangeness of strange attractors. *Physica. 9D,* 183-208.

Gray, C.M., Konig, P., Engel, A.K., & Singer, W. (1989). Oscillatory response in cat visual cortex exhibit inter-columnar synchronization which reflects global stimulus properties. *Nature, 338,* 334-337.

Gray, C.M., & Singer, W. (1989). Stimulus specific neuronal oscillations in orientation columns of cat visual cortex. *Proceedings of the National Academy of Sciences,* USA, *86,* 1968-1702.

Guevara, M.R., Glass, L., & Shrier. A. (1981). Phase locking, period-doubling bifurcations, and irregular dynamics in periodically stimulated cardiac cells. *Science, 214,* 1350-1353.

Haken, H. (1983). *Advanced synergetics.* New York: Springer-Verlag.

Hull, S.S., Evans, A.R., Vanoli, E., Adamson, P.B., Stramba-Badiale, M., Albert, D.E., Foreman R.D., & Schwartz P.J. (1990). Heart rate variability before and after myocardial infarction in conscious dogs at high and low risk of sudden death. *Journal of the American College of Cardiology, 16,* 978-985.

Karmos, G., Molnar, M., & Csepe, V. (1986). Intracortical profiles of evoked potential components related to behavioural activation in cats. In W.C. McCallum, R. Zappoli, & F. Denoth (Eds.), *Cerebral psychophysiology: Studies in event-related potentials* (pp. 555-557). EEG Suppl. 38. Amsterdam: Elsevier Science Publishers B.V.

Kleiger, R.E., Miller, J.P., Bigger, J.T., & Moss, A.J. (1987). Multicenter post-infarction research group: Decreased heart rate variability and is association with increased mortality after acute myocardial infarction. American Journal of Cardiology, *59,* 256-262.

Kleiger, R.E., Miller, J.P., Krone R.J., & Bigger, J.T. (1990). Multicenter postinfarction research group: The independence of cycle length variability and exercise testing on predicting mortality of patients surviving acute myocardial infarction. *American Journal of Cardiology, 65,* 408-411.

La Rovere, M.T., Specchia, G., Mortara, A., & Schwartz, P.J. (1988). Baroreflex sensitivity, clinical correlates and cardiovascular mortality among patients with a first myocardial infarction: A prospective study. *Circulation, 78,* 816-824.

Lombardi, F., Sandrone, G., Pempruner, S., Sala, R., Garimoldi, M., Cerutti, S., Baselli, G., Pagani, M., &

52   SKINNER ET AL.

Malliani, A. (1987). Heart rate variability as an index of sympathovagal interaction after acute myocardial infarction. *American Journal of Cardiology, 60,* P1239–1245.

Mandelbrot, B.B. (1983). *The fractal geometry of nature.* New York: Freeman and Co.

Martin, G.J., Magid, N.M., Myers, G., Barnett, P.S., Schaad, J.W., Weiss J.S., Lesch, M., & Singer, D.H. (1987). Heart rate variability and sudden death secondary to coronary artery disease during ambulatory electrocardiographic monitoring. *American Journal of Cardiology, 60,* 86–89.

Mayer-Kress, G., Yates, F.E., Benton, L., Keidel, M., Tirsch, W., Poppl, S.J., & Geist, K. (1988). Dimensional analysis of non-linear oscillations in brain, heart and muscle. *Mathematical Biosciences, 90,* 155–182.

Mitra, M., & Skinner, J.E. (in press). Low-dimensional chaos in the olfactory bulb of the conscious rabbit: A novel odor evokes spatially-uniform increases in the correlation dimensions of surface potentials. *Behavioral Neuroscience.*

Molnar, M., Karmos, G., Csepe, V., & Winkler, I. (1988). Intracortical auditory evoked potentials during classical aversive conditioning in cats. *Biological Psychology, 26,* 339–350.

Molnar, M., & Skinner J. (in press). Low-dimensional chaos in event-related potentials. *International Journal of Neuroscience.*

Multicenter Postinfarction Research Group. (1983). Risk stratification and survival after myocardial infarction. *New England Journal of Medicine, 309,* 31–336.

Myers, G.A., Martin, G.J., Magid, N.M., Barnett, P.S., Schaad, J.W., Weiss, J.S., Lesch, M., & Singer, D.H. (1986). Power spectral analysis of heart rate variability in sudden cardiac death: Comparison to other methods. *IEEE Transactions on Biomed Eng,* BME-33, *12,* 1149–1157.

Naatanen, R. (1987). Event-related potentials in research of cognitive processes—A classification of components. In E. van der Meer, J. Hoffmann (Eds.), *Knowledge aided information processing* (pp. 241–273). Amsterdam: Elsevier.

Ott, E., Grebogi, C., & Yorke, J.A. (1990). Controlling chaos. In D.K. Campbell (Ed.), *Chaos* (pp. 153–172). New York: American Institute of Physics.

Packard, N.H., Crutchfield, J.P., Farmer, J.D., & Shaw, R.S. (1980) Geometry from a time series. *Physical Review Letters, 45,* 712–716.

Parker, G.W., Michael, L.H., Hartley, C.J., Skinner, J.E., & Entman, M.L. (1990). Central beta-adrenergic mechanisms may modulate ischemic ventricular fibrillation in pigs. *Circulation Research, 66,* 259–279.

Pratt, C.M., Theroux, P., Slymen, D., Riordan-Bennett, A., Morisette, D., Galloway, A., Seals, A.A., & Holstrom, A. (1987). Spontaneous variability of ventricular arrhythmias in patients at increased risk for sudden death after acute myocardial infarction: Consecutive ambulatory electrocardiographic recordings in 88 patients. *American Journal of Cardiology, 59,* 278–283.

Rapaport, E. (1988). Sudden cardiac death. *American Journal of Cardiology, 62,* 31–61.

Rapp, P.E., Bashore, T.R., Martineire, J.M., Albano, A.M., Zimmerman, I.D., & Mees, A.I. (1989). Dynamics of brain electrical activity. *Brain Topography, 2,* 99–118.

Rapp, P.E., Bashore, T.R., Zimmerman, I.D., Martinerie, J.M., Albano, A.M., & Mees, A.I. (1990). Dynamical characterization of brain electrical activity. In S. Krasner (Ed.), *The ubiquity of chaos* (pp. 10–22). Washington, DC: American Association for the Advancement of Sciences.

Rich, M.A.W., Saini, J.S., Kleiger, R.E., Carney, R.M., teVelde, A., & Freedland, K.E. (1988). Correlation of heart rate variability with clinical and angiographic variables and late mortality after coronary angiography. *American Journal of Cardiology, 62,* 714–717.

Roschke, J., & Basar, E. (1990). The EEG is not a simple noise: Strange attractors in intracranial structures. In E. Basar (Ed.), *Chaos in brain function* (pp. 49–62). New York: Springer-Verlag.

Schuster, H.G. (1988). *Deterministic chaos.* VCH: Weinheim.

Skinner, J.E., Carpeggiani, C., Landisman, C.E., & Fulton, K.W. (1991a). The correlation-dimension of the heartbeat is reduced by myocardial ischemia in conscious pigs. *Circulation Research, 68,* 966–976.

Skinner, J.E., Goldberger, A.L., Mayer-Kress, G., & Ideker, R.E. (1990a). Chaos in the heart: Implications for clinical cardiology. *Biotechnology, 8,* 1018–1024.

Skinner, J.E., Lie, J.T., & Entman, M.L. (1975). Modification of ventricular fibrillation latency following coronary artery occlusion in the conscious pig: The effects of psychological stress and beta-adrenergic blockade. *Circulation, 51,* 656–667.

Skinner, J.E., Martin, J.L., Landisman, C.E., Mommer, M.M., Fulton, K., Mitra, M., Burton, W.D., & Saltzberg, B. (1990b). Chaotic attractors in a model of neocortex: Dimensionalities of olfactory bulb surface potentials are spatially uniform and event related. In E. Basar (Ed.), *Chaos in brain function* (pp. 119–134). New York: Springer-Verlag.

Skinner, J.E., Mitra, M., & Fulton, K. (1991b). Low-dimensional chaos in a simple biological model of neocortex:

Implications for cardiovascular and cognitive disorders. In J.G. Carlson, & A.R. Seifert (Eds.), *An international perspective on self-regulation and health* (pp. 95-117). New York: Plenum.

Skinner, J.E., Molnar, M., & Harper, R.M. (in press). Higher cerebral regulation of cardiovascular and respiratory function. In M.H. Kryger, T. Roth, & W.C. Dement (Eds.), *Principles and practice of sleep medicine* (2nd ed). Philadelphia: W.B. Saunders Co.

Skinner, J.E., Pratt, C.M., & Vybiral, T. (in press). Low-dimensional chaos in heartbeat intervals predicts sudden arrhythmic death in cardiac patients. *Circulation Research.*

Skinner, J.E., & Reed, J.C. (1981). Blockade of a frontocortical-brainstem pathway prevents ventricular fibrillation of the ischemic heart in pigs. *American Journal of Physiology, 240,* H156-H163.

Skinner, J.E., & Yingling, C.D. (1977). Central gating mechanisms that regulate event-related potentials and behavior: A neural model for attention. In J.E. Desmedt (Ed.), *Progress in Clinical Neurophysiology, Vol. I* (pp. 30-69). Brussels: Karger-Basel.

Takens, F.(1981). Detecting strange attractors in turbulance. *Lecture Notes in Mathematics, 898,* 366-381.

Takens, F. (1985). On the numerical determination of the dimension of an attractor. *Lecture Notes in Mathematics, 1125,* 99-106.

Theiler, J. (1988). Quantifying chaos: Practical estimation of the correlation dimension. Unpublished thesis. California Institute of Technology, Pasadena, California.

Verrier, R.L., & Lown, B. (1981). Autonomic nervous system and malignant cardiac arrhythmias. In H. Weiner, M.A. Hofer, A.J. Stunkard (Eds.), *Brain, behavior, and bodily disease* (pp. 273-291). New York: Raven.

Vaughan, H.G., & Arezzo, J.C. (1988). The neural basis of event-related potentials. In T.W. Picton, (Ed.), *Human event-related potentials.* (pp. 45-96). EEG Handbook Revised Series, Vol. 3. Amsterdam: Elsevier Science Publishers B.V.

Wilson, D.A., & Leon, M. (1988). Spatial patterns of olfactory bulb single-unit responses to learned olfactory cues in young rats. *Journal of Neurophysiology, 59,* 1770-1782.

Winfree, A.T. (1987). *When time breaks down: The three-dimensional dynamics of electrochemical waves and cardiac arrhythmias.* Princeton, NJ: Princeton University Press.

Wood, C.C., McCarthy, G., Squires, N.K., Vaughan, H.G., Woods, D.L., & McCallum, W.C. (1984). Anatomical and physiological substrates of event-related potentials. In R. Karrer, & P. Tueting (Eds.), *Brain and information: Event-related potentials* (pp. 681-721). Annals of the New York Academy of Sciences, Vol. 425. New York: New York Academy of Sciences.

Biosensors & Bioelectronics **9** (1994) 45–55

A fractal analysis of external diffusion limited first-order kinetics for the binding of antigen by immobilized antibody

Ajit Sadana* & Amarendra Madagula

Chemical Engineering Department, University of Mississippi, MS 38677–9740 USA.
Tel: [1] (601) 232 5349. Fax: [1] (601) 232 7023

(Received 6 November 1992; revised version 27 August 1993; accepted 31 August 1993)

Abstract: A fractal analysis of external diffusion limited first-order kinetics for the binding of antigen in solution by immobilized antibody on a fibre-optic biosensor indicates that as the fractal parameter (measure of "disorder" on the surface) increases the rate of binding and the amount of antigen bound to the antibody on the surface decreases. The fractal analysis and exponential type binding rate coefficients are used to analyze the influence of time-dependent binding rate coefficients on external diffusion limited kinetics. A decrease in the binding rate coefficients with time decreases the Damkohler number (decrease in the mass transfer limitations) leading to an increase in the rate of binding and the amount of antigen bound to the antibody on the surface, as expected. An increase in the (exponential) binding rate coefficient with time leads to unusual shapes of the binding curves. The time-dependent binding rate coefficients provide a more realistic picture of the binding of antigen in solution to the antibody covalently attached to the surface, and should assist in the control and manipulation of these interactions at the surface. A value of the fractal dimension of the surface of 2·96 to 2·97 obtained for our system characterizes the anomalies in the reaction-diffusion system and the heterogeneity of the surface.

Keywords: antigen, binding rate coefficient, fractal dimension, reaction-diffusion.

INTRODUCTION

There is an ever increasing need for sensitive detection systems (or sensors) capable of distinguishing a wide range of substances. Sensors

find applications in the areas of physics, chemistry, medicine, aviation, oceanography, and environmental control. A sensor should be reliable, rapid in its measurement, and be able to detect concentrations of substances at low levels, sometimes even in a mixture of similar substances. Besides, the sensor should be reasonably inexpensive and relatively simple to operate.

Biosensors, as the name indicates, use biologi-

---

* Author to whom correspondence should be addressed.

cally-derived molecules as sensing elements. Biosensors should be sensitive, specific, and stable (Scheller *et al.*, 1991). Their sensitivity and stability can be improved by a better understanding of their mode of operation. Eddowes (1987) emphasizes the "balance" inherent in the practical utility of biosensor systems. He estimates that though acceptable response times of the order of minutes or less should be obtainable at μM concentration levels, inconveniently lengthy response times will be found at nM or lower concentrations. The success of the detection scheme will be significantly enhanced if one obtains physical insights into the different steps that are involved in the "sensing" process. One such detection scheme is the solid-phase immunoassay technique that has already gained importance.

The solid-phase immunoassay technique provides a convenient means for the separation of reactants (for example, antigen) in a solution. Such a separation is possible because of the high specificity of the analyte for the immobilized antibody. External diffusional limitations play a role in the analysis of such assays (Giaver, 1976; Eddowes, 1987; Bluestein *et al.*, 1991; Place *et al.*, 1991). The influence of diffusion in such systems has been analyzed to some extent (Stenberg *et al.*, 1982; Nygren and Stenberg, 1985; Stenberg and Nygren, 1982; Sadana and Sii, 1992a,b).

Stenberg *et al.* (1986) have analyzed in great detail the effect of external diffusion on solid-phase immunoassay where the antigen is immobilized to a solid surface and the antibodies are in solution. These authors noted that diffusion plays a significant part when high concentrations of antigens (or binding sites) are immobilized on the surface. The above analysis is a general description of diffusion limitations. The "reverse" system wherein the antibody is immobilized on the surface and the antigen is in solution is also of interest.

In protein adsorption systems, which exhibit behaviour similar to that of antibody-antigen systems at the solid-liquid interface (Stenberg and Nygren, 1988), the influence of the surface-dependent intrinsic adsorption and desorption rate constants on the amount of protein adsorption has been analyzed (Cuypers *et al.*, 1987; Nygren and Stenberg, 1990). Cuypers *et al.* (1987) basically analyzed the influence of a variable adsorption rate coefficient on protein adsorption.

Nygren and Stenberg (1990), while studying the adsorption of ferritin from a water solution to a hydrophobic surface, noted that initially the adsorption rate coefficient of new ferritin molecules increased with time. Nygren and Stenberg (1985) also noted a decrease in binding rate with time while studying the kinetics of antibody binding to surface-immobilized bovine serum albumin (antigen) by ellipsometry. They indicated that the decrease in binding rate with time is probably due to a saturation through steric hindrance at the surface.

Kopelman (1988) indicates that surface diffusion-controlled reactions that occur on clusters or islands are expected to exhibit anomalous and fractal-like kinetics. These fractal kinetics exhibit anomalous reaction orders and time-dependent rate (for example, binding) coefficients. Fractals are disordered systems, and the disorder is described by non-integral dimensions (Pfeiffer and Obert, 1989). The time-dependent adsorption rate coefficients observed experimentally (Cuypers *et al.*, 1987; Nygren and Stenberg, 1990) may also be due to non-idealities or heterogeneity on the surface. Antibodies are heterogeneous and their immobilization on a fibre-optic surface, for example, will definitely exhibit a degree of heterogeneity. This is a good example of a "disordered system," and a fractal analysis is appropriate for such systems. Besides, the antibody-antigen reaction on the surface is a good example of a low dimension reaction system in which the distribution tends to be "less random" (Kopelman, 1988), and a fractal analysis would provide novel physical insights into the diffusion-controlled reactions occurring at the surface. Furthermore, Matuishita (1989) indicates that the irreversible aggregation of small particles occurs in many natural processes, such as polymer science, material science, immunology, etc. These aggregation processes frequently result in the formation of complex materials which can be described by fractals (Mandelbrot, 1982). Daccord (1989) emphasizes that when too many parameters are involved in a reaction, the fractal dimension for reactivity may be a useful global parameter. Since biosensor performance is constrained by chemical binding kinetics, equilibrium, and mass transport of the analyte to the biosensor surface, it behooves one to pay particular care to the design of such systems, and to explore new avenues by which further insight or knowledge may be obtained in these systems.

We present in this paper a fractal analysis for the binding of an antigen molecule in solution to a single binding site of an antibody on the surface (first-order kinetics). This is when external diffusional limitations are present. The fractal analysis is one means to elucidate time-dependent binding rate coefficients, and the influence of these time-dependent rate coefficients on first-order binding kinetics is examined. The role of exponential-type time-dependent adsorption binding coefficients is also analyzed for first-order systems.

THEORY

Figure 1 describes the steps that are involved in the binding of the antigen in solution to the antibody covalently attached to a surface. The

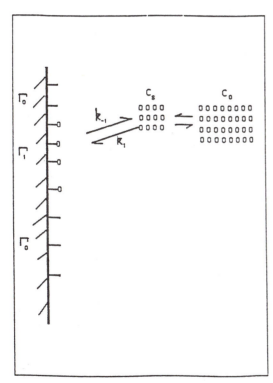

Fig. 1. Elementary steps involved in the binding of the antigen to the antibody covalently attached to the surface. Each arm of the antibody molecule reacts with an antigen molecule independent of the other arm.

rate of binding of a single antigen by an antibody is given by (Fig. 1):

$$\frac{d\Gamma_1}{dt} = 2k_1 C_s(\Gamma_0 - \Gamma_1) - k_{-1}\Gamma_1, \qquad (1)$$

where Γ_0 is the total concentration of the antibody sites on the surface; Γ_1 is the surface concentration of antibodies that are bound by antigens at any time, t; c_s is the concentration of the antigen close to the surface; k_1 is the forward reaction rate constant; and k_{-1} is the reverse reaction rate constant. Even though the antibody molecule has two binding sites, for all practical purposes we believe that an antigen molecule reacts with the antibody as if it had only one binding site. The stoichiometric coefficient 2 reflects the possibility that either of the "two" binding sites of the antibody may interact with the antigen. The simplified reaction scheme, then, is:

$$Ab + Ag \underset{k_{off}}{\overset{k_{on}}{\rightleftharpoons}} Ab \cdot Ag \qquad (2a)$$

where Ab is the antibody binding site and Ag is the antigen.

Note that though eqn (2a) is experimentally found to represent the overall binding of haptens to immunoglobulins (antibodies) in different investigated systems, Pecht and Lanchet (1976) and Shoup and Szabo (1982) indicate that the mechanism is:

$$Ab + Ag \underset{k_{-1}}{\overset{k_1}{\rightleftharpoons}} Ab \cdots Ag \underset{k_{-2}}{\overset{k_2}{\rightleftharpoons}} Ab \cdot Ag \qquad (2b)$$

Here $Ab \ldots Ag$ is the encounter step while the second step is the actual binding step. Making the steady-state approximation for the encounter complex yields:

$$k_{on} = \frac{2k_1 k_2}{k_{-1}+k_2} \text{ and } k_{off} = \frac{k_{-1}k_{-2}}{k_{-1}+k_2} \qquad (2c)$$

Under diffusion-controlled conditions $k_2 \gg k_{-1}$ (Pecht and Lancet, 1976). Then $k_{on} = 2k_1$ and $k_{off} = k_{-1} k_{-2}/k_2$. For all practical purposes. $k_{off} \approx 0$ since we are examining initial binding kinetics.

Since we are interested in initial binding kinetics, $\Gamma_1 \ll \Gamma_0$. Also, $k_1 c_s \Gamma_0 \gg k_{-1} \Gamma_1$. Physically, even if there is some desorption. the antigen quickly re-adsorbs. These two conditions simplify eqn (1) to:

$$\frac{d\Gamma_1}{dt} = 2k_1 c_s \Gamma_0 = \frac{d\Gamma_{Ag}}{dt}, \qquad (3)$$

where Γ_{Ag} is the surface concentration of the bound reactant or antigen. The first-order dependence on antigen concentration close to the surface is expected if one antigen molecule in solution binds to a single binding site on the surface. For first-order reaction kinetics, note that k_{on} and k_{off} are equal to k_1 and k_{-1}, respectively.

The diffusion limitation of the reaction scheme can be determined by considering the equation:

$$\frac{\partial c}{\partial t} = D\nabla^2 c = \frac{\partial^2 c}{\partial x^2}. \tag{4a}$$

Equation (4a) may be rewritten in dimensionless form as:

$$\frac{\partial y}{\partial \theta} = \frac{\partial^2 y}{\partial z^2}, \tag{4b}$$

where $y = c/c_o$, $z = x/L$, where L is a characteristic length dimension, for example, the diameter of a fibre-optic biosensor, and $\theta = t/(L^2/D)$.

The information presented above can be used in the development of sensors. In sensor applications, fibre-optic sensors are finding considerable application. These sensors are cylindrical in nature and have diameters that are typically 400–600 μm. For all practical purposes, the analysis that assumes single-dimension diffusion on a flat-plate is appropriate considering the dimensions of the molecule, the diffusion coefficient of the reactant in the solution, and the radius of the fibre-optic sensor. Place *et al.* (1991) in their recent review of immunoassay kinetics at continuous surfaces have utilized diffusion coefficients in the range 10^{-7} to 10^{-6} m²/sec for diffusing species of molecular weight 10^5 to 10^2 daltons, respectively, to estimate the effect of the molecular weight of the diffusing species on the equilibration time with a cell dimension of 1 mm. Assuming a typical value for the diffusion coefficient, D, equal to 4×10^{-7} cm²/sec, and a reaction period of 100 sec, yields $\sqrt{Dt}$ equal to 0·0063 cm. Since $\sqrt{Dt}$ is much smaller than the diameter of the fibre-optic sensor (0·06 cm), the cylindrical surface may be approximated by a plane surface.

The boundary condition for eqn (4a) is:

$$\frac{d\Gamma_{Ag}}{dt} = D\frac{\partial c}{\partial x}\bigg|_{x=0}. \tag{5a}$$

Here $x = 0$ represents the origin of the Cartesian coordinate system and is physically the surface

of, for example, the fibre to which the antibody is attached. Equation (5a) arises because of mass conservation, wherein the flow of antigens to the surface must be equal to the rate of antigen reacting with antibodies at the surface of the fibre.

From eqns (3) and (5a):

$$\frac{dc}{dx}\bigg|_{x=0} = \frac{k_1\Gamma_0 c(0,t)}{D}. \tag{5b}$$

Equation (5b) may be rewritten in dimensionless form as:

$$\frac{\partial y}{\partial x}\bigg|_{x=0} = Da\, u, \tag{5c}$$

where $y = c/c_0$, $z = x/L$, $u = c(0,t)/c_o$, and Da is the Damkohler number and is equal to $Lk_1\Gamma_0/D$. The Damkohler number is the ratio between the maximum reaction rate and the maximum rate of external diffusional mass transport.

Prior to solving eqn (4a), it is instructive to estimate the Damkohler number for typical antibody-antigen systems. For fibre-optic biosensors' some typical values are as follows: L, the diameter of the fibre-optic biosensor = 0·06 cm; D, the diffusion coefficient for the antigen = 4×10^{-7} cm²/sec (a typical value, Place *et al.*, 1991); and k_1, the forward association constant = 10^9 cm³/(mol-s) (DeLisi, 1976). The concentration of the antibody attached to the fibre-optic surface = 0·96 ng/mm², and the molecular weight of the antibody is 160 000 (Bhatia *et al.*, 1989). Then, $\Gamma_0 = 6·3 \times 10^{-12}$ g mol/cm². Substituting these values into the Damkohler number yields $Da = 900$. This is a high value for the Da and should lead to significant external diffusional limitations.

Another parameter of interest that defines the diffusional mass transport in these systems is ϕ_t (Stenberg *et al.*, 1986), which is equal to $\sqrt{\pi\Gamma_0}/(2c_o \sqrt{Dt})$. Here c_o is the initial concentration of the antigen in solution. A typical value of c_o is 50 μg/ml. Using the numbers presented yields a value of $\phi_t = 2·82$. It is estimated that ϕ_t should be less than 0·5 for the system to be away from external diffusional limitations (Stenberg *et al.*, 1986). The high estimated values of Da and ϕ_t indicate the presence of external diffusional limitations.

The above estimates of Da and ϕ_t are made with a stagnant fluid model. In this model to simplify the calculations we postulate that near the surface is a stagnant film in which the entire resistance to diffusion resides. It is assumed that there is a sharp transition between a stagnant film and a well-mixed fluid in which concentration gradients are negligible. The molecule (antigen in our case) diffuses through the film by molecular diffusion as predicted by Fick's law. One may be tempted to reduce diffusional effects by increasing convection. This is impractical in these types of systems because one is usually dealing with small volumes (antigens and antibodies are expensive) which are difficult to stir. However, as the sample is introduced (for example, the immersion of the fibre-optic biosensor in a solution of antigen), there is always some motion of fluid in the droplets which would enhance mass transfer significantly over the values obtained by the stagnant film model.

An estimate of the local stirring required to enhance the antibody–antigen interactions is instructive. The following argument is adapted from Berg and Purcell (1977). Transport by stirring in our case is given by some velocity, V_s, and by a length, l, the distance of travel. The characteristic time in this case is given by l/V_s. A good approximation for l is the diameter of the antigen molecule. Let $l = 100 \times 10^{-9}$ m (Humphrey, 1972). Movement of molecules over distance l by diffusion alone is characterized by l^2/D. Stirring is effective only if $l/V_s < l^2/D$. In this case $V_s > D/l = 4 \times 10^{-2}$ cm/sec. Thus, stirring is effective for speeds of the order of 10^{-1} cm/sec.

The appropriate initial condition for eqn (4a) is:

$$c(x,0) = c_o \, for \, x > 0, t = 0,$$
$$c(0,0) = 0 \, for \, x = 0, t = 0. \qquad (5d)$$

The above initial condition is equivalent to the rapid immersion of a sensor into a solution with antigens.

The solution for eqns (4a), (5b) and (5d) may be obtained from Carslaw and Jaeger (1959), which describes a semi-infinite solid, initially at temperature zero, heated at $x = 0$ by radiation from a medium at a particular temperature. Our equations for the binding of the antigen to the antibody binding site and the heat transfer case correspond exactly. Transforming the solution from Carslaw and Jaeger (1959) to our notation yields:

$$u = \frac{c(0,t)}{c_o} = 1 - e^{\frac{t}{\tau}} erfc(Da\gamma). \qquad (6)$$

Here $\tau = D/(k_1^2 \Gamma_o^2)$ and $\gamma = \sqrt{Dt}/L$.

Starting with $\Gamma_{Ag} = 0$ at time $t = 0$, and integrating eqn (3) yields:

$$\Gamma_{Ag}(t) = k_1 \Gamma_0 \int_0^1 c(x=0,t')dt'. \qquad (7a)$$

The solution of the above integral can be obtained by integration by parts. The solution may be adapted from the solution given earlier (Stenberg et al., 1986). Then:

$$\Gamma_{Ag}(t) = c_0 \sqrt{D\tau} \left[2\sqrt{\frac{\bar{t}}{\pi}} + \exp(\bar{t}) \, erfc(\sqrt{\bar{t}}) - 1 \right]. \qquad (7b)$$

where $\bar{t} = t/\tau$.

Equation (7b) may be utilized to model the concentration of the antigen bound to the antibodies which are, for example, covalently attached to an optical fibre. Equation (7b) may be rewritten in dimensionless form as:

$$v = \frac{\Gamma_{Ag}}{C_o \sqrt{D\tau}} = 2\sqrt{\frac{\bar{t}}{\pi}} + \exp(\bar{t}) \, erfc(\sqrt{\bar{t}}) - 1. \qquad (7c)$$

Note that eqn (7c) is applicable to both types of systems wherein the antibody is non-covalently or covalently attached to the biosensor surface and the antigen is in solution, or the antigen is covalently or non-covalently attached to the biosensor surface and the antibody is in solution. Surely, heterogeneity of adsorption is a more realistic picture of the actual situation and should be carefully examined to determine its influence on external mass transfer limitations and on the ultimate analytical procedure. In general, a heterogeneity of the antibody (or antigen) immobilization on the solid surface should yield lower specific rates of binding, thereby alleviating the diffusional constraints to a certain extent. Heterogeneity in the covalent attachment of the antibody to the surface can probably be accounted for by considering an appropriate distribution of covalent energies for attachment, and needs to be considered in the analysis. However, such an attempt is beyond the scope of this paper.

Heterogeneity may arise due to different factors. The antibodies, especially polyclonal antibodies, possess an "inherent heterogeneity" in that the antibodies in a particular sample are not

74 • Chapter 8

A. Sadana & A. Madagula

Biosensors & Bioelectronics

identical. Furthermore, different sites on the antibody may become covalently bound to the surface. As a result, especially in large antibodies, steric factors will play a significant role in determining the Ag/Ab ratio. It is of interest to make the influence of heterogeneity on the kinetics of antibody-antigen interactions more quantitative.

Fractal Analysis

One way of introducing heterogeneity into the analysis is to consider a time-dependent adsorption rate coefficient. Kopelman (1988) has recently indicated that classical reaction kinetics is sometimes unsatisfactory when the reactants are spatially constrained on the microscopic level by walls, phase boundaries, or force fields. These types of "heterogeneous" reactions, for example, bio-enzymatic reactions, that occur at interfaces of different phases exhibit fractal orders for elementary reactions and rate coefficients with temporal memories. In these types of reactions the rate coefficient exhibits a form given by:

$$k = k't^{-b}, 0 \leq b \leq 1 \ (t \geq 1). \qquad (8a)$$

Note eqn (8a) fails at short times. In general, k depends on time, whereas $k' = k(t = 1)$ does not. Kopelman (1988) indicates that in three dimensions (homogeneous space), b equals zero. This is in agreement with the results obtained in classical kinetics. Also, with vigorous stirring, the system is made homogeneous, and b again equals zero. However, for diffusion-limited reactions occurring in fractal spaces, $b>0$; this yields a time-dependent rate coefficient.

It is instructive to plot eqn (7c). τ in eqn (7c) is the time taken by the diffusional limitations to "set-in." On utilizing the values for k_1, D, and Γ_o mentioned earlier, one obtains a τ value of 1 second. This compares favourably with $\tau = 0.25$ second (Place $et\ al.$, 1991).

The time-dependence of the adsorption rate coefficient, k_1, may be due to a "mathematical" poisoning that is created through self-ordering (Kopelman, 1988). This is due to the compactness of the random walk. Kopelman (1988) emphasizes that eqn (8a) fails at short times. Equation (8a) may be rewritten as:

$$k_1 = \frac{k_1'}{(t+1)^b} \quad t \geq 0. \qquad (8b)$$

where k_1' is $10^9/(gmol) (sec)^{1-b}/cm^3$. For example,

when $b = 0.5$, then $k_1' = 10^9 \ cm^3/(gmol)(sec)^{\frac{1}{2}}$, and at time t equal to zero second. k_1 equals 10^9 $cm^3/(gmol)(sec)$, our initially selected value of the forward adsorption rate (constant) coefficient. Substituting eqn (8b) in eqn (7c) yields:

$$\frac{\Gamma_{Ag}}{c_o\sqrt{D\tau}} (1+\bar{t})^{-b} = 2 \sqrt{\frac{\bar{t}(1+\bar{t})^{-2b}}{\pi}}$$
$$+ \exp[\bar{t}(1+\bar{t})^{-b}] \, erfc \, [\sqrt{\bar{t}(1+\bar{t})^{-b}}] - 1 \qquad (9a)$$

Equation (9a) is in non-dimensional form. Even though it is apparently "fashionable" to present dimensionless plots, it is appropriate in this case to present dimensional plots of Γ_{Ag}/c_o versus t. Then eqn (9a) yields:

$$\frac{\Gamma_{Ag}}{c_o} = \sqrt{D\tau}\Bigg[2 \sqrt{\frac{\bar{t}}{\pi}}$$
$$+ (1+\bar{t})^b \exp\{\bar{t}(1+\bar{t})^{-2b}\} \, erfc \, \{\sqrt{\bar{t}(1+\bar{t})^{-b}}\}$$
$$- (1+\bar{t})^b\Bigg] \qquad (9b)$$

Note that for a time-invariant adsorption rate coefficient, k_1, b equals zero and eqn (9a) reduces to eqn (7c) as it should. Note that in eqn (9a), since τ is a function of k_1, then $\bar{t}$ equals t/τ_o. Here τ_o is the initial value (equal to 1 second, when k_1 (is a constant) equals $10^9 \ cm^3/(gmol)(sec)$. The coefficient b in eqn (9a) is the fractal dimension of the system, and is the non-integral dimension that represents the "disorder" of the system. The higher the value of b the more the "disorder" of the system.

Figure 2 provides plots of Γ_{Ag}/c_o versus t for different values of b between b equals zero and one. Note that as the fractal parameter b increases, Γ_{Ag}/c_o decreases as expected. For example, as b increases from zero to one for say, $t = 100$, Γ_{Ag}/c_o decreases from 0.00065 to 0.000065 $(g/cm^2)/(gmol/cm^3)$. This is almost an order of magnitude in reduction of the amount of antigen attached to the antibody on the surface, owing to the "disorder" of the system or the fractal nature of the surface. The non-random nature or the "disorder" of the system prevalent in the low dimensions hinders (predicts) a lower attachment of the antigen in solution to the antibody on the surface.

The range of b chosen was from 0 to 1 as indicated by Kopelman (1988). It is possible that for the reactions occurring at the interface, the

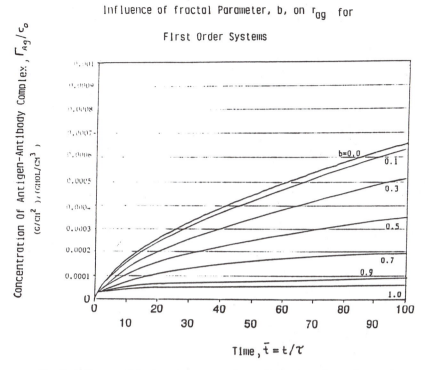

Fig. 2. *Influence of the fractal parameter, b, on Γ_{Ag}/c_0 for a first-order reaction.*
$$0 \leq b \leq 1$$

values of b may be greater than one, for antibody-antigen interactions.

For the A + A type of reactions, Kopelman (1988) indicates that $b = 1-d_s/2$ (Kopelman, 1986; Klymko and Kopelman, 1982, 1983) where d_s is the spectral (or random-walk occurrence) dimension and is defined by:

$$p \sim t^{-d_s/2} \tag{10}$$

Here p is the probability of the random walker returning to its origin after time t. Kopelman (1988) emphasizes that for the whole class of random fractals, in all embedded euclidean dimensions (two, three, or higher), d_s is always ~ 1·33 (Kopelman, 1986; Alexander and Orbach, 1982). Then, b equals 0·33 for $A + A$ reactions. The self-ordering effect is much more prominent for the two reactant case ($A + B$), which is closer to our case.

For the diffusion-limited case, Kopelman (1986) indicates that the reaction order, n, is given by:

$$n = 1 + \frac{2}{d_s} \tag{11}$$

Then, a d_s value of 4/3 yields a value of 5/2 for n. Kopelman (1988) emphasizes that, semantically, any binary reaction kinetics with $b > 0$ or $n > 2$ may be referred to as "fractal-like" kinetics. The b equal to zero plot in Figure 2 represents first-order kinetics (or pseudo-second order, since Γ_o is constant for initial time studies). As b increases from 0 to 1, then n increases slowly at first, but more rapidly as $b \rightarrow 1$. For b equal to 0·25, 0·5 and 0·75, n equals 2·33, 3 and 5 respectively. In eqn (3), if we subtract the first-order dependence on Γ_o, then the order dependence of the c_s term is 1·33, 2 and 4, respectively.

Reactions such as antibody-antigen interactions on a fibre-optic surface will be diffusion-controlled, and may be expected to occur on clusters or islands (indicating some measure of heterogeneity at the reaction surface). This leads to anomalous reaction orders and time-dependent adsorption rate coefficients. It appears that the non-randomness of the reactant distributions in low dimensions leads to an apparent "disguise" in the reaction kinetics. This disguise in the diffusion-controlled reaction kinetics is manifested through changes in both the rate coefficient as well as in the "order" of the reaction. Examples of "reaction-disguised" and "deactivation-disguised" kinetics (Malhotra and Sadana, 1989; Sadana, 1988; Sadana and Henley, 1987) due to diffusion are available in the literature.

It would be of interest to obtain a value for the fractal parameter, b (or perhaps a range for b) for fibre-optic systems involving antibody-antigen interactions that is characteristic of these systems. This would be of tremendous help in analyzing these systems, besides providing novel physical insights into the reactions occurring at the interface. Techniques for obtaining values of fractal parameters from reaction systems are available (Schmidt, 1989), though they may have to be modified for fibre-optic biosensor systems. If one can find ways to relate the fractal parameter to a "measure" of heterogeneity at the reaction interface, then one could facilitate the manipulation of the interface reaction in desired directions. Kopelman (1988) emphasizes that in a classical reaction system the distribution stays uniformly random, and in a fractal-like reaction system the distribution tends to become "less random," that is it is actually more ordered. Also, initial conditions that are usually of little importance in "re-randomizing" classical kinetics may become important in fractal kinetics. This aspect is beyond the scope of the present paper, but studies are in progress that examine the effect on fractal-like systems of Gaussian and other distributions.

Fractal-like kinetics are not the only way to obtain time-dependent adsorption rate coefficients in antibody-antigen (or more generally speaking, protein) interactions at the interface. The next section analyzes the influence of decreasing and increasing adsorption rate coefficients on external diffusion limited kinetics.

Time-Dependent Exponential-Type Adsorption Rate Coefficients

The decreasing and increasing adsorption rate coefficients are assumed to exhibit the exponential forms (Cuypers *et al.*, 1987):

$$k_1 = k_{1,0} \exp(-\beta t) \tag{12a}$$

and:

$$k_1 = k_{1,0} \exp(\beta t) \tag{12b}$$

Here β and $k_{1,0}$ are constants.

Cuypers *et al.* (1987) proposed only a decreasing adsorption rate coefficient with time. Substituting eqns (12a) and (12b) in eqn (7c) yields:

$$\frac{\Gamma_{Ag}}{C_o\sqrt{D\bar{\tau}}} \exp(-\beta\bar{t}) = 2\frac{\sqrt{\bar{t}}}{\pi} \exp(-\beta\bar{t})$$
$$+ \exp[\bar{t}\exp(-\beta\bar{t})]\, erfc[\sqrt{\bar{t}\exp(-2\beta\bar{t})}] - 1 \tag{13a}$$

and:

$$\frac{\Gamma_{Ag}}{C_o\sqrt{D\bar{\tau}}} \exp(\beta\bar{t}) = 2\sqrt{\frac{\bar{t}}{\pi}} \exp(\beta\bar{t})$$
$$+ \exp[\bar{t}\exp(\beta\bar{t})]\, erfc[\sqrt{\bar{t}\exp(2\beta\bar{t})}] - 1 \tag{13b}$$

Equations (13a) and (13b) in dimensional form are:

$$\frac{\Gamma_{Ag}}{C_o} = \sqrt{D\bar{\tau}}\left[2\sqrt{\frac{\bar{t}}{\pi}}\right.$$
$$+ \exp[\bar{t}\exp(-\beta\bar{t})]\exp(\beta\bar{t})\, erfc[\sqrt{\bar{t}\exp(-2\beta\bar{t})}]$$
$$\left. - \exp(\beta\bar{t})\right] \tag{14a}$$

and:

$$\frac{\Gamma_{Ag}}{C_o} = \sqrt{D\bar{\tau}}\left[2\sqrt{\frac{\bar{t}}{\pi}}\right.$$
$$+ \exp[\bar{t}\exp(\beta\bar{t})]\exp(-\beta\bar{t})\, erfc[\sqrt{\bar{t}\exp(2\beta\bar{t})}]$$
$$\left. - \exp(-\beta\bar{t})\right] \tag{14b}$$

respectively.

Figure 3a provides plots of Γ_{Ag}/c_o versus t for different values of β for a decreasing (exponential-type) adsorption rate coefficient. As β increases Γ_{Ag}/c_o increases as expected (Sadana and Sii, 1992b). As the adsorption rate coefficient, k_1, decreases with time, the Damkohler number decreases. This alleviates the mass transfer limitation, and increases not only Γ_{Ag}/c_o but also the rate of attachment of the antigen in solution to the antibody on the surface. For $t = 100$, as β increases from 0 to 0.009, Γ_{Ag}/c_o increases from 0.00066 to 0.00072. This represents an increase of about 9 percent.

Figure 3b provides plots of Γ_{Ag}/c_o versus t for

(a)

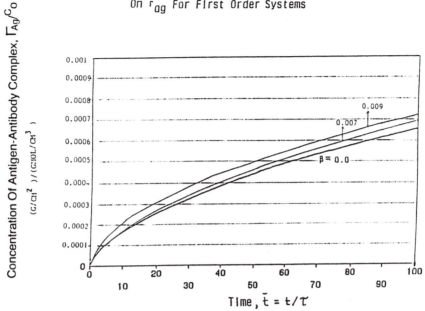

(b)

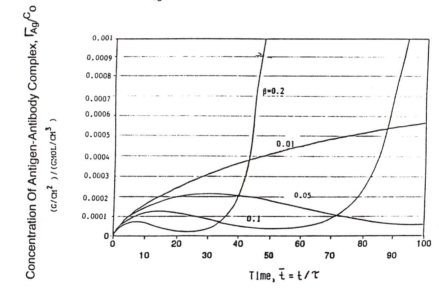

Fig. 3. *Influence of a time-dependent (exponential type) adsorption rate coefficient on the amount of antigen* Γ_{Ag} *attached to the antibody on the surface for a first-order reaction:*
(a) $k_1 = k_{1,0} \exp(-\beta t)$
(b) $k_1 = k_{1,0} \exp(\beta t)$

different values of β from β equal to zero to β equal to 0·2. The curve exhibits an interesting increase followed by a decrease in Γ_{Ag}/c_o for β = 0·05. Note the sharp increase in Γ_{Ag}/c_o for β = 0·1 and 0·2. This is an interesting exhibit of the influence of a time-dependent adsorption rate coefficient on the amount of antigen in solution attached to the antibody on the surface. This demands careful study prior to offering an explanation. A better understanding of the shape of the curve, besides the applicability of fractals, will provide novel physical insights into the reactions occurring at the interface, and should assist in the control and manipulation of the antigen-antibody interaction at the interface.

CONCLUSIONS

The analysis of time-dependent binding of antigen in solution to antibody immobilized on a fibre-optic biosensor surface is a more realistic approach to the problem and provides novel insights into the influence of the external diffusion limited reaction. The time-dependence of binding rate coefficients for a first-order reaction is analyzed using "fractal concepts" and an exponential type, increasing or decreasing binding rate coefficient. The fractal approach is conducive to analyzing reactions in a low-dimensional (constrained) environment and results in anomalous reaction orders that help elucidate the "disorder" or the "geometrical constraints" of the system.

An increase in the fractal parameter from 0 ("fractal free" kinetics) to 1 decreases the rate of the antigen binding and the amount of antigen bound (by about an order of magnitude for t = 100). As expected, the constrained environment (owing to heterogeneity and otherwise) leads to this decrease in antigen bound and also in the rate of binding. A value of fractal dimension of the surface of 2·96 to 2·98 obtained for our system characterizes the anomalies in the reaction-diffusion systems and the heterogeneity of the surface. It would be of interest to obtain a value(s) of the fractal parameter for other antibody-antigen interactions on a fibre-optic surface. One would then compare the results of different workers under a "common framework," which would then help formulate general directions to better understand and control these difficult and "fast" reactions. The magnitude of the fractal

dimension should also provide physical insights into the reactions occurring at the interface. Furthermore, Kaye (1989) emphasizes that fractal dimensions are useful summaries of data which may often be unmanageable. A decrease in the binding rate (exponential type) coefficient with time decreases the Damkohler number leading to the increased antigen bound to the antibody and an increase in the rate of binding, as expected. The increase in binding rate (exponential type) coefficient with time leads to peculiar shapes in the binding curves with time. This aspect needs to be analyzed further.

The analysis provides a framework for quick estimates of the effects of external diffusional limitations and a variable adsorption rate coefficient on the rate of attachment and the amount attached in antigen-antibody first-order systems. A variable rate coefficient for binding provides a more realistic picture of the events occurring in antigen-antibody reaction systems, for example, on the fibre-optic surface.

REFERENCES

Alexander, S. & Orbach, R. (1982). *J. Phys. (Paris) Lett.*, **43**, L625-L628.

Berg, H.C. & Purcel, E.M. (1977). *Biophys. J.*, **20**, 193–203.

Bhatia, S.K., Shriver-Lake, L.C., Prior, K.J., Georgerm, J.H., Calvert, J.M., Bredehorst, R. & Ligler, F.S. (1989). *Anal. Biochem.*, **178**, 408–413.

Bluestein, B.I., Craig, M., Slovacek, G., Stundtner, L., Urciouli, C., Walczak, I. & Luderer, A. (1991). in "Biosensors With Fiber-Optics." D. Wise and L.B. Wingard, Jr., eds., p. 181, Humana, New York.

Carslaw, H.S. & Jaeger, J.C. (1959). "Conduction Of Heat In Solids." 2nd ed., p. 72, Clarendon, Oxford.

Cuypers, P.A., Willems, G.M., Hemker, H.C. & Hermans, W.T. (1987). in "Blood In Contact With Natural And Artificial Surfaces." E.F. Leonard, V.T. Turitto and C. Vroman, eds. *Annals N.Y. Acad. Sci.*, **516**, 244–252.

Decord, G. (1989). *Dissolutions, Evaporations, Etchings*. In Avnir, D., ed., "The Fractal Approach To Heterogeneous Chemistry. Surfaces, Colloids, Polymers." J. Wiley, New York, pp. 181–197.

De Lisi, C.A. (1976). "Antigen-Antibody Interactions." Lecture notes in Biomathematics, Vol. 8, Springer, Verlag, Berlin.

Eddowes, M.J. (1987). *Biosensors*, **3**, 1–15.

Giaver, I. (1977). German Patent 2,638,207, March 10.

Biosensors & Bioelectronics

Humphrey, A.E. (1972). "Lecture Notes In Biotechnology." University of Pennsylvania Press, Philadelphia, PA.

Klymko, P. & Kopelman, R. (1982). *J. Phys. Chem.*, **86**, 3686–3688.

Klymko, P. & Kopelman, R. (1983). *J. Phys. Chem.*, **87**, 4565–4567.

Kopelman, R. (1986). *J. Stat. Phys.*, **42**, 185–192.

Kopelman, R. (1988). *Science*, **241**, 1620–1626.

Malhotra, A. & Sadana, A. (1989). *Biotech. Bioeng.*, **34**, 725–730.

Mandelbrot, B.B. (1982). "The Fractal Geometry Of Nature." Freeman, San Francisco, CA.

Matsushita, M. (1989). "Experimental Observations Of Aggregates" in Avnir, D., ed., "The Fractal Approach To Heterogeneous Chemistry. Surfaces, Colloids, Polymers." J. Wiley, New York, pp. 161–179.

Nygren, H. & Stenberg, M. (1985). *J. Immunol. Methods*, **80**, 15–24.

Nygren, H. & Stenberg, M. (1990). *Biophys. Chem.*, **38**, 67–75.

Pecht, I. & Lancet, D. (1976). "Kinetics Of Antibody-Hapten Interactions." in *Chemical Relaxation In Molecular Biology*, I. Pecht and R. Rigler, eds. Springer-Verlag, Heidelberg, pp. 306–338.

Pfeiffer, P. & Obert, M. (1989). "Fractals: Basic

First-order kinetics for the binding of antigen

Concepts And Terminology." in Avnir, D., ed., "The Fractal Approach To Heterogeneous Chemistry. Surfaces, Colloids, Polymers." J. Wiley, New York, pp. 11–44.

Place, J.F., Sutherland, R.M., Riley, A. & Mangan, C. (1991). in "Biosensors With Fiberoptics." D. Wise and L.B. Wingard, Jr., eds., p. 253, Humana, New York.

Sadana, A. (1988). *Trends In Biotechnology*, **6**(5), 84–89.

Sadana, A. & Henley, J.P., Jr. (1987). *J. Biotech.*, **5**, 67–73.

Sadana, A. & Sii, D. (1992a). *J. Colloid Interface Sci.* **151**(1), 166–177.

Sadana, A. & Sii, D. (1992b). *Biosensors and Bioelectronics*. **7**, 559–568.

Scheller, F.W., Hintsche, R., Pfeiffer, D., Schubert, F., Rebel, K. & Kindervater, R. (1991). *Sensors and Actuators*, **4**, 197–206.

Shoup, D. & Szabo, A. (1982). *Biophys. J.*, **40**, 33–39.

Stenberg, M. & Nygren, H. (1982). *Anal. Biochem.*, **127**, 183–192.

Stenberg, M. & Nygren, H. (1988). *J. Immunol. Methods*, **113**, 3–15.

Stenberg, M., Stiblert, L. & Nygren, H. (1986). *J. Theor. Biol.*, **120**, 129–140.

Physiological Heterogeneity: Fractals Link Determinism and Randomness in Structures and Functions

James B. Bassingthwaighte

Spatial variation in concentrations or flows within an organ and temporal variation in reaction rates or flows appear to broaden as one refines the scale of observation. How can we characterize heterogeneity independently of scale? Fractals come to our rescue! A system is fractal if its features adhere to the same rules through a succession of different scales. Fractals efficiently describe many types of observations, geometric and kinetic, and help to integrate physiological knowledge.

Introduction

Scatter in physiological observations is real and is more than can be accounted for by measurement error. It is a natural phenomenon; there is spatial variation in the densities of stars in various parts of the universe, in regional flows within an organ, or in regional enzyme or receptor concentrations. There is temporal variation in the intensity of the

wind, the rates of opening and closing of ion channels, and of velocities of blood in capillaries.

There is a problem in knowing how to describe such variation. For example, consider the variation in local concentrations of a substance within an organ. If the organ is divided into regions, then for 16, 64, or 256 pieces we have only one estimate of the mean, but three different measures of variance. The largest estimate is that for the largest number of pieces, which is for the most refined observations on the smallest sized pieces. Likewise for

channel fluctuations: when the duration of openings of an ion channel is measured, the variation is broader when the observations are made over short intervals with high-resolution instrumentation and narrower when made over long intervals with lower fidelity. While this problem seems obvious when considered directly, no standard method of handling it has evolved. In response to a question such as "What is the variance of population densities in this country?", it is traditional for the statistician to ask, quite reasonably, "What is the size of the domain you wish to consider?" Given an arbitrary choice for size, one can calculate a variance. But our real question is, "How can we describe the system in a fashion that is independent of the magnitude of the domain or period of observation?" This is where Mandelbrot's fractal concept comes to the rescue.

What are fractals?

Mandelbrot's coined word "fractal," like "fraction," comes from the Latin adjective fractus, from the verb frangere, to break into (irregular) pieces, to fragment. Fractal systems or sets are those whose characteristic form or variation of form or degree of irregularity is the same through a succession of magnifications of scale.

Dr. Bassingthwaighte is in the Center for Bioengineering, University of Washington WD-12, Seattle, WA 98195, USA.

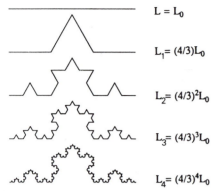

$L = L_0$

$L_1 = (4/3)L_0$

$L_2 = (4/3)^2 L_0$

$L_3 = (4/3)^3 L_0$

$L_4 = (4/3)^4 L_0$

FIGURE 1. Recursive extension of a line... a simple fractal system. If started from an equilateral triangle, this forms the traditional fractal snowflake. On iteration the length increases by 1/3, i.e., $L_{N+1}/L_N = 4/3$, going to infinity; the fractal dimension D is 1.262.

A simple example is a fractal line, shown in Fig. 1. Beginning with a straight line of length L_0, the middle third of the line is replaced by two sections of length $L_0/3$, so that the new total length is $L_0 \cdot 4/3$. For the next generation each straight line segment is replaced by four segments in the identical fashion so that the total length is $L_0 \cdot (4/3)^2$. With each succeeding generation the length increases in the same proportion so that by the Nth generation the length L_N has grown to $L_0 \cdot (4/3)^N$. The step-by-step iteration for the $N + 1^{th}$ step from the Nth is

$$L_{N+1} = L_N \cdot 4/3$$

and the overall expression is

$$L_N = L_0(4/3)^N$$

As $N \to$ infinity, the length L_N does also.

Now let us turn our viewpoint around and attempt to measure the length of the fractal profile produced as $N \to$ infinity. This is the same kind of problem as is measuring the variance in population densities or the length of a coastline: the apparent length of the contour depends on the length of the measuring stick that is used. Consider a pair of calipers set at the fixed length L_0: the apparent length of each of the crooked lines in Fig. 1 (and all higher-order lines) is L_0 because the calipers cannot measure the outcropping irregularities. When the calipers are set at length $L_0/3$, then the length for all lines except the first appears to be $4L_0/3$. And so on,

the shorter the caliper setting the longer the measured length of the infinitely long fractal profile. If we call the length of the measuring stick ϵ, and $\epsilon = 1$ is the initial reference length, then there is an expression that gives the length measured with each particular stick length

$$L(\epsilon) = L(\epsilon = 1) \cdot \epsilon^{1-D} = L_0 \epsilon^{1-D}$$

where D is the fractal dimension. Take a particular case, when ϵ is reduced from 1 to 1/3 and the measure of L is increased by 4/3. Now take logarithms of both sides

$$\log \frac{L(\epsilon = 1/3)}{L(\epsilon = 1)} = (1 - D)\log \epsilon$$

or, substituting in the actual lengths

$$\log(4/3) = (1 - D)\log 1/3$$

From this, a little algebra gives the fractal dimension, D

$$D = 1 - \log(4/3)/\log(1/3) = 1.262$$

In other words

$$D = 1 -$$

$$\frac{\log(L_A \text{ with stick } A/ \quad L_B \text{ with stick } B)}{\log(\text{length of stick } A/ \quad \text{length of stick } B)}$$

Thus a fractal description of the length of the contour in Fig. 1 is

$$L(\epsilon) = L(\epsilon = L_0) \cdot \epsilon^{-0.262}$$

D is a measure of the irregularity of the system. It is always greater than one in the one-dimensional situations that we consider here. The general statement is that D must equal or exceed (the usual case) the topological dimension (0 for a point, 1 for a line, 2 for a surface, etc.). (Note that the numerator in the fraction of the "word equation" is the log of a number >1, therefore positive, whenever the ratio in the denominator is <1, having a negative log, with the result that the fraction itself is always negative.) A value of $D <1$ would mean that the measured length of the line gets shorter as the measuring stick gets shorter, which is absurd. A value of 1 means that the exponent $1 - D$ (or $D - 1$, see below) is 0, and the measured length is independent of the length of the measuring stick; i.e., there is no irregularity. As the irregularities increase, D also increases, so it serves

as a measure of irregularity, roughness, and variation.

When this D is found to be constant over a succession of different measuring stick lengths, as it is for this example, one can say that the system is fractal over the range of the observations. (This would be true for the contour in Fig. 1 even if different ϵ's and different fractional ϵ's were used, but it would take a series of measurements to get D accurately.) Since real systems are probably never infinitely fractal, extrapolation beyond the observed range entails risk but may nevertheless be advantageous, as discussed below.

In general, fractal systems are those that follow simple rules of recursion, that is, undergo an iterative process by which a feature is changed generation by generation, in discrete steps. The process is "discrete" or discontinuous, as opposed to the usual continuous processes that we consider in physiology. (But the dividing line can be subtle when intervals or the degrees of change are small.) In general, the next generation, the $N + 1^{th}$, is derived from the present one, the Nth, in a recursive fashion

$$x_{N+1} = f(x_N) + c$$

where $f(x_N)$ is some function of x_N and c may be a constant or a random number. Mandelbrot showed that an infinite variety of patterns can be derived solely from $z_{N+1} = z_N^2 + c$, where c is a complex number. The phenomena are wonderfully portrayed by Peitgen and Richter (10), who also give an excellent introduction to fractals.

The structure of natural systems is often fractal

Mandelbrot's (8) book, *The Fractal Geometry of Nature*, gives numerous examples of biological and other systems that appear to behave in a fractal fashion. Log-log plots have slopes of $D - 1$ or $1 - D$ depending on whether the "measure" is proportional to or reciprocally related to the "measuring stick length." The diameters of successive branches of the bronchial tree (15) and of the arteries of an organ (13) show log-log relationships with branch length. Fractal rules have been used to construct "trees" (1).

The rules for fractal recursions can be probabilistic as well as deterministic. Random and algebraic relationships can both be encompassed. This is probably what occurs in nature. For example, the length of an unbranched arteriole may equal N diameters, with some scatter in N. If the geometry of the vascular bed is more or less fractal in nature, is it not likely that physiological functions be fractal also? Flow, being governed by the physical geometry and perfusion pressure, is a likely possibility.

Given that the vascular system has the duty to deliver nutrients to every cell in the tissue and that the bronchial tree needs to deliver gas to every alveolus, a space-filling fractal system can be expected to develop naturally. Capillaries can be expected to bud and develop as tissue grows and the vessels supplying them to enlarge as required to provide the flow, so that the end result is a network supplying the whole of the organ.

A space-filling system of branches analogous to the bronchial tree is shown in Fig. 2, a plane-filling recursion of straight line segments. The left side of the repetitive branching system has undergone one less division than the right side. The provision for a limit at a given element size, or when the residual uninvaded space reaches a minimum area or volume, renders the

system "pseudofractal," for it does not divide indefinitely to infinitely small elemental dimension. Lefèvre (6) used a finite iterative scheme to synthesize an "optimal" form of the pulmonary arterial system. No real system is infinitely fractal, but this does not create a problem in using the fractal concept over an appropriate range.

Fractals and heterogeneity of regional properties in an organ

Consider any intrinsic characteristic of a system, the brightness of regions in the sky, the densities of dwellings across a land, or, within an organ, the local concentrations of an enzyme or the magnitudes of regional flows. How to measure the variances of these features is the same problem as how to measure variance in population densities, namely, how to define the variance in a fashion that is independent of the size of the unit chosen for making the measurement. When the system is fractal there is a precise answer.

The measurement of variation in regional flows throughout an organ is our example problem. The mean flow per gram of tissue is simply the total flow divided by the mass of the organ. Consider the flows everywhere to be steady, setting aside consideration of fluctuations for later. The organ is divided into

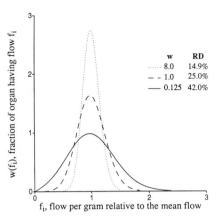

FIGURE 3. Diagram of distribution of blood flows in a 64-g sheep heart. Flows (*abscissa*) are relative to mean flow for the heart, and *ordinate* is fraction of the mass of the heart with a given local flow per gram of myocardium. Area of each curve is unity, as for any probability distribution. Fractal description is $RD(w) = 25 \, w^{-0.25}$; with w, sample size in grams; RD, relative dispersion, equal to standard deviation divided by the mean; and fractal $D = 1.25$.

weighed pieces, and the flow to each piece is measured (from the deposition of indicator or microspheres, e.g., Ref. 3), giving us estimates of the flow per gram in each piece. When the organ has been divided into eight pieces, we have, of course, the same estimate of the total organ flow that we started with, but we have the additional information on the variability of regional flows. The relative dispersion (RD) of the regional flows is given by the standard deviation divided by the mean, which is merely the usual coefficient of variation. When each of the 8 pieces is further divided into 8, making 64 pieces, we find that the original 8 pieces were not internally uniform, so that the relative dispersion is larger, as depicted in Fig. 3. Dividing each of these 64 pieces into 8, to a total of 512 pieces in the hypothetical example, broadens the distribution yet further. Now we have three estimates of the variation. How do we compare our results with those found in other laboratories? Which one do we use to report the "true variation?"

This is where the fractal approach solves our problem. In Fig. 4, the relative dispersion is plotted versus the number of pieces into which the tissue has been divided to make the measurement of variability. What is

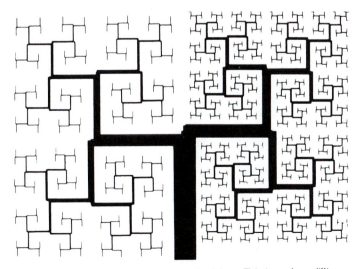

FIGURE 2. A pseudofractal analog to the bronchial tree. This is a plane-filling recursion in which line thicknesses (diameters) and lengths are not quite self-similar with division: the ratio of line thickness to length decreases with each iteration, going to zero. Ratio was decreased more rapidly for the left side than the right. (From Mandelbrot (8), plate 164.)

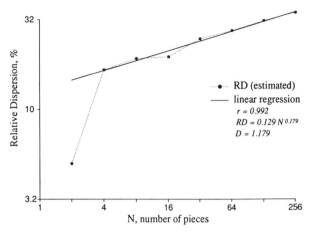

FIGURE 4. Apparent variation in regional myocardial blood flow as a function of the number of pieces into which the heart is cut. RD, relative dispersion, is standard deviation divided by mean. Microsphere distributions in baboon hearts. Data from King et al. (6).

interesting, and perhaps even remarkable, is that the relative dispersion is so precisely fractal. The sizes of the pieces range from 16 g (for N = 4) to ~250 mg. Over this range the fractal expression that fits the data is

$$RD = RD(N = 1) \cdot N^{D-1}$$

where RD is in %, the extrapolated value of RD(N = 1) = 12.9%, and the fractal dimension D is 1.18. The real value of RD(N = 1) can only be zero, and by definition it cannot be on the fractal curve; thus the use of the intercept obtained by linear extrapolation of the plot to the ordinate, where log 1 = 0, is arbitrary.

Translation into the size of the tissue pieces is a more general way of expressing the data

$$RD(w) = RD(w = 1 G) \cdot w^{1-D}$$

where w is the mass of the observed pieces of tissue and the fractal D is again 1.18. The exponent is $1 - D$ rather than $D - 1$, because the mass of the individual pieces is the heart mass divided by N, which is thus the reciprocal. The plot of the data expressed in this way is the mirror image of Fig. 4, and, of course, the slope is negative. The reference value of RD is arbitrarily taken to be that for 1-G pieces; this is ~17% in the normal heart.

How can we put this information to work? One application is in relating estimates from one lab to another. Each lab should calculate the fractal D and RD(w = 1 G) to describe the data. Failing that, we might as-

sume that our D applies to their hearts and estimate a value for RD (w = 1 G) for each set of data.

What is the "true" heterogeneity?

Orbach (9) has persuasively argued that systems can be fractal over only a limited range. The concept of flow heterogeneity will not apply to single cardiac cells, because many are supplied by one capillary. At the extremes the system either appears unmeasured (whole heart) or further division is meaningless (single capillary). It is this latter issue that invites debate. When has the system been examined closely enough to reveal the ultimate heterogeneity?

The answer is not an arbitrary one but depends on the function or structure that is being studied. Obviously, the vascular tree cannot be fractal beyond the dimensions of the capillary. A more subtle question is, "What is the size of the functional unit beyond which further refinements in the measurement of local flow are useless?" The answer will depend on further questions. Flow for the delivery of substrate? For the removal of metabolites? For delivery of humoral vasodilators? For the latter, delivery to the arteriole will do, but other solutes have to go farther. Substances with higher diffusion coefficients will have more uniform distributions within the tissue, in spite of differences in flows in neighboring capillaries, than will solutes with low diffusion coefficients or with lipid solubility so low that they do not cross membranes. Presum-

ably, also, flows in immediately adjacent regions will tend to be similar, and flows in widely separated regions less similar. Similarity with proximity, delivery from a common parent artery, diffusional spreading, etc., all have the same effect on the dispersion, namely, to tend toward uniformity within a small region. The curve of Fig. 4 must bend toward a plateau, becoming convex upward and deviating from the purely fractal relationship. Rigaut (11) has observed such curvature in fractal plots of alveolar boundary lengths. The explanation is simply that when regions are so small that they are internally uniform, further magnification or refinement of scale produces no further variance.

From the estimates of interarteriolar distances, one might estimate the size of a functional microvascular unit in the heart to be 0.2–1 mg. By extrapolating the fractal relationship down to this dimension, correcting for the increasing methodological error as the size of the pieces diminishes, we estimate the "true" heterogeneity of local flows at the functional unit level to be near 60%. This is the result we had been seeking.

This large variation has important influences on the net arteriovenous extraction of solutes. Since solute extraction across an organ is most efficient when the flow is uniform, internal nonuniformity might be inefficient unless it is primarily related to local metabolic needs. Heterogeneity partly explains the observation that coronary sinus oxygen concentrations are higher than the mean capillary concentration. Failure to account for this broad heterogeneity in calculating capillary permeability-surface area products (the conductivity of the walls of the capillary for solutes) from tracer extractions results in underestimation by >70% (2). We take advantage of the fractal nature of flow heterogeneity to estimate the true heterogeneity approximately and to use it in the modeling analysis of tracer dilution curves to avoid the systematic errors.

Structural and dynamic fractals

It seems likely that all neural, epithelial, and endothelial branching systems are fractal in one or more features. If the fractal approach is so widely applicable, so fundamental to biological phenomena, it should be regarded as a primary and basic model for many systems. As such, it may be a replacement for more complex models that are less fundamental. At least, the fractal model should be considered and tested before being rejected in favor of more complicated models. It is very early to say how widespread the applications may be, but at least two classes of fractal phenomena in biology can be identified, structural and dynamic. The fractal structure of the vascular system seems evident from the work of Suwa and Takahashi (13). Similar work is required to describe other branching networks in blood vessels, neural networks, and excretory ducts in organs. Growth patterns are well structured (14) but nevertheless irregular and usually fill the boundaries of their space quite precisely. It is interesting to speculate on whether the basic fractal nature of growth provides some basis for the logarithmic relationship between metabolism and animal size so comprehensively portrayed by Schmidt-Nielsen (12) in his monograph, "Scaling. Why is animal size so important?"

Fractal dynamics may be seen in well-integrated systems as well as in molecular phenomena. In a case as complicated as pulmonary ventilation-perfusion ratios, the basis is in the anatomy of both the vascular and bronchial trees and in the dynamics of local flows and ventilation. Such a system will be difficult to work out in detail because of the difficulties in making refined measurements in both space and time. The fractal analysis of temporal fluctuations in local flow is accomplished by using time as the variable rather than space. Temporal heterogeneity of flow, the standard deviation of the flows over a given interval, τ, divided by the mean over a long time, is broader the shorter the interval τ over which the flow is measured. It is analogous to the spatial heterogeneity, even to the form of the equation

$$\mathrm{RD}(\tau) = \mathrm{RD}(\tau = 1 \ \mathrm{s}) \cdot \tau^{1-D_\tau}$$

where the choice of the reference interval at 1 s is arbitrary. The value of D_τ in preliminary analyses of capillary flow fluctuations appears to be ~1.3. As with spatial fluctuations, there must be a deviation from the fractal relationship to a plateau at very short intervals. For flow this must be due in part to the inertia of a moving column of fluid: it cannot be stopped or reversed at infinitely high frequencies without an infinite expenditure of energy.

At the molecular level, the simplest and most fundamental fractal phenomenon is molecular diffusion. Brownian movement by random molecular collisions was described mathematically by Einstein in 1905. For one-dimensional diffusion the fractal D is 2; the spread (standard deviation) of a group of molecules increases in proportion to time; i.e., $\mathrm{RD}(\tau)$ is proportional to τ^{D-1}. Solute diffusion in fractal meshes of fibers is hindered by collision with the fibers and by reduced fluid mobility in narrow passages. For transcapillary permeation through the interendothelial clefts we should consider the process to be hindered diffusion within a fractal fiber mesh with additional hindrance imposed by proximity to the endothelial cell surfaces on either side.

Solute interactions with proteins are probably fractal phenomena. For fatty acid binding to albumin or calcium binding to aequorin, a wide range of rate constants has been observed; the reported rate constants vary severalfold, deviating markedly from a simple first-order process. A possible cause is that multiple collision of the solvent molecules with the protein causes enough flexing of the protein to allow the solute to gain access to the binding site intermittently or with varying ease.

That ion channels are fractal has been demonstrated by Liebovitch et al. (7). Their patch-clamp data show that the durations of channel openings or closings follow a fractal model better than one with mono- or multiexponential rate constants. Their data were for a channel in lens epithelial cells. The time- and voltage-dependent potassium channel in excitable cells is probably fractal; Cole and Moore (4) observed that raising the conductance variable to a power of 25 gave a better fit to the current time course on depolarization than did the power of 4 originally assigned by Hodgkin and Huxley in 1952. Such a high exponent implies a many-level process, probably fractal.

Conclusion

The use of fractals in providing quantitative summarizing descriptions of biological systems is in its infancy. Fractal models of many forms are possible, and they can be applied widely. Their development must proceed as with any other type of model, deterministic or stochastic. This essay illustrates one of the simplest examples of application of fractals to the characterization of a system and may be useful in suggesting others.

The author has appreciated the discussions with Dr. Barry Gray (University of Oklahoma) and Dick Slaaf (Limburg University, Maastricht, the Netherlands) in the development of this approach.

This work was supported by Grants HL-19135, HL-19139, and RR-01243 from the National Institutes of Health.

References

1. Barnsley, M. F., P. Massopust, H. Strickland, and A. D. Sloan. Fractal modeling of biological structures. *Ann. NY Acad. Sci.* 504: 179–194, 1987.
2. Bassingthwaighte, J. B., and C. A. Goresky. Modeling in the analysis of solute and water exchange in the microvasculature. In: *Handbook of Physiology. The Cardiovascular System. Microcirculation.* Bethesda, MD: Am. Physiol. Soc., 1984, sect. 2, vol. IV, chapt. 13, p. 549–626.
3. Bassingthwaighte, J. B., M. A. Malone, T. C. Moffett, R. B. King, S. E. Little, J. M. Link, and K. A. Krohn. Validity of microsphere depositions for regional myocardial flows. *Am. J. Physiol.* 253 (*Heart Circ. Physiol.* 22): H184–H193, 1987.
4. Cole, K. S., and J. W. Moore. Potassium ion current in the squid giant axon: dynamic characteristic. *Biophys. J.* 1: 1–14, 1960.
5. King, R. B., J. B. Bassingthwaighte, J. R. S. Hales, and L. B. Rowell. Stability of heterogeneity of myocardial blood flow in normal awake baboons. *Circ. Res.* 57: 285–295, 1985.
6. Lefèvre, J. Teleonomical optimization of a fractal model of the pulmonary arterial bed. *J. Theor. Biol.* 102: 225–248, 1983.
7. Liebovitch, L. S., J. Fischbarg, J. P. Koniarek, I. Todorova, and M. Wang. Fractal model of ion-channel kinetics. *Biochim. Biophys. Acta* 896: 173–180, 1987.
8. Mandelbrot, B. B. *The Fractal Geometry of Nature.* San Francisco, CA: Freeman, 1983.
9. Orbach, R. Dynamics of fractal networks. *Science Wash. DC* 231: 814–819, 1986.

10. Peitgen, H. O., and P. H. Richter. *The Beauty of Fractals: Images of Complex Dynamical Systems.* Berlin: Springer-Verlag, 1986.

11. Rigaut, J. P. An empirical formulation relating boundary lengths to resolution in specimens showing non-ideally fractal dimensions. *J. Microsc.* 133: 41–54, 1984.

12. Schmidt-Nielsen, K. *Scaling. Why Is Animal Size So Important?* New York: Cambridge Univ. Press, 1984.

13. Suwa, N., and T. Takahashi. *Morphological and Morphometrical Analysis of Circulation in Hypertension and Ischemic Kidney.* Munich, FRG: Urban & Schwarzenberg, 1971.

14. Thompson, D. A. W. *On Growth and Form.* Cambridge, UK: Cambridge Univ. Press, 1961.

15. Wilson, T. A. Design of the bronchial tree. *Nature Lond.* 213: 668–669, 1967.

BioSystems, 30 (1993) 137–160
Elsevier Scientific Publishers Ireland, Ltd.

137

Fractal graphical representation and analysis of DNA and protein sequences

Victor V. Solovyev [1]

Institute of Cytology and Genetics, Russian Academy of Science, Novosibirsk, 630090, Russia.

1. Introduction

1.1. The use of oligonucleotide and oligopeptide dictionaries in the analysis of genetic texts

The huge amount of sequence data generated by the ongoing genome sequencing project requires a major advance in approaches capable of characterizing and analyzing new sequences. Methods capitalizing on general sequence properties, such as analysis of sequence oligonucleotide composition, i.e. the set of oligonucleotides contained in the sequences under analysis, are currently being developed. It is assumed that an excess of oligonucleotides of some type over the number expected for random sequences can be taken as an evidence for their functional significance. For revealing such functionally significant oligonucleotides, Trifonov and coauthors (Brendel et al., 1986; Beckmann et al., 1986) introduced the notion of *contrast words*. Functionally or evolutionary different sequences were shown to have different vocabularies of contrast words. A good classification of macromolecules, such as 16S rRNA, 23S rRNA, tRNA and others, based on the vocabularies of contrast words, was given in (Trifonov, 1990; Pietrokovsky et al., 1990). Powerful mathematical tools for assessing statistical significance of oligomer patterns in the symbol sequences were developed by Guibas and Odlyzko (1981), Karlin et al.(1989), Gentleman and Mullin (1989), Pevzner et al.(1989).

Investigation of differences in the oligonucleotide composition of exons and introns of eukaryotic genes and the application of these differences to prediction of the exon–intron structure of new sequences are being pursued (Claverie and Bougueleret, 1986). These authors suggest a simple discriminant measure to identify protein-coding regions in a given DNA fragment. In particular, they process a sequence $\mathcal{S} = \{ S_i \mid i = 1, \ldots, N \}$ where N is its length, and produce an oligonucleotide set: $\mathcal{S}_L = \{ S_{L,i} \mid i = 1, \ldots, N - L + 1 \}$ (here L is the oligonucleotide size). In this way, the oligonucleotide frequencies are tabulated.

For example, having tabulated the frequencies of oligonucleotides (F_{ex}) and (F_{in}) for a set of vertebrate exons and introns respectively, it is possible to construct the discriminant profile of a given nucleotide sequence:

$$D_i = \frac{F_{\text{ex}}(S_{L,i})}{F_{\text{ex}}(S_{L,i}) + F_{\text{in}}(S_{L,i})},$$

where i is the position along the sequence.

This profile is to be interpreted as the probability of the sequence position i to belong to an exon. The authors of the paper demonstrated the discrimination between introns and exons when $L = 6$ and D_i

---

[1]   Present address: Department of Cell Biology, Baylor College of Medicine, Houston, TX 77030

was averaged over 30–40 nucleotide positions. However, the accuracy of the method was not estimated by analysis of a sufficient number of genes.

Several approaches to construction of phylogenetic tree by analysis of oligonucleotide frequencies have been suggested (Blaisdell, 1986, 1989; Solovyev and Seledtsov, 1991). Taking into account uneven distribution of mutations in nucleotide sequences in the course of evolution, the latter authors assumed that it is possible to reconstruct the true phylogeny, based on the relatively conservative oligonucleotides (unchanged by mutations in many sequences). Such oligonucleotides usually correspond to functionally significant regions when considered in a set of homologous sequences. The trees constructed for 5S rRNA genes and globin amino acid sequences agree with the expected phylogeny and are not worse than the corresponding reconstruction using more traditional methods based on the principle of maximal parsimony. The phylogenetic tree for 87 globin genes permitting the analysis of their duplication was constructed. Important applications of the approach to the classification of functional sites in eukaryotic genomes were presented also (Solovyev and Seledtsov, 1991).

Analysis of oligonucleotides in 5'-regions of eukaryotic genes allows one to reveal the laws of location and context characteristics of such important promoter elements as CCAAT–box and GC–box (Bucher and Trifonov, 1988). It should be emphasized also that TATA–box, often necessary for the initiation of transcription by polymerase II, occurs in non-coding gene regions 10 times more often than in coding gene regions (Volinia et al., 1989). In addition, it has been shown that oligonucleotides which are rare in other parts of a eukaryotic genome are frequently encountered in the regulatory sequences (Volinia et al., 1988).

A number of interesting features independent on a gene type or species have been revealed. For example, introns are saturated with mirror symmetrical repeats (Beckmann, et al., 1986), but are not rich in complementary repeats. Ohno and Yomo (1991) demonstrated an excess of TG, CT, CA and a deficiency of CG, TA dinucleotides in genomic DNA of eukaryotes. Ohno mentioned also the existence of certain "ubiquitous" oligopeptides in all proteins (Ohno, 1991).

Thus, application of oligonucleotide dictionaries is a useful approach to analysis of nucleotide sequences. They can also be used in a number of powerful methods for fast homology search in databases (Wilbur and Lipman, 1983; Torney et al., 1990; Pearson, 1990), multiple alignment (Zharkikh et al., 1991; Solovyev et al., 1992) and in the classification of proteins (Gibbs et al., 1971). Such dictionaries turned out to be very useful for locating the boundaries of functional domains and identification of functional sites in globular proteins (Solovyev and Makarova, 1992).

Unfortunately, it is almost impossible to perceive visually sets of oligonucleotides. Thus, methods of graphic representation of genetic texts can not only be used to obtain visual images of global features of a sequence (or a group of sequences), but also can be used to analyze the regularities and classification of genetic texts. This is especially timely for investigating the huge amount of sequences produced from the ongoing human DNA sequencing.

1.2. Fractal representation (chaos game) of a nucleotide sequence

1.2.1. Chaos game (CG)

A remarkable representation of nucleotide sequences on a plane using methods of non-linear dynamics (or chaotic dynamic systems) was suggested by Jeffrey (1990). First we perform a cursory review of the original work to pave way for extensions that are the subject of the present contribution.

The technique is based on a simple *chaos game (CG)* algorithm which can produce pictures of fractal structures (Barnsley, 1988). This algorithm proceeds as follows:

(i) Locate n dots on a piece of paper and label them with numerals.

(ii) Plot an arbitrary point and denote it by (X, Y).

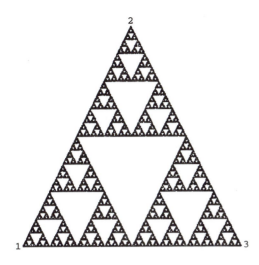

Fig. 1. Fractal representation of the Sierpinsky triangle.

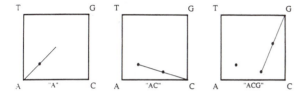

Fig. 2. Fractal graphic representation of the sequence "ACG". The lines are fictious and are used to present the process of generation of the image.

(iii) Roll an n-sided die, each side of which corresponds to one of n transformations $V_1, V_2, \ldots, V_n$ of coordinates that set the fractal structure. Apply the obtained transformation to the point generated at the previous step. Repeat the process the required number of times. Mathematically, the CG is described by an iterated function system (IFS) of linear equations:

$$X' = a_1 X + a_2 Y + a_3; \qquad Y' = b_1 X + b_2 Y + b_3.$$

For instance, if three non-collinear points are selected and each roll of a "3-sided" die produces the midpoint between the current point and the vertex corresponding to the toss, then irrespective to the initial point a fractal structure known as *Sierpinsky triangle* (Fig. 1) is obtained (Jeffrey, 1990). Jeffrey remarked that an analogous chaos game (CG) for 5, 6 or more points (and sides of a die) also produces a distinctive fractal structure, but a CG for a 4-sided polygon produces a uniformly filled square.

1.2.2. Graphic representation of nucleotide sequence

We label the four corners of a square with the symbols of the nucleotide alphabet (A, T, G, and C) and plot the points corresponding to the nucleotides in a DNA sequence according to the following algorithm: the imaginary zero point is positioned in the center, and each consecutive point is placed in the middle of the segment between the last plotted point and the corner corresponding to the current nucleotide in a sequence (Fig. 2).

Drawn in this way, a random sequence would uniformly fill the square (Fig. 3). Uneven filling of the square with points indicates a certain structure in the sequences plotted. Jeffrey pointed out a number of characteristics of fractal representation of the sequences and alluded to their biological significance:

(i) Continuous subsequences of the plotted sequence are in one-to-one correspondence to points of the GR (graphic representation);

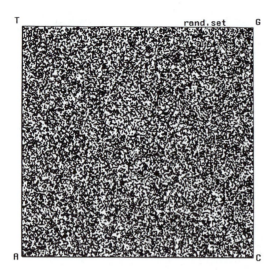

Fig. 3. Fractal representation of 88 random sequences of equiprobable nucleotides, of total length 39099 bp.

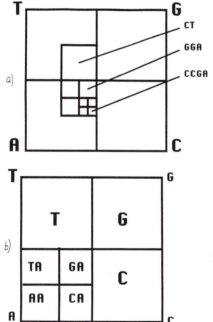

Fig. 4. (a) Correspondence between oligonucleotides and subsquares. (b) Subdivision of the primary square into quadrants of mononucleotides and subquadrants of dinucleotides. The process can be continued to get subquadrants of trinucleotides, tetranucleotides and so on.

(ii) If the side of the square is 1, two sequences having k identical terminal nucleotides will always be in the same subsquare of side 2^{-k}. Thus if the square is divided into subsquares with suitable side (Fig. 4), identical oligonucleotides of the gene will appear in the same subsquare.

Jeffrey constructed fractal representations of a number of pro- and eukaryotic sequences, demonstrated the existence of a non-random structure in them, and set up a number of problems, the most important of which was how to use fractal representation in order to identify biologically interesting characteristics of

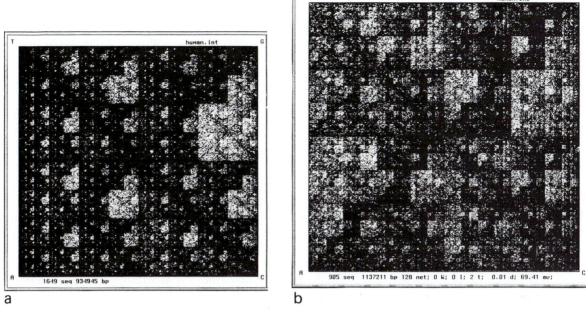

Fig. 5. Fractal representation of 1649 intron sequences (a) and exons from 905 genes of *Homo sapiens* (b). All sequences are from GenBank, Release 65 (Cinkosky et al., 1991).

a sequence or a group of sequences.

2. Use of fractal representation for analysis of nucleotide sequences

2.1. Classification of functional regions

A family of sequences performing a particular function contains both a relatively conservative set of oligonucleotides (providing fulfillment of the function) and oligonucleotides which vary from one sequence to another. It is clear that as a rule only sufficiently long oligonucleotides can be functionally significant. Also, some sequences can have higher occurrences of some types of oligonucleotides as a consequence of their generation by amplification or duplication mechanisms in the course of evolution. Therefore if one draws all sequences from such set, the *fractal representation of a set (FRS)* will be characterized by uneven density of points. A high density should be observed in square regions corresponding to conservative regions of the sequences, while a low density would be observed in regions of non-specific oligonucleotides. In Fig. 5 FRS patterns of human coding and intron sequences are presented. The latter is characterized not only by clear nonhomogeneity of the point density, but also by a certain repetitive structure (self-duplication), which is intrinsic to fractals.

Based on FRS, Solovyev, Korolev and Lim (1991, 1992) suggested an approach to nucleotide sequence classification which is reviewed in this paragraph. We consider the square with sides of length 1. If it is subdivided into $n \times n$ cells (subsquares), the sides of a cell will be $1/n$. Hence, if the square is subdivided into 4 cells ($n = 2$), each cell will correspond to a particular nucleotide. For $n = 4, 8, \ldots, 2^k$, each subsquare will correspond to a dinucleotide, trinucleotide, tetranucleotide, $\ldots$, k-nucleotide, respectively. Let the number of points of FRS in a certain cell, i.e. the density of points, be P_{ij}, where $i, j = 1, \ldots, n$ are the indices of row and column of the cells in the square, respectively. To identify common oligonucleotides, cells with density lower than a certain threshold level can be eliminated. In particular, it is possible to introduce a threshold value derived from FRS of random sequences. Given a set of S sequences of lengths $(L_1, \ldots, L_s)$ with the total length $L = \sum_{m=1}^{s} L_m$, it is possible to generate a set of k random sequences S_k^r with matching lengths. If the average density of FRS is denoted by $P = L/n^2$, then the standard deviation is computed using the following equation:

$$\delta = \sqrt{\frac{1}{(n^2 - 1)} \sum_{i,j=1}^{n} (P_{ij} - P)^2}, \tag{1}$$

where P_{ij} is the number of points in the (i, j)-th cell.

The collection of cells of FRS satisfying the condition $P_{ij}^m > P + m\delta$ is called the *mask* M_n^m. $m = 0, 1, 2, \ldots$ is a variable parameter that determines the threshold level for elimination of non-specific oligonucleotides. Non-specific nucleotides can be eliminated either by a statistical criterion (1), or by a simple condition which rejects cells containing less than $1, 2, \ldots, l$ ($l \ll L$) nucleotides.

It has been shown above that certain parts of the mask correspond to similar oligonucleotides in a set of sequences when the basic square is subdivided into cells. The more frequent is an oligonucleotide, the higher is the value P_{ij} in the corresponding cell. So it is natural to plot P_{ij} as a third coordinate. Maxima in such a plot will correspond to conservative (highly represented) oligonucleotides for the family. It is possible to present this coordinate with different colors. Masks for sets of globins, actins and other genes were constructed (Solovyev et al., 1992). On Fig. 6 a globin mask is presented as an example. We applied FRS masks to classification of sequences using a simple definition of similarity. For example, a measure F can be defined as

$$F = \sum_{i,j=1}^{n} P_{ij}, \tag{2}$$

where the summation is performed over all cells in the square in which the points (nucleotides) of the sequence under investigation are plotted. Analogously, one can consider only those cells that correspond to the specific masks M_n^m:

$$F = \sum_{i,j=1}^{n} a_{ij}, \tag{3}$$

where $a_{ij} = P_{ij}$ if a cell belongs to the mask M_n^m and $a_{ij} = 0$ otherwise. In addition, instead of P_{ij}, it is possible to use other weight functions, in particular, $\log(P_{ij})$ or 1. In some cases, one can use $\log(P_{ij})$ to suppress unusually high weights of some cells. On the other hand, the constant weight 1 can be used in cases when the densities are not very high and the statistical differences between cells cannot be determined accurately.

To select the optimal parameters (n, m, a) for identification of a sequence set, the following "jack-knife" procedure (Manly, 1991) is used. Each p-th sequence ($1 \le p \le k$) is eliminated one at a time from the set of k sequences to serve as the control, and a mask $\tilde{M}_n^m$ is constructed from the remaining $(k - 1)$ sequences (the learning set). Then the similarity of the p-th sequence to the (remaining) set is estimated for all $p = 1, \ldots, k$ based on the measure F, and a histogram of F values is constructed. The histogram for the corresponding set of random sequences is also constructed using the mask for the full set M_n^m. The larger is the difference between these histograms, the better the mask recognizes the sequences of the considered type (Fig. 7). Sample histograms which show distinct separation between random sequences and globin

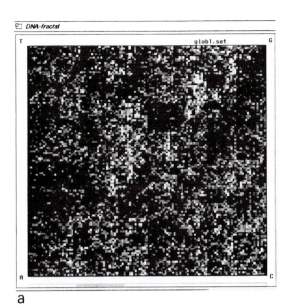

a

Fig. 6. The mask M_{128}^1 for 88 coding regions of globin genes. The larger is the number of dots, the brighter is the cell.

genes and between globin and actin genes are presented in Fig. 8. In (Solovyev et al., 1992), other examples have been considered, which demonstrate that masks of FRS not only produce a good classification of sequences for diverse gene families, but can also discriminate between subfamilies such as α- and β-actin genes.

2.2. Search for functional regions

Having constructed the mask pertaining to a particular set of sequences, we write down the corresponding matrix and use it to identify sequences of the given type in a genetic text. A sliding window technique is used. The window has a fixed length, which equals the average or the minimum length $\bar{L}$ of sequences in the learning set. It is moved along a sequence and the values of F (equation (2) or (3)) for sequences of length $\bar{L}$ are calculated for each window position. For selecting regions of interest (for example, globin genes), we use the threshold $F_{\min}$ defined as the minimum value of F for sequences from the learning set (globin genes in this example) based on the matrix $\tilde{M}_m^n$. In this way, for any window position which gives $F > F_{\min}$, it is reasonable to assume existence of a desired sequence somewhere nearby. Predicted location of the sequence is assumed to coincide with the position of the window when a maximum of F is obtained. Performance of this algorithm is exemplified with the human globin DNA region from chromosome 11, whose length is 73,323 bp (GenBank entry HUMHBB). The mask M_m^n is created based on 86 globin sequences (human globin genes were excluded). Using this mask, the entire region is processed with a 50 bp window (the approximate size of a small exon). Five peaks corresponding to globin genes are clearly visible. A pseudo-gene globin region is found also (positions 45,728–47,142), but the peak is less pronounced (Fig. 9). It is interesting that the exon structure is visible. Other examples of successful application of FRS masks for various gene families are presented in (Korolev et al., 1992). In particular, we successfully tested the algorithm on such nontraditional (for oligonucleotide-based recognition) sequences (in contrast to protein-coding regions) as long terminal repeats (LTR) of retroviral DNA.

144

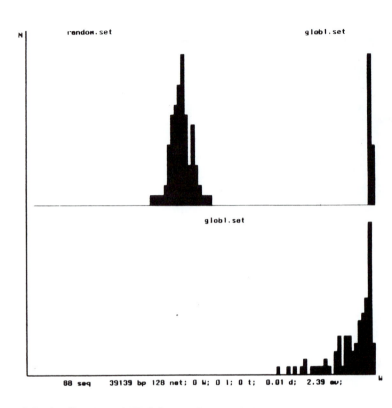

Fig. 7. Histograms of the discriminant functional for globin genes and random sequences constructed using the mask M_{128}^1 for globin genes. On the bottom histogram weights of globin genes after jack-knife procedure are presented. Abscissa — the value of the discriminant function, ordinate — the number of sequences. Only coding regions of globin genes are considered.

2.3. Application of FRS for analysis and delineation of gene structure

The more abundant is an oligonucleotide, the higher is the number of dots P in the corresponding cell. So it is natural to plot P as a third coordinate (we call the resulting picture *fractal representation of oligonucleotide composition (FRC)*). Maxima in FRC's correspond to frequent oligonucleotides, while minima correspond to rare ones. FRC's of human introns and coding regions extracted from GenBank (1992) are presented in Fig. 10, where each column corresponds to the number of occurrences of some oligonucleotide in these sets. In Fig. 11 FRC of 100 bp fragments located immediately upstream of the start codon (5′-regions of human genes) and those located downstream of stop codon (3′-regions of human genes) are presented. The peculiarities of oligonucleotide composition can be applied to recognition of these regions.

FRC's for regions upstream of transcription start points of human genes are presented in Fig. 12. We can see that the composition of the regions (-300)–(-201), (-200)–(-101) and (-100)–(-1) is generally similar, but the concentration of specific oligonucleotides increases towards the promoter region (-100)–(-1).

Correlation coefficient $R_L^{1,2}$ between matrices corresponding to the masks of FRS's of different DNA regions is an estimate of the sets similarity. Consider two FRS matrices M_1 and M_2, whose elements $P_{i,j}^1$ and $P_{i,j}^2$ equal to the number of FRS dots in the corresponding cells ($1 \le i \le n$, $1 \le j \le n$). Then

$$R_L^{1,2} = \frac{1}{n^2} \left(\sum_{i,j=1}^{n} (P_{i,j}^1 - P^1)(P_{i,j}^2 - P^2) \right) \bigg/ \left(\sum_{i=1}^{n} \left(P_{i,j}^1 - P^1\right)^2 \left(P_{i,j}^2 - P^2\right)^2 \right)^{1/2},$$

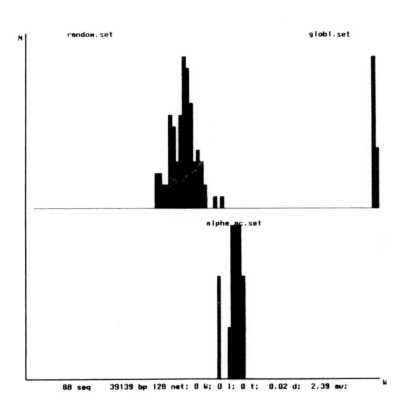

Fig. 8. Histograms of the discriminant functional for globin and α-actin genes constructed using the mask M_{128}^1 of globin genes. Other details as in Fig. 7.

where the superscripts 1 and 2 denote the sequence sets under comparison, L is the oligonucleotide size, P^1 and P^2 are the average numbers of dots in a cell for M_1 and M_2, respectively.

Based on values of R it is possible to distinguish between functional and duplicational similarity (though both may occur simultaneously). Functional similarity is characterized by existence of a group of over-represented oligonucleotides against weak similarity in other regions of sequences. To identify such similarity, we suggest to use $R_L^{1,2}$ where only nucleotides satisfying $P_{i,j}^1 \gg \max(P^1, P^2)$ or $P_{i,j}^2 \gg \max(P^1, P^2)$ are considered.

We investigated the value of $R_L^{1,2}$ for various parts of 5'-flanking regions. Results presented in Table 1 support the visual observation that the concentration of specific oligonucleotides increases towards the promoter region. Such structure of the 5'-region can have a functional value, related to organization of chromatin or providing high concentration of regulatory proteins in this region. The observed trend can provide effective interaction of the region with the universal protein complex and promote initiation of transcription (Solovyev, 1991). Among oligonucleotides typical for these 5'-regions are known sites of transcription initiation: TATA-box, CCAAT-box, GC-box (Table 2).

During the last few years some complex systems for prediction of the gene structure were created (Gelfand, 1990; Fields and Soderlund, 1990; Uberbacher and Mural, 1992; Guigo et al.,1992). These systems combine information about functional signals and statistical properties of coding and intron regions. On this basis potential first, internal and terminal exons are generated and the best combination of them provides the predicted gene structure. However, the problem requires further investigation. For example, the testing of the last algorithm (Guigo et al., 1992) on an independent data set demonstrated that correct exons with the correct boundaries were predicted only in 54% of cases (Guigo et al., 1992). It should be

146

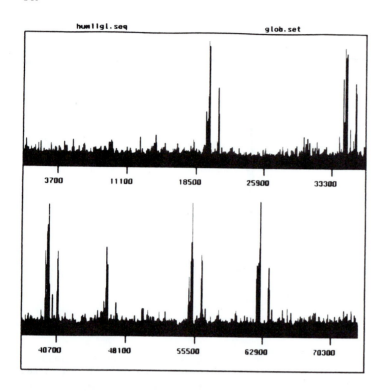

Fig. 9. Search for globin genes using the fractal image of the globin family in human chromosome 11. Five dominant peaks correspond to globin genes, smaller peaks correspond to pseudogenes (marked). The exon structure is also visible.

Table 1

The correlation coefficient values between FRS masks for (-1)–(-100), (-101)–(-200) and (-201)–(-300) 5′-regions of human genes. The denominator values are computed for all oligonucleotides, and numerators are computed for oligonucleotides which occur more than 10 times.

-100/-200	-100/-300	-200/-300
0.615/0.330	0.519/0.253	0.704/0.282

mentioned that 84% of coding regions predicted by this system are actually coding.

Now we describe the implementation of the simplest variant of the program for prediction of coding regions based on fractal representation. We calculate the FRS masks (matrices) for human coding (M_c), intron (M_{in}), 5′ ($M_{5'}$) and 3′ ($M_{3'}$) sequences extracted from GenBank.

For discrimination between coding and intron regions we follow the work by Claverie and Bougueleret (1990). They considered *in-phase* (starting in the 1-st codon position) hexanucleotides (dicodons) and a window of size 40 bp. For the discrimination between coding and intron regions we use the following measure:

$$F(\mathbf{s}) = \frac{F_{M_c^p}(\mathbf{s})}{F_{M_c^p}(\mathbf{s}) + F_{M_{in}}(\mathbf{s})}, \qquad (4)$$

where $F_{M_c^p}(\mathbf{s})$ and $F_{M_{in}}(\mathbf{s})$ are the values of function for a sequence fragment s corresponding to the current window position, computed for the coding and intron FRS masks M_c^p and M_{in} respectively (with

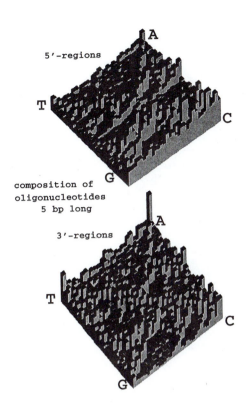

Fig. 10. FRC (Fractal Representation of Composition) of 3917 human coding sequences (bottom) and 4963 human intron sequences (top) for hexanucleotides.

oligonucleotides in only one of the three phases are taken into account).

In (Solovyev and Lawrence, 1992) we considered 9-nucleotides and obtained 87% accuracy for 25575 coding and 45798 noncoding test windows of length 54 bp, and 91.5% accuracy for 108 bp windows. When intron sequences were used as the noncoding sample, the accuracy for 54 bp windows was 91%, and for 108 bp windows it was 95.5%.

For prediction of the gene structure the value F is calculated for each window position using fractal matrices of coding, intron, 5'- and 3'-regions. For prediction of 5'- and 3'-regions we used the function similar to (4), where instead of $F_{M_c^p}(s)$ F-values based on octanucleotide frequencies in 5'- or 3'-regions, respectively, were considered, while $F_{M_{in}}(s)$ were octanucleotide frequencies in introns. On Fig. 13 we present as an example analysis of the human β-globin gene. We can see that this approach allows us to distinguish different genic functional regions: 5'-leader, exons, introns and 3'-region. It should be noted that we do not take into account information about site splicing position, which would be used in the further development of this graphical system.

3. Fractal representation of amino acid sequences

From the above consideration of nucleotide sequences it is clear that the graphical representation (GR) of a genetic text in an arbitrary alphabet should satisfy two conditions:

(i) a set of random sequences should generate a plot of uniform point density,

(ii) points of identical oligomers of genetic texts (oligopeptides, oligonucleotides) should concentrate in same regions of FRS plots.

148

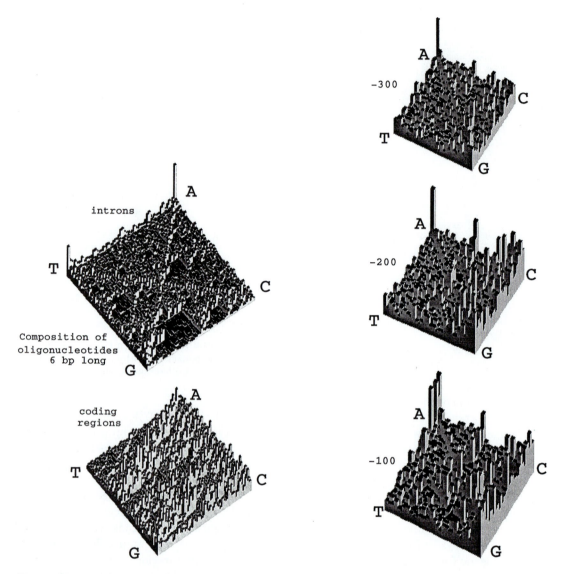

Fig. 11. FRC for 1993 upstream 100 bp regions (top) and 2092 downstream 100 bp regions of human genes for pentanucleotides.

Fig. 12. FRC of 5′-flanking regions: (a) (−300)–(−201), (b) (−200)–(−101), (c) (−100)–(−1).

For fractal representation of amino acid sequences (FRA) consider a rectangle $5a_x \times 4a_y$, where a_x, a_y are scaling factors, subdivided into 20 cells corresponding to the twenty amino acids (Fig. 14). Let the amino acids be numbered from 1 to 20 in the following order: (A, V, L, I, C, M, P, F, Y, W, D, N, E, Q, H, S, T, K, R, G). The correspondence between the cells and the amino acids is defined by the following equations:

Table 2
Oligonucleotides which occur more than 13 times in (-300)–(-201), (-200)–(-101) and (-100)–(-1) 5′-regions of human genes.

==========	-100	===============	===== -200	===============
GGGCGGGG 52	AGCAGCCA 15	GGCCCTTT 13	GGGAGGAG 16	GGGGGCGG 15
GAGGAGGG 15	GAGGGAGG 15	GCCCTTTA 13	AAAAAAAA 58	CCCGCCCC 14
GGGGCGGG 52	GGCGGGGG 23	GGGGTGGG 13	TGTGTGTG 21	GGCGGGGG 13
GGGGAGGG 24	GCGGGGGC 16	GTGGGGGA 14	GTGTGTGT 20	CCTCCCGG 13
TATAAAAA 20	CGGCCGGC 13	GCCCGGCC 13	TCCCCACC 34	CTCCCTCC 13
AGGAGGAG 16	CCTTTATA 15	GCGGCCGG 13	CCCTCCCC 35	
GGAGGAGG 17	GCAGAGGG 17	GCCGGGCG 13	CCCCACCC 30	== -300 ===
AAAAAAAG 37	AGGGCAGG 17	GCGGGGCC 13	CCTCCCCA 34	
ATAAAAGG 23	GCCCCGCC 19	GGGGCCGG 13	CCACCCTC 24	AAAAAAAA 45
GGCGGGGC 32	CCCTCCCC 14	CTGATTGG 13	CTCCCCAC 21	TGTGTGTG 23
CGGGGCGG 27	GGTATAAA 15	CTATAAAG 13	ACCCTCCC 22	GTGTGTGT 21
CCCGCCCC 22	AAAAAGGG 14	CCTCCCCC 13	CCCACCCT 21	GGGTGGGG 14
GGGGGCGG 30	CCGCGCCC 13	CCTCCTCC 13	CACCCTCC 23	AAAAGAAA 20
GGGCCGGG 15	CGCCCACC 14	CCCCCTCC 13	CCTTCCCC 16	AAAGAAAA 18
GGCCAGGG 15	AGGCGGGG 13	CCCCTCCT 13	CCCCTCCC 23	TTTGTTTT 20
CCCCGCCC 28	GGGAGGGG 18	GGCTGGGC 13	GTGCTCGG 15	TTGTTTTG 23
GCGGGGCG 22	AAAAGAAA 14	GCAGGGAG 13	CTCCTCCC 19	TTTTGTTT 17
GTATAAAA 35	CAAAGCAG 14	TATATAAG 14	TCCTCCCC 17	GTTTTGTT 14
CCCCACCC 15	GGGAGGGC 14	CGCGCCCC 13	GCTCGGCT 16	GGGCGGGG 16
CACCCCCA 14	CCCTCCTC 17	GAGGGAGA 13	CCCCACCT 14	AGAGGGAG 13
ATAAAAAG 17	AAAGCAGA 13	CACCGGCC 13	TTCCCCAC 15	TGTTTTGT 13
GGGCCAGG 15	AGAGGGCG 13	CCTATAAA 14	GTGGGAGG 17	GGGAGAGG 13
AGTATAAA 24	GGCGTGGG 13		CCCCAGGG 13	
TATAAAAG 26	AAGAAAAA 13		CCCAGCCC 13	
GGAGGGAG 18	GAAAAAAG 13		CCCTCCCG 14	
ATAAAAGC 21	AAAAAAGA 13		GTGTGGGA 13	
TCCTCTCT 15	ATCCTCTC 13		TGTGGGAG 14	
CTCCGCCC 21	CCTCTCTC 15		GGGAGGGG 15	
CTTTATAA 18	CCGGCCCT 14		TGCTCGGC 14	
GGGCAGGG 22	CCCTTTAT 14		TCTCCTCC 14	
AGGGAGGG 19	AGGGTCTG 15		GCCCCTCC 14	
GGGAGGGA 15	CAGGGCAG 14		CCAGCCCC 14	
GGGCGGGC 18	CAGAGGGC 13		CTCCCCAT 13	
AAAGAAAA 14	GAGAAGGG 13		GGGCGGGG 18	
TAAAAAGG 16	AGCAGAGG 15		CTCGGCTG 13	
AGAAAAAA 17	GGGGCTTT 14		CCCCGCCC 17	
TGAGTATA 15	AAAAGGGC 13		CCCGGCTG 13	
GAGTATAA 15	CCCAGCCC 16		GGGGCGGG 16	
TAAAAGCC 15	CGGGGGCG 14		TTTTTTTT 13	

$$x^J = \text{Int}((J-1)/4) + 1,$$
$$y^J = J - 4(n_x - 1), \qquad (5)$$

where $x^J = 1, \ldots, 5$, $y^J = 1, \ldots, 4$ are the coordinates of the lower left vertex of the rectangular cell (of size $a_x \times a_y$) corresponding to the amino acid J.

We construct FRA as follows:

(i) Plot the first amino acid of the sequence as a point in the center of the rectangular cell associated with this amino acid;

(ii) Plot the current amino acid by projecting *conformally* the location of the last plotted point in the $5a_x \times 4a_y$ rectangle into the $a_x \times a_y$ rectangular cell associated with the current amino acid. Other points, which have been plotted earlier in the iterative process, are untouched;

(iii) Repeat step (2) until the amino acid sequence is exhausted.

Computation of the coordinates of the point corresponding to the current amino acid J is performed as follows. Let (x, y) be the coordinates of the last plotted point in the rectangle $(0, 0; 0, 4a_y; 5a_x, 4a_y; 0, 5a_x)$

150

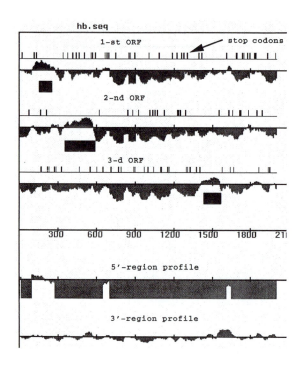

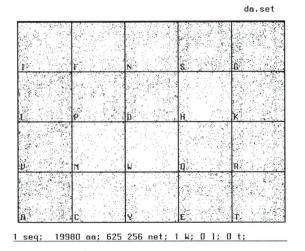

1 seq; 19980 aa; 625 256 net; 1 W; 0 1; 0 t;

Fig. 14. Fractal representation of a random sequence with amino acid probabilities coinciding with those in the PIR data bank (Barker et al., 1990). Note that 20 amino acid are numbered consistently in course of creation of a FRS.

Fig. 13. Analysis of the human β-globin gene by fractal matrices for different gene regions. The dominant peaks in the 1-st, 2-nd and 3-rd reading frames correspond to real codon positions. The approach allows us also to see 5'- and 3'-regions.

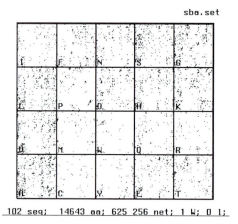

102 seq; 14643 aa; 625 256 net; 1 W; 0 1;

Fig. 15. Fractal representation of globin sequences.

and let the coordinates of the left bottom corner of the cell corresponding to the amino acid J be (x^J, y^J). Then the coordinates in question are

$$x = x^J + x/5,$$

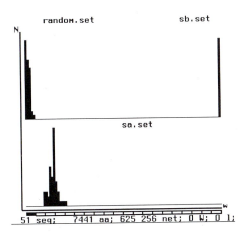

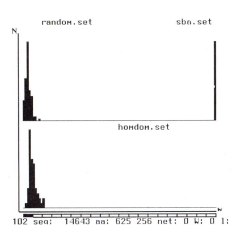

Fig. 16. Histograms of fractal weights of random sequences, 51 α-globin and 51 β-globin sequences constructed using mask $M125 \times 61$ of β-globins.

Fig. 17. Histograms of fractal weights of random sequences, 102 globin and 51 homeo-domain sequences constructed using mask $M125 \times 61$ of β-globins.

$$y = y^J + y/4.$$

It is clear that representation of random sequences of equiprobable amino acids produces a uniformly filled rectangle.

As for protein families, each of them has a specific FRA (Fig. 15). When $n_x = 1, 2$ and $n_y = 1, 2$, the representation essentially coincides with the one suggested by Jeffrey (1990) for nucleotide sequences, except that x^J, y^J are chosen as the left bottom corners of the subsquares of the corresponding nucleotide and are not the corners of the main square. The main principle of construction of the graphic representation, applied in the work, is: *Area of the GR, where dots corresponding to the current letter can occur, should decrease $(1/\alpha)$-fold at each iteration, where α is the alphabet size.* This principle permits to satisfy the conditions considered at the beginning of Section 3.

The approach for construction of FR's of nucleotide and amino acid sequences can be simply generalized so that it would be applicable for genetic texts with other number of monomers (e.g. when classes of amino acids with similar physical properties are considered) (Solovyev, 1991). The only requirement is that the alphabet size (L) is not a prime number: $L = k \times m$, where k and m may be used in the above equations instead of numbers 4 and 5.

3.1. Classification of amino acid sequences on the base of FRA

To determine whether FRA is suitable for identification and classification purposes, we used the approach similar to one described above for nucleic acids. Now the rectangle of FRA $(5a_x, 4a_y)$ is broken into $m \times n$ cells. If we take $m = 5^k$, and $n = 4^k$, each cell would correspond to a k-peptide. This division generates a mask M_k^m, where m is the threshold for elimination of non-specific peptides. The weight histograms for several protein sequences constructed by FRA masks are presented in Figs. 16 and 17. A good separation occurs not only between the random sequences and proteins of particular families, but also between protein subfamilies performing similar function as exemplified by α- and β-globins.

Visual difference of the corresponding histograms is not the only criterion of the separation quality. A more formal estimate is provided by the Mahalonobis distance defined as

152

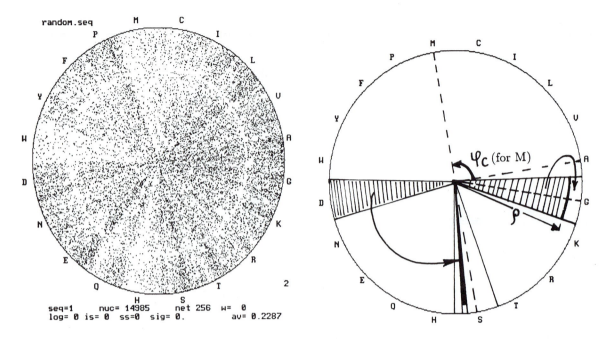

Fig. 18. Circular graphic representation (CGR) of a random sequence with amino acid frequencies corresponding to those in PIR data bank (Barker et al., 1990).

Fig. 19. Projection of CGR points to the sector corresponding to the current letter (if the current letter S does not coincide with the previous one D, and if both the previous and the current letters are G).

$$MD = \frac{(F_e - F_t)^2}{\sigma_e^2 + \sigma_t^2}$$

where F_e and F_t are means and σ_e^2 and σ_t^2 are variances of two distributions.

4. Circular graphic representation of genetic texts with an arbitrary alphabet

FR of genetic texts with the alphabet size $\alpha = l \times k$ where $l > 1$ and $k > 1$ was presented in section 3. However, it is not appropriate for prime α. A circular graphic representation of genetic texts (CGR) considered in this section does not have this restriction. Let the letters of the alphabet be numbered by $i = 1, 2, \ldots, \alpha$. Divide a circle of radius R into α sectors, so that the letter i is set in correspondence with the sector whose central radius has the angle

$$\varphi_c = (i-1)u + U/2,$$

where $U = 2\pi/\alpha$ (Fig. 18).

Let the polar coordinates of the dot corresponding to the last processed letter be (r, φ), and those of the current letter J be $(r_{\text{new}}, \varphi_{\text{new}})$. Further construction is based on the main principle stated in the end of Section 3. Thus the circle is projected into the sector corresponding to the current letter, while each sector is projected into a subsector of width $2\pi/\alpha^2$ (Fig. 19).

Movement of dots corresponding to poly-N sequences towards the external arc is achieved by the following trick. Dots from the sectors corresponding to non-J letters are projected into the central part of the J-

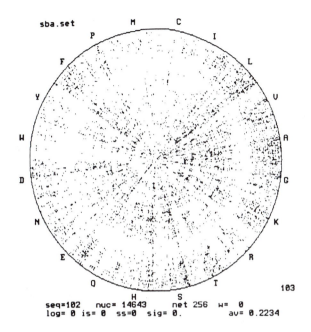

Fig. 20. Circular graphic representation (CGR) of 102 globin sequences.

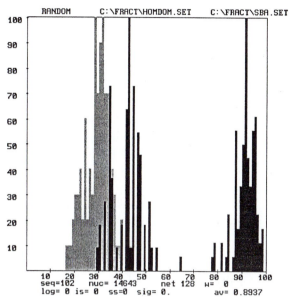

Fig. 21. Histograms of CGR weights for random sequences, 102 globin and 66 homeo-domain sequences constructed using the mask $M128 \times 128$ of globins.

sector having the radius ρ, while dots from the J-sector are projected into the external ring sector with the internal radius ρ and the external radius R, where ρ is defined by the condition that the ring area is α times smaller than the area of the entire sector (Fig. 19):

$$(1/\alpha)R^2 2\pi/\alpha = \pi(R^2 - \rho^2)2\pi/\alpha.$$

Thus $\rho = R\sqrt{1 - 1/\alpha}$.

The projection of dots from the J-sector is performed by the following procedure that satisfies the main principle. Let $\varphi_m = 1/4 \cdot 2\pi/\alpha$ (Fig. 19). Then for dots of the left semicircle (relative to the line corresponding to the central radius of the J-sector whose angle is φ_c) we write:

$$\varphi_{\text{new}} = \varphi_c - \varphi_m - (\varphi_m - u + \varphi_s)d,$$

where $u = (\varphi_c - \varphi)/\alpha$ is a term related to α-fold decrease of the area, $\varphi_s = \varphi_m/\alpha$, and $d = \alpha/(\alpha - 1)$ is the increase of the area of non-J sectors. Similarly, for the right semicircle:

$$\varphi_{\text{new}} = \varphi_c + \varphi_m - (\varphi_m - u + \varphi_s)d,$$

The radius of the dot is computed based on the condition that the larger has been the radius of the last plotted point, the smaller should be the current radius (if the previous letter does not coincide with the current one). Thus r_{new} is found from the condition of the α-fold decrease of the letter area (Fig. 19):

$$\pi r_{\text{new}}^2 (2\pi/\alpha^2)(\alpha/(\alpha - 1)) = (1/\alpha)\pi(R^2 - r^2)(2\pi/\alpha)$$

Then $r_{\text{new}} = \sqrt{R^2 - r^2}\sqrt{1 - 1/\alpha}$.

154

If the current letter J coincides with the previous one, the dots from the sector J are projected into the outer ring of the same sector. At the first occurrence of the letter J the dots are located within the inner subsector $0 \leq r \leq \sqrt{1 - 1/\alpha} \cdot R = \rho$. Thus this subsector, whose area is $\sim \pi\rho^2$, is projected into the corresponding part of the outer ring. From consideration of the proportion of the initial and terminal projection areas

$$\frac{\pi(r_{\text{new}}^2 - \rho^2)2\pi/\alpha}{\pi(R^2 - \rho^2)2\pi/\alpha} = \frac{r^2}{R^2},$$

it follows that $r_{\text{new}} = \sqrt{r^2/\alpha + \rho^2}$ and $\varphi_{\text{new}} = \varphi$. If the run of J persists, the outer J-ring is projected into its outer subring of the area decreased α-fold. At each step we should know two radii: ρ_1 (the minimum radius, where dots of previous level are located) and ρ_2 (the current minimum radius). The ratio of the areas of the rings of potential location of dots for two successive transformations is, as usual, $1/\alpha$:

$$(1/\alpha)\pi(R^2 - \rho_1^2)2\pi/\alpha = \pi(R^2 - \rho_2^2)2\pi/\alpha,$$

thus

$$\rho_2^2 = R^2(1 - 1/\alpha) + (1/\alpha)\rho_1^2, \tag{6}$$

Since $\rho_1^2 = (1 - 1/\alpha)R^2$,

$$\rho_2^2 = (1 - 1/\alpha)R^2 + (1/\alpha)(1 - 1/\alpha)R^2 = R^2(1 - 1/\alpha^2), \tag{7}$$

It is clear from equations (6) and (7) that the inner radii of the rings at each step can be computed iteratively:

$$\rho_1 = R\sqrt{1 - (1/\alpha)^{k-1}} \quad \text{and} \quad \rho_2 = R\sqrt{(1 - (1/\alpha)^k)},$$

where k is the run length (the number of identical successive letters).

The proportion of the areas when projecting is:

$$\frac{\pi(r_{\text{new}}^2 - \rho_2^2)2\pi/\alpha}{\pi(R^2 - \rho_2^2)2\pi/\alpha} = \frac{\pi(r^2 - \rho_1^2)2\pi/\alpha}{\pi(R^2 - \rho_1^2)2\pi/\alpha},$$

and thus

$$r_{\text{new}} = \frac{(r^2 - \rho_1^2)(R^2 - \rho_2^2) + \rho_2^2(R^2 - \rho_1^2)}{R^2 - \rho_1^2}.$$

We can simplify this equation, using (6):

$$r_{\text{new}} = \sqrt{(r^2 - \rho_1^2)/\alpha + \rho_2^2}.$$

For all cases of projection of letter runs $\varphi_{\text{new}} = \varphi$.

Thus we have equations for construction of circular graphic representation of a text over an alphabet of arbitrary size. Below we exemplify this technique with amino acid sequences.

Random amino acid sequences fill the circle uniformly (not shown), while the sequences with frequencies of amino acids typical for real proteins taken from the data base (Barker et al., 1990) are characterized by unhomogeneous image (Fig. 18). In this case text sequences were generated with random distribution of amino acids along a sequence.

CGR of globins and homeo-domain proteins have their own specific images (Fig. 20; homeo-domain proteins data not shown). These images can be used to identify the family and discover regularities of its structure. A mask-based method similar to one for classification of nucleic acid sequences can be applied in this case also. Histograms of globin sequences classification by the CGR mask of globin family is presented in Fig. 21. The quality of separation is quite high.

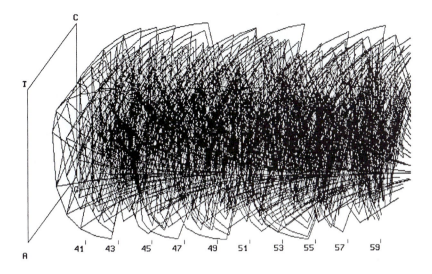

Fig. 22. Three-dimensional fractal representation (TFRS) of random sequences.

5. Three-dimensional representation of sequences on the base of FRS

FRS does not allow one to see clearly differences between sequences within a group. To analyze these peculiarities the following three-dimensional fractal representation of a set of sequences (TFRS) is suggested. When an ordinary FRS is constructed, each i-th letter is described by two coordinates (X, Y). Now introduce the third coordinate $Z = ih$, where h is a scaling factor. The coordinates of the first letter are $X = 0.5$, $y = 0.5$ and $Z = 0$.

TFRS for random sequences is presented on Fig. 22 and that for a sample of 3′-splicing sites of human genes, on Fig. 23. This representation delineates conservative sequence regions and their location. If there is no unique consensus for a site, the image separates can into clusters. It should be noted that TFRS analysis requires alignment of conservative regions. A measure of the proximity of plotted sequences may be constructed based on this representation, and alignment algorithm can be realised by shifting one of the sequence along Z-axis to maximize the value of the measure.

6. Three-dimensional graphic representation of a sequence set based on H-curves

A nucleotide sequence can be represented as a three-dimensional H-curve (Hamori, 1985). First a system of four base vectors corresponding to nucleotides is defined (Fig. 24). Then the vectors corresponding to nucleotides of a sequence are attached consecutively in the head-to-tail manner (Varga et al., 1991). When H-curves for a set of functionally similar sequences are constructed simultaneously, we obtain a HRS. Examples are presented on Figs. 25 (random sequences) and 26 (human 3′-splice sites). It can be seen that HRS for the conservative part of the latter image is much more compact. It is interesting to note that the one-to-one map of the nucleotide sequence onto a DNA walk, suggested recently (Peng et al., 1992) for analysis of long range correlations in nucleotide sequences, is the simplified case of the H-curve representation with 2 types of nucleotides.

156

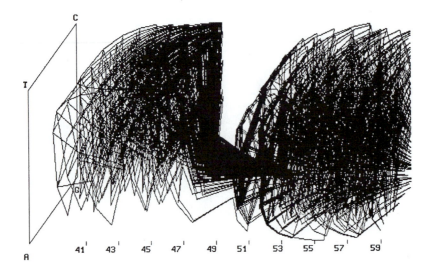

Fig. 23. There-dimensional fractal representation (TFRS) of human 3′-splice sequences.

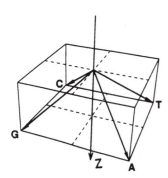

Fig. 24. Four three-dimensional vectors corresponding to nucleotides used for construction of H-curves.

Conclusion

This paper describes new pattern recognition approaches to classification and search for particular genome functional regions. The approaches are based on graphical representation of sequence sets and can present a global view on the sequence features. In practice analytical possibilities of graphical representations are similar to the application of usual oligonucleotide counts, and they can be employed in a manner similar to the use of dot-matrices in sequence alignments.

Graphical images of sequence sets can be easily compared both visually and by computer procedures. They are useful not only for analysis of a particular sequence, but for representation of the global oligonucleotide (or oligopeptide) composition of a given set, which can itself provide basis for further application of analytical methods. Taking into account fractal representation of amino acid sequences and graphical representation of genetic texts with the arbitrary size of an alphabet (Solovyev, 1991), we can say that these approaches provide a general graphical apparatus for investigation of both nucleic acid and protein genetic texts. They can be applied in different studies of structural and functional organization of genomes. Finally, fractal geometry, according to Mandelbrot (1982), is the "Geometry of Nature", and it

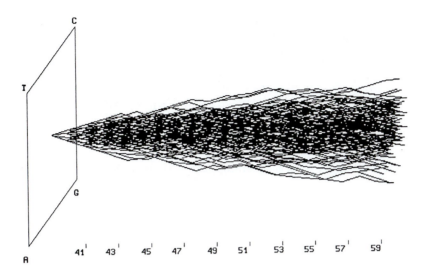

Fig. 25. Three-dimensional H-curve representation of random sequences.

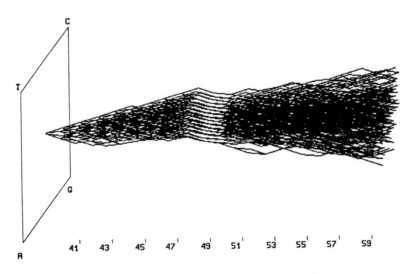

Fig. 26. Three-dimensional H-curve representation of human 3'-splice sequences.

is really everywhere (Barnsley, 1988), since current applications of it range from description of structural environment characteristics of catalytic processes in chemistry (Anvir, 1991) and to analysis of structural characteristic of nucleotide sequences, as described in the present contribution.

158

Acknowledgements

The author would like to thank I.A. Seledtsov for the assistance in organization of the graphic library for IBM PC, I.N. Klikunova and K.S. Makarova for preparation of some sequence sets, and Drs. S. Korolev, H.A. Lim, L. Milanesi and C. Lawrence for helpful discussions.

References

Avnir, D., 1991, Fractal geometry — A new approach to heterogeneous catalysis. Chemistry & Industry 24, 912–916.

Barker, W.C., George, D.G. and Hunt, L.T., 1990, Protein sequences database. Meth. Enzymol. 183, 31–60.

Barnsley, M.F., 1988, Fractals Everywhere (Academic Press, San Diego).

Beckmann, J.S., Brendel, V. and Trifonov, E.N., 1986, Intervening sequences exhibit distinct vocabulary. J. Biomol. Struct. Dynam. 4, 391–400.

Blaisdell, B.E., 1986, A measure of the similarity of sets of sequences not requiring sequence alignment. Proc. Natl. Acad. Sci. USA 53, 5155–5159.

Blaisdell, B.E., 1989, Effectiveness of measures requiring and not requiring prior sequence alignment for estimating the dissimilarity of natural sequences. J. Mol. Evol. 29, 526–537.

Brendel, V., Beckmann, J.S. and Trifonov, E.N., 1986, Linguistics of nucleotide sequences: morphology and comparison of vocabularies. J. Biomol. Struct. Dynam. 4, 11–21.

Bucher, P. and Trifonov, E.N., 1988, CAAT–box revisited. Bidirectionality, location and context. J. Biomol. Struct. Dynam. 5, 1231–1236.

Cinkosky, M.J., Fickett, J.W., Gilna, P. and Burks, C., 1991, Electronic data publishing and GenBank. Science 252, 1273–1277.

Claverie, J.M. and Bougueleret, L., 1986, Heuristic information analysis of sequences. Nucl. Acids Res. 14, 179–196.

Claverie, J.M., Sauvaget, I. and Bougueleret, L. 1990, K-tuple sequence analysis: from exon–intron discrimination to T–cell epitope mapping. Meth. Enzymol. 183, 237–252.

Fields, C. and Soderlund, C.A., 1990, gm: a practical tool for automating DNA sequence analysis. Comput. Appl. Biosci. 6, 263–270.

Gelfand, M.S., 1990, Computer prediction of the exon–intron structure of mammalian pre-mRNAs. Nucl. Acids. Res. 18, 5865–5869.

Gentleman, J.F. and Mullin, R.C., 1989, The distribution of the frequency of occurrence of nucleotide subsequences, based on their overlap capability. Biometrics 45, 35–52.

Gibbs, A.J., Dale, M.B., Kinns, H.R. and MacKenzie, H.G., 1971, The transition matrix method for comparing sequences; its use in describing and classifying proteins by their amino acid sequences. Syst. Zool. 20, 417–425.

Guibas, L.J. and Odlyzko, A.M., 1981, String overlaps, pattern matching, and nontransitive games. J. Combinatorial Theory, ser. A, 30, 188–208.

Guigo, R., Knudsen, S., Drake, N. and Smith, T., 1992, Prediction of gene structure. J. Mol. Biol. 225 (in press).

Hamori, E., 1985, Novel DNA sequence representation. Nature 314, p. 585.

Jeffrey, H.J., 1990, Chaos game representation of gene structure. Nucl. Acids Res., 18 2163–2170.

Karlin, S., Ost, F. and Blaisdell, E.B., 1989, Patterns in DNA and amino acids sequences and their statistical significance, in: Mathematical Methods for DNA Sequences (M.S.Waterman, ed.) (CRC Press, Boca Raton FL) pp. 133–157.

Korolev, S.V., Solovyev, V.V. and Tumanyan, V.G., 1992, A new global method for searching functional region of DNA based on fractal geometry representation of nucleotide sequences. Comput. Appl. Biosci. (in press).

Mandelbrot, B., 1982, The Fractal Geometry of Nature (W.H. Freeman, San Francisco).

Manly, B.F., 1991, Randomization and Monte-Carlo Methods in Biology (Chapman and Hall, New York).

Ohno, S., 1991, Many peptide fragments of alien antigens are homologous with host proteins, thus canalizing T–cell responses. Proc. Natl. Acad. Sci. USA 88, 3065–3068.

Ohno, S. and Yomo, T., 1991, The grammatical rule for all DNA: link and coding sequences. Electrophoresis 12, 103–108.

Pearson, W.R., 1990, Rapid and sensitive sequence comparison with FASTP and FASTA. Meth. Enzymol. 183, 63–98.

Pevzner, P.A., Borodovsky, M.Y. and Mironov, A.A., 1989, Linguistics of nucleotide sequences. I. The significance of deviations from mean statistical characteristics and prediction of the frequencies of occurrence of words. J. Biomol. Struct. Dynam. 6, 1013–1026.

Peng, C.-K., Buldyrev, S.V., Goldberger, A.L., Halvin, S., Sciortino, F., Simons, M. and Stanly, H.E., 1992, Long-range correlations in nucleotide sequences. Nature 356, 168–170.

Pietrokovsky, S., Hirshon, J. and Trifonov, E.N., 1990, Linguistic measure of taxonomic and functional relatedness of nucleotide sequences. J. Biomol. Struct. Dynam. 7, 1251–1268.

Solovyev, V.V., 1991, Graphic methods of representation and analysis of the DNA and protein sequences (Institute of Cytology and Genetics, Russian Acad. Sci., Novosibirsk) (in Russian).

Solovyev, V.V., Korolev, S.V. and Lim, H.A., 1992, A new approach for the classification of functional regions of DNA sequences based on fractal representation. Int. J. Genomic Res. 1, 108–127.

Solovyev, V.V., Korolev, S.V., Tumanyan, V.G. and Lim, H.A., 1991, A new approach to classification of DNA regions based on fractal representation of functionally similar sequences. Dokl. Biochem. 319, 1496–1500.

Solovyev, V.V. and Lawrence, C., 1992 Identification of human gene structure in larger scale sequencing project, in: Abstr. 3-rd Keck Symp. on Computational Biology, Houston.

Solovyev, V.V. and Makarova, K.S., 1992, A novel method of protein sequences classification based on oligopeptide frequency analysis and its application to search for functional sites and to domain localization.

160

Comput. Appl. Biosci. (in press).

Solovyev, V.V. and Rogozin, I.B., 1986, Program package of context analysis of DNA, RNA and protein sequences "CONTEXT" (Institute of Cytology and Genetics, Russian Acad. Sci., Novosibirsk) (in Russian).

Solovyev, V.V. and Seledtsov, I.A., 1991, Phylogenetic tree construction based on the analysis of the relatively conservative regions of the nucleotide and amino acid sequences. Proc. Acad. Sci. of Russia 321, 1109–1114 (in Russian).

Solovyev, V.V., Streletc, V.B. and Milanesi, L., 1992, Multiple sequence alignment based on new approaches of tree construction and sequences comparison, in: Abstr. 2-nd Int. Conf. on Bioinformatics, Supercomputing, and Complex Genome analysis (St. Petersburg, FL) p. 64.

Torney, D.C., Burks, C., Davison, D. and Sirotkin, K.M., 1990, Computation of d^2: a measure of sequence dissimilarity, in: Computers and DNA (G.Bell and T.Marr, ed.) (Addison–Wesley) pp. 109–125.

Trifonov, E.N., 1990, in: Structures and Methods, vol. 1. Human Genome Initiative and DNA Recombination (H.Ramaswamy and M.Sarma, eds.).

Uberbacher, E.C. and Mural, R.J., 1991, Locating protein coding regions in human DNA sequences using a multiple sensor — neural net approach. Proc. Natl. Acad. Sci. USA 88, 11261–11265.

Varga, G., Carrol, T., Hamori, E. and Lim, H.A., 1991, Computer graphics algorithm for abstract representation of protein and DNA sequences. Preprint (SCRI, Florida State University).

Volinia, S., Bernardi, F., Gambari, R. and Barrai, I., 1988, Co-localization of rare oligonucleotides and regulatory elements in mammalian upstream gene regions. J. Mol. Biol. 203, 385–390.

Volinia, S., Gambari, R., Bernardi, F. and Barrai, I., 1989, The frequency of oligonucleotides in mammalian genic regions. Comput. Appl. Biosci. 5, 33–40.

Wilbur, W.J and Lipman, D.J., 1983, Rapid similarity searches of nucleic and protein data banks. Proc. Natl. Acad. Sci. USA. 80, 726–730.

Zharkikh, A.A., Rzhetsky, A.Y., Morosov, P.S., Sitnikova, T.L. and Krushal, J.S., 1991, VOSTORG: a package of microcomputer programs for sequence analysis and construction of phylogenetic trees. Gene 101, 251–254.

Fractal analysis of protein chain conformation

Houqiang Li*, Ying Li and Huaming Zhao

Department of Chemistry, Sichuan University, Chengdu 610064, People's Republic of China
(Received 30 May 1989; revised 12 September 1989)

This paper presents a simple practical method for characterizing conformation of protein chains. A single number D_f, as the fractal dimension, is assigned to each chain. $D_f = L_n(N)/L_n(N \cdot d/L)$, where N is the number of the amino acid residues in the chain, L and d are the total length and the planar diameter of the chain, respectively. In general, $1 < D_f \leqslant 2$, which is related to the shape of the protein chain. These values are different from those of Stapleton's group, but in agreement with computer simulations.

Keywords: Protein; conformation; fractal; fracton; simulation

Introduction

The catalysis of enzymes has been one of the most fascinating phenomena on which studies have, over the years, been challenging problems. Various concepts and techniques have been developed in this field. As is well known, enzymes are, generally, protein molecules, and their catalysis is of relevance to protein conformations. Stapleton and coworkers[1] introduced a fractal model to characterize the anomalous temperature dependence of the Raman electron spin relaxation rates in proteins containing iron. The model explains the observed T^n temperature dependence ($5 \leqslant n \leqslant 7$) of the Raman spin-lattice relaxation rate[2]. The exponent n equals $(3 + 2d_f)$, where d_f is the fracton or spectral dimension[3]. In general, $1 \leqslant d_f \leqslant D_f \leqslant 2$ for a given biopolymer, D_f being the fractal dimension. As is well known, a fractal implies a complex pattern[4,5] with the self-similarity (or self-affinity), and its natural dimension, i.e. fractal dimension, can be used to characterize its shape and irregularity. Mandelbrot[4] has found extensive potentialities of its applications to natural phenomena. The fractal description of the protein has developed so rapidly and is so widespread in recent years[6 8], that fractal geometry has become a powerful tool in dealing with this problem. However, recently Yang[9] and Krumhans[10] pointed out that Stapleton's method is not satisfactory since the fracton dimension (d_f) is in general different from the fractal dimension (D_f) and the Euclidean space dimension (d). D_f reflects the geometrical structure of the fractals, and d_f reflects the topological structural properties of the fractals. Moreover, based on the Alexander–Orbach conjecture[3], the fracton dimension equals 4/3 for the percolation, and $d_f = 1$ for the linear protein chain[11]. In this communication, a simple method is proposed to calculate the fractal dimensions of the protein chains.

Theory and methods

The protein molecules are long chain copolymers, though no bifurcation or branch is involved, usually folded through cross-linking as a consequence of the interaction

of the contiguous amino acid residues by hydrogen bonding, Van der Waals force, etc. Protein strands are neither regularly recurrent nor strictly random fabrication of the copolymers, yet they have statistical self-similarities and can, therefore, be characterized by an average fractal dimension.

First, a protein molecular chain may be regarded as a space curve in three dimensions, and being a planar curve in two-dimensional space. Since it is a fractal object the conformation may be characterized by fractal dimension (D_f). We will first look into the fractal property of a protein chain in a plane, then extend the results to three-dimensional space based on the principle of fractal geometry. Second, according to Mandelbrot's theory[4], the general form of a fractal dimension of a planar curve is

$$(\text{length})^{1/D_f} = k(\text{area})^{1/2} \qquad (1)$$

where 'length' signifies the total length of the curve, 'area' is the maximum potential area the curve fills, and k is a constant.

To use fractals practically, three decisions must be made from outside information. First, the appropriate size and shape of limiting planar area must be determined. In the present case, the limiting area should be what is filled by a self-avoiding random walker. A random walk chain in a plane tends to fill a circular area, so that we can choose a circle as the appropriate profile of the area. Second, the appropriate units of measurement must be chosen well and made explicit because the estimates of fractal dimensions vary with the scale of measurement. We should choose the average step size as the appropriate unit. Third, the constant k is so chosen as to ensure that the right-hand side of equation (1) yields a true one-dimensional characteristic of the area. This straight-line characteristic can be the 'linear size' or 'linear scale' of the area. We can choose the diameter of the circle as the straight-line characteristic of the chosen area profile. Such choices should lead to the following general equation

$$(L/b)^{1/D_f} = (k/b)A^{1/2} \qquad (2)$$

where L is the total length of the curve, b is the average step length ($b = L/N$, N being the total number of steps), $k = 2\pi^{-1/2}$, and A is the area of the circle potentially

* To whom all correspondence should be addressed.

0141-8130/90/010006-03

	$a_1 = a = 45$ (A)	1.432		
	$d_2 = b = c = 30$ (Å)	1.615		
	$d = 35$ (Å)	1.536	1.54 ± 0.02	1.76
Carboxypeptidase $A(Z_n^{2+})$	$N = 307,\ V = 50 \times 42 \times 38$			
	$d_1 = a = 50$	1.627		
	$d_2 = c = 38$	1.765		
	$d = 43$	1.696	1.68 ± 0.02	1.56
Chymotrypsin (α)	$N = 245,\ V = 51 \times 40 \times 40$			
	$d_1 = a = 51$	1.416		
	$d_2 = b = c = 40$	1.668		
	$d = 44$	1.625	1.63 ± 0.03	1.36
Myoglobin	$N = 153,\ V = 43 \times 35 \times 23$			
	$d_1 = a = 43$	1.493		
	$d_2 = c = 23$	1.834		
	$d = 34$	1.605	1.62 ± 0.03	1.66
Haemoglobin (β)	$N = 146,\ d \approx 55$ (Å)	1.378	1.40 ± 0.03	1.64

filled by a self-avoiding random walker. Thus, the fractal dimension (D_f) is given by

$$D_f = \ln(L/b)/\ln[(k/b)A^{1.2}] = \ln(N)/\ln(Nd/L) \qquad (3)$$

For a protein molecular chain, N is the number of amino acid residues in the chain, d is the diameter of the protein, and L is the chain length. Then, $L = N \cdot b$, here b is the average bond length of C—C, C—O and C—N bonds, and its value is 1.48 Å.

To test the calculated results, computer simulations were carried out using the Monte Carlo method. The Monte Carlo method is a computational technique in which various states of a system are generated with random numbers and weighted with appropriate probabilities. As models, Monte Carlo simulations are useful in analysis of protein chain conformations. For our model, we considered a self-avoiding random walk model with massless bonds[12] and used the s-p enrichment technique on an IBM 3081 computer. Further details of this method may be found in Refs 12 to 14. In the present communication, we have utilized the Monte Carlo method to compute the fractal dimension of a protein chain. The number of monomers $N(R)$ are counted as a function of the radial distance (R) from an arbitrary origin, and fit $N(R)$ to $R^{\bar{D}}$ (Refs 15, 16); such fits need to be done at several places within the structure. The average fractal dimension is obtained as the best fit of $N(R) \propto R^{\bar{D}}$, by a least-squares linear fit of $\ln(N)$ to $\ln(R)$. In the above calculations, the key procedure is to assess the appropriate planar diameter (R) of the protein chain. The simplest way to estimate this value is to find first the largest distance between two points on the curve.

Results and discussion

Based on the data determined by X-ray crystallography[17] from the literature, the fractal dimensions of some protein molecular chains are calculated by equation (3) and the results are listed in Table 1. It is shown that D_f is the reflection of the profile of the protein molecule. Generally, a real protein molecule is an ellipsoid with three diameters, a, b, c and its volume $V = a \times b \times c$. The D_f

values are calculated by the average diameter (d) and are in agreement with the results of computer simulations. The deviation of our results from those of the Stapleton group[2] is conceivable since the latter is the fracton dimension of the backbone of protein.

The fracton dimension concept was first introduced by Alexander and Orbach[3], and at low frequencies (ω) is defined by

$$\rho(\omega) \sim \omega^{d_f - 1} \qquad (4)$$

or

$$Nt \propto t^{d_f/2} \qquad (5)$$

where $\rho(\omega)$ is the density of state, Nt is the number of distinct sites in the fractal visited by a random walker up to time t. The fracton dimension (d_f) was originally introduced through a consideration of the scaling properties of both the volume and the connectivity in calculating the density of states on a fractal. It differs in general from D_f because d_f reflects the geometrical structure of the fractal and D_f reflects the topological structural properties of the fractal. For example, with the Sierpinski gasket in d-dimension Euclidean space, its fractal dimension is easily found as $D_f = \ln(d + 1)/\ln 2$, and the fracton dimension $d_f = 2\ln(d + 1)/\ln(d + 3)$[11]. In addition Alexander and Orbach pointed out[3], that the fracton dimension of percolation in any dimension d, $1 < d \leqslant 6$, seems to be close to 4/3. For a linear chain, it is $d_f = 1$, no matter what its fractal dimension is. Thus, if only the backbone of the protein is taken into account, it results in $d_f = 1$ (Ref. 12).

Stapleton and co-workers[1,2,8] have found that in the temperature range between 4 and 20 K the electron-spin relaxation rate ($1/T_1$) of low-spin ferric iron in a number of haem and iron-sulphur proteins is dominated by a two-phonon (Raman) process, of which the temperature dependence is given by

$$1/T_1 \propto T^{3 + 2d_f} f(T/\theta, d_f) \qquad (6)$$

where θ is the Debye temperature, f is a smooth analytic function of T/θ, and T is the absolute temperature. The experiment indicates that the low-temperature (4 ~ 20 K) behaviour of $1/T_1$ is best described by a non-integer power law of the form

$$1/T^1 \propto T^{3+2d_i} \propto T^n \tag{7}$$

with $n \approx 6.3$ for haemoproteins[1] and $n \approx 5.67$ for ferredoxin[2]. Stapleton et al.[1] obtained for different proteins values of d_f between 1 and 2 using equation (7). Alexander and Orbach[3] also established the relationship between the fractal and fracton dimensions as follows

$$d_f = 2D_f/dw \tag{8}$$

where dw is the exponent connecting the root-mean-square displacement Rw of a random walker on the fractal with the number of steps $N_w \propto R^{dw}$, dw is called the fractal dimension of the walk. Similar to dw, many other fractal dimensions may be defined.

In general, we have $1 < D_f \leqslant 2$ for a protein in a plane. For a protein in three-dimensional space, its fractal dimension is $D_{ft} = (D_f + \Delta D_f)$, where ΔD_f, the increment of fractal dimension, can be calculated by the transformation of the projection[18], and its value $\Delta D_f \approx 1$ for the self-affine structure[19,20]. Therefore, the D_{ft} values of the protein molecular chains with three-dimensional structure may be estimated through the self-affine fractals.

The fractal dimensions are useful in the interpretation of certain thermodynamic properties[21,22], reaction kinetics[23], and catalysis of the protein molecules, particularly enzymes. In our other paper[24], we have discussed the applications of fractal dimensions to the Hill coefficients of the allosteric enzymes.

Acknowledgements

The authors wish to thank Dr M. Xiang for computer simulation. This research is supported by Science Fund of the Chinese Academy of Sciences.

References

1   Stapleton, H. J., Allen, J. P., Flynn, C. P., Stinson, D. G. and Kurtz, S. R. Phys. Rev. Lett. 1980, 45, 1456
2   Allen, J. P., Colvin, J. T., Stinson, D. G., Flynn, C. P. and Stapleton, H. J. Biophys. J. 1982, 38, 299
3   Alexander, S. and Orbach, R. J. Phys. (Paris), Lett. 1982, 43, L625
4   Mandelbrot, B. B. 'The Fractal Geometry of Nature', Freeman, San Franciso, New York, 1982
5   Mandelbrot, B. B., 'Fractals and Multifractals: Noise, Turbulence and Galaxies', Springer, New York, 1988
6   Lewis, M. and Rees, D. C. Science 1985, 230, 1163
7   Liebovitch, L. S., Fischbarg, J., Koniarek, J. P., Todorova, I. and Wang, M. Biochim. Biophys. Acta 1987, 896, 173
8   Wagner, G. C., Colvin, J. T., Allen, J. P. and Stapleton, H. J. J. Am. Chem. Soc. 1985, 107(20), 5589
9   Yang, Y. S. 'Fractals in Physics', (ed. L. Pietronero and E. Tosatti) North-Holland, Amsterdam, 1986, 119
10 Krumhansl, J. A. Phys. Rev. Lett. 1986, 56(25), 2696
11 Rammal, R. and Toulouse, G. J. Phys. (Paris) Lett. 1983, 44, L13
12 Helman, J. S., Coniglio, A. and Tsallis, C. Phys. Rev. Lett. 1984, 53(12), 1195
13 Fichthorn, K. A., Ziff, R. M. and Gulari, E. 'Catalysis' (ed. by J. W. Ward), Elsevier Science Publishers, B.V. Amsterdam, 1988, 883
14 Binder, K. 'Monte Carlo Methods in Statistical Physics', Springer-Verlag, Berlin, 1979
15 MacDonald, M. and Jan, N. Can. J. Phys. 1986, 64, 1353
16 Pfeifer, P., Wetz, U. and Wippermann, H. Chem. Phys. Lett. 1985, 113(6), 535
17 Blundell, J. L. and Johnson, L. N. 'Protein Crystallography', Academic Press, New York, 1976
18 Falconer, K. J. 'The Geometry of Fractal Sets', Cambridge University Press, 1985, 80
19 Mandelbrot, B. B. in 'Fractal in Physics' (ed. by L. Pietronero and E. Tosatti), North-Holland, Amsterdam, 1986, 3-28
20 Li, H. Q. 'Fractals and Fractal Dimensions', Sichuan Education Press, Chengdu, 1989
21 Katzen, D. and Procaccia, I. Phys. Rev. Lett. 1987, 58(12), 1169
22 Kohmoto, M. 'Entropy Function for Multifractals', University of Utah, Preprint, 1988
23 Kopelman, R. J. J. Stat. Phys. 1986, 42(1/2), 185
24 Li, H. Q. and Zhao, H. M. 'Fractal Theory and its Application', Proceedings of the National Scientific Congress on Theory and Application of Fractals. July 13-16, Chengdu, China. Sichuan University Press, 1989, p 62

Fractal analysis of photolysis of nitrosyl haemoglobin at low temperatures

Léa J. El-Jaick* and Eliane Wajnberg

CBPF/CNPq, Rua Dr Xavier Sigaud 150, Urca, CEP 22290, Rio de Janeiro, Brazil
(Received 14 August 1992; revised 12 November 1992)

Photolysis of nitrosyl haemoglobin (HbNO) has been studied from 5.9 K to 20 K for R, T and RT conformations. It was observed that the experimental curves have two different behaviours at a given temperature in a particular conformation. At shorter time scales the data are well reproduced by a model based on fractal concepts, where the relevant parameter is the difference between the fractal dimension and the fracton. For simplicity at longer time scales a simple exponential was used to fit the curves.

Keywords: Photolysis; nitrosyl haemoglobin; fractal

Introduction

The dynamic aspects of protein have already been well demonstrated from experimental and theoretical studies[1-4]. Several models have been proposed to describe the structural fluctuations: few state exponentials[5], conformational substates with different distributions[6,7], spin glasses[8], etc.[9,10]. But unfortunately photolysis experiments at low temperatures cannot distinguish the physical differences among the majority of these models[10-12].

Protein kinetics has been represented since 1950 by a few discrete states Markov model which assumes that there are small numbers of discrete conformational states linked by a kinetic rate constant independent of the time scale. This means that the transition probability per unit time to change their conformational states depends only on the latest state and not on the history of previous states. The probability distributions are therefore expressed as exponentials or sums of exponentials. However since 1970 many experiments (flash photolysis[1,4], Mössbauer spectroscopy[13], X-rays[14], fluorescence[15], etc.) have shown that protein kinetics can also be well reproduced by continuous functions, which implies that assumptions of Markov states are not consistent with the dynamics of protein conformations. The good fit of experimental data with the Markov model can be due to its large number of parameters, not to the existence of discrete states[16-18].

Proteins can be characterized by a fractal dimension because they exhibit a statistical self-similarity structure. The fractal concept can be related to photodissociation processes since these processes require multiple statistical paths. This concept has been used both in the function–structure relation of different biological systems[19] and in the interpretation of experimental results where dynamic aspects of proteins are relevant[5,10,20,21]. It has particularly been evoked to describe the anomalous behaviour of the temperature dependence of the

spin-lattice relaxation time in haemoproteins[20,22,23]. Powers and Blumberg[10] have introduced the fractal concept in the analysis of photodissociation experiments by including a periodic factor to the power law model[1], but the fractal dimension is not explicit in this model. Liebovitch et al.[5] have used fractal models to develop new methods to analyse the kinetics of ion channels of membrane. The fractal model differs from the Markov model in the assumption that proteins exhibit motion and conformational dynamics over many time scales. Because of that the kinetic rate constants which link these states depend on the time scales.

In a previous paper[24] we have shown that the kinetic curves of the photolysis of nitrosyl haemoglobin (HbNO) obtained by electron paramagnetic resonance (e.p.r.) at low temperatures are fitted equally well by a biphasic exponential and a distribution of activation energies. To obtain better understanding of the HbNO dynamics we used, in the present work, fractal concepts from the model proposed by Liebovitch et al.[5] to analyse the same experimental kinetic curves.

Experimental

The experimental curves analysed were those used in our previous paper[24] where experimental procedures are given in detail. It is important to call attention to the fact that the experiments are performed under continuous illumination in contrast to the majority of papers where the kinetics is followed after a laser pulse[1].

Results and discussion

Our experimental data are the result of the competition between dissociation and recombination of NO to human haemoglobin during continuous illumination at temperatures below 20 K.

As described in the preliminary paper[24] these data are equally well fitted by two exponentials and by an energy distribution, but both models demand a large number of parameters.

---

*To whom correspondence should be addressed.

0141–8130/93/020119–05
© 1993 Butterworth-Heinemann Limited

Photolysis of nitrosyl haemoglobin: L. J. El-Jaick and E. Wajnberg

The model of Liebovitch *et al.*[5] for dynamics of proteins based on fractal concepts supposes that proteins have to be in a single conformation for a time sufficiently long to be measured. This time defines an effective time scale t_{eff}. The effective kinetic rate constant, k_{eff}, defined as the probability per unit time to change the conformational states of proteins, can thus be expressed in terms of $P(t)$, which is the probability distribution that the state remains in a particular conformation during the time t. Thus

$$k_{eff}(t_{eff}) = -\frac{d}{dt}\{\ln P(t)\}_{t=t_{eff}} \quad (1)$$

Liebovitch *et al.*[5] used the self-similarity of fractals to write k_{eff} as a function of the time scale as

$$k_{eff}(t_{eff}) = A t_{eff}^{d_f - d} \quad (2)$$

where A is a constant (frequency factor), d is the fractal dimension and d_f is the topological dimension (or fracton).

Equation (2) implies that the probability distribution $P(t)$ is

$$P(t) = \exp\left[-\frac{A}{1+d_f-d} t^{1+d_f-d}\right] \quad (3)$$

Applying the fractal model to our results, and keeping in mind that the e.p.r. technique measures only the NO bound to Hb, we can identify the normalized fractions of unbound molecules of the ligands, $N(t)$, with $1 - P(t)$, where $P(t)$ is the fraction of NO bound.

The experimental curves log $P(t) \times t$ of HbNO, for R, T and RT conformations, show clearly two different behaviours at short and long time scales (*Figure 1*). As a result the attempt to fit the kinetic curves using equation (3) of the fractal model was unsuccessful when performed over the whole range of time.

Using a Monte Carlo-like method (random numbers) we fitted in the present paper the logarithm of our data to equation (3) for short time scales. For long time scales

Table 1 Parameters obtained with a fractal model (D and A) and exponential model (B and k_e)

Temp. (K)	$D = d - d_f$	A (s^{-1})	B (s^{-1})	k_e (s^{-1})
R conformation				
5.9		0.140	0.965	0.023
7.0		0.128	0.774	0.020
	0.65 ± 0.03			
9.1		0.132	0.565	0.160
12.3		0.205	0.893	0.035
RT conformation				
6.5		0.116	0.470	0.010
10.1		0.147	1.501	0.023
	0.61 ± 0.01			
13.4		0.174	4.289	0.038
15.5		0.162	1.476	0.030
T conformation				
10.4		0.165	3.344	0.064
16.2		0.203	0.283	0.027
	0.56 ± 0.04			
17.4		0.194	0.476	0.035
19.6		0.216	0.150	0.010

we used a simple exponential model

$$P(t) = B \exp[-k_e t] \quad (4)$$

where B is a constant (frequency factor) and k_e is the time independent kinetic rate constant. The choice of the time where the behaviour changes was made by visual inspection. This time is temperature independent for each conformation.

The fits were made for each temperature with no restriction on the parameters. We have called D the difference between the fractal and fracton dimension, $d - d_f$. The values obtained for D are identical within the experimental error for the different temperatures of each conformation. The fitting was then repeated fixing D as the average of those values to recalculate the frequency factor A.

Table 1 shows the results obtained from equations (3) and (4).

Figure 1 shows the logarithmic plot of the NO bound for the HbNO in the RT conformation at two temperatures. The solid lines were obtained using the results of *Table 1*. The change of the behaviour happens at about 100 s.

This change of the behaviour of $N(t)$ with time scale was not noted in our previous paper[24] because it is only evident with the logarithmic plots of the number of NO molecules bound, which was not used there.

As we can see in *Figure 2*, where $F(t)$ is the non-normalized fraction of NO unbound under illumination, at 16.2 K for T conformation, it is, in fact, very difficult to observe that the curve changes at about 70 s. Although the fitting parameters are obtained from the logarithmic form of $N(t)$, *Figure 2* shows that the non-logarithmic curve $F(t)$ is well reproduced.

A comparison between the fits of log $N(t) \times t$ for R conformation at 5.9 K is shown in *Figure 3*. The top curve is fitted with the fractal and exponential models using the parameters of *Table 1*, the bottom curve with the conformational substates model using parameters of *Table 3* of Ref. 24.

The difference between these fits is better observed from both residuals (differences between experimental

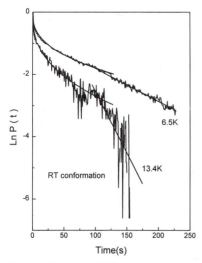

Figure 1 Fraction of NO molecules bound to the Hb in the RT conformation at two temperatures. Solid lines are obtained with parameters of *Table 1*. Below about 100 s a fractal model was used. For longer times, a simple exponential model was used

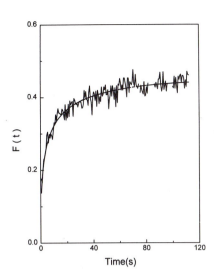

Figure 2 Non-normalized fraction of unbound NO under illumination, at 16.2 K for T conformation. The solid line is obtained with parameters of *Table 1*. Below about 70 s a fractal model was used. For longer times, a simple exponential model was used

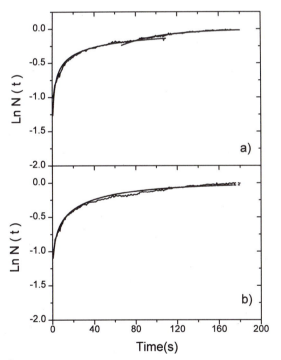

Figure 3 Comparison between the normalized fraction of unbound NO, at 5.9 K for R conformation, fitted with: (a) fractal and simple exponential model, with parameters of *Table 1*; (b) distribution of activation energies with parameters of *Table 3* of Ref. 24

and calculated values of $\ln P(t)$ in *Figure 4a*. Other residuals curves are shown in *Figures 4b, 4c* and *4d*.

The good fits previously published[24] may have been fortuitous because in that paper they were obtained from non-logarithmic curves which hide the electronic noise. The large noisy data do not allow us to extract the

experimental values of the kinetic rate constant from the kinetic data.

Observing the logarithmic plot of the fraction of NO molecules bound, the high electronic noise is obvious mainly at temperatures above 10 K. But it is also evident that these curves have two different behaviours, at short and large time scales.

At large time scales we cannot affirm if the curves behave as a simple exponential, because it is very difficult to fit them due to the experimental noise, but we have seen that the fractal model is not able to fit the curves over the whole time range. For simplicity we considered the exponential dependence in the figures.

At short time scales the curves are well reproduced by the fractal model. The value of the fractal dimension cannot be directly determined from this fitting procedure because the difference $D = d - d_f$ is the relevant parameter. To determine d we should look for a reasonable value for the protein fracton dimension but there is a strong divergence about this value in the literature. Some authors claim that $d_f = d$ but others take $d_f = 1$ if connecting bridges are not considered in a self-avoiding walk (SAW) model[5,22,25–28].

In the present paper we can not take $d_f = d$ ($D = 0$) since equation (3) has resulted in a good fit. If $d_f = 1$ our D values yield the fractal dimensions of 1.65 ± 0.03, 1.61 ± 0.01 and 1.56 ± 0.04 for R, RT and T conformations. The value for R state is consistent with the experimental results obtained from X-ray data by Stapleton *et al.* for the chain fractal dimension of haemoproteins, which varies from 1.48 to 1.68[26,29]. If we take d_f as determined from relaxation experiments[20,26,29,30], it varies from 1.18 to 1.65 depending on the protein, ligand and solvent. Then d of the R conformation varies from 1.83 to 2.3, which tends to the value range of the re-entrant fractal dimension, calculated from the X-ray data[26]. Unfortunately our results can not elucidate that divergence, but they yield a new insight into the problem.

The results of D for RT and T conformations can not be compared because they do not exist in the literature. However the most encouraging finding from our analysis is that the fractal dimension d decreases from 1.65 to 1.56 going from R to T conformation if the fracton does not depend on the protein conformation. This decrease implies a less open R structure than that of T. This result is consistent with the relative movement of subunits that brings closer together the carboxyl ends of β chain in the transition from T to R[31].

The fact that our results can be consistent with the hypothesis that $d_f = 1$ suggests that, in the photo-dissociation phenomenon the haemoprotein can be considered as a linear chain, while the relaxation mechanism requires that $d_f \not\equiv 1$.

Conclusions

Fractal dimensions of haemoproteins have been obtained by different approaches. It was first introduced to explain the anomalous temperature dependence of the Raman spin-lattice relaxation measured by e.p.r.[29,30]. A fractal model of low frequency vibrational modes for these proteins stimulated the computation of the fractal dimension from the C_α coordinates in the chain[26]. The geometrical data and coordinates were provided by a databank based on X-ray crystallographic results. The

Photolysis of nitrosyl haemoglobin: L. J. El-Jaick and E. Wajnberg

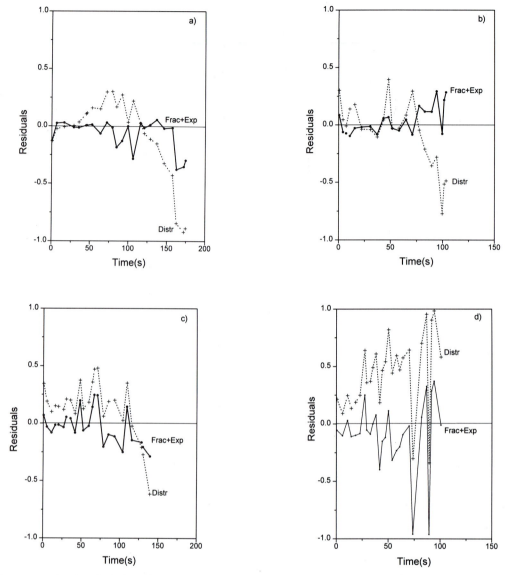

Figure 4 Residuals of the fits of the fractal and simple exponential model (□) and distribution of activation energies model (*) for: (a) R state at 5.9 K; (b) R state at 12.3 K; (c) RT state at 15.5 K; (d) T state at 17.4 K

calculated values of the fractal dimension agree well with those determined experimentally, as was shown earlier.

Nevertheless e.p.r. is practically restricted to the R conformation of haemoproteins. The nitrosyl human haemoglobin is one of the very few haemoproteins in which the R ↔ T equilibrium can be displaced to T and e.p.r. measurements are still possible, as well as relaxation measurements. As the spin-lattice relaxation temperature dependence in HbNO is not dominated by a Raman relaxation mechanism, it therefore is not related to the fractal character of the protein, as well as in the nitrosyl myoglobin[32,33].

We have shown in this paper that photodissociation experiments can be interpreted on the basis of a fractal model and so we can perceive that the fractal dimension is sensitive to the quaternary conformation of the protein[5,16,18].

To further understand photodissociation results it is necessary to enhance the signal-noise ratio for long time scales.

The use of the fractal model in the analysis of the photodissociation experiments is consistent with other uses of kinetic experiments with proteins.

The results given here confirm that the fractal model provides a framework within which protein dynamics can be understood.

Acknowledgements

We are grateful to Dr M. P. Linhares who performed the experiments and Dr R. Charlab and E. Mavropolous for technical assistance in sample preparation as described in the previous paper. We also thank Professor G. Bemski for his

Photolysis of nitrosyl haemoglobin: L. J. El-Jaick and E. Wajnberg

critical reading and Maria Antonia Muniz for her suggestions on the manuscript.

References

1   Austin, R. H., Beeson, K. W., Eisenstein, L., Frauenfelder, H. and Gunsalus, I. C. *Biochemistry* 1975, **14**, 5355
2   Powers, L., Chance, B., Chance, M., Campbell, B., Friedman, J., Khalid, S., Kumar, C., Naqui, A., Reddy, K. S. and Zhou, Y. *Biochemistry* 1987, **26**, 4785
3   Jortner, J. and Ulstrup, J. *J. Am. Chem. Soc.* 1979, **101**, 3744
4   Levy, R. M., Perhia, D. and Karplus, M. *Proc. Natl. Acad. Sci. USA* 1982, **79**, 1346
5   Liebovitch, L. S., Fischbarg, J., Koniarek, J. P., Todorova, I. and Wang, M. *Biochem. Biophys. Acta* 1987, **896**, 173
6   Young, R. D. and Bowne, S. F. *J. Chem. Phys.* 1984, **81**, 3730
7   Agmon, N. and Hopfield, J. J. *J. Chem. Phys.* 1983, **79**, 2042
8   Stein, D. L. *Proc. Natl. Acad. Sci. USA* 1985, **82**, 3670
9   Bialek, W. and Goldstein, R. F. *Biophys. J.* 1985, **48**, 1027
10   Powers, L. S. and Blumberg, W. E. *Biophys. J.* 1988, **54**, 181
11   El-Jaick, L. J., Wajnberg, E., Bemski, G. and Linhares, M. P. *Int. J. Biol. Macromol.* 1988, **10**, 185
12   Plonka, A., Kroh, J. and Berlin, Y. A. *Chem. Phys. Lett.* 1988, **153**, 433
13   Hartman, H., Parak, F., Steigmann, W., Petsko, J. A., Ponzi, D. R. and Frauenfelder, H. *Proc. Natl. Acad. Sci. USA* 1982, **79**, 4967
14   Chance, B., Fischetti, R. and Powers, L. *Biochemistry* 1983, **22**, 3820
15   Di Iorio, E.E., Hiltpold, U. R., Filipovic, D., Winterhalter, K. H. and Gratton, E. *Biophys. J.* 1991, **59**, 742
16   Liebovitch, L. S. and Sullivan, J. M. *Biophys. J.* 1987, **52**, 979
17   Condat, C. A. and Jäckel, J. *Biophys. J.* 1989, **55**, 915
18   Liebovitch, L. S. *Biophys. J.* 1989, **55**, 373
19   West, B. J. and Goldberg, A. L. *Am. Sci.* 1987, **75**, 354
20   Stapleton, H. J., Allen, J. P., Flynn, C. P., Stinson, D. G. and Kurtz, S. R. *Phys. Rev. Lett.* 1980, **45**, 1456
21   Liebovitch, L. S. and Tóth, T. *Ann. NY Acad. Sci.* 1990, **591**, 375
22   Helman, J. S., Coniglio, A. and Tsallis, C. *Phys. Rev. Lett.* 1984, **53**, 1195
23   Wajnberg, E. and Bemski, G. *Phys. Lett. A* 1988, **132**, 4
24   El-Jaick, L. J., Wajnberg, E. and Linhares, M. P. *Int. J. Biol. Macromol.* 1991, **13**, 289
25   Rammal, R. and Toulouse, G. *J. Phys. (Paris) Lett.* 1983, **44**, L13
26   Colvin, J. T. and Stapleton, H. J. *J. Chem. Phys.* 1985, **82**, 4699
27   MacDonald, M. and Jan, N. *Can. J. Phys.* 1986, **64**, 1353
28   Cates, M. E. *Phys. Rev. Lett.* 1985, **54**, 1733; Stapleton, H. J. *Phys. Rev. Lett.* 1985, **54**, 1734; Helman, J. S. *Phys. Rev. Lett.* 1985, **54**, 1735
29   Wagner, G. C., Colvin, J. T., Allen, J. P. and Stapleton, H. J. *J. Am. Chem. Soc.* 1985, **107**, 5589
30   Allen, J. P., Colvin, J. T., Stinson, D. G., Flynn, C. P. and Stapleton, H. J. *Biophys. J.* 1982, **38**, 299
31   Dickerson, R. E. and Geis, I. 'Hemoglobin' The Benjamin/Cummings, Menlo Park, CA, 1983
32   Wajnberg, E., Linhares, M. P., El-Jaick, L. J. and Bemski, G. *Eur. Biophys. J.* 1992, **21**, 57
33   Nascimento, O. R., Martin Neto, L. and Wajnberg, E. *J. Chem. Phys.* 1991, **95**, 2265

FRACTAL ANALYSIS OF A VOLTAGE-DEPENDENT POTASSIUM CHANNEL FROM CULTURED MOUSE HIPPOCAMPAL NEURONS

LARRY S. LIEBOVITCH* AND J. MICHAEL SULLIVAN‡

*Department of Ophthalmology, Columbia University, College of Physicians and Surgeons, New York, New York 10032; and ‡Departments of Physiology-Biophysics and Anesthesiology, Mt. Sinai School of Medicine, New York, New York 10029

ABSTRACT   The kinetics of ion channels have been widely modeled as a Markov process. In these models it is assumed that the channel protein has a small number of discrete conformational states and the kinetic rate constants connecting these states are constant. In the alternative fractal model the spontaneous fluctuations of the channel protein at many different time scales are represented by a kinetic rate constant $k = At^{1-D}$, where A is the kinetic setpoint and D the fractal dimension. Single-channel currents were recorded at 146 mM external K^+ from an inwardly rectifying, 120 pS, K^+ selective, voltage-sensitive channel in cultured mouse hippocampal neurons. The kinetics of these channels were found to be statistically self-similar at different time scales as predicted by the fractal model. The fractal dimensions were ~2 for the closed times and ~1 for the open times and did not depend on voltage. For both the open and closed times the logarithm of the kinetic setpoint was found to be proportional to the applied voltage, which indicates that the gating of this channel involves the net inward movement of approximately one negative charge when this channel opens. Thus, the open and closed times and the voltage dependence of the gating of this channel are well described by the fractal model.

INTRODUCTION

Ions can cross the hydrophobic cell membrane through the hydrophilic interior of ion channels. Everpresent thermal fluctuations provide the energy for these channels to spontaneously change their conformation so that they are continuously fluctuating between open and closed states. The patch clamp technique can resolve the open and closed durations of an individual channel by measuring the picoamp currents across a small membrane patch with a few such channels (1, 2). Thus, the sequence and duration of the conformational states of the channel are obtained. This provides a unique opportunity to study the kinetics of the spontaneous conformational changes of a single molecule at a time.

The kinetics of these channels have been widely modeled, and experimental results from single channel and noise analysis experiments interpreted, by assuming that the channel has a small number of discrete conformational states, such as closed $\rightleftharpoons$ closed $\rightleftharpoons$ open, and that the transition probabilities between these states can be described by a Markov process (1–14). That is, it is assumed that the transition probabilities per unit time, the kinetic rate constants, are independent of the time spent in the current state and also independent of the history of the previous sequence of states of the channel. However, these assumptions may not be consistent with the physical chemistry of the dynamics of the conformational changes in proteins. Many proteins have large numbers of conformational states that are separated by only small energy barriers. Moreover, changes in protein conformation occur over many time scales from picosecond rotations around bonds to unfolding modes that last minutes (15–23). Thus, a channel would be expected to have a continuum of many conformational states, rather than a few discrete states, and have dynamic processes and thus "memory" at all time scales.

A new model of channel kinetics, consistent with these ideas, has recently been proposed (24–26). In the fractal model, the closed and open states are each represented as a continuum of many conformational states. The kinetic rate constant for leaving the closed or open states is then a mixture of the rate constants for leaving this collection of states. The fractal model proposed that this effective rate constant has the form At^{1-D}, where A is the kinetic setpoint, t is the time the channel has resided in the current state, and D is the fractal dimension. This form was chosen because many other physical systems composed of processes that occur over a large range of spatial or temporal scales display this type of scaling.

We will first review the fractal model and then use it to analyze and interpret the single channel currents recorded from a K^+-selective channel in cultured mouse hippocampal pyramidal cells. This is a large conductance inward rectifying channel. Its activity is voltage dependent in that the fractional time it remains open decreases as the cell is hyperpolarized. Channels of this type were studied by Wong and Clark (27) and later by Sullivan and Cohen (28), Huguenard and Alger (29), and Sullivan (30, 31).

FRACTAL MODEL OF ION CHANNEL KINETICS

Building on a long history of mathematical ideas, Mandelbrot developed, organized, and expanded the concept he named "fractals" (32–40). A fractal object has a similar appearance when viewed at different scales of magnification. This property of fractals is called statistical self-similarity. For example, the coast of Britain looks just as "wiggly" on maps of different scales (40). Although the wiggles are of similar size when measured in centimeters on the map, they will correspond to different lengths in kilometers because the maps have different scales of centimeters to kilometers.

The total length of the coast depends on the scale of the map on which it is measured. As the measurement is done on maps of finer scale, the irregularities resolved will be finer, so that the length measured in kilometers is therefore longer. For coastlines and many other objects the value L measured for a property is proportional to a power of the scale ϵ at which it is measured, namely that $L = A\epsilon^{D_T - D}$, where A is a constant, D_T is the topological dimension, and D is the fractal dimension. This scaling relationship is an important property of fractals. For the west coast of Britain where $D_T = 1$, Richardson (41) found that the fractal dimension $D = 1.25$. These intuitive notions of self-similarity and scaling are both contained in the formal definition that a set in a metric space is fractal if the Hausdorff-Besicovitch dimension exceeds the topological dimension (33, p. 361).

In the last few years there has been an explosive growth in the objects and processes that have been found to have fractal properties. For example a small sampling of fractals found in nature include: the perimeters of clouds (42); the surface area of proteins (43); the surface area within bulk samples of minerals (44); the surface areas of the membranes of intracellular organelles (45); Brownian motion (33, 46); the intensity of earthquakes (47); the branching pattern of the bronchial tree (48); the patterns formed when water is injected into clay (49, 50), or lipids into lipids (51), or the pathway of sparks in dielectric breakdown (50); the motions induced by photodissociation of CO-myoglobin (52); the shape of soot particles (53); the vibrations in solid state materials (54); and the dielectric relaxation of glasses and polymers (55–57).

To formulate a channel model where the kinetics have the fractal properties discussed above we describe the channel as having one open and one closed state,

$$\text{closed} \underset{k_c}{\overset{k_o}{\rightleftharpoons}} \text{open} ,$$

where the kinetic rate constants $k_o(t)$ and $k_c(t)$ are the probabilities per unit time of leaving the closed and open states. We will derive the properties of the closed state. The equations for the open state are analogous with $k_o(t)$ replaced by $k_c(t)$. Let $P(t)$ be the probability that the channel remains closed over the interval $[0, t]$. The probability that the channel remains closed over the interval $[0, t + \Delta t]$ is then equal to the probability that the channel is closed up to time t and that it does not open in the next Δt interval. Taking the limit $\Delta t \rightarrow 0$ and integrating yields the result (see for example reference 26) that

$$\int \frac{dP(t)}{P(t)} = - \int k_o(t)\, dt . \tag{1}$$

The probability per unit time that the channel is closed for duration t is given by the probability density function

$$f(t) = - \frac{dP(t)}{dt} . \tag{2}$$

For a channel with fractal kinetics, the faster we look, the faster the channel will flicker open and closed. Just as the coast of Britain is longer when we measure it at finer spatial resolution, the effect kinetic rate constant of the channel is larger when we measure it at finer temporal resolution. Let the smallest time interval that we can resolve define the effective time scale t_{eff}. We can only detect channel closings of duration $t > t_{eff}$. Thus, the meaningful measurement of channel kinetics is not the kinetic rate constant, which is the probability that a closed channel will open; but rather the effective kinetic rate constant, k_{eff}, which is the conditional probability that a channel that has been closed for at least duration t_{eff} will open.

Let $\mathcal{A}$ be the probability that a closed channel will open at time T in the interval $t_{eff} < T \le t_{eff} + \Delta t$ and $\mathcal{B}$ the probability that the channel will remain closed for at least duration $T > t_{eff}$. The effective kinetic rate constant k_{eff} evaluated at t_{eff} is thus probability per unit time for event $\mathcal{A}$ given that event $\mathcal{B}$ has already occurred, namely $k_{eff} = \lim_{\Delta t \rightarrow 0} \text{prob}(\mathcal{A}|\mathcal{B})/\Delta t$. The definition of the conditional probability is that prob $(\mathcal{A}|\mathcal{B}) = \text{prob}(\mathcal{A}$ and $\mathcal{B})/\text{prob}(\mathcal{B})$. Note that $\mathcal{A} \cap \mathcal{B} = \mathcal{A}$, that is, the event $t_{eff} < T \le t_{eff} + \Delta t$ and the event $t_{eff} < T$, is the same as the event $t_{eff} < T \le t_{eff} + \Delta t$. Hence prob $(\mathcal{A}$ and $\mathcal{B}) = \text{prob}(\mathcal{A})$. Thus, we find that

$$k_{eff}(t_{eff}) = \frac{f(t_{eff})}{P(t_{eff})} = - \frac{d[\ln P(t)]}{dt}\bigg|_{t = t_{eff}} . \tag{3}$$

In renewal theory k_{eff} is called the "age-specific failure rate" and it gives the conditional probability that a component (e.g., a light bulb) that has survived to age t_{eff} will fail in the next Δt interval. The derivation of k_{eff} given above is from the monograph on renewal theory by Cox (58, pp. 3–5). The function k_{eff} is also widely used in actuarial work, for example, in determining premiums for life insurance policies.

To formulate a model of ion channel kinetics having fractal properties we assume that the effective kinetic rate constant for leaving the continuum of protein conformations that constitute the closed state is given by

$$k_{\text{eff}}(t_{\text{eff}}) = A \, t_{\text{eff}}^{1-D} \, . \tag{4}$$

This effective kinetic rate constant summarizes the information about the processes that happen at many different time scales. The fractal dimension D determines how sensitive k_{eff} is to changes in temporal scale. The kinetic setpoint A determines if all the processes happen slowly or rapidly. Note that since the current through the channel depends only on a single variable, that is time, the topological dimension $D_T = 1$.

The definition of the effective rate constant (Eq. 3) and the fact that it satisfies a fractal scaling relationship (Eq. 4) requires that the microscopic kinetic rate constant $k_o(t)$ is given by

$$k_o(t) = At^{1-D} \, . \tag{5}$$

Note that t is the time the channel has spent in its current state and k_o is the transition probability per unit time out of that state. When $D > 1$, the longer the channel resides in any state, the less likely it is to exit that state in subsequent time intervals.

The kinetic rate constant $k_o(t)$ from Eq. 5 can be substituted into Eq. 1 to find that

$$P(t) = e^{-[A/(2-D)]t^{2-D}} \tag{6}$$

This form is known as the Weibull distribution (58, pp. 20–22). Since it was first used by Kohlrausch in 1864 to describe mechanical creep it has been used to model many different physical processes (57). In the study of the dielectric relaxation of glasses and polymers it is known as the stretched exponential or Williams-Watts law (55–57). From Eqs. 2 and 6 we find that the frequency histogram of closed times is given by

$$f(t) = A \, t^{1-D} e^{-[A/(2-D)]t^{2-D}} \tag{7}$$

The rate of channel openings and closings should depend inversely on the time scale, so that $D \geq 1$. To normalize the probability distribution requires that $\lim_{t \to 0} P(t)$ exist, which is true only if $D < 2$. Thus, the fractal dimension D is restricted to the range $1 \leq D < 2$. (Actually, this upper bound is only a weak restriction because the probability distribution can be renormalized using the number of observed closed durations rather than the total number of closed durations when $D \geq 2$.)

METHODS

Experimental Techniques

Mouse embryonic hippocampal neurons (14–16 d gestation) were maintained in primary dissociated culture according to established protocols

(59). Briefly, embryonic mouse hippocampi from Swiss Webster mice (Buckberg Laboratory Animals, Tompkins Grove, NY) were isolated and cut into small clumps in dissecting solution (Eagle's minimum essential medium [MEM-GG] supplemented with 6 g/liter glucose, 2 mM L-glutamine, and 15 mM Hepes), and treated with trypsin (100 μg/ml for 20 min at 35°C under 5% CO_2/95% air [vol/vol]. After pelleting of tissue and resuspension in MEM-GG supplemented with 5% (vol/vol) fetal bovine serum (FBS) and 5% (vol/vol) horse serum (HS)(MEM-GG-BH), the suspension was triturated four times with a 25-gauge needle on a 5-ml syringe and plated on 18-mm collagen-coated (60) or poly-L-lysine (61, 62) coverslips (Carolina Biological Supply Co., Burlington, NC) in 35- or 60-mm Falcon culture dishes (Becton, Dickinson & Co., Oxnard, CA) on a drop of MEM-GG-BH. About 1/4 to 1/2 hippocampus was plated per coverslip overnight under 5% CO_2/95% air (vol/vol) at 35°C. The next day 1.5 ml of MEM-GG-BH was added or coverslips were transferred to dishes where whole brain cultures (minus hippocampus) had been grown over the previous 7–9 d in MEM-GG supplemented with 20% FBS and 2% HS. At the time of transfer to whole brain co-culture, serum-containing medium was totally replaced with a serum-free chemically defined medium (63–65) consisting of MEM-GG supplemented with insulin (5 μg/ml), human transferrin (100 μg/ml), sodium selenite (30 nM), triiodothyronine (0.3 nM), hydrocortisone (20 nM), and progesterone (20 nM). All cultures were maintained at 5% CO_2/95% air (vol/vol) at 35°C and media was changed weekly for both serum-containing and "serum-free" cultures. All media formulations, sera, and L-glutamine were obtained from Gibco (Grand Island, NY). All hormones and supplements were obtained from Sigma Chemical Co. (St. Louis, MO) except dextrose (Fisher Scientific Co., Pittsburgh, PA). Pyramidal cells maintained in serum-containing or serum-free medium had similar shapes with well developed dendritic arborizations after a few days in culture. Hippocampal pyramidal cells used for electrophysiological analysis had been maintained in cultures for 4 d to longer than 2 wk and were selected solely on the basis of morphological criteria (31).

Coverslips containing pyramidally shaped neurons were washed two to three times in the extracellular electrophysiological recording solution containing (in mM): 145 NaCl, 5.6 KCl, 1.0 CaCl$_2$, 0.8 MgCl$_2$, 5.6 glucose, and 4.0 Hepes-KOH, pH 7.2. Coverslips were then transferred to a specially designed chamber and viewed under 400× Nomarski (Diaphot) optics (Nikon Inc., Garden City, NY).

Patch electrodes were fabricated from Corning 7052 glass (Garner Glass Co., Clairmont, CA) according to the method of Corey and Stevens (66) and coated with Sylgard 184 elastomer (Dow Corning Corp., Midland, MI) to within 100 μm of the tip, and firepolished to resistances of 5–10 MΩ when filled with cell-attached patch recording fluids. Electrodes were secured in a specially designed holder (EW Wright, Guilford, CT) which was plugged directly into the headstage BNC. Patch clamp recording was used according to the method of Hamill et al. (9) using a Dagan 8900 Patch-Whole-Cell Clamp with a selected low noise 10 GΩ headstage (Dagan Corp., Minneapolis, MN; headstage 8930A). The ground and pipette electrodes were Ag/AgCl junctions. Electrode tips were initially filled by suction and finally filled to about a 1-cm column of fluid by backfilling with fine polystyrene needles attached to a syringe with a 0.22-μm filter (No. 4192; Gelman Sciences, Inc., Ann Arbor, MI). The experiments reported here were done with a pipette filling solution containing (in mM): 145.6 KCl, 1.0 CaCl$_2$, 1.0 MgCl$_2$, and 4.0 Hepes-KOH, pH 7.2. Electrodes were placed onto the surface of the cultured hippocampal neuron cell bodies (Leitz manipulators) and positioned until a slight dimpling of the surface was noted under 400× Nomarski. Slight suction (10–20 cm water) was applied to the pipette interior to obtain gigaohm seals while constantly adjusting the junction potential and was followed by electronic subtraction of pipette/patch input capacitance using a three time constant correction circuit.

Using conditions employed previously to identify single, inward rectifying K$^+$ channels in nonneuronal preparations (67–70) or in hippocampal neurons (27) with high concentrations of K$^+$ in the pipette it was often possible (~10–20% of patches) under conditions of stable, gigaohm seals to identify a high conductance, K$^+$ selective channel with inward rectifying I-V curves (28, 30, 31). Detailed analysis of the conductance properties of these channels indicates apparent ideal selectivity for K^+ permeation, a square root dependence of extracellular K^+ on conductance, apparent block by Cs^+ and Ba^{2+}, and saturation of inward current with increasing K^+ at constant voltage in apparent violation of the Goldman-Hodgkin-Katz equation (31). In addition these channels also exhibit submaximal current levels, which have properties consistent with subconductance states (28, 30, 31).

Single channel currents from cell attached patches with command potentials at hyperpolarizing voltages of 0, 22, 41, and 60 mV (relative to the resting membrane potential) were recorded on FM tape (model B, 4 track tape recorder; A. R. Vetter Co., Rebersburg, PA) at 7½ in./s (~2.25 kHz). Single channel open and closed times were measured in two ways:)(a) by playback of tape records at ⅛ recording speed (15/16 ips) onto a paper recorder (frequency response ~100 Hz; Gould Inc., Cleveland, OH) and then manual measurement of the duration of events, or (b) digitization of analog data from tape at 10 kHz on a Data General Eclipse System (Westboro, MA) and analysis using the IPROC automated pattern recognition program (71) employing half-maximal current amplitude event detection criterion and a pattern recognition algorithm for noise rejection (72, 73).

Markov Analysis

Open and closed time duration histograms were fitted to single and multiple exponential functions using a Marquardt-Levinberg algorithm (74) that does not require analytical derivatives and incorporates subroutine ZXSSQ by International Mathematical and Statistical Libraries Inc. (Houston, TX). The open time distributions could always be fit by a single exponential while triple exponentials were necessary to fit the closed time distributions. These distributions were interpreted in terms of a

$$\text{closed} \underset{k_{21}}{\overset{k_{12}}{\rightleftharpoons}} \text{closed} \underset{k_{32}}{\overset{k_{23}}{\rightleftharpoons}} \text{closed} \underset{k_{O3}}{\overset{k_{34}}{\rightleftharpoons}} \text{open}$$

kinetic model. This model was chosen because of its relative simplicity and because of its useful application to other K^+ channels (75). The rate constant k_{O3} is equal to the inverse of the time constant of the open time distribution. The other rate constants were calculated by solving the nonlinear equations (3.65, 3.66, 3.67, and 3.70) of Colquhoun and Hawkes (11) with the time constants and amplitudes of the total closed distribution function as input. A program called 4STATE (incorporating IMSL subroutine ZSPOW) was used to solve the system of nonlinear algebraic equations at each voltage in each patch.

Fractal Analysis

Liebovitch et al. have shown that a plot of log k_{eff} vs. log t_{eff} is a sensitive method to analyze ion channel kinetics (24–26). If there are multiple plateaus on this plot, then the channel has multiple, discrete states that can be well represented by a Markov process. However, if the kinetics of the channel are fractal, then this plot will be a straight line of the form log $k_{eff} = (1 - D) \log t_{eff} + \log A$. Thus, the two parameters of the fractal model, the fractal dimension D and the kinetic setpoint A, can be determined from the slope and intercept of this plot.

The analytic definition k_{eff} (Eq. 3) can be recast into a form more useful for analyzing the experimentally measured closed durations. For a two-state closed $\rightleftharpoons$ open Markov process, that is, the fractal model with $D = 1$, then $P(t) = \exp(-k_o t)$, $f(t) = k_o \exp(-k_o t)$, and $k_o = -d/dt[\ln P(t)]$ where k_o is a constant. Note the similarity of this form for k_o to that for the effective kinetic rate constant $k_{eff} = -d/dt[\ln P(t)]|t = t_{eff}$. Thus, over a small range of times the kinetics of any channel are locally of the form of a closed $\rightleftharpoons$ open Markov process with $k_{eff} = k_o$.

Thus, k_{eff} is equal to minus the slope of $\ln f(t)$ vs. t evaluated over a small range of closed durations. To do this, we construct frequency histograms of closed times each with a different bin size. The bin size t_b determines the effective time scale of the analysis and thus $t_b = t_{eff}$. Then,

for each histogram, we use least squares to determine the slope over the second through fourth bins. We must exclude the first time bin that includes the closings $t \ll t_b$ that are much less than the time scale t_b, and the longer time bins that include all the closings $t \gg t_b$ that are much longer than the time scale t_b. This procedure thus determines k_{eff} as a function of t_{eff}. We have previously validated this procedure by comparing k_{eff} determined analytically from fractal and multistate Markov models using Eq. 3 with k_{eff} determined by constructing the closed time histograms from finite difference simulations of single channel currents from those same models (26). The effective kinetic rate constants determined by both methods were very similar. However, for the channel models with fractal kinetics, the plots of log k_{eff} vs. log t_{eff} based on this fitting procedure overestimated the fractal dimension D by ~10%.

Once the fractal dimension D and the kinetic setpoint A have been determined from the plot of log k_{eff} vs. log t_{eff} it is simple to fit the fractal model to the experimentally measured distribution of closed times. The number of closings of duration t to $t + \Delta t$ is given by $N(t) = N_T \Delta t f(t)$. Since $f(t)$ depends only on D and A it is already completely known. To determine N_T we minimize the residuals $S = \Sigma_{i-1,n}\{\ln [N_T f(t_i)] - \ln [N(t_i)/\Delta t]\}^2$, where n closed durations were observed. We use the logarithms because for the limiting case $D = 1$ this reduces to a semilogarithmic fit, which can be done analytically and because $f(t)$ often extends over several decades so that if the logarithms are not used then only the few highest values of $f(t)$ would actually influence the fitting procedure. Minimizing the residuals, $\partial S/\partial N_T = 0$, we find that $N_T = \exp \{(-1/n)\Sigma_{i-1,n} \ln [f(t_i)\Delta t/N(t_i)]\}$.

A Macintosh microcomputer (Apple Computer Inc., Cupertino, CA) was used for the data analysis. The open and closed times were stored in a spreadsheet (Microsoft Excel), the mathematics performed by programs in Microsoft BASIC, and the results plotted with Cricket Graph. Using Switcher to load several programs in memory at once it is very easy to transfer data and results between programs by using the buffer (the clipboard) which can be accessed by all programs on the Macintosh.

Note that this fractal analysis uses only a least squares fit of a straight line which can be done analytically to determine D and A and a sum to determine N_T. These are closed (and not iterated) procedures and considerably simpler than the much more complex and often numerically delicate techniques required to determine the kinetic rate constants of the multiple state Markov models.

RESULTS

Markov Model

At least one open and three closed states were required to fit the distributions of open and closed durations. The details of the fitting procedure and the results are described by Sullivan (31) and Sullivan and Cohen (manuscript in preparation). A very complex picture emerges of the voltage dependence of this channel. The variation of the time constants for leaving the open and closed states are shown in Fig. 1. The time constant from the open state decreases with hyperpolarization while for the closed states, the short time constant remains approximately constant, the medium time constant decreases, and the long time constant increases with hyperpolarization. As shown in Fig. 2 the kinetic rate constants of this Markov model show no consistent changes that can be interpreted in a simple clear physical model.

Markov models cannot be uniquely determined from just the distributions of the open and closed durations. Thus, it is possible that another Markov model (that we were unable to find) might prove easier to interpret in

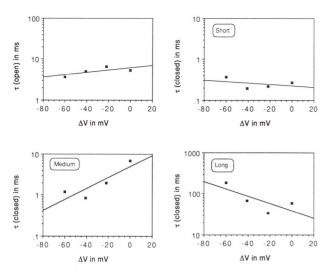

FIGURE 1 The open times could be fit by a single exponential and the closed times by the sums of three exponentials. The variation of those time constants with voltage is shown above. The data shown here are the average from two patches.

terms of a physical model. It is also possible that the data here are insufficient to produce good estimates of all the parameters that a multi-state Markov model requires. However, the data were sufficient to produce good estimates of the fractal parameters.

Fractal Model

The open and closed durations measured from the single channel records were used to construct histograms of bin sizes 1, 2, 4, 8, 16, 32, 64, 128, 256, and 512 ms. Only histograms with enough statistical accuracy to have monotonically decreasing nonzero numbers of durations in the first four bins were used for further analysis. A sample of these histograms, when 0 mV was applied, is shown in Figs.

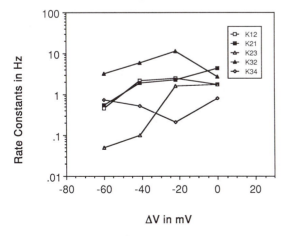

FIGURE 2 The variation of the kinetic rate constants with voltage calculated from the Markov model

$$\text{closed} \underset{k_{21}}{\overset{k_{12}}{\rightleftharpoons}} \text{closed} \underset{k_{32}}{\overset{k_{23}}{\rightleftharpoons}} \text{closed} \underset{k_{O3}}{\overset{k_{34}}{\rightleftharpoons}} \text{open}.$$

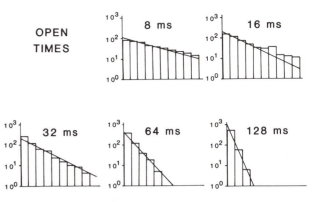

FIGURE 3 The open times recorded at 0 mV were used to construct frequency histograms of bin width 8, 16, 32, 64, and 128 ms. The lines are the least squares fit of a single exponential using the second through fourth bins. The negative of the slopes of these lines equals the effective kinetic rate constant k_{eff} for leaving the open state at the effective time scale t_{eff} equal to the bin size.

3–4. The lines on these figures are a least squares fit using the second through fourth bins. The negative values of the slopes of these lines are the effective rate constants k_{eff} shown in Fig. 5. These plots of log k_{eff} vs. log t_{eff} for both the open and closed times do not have the plateaus that would indicate the existence of the multiple discrete states predicted by the Markov models. Rather, they are approximately straight lines, indicating that these channels can be represented by a model with fractal kinetics.

As shown in Fig. 6, the fractal dimension D for both the open and closed times does not vary with the applied voltage. We found that $D(\text{open}) = 1.34 \pm 0.11$ (mean ± SEM) and that $D(\text{closed}) = 2.07 \pm 0.12$. The fractal model of ion channel kinetics predicts that the fractal dimension D should be within the range $1 \leq D < 2$. The values found for $D(\text{open})$ and $D(\text{closed})$ are within this range. The value of $D(\text{open})$ is greater than one (*t* test, $P < 0.025$) and the value for $D(\text{closed})$ is not greater than two (*t* test, $P < 0.3$). Because the fitting procedure tends to overestimate the fractal dimension by ~10%, we believe

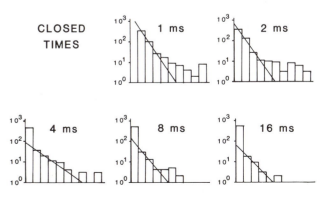

FIGURE 4 The closed times recorded at 0 mV were used to construct frequency histograms of bin width 1, 2, 4, 8, and 16 ms. The lines are the least squares fit of a single exponential using the second through fourth bins. The negative of the slopes of these lines equals the effective kinetic rate constant k_{eff} for leaving the closed state at the effective time scale t_{eff} equal to the bin size.

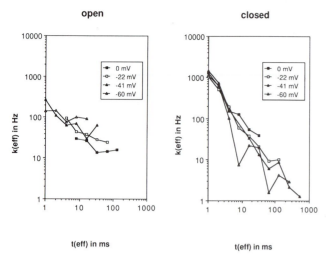

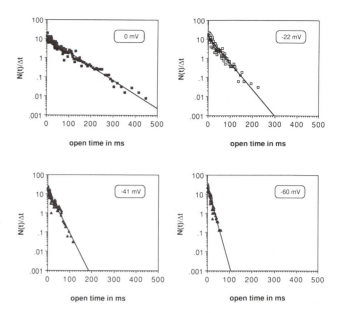

FIGURE 5 The effective kinetic rate constants k_{eff} for leaving the open and closed states are plotted versus the effective time scale t_{eff} for patches that were voltage clamped at hyperpolarizing voltages of 0, 22, 41, and 60 mV. There are no plateaus in the plot that would indicate the existence of multiple, discrete conformational states predicted by the Markov models of ion channel kinetics. The linearity of the data at each voltage is consistent with the fractal model of ion channel kinetics. The slope and intercept of the lines on these plots determines the fractal dimension D and the kinetic setpoint A.

FIGURE 7 Semilogarithmic plot of the open time histograms. The lines are the best fit of a single exponential to the data.

that $D(\text{open}) \approx 1$ and $D(\text{closed}) \approx 2$. The kinetic setpoint A was strongly dependent on voltage. As also shown in Fig. 6, $-\log[A(\text{open})]$ and $\log[A(\text{closed})]$ are proportional to voltage with approximately the same constant of proportionality.

When $D \approx 1$, the probability density function $f(t) = A\exp(-At)$. Hence, $D(\text{open}) \approx 1$ implies that the histogram of open times should be well fit by a single exponential. Thus, on a semilogarithmic plot the open times should

be well fit by a straight line and this is indeed true as seen in Fig. 7. The closed times, also presented on semilogarithmic plot in Fig. 8, are also well represented by the fractal model.

When $D \approx 2$, then $t^{2-D} = e^{(2-D)\ln t} \approx 1 + (2 - D)\ln t$, thus the probability density function $f(t) \approx A\exp\{-[A/(2 - D)]\}t^{1-D-A}$. That is, when $D \approx 2$, the frequency histogram of the fractal model is no longer a stretched exponential, but becomes a power law where $f(t) \propto t^{1-D-A}$. Hence, $D(\text{closed}) \approx 2$ implies that the histogram of closed times should be well fit by a straight line on a log-log plot. This is indeed the case as shown in Fig. 10. For comparison a log-log plot of the open times is shown in Fig. 9. Since

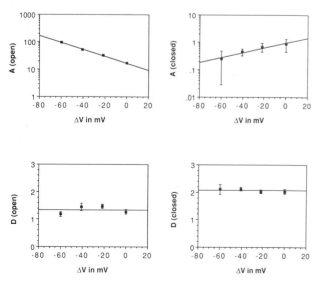

FIGURE 6 The dependence of the kinetic setpoint and fractal dimension on voltage are shown. The fractal dimension does not depend on voltage. The logarithms of the kinetic setpoint for the open and closed times are proportional to voltage with approximately the same constant of proportionality.

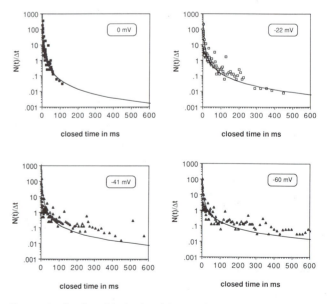

FIGURE 8 Semilogarithmic plot of the closed time histograms. The lines are the best fit of the fractal model to the data.

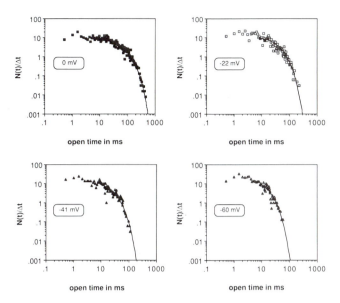

FIGURE 9 Logarithmic-logarithmic plot of the open time histograms. The lines are the best fit of a single exponential to the data.

D(open) is not close to 2, the open times are not a straight line on a log-log plot.

DISCUSSION

Ion channels open and close spontaneously. The mathematical model known as a Markov process, which has been widely used to represent the kinetics of these channels and interpret the results from single channel and noise analysis experiments, assumes that the channel proteins have only a few discrete conformational states. However, it is known that the spontaneous fluctuations in the conformation of

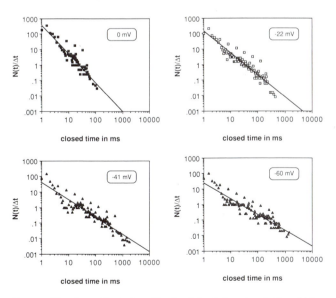

FIGURE 10. Logarithmic-logarithmic plot of the closed time histograms. As determined from the plot of log k_{eff} vs. log t_{eff} in Fig. 5, D(closed) = 2.07 ± 0.12. When the fractal dimension $D \approx 2$, the fractal model predicts that the closed time histogram is a power law and thus a straight line on such a log-log plot. The lines are the best fit of such a power law to the data.

proteins involve many different processes that occur over many different time scales from 10^{-15} to 10^3 s (15–23). This suggests that the fluctuations of the channel protein pass through a very large number of conformational states. To reflect this behavior Liebovitch et al. (24–26) proposed a new model of ion channel kinetics where the channel is represented by a continuum of many conformational states. In this fractal model the dynamic processes that take place over many different time scales are represented by a kinetic rate constant that has the fractal form $k = At^{1-D}$. This form was chosen because many other systems (from the length of the coast of Britain to dielectric relaxation in glasses) that are composed of processes that occur over a large range of spatial or temporal scales have this type of scaling behavior (32–57). The fractal dimension D determines the relative contribution of processes at different time scales and the kinetic setpoint A determines if all the processes happen slowly or rapidly.

We used both the Markov and fractal models to interpret single channel currents recorded from a K^+-selective, voltage-dependent channel in cultured neurons from the mouse hippocampus. The histograms of the durations of the open and closed times are well fit by both models. The fractal model is more parsimonious about its assumptions than the Markov model. The fractal model depends on four parameters while the Markov closed ⇌ closed ⇌ closed ⇌ open model depends on six kinetic rate constants. Also, the mathematical analysis needed to determine the parameters of the fractal model is much simpler than that required to determine the parameters of the Markov model.

The voltage dependence of the kinetic rate constants of the Markov model is complex. Each of the many kinetic rate constants are independent parameters having a unique and independent variation with voltage. However, in the fractal model, it is seen that the entire voltage dependence of all the short, medium, and long closed and open times of the channel can be understood entirely in terms of how the kinetic setpoint, varies with voltage. As seen in Fig. 6 the fractal dimensions of both the open and closed states does not depend on voltage. However, $-\log[A(\text{open})]$ and $\log[A(\text{closed})]$ are proportional to voltage with approximately the same constant of proportionality. This suggests

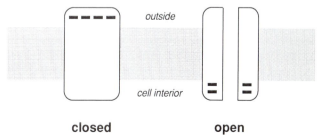

FIGURE 11. When the ion channel opens or closes there is a net movement of charge across the channel protein. Based on the voltage dependence the fractal model suggests that approximately one net negative charge moves inward when the channel opens and one net negative charge moves outward when the channel closes.

that, as shown in Fig. 11, there is a net movement of negative charge inward when the channel opens and an identical movement of net negative charge outward when the channel closes. If the voltage simply adds to the existing energy barriers then the kinetic setpoints will have the form $A = A_o e^{zeV/kT}$ where A_o is a constant, z the net gating charge, e the charge on an ion, V the voltage, k the Boltzmann constant, and T the absolute temperature. From that relationship and the slope of the plots of $\log[A]$ vs. voltage we estimate that 0.53 ± 0.06 net negative charges move inward when the channel opens and that 0.74 ± 0.01 net negative charges move outward when the channel closes. Considering both the possible systematic and random errors involved in this determination, the near equality of these two numbers is important. The number of gating charges calculated from the data depends on the analysis used. Thus, unlike the Markov model, the fractal analysis leads to a consistent number of gating charges for both opening and closing, which provides strong support for the fractal interpretation of ion channel kinetics.

The variation of the time constants of the multiexponential fits to the frequency histograms of the closed and open times and the kinetic rate constants of the Markov model suggest no physical interpretation of the voltage dependence. On the other hand, the variation of A and D of the fractal model described above leads to a clear, simple, physical interpretation of the voltage dependence; namely, that the energy to open or close the channel $\Delta E = (\Delta E)_o + (\Delta E)_g$, where $(\Delta E)_o$ is the intrinsic energy difference between the open and closed conformation of the channel and $(\Delta E)_g$ is the energy required to move the gating charges through the voltage applied across the patch. This simple model explains the variation of $\log[A]$ vs. voltage and thus the voltage dependence of all the short, medium, and long closed and open times of the channel.

Moreover, as shown above when $D \approx 2$, the probability density of the open or closed times has the form $f(t) \approx A \exp\{-[A/(2-D)]\}t^{1-D-A}$. For this K$^+$ channel we found that the fractal dimension D does not vary with voltage while the kinetic setpoint A does indeed depend on the voltage. For any channel with a similar form for the voltage dependence of D and A, when $D \approx 2$ the exponential term will be exquisitely sensitive to small changes in A. Hence, when $D \approx 2$ small changes in the voltage-dependent kinetic setpoint A will dramatically change the open or closed time distribution. Thus, if the fractal model is correct, then the fractal dimension measured at a single voltage can be used to predict the voltage sensitivity of an ion channel. For the K$^+$ channel we observed, $D(\text{closed}) \approx 2$ and so the voltage dependence of $A(\text{closed})$ greatly increases the probability of the channel remaining closed for long durations as the patch is hyperpolarized, effectively turning the channel off.

The frequency histograms of the open and closed durations of many ion channels have been quite successfully fit by multiple state Markov models (1, 2). Does this exten-sive literature contradict the fractal model? It is too early to tell. The extant data will have to be re-analyzed from the fractal viewpoint and the fractal and Markov models compared. This will require the original data, because it is almost impossible to do from the published results. Nonetheless, some of the published results are quite suggestive. For example, Blatz and Magleby (76) found that the distribution of closed times of a chloride channel is overall a power law, which to us suggests that the kinetics is fractal with fractal dimension ≈ 2. The small scale features of this data could be interpreted either as (a) a fractal continuum of states, separated by small energy barriers, some of which are longer lived than others, or (b) as due to the sum of discrete Markov states separated by steep energy barriers. The resolution of this issue will depend on future biophysical measurements of ion channel protein dynamics. Qualitatively, a stretched exponential form, characteristic of fractals, is the form most often seen for the distribution of open and closed times in published single channel papers. Nonetheless, qualitative judgments are not conclusive. The data must be rigorously re-analyzed to determine if it is consistent with or contradicts the fractal model.

The two channels that we have analyzed, the K$^+$ channel in an excitable cell presented here and a nonselective channel in an epithelium (24–26), are well fit by the fractal model. If the fractal model applies to other channels as well then the fractal dimension D and the kinetic setpoint A may serve as a useful phenomenological classification scheme of ion channel types. If that is true, then we will be faced with the entertaining challenge of trying to derive D and A from ion channel structure and dynamics.

We thank Dr. Fred Sachs for the opportunity for one of us (J. M. Sullivan) to visit his laboratory and Anthony Auerbach and Jim Neal for their assistance in using the patch clamp and Markov analysis software developed in that laboratory. J. M. Sullivan also thanks his Ph.D. thesis committee and specifically Dr. Stephen Cohen for the use of his laboratory facilities and the aid of his technical personnel who provided cultured hippocampal cells. We also thank Ms. Mei Wang who assisted in this work and measured 1,551 closed and 1,551 open durations from the chart recordings. The development of the fractal model of ion channel kinetics has benefited from helpful discussions with Leo Levine, Michael Shlesinger, Howard Eggers, Raúl Chiesa, Lu-Ku Li, Stefan Machlup, Jorge Fischbarg, and Jan Koniarek. Healthy and helpful criticisms were also provided by Watt Webb, Fred Sachs, and Karl Magleby.

This work was supported in part by National Institutes of Health grants EY6234, EY1080, EY6178, GM7280, and NIDA3613.

Received for publication 5 June 1987 and in final form 5 August 1987.

REFERENCES

1. Sakmann, B., and E. Neher, editors. 1983. Single Channel Recording. Plenum Publishing Corp., New York.

2. Hille, B. 1984. Ionic Channels of Excitable Membranes. Sinauer Associates Inc., Sunderland, MA.

3. Stevens, C. 1972. Inferences about membrane noise from electrical measurements. *Biophys. J.* 12:1028–1047.

4. Verveen, A. A., and L. J. DeFelice. 1974. Membrane noise. *Prog. Biophys.* 28:189–265.

BIOPHYSICAL JOURNAL VOLUME 52 1987

5. Conti, F., and E. Wanke. 1975. Channel noise in nerve membranes and lipid bilayers. *Q. Rev. Biophys.* 8:451–506.

6. van Driessche, W., and K. G. Gullentops. 1978. Conductance fluctuation analysis in epithelia. *Tech. Cell Physiol.* P123:1–13.

7. Lindemann, B. 1980. The beginning of fluctuation analysis of epithelial ion transport. *J. Membr. Biol.* 54:1–11.

8. DeFelice, L. J. 1981. Introduction to Membrane Noise. Plenum Publishing Corp., New York.

9. Hamill, O. P., A. Marty, E. Neher, B. Sakmann, and F. J. Sigworth. 1980. Improved patch-clamp techniques for high-resolution current recording from cells and cell-free membrane patches. *Pfluegers Arch. Eur. J. Physiol.* 391:85–100.

10. Colquhoun, D., and A. G. Hawkes. 1977. Relaxation and fluctuations of membrane currents that flow through drug-operated channels. *Proc. R. Soc. Lond. B. Biol. Sci.* 199:231–262.

11. Colquhoun, D., and A. G. Hawkes. 1981. On the stochastic properties of single ion channels. *Proc. R. Soc. Lond. B. Biol. Sci.* 211:205–235.

12. Colquhoun, D., and A. G. Hawkes. 1982. On the stochastic properties of single ion channel openings and clusters of bursts. *Philos. Trans. R. Soc. Lond. B. Biol. Sci.* 300:1–59.

13. FitzHugh, R. 1983. Statistical properties of the asymmetric random telegraph signal, with applications to single-channel analysis. *Math. Biosci.* 64:75–89.

14. Jackson, M. B. 1985. Stochastic behavior of a many-channel membrane system. *Biophys. J.* 47:129–137.

15. Careri, G., P. Fasella, and E. Gratton. 1975. Statistical time events in enzymes: a physical assesment. *CRC Crit Rev. Biochem.* 3:141–164.

16. Gurd, F. R. N., and T. M. Rothgeb. 1979. Motions in proteins. *Adv. Prot. Chem.* 33:73–165.

17. Williams, R. J. P. 1979. The conformational properties of proteins in solution. *Bio. Rev.* 54:389–437.

18. Karplus, M., and J. A. McCammon. 1981. The internal dynamics of globular proteins. *CRC Crit. Rev. Biochem.* 9:293–349.

19. Karplus, M., and J. A. McCammon. 1983. Dynamics of proteins: elements and function. *Annu. Rev. Biochem.* 52:263–300.

20. Levitt, M. 1983. Molecular dynamics of native protein I. computer simulation of trajectories. *J. Mol. Biol.* 168:595–620.

21. Levitt, M. 1983. Molecular dynamics of native protein II. analysis and nature of motion. *J. Mol. Biol.* 168:621–657.

22. Ringe, D., and G. A. Petsko. 1985. Mapping protein dynamics by X-ray diffraction. *Prog. Biophys. Mol. Biol.* 45:197–235.

23. Karplus, M., and J. A. McCammon. 1986. The dynamics of proteins, *Sci. Am.* April 1986:42–51.

24. Liebovitch, L. S., J. Fischbarg, and J. P. Koniarek. 1986. Fractal model of ion channel kinetics. *J. Gen. Physiol.* 88:34a–35a. (Abstr.)

25. Liebovitch, L. S., J. Fischbarg, J. P. Koniarek, I. Todorova, and M. Wang. 1987. Fractal model of ion channel kinetics. *Biochim. Biophys. Acta.* 896:173–180.

26. Liebovitch, L. S., J. Fischbarg, and J. P. Koniarek. 1987. Ion channel kinetics: a model based on fractal scaling rather than multistate Markov processes. *Math. Biosci.* 84:37–68.

27. Wong, R. K. S., and R. B. Clark. 1983. Single K⁺ channel currents from hippocampal pyramidal cells of adult guinea pig. *Soc. Neurosci. Abstr.* 9:602.

28. Sullivan, J. M., and S. A. Cohen. 1985. Single ion channels in cultured hippocampus show inward rectification. *Biophys. J.* 47:385a. (Abstr.)

29. Huguenard, J. R., and B. E. Alger. 1985. Properties of the inward rectifying potassium channel in acutely dissociated hippocampal pyramidal cells. *Soc. Neurosci. Abstr.* 11:786.

30. Sullivan, J. M. 1987. A voltage- and calcium-sensitive inward rectifying potassium channel active in the resting membrane of cultured mouse hippocampal neurons. *Biophys. J.* 51:54a. (Abstr.)

31. Sullivan, J. M. 1987. Patch clamp study of a large conductance, inward rectifying potassium channel in cultured mouse hippocampal neurons. Ph.D. Dissertation, City University, New York.

32. Mandelbrot, B. B. 1977. Fractals: Form, Chance, and Dimension. W. H. Freeman & Co. Publishers, San Francisco.

33. Mandelbrot, B. B. 1983. The Fractal Geometry of Nature. W. H. Freeman & Co. Publishers, San Francisco.

34. Barcellos, A. 1984. The fractal geometry of Mandelbrot. *College Math. J.* 15:98–114.

35. Gardner, M. 1976. In which "monster" curves force redefinition of the word "curve." *Sci. Am.* Dec. 1976:124–133.

36. Gardner, M. 1978. White and brown music, fractal curves and one-over-f fluctuations. *Sci. Am.* April 1978:16–32.

37. Gleick, J. 1985. The man who reshaped geometry. *N. Y. Times Sec. 6 (Mag.).* Dec. 5, 1985:64.

38. Anon. 1986. Mathematics with a twist. *Compressed Air Mag.* Aug. 1986:7–13.

39. Peitgen, H.-O., and P. H. Richter. 1986. The Beauty of Fractals. Springer-Verlag, New York.

40. Mandelbrot, B. B. 1967. How long is the coast of Britain? Statistical self-similarity and fractal dimension. *Science (Wash. DC).* 156:636–638.

41. Richardson, L. F. 1961. The problem of contiguity: an appendix to *Statistics of Deadly Quarrels. General Systems Yearbook.* 6:139–187.

42. Lovejoy, S. 1982. Area-perimeter relation for rain and cloud areas. *Science (Wash. DC).* 216:185–187.

43. Lewis, M., and D. C. Rees. 1985. Fractal surfaces of proteins. *Science (Wash. DC).* 230:1163–1165.

44. Avnir, D., D. Farin, and P. Pfeifer. 1984. Molecular fractal surfaces. *Nature (Lond.).* 308:261–263.

45. Paumgartner, D., G. Losa, and E. R. Weibel. 1981. Resolution effect on the sterological estimation of surface and volume and its interpretation in terms of fractal dimensions. *J. Microsc.* 121:51–63.

46. Lavenda, B. H. 1981. Brownian motion. *Sci. Am.* Feb. 1985:70–84.

47. Kagan, Y.Y., and L. Knopoff. 1981. Stochastic synthesis of earthquake catalogs. *J. Geophys. Res.* 86:2853–2862.

48. West, B., V. Bhargava, and A. L. Goldberger. 1986. Beyond the principle of similitude, renormalization in the bronchial tree. *J. Appl. Physiol.* 60:1089–1097.

49. Damme, H. V., F. Obrecht, P. Levitz, L. Gatineau, and C. Laroche. 1986. Fractal viscous fingering in clay slurries. *Nature (Lond.).* 320:731–733.

50. Stanley, H. E., and N. Ostrowksy, editors. 1986. On Growth and Form, Fractal and Non-Fractal Patterns in Physics. Martinus Nijhoff Publishers, Boston.

51. Miller A., W. Knoll, and H. Möhwald. 1986. Fractal and non-fractal crystalline phospholipid domains in monomolecular layers. *Biophys. J.* 49:317a. (Abstr.)

52. Ansari, A., J. Berendzen, S. F. Bowne, H. Frauenfelder, I. E. T. Iben, T. B. Sauke, E. Shyamsunder, and R. D. Young. 1985. Protein states and proteinquakes. *Proc. Natl. Acad. Sci. USA.* 82:5000–5004.

53. Sander, L. M. 1986. Fractal growth processes. *Nature (Lond.).* 322:789–793.

54. Orbach, R. 1986. Dynamics of fractal networks. *Science (Wash. DC).* 231:814–819.

55. Williams, G., and D. C. Watts. 1970. Non-symmetrical dielectric relaxation behavior arising from a simple empirical decay function. *Trans. Faraday Soc.* 66:80–85.

56. Shlesinger, M. F. 1984. Williams-Watts dielectric relaxation: a fractal time stochastic process. *J. Stat. Phys.* 36:639–648.

57. Klafter, J., and M. F. Shlesinger. 1986. On the relationship among the three theories of relaxation in disordered systems. *Proc. Natl. Acad. Sci. USA.* 83:848–851.

58. Cox, D. R. 1962. Renewal Theory. Science Paperbacks, London.

59. Peacock, J. H., D. F. Rush, and L. H. Mathers. 1979. Morphology of dissociated hippocampal cultures from fetal mice. *Brain Res.* 169:241–246.

60. Bornstein, M. B. 1958. Reconstituted rat tail collagen used as a substrate for tissue cultures in Maximov slides and roller tubes. *Lab. Invest.* 7:134–137.

61. Yavin, E., and Z. Yavin. 1974. Attachment and culture of dissociated cells from rat embryo cerebral hemispheres on polylysine-coated surface. *J. Cell Biol.* 62:540–546.

62. Letourneau, P. C. 1975. Possible roles for cell-to-substrate adhesion in neuronal morphogenesis. *Dev. Biol.* 44:77–91.

63. Bottenstein, J. E., and G. H. Sato. 1979. Growth of a rat neuroblastoma cell line in serum-free supplemented medium. *Proc. Natl. Acad. Sci. USA.* 76:514–517.

64. Bottenstein, J. E. 1983. Defined media for dissociated neural cultures. *In* Current Methods in Cellular Neurobiology. Volume IV. Model Systems. J. L. Barker and J. F. McKelvy, editors. John Wiley & Sons, Inc., New York. 107–127.

65. Seifert, W., B. Ranscht, H. J. Fink, F. Forster, S. Beckh, and W. H. Muller. 1983. Development of hippocampal neurons in cell culture: a molecular approach. *In* Neurobiology of the Hippocampus. W. Seifert, editor. Academic Press, Inc., New York. 7.

66. Corey, D. P., and C. F. Stevens. 1983. Science and technology of patch recording electrodes. *In* Single Channel Recording. B. Sakmann, and E. Neher, editors. Plenum Publishing Corp., New York. 53–68.

67. Fukushima, Y. 1981. Single channel potassium currents of the anomalous rectifier. *Nature (Lond.).* 294:368–371.

68. Fukushima, Y. 1982. Blocking kinetics of the anomalous potassium rectifier of tunicate egg studied by single channel recording. *J. Physiol. (Lond.).* 331:311–331.

69. Ohmori, H., S. Yoshida, and S. Hagiwara. 1981. Single K^+ channel currents of anomalous rectification in cultured rat myotubes. *Proc. Natl. Acad. Sci. USA.* 78:4960–4964.

70. Sakmann, B., and G. Trube. 1984. Voltage-dependent inactivation of inward rectifying single-channel currents in the guinea pig heart cell membrane. *J. Physiol. (Lond.).* 347:659–683.

71. Sachs, F., J. Neil, and N. Barkakati. 1982. The automated analysis of data from single ionic channels. *Pfluegers Arch. Eur. J. Physiol.* 395:331–340.

72. Auerbach, A., and F. Sachs. 1983. Flickering of a nicotinic ion channel to a subconductance state. *Biophys. J.* 42:1–10.

73. Auerbach, A., and F. Sachs. 1984. Single-channel currents from acetylcholine receptors in embryonic chick muscle: kinetic and conductance properties of gaps within bursts. *Biophys. J.* 45:187–918.

74. Press, W. H., B. P. Flannery, S. A. Teukolsky, and W. T. Vtterling. 1986. Numerical Recipes. Cambridge University Press, London.

75. Guharay, F., and F. Sachs. 1984. Stretch-activated single ion channel currents of tissue-cultured embryonic chick skeletal muscle. *J. Physiol. (Lond.).* 352:685–701.

76. Blatz, A. L., and K. L. Magleby. 1986. Quantitative description of three modes of activity of fast chloride channels from rat skeletal muscle. *J. Physiol. (Lond.).* 387:141–174.

Journal of Neuroscience Methods, 27 (1989) 173–180
Elsevier

173

NSM 00913000

A Fractal Analysis of Cell Images

T.G. Smith Jr.[1], W.B. Marks[2], G.D. Lange[3], W.H. Sheriff Jr.[3] and E.A. Neale[4]

[1]*Laboratory of Neurophysiology, NINDS, National Institutes of Health, Bethesda, MD 20892 (U.S.A.),*
[2]*Laboratory of Neural Control, NINDS, National Institutes of Health, Bethesda, MD 20892 (U.S.A.),*
[3]*Instrumentation and Computer Section, NINDS, National Institutes of Health, Bethesda, MD 20892 (U.S.A.)*
and [4]*Laboratory of Developmental Neurobiology, NICHD, National Institutes of Health, Bethesda, MD 20892 (U.S.A.)*

(Received 19 May 1988)
(Revised 17 October 1988)
(Accepted 21 October 1988)

Key words: Cultured neuron; Dendritic branching; Dendritic contour; Fractal geometry; Fractal dimension

Methods of digital image analysis have been adapted to measure the fractal dimension of cellular profiles. The fractal dimension is suggested as a useful measure of the complexity of a contour. Three methods produce similar results when applied to constructed, near-ideal fractal figures. Comparison of the measurements for a variety of image types indicates the measurement accuracy in each case and may help in interpreting the results when applied to real, non-ideal cell images of unknown fractal dimension. Two of the methods are currently adopted as appropriate for use on neuronal contours. A correlation exists between the complexity of these contours and the magnitude of the estimated fractal dimension.

INTRODUCTION

The purpose of this paper is to report that the morphological shapes of the borders of vertebrate central nervous system neurons, grown as a monolayer in cell culture, can be characterized by Mandelbrot's 'fractional dimension' (*D*), which is a measure of complexity (Mandelbrot, 1982; Kaye, 1985, 1987; Stanley and Ostrowsky, 1985; Damme et al., 1986). Moreover, the results are as expected, viz., cells with simple, uncomplicated structures have a small fractal dimension, while cells with complex structures have a large fractal dimension. Thus, the measurement of the fractal dimension as a dependent variable may be a useful 'tool' in experiments concerned with quantitative morphological complexity.

The border of a neuron can be fully specified as a series of Cartesian coordinates. Most of the process of border specification can be automated (Smith et al., 1988). The next logical step of analysis is reduction of

the data to a few numbers relevant to morphological classification and/or physiological processes. One fruitful approach to the latter problem has been to represent a neuron as a concatenation of simple geometrical objects (e.g. cylinders and cones) for the purpose of establishing the macroscopic electrical properties of the cell in the form of equivalent electrical circuits (Rall, 1985). This has been a productive approach, but it has limitations. For example, in questions dealing with important differences in the details of morphology between classes of neurons, some other mode of description is in order.

One possibility is the formalism of fractal geometry. Since the concepts of fractal geometry were introduced in the mid-1970's (Mandelbrot, 1982), they have contributed significantly to many areas of the arts and sciences. Much effort has been directed toward the generation of natural-looking scenes (so-called 'fractal forgeries'; Voss, 1985; Pietgen and Richter, 1986). Less effort has been directed to the analytic use of fractal geometry on real images. Strategies for measuring the *D* of images have been slow to develop and difficult to implement on computers or image processors and analyzers. Although the concepts of fractal geometry have been used in basic research (Rigaut, 1984; Morse et al., 1985; Stanley and Ostrowsky, 1985; Damme et

Correspondence: T.G. Smith, Laboratory of Neurophysiology, NINDS, National Institutes of Health, Building 36, Room 2602, Bethesda, MD 20892, U.S.A.

al., 1986; Rigaut et al., 1987; Sernetz et al., 1988) the main use of fractal geometry in morphometry has been in the area of fine-particle and powder technology (Flook, 1978; Kaye, 1978, 1984, 1985, 1987).

The basic concepts of fractal geometry hold that we do not live in a Euclidian world of points, straight lines, rectangles and cubes, except as largely created by man. Natural objects are often rough and are not well described by the ideal constructs of Euclidian geometry. In many cases, the natural roughening processes work over a wide range of scales: craters may have smaller craters, etc. Thus, an important defining characteristic of fractal geometry is the property of 'self-similarity'. Fractal images are similar, in a statistical sense, at all levels of magnification or scale. As a fractal image is viewed at higher and higher magnifications, the amount of detail is constant. This is equivalent to stating that any measured length is proportional to the resolvable length raised to a power. This exponent is zero for a Euclidian line and -1 for a Euclidian surface. D is equal to 1 minus this exponent. D is called the fractal dimension: *fractal* because it is not necessarily an integer, and *dimension* because it has the property described above that the 'measure', or 'size' of a set of points, is proportional to length to a power of D, a property of dimensionality, as in volume $=$ length^3 (Mandelbrot, 1982, p. 36).

In principle, a theoretical or mathematically generated fractal is self-similar over an infinite range of scales. Natural fractal images, however, have a limited range of self-similarity. With real-world objects the range is usually between two and four decades (Peitgen and Richter, 1986). On the other hand, in some instances the D of a natural object can change with changes of scale. Kaye (1984, 1985; see also Rigaut, 1984) has found that analysis of carbon-black particles with Richardson plots (see Methods) can yield as many as 3 distinct slopes. The two regions of highest slope represent different aspects of the ruggedness of these particles, while the third, with the smallest rulers, converges to a slope of zero ($D = 1$). This zero slope measures the circular outlines of the basic spheres that comprise these particles and is, therefore, a topological or Euclidian dimension as well as a fractal dimension.

In the above formulation, ideal points still have a dimension of zero, ideal lines a dimension of one, perfectly flat planes dimensions of two, etc., just as they do in Euclidean geometry. However, collections of real points have dimensions greater than 0, real lines greater than 1, real surfaces greater than 2, etc. At each level, as the dimensions of an object move from one integer to the next, the complexity of the object increases; it becomes more area-filling from 1 to 2, more volume-filling from 2 to 3, etc.

Strategies have been developed for measuring the Ds of images (Flook, 1978, 1982; Kaye, 1978, 1984, 1985,

1987) and the purpose of this paper is to review and explain them. We have restricted the results to measurements of closed perimeters on flat surfaces, which have a D between one and two. In order to test these methods, we have used computer-generated fractal images based on the methods of Mandelbrot (1982). These are, for the most part, Koch triadic and quadric fractals (Mandelbrot, 1982, p. 34), as well as fractal 'rivers' (Mandelbrot, 1982 pp. 255–256). In the methods we shall discuss here, we have found it best to start with binary (Black = 0; White = 1) representations of the closed and unbroken edges of our images. Our constructed images are already binary. For natural gray scale objects we have discussed elsewhere (Smith et al., 1988) how we produce binary images using a modification of an edge-detecting algorithm developed by Marr and Hildreth (1980).

METHODS

Measurements using calipers ('TRA')

This method of determining the fractal dimension of a border is connoted in Richardson's classical problem of the measurement of the length of the coastline of Great Britain (Mandelbrot, 1982). One finds that the coastline length is a function of the span of the caliper employed in the measurement. That is, the length does not converge to a stable value. Therefore, if one plots the logarithm of the coastline length vs. the logarithm of the ruler length, one obtains a straight line over at least part of the plot. Thus, the coastline is self-similar over a limited range of scale. The slope, S, of that line is related to the fractal dimension by $D = 1 - S$.

We have automated the measurement of border length to produce a file of X, Y coordinates. The file is scanned along the border, in a clock-wise manner, until a point is found whose vector distance from the starting point is equal to the caliper span. Roundoff can be dealt with by small adjustments of the caliper span at each step. The procedure is continued until the border has been traversed. The perimeter $L(\epsilon)$ is given by $L(\epsilon) = \epsilon \times$ number of caliper spans.

This algorithm is repeated for a range of caliper spans (ϵ) and log $L(\epsilon)$ is plotted against log ϵ. Fig. 1A illustrates a Koch quadric island of $D = 1.50$ and Fig. 1B-TRA is a Richardson plot of log L vs. log ϵ. The measured $S = -0.48$; therefore, the estimated $D = 1.48$.

Pixel dilation method ('DIL')

This method of determining D was devised by Flook (1978) to study the profiles of rugged mineral particles and begins with a binary border-image of the particle. Our implementation of dilation is by a structuring element approximating a circle (Flook, 1978; Mandelbrot, 1982). Each pixel is replaced by a disc with a diameter

KOCH 1.50

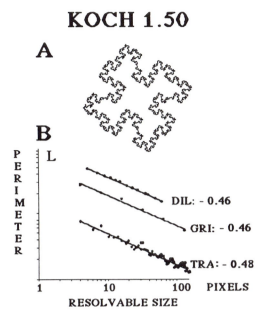

Fig. 1. A: Koch quadric island of fractal dimension 1.5 B: log-log plots of measurements taken on 'A' to determine fractal dimension with Dilation (DIL), Grid (GRI) and Trace (TRA) methods (see text). 'L' of ordinate equals perimeter length in arbitrary units. Abscissa equals resolvable length in pixels. Numbers to right of labels represent slopes (S). Estimated fractal Dimension (D) is given by $D = 1 - S$.

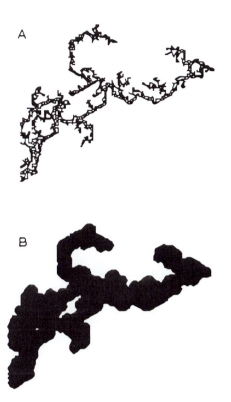

Fig. 2. A: artificial image generated by using Mandelbrot's (1982) rules for generating branching rivers (p. 255–6). B: Minkowski 'sausage' created by the application of Dilation method to A. The perimeter is calculated as the area of this figure divided by the diameter of the dilating disc.

varying from 3 to 61 pixels. In our image processor this operation is a convolution procedure. The effect of the method is to widen the border by widths E equal to the diameter. This reduces or 'filters' shape-details of size less than E. The length of the widened outline (Fig. 2 A, B), is estimated as its area A divided by its width E. (Minkowski, see Mandelbrot, 1982). The length decreases as E increases.

The lengths (A/E) are plotted against the diameters (E) on a log-log scale. The slope of the line (S) is related to D by $D = 1 - S$. Fig. 1B-DIL illustrates the Flook plot of the Koch island shown in Fig. 1A. The measured slope is –0.46 and estimated $D = 1.46$.

Tile-counting or mosaic-amalgamation methods ('Grid')

Voss (1985) has discussed this method as a good general technique for determining the fractal dimension of borders. The binary border-image to be analyzed is superimposed on a succession of square grids of increasing edge lengths. The number of 'tiles' in the grid that the border contacts are counted. A tile is counted only once if it is encountered by the border, irrespective of the number of pixels that encounter it. Then, the log of the number of tiles encountered is plotted against the log of the tile edge length. As before, $D = 1 - S$. Fig. 1B-GRI illustrates the result of this method when applied to Fig. 1A; D is estimated at 1.46.

In summary, we have adopted or modified methods which give estimates of fractal dimension of images that are binary silhouettes or closed border-images lying in a flat plane; i.e. they have a D between one and two. We have tested and calibrated these methods with thirteen computer-generated images of known D. These Koch and river images were generated by methods discussed by Mandelbrot (1982, p. 34, p. 225).

Fig. 3A tabulates fractal dimensions used to construct the different, test fractal images of known D (CON). The D's obtained when measuring these images with Dilate (DIL), Grid (GRI) and Trace (TRA) are also tabulated. In Fig. 3B we plot the constructed values on the abscissa and the measured values on the ordinate for each of the methods. The scatter of the Koch plots is caused by their periodicity. The river plots avoid this by their random method of construction, but this introduces scatter. Thus, the estimated D of the constructed figures may deviate somewhat from their nominal values.

With more experience, one of the measures may ultimately prove superior. Since the methods may be measuring somewhat different properties related to the fractal dimension of the structures, it is not legitimate to average them. Instead we often examine the

176

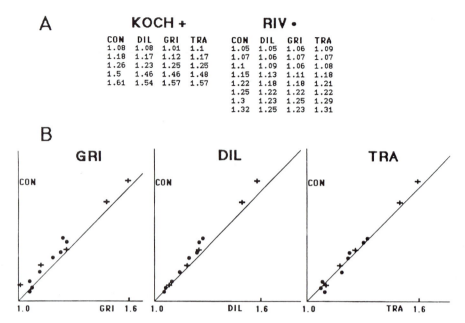

Fig. 3. A: columns CON show the nominal fractal dimension of computer constructed Koch and river fractal images. Columns DIL, GRI, and TRA show fractal dimensions estimated by the Dilate, Grid and Trace methods, respectively. B: plots of the numbers in A. Estimates by Grid, Dilate and Trace plotted horizontally against constructed values vertically. Estimates of Koch islands: +; of rivers: '·'. The lines have the ideal slope of one.

curves from our three methods and chose a value of D from one or more of them.

Biological methods

The 27 neurons studied in this research were vertebrate CNS neurons grown in cell culture. Each had been injected with horseradish peroxidase via a micropipette, so as to increase its contrast over other, background neurons and other structures (Neale et al. 1978). After fixation, enzyme development and embedding in plastic, the cells were visualized with an inverted brightfield light-microscope. Images of the cells were collected on a video camera, digitized and analyzed with an image processor. Binary silhouettes of the neurons were obtained by using a modified Marr-Hildreth filtering–convolution scheme (Marr and Hildreth, 1980; Smith et al., 1982). Details of the microscope, image processor etc. have been reported elsewhere (Smith et al., 1982).

RESULTS

The 3 methods (Trace, Dilate and Grid) yielded consistent results when applied to constructed fractal images of known dimension. Similar results were also found with a few of the 27 neurons studied here. More typically, however, we find that Dilate and Grid give straight lines over a range of values on the Richardson

plots (DIL and GRI in Fig. 4B). The Trace plots are usually curved and have no clear straight line slope (TRA in Fig. 4B). Therefore, the results reported here are limited to those from the Grid and Dilate methods.

While the results of the two methods closely agreed in value on each of the individual neurons, the D's of the group varied between 1.14 and 1.60. A typical result is illustrated in Fig. 4. Fig. 4A shows a silhouette of the neuron, while Fig. 4B illustrates the Richardson plots. If the plot results in a straight line, then the image is 'fractal' over that span of dimension. As can be seen in Fig. 4, the slope is constant over about two orders of magnitude and a value of D = 1.30 to 1.33. Similar fits of data to a straight line were obtained with the other neurons with slopes of −0.14 to −0.60. Fig. 5 illustrates examples of border silhouettes of those neurons with a line drawn from them to their D value on the D-axis.

DISCUSSION

It is apparent in Fig. 5 that as the neuronal shape progresses from relatively simple (A, B) to more complex (C–H), the value of D increases. It is also clear that while neurons with similar D's (C and D) may appear similar in structure, this is not always the case (cf. G and H). This raises the question of what aspect of the cell's 'complexity' is the D actually 'measuring'? From

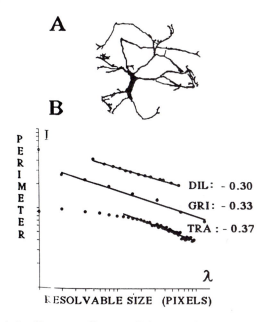

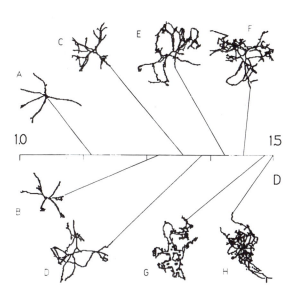

Fig. 4. A: silhouette of horseradish peroxidase injected spinal cord neuron which has been grown in tissue culture. B: log–log Richardson plots of data obtained by the Dilation (DIL), Grid (GRI) and Trace (TRA) methods of determining fractal dimension (see text). '*L*' of ordinate equals perimeter length. 'λ' of abscissa equals resolvable length in pixels. The numbers represent the slopes (*S*) of the lines. The fractal dimension (*D*) is given by $D = 1 - S$.

Fig. 5. Composite of typical border silhouettes (A–H) of neurons studies. A line connects each silhouette to its *D* value on the *D* axis. See text.

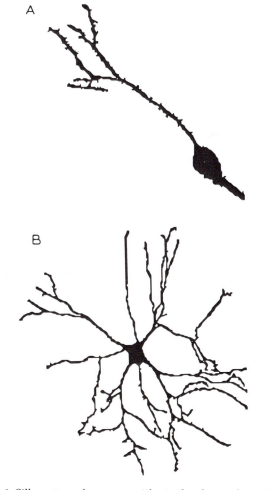

studies we have undertaken on 'test' images, it appears that two important characteristics are the ruggedness of the border and the profusion of the dendritic branching, with *D* increasing as these increase. These two characteristics seem to represent complexity properties at the ends of a range of scales with no precise dividing line between them. Of course, a rugged border might appear branched at higher magnification and branches appear as ruggedness at lower magnification. This is consistent with the concept of self-similarity.

For any given neuron it is not entirely clear whether one or the other or both of these (or other) factors are contributing to *D*. We have found examples, however, where each appears dominant. The two cells illustrated in Fig. 6 have similar, small *D*'s but it would appear that border ruggedness contributes more to *D* than dendritic branching in A, while the opposite is true in B. Similar results for cells with large *D*'s are shown in Fig. 7. Clearly, therefore, *D* does not uniquely specify a cell's shape, nor was it expected to do so. It is, nonetheless, a quantitative, distinguishing characteristic that connotes the bounds of morphological possibilities. Finally, *D* may provide a quantitative dependent variable in experiments where an independent variable may be expected to affect neuronal morphological complexity.

Fig. 6. Silhouettes of neurons with similar, low values of *D*. Complexity of A is due to rugged border, while that of B is from profuse branching.

178

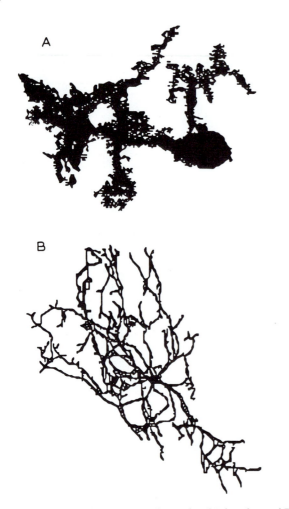

Fig. 7. Silhouettes of neurons with similar, high values of D. Complexity of A is due to rugged border, while that of B is from profuse branching.

We have demonstrated that the concepts of fractal geometry can be applied to neuronal morphology and that fractal dimension of a neuronal border may be a useful descriptor of a cell's complexity. The question of how useful may be estimated by comparing D with other quantitative measures of complexity. One common measure of complexity used in stereology is the aspect ratio (perimeter^2/area) (Russ, 1986). The correlation coefficient of the log of aspect ratios of the 27 neurons with the D's of those neurons is 0.68. This suggests that there is some correlation between what they are measuring, at least part of which is complexity.

Other, psychological studies have shown that there is a high degree of correlation between fractal dimension and the perceived complexity by human subjects (Cutting and Garvin, 1987). Indeed, the fractal dimension correlated much better than most other quantitative methods of measuring complexity.

In the context of these results, it is legitimate to inquire into the utility and insights gained from knowing D. At the simplest level, a cell's D can be considered as a quantitative descriptor whose magnitude gives some 'feel' for its structural complexity. At the next level, D may be useful as a classifying variable. For example, it is not known whether all members of a cell type (e.g., Purkinje cells) have similar D's, what their variations are, or how their D's compare with other cell types.

There have been other areas of biology to which the concepts of fractal geometry have been applied with some utility (Bassingthwaighte, 1988). An intriguing question in this regard has been the relevance of these findings to physiological function. This has been partially determined in the areas of the cardiovascular (Bassingthwaighte, 1988) and pulmonary (Rigaut et al., 1987; West and Goldberger, 1987) systems with respect to the flow of fluids. There has also been progress in studies of metabolism (Sernetz et al., 1985), field biology (Morse et al., 1985) and protein structure (Stapleton et al., 1980). The relevance of D to neuronal function is unknown at this time; however, a few suggestions may be offered. In general, it is known that the fractal dimension '. . . provides some measure about how many relevant degrees of freedom are involved in the dynamics of the system under consideration. And naturally a system with many degrees of freedom is generally considered to be more complex than one with only a few degrees of freedom' (Mayer-Kress, 1985, p. 2). The most obvious is that it is related to the growth of various forms of neuronal structure. Fractal dimension is possibly a reflection of the degree of synaptic connectivity, i.e., the greater the irregularity of the border, the greater the opportunity for synaptic contacts. Finally, it might represent some aspect of the flow of intracellular material or the spread of membrane potential in time and space over the somatic-dendritic surface.

Perhaps the most important practical aspect of fractal dimension may be its use as a quantitative variable, which morphologists can study as a dependent variable in the context of many independent variables. Consider an experiment where the question is the nature of the increase in complexity with cellular maturation. It is generally known that neuronal structure becomes more complex with development, but the question is how? By plotting D as a function of time, one may be able to determine the functional relationship between age and complexity.

While fractal dimension alone does not completely specify a cell's morphology, it, in combination with other measures, may contribute to the development of a new branch of science that might be called 'quantitative cellular morphometry'.

In conclusion, this paper may be looked upon as the provision of a set of tools employed to measure the complexity of cellular structure. These techniques are generalizable to two and three dimensional spaces to investigate surfaces and volumes of cellular structural complexity.

REFERENCES

Bassingthwaighte, J.B. (1988) Physiological heterogeneity: fractals link determinism and randomness in structures and functions. News Physiol. Sci., 3: 5–10.

Cutting, J.E. and Garvin, J.J. (1987) Fractal curves and complexity, Percept, Psychophys., 42: 365–370.

Damme, H.V., Oberecht, F., Levitz, P., Gatineau, L. and Laroche, C. (1986) Fractal viscous fingering in clay slurries, Nature (London), 320: 731–733.

Flook, A.G. (1978) The use of dilation logic on the quantimet to achieve fractal dimension characterisation of textured and structured profiles, Powder Technol., 21: 295–298.

Flook, A.G. (1982) Fractal dimensions: their evaluation and significance in stereological measurements, Acta Stereol., 1: 79.

Kaye, B.H. (1978) Specification of the ruggedness and/or texture of a fine-particle profile by its fractal dimension, Powder Technol., 21: 1–16.

Kaye, B.H. (1984) Multifractal description of a rugged fine-particle profile, Part. Charact., 1: 14–21.

Kaye, B.H. (1985) Applications of recent advances in fine-particle characterization to mineral processing, Part. Charact., 2: 91–97.

Kaye, B.H. (1987) Fractal dimension and signature waveform characterization of fine-particle shape, Am. Lab., 19: 55–63.

Mandelbrot, B.B. (1982) The Fractal Geometry of Nature, Freeman, New York.

Marr, D. and Hildreth, E. (1980) Theory of edge detection, Proc. Roy. Soc. Lond., B, 207: 187–217.

Mayer-Kress, G. (1985) Introductory remarks. In G. Mayer-Kress (Ed.), Dimensions and Entropies in Chaotic Systems, Springer, New York.

Morse, D.R., Lawton, J.H., Dodson, M.M. and Williamson, M.H. (1985) Fractal dimension of vegetation and the distribution of arthropod body lengths, Nature (Lond.), 314: 731–733.

Neale, E.A., Macdonald, R.L. and Nelson, P.G. (1978) Intracellular horseradish peroxidase injection for correlation of light and electron microscopic anatomy with synaptic physiology of cultured mouse spinal cord neurons, Brain Res., 152: 265–282.

Peitgen, H.O. and Richter, P.H. (1986) The Beauty of Fractals, Springer, New York.

Rall, W. (1985) Time-constants and electrotonic length of membrane cylinders and neurons, Biophys. J., 9: 1483–1508.

Rigaut, J.P. (1984) An empirical formulation relating boundary lengths to resolution in specimens showing 'non-ideally fractal' dimensions, J. Microsc., 133: 41–54.

Rigaut, J.P., Berggren, P. and Robertson, B. (1987) Stereology, fractals and semifractals: the lung alveolar structure studied through a new model, Acta Stereol., 6: 63–67.

Russ, J.C. (1986) Practical Stereology, Plenum Press, New York.

Sernetz, M., Gelle'ri, B. and Hoffman, J. (1985) The organism as bioreactor. Interpretation of the reduction law of metabolism in terms of heterogeneous catalysis and fractal structure, J. Theor. Biol., 117: 209–230.

Sernetz, M., Bittner, H.R. and Wlczek, P. (1988) Fraktale biologische Strukturen-Bildanalyse und Bildsynthese, Spiegel Forsch., 5: 8–11.

Smith, Jr. T.G., Marks, W.B., Lange, G.D., Sheriff, Jr. W.H. and Neale, E.A. (1988) Edge detection in images using Marr-Hildreth filtering techniques, J. Neurosci. Methods, 26: 75–82.

Stanley, H.E. and Ostrowsky, N. (Eds.) (1985) On Growth and Form, Nijhoff, Amsterdam.

Stapleton, H.J., Allen, J.P., Flynn, C.P., Stinson, D.G. and Kurtz, S.R. (1980) Fractal form of proteins, Phys. Rev. Lett., 45: 1456–1459.

Voss, R.F. (1985) Random fractal forgeries. In: R.A. Earnshaw (Ed.), Fundamental Algorithms for Computer Graphics. NATO ASI Series, Vol. F17, 805–835, Springer, Berlin.

West, B.J. and Goldberger, A.L. (1987) Physiology in fractal dimensions, Am. Sci., 75: 354–365.

brief review

Applications of fractal analysis to physiology

ROBB W. GLENNY, H. THOMAS ROBERTSON, STANLEY YAMASHIRO,
AND JAMES B. BASSINGTHWAIGHTE
*Department of Medicine and Center for Bioengineering, University of Washington,
Seattle, Washington 98195*

GLENNY, ROBB W., H. THOMAS ROBERTSON, STANLEY YAMASHIRO, AND JAMES B. BASSINGTHWAIGHTE. *Applications of fractal analysis to physiology.* J. Appl. Physiol. 70(6): 2351–2367, 1991.—This review describes approaches to the analysis of fractal properties of physiological observations. Fractals are useful to describe the natural irregularity of physiological systems because their irregularity is not truly random and can be demonstrated to have spatial or temporal correlation. The concepts of fractal analysis are introduced from intuitive, visual, and mathematical perspectives. The regional heterogeneities of pulmonary and myocardial flows are discussed as applications of spatial fractal analysis, and methods for estimating a fractal dimension from physiological data are presented. Although the methods used for fractal analyses of physiological data are still under development and will require additional validation, they appear to have great potential for the study of physiology at scales of resolution ranging from the microcirculation to the intact organism.

mathematical analysis; heterogeneity; spatial correlation; temporal correlation; microcirculation; morphology; blood flow distribution

THE INTENT OF THIS REVIEW is to provide physiologists with the basic tools for working with fractals, by use of intuitive, visual, and formal mathematical definitions of the concepts of fractal geometry, self-similarity, scale independence, and fractal dimensions. Although the concepts underlying fractals are new, mathematical sophistication is not a prerequisite for a working knowledge of fractal applications. Applications of fractal analysis in physiology will be reviewed with examples from pulmonary morphology, pulmonary and cardiovascular circulation, and time-dependent analysis of physiological measurements. APPENDICES A and B include a glossary of terms and variables, a listing of the equations, and an illustrative analysis of a simple data set.

Fractal analysis is still in the formative stages of development, and its ultimate importance as an investigative tool in physiology is not fully established. Nevertheless, it is providing new perspectives into the physiology of cells, organs, and intact organisms, with mathematical models of branching structures and with descriptors of spatial and temporal correlation. The robust descriptive properties of this approach in the analysis of physiological variability suggest that it may signal the development of a new paradigm (16) compelling the attention of investigators from diverse areas of physiological inquiry.

Self-Similarity and Fractal Dimensions

A fractal structure or fractal process can be loosely defined as having a characteristic form that remains constant over a magnitude of scales. A structure is fractal if its small-scale form appears similar to its large-scale form. Similarly, a process is fractal if a variable as a function of time undergoes characteristic changes that are similar regardless of the time interval over which the observations are made. In the parlance of fractal analysis, this is the quality of self-similarity, also termed scale independence. Because fractal analysis is not a familiar tool to most physiological investigators, we will systematically develop these principal definitions and concepts. Concurrently we will derive numerical methods to determine whether a structure or process is fractal and to estimate a fractal dimension.

The Koch curve (Fig. 1), created by the Swedish mathematician Helge von Koch in 1904, is a fractal structure that provides a simple introduction to the concepts of self-similarity and fractal dimensions. This curve is defined by the following iterative transformations. Beginning with a straight line of length l_0 (Fig. 1, top line), the middle third of the line is replaced with two segments of length $1/3\ l_0$, forming part of an equilateral

2352

triangle (Fig. 1, second line). The next iteration repeats the same procedure on each of the four resultant straight-line segments. Subsequent generations are formed in an identical fashion, and the completed figure represents the infinite expression of this iterative procedure. The completed Koch curve exemplifies the properties of self-similarity because, regardless of the scale used to examine any portion of the Koch curve, it maintains its characteristic form.

Examples of self-similar structures abound in the natural world. A tree maintains a quality of self-similarity independent of the perspective or scale from which it is viewed. The branching angles and proportionate diameters of branches appear to remain constant regardless of whether we are looking at the main trunk or the terminal branches. Clouds are fractal, with each billowing appendage similar in form to its entirety. In fact, without a reference scale, it is not possible to estimate the size of a cloud from a photograph (4). The classic example of fractal structures is a coastline, which appears to maintain the same degree of irregularity regardless of the size or detail of the map studied (23).

The bronchial tree can be visualized as a fractal structure, the final form of which is generated by an iterative process akin to that described above for the Koch curve (8, 24, 28, 42). The primordial lung bud initially under-

goes a bifurcation to form the right and left bronchi, and subsequent generations are formed by a repetitive bifurcation of the most distal airways (18). In this manner, a dichotomously branching network is produced, filling the available space. In his initial description of potential fractal structures in nature, Mandelbrot (24) described a simple rectangular branching algorithm that bore a striking resemblance to the bronchial tree (Fig. 2, *left*). Since that first model, more realistic two-dimensional iterative transformation algorithms have been implemented on computers to simulate the growth and geometry of the bronchial tree (29). All these models exhibit the necessary quality of self-similarity to be deemed fractal, in that each generation appears similar to previous generations, regardless of the level of bifurcation examined.

Contour-measuring method. A second principle of fractal structures and processes is a corollary of self-similarity: because the underlying form of a structure or process remains similar through successive magnifications of scale, it follows that a measured length of its form cannot approach a limit. Remembering the Koch curve, we can expand indefinitely the set of segments that contributes to its length. Although this property is a necessary requirement for a structure or process to be fractal in a strict mathematical sense, it is possible to discuss fractal properties of natural objects over a limited range of scales.

The Koch curve (Fig. 3, *left*) is a good model to formally examine the characteristic of the scale-dependent length of fractal structures. Because of its jaggedness, the apparent length $[L(l)]$ of the curve will be dependent on the length (l) of the measuring device chosen. If we use a stick of length l_0, equal to the straight-line distance from one end to the other of the curve, none of the protruding structures will be measured and the apparent length of the entire line is l_0. If the measuring stick length l is decreased to $1/3\, l_0$ and then $1/9\, l_0$, the apparent contour length increases to $4/3\, l_0$ and $16/9\, l_0$, respectively. Generalizing this process for n iterations and a measuring stick of length $l = (1/3)^n l_0$, the corresponding measured length would be $(4/3)^n l_0$. Therefore, as l becomes infinitely small, or as $n \rightarrow \infty$, the apparent contour length of the Koch curve becomes infinite. As increasing magnification reveals more detail, the overall appearance of the new segment examined remains similar to that of the previous segment.

Mandelbrot (23) derived an "exponent of similarity," which he later renamed the fractal dimension (D), to characterize the complexity of fractal figures. D can be related to the Euclidean dimension (E). A line segment of $E = 1$ can be cut into N identical pieces. The ratio of the piece lengths (l) to l_0 is $l/l_0 = N^{-(1/1)}$. A square of $E = 2$ can be partitioned into N identical squares, and in an analogous fashion the ratio of the side lengths of the smaller squares to the initial square will be expressed by $l/l_0 = N^{-(1/2)}$. By the same process, a solid divided into N identical cubes will have side lengths that are scaled down from the original by a factor $l/l_0 = N^{-(1/3)}$. In each case, the ratio of the lengths is scaled down by $l/l_0 = N^{-(1/E)}$, where E represents the Euclidean dimension of the subdividing unit.

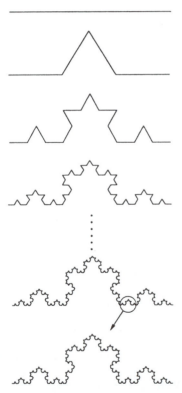

FIG. 1. Generation of Koch curve produced by a simple iterative transformation beginning with a straight line (*top*). At each step, middle third of each line segment is replaced with 2 segments, one-third of the length of the line, forming part of an equilateral triangle. Completed curve has an infinite number of iterations. Regardless of magnification of scale, any part of the curve resembles the whole (*bottom*). [From Glenny and Robertson (5).]

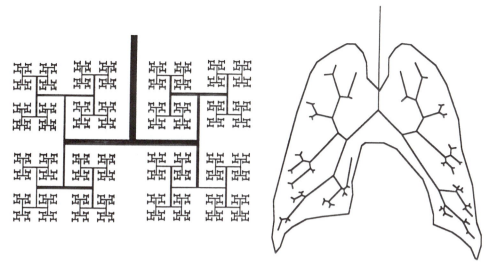

FIG. 2. Two-dimensional representations of bronchial tree. *Left*: symmetrical bifurcating network with 90° branching angles and length segments scaled proportionally from parent branch (similar to Mandelbrot's model of the lung). *Right*: more realistic model in which branching segments fill a predetermined boundary. [From Nelson and Manchester (29).]

Similarly, a fractal figure will have a constant relationship between the number of pieces into which the figure is cut (N) and the ratio of the piece length to the total length measured at that particular choice of l, expressed again by

$$\frac{l}{l_0} = N^{-(1/D)} \qquad (1)$$

where in this instance D is a fractal dimension (39). If N is expressed as $[L(l)/l]/[L(l_0)/l_0]$ in *Eq. 1* and both sides of the equation are raised to the D power, *Eq. 1* can be rewritten as $(l_0/l)^D = [L(l)/l]/[L(l_0)/l_0]$ or

$$\frac{L(l)}{L(l_0)} = \left(\frac{l}{l_0}\right)^{1-D} \qquad (2)$$

For the Koch curve, in which $L(l)/L(l_0) = 4/3$ and $l/l_0 = 1/3$ for each iteration, D can be determined by substitution and solving the equation $1 - D = \ln(4/3)/\ln(1/3)$. The Koch curve therefore has a D = $\ln(4)/\ln(3) = 1.261$. . . . Unlike E, D is not usually an integer, but a fractal structure will always have a dimension equal to or less than the space in which the structure is defined (D < E).

Taking the logarithm of both sides of *Eq. 2* and rearranging the terms yields

$$\ln L(l) = (1 - D) \ln\left(\frac{l}{l_0}\right) + \ln L(l_0) \qquad (3)$$

In this form, a log-log plot of $L(l)$ vs. l/l_0 produces a line with a slope of $(1 - D)$ and an intercept of $\ln[L(l_0)]$. Figure 3, *right*, shows such a plot for the Koch curve, demonstrating a slope of -0.261 . . . or D = 1.261. . . . The value of the intercept is dependent on the arbitrary choice of l_0 and does not affect the determination of D. *Equation 3* thus provides a working definition of a fractal process or structure. A process or object may be fractal if

the logarithm of the measured value is linearly related to the logarithm of the scale of measurement. D is 1.0 minus the slope of this linear relationship.

An intuitive grasp of the meaning of a fractal dimension can be obtained from examination of some different fractal figures. A straight line has properties of self-similarity, in that at higher and higher resolutions it continues to show its same straight shape. It has a topological, fractal, and Euclidean dimension of 1. For different fractal line algorithms generated in two space, a topological dimension of 1 and a Euclidean dimension of 2 are maintained, but the more complex line figures have progressively increasing fractal dimensions. When the line becomes so complex that it nearly fills the plane, D_s approaches 2.0. Figure 4 illustrates some fractal curves that are iteratively produced by different rules, yielding different fractal dimensions (38). Even at the limited level of iteration illustrated in Fig. 4 the curves with higher fractal dimensions are more space filling. The fractal dimension therefore serves as a measure of complexity that is independent of the scale of magnification. As we will show later, this measurement of complexity can be used to characterize physiological structures and processes that have fractal properties.

Objects described by Euclidean geometry are not fractal. For example, a semicircle has no repeating characteristic form at different scales of inspection. Application of the contour-measuring method described for the Koch curve to the semicircle (Fig. 5, *left*) demonstrates that a semicircle is not fractal. For an initial measuring stick of l_0, if the distance around the semicircle is cut in half at each iteration (n), the apparent contour of the semicircle, $L(n)$, is dependent on n by the relationship

$$L(n) = l_0 / [\prod_{i=1}^{n} \cos(\pi/2^{i+1})]$$

As $n \rightarrow \infty$, $L(n) \rightarrow \pi l_0/2$. Hence the semicircle is not fractal because its length approaches a limit as the scale

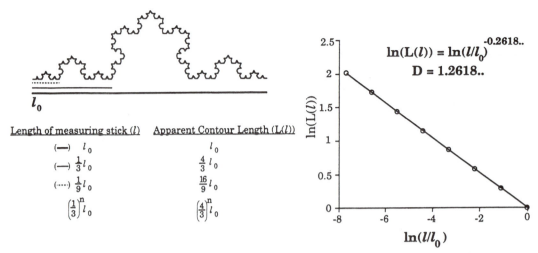

FIG. 3. Apparent contour length of Koch curve is dependent on length of measuring stick. *Left*: the finer the scale (greater magnification), the greater the apparent length of the curve. *Right*: fractal (log-log) plot of apparent length, $L(l)$, of Koch curve as a function length of measuring device, l relative to l_0. Line through points represents least-squares linear regression fit. Relationship appears linear with a slope of $-0.2618\ldots$ and thus a fractal dimension (D) of $1.2618.\ldots$

of measurement decreases. Applying the log-log plot of contour length vs. measuring stick length (see Fig. 3) to the example of the semicircle shows that the slope of the plot rapidly approaches zero and therefore is not fractal (Fig. 5, *right*).

A measuring stick of length $(1/3)^n l_0$ was initially chosen to measure the Koch curve because it produces easily

Topological Dimension		Fractal Dimension
1	————————	1.0
1		1.26
1		1.50
1		1.82

FIG. 4. Lines of topological *dimension 1* with different fractal dimensions. Fractal dimension is bounded by topological dimension and Euclidean dimension (in this case, *dimensions 1* and *2*). The greater the irregularity of the line, or the more space it fills, the greater the fractal dimension. [From Glenny and Robertson (5).]

analyzed contour lengths. Another choice of measuring stick length would have been $(1/3)^{(n-1/2)}l_0$, which produces apparent contour lengths of $4^{(n-1/2)}l_0$ and D = $1.262.\ldots$ A less optimal choice of measuring stick length yields a less accurate estimate of D. For example, measuring stick lengths of $(1/2)^n l_0$ and $(2/3)^n l_0$ produce estimated D of $1.216\ldots$ and $1.262\ldots$, respectively. Figure 6 demonstrates the measurements on a Koch curve obtained from a stick length of $(2/3)^n l_0$, with the results plotted on a log-log plot as was done in Fig. 3. Note that, particularly at the larger stick lengths, more scatter is produced if only the first eight measurements of the apparent contour length are utilized. The least-squares estimate of D is accordingly incorrect, although it is apparent that this error will become less important if the measurements are continued with smaller measuring sticks. If finer measurements are made with smaller measuring stick lengths, the estimate of D will approach the theoretical D of $1.262.\ldots$

The accuracy of the measured contour length of a fractal line improves as the measuring stick gets smaller. The best estimate of D therefore should be determined from the measurements obtained using the smaller measurement segments, particularly in those circumstances where the optimal length of subdivision of the measuring stick is not known. Thus when working with experimental data, there is a rationale for excluding those measurements that were obtained using the largest measuring sticks and then fitting a least-squares regression line to the log-log plot of $L(l)$ vs. l/l_0. This approach ignores the information present in the larger measurements. Another approach is to fit a weighted least-squares linear regression to the entire data set. By weighting those measurements obtained using the smaller measuring sticks more heavily, a better estimate of D is obtained.

The confidence in an estimated value of D is dependent on the fit of the data to the regression line and the number of data points determining the line. Increasing

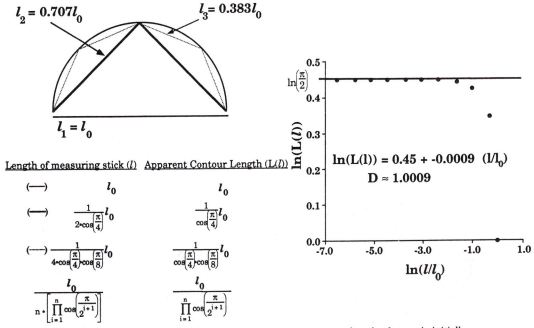

FIG. 5. Fractal analysis of a semicircle, which is not fractal. *Left*: apparent contour length of curve is initially determined by a measuring stick of length l_0 equal to diameter of semicircle. Measuring stick is then repeatedly shortened so that at each iteration (n) it bisects distance around curve between prior cords. Apparent length of curve, $L(l)$, at each iteration can be determined, and as n increases, $L(l)$ goes to $\pi l_0/2$. *Right*: fractal plot of $L(l)$ as a function of length of measuring stick, l relative to l_0. Line represents weighted least-squares fit to data; slope of this line is -0.0009.

the number of observations will improve the estimate of D by decreasing the variability in the measurement as the scale of measurement decreases. A statistical description of our confidence in the slope of the regression line can be determined from the standard deviation (SD) from the regression and arbitrary confidence intervals. The SD from the regression will actually be underestimated in these analyses because the observations are not independent of each other. When a measuring stick

length of $(1/3)^n l_0$ is used to measure the Koch curve as in Fig. 3, *right*, we are certain that the slope of this line is -0.262 because of the perfect fit of the data to the line. However, we are only 95% confident that the slope of the line in Fig. 6 lies between -0.365 and -0.165 and that D is between 1.165 and 1.365. These issues emphasize two important points about the experimental estimation of D. First, even for measurements on theoretically constructed fractal figures, the estimate of D is dependent on measurement sampling. Second, the confidence in the estimate of D can be strengthened by increasing the number of measurements obtained or using the optimal measuring stick, which decreases the variation of the measurements.

Finally in any real system, there will be measurement error, and this error will become more troublesome at the smaller measuring stick lengths. The effect of random noise superimposed on a fractal signal is to reduce the correlation. How this affects the estimate of D depends on the noise characteristics.

A relatively good linear fit between a variable and a measuring scale length on a log-log plot is not adequate proof that the variability of a process is explained only by its fractal properties. Such an observation does not exclude other nonfractal models, and it cannot establish whether a fractal model is better than any other. It is also important to recognize that a nonlinear relationship between two variables on a log-log plot does not prove that the relationship is not fractal. As shown in Fig. 6, a poor choice of measuring stick lengths or scale of measurements for a fractal structure may produce observations that do not appear linear. Rigaut (32) has proposed an

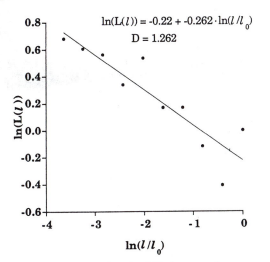

FIG. 6. Apparent contour length of Koch curve where measuring stick, l, is two-thirds the length of previous measuring stick. Linear fit to log-log data of apparent contour length $L(l)$ as a function of measuring stick length is not as good as in Fig. 3 (*right*), where a different measuring stick length was used.

2356

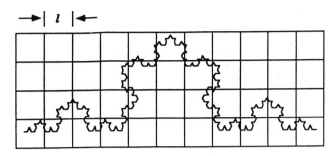

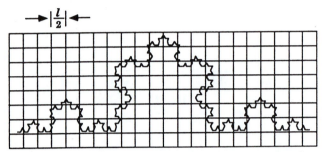

FIG. 7. Box or grid approach to determining fractal dimension of an object. Number of boxes containing a portion of curve, $N_{box}(l)$, is determined for progressively smaller box dimensions, l. *Top:* $N_{box}(l) = 23$ of the 44 boxes. *Bottom:* when l is decreased by one-half, $N_{box}(l/2) = 56$ of the 176 boxes. Fractal dimension can be determined from log-log plot of $N_{box}(l)$ as a function of l.

alternative method for determining the D of log-log plots that are not linear. When the log-log plot is linear, Rigaut's method provides the same D as the least-squares regression method. However, if the line is curved, Rigaut's approach invokes a continuum of D values. The utility of his approach needs further exploration.

Box-counting method. Other methods for determining D use similar iterative scaling algorithms. A common method is the box or grid approach in which a fractal figure is covered with a grid or boxes of side length l (Fig. 7) and the number of boxes in which part of the figure is present is $N_{box}(l)$. By use of this technique, D can be determined from the slope of the log-log plot of $N_{box}(l)$ as a function of l. The advantage of this approach is that it can be efficiently coded as a computer algorithm and adapted to measure objects or processes in multiple (Euclidean) dimensions (20a). In practice, as was apparent with the measuring stick method, it is useful to examine as large a range of l as possible and to average D over a number of different placements of the grid or boxes (39). D is again usually determined from the slope of a log-log plot (L. S. Liebovitch and T. I. Toth, unpublished observations). The boxes do not have to be arranged on the rectangular grid but can be slid to minimize the number of boxes used at each level. This will merely shift the position of the line on the log-log plot and will not affect the estimate of D. Using this approach to determine D for the Koch curve in Fig. 7 yields an estimate of 1.23. Although close, this estimate differs from the theoretical value of 1.261 . . . because only a finite number of boxes and sizes can be used to measure a line that has infinite length.

A strict mathematical definition of a fractal structure has been offered by Mandelbrot (24) as a set for which the Hausdorff-Besicovitch dimension strictly exceeds the topological dimension. It is impossible to apply this definition to a set of physiological measurements where the mathematical structure of the variable of interest is not known. We have therefore chosen to define a structure or process as potentially fractal if it maintains a characteristic form over many orders of magnitude of scale. A fractal structure or process can be tested for self-similarity by using the contour-measuring or box-counting method to determine whether there is a linear relationship obtained from *Eq. 3*. Although this definition cannot prove that a structure or process is fractal, it provides an estimate of D that can be used to characterize the irregularity or spatial and temporal correlation of a structure or process.

Although this approach using log-log plots provides an easily implemented means of testing whether a structure or process is fractal, uncertainties concerning the procedure remain. How sure are we that the structure or process is truly fractal as opposed to some other model such as an exponential decay process? There are not necessary and sufficient conditions to prove that the variability in real data sets is only fractal. A log-log linear relationship may be a necessary but insufficient requirement for some structures or processes to be characterized as fractal. Theoretical fractal structures have been described that have curved log-log plots, and the significance of this curvature and other nonlinear forms of these plots is not known. These issues are not resolved and will obviously be central to the future development of these approaches as a means of testing experimental hypotheses. Nevertheless, interesting preliminary results have been obtained in a number of physiological examples, as will be shown in subsequent sections.

Fractal Structures, Spatial Heterogeneity, and Spatial Correlation

Fractal analysis of morphology. Tree structures display self-similar characteristics, with their small-scale structures branching in a manner similar to their large-scale form. The mammalian bronchial and pulmonary vascular trees are richly arborizing structures that, despite their complexity, have a simple underlying order that spans many orders of magnitude in scale. A number of investigators have attempted to characterize this complexity and order in mathematical models with limited success. The self-similar nature of the bronchial and vascular trees suggests that fractal analysis may afford better mathematical models and provide some insight into their structure and morphogenesis.

Weibel and Gomez (41) used a simple exponential model to describe a unifying scaling relationship between the change in airway dimension and branch order. They collected morphometric data from casts of human lungs and found that an exponential relationship fit their data well up to the 10th generation but deviated significantly thereafter. The data of Weibel and Gomez have been reanalyzed by West et al. (42) using fractal analysis to show that their data can be better fit over the entire range of measurements by a fractal relationship between branch generation and branch diameter. Independent of scale or branch generation, the relationship of diameters between parent and daughter branches remains similar throughout all levels of the bronchial tree, demonstrating fractal properties of the airways. Fractal analysis in this particular example clearly provides a superior model in comparison to the original exponential model, inasmuch as the bronchial tree is more accurately represented over the entire range of the morphometric data.

Nelson and Manchester (29) have also used fractal analysis to explore the morphometric data obtained by others on the human airways. They used an approach similar to the contour-measuring method in which their scale of measurement was the average branch length at a given level of the tree and the contour length was the total branch length of all segments for that level. Using data from Horsfield and Cumming (11) and Raabe et al. (31), they estimated D to be 2.64 and 2.76, respectively. In their analysis, the bronchial tree was modeled as a stick figure with no volume (topological dimension of 1) filling a three-dimensional space (E = 3). D = 2.64 and 2.76 therefore appear to be appropriate, inasmuch as these values lie between the topological and Euclidean dimensions.

Self-similarity has been recognized within the topology of the bronchial and pulmonary vascular trees for some time (9, 12, 22, 34). Using topological branching and ordering schemes developed for geographical stream analysis (Strahler ordering), Horsfield has shown that the ratio of mean diameters and lengths between parent and daughter branches remains relatively constant throughout all generations of the bronchial and pulmonary vascular trees. Excluding the 3 initial generations of 17 total generations in a human pulmonary vascular tree, the mean ratio of diameters between parent and daughter branches was 1.60 with a SD of only 0.056 (9).

With the advent of fractal analysis, Horsfield has reanalyzed his own data and confirmed that the bronchial tree is fractal; with the diameter and lengths of branches related to the branch generation by a log-log relationship (10). He compared fractal analysis of the bronchial tree with an exponential fit and concluded that the differences in the models are due primarily to the ordering system used to identify the branch generations. He also compared his analysis with West's and noted a difference in the linearity of their fractal models. West and associates (42) noted a sinusoidal variation in their data about a linear log-log relationship between the generation and the branch diameter and introduced a variable with a harmonic oscillation to improve the fit of their data. On the other hand, Horsfield found that his data nicely fit a linear relationship between the generation and the branch diameter. Horsfield (9) again ascribed this difference to the ordering system used to identify branch generations. The Strahler ordering system used by Horsfield is believed to be more correct for asymmetrically branching trees, and the fact that the fractal model provides a better fit to this ordering scheme may be evidence for this assertion (22).

Another interesting observation from Horsfield's data (9) and from Nelson's analysis of bronchial tree morphometric data (28) is that the first three generations of the trees do not conform to the fractal pattern of the rest of the lung. This suggests that the initial branchings of the pulmonary vasculature and bronchial tree are either not fractal or may have a different fractal dimension. Recent embryologic observations by Massoud and associates (26) have demonstrated that in fact there are two different branching patterns in the rat fetal lung, peripheral and central. The central branches of the pulmonary bronchial tree exhibit monopodial branching, while the rest of the tree divides dichotomously. This does not mean that the initial branches of the bronchial tree are not fractal, but rather they may follow a different fractal pattern of growth with a different fractal dimension.

Nelson and Manchester (29) have applied the concepts of fractal growth patterns to the embryologic development of the pulmonary vascular tree. They have developed two-dimensional models to study the effects of boundaries that limit the growth of the vascular tree. They have shown that the development of the vascular tree can be modeled by fractal branching algorithms and boundaries that change as the embryo develops. These models develop strikingly realistic vascular patterns as shown in Fig. 2, *right*. With these models, simulations can be performed to study the effects of varying boundaries on developmental and morphologic structures (29). All these models are limited to two-dimensional space. More realistic models will have to branch into three dimensions. Although the computational effort will be greatly increased, the same fractal concepts that have been developed for two dimensions will be applicable to three dimensions.

Fractal structures are not confined to the pulmonary bronchial and vascular trees. Rigaut and associates (32) have used various magnifications and measuring lengths to estimate the boundary lengths of alveoli and found them to be fractal over a certain range. They also noted that their log-log plots of boundary lengths were not linear but tended to be convex upward. They interpreted this to show that the alveolar boundaries did not have a constant fractal dimension but rather what they termed a continuous fractal dimension transition (32). Fractal patterns have been used to characterize the complexity of neuronal cellular profiles (35). Smith and associates (35) used methods similar to the box-counting algorithm described above to characterize the contours of spinal cord neurons at different stages of maturity. They found that as the cells developed, they became more complex with D progressively increasing from 1.1 to 1.5. Sander (33) has shown that crystal growth patterns can be modeled and characterized by fractal analysis. In a process called diffusion-limited aggregation, a crystal starts as a seed point in the middle of a space. Particles are then introduced into the space and allowed to randomly move through the space until they touch the initial seed or a new part of the crystal. They stick to the crystal wherever they touch it and thus cause the crystal to grow. The structure of the resultant crystal can be characterized by fractal analysis. Other authors have used fractal growth

2358

patterns or diffusion-limited aggregation to describe the growth of the microvascular system (27, 36).

Fractal characterization of spatial heterogeneity using relative dispersion (RD) analysis. The observation that the vascular structures distributing flow to an organ are fractal suggests that the distribution of flow within the organ may be fractal as well. Although the small-scale variability in organ flow has been described as random, the branching structure of vascular anatomy suggests that regional flow is also best described by fractal measures. Heterogeneity of regional blood flow in an organ can be characterized by measuring the RD (SD/mean) of the regional flows when the organ is divided into a number of pieces. The observed RD is a sum of the spatial variation and the fluctuation of local flows over time (1, 3). When the distribution of flows is measured by a single rapid injection of a deposited flow marker, there is little contribution from the temporal fluctuations to the total heterogeneity.

When the heterogeneity of organ blood flow is characterized by this means, the calculated spatial RD (RD_s) is dependent on the size of the sampled pieces (1). If the blood flow in each of four pieces of an organ is measured, one can obtain the mean, SD, and hence RD of flow in the organ. If these same pieces are progressively subdivided, then for 8, 16, 32, 64, or more regions, the mean remains constant but the estimate of the SD and RD increases. Even after appropriate corrections for experimental error, the largest estimate of RD_s will be obtained from the finest subdivisions of the organ (1).

The heterogeneity of organ blood flow can be characterized independently of scale by employing fractal analysis (1, 3, 5). The fractal equation describing the RD of flows for a given spatial resolution (piece size) is given by rephrasing *Eq. 2*, using RD_s as a function of a volume of size v

$$\frac{RD_s(v)}{RD_s(v_0)} = \left(\frac{v}{v_0}\right)^{1-D_s} \tag{4}$$

Here $RD_s(v)$ is the measured relative dispersion when the organ is partitioned into regions of volume v, $RD_s(v_0)$ is the RD_s found for an arbitrarily chosen piece size, and D_s is the derived spatial fractal dimension. Multiplying both sides of *Eq. 4* by RD_s and taking the logarithms, we obtain

$$\ln RD_s(v) = (1 - D_s) \ln\left(\frac{v}{v_0}\right) + \ln RD_s(v_0) \tag{5}$$

If the slope of log $RD_s(v)$ vs. log (v/v_0) is constant over a range of partitions, the system is said to behave fractally within that range. The greater the rate of increase in observable heterogeneity with an increase in resolution, the greater is the fractal dimension. The fractal dimension therefore serves as a measure of the scale-independent irregularity, roughness, or variation of a system (1). An advantage of this analytic approach is that it provides an estimate of D_s from easily obtained measurements of the RD_s of regional organ flow during successive subdivisions of the tissue pieces down to v_0.

Although regional blood flow to an organ is distributed in three-dimensional space, when characterized as a RD, the heterogeneity of flow is one dimensional (1, 3, 5). The limits of RD_s that are imposed by the analytic procedure can be explored by inspecting the two extremes of blood flow distribution: uniform flow and randomly distributed flow. In the instance of complete homogeneity, $RD_s(v) = 0$. Solving for D_s in *Eq. 4* provides us with the lower boundary of 1.0 for D_s. For the case of random flow distribution, let there be distinct regions of flow that are distributed with a SD σ and mean μ. If the whole organ is partitioned into m pieces of volume $v_0 = v/m$, where v is the volume of the entire organ, the calculated $RD_s(m) = \sqrt{\sigma^2}/\mu$. If the organ had been divided into n larger pieces of volume, $v = m/n \cdot v_0$, $RD_s(n) = [\sqrt{(v_0/v) \cdot \sigma^2}]/\mu$, or $RD_s = (v/v_0)^{-1/2}(\sigma/\mu)$. Taking the logarithm of both sides yields the fractal form of the equation for a random flow distribution with a slope of −0.5 and thus a D_s of +1.5. In RD analysis a D_s of 1.0 indicates totally correlated magnitudes of flow between neighboring regions of the organ in that the flow is the same everywhere, while a D_s of +1.5 indicates that the magnitude of flow is uncorrelated or randomly distributed among neighboring pieces of the organ. D_s values ≥ 1.5 indicate inversely or negatively correlated flows.

Pulmonary blood flow distribution can be characterized by fractal methods (5). A composite fractal plot of the $RD_s(v)$ for six supine dogs is presented in Fig. 8. D_s for these animals ranged from 1.07 to 1.12 with an average of 1.09. The data fit the fractal model well, with an average correlation coefficient (r) of 0.98. It is interesting to note that the observed measures of RD_s appear to oscillate about the linear regression line. As discussed earlier, this may be due to the fact that the lung pieces (measuring stick) are not the proper shape or orientation for our measurement. The appropriate sectioning of the organ would be along the vascular tree, with regions of common

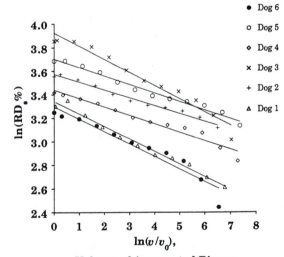

Volume of Aggregated Pieces

FIG. 8. Relative dispersion (RD) of regional pulmonary blood flows plotted as a function of volume of aggregated lung pieces. Smallest regions (v_0) are "voxels" from a planar gamma camera in which voxels are $1.5 \times 1.5 \times 11.5$ mm or 24 mm³. [From Glenny and Robertson (5).]

TABLE 1. *Spatial heterogeneity of cardiac blood flow and fractal dimensions for pulmonary blood flow*

	No. of Animals	D_s	Mean r_s
Baboon hearts	10	1.21 ± 0.04	0.49
Sheep hearts	11	1.17 ± 0.06	0.58
Rabbit hearts	6	1.25 ± 0.07	0.41
Dog lungs	6	1.09 ± 0.02	0.76

perfusion being grouped together. The data points shown in Fig. 8 do not include the first four subdivisions of the lungs, because those measurements are disproportionately smaller.

The heterogeneity of myocardial blood flow has been characterized by fractal analysis as well (2, 3). The distribution of radiolabeled microspheres to the heart was analyzed by progressively subdividing the heart into finer pieces. In this original application of the RD approach, regional flows were normalized to mass rather than to volume. The spatial heterogeneity of cardiac blood flow in baboons, sheep, and rabbits, as characterized by the fractal dimension, is shown in Table 1, along with the fractal dimensions for pulmonary blood flow in dogs. Although the number of pieces in the cardiac data sets is relatively small, the fractal dimensions are significantly different between some of the species and organs. This indicates that the spatial distribution of flow is different among these organs and suggests that this is necessary for their different functions or is due to dissimilar morphogenesis.

This comparison demonstrates an advantage of fractal analysis in that comparisons of measurements can be made between experiments, species, and laboratories, regardless of units or scales of measure. The heterogeneity of blood flow in the hearts of baboons and sheep measured by one technique can be compared with the heterogeneity of blood flow in dog lungs measured in another laboratory by use of very different methods.

Blood flow heterogeneity can be fractal only over a limited range. If smaller and smaller pieces are used to measure flow to a region of tissue, eventually the flows will become more similar as the anatomic limit of a capillary is reached (1). As long as heterogeneity is fractal, the log of RD_s will remain linear with respect to the log of the volume of pieces. However, as the functional unit of perfusion is approached with smaller piece sizes, RD will stabilize, causing a plateau in the fractal plot (1). Theoretically, fractal analysis could identify the size of the functional unit of flow in a lung by finding the piece size where there is an inflection in the slope of the fractal plot (1). The method we used to measure regional blood flow distributions could be used to examine 24-mm³ pieces of lung. No inflection point could be detected, suggesting that the unit of uniform perfusion is <24 mm³. However, registration error between the true vascular boundaries and the imposed partitioning may cause the plateau to be slurred and produce an underestimate of the size of the unit of perfusion (5).

Fractal analysis of spatial correlation. The measurement of spatial blood flow heterogeneity implies a mea-

sure of correlation as well. The fractal dimensions of regional pulmonary and myocardial blood flow indicate that flow is not randomly distributed but rather has some spatial organization. The spatial correlation of flow is a measure of the similarity of flow magnitudes between neighboring regions of the organ. This spatial correlation is apparent when the local blood flow distributions are examined in isogravitational lung slices (5), in that high-flow regions tend to be near areas of high flow and low-flow regions usually are adjacent to other low-flow areas. The RD method used to characterize the spatial heterogeneity of organ blood flow maintains spatial information by always aggregating nearest neighbors. Van Beek et al. (37) have shown that the spatial correlation of flows within an organ can be determined from D_s.

The relationship between the spatial correlation of blood flow and D_s can be ascertained by exploring the expected RD of flow to combined neighboring regions of an organ. If adjacent pieces, Y_1 and Y_2, are combined, the expected flow, $\overline{(Y_1 + Y_2)} = 2\mu$, and the variance of the aggregated regions, $Var(Y_1 + Y_2) = Var(Y_1) + Var(Y_2) + 2 Cov(Y_1, Y_2)$, where Cov is the covariance. Because $Var(Y_1) = Var(Y_2) = Var(Y)$ the RD of the combined pieces is

$$RD_s(Y_1 + Y_2) = \frac{1}{\sqrt{2}} \cdot \frac{\sqrt{Var(Y) + Cov(Y_1, Y_2)}}{\mu} \quad (6)$$

$RD_s(Y_1 + Y_2)$ can also be defined by the fractal *Eq. 4*

$$\frac{RD_s(Y_1 + Y_2)}{RD_s(Y)} = \left(\frac{Y_1 + Y_2}{Y}\right)^{1-D_s} = 2^{1-D_s} \quad (7)$$

If the correlation of flows between adjacent regions is the same correlation used for the linear regression of two

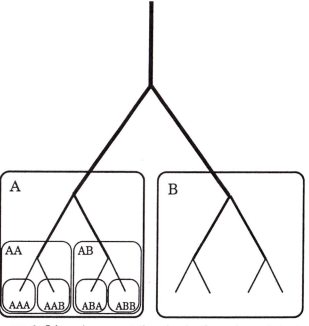

FIG. 9. Schematic representation of regional vascular perfusion to an organ. If blood flow distribution is fractal, then blood flow in adjacent pieces will have the same correlation regardless of size.

2360

variables, then the spatial correlation $r_s = \text{Cov}(Y_1, Y_2)/\text{Var}(Y)$. *Equations 6* and *7* can be rewritten in terms of r_s

$$r_s = 2^{3-2D_s} - 1 \qquad (8)$$

where D_s is bounded by 1.0 and 1.5.

As predicted by *Eq. 8*, a uniform blood flow distribution to neighboring pieces of tissue ($D_s = 1.0$) is perfectly correlated with $r_s = 1.0$, while a random blood flow ($D_s = 1.5$) is completely uncorrelated with $r_s = 0.0$. When the D for baboon heart, sheep heart, and dog lung blood flows are substituted into this equation, regional $r_s = 0.49, 0.58,$ and 0.76, respectively, (Table 1).

Equation 8 tells us that if blood flow distribution in an organ is fractal, then, regardless of the location of the region examined, blood flow to neighboring regions of tissue is also correlated. In Fig. 9, a schematic representation of regional vascular perfusion to an organ, the correlation of blood flow between pieces *AAA* and *AAB*, is the same as between pieces *ABA* and *ABB*. A second consequence of *Eq. 8* is that if the blood flow distribution is fractal, blood flow to neighboring pieces of an organ is correlated regardless of the size of the pieces. This means that in Fig. 9 the correlation of blood flow between pieces *A* and *B* is the same as between *AA* and *BB* as well as between *AAA* and *AAB*.

A similar derivation of r_s can be done for pieces of tissue formed by aggregating more than two neighboring pieces. This is the extended-range correlation technique of Bassingthwaighte and Beyer (unpublished observations), which is given as the last equation in the APPENDIX and can be applied to isotropic or anisotropic spatial intensities. The correlation between regions falls off with increasing separation between them. The rate of fall off of r_s is exactly the same for all sample sizes, a fractal "self-similarity," and asymptotically follows a power law with a log-log slope of $2.0(1 - D)$ for $1.0 \le D \le 1.5$. The fall off is less rapid than an exponential; i.e., the correlation extends over a longer range of separation.

Fractal modeling of vascular trees. Let us return to our original assertion that the regional distribution of organ

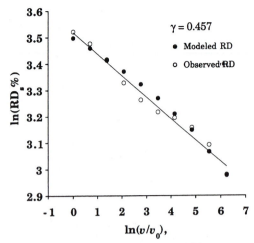

FIG. 11. Optimized fit of modeled data to actual RD data from a dog lung. Best fit of branching network model to data yields a γ of 0.457. Note slight downward concavity of dichotomously branching network model (v_0 = voxel size = 24 mm³).

blood flow may be fractal because the vascular structures distributing the flows are fractal themselves. We can test this hypothesis by modeling the pulmonary vasculature as a fractal structure and examining the distribution of flows produced by such a model.

A simple vascular model can be depicted by a main stem vessel with repetitively bifurcating daughter branches (Fig. 10). At each generation the number of branches doubles, producing 2^n terminal branches after n generations. If the diameters and lengths of daughter branches are recursively defined by the parent branch, the vascular structure will be fractal with respect to the diameters and lengths (37). If the relative fraction of flow distributed to each of the daughter branches remains constant throughout all generations, the fraction of flow to one daughter branch can be represented by γ and the fraction of flow to the other branch is therefore $1 - \gamma$. If the flow in the main stem vessel is F_0, the flow at any branch can be determined and the flows emerging after n generations have the values

$$F = \gamma^k (1 - \gamma)^{n-k} F_0 \qquad (9)$$

where k assumes integer values from 0 to n. The flow distribution in this model is skewed to the right and is similar to that seen in hearts and lungs. If $\gamma = 0.5$, the branching is symmetrical and flows are uniform, while deviations of γ away from 0.5 produce heterogeneity. Fixed values of γ differing by 0.03 or 0.04 from 0.5 and random values for $\gamma = 0.5 \pm 0.04$ give good fits to organ flow data. All these values are slightly curved on log-log plots. As noted previously, the significance of this curvature is a theoretically fractal structure is not clear.

When the observed distributions of blood flow in an organ are modeled by this asymmetrically bifurcating network, a γ can be determined for the best fit to the actual RD data. The observed RD and the theoretical RD for the best-fitting γ are shown in Fig. 11 as a function of the piece size for a given dog lung. The mean coefficient

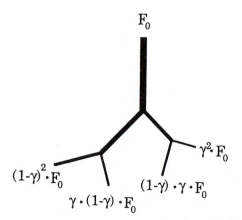

FIG. 10. Asymmetric fractal branching network in which relative fraction of blood flow from parent segment to daughter branches is γ and $1 - \gamma$. Flow at each segment of network can be determined given flow into network (F_0), and RD of blood flow can be calculated as a function of γ.

of variation between this model and the experimental data was 0.070 ± 0.042 (6). The γ that best fit the RD data for baboon hearts, sheep hearts, and dog lungs are 0.461 ± 0.007, 0.451 ± 0.022, and 0.459 ± 0.009, respectively (37). It is evident that this simple fractal network accurately models the observed RD values over a large range of piece sizes.

The estimated branching asymmetry of this fractal network can be compared with the branching asymmetry of the human pulmonary vasculature quantitated by morphological techniques. Horsfield and Woldenberg (13) measured the diameters of parent and daughter branches at 1,937 bifurcations in casts of saline-filled fully inflated lungs. They determined that the mean ratio of daughter diameters was 1.274. Using Poiseuille's law, this would be equivalent to $\gamma = 0.365$. This degree of asymmetry would produce a flow distribution with RD = 136% after only 15 generations. This appears to be unreasonably large compared with the measured RD of ~35% in dog lungs after a similar number of generations (5). A possible explanation for this discrepancy is that the morphological measurements were made on saline-filled fully inflated lungs with casting resin injected at a pressure of 40 cmH$_2$O, while the measurement of flow distributions in the dogs was made on intact animals at functional residual capacity. The observation that the physiologically measured heterogeneity of flow is less than predicted by anatomic measurements may also suggest that, in intact animals, local regulatory mechanisms could limit the heterogeneity of blood flow.

The fractal branching model is not meant to be a precise representation of anatomic structures. Rather it emphasizes the concept of how small degrees of asymmetry in flow can produce heterogeneous blood flow distributions similar to those seen in experimental studies. The precise value of γ or σ is of little importance relative to this idea. The fractal branching model offers a possible mechanism to explain the observed heterogeneity of pulmonary blood flow within isogravitational planes. By use of the concepts of fractals, this model is able to relate the function and structure of the pulmonary vascular tree and offer an explanation for the spatial distribution and gravity-independent heterogeneity of blood flow.

Fractal Process, Temporal Heterogeneity, and Temporal Correlation

The concepts of self-similarity and fractal dimensions can also be applied to observations made over time. Examples of appropriate time-dependent variables abound in physiological studies, including fluctuating ionic currents, blood flows and pressures, and ventilatory excursions. Several methods of eliciting the underlying dimensionality of such measurements have been developed for time series data. These fall into two classes: *1*) dispersion analysis, which gives a measure of local correlation, and *2*) minimal order analysis, which defines the minimal order of a set of differential equations describing the chaotic dynamic behavior of the system that is fluctuating unpredictably while remaining bounded and self-

correlated. Although each of these approaches defines fractal measures, described by a fractal dimension, they are quite different. Dispersion analysis reduces the complexity of the system, regarding it as one-dimensional, while the time series analysis for the dimension of a chaotic signal attempts to define the minimal degree of complexity or order of the system. Minimal order analysis is not discussed here.

Dispersion analysis. Three basic methods of dispersion analysis can be applied to temporal observations, one using the RD (RD$_r$), the second using Hurst's rescaled range, and the third being the measure of extended-range correlation. The simplest analysis is the application of RD described above for spatial variation (3). The application to a signal V(t) is shown in Fig. 12, where V(t) may be any measure such as voltage, velocity, or position. A digitized signal measured at uniform intervals (τ_0) can be considered as a population of observations in one dimension. RD$_r(\tau_0)$ is initially calculated for all the sampled data in the upper row of Fig. 12. Pairs of neighboring points are then averaged to obtain the second row, and RD$_r(2\tau_0)$ is calculated. Recursive pairing to double the interval length and recalculation of the SD on the combined data points gives RD$_r(4t_0)$, RD$_r(8t_0)$, . . . RD$_r(N\tau_0)$ for each row of "observations" in Fig. 12. When RD$_r(N\tau_0)$ and N are plotted on logarithmic scales, they are well characterized by a fractal relationship, which is a straight line

$$RD_r(N\tau_0) = RD_r(\tau_0)N^{1-D_r} \qquad (10)$$

D$_r$ for this random signal is 1.5, so the exponent of N is -0.5. This result indicates that with each doubling of the averaging interval to $2t_0$, $4t_0$, etc., the RD$_r$ scales down by $1/\sqrt{2}$, i.e., to 0.707 of the RD$_r$ at the next smaller interval duration. As was the case with the measuring stick length

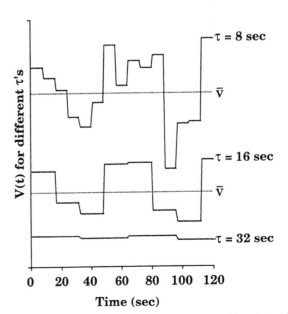

FIG. 12. *Top curve:* V(t) as a function of time at uniform intervals, $\tau = 8$ s. *Bottom 2 curves:* successive averages over intervals (τ) of double the length. Note diminution in dispersion with successive lumpings.

for the contour length method, there is no particular need to use interval doubling, because any increment will give a similar D_r, provided enough data points are available. The D_r of 1.5 is that expected for any random signal. In this case, the random signal was Gaussian with a mean of 1.0 and an SD of 0.3. The r, given by *Eq. 8*, is zero in this case. The same D_r would be found for other random signals, uniform over an interval such as Poisson or random walk. The information from this analysis is limited to the variance and does not characterize the form of the distribution or higher moments such as skewness and kurtosis.

Fractal analysis of time-dependent observations provides a means for characterizing temporal correlation in a fashion similar to that of spatial correlation. Correlation over time is also described as memory. If a fractal process with positive correlation is trending upward, adjacent observations in time will also tend to increase, and similarly if the process is trending downward, neighboring observations in time will likely be decreasing as well. In other words, the state or position of a process, $V(t)$, is influenced by its previous values $V(t - 1)$. Negative temporal correlation signifies that adjacent values in time tend to move away from each other.

When the RD_r analysis was applied to the time series data on erythrocyte velocities from Kislyakov et al. (15), a D_r of 1.37 was found. The more extensive data of Oude Vrielink et al. (30), shown in Fig. 13, *left*, allow a more accurate test for a fractal relationship. The RD_r vs. τ relationship (Fig. 13, *right*) gives a D_r of 1.16, indicating correlation with the coefficient $r = 0.60$. The fact that there is correlation is intriguing and invites further experimental work and other analyses to determine the basis of the correlation. It is important to emphasize that this similarity of adjacent observations over time holds true over the entire range of the time intervals examined. The statement that observations adjacent in time are similar is not the important conclusion of this analysis but, rather, that this is a fractal process in which the relationship between successive measurements is consistent on all time scales.

Hurst's (14) "rescaled range analysis" is similar to the RD analysis and can be applied to spatial as well as temporal data. In the simplest version of this method (4), the SD is normalized by dividing it into the local range (R) of the cumulative differences from the mean over the interval of length τ, rather than by the mean as in the RD analysis. R generally increases with the interval duration, but SD changes little. The approach is to plot the log R/SD vs. log τ. The slope is H − 1, where H is the Hurst coefficient

$$\frac{\text{R/SD for interval } \tau}{\text{R/SD for interval } \tau_0} = \left(\frac{\tau}{\tau_0}\right)^{H-1} \tag{11}$$

The R/SD grows with the interval length τ, as might be expected because the dispersion is in the denominator. The values of R/SD are very scattered for short τ or few observations, but the information content is very similar to that provided by the RD analysis, and H is related to D

$$H = 2 - D \tag{12}$$

The approach is good when H = 0.5 (random, no correlation) and when H > 0.5 (correlated functions with "memory"). The r between adjacent intervals is $2^{2H-1} - 1$, the same as in *Eq. 8*.

Both the RD analysis and rescaled range analysis need to be carefully evaluated by extensive testing. The RD analysis appears more robust, particularly for smaller data sets, and may be less subject to the skewing attendant on dividing by individual values of SD within each interval, as in the rescaled range analysis. Hurst's original method is more precise than described above or by Feder (4) in that it accounts for local trends in the data.

The extended-range correlation technique of Bassingthwaighte and Beyer (unpublished observations) is a test of the fractal nature of a time series. The two-point autocorrelation is determined for units separated by n units, giving a statistical measure of $r(n)$ for any n

$$r(n) = \frac{\sum x_i(\tau) x_i(\tau + n\tau)}{\text{Var}(x)} \tag{13}$$

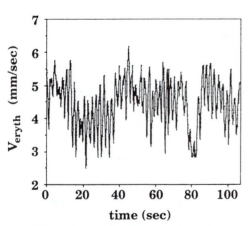

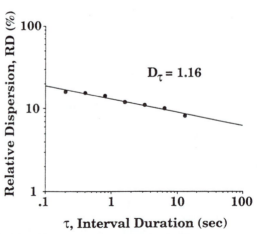

FIG. 13. Fractal (RD) analysis of vasomotion. *Left*: erythrocyte velocities (V_{eryth}) in a 7-μm arteriole of rabbit tenussimus muscle with $\Delta t = 0.1$ s. [Data from Oude Vrielink et al. (30).] *Right*: RD of velocities averaged over intervals of length τ decreases with increasing τ and has an apparent D of 1.162.

The theoretical fractal curve for the correlation is

$$r(n) = \tfrac{1}{2}[\,|n+1|^{2H} - 2n^{2H} + |n-1|^{2H}\,] \qquad (14)$$

which for $n > 3$ follows a simple relationship that is a straight line on a log-log plot, $r(n)/[r(n-1)] = [n/(n-1)]^{2H-2}$. Thus H can be calculated directly from the slope, H = (slope + 2)/2.

These methods bear a relationship to Fourier analysis where one obtains the relative power and phase at each frequency. When the logarithm of the amplitude of the individual frequency components of the signal vs. the logarithm of the frequency is plotted for fractal signals, the slope of the relationship between the two components can be a straight line with slope $-\beta$ (39). The fractal self-similarity demonstrated in this analysis is the constant ratio of power at any two frequencies, independent of the resolution (the position of the frequency scale). In this context, white random noise (all frequencies with equal power) has $\beta = 0$ and so-called Brownian noise has $\beta = 2$. Sets of noise with amplitude proportional to $f^{-\beta}$ exhibit memory. Over this limited range

$$\beta = 2H - 1 = 3 - 2D_r, \qquad (15)$$

Goldberger et al. (7) have used frequency analysis to characterize the fractal nature of the electrocardiographic signal. They argued that an electrical stimulus passed through a fractal network should result in a voltage-time pulse with a power spectral density that has a linear relationship on a log-log plot. They asserted that the His-Purkinje conduction network is a fractal structure and should therefore produce a fractal process. In testing this hypothesis, using a fast Fourier transformation, they examined a single QRS complex from 21 resting subjects. When they plotted the logarithm of the mean square of the amplitudes against the logarithm of the frequency for the mean data of 21 subjects, they found a power-law relationship.

Many natural signals including ionic channel noise (20), speech intensities (39), Nile River flood levels (14, 25), and rain (21) are analogous to correlated noise, with $0.5 < \beta < 1.5$. Most interestingly, music of almost all cultures (40) shows frequency and intensity changes with $\beta = 1$. These have been characterized by how the amplitude of V(t) varies between points in time, such that

$$\Delta V = k\Delta t^{H} \qquad (16)$$

For H = 0.5, ΔV is typical Brownian motion, and for $0.5 < H < 1.0$, there is positive correlation between neighboring points. Commonly, natural phenomena show H's of 0.7–0.8 (14).

Utility of Fractal Analysis, Structures, and Processes

One advantage of applying fractal analysis to biological systems relates to the analogy between the mathematical structure of fractals and the patterns of growth of the neural, vascular, and airway pathways. The evolution of multicellular organisms has mandated the development of connections between the environment and each individual cell. These branching connections must make the transition from large to small and simple to complex as efficiently as possible. An example is the transport of respiratory gases between the environment and alveoli along the dichotomous fractal branching of the airways, which transforms a simple 3-cm² tracheal cross section to a complex 70-m² alveolar surface area. The blood reaching the alveolar capillaries undergoes a similar transformation from a single large vessel to a complex capillary network by means of fractal branching. The fractal description of these network patterns is logical and based on the scale-independent similarity of these systems over several orders of magnitude.

With increasingly greater spatial and temporal resolution of physiological measurement, it is becoming evident that biologic systems are not smooth continuous processes. They do, however, maintain a degree of spatial and temporal correlation. Fractal analysis permits the characterization of these processes or structures that are not easily represented by the traditional analytic tools. By providing a geometric framework for the description of apparently irregular patterns, fractal analysis is able to characterize natural structures (36). Biological structures as diverse as protein surfaces, neuronal cell contours, and the bronchial tree can be succinctly characterized by fractal analysis (19, 35, 42). This unifying strategy allows characterization and comparison of a vast array of physiological systems.

The construction of self-similar structures reveals a potential advantage in coding for the growth and development of the necessarily complex vascular, neural, and airway networks. Complex mathematical fractal figures can be constructed from simple recursive algorithms (39). This recursive quality of the mathematical kernel permits a concise description of remarkably complex structures (43). Because there cannot possibly be a complete genetic description for the construction of every alveolus and capillary, it seems logical to propose that there are elementary recursive rules to guide their construction. These construction codes are probably not fractal themselves but are likely deterministic rules defining basic elements that are influenced by the environment in which the structure grows. The branching structures of the vascular system and the bronchial tree are such examples, where it is not known whether the branching angles and diameters are determined by the parent branch or by the similar environment in which they are constructed. Although the mechanisms by which these rules operate are speculative, a coding for self-similar structures is clearly the most efficient and appropriate algorithm to explain both the order and complexity of ontogeny. The efficiency of the finalized structures is also of importance to the organism. Lefèvre (18) has shown that a self-similar branching model of the pulmonary vascular system optimizes the cost-function (energy-materials) relationship while closely approximating physiological and morphometric data. Tsonis and Tsonis (36) have related fractal patterning to minimal energy consumption as well. If the development of biologic trees such as the bronchial and vascular systems can be modeled by fractal structures, then these models can also be used to investigate the effects of boundary limitation on these trees (29).

With these new analytic methods for characterizing physiological systems, physiologists are faced with a problem similar to that in the parable of the blind men attempting to describe an elephant. Although we can accurately describe single characteristics, we lack the perspective to determine the best approach for characterizing complete systems. Fractal analysis using the RD or frequency domains can be applied to any spatial or temporal physiological measurement. At present, we need to explore each of the different techniques to determine the relative advantages and limitations of each when applied to physiological systems. Our recommendations to those wishing to use these methods is to try them all, because each approach may provide unique information. From a practical standpoint, the limiting factor with these analytic methods is data set size. As a first approximation, at least a few hundred data points are required for the dispersional analysis and more would obviously improve the dimensional estimates obtained.

In this review we have focused on the various fractal measures of correlation in spatial properties and temporal fluctuations. Physiologists seek insight into biological mechanisms from the variable signals of life processes such as measurements of pressures, frequencies, and flows. The traditional analytic tools have been measures of means and variances with statistical approaches based on the assumption of random error in the measurements. The fractal revolution has brought the realization that this "error" can be analyzed as a fundamental property of the biological system that may include complex information with structure defined by these new analytic techniques.

APPENDIX A
Definitions

Box measurement	A method of estimating fractal dimension by covering the structure to be analyzed with boxes of various side lengths
Contour measurement	A method of estimating fractal dimension using measuring sticks of various lengths
Euclidean dimension	Integer representing the fewest coordinates required to represent an object in traditional Euclidean geometry. Euclidean dimension of a straight line is 1, that of a curved line or plane is 2, and that of a curved surface or sphere is 3
Fractal dimension	An estimate of the scale-independent complexity or irregularity of a system over space or time. It can assume all real values greater than or equal to the topological dimension and less than or equal to the Euclidean dimension
Fractal structure	An object that has a characteristic form that remains constant over a magnitude of scales, an object with small-scale structure similar to its large-scale structure
Fractal process	A variable as a function of time with fluctuations over a short time scale similar to those over a longer time scale
Heterogeneity	A measure of nonuniformity
Hurst exponent	A measure of complexity or irregularity of a system over space or time determined from rescaled range analysis. It can assume all real values between 0.5 and 1.0 and is related to the fractal dimension (D) by the equation $H = 2 - D$, where D is either D_s or D_r
Koch curve	A self-similar geometric structure defined by a series of repeated transformations first described by Helge von Koch in 1904 (see Fig. 1)
Memory	Characteristic of a time-dependent variable that has temporal correlation. It signifies that a positively correlated process will tend to continue moving in the same direction. $V(t)$ is influenced by $V(t - 1)$
RD analysis	A method of estimating a fractal dimension using the measure of relative dispersion (RD) of a variable for varying scales of space or time
Relative dispersion	A measure of heterogeneity of a distribution (SD divided by mean of distribution)
Rescaled range analysis	Method of determining whether a structure or process is fractal and estimating the Hurst exponent. It is similar to RD analysis, in which the scale of measurement is a time period (τ) and the observed measurement is the local range divided by SD (R/SD) of observations. Hurst exponent is slope of log-log plot of τ vs. R/SD
Scale independence	A characteristic of fractal structures or processes where characteristic forms or fluctuations remain constant independent of the scale of measurement (self-similarity)
Self-similarity	A characteristic of fractal structures or processes where characteristic forms or fluctuations on a small scale of measurement are similar to those on a larger scale of measurement (scale independence)
Spatial correlation	A measure of the similarity in an observed variable between 2 adjacent regions. It can assume all real values between −1.0 and 1.0. A value of −1.0 indicates complete negative correlation, 0.0 represent a random relationship, and 1.0 indicates complete uniformity.
Temporal correlation	A measure of similarity in an observed variable between 2 adjacent observations in time. It can assume all real values between −1.0 and 1.0. A value

t	V(t)					
1	10.31					
2	19.03	14.67				
3	34.7					
4	19.26	26.98	20.83			
5	65.42					
6	34.79	50.11				
7	19.07					
8	35.34	27.21	38.66	29.74		
9	34.82					
10	18.80	26.81				
11	18.69					
12	10.28	14.49	20.65			
13	19.03					
14	10.12	14.58				
15	5.58					
16	10.07	7.83	11.20	15.92	22.83	
17	35.52					
18	19.28	27.4				
19	35.88					
20	64.40	50.14	38.77			
21	66.83					
22	35.61	51.22				
23	121.34					
24	64.34	92.84	72.03	55.4		
25	19.35					
26	35.78	27.57				
27	35.77					
28	64.38	50.08	38.82			
29	10.04					
30	19.10	14.57				
31	18.82					
32	35.52	27.17	20.87	29.85	42.62	32.73
33	35.36					
34	19.28	27.32				
35	19.00					
36	10.06	14.53	20.93			
37	35.78					
38	18.94	27.36				
39	66.09					
40	34.90	50.50	38.93	29.93		
41	64.76					
42	34.91	49.84				
43	35.16					
44	18.89	27.03	38.43			
45	64.39					
46	35.09	49.74				
47	66.18					
48	121.58	93.88	71.81	55.12	42.52	
49	122.48					
50	229.45	175.97				
51	120.93					
52	66.25	93.59	134.78			
53	66.75					
54	34.95	50.85				
55	119.86					
56	64.75	92.31	71.58	103.18		
57	121.15					
58	65.03	93.09				
59	64.8					
60	36.00	50.4	71.75			
61	64.91					
62	35.59	50.25				
63	19.33					
64	35.71	27.52	38.89	55.32	79.25	60.88
Mean	46.81	46.81	46.81	46.81	46.81	46.81
SD	38.97	35.05	31.19	27.28	23.54	19.91
RD%	83.25	74.88	66.63	58.28	50.29	42.53
ln(RD%)	4.42	4.32	4.20	4.07	3.92	3.75
N	64	32	16	8	4	2
Size (τ)	1	2	4	8	16	32
ln(τ)	0	0.69	1.39	2.08	2.77	3.47

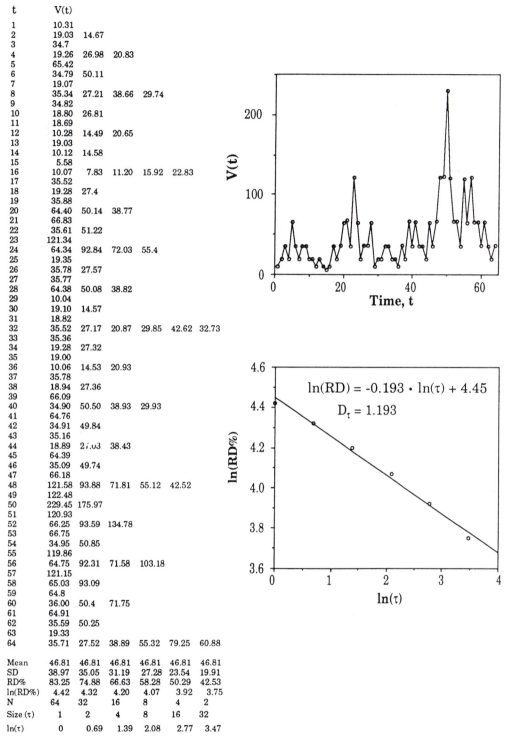

$$\ln(RD) = -0.193 \cdot \ln(\tau) + 4.45$$

$$D_\tau = 1.193$$

FIG. 14. RD method of fractal analysis for a time course signal. Columns t (in arbitrary units) and $V(t)$ (value of signal at *time t*) represent original time course signal sampled at given temporal resolution. *Top right*: 64 observations presented in graphical form. *Bottom right*: mean, SD, RD (RD% = 100·SD/mean), and other necessary calculations. Column to the right of $V(t)$ is obtained by averaging 2 adjacent measurements of original data to make 1 observation. N has now been reduced to 32, and time interval has increased to 2. Mean, SD, and RD are again calculated for a new grouping of data with RD = 74.88%. If scale of time interval is increased again by averaging every 2 points of the new data set ($\tau = 4$), a new RD can be calculated. This process is continued until there are only 2 data points and $\tau = 32$, which results in 6 measurements of RD at 6 different scales of resolution.

2366

Topological
dimension

of -1.0 indicates complete negative correlation, 0.0 represents a random relationship, and 1.0 indicates complete uniformity

Smallest Euclidean dimension that an object can be reduced to by a 1:1 continuous point mapping (i.e., stretching but not tearing), e.g., a curved line can be reduced to a straight line of 1 dimension, and a curved surface can be reduced to a flat plane of 2 dimensions. It can assume only integer values. A branching line is topologically 1-dimensional but may require embedding in a plane or 3-dimensional space to reveal its form

Variables

β	Power spectrum exponent as measured by spectral analysis; $\beta = 0.0$ for white noise and $\beta = 2.0$ for Brownian motion
D_s	Spatial correlation as measured by RD analysis; $1.0 \leq D_s \leq 1.5$
D_τ	Temporal correlation as measured by RD analysis; $1.0 \leq D_\tau \leq 1.5$
E	Euclidean dimension
H	Hurst exponent
l	Measuring stick of a given length, l
l_0	Initial measuring stick length
$L(l)$	Apparent contour length of a structure using a measuring stick of length l
m	Mass of observed piece
m_0	Mass of reference piece, arbitrarily chosen
$N_{box}(l)$	Number of boxes of side length l covering the structure
R	Local range in Hurst analysis
RD_s	Relative dispersion of spatially oriented observations
RD_τ	Relative dispersion of temporally oriented observations
r_s	Spatial correlation between adjacent regions; $-1.0 \leq r_s \leq 1.0$.
r_τ	Temporal correlation between observations adjacent in time; $-1.0 \leq r_\tau \leq 1.0$
$r(n)$	Correlation between observations separated by n units of space or time
SD	Standard deviation of observations
ν	Volume of observed region
ν_0	Volume of reference region, arbitrarily chosen

Equations

$$\frac{L(l)}{L(l_0)} = \left(\frac{l}{l_0}\right)^{1-D}$$

$$\ln L(l) = (1 - D) \ln\left(\frac{l}{l_0}\right) + \ln L(l)$$

$$\ln RD_s(\nu) = (1 - D_s) \ln\left(\frac{\nu}{\nu_0}\right) + \ln RD_s(\nu_0)$$

$$\frac{RD_s(\nu)}{RD_s(\nu_0)} = \left(\frac{\nu}{\nu_0}\right)^{1-D_s}$$

$$\frac{RD_s(m)}{RD_s(m_0)} = \left(\frac{m}{m_0}\right)^{1-D_s}$$

$$r_s = 2^{3-2D_s} - 1$$

$$F = \gamma^k (1 - \gamma)^{n-k} F_0$$

$$\frac{R/SD \text{ for interval } \tau}{R/SD \text{ for interval } \tau_0} = \left(\frac{\tau}{\tau_0}\right)^{H-1}$$

$$r(n) = \frac{\sum x_i(\tau) x_i(\tau + n\tau)}{Var(x)}$$

$$r(n) = \frac{1}{2}[|n + 1|^{2H} - 2n^{2H} + |n - 1|^{2H}]$$

APPENDIX B

Figure 14 is an example of the RD method of fractal analysis for a time course signal. The demonstration data set is smaller than the recommended minimal size to facilitate working through the example with a hand calculator.

This study was supported by National Heart, Lung, and Blood Institute Grants HL-08155, HL-38736, and RR-1243 and by Grant 89-WA-515 from the American Heart Association—Washington Affiliate.

Address for reprint requests: J. B. Bassingthwaighte, University of Washington, WD-12, Seattle, WA 98195.

REFERENCES

1. BASSINGTHWAIGHTE, J. B. Physiological heterogeneity: fractals link determinism and randomness in structures and functions. *News Physiol. Sci.* 3: 5–10, 1988.
2. BASSINGTHWAIGHTE, J. B., R. B. KING, AND S. A. ROGER. Fractal nature of regional myocardial blood flow heterogeneity. *Circ. Res.* 65:578–590, 1989.
3. BASSINGTHWAIGHTE, J. B., AND J. H. G. M. VAN BEEK. Lightning and the heart: fractal behavior in cardiac function. *Proc. IEEE* 76: 693–699, 1988.
4. FEDER, J. *Fractals.* New York: Plenum, 1988.
5. GLENNY, R. W., AND H. T. ROBERTSON. Fractal properties of pulmonary blood flow: characterization of spatial heterogeneity. *J. Appl. Physiol.* 69: 532–545, 1990.
6. GLENNY, R. W., AND H. T. ROBERTSON. Fractal modeling of pulmonary blood flow heterogeneity. *J. Appl. Physiol.* 70: 1024–1030, 1991.
7. GOLDBERGER, A. L., BHARGAVA, B. J. WEST, AND A. J. MANDELL. On a mechanism of cardiac electrical stability. The fractal hypothesis. *Biophys. J.* 48: 525–528, 1985.
8. GOLDBERGER, A. L., D. R. RIGNEY, AND B. J. WEST. Chaos and fractals in human physiology. *Sci. Am.* 262: 42–49, 1990.
9. HORSFIELD, K. Morphometry of the small pulmonary arteries in man. *Circ. Res.* 42: 593–597, 1978.
10. HORSFIELD, K. Diameters, generations, and orders of branches in the bronchial tree. *J. Appl. Physiol.* 68: 457–461, 1990.
11. HORSFIELD, K., AND G. CUMMING. Morphology of the bronchial tree in man. *J. Appl. Physiol.* 24: 373–383, 1968.
12. HORSFIELD, K., F. G. RELEA, AND G. CUMMING. Diameter, length, and branching ratios on the bronchial tree. *Respir. Physiol.* 26: 351–356, 1976.
13. HORSFIELD, K., AND M. J. WOLDENBERG. Diameters and cross-sectional areas of branches in the human pulmonary arterial tree. *Anat. Rec.* 223: 245–251, 1989.
14. HURST, H. E., R. P. BLACK, AND Y. M. SIMAIKI. *Long-Term Storage: An Experimental Study.* London: Constable, 1965.
15. KISLYAKOV, Y. Y., Y. I. LEVKOVITCH, T. E. SHUYMILOVA, AND E. A. VERSHININA. Blood flow fluctuations in cerebral cortex microvessels. *Int. J. Microcirc. Clin. Exp.* 6: 3–13, 1987.
16. KUHN, T. S. The structure of scientific revolutions. In: *International Encyclopedia of Unified Science.* Chicago: University of Chicago Press, 1970.

17. LANGMAN, J. *Medical Embryology. Human Development—Normal and Abnormal* (3rd ed.). Baltimore, MD: Williams & Wilkins, 1975.

18. LEFÈVRE, J. Teleonomical optimization of a fractal model of the pulmonary arterial bed. *J. Theor. Biol.* 102: 225–248, 1983.

19. LEWIS, M., AND D. C. REES. Fractal surfaces of proteins. *Science Wash. DC* 230: 1163–1165, 1985.

20. LIEBOVITCH, L. S., J. FISCHBARG, J. P. KONIAREK, I. TODOROVA, AND M. WANG. Fractal model of ion-channel kinetics. *Biochim. Biophys. Acta* 896: 173–180, 1987.

20a. LIEBOVITCH, L. S., AND T. I. TOTH. A fast algorithm to determine fractal dimensions by box counting. *Phys. Lett. A* 141: 386–390, 1989.

21. LOVEJOY, S., AND B. B. MANDELBROT. Fractal properties of rain, and a fractal model. *Tellus* 37A: 209–232, 1985.

22. MACDONALD, N. *Trees and Networks in Biological Models.* New York: Wiley, 1983.

23. MANDELBROT, B. B. How long is the coast of Britain? Statistical self-similarity and fractional dimension. *Science Wash. DC* 156: 636–638, 1967.

24. MANDELBROT, B. B. *The Fractal Geometry of Nature.* San Francisco: Freeman, 1983.

25. MANDELBROT, B. B., AND J. R. WALLIS. Some long-run properties of geophysical records. *Water Resour. Res.* 5: 321–340, 1969.

26. MASSOUD, E. A. S., A. ROTSCHILD, R. MATSUI, H. S. SEKHON, AND W. M. THURLBECK. In vitro airway branching morphogenesis of the fetal rat lung. (Abstract) *Am. Rev. Respir. Dis.* 141: A340, 1990.

27. MEAKIN, P. A new model for biological pattern formation. *J. Theor. Biol.* 118: 101–113, 1986.

28. NELSON, T. R. Morphological modeling using fractal geometries. In: *Medical Imaging II: Image Formation Detection, Processing, and Interpretation/Image Data Management and Display.* Bellingham, WA: SPIE-Int. Soc. Opt. Eng., 1988, p. 326–333.

29. NELSON, T. R., AND D. K. MANCHESTER. Modeling of lung morphogenesis using fractal geometries. *IEEE Trans. Med. Imaging* 7: 321–327, 1988.

30. OUDE VRIELINK, H. H. E., D. W. SLAAF, G. J. TANGELDER, S. WEIJMER-VAN VELZEN, AND R. S. RENEMAN. Analysis of vasomotion waveform changes during pressure reduction and adenosine application. *Am. J. Physiol.* 258 (*Heart Circ. Physiol.* 27): H29–H37, 1990.

31. RAABE, O. G., H. C. YEH, G. M. SCHUM, AND R. F. PHALEN. *Tracheobronchial Geometry: Human, Dog, Rat, Hamster.* Washington DC: US Govt. Printing Office, 1976.

32. RIGAUT, J. P. An empirical formulation relating boundary lengths to resolution in specimens showing non-ideally fractal dimensions. *J. Microsc.* 133: 41–54, 1984.

33. SANDER, L. M. Fractal growth. *Sci. Am.* 256: 94–100, 1987.

34. SINGHAL, S., R. HENDERSON, K. HORSFIELD, K. HARDING, AND G. CUMMING. Morphometry of the human pulmonary arterial tree. *Circ. Res.* 33: 190–197, 1973.

35. SMITH, T. G., JR., W. B. MARKS, G. D. LANGE, W. H. SHERIFF, JR., AND E. A. NEALE. A fractal analysis of cell images. *J. Neurosci. Methods* 27: 173–180, 1989.

36. TSONIS, A. A., AND P. A. TSONIS. Fractals: a new look at biological shape and patterning. *Perspect. Biol. Med.* 30: 355–361, 1987.

37. VAN BEEK, J. H. G. M., S. A. ROGER, AND J. B. BASSINGTHWAIGHTE. Regional myocardial flow heterogeneity explained with fractal networks. *Am. J. Physiol.* 257 (*Heart Circ. Physiol.* 26): H1670–H1680, 1989.

38. VAN ROY, P., L. GARCIA, AND B. WAHL. *Designer Fractal. Mathematics for the 21st Century.* Santa Cruz, CA: Dynamic Software, 1988.

39. VOSS, R. F. Fractals in nature: from characterization to simulation. In: *The Science of Fractal Images,* edited by H. O. Peitgen and D. Saupe. New York: Springer-Verlag, 1988, p. 21–70.

40. VOSS, R. F., AND J. CLARK. "1/f Noise" in music and speech. *Nature Lond.* 258: 317–318, 1975.

41. WEIBEL, E. R., AND D. M. GOMEZ. Architecture of the human lung. *Science Wash. DC* 137: 577–585, 1962.

42. WEST, B. J., V. BHARGAVA, AND A. L. GOLDBERGER. Beyond the principle of similitude: renormalization in the bronchial tree. *J. Appl. Physiol.* 60: 1089–1097, 1986.

43. WEST, B. J., AND A. L. GOLDBERGER. Physiology in fractal dimensions. *Am. Sci.* 75: 354–365, 1987.

Fascinating rhythm: A primer on chaos theory and its application to cardiology

Recent advances in nonlinear mathematics have led to the development of a science called "chaos" and its application to biology and cardiology. We discuss the basics of chaotic behavior, comparing and contrasting it with periodic and random behavior. Also discussed is the way in which nonlinear systems can become chaotic and the applications of chaos to cardiac arrhythmias. Finally, we describe the methods used to study nonlinear systems and seemingly random behavior. Five tools of nonlinear dynamics are described (phase plane plots, return maps, Poincaré sections, fractal dimensions, and spectral analysis). A glossary is included that explains much of the basic vocabulary of chaos theory.

Timothy A. Denton, MD, George A. Diamond, MD, Richard H. Helfant, MD, Steven Khan, MD, and Hrayr Karagueuzian, PhD. *Los Angeles, Calif.*

"Somehow, a myth has arisen . . . that detailed mathematical and theoretical analysis are not appropriate in biology . . . Yet if the complex dynamic phenomena that occur in the human body were to arise in some inanimate physical system . . . they would be subjected to the most sophisticated experimental and theoretical study."[1]

PROLOGUE

While caring for a patient with a large pericardial effusion, a physician notes that each electrocardiographic R wave and each peak systolic pressure wave is of a different amplitude (Fig. 1, *A* and *B*). Although the phenomenon disappears following pericardiocentesis, the physician wonders if there might be a hidden pattern underlying this seemingly random behavior, and therefore plots the height of each wave against the height of the succeeding wave. To the physician's surprise, the relation for R wave amplitude is highly structured (Fig. 1, *C*), but that for systolic pressure is not (Fig. 1, *D*).

Although this particular example is completely fanciful, many scientists have made precisely analo-

gous observations over the last 20 years. The explanation for these puzzling findings lies in a new science called chaos. In recent years, this new discipline, based on the mathematics of nonlinear dynamics, has been applied to many areas of physical and biological science.[1-7] Its application to cardiology may provide an innovative tool to aid our understanding of many physiologic phenomena that heretofore were deemed inexplicable using conventional methodologies. Specifically, a better understanding of the mathematical physiology of cardiac rhythms may allow us to predict the onset of lethal arrhythmias, and intervene prior to the development of catastrophic clinical events.

This essay is a primer on the priciples of chaos—what it is, what causes it, and how to detect it. As much as possible, we have attempted to write the text in non-mathematical form. We have used a variety of metaphors and hypothetical examples as pedagogic aids to a deeper understanding of the underlying concepts. Our purpose is to provide appreciation without intimidation. Those interested in a more comprehensive review of the subject are referred to a number of excellent books and articles. Gleick[7] and Stewart[8] have written superb nontechnical descriptions of chaos theory, and concise accounts are also available.[3, 9-12] Moon[6] offers a highly accessible technical discussion of the theory, while Thompson and Stewart[13] and Bergé et al.[14] provide more mathematically rigorous expositions. Those interested in biological aspects of the theory are referred to a technical review by Olsen and Degn,[4] and to books by Holden,[5] Glass and Mackey,[1] and Winfree.[15]

From the Divisions of Cardiology, and Thoracic and Cardiovascular Surgery, Cedars-Sinai Medical Center, and the School of Medicine, University of California, Los Angeles.

This work was supported in part by a National Heart, Lung, and Blood Institute Training Grant (No. 2T32HL07380) from the National Institutes of Health, Bethesda, Md.

Received for publication May 4, 1990; accepted June 20, 1990.

Reprint requests: Timothy A. Denton, MD, Division of Thoracic and Cardiovascular Surgery, Room 6215, Cedars-Sinai Medical Center, 8700 Beverly Blvd., Los Angeles, CA 90048.

4/1/24333

1420 *Denton et al.*

December 1990
American Heart Journal

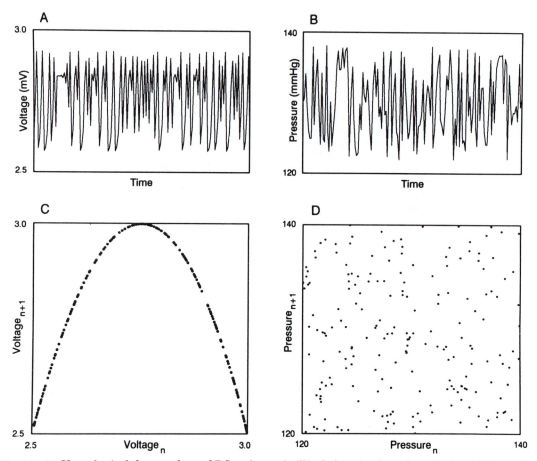

Fig. 1. A, Hypothetical beat-to-beat QRS voltage (millivolts) as a function of time (200 cycles). **B,** Hypothetical simultaneous beat-to-beat peak systolic blood pressure in millimeters of mercury as a function of time. **C,** QRS voltage of each beat (n) on the x axis versus QRS voltage of the subsequent beat (n + 1) on the y axis based on the data in **panel A. D,** Peak systolic blood pressure of each beat (n) on the x axis versus peak systolic blood pressure of the subsequent beat (n + 1) on the y axis based on the data in **panel B.**

The present discussion is divided into three sections. The first is an introduction to nonlinear dynamics and chaos, the second reviews the current status of its application to cardiology, and the third describes some of the methods used to study chaotic activity. A glossary of unfamiliar technical terms is provided as an appendix, and the terms themselves are highlighted in *italic* lettering when they first appear in the text. The glossary also contains terms not used in this text, but encountered often enough in the references cited to warrant their brief definition here.

AN INTRODUCTION TO NONLINEAR DYNAMICS AND CHAOS

What is chaos? *Chaos* is best understood by comparing it to two other behaviors with which we are more familiar— *randomness* and *periodicity*. Random behavior never repeats itself, and is inherently unpredictable and disorganized except in a very special way. We can predict the average behavior of a collection of gas molecules with absolute precision, but we can never predict the individual behavior of a single molecule. Similarly, we can predict the average change in heart rate as we administer digoxin to a patient in atrial fibrillation, but we cannot predict the individual pattern of R-R intervals. A very simple random series is represented by the number of letters in the first word of each sentence of this paragraph—5, 6, 2, 9, 1, 5, 8. There is no rule for predicting the seventh number in this series from the preceding six numbers—if there were, the series would not be random. Although one might think otherwise, very few biologic processes are considered fundamentally random (genetic translocation, ovulation, fertilization, receptor binding).

Periodic behavior, on the other hand, is highly

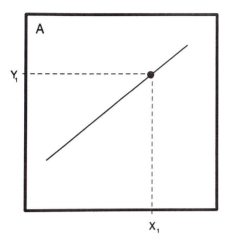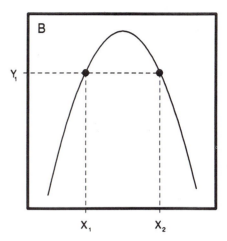

Fig. 2. A, A typical linear function. For every value of Y, there is a unique value of X. **B,** A typical nonlinear function. In this example, for any single value of Y (except its maximum) there are two possible values of X.

predictable because it always repeats itself over some finite time interval. A mathematical sine wave and electrocardiographic normal sinus rhythm are typical examples. Systems exhibiting periodic behavior are governed by an underlying *deterministic* process. Thus if we know the amplitude, frequency, and phase of a sine wave at any instant, we can predict the amplitude at any other point in time. An example of periodic behavior is given by the following simple mathematical system: $x_{n+1} = |x_n - 7|$. The next number in this series is the absolute value of the preceding number minus seven. With an initial value of 2, we obtain the following series of numbers: 2, 5, 2, 5, 2, 5... The next number in the series—2—can be predicted because one knows the rule. Periodic behavior in biological systems is generally considered normal (diurnal variation, sinus rhythm, menstruation, peristalsis), but at least two examples are decidedly abnormal (ventricular tachycardia and petit mal seizures).

Chaos is distinct from periodicity and randomness, but has characteristics of both. Although chaotic behavior looks disorganized (like random behavior), it is really deterministic (like periodic behavior). The Bernoulli map[6] is a simple example of a chaotic system: $x_{n+1} = 2x_n$ (mod 1). The mod 1 means that the integer value of the number x is subtracted from the number to leave only the decimal value (example: mod 1 of 1.73 = 0.73). With an initial value of 0.85, we obtain the following series of numbers—0.85, 0.7, 0.4, 0.8, 0.6... Although the series seems random, it is completely determined by a very simple rule. If one knows the rule, one can predict the next number in the series—0.2—with complete confidence.

A number of physical processes are known to be chaotic (some chemical reactions,[15, 16] fluid turbulence,[18] the orbit of Pluto,[19] solar radio emissions,[20, 21] atomic motion,[22] weather,[2, 23] polar ice[24]), and a few biological examples have been reported (measles epidemics,[4, 25] population biology models,[26-30] evolution models,[31] stretch reflex,[32] models of cardiac behavior,[33, 34] cardiopulmonary interactions,[35, 36] embryology,[37, 38] sociology of war models,[39] hematopoiesis,[35, 36] some biochemical reactions,[40-42] and the electroencephalogram[43-46]).

What causes chaos? Conventional biologic systems are often viewed as *linear*. A familiar example of a linear system is a straight line graph of some independent variable on the x axis plotted against a dependent variable on the y axis—"the more the merrier" is a prosaic representation.[7] The simplicity of linear systems is so attractive that investigators routinely attempt to "linearize" complex sets of data by various transformations of the axes (plotting the logarithm of x against the reciprocal of y, for example). This practice, however, may misrepresent the true state of the system; as a result, the underlying pathologic process, or mechanism, may be overlooked.

The classical Starling curve describing the relation between cardiac output and ventricular filling pressure is one such case. Initially, cardiac output rises as filling pressure is increased, but at some point further increases in filling pressure result in a fall in cardiac output. This classical *nonlinear* behavior is readily explained at a molecular level by the physical relation between actin and myosin filaments in the sarcomere. At low levels of resting tension there is only a small

1422 *Denton et al.*

December 1990
American Heart Journal

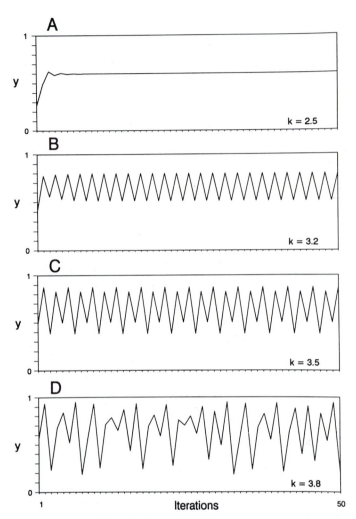

Fig. 3. Iterative solutions of the logistic map. **A,** When k = 2.5 the output of the system *(y)* exhibits a single state after a brief initial period of oscillation. **B,** When k = 3.2 the system alternates between two states. **C,** When k = 3.5 the system has four states. **D,** When k = 4, the system has an infinite number of states.

stretch on the sarcomere, and little interaction between active sites on the actin and myosin filaments. As tension rises, the sarcomere stretches, interaction between actin and myosin increases, and developed force thereby increases. As tension rises still further, the sarcomere stretches to a point where the overlap between actin and myosin and the attendant developed force begin to fall off.

With linear equations, there is always a one-to-one correspondence between values on the x and y axes (Fig. 2, *A*). This is often not the case with nonlinear equations. Nonlinear equations are of two types, monotonic and folded. Monotonic equations (those that are always increasing or always decreasing), such as $y = e^x$, always have a one-to-one correspondence between values on the x and y axes. In contrast, folded nonlinear equations (those that change direc-

tion), like the Starling curve, exhibit local maxima or minima. As a result, a single value of y can be associated with two (or more) values of x (Fig. 2, *B*). As we shall see, this ambiguity gives rise to chaos under some conditions.

Many nonlinear systems can be represented by simple equations. Consider the so-called *logistic map*[3, 9, 26, 47-49] based on the simple equation for a parabola: $y = k \cdot x \cdot (1 - x)$; where x is a variable ($0 \leq x \leq 1$) and k is a parameter ($0 \leq k \leq 4$). The logistic equation contains both linear and nonlinear components that are better seen when the equation is expressed in another form: $y = kx - kx^2$. The kx term is the linear portion of the equation, and the kx^2 term is the nonlinear portion. If we choose particular values for k and x, we can plug them into the equation and get a value for y. If we now substitute y as

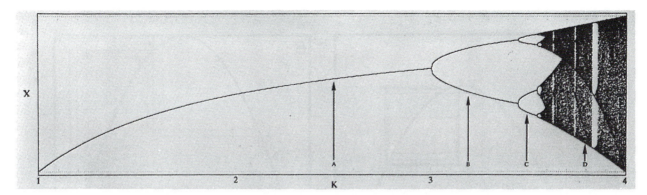

Fig. 4. Bifurcation diagram for the logistic map. The x axis represents values of the parameter k from 1 to 4, and the y axis represents 100 iterated values of the variable x at each fixed value of k. Starting with k = 1, the system has only one state (Fig. 3, *A*). At k = 3.0, a bifurcation occurs and the system now has two states (as in Fig. 3, *B*). At k = 3.45, another bifurcation occurs and the system now has four states (as in Fig. 3, *C*). At k > 3.57, the system develops an infinite number of states (chaos). The letters in the diagram correspond to the four behaviors seen in Fig. 3.

the new value for x, we obtain a new value for y (k remains the same). This repetitive process of substituting the solution to an equation back into the same equation to obtain the next solution is called *iteration*. If we iterate the equation many times and plot each new value of y on the vertical axis against the number of iterations on the horizontal axis, we will have constructed a graph that represents the *dynamic* behavior of the system. Depending on the value of k, the behavior can be quite spectacular.

As a specific example, if we choose an initial condition x = 0.05, k = 2.5, and iterate the equation 50 times, we see that after a short oscillation, the system settles into a predictable and stable output—a flat line (Fig. 3, *A*). The system is stable because the linear portion of the equation is dominant. By increasing k to 3.2 and keeping the initial value of x the same, a sudden qualitative change in behavior of the system occurs—it begins to oscillate between two different states as the nonlinear portion of the equation becomes manifest (Fig. 3, *B*). This abrupt transition, based in this case on a small change in a parameter, is called a *bifurcation*. Increasing k still further to 3.5 causes another bifurcation to four states (Fig. 3, *C*). Suddenly, as we increase k to 3.8, the system begins to exhibit strikingly *aperiodic*, seemingly random, behavior—chaos—as the nonlinear term becomes dominant (Fig. 3, *D*). The entire range of behavior for the logistic map is summarized in the *bifurcation diagram* illustrated in Fig. 4.

This behavior may be better understood by a graphic demonstration (Fig. 5). Let us start with a parabola. The height of this parabola is directly proportional to the parameter k. Then we choose an initial value for x (0.05) and find the next value by

drawing a horizontal line between x and a diagonal line of identity. From that point on the line of identity, we draw a vertical line to the parabola. That new value (y) then becomes the next value for x. We can repeat this process as long as we like.

In our earlier numeric example, after some initial instability, the system oscillated between two values, a and b (Fig. 3, *B*). Fig. 5, *A* demonstrates that with k = 3.2, a transient period of instability, only two points on the parabola are visited (a and b). Fig. 5, *B* demonstrates what happens when the parabola height (k) is increased to 4. Note that there is no stability, and that each intersection of the parabola is at a different point.

Nonlinear systems such as the logistic map can pass through a variety of identifiable stages before they become chaotic,[50-57] and the identification of these stages might have important clinical implications. Imagine a completely hypothetical example, wherein a pateint undergoing coronary artery bypass surgery develops sinus arrest (a logistic map with k = 0) in response to hypothermia, but as body temperature returns to normal, so too does normal sinus rhythm (k = 2.5). On the second postoperative day, atrial bigeminy occurs (k = 3.2), followed by atrial fibrillation (k = 3.8) on the third day. Had the atrial bigeminy been recognized as a harbinger of chaos, and a suitable drug been administered capable of reducing the value of k, the arrhythmia might have been abolished, and the subsequent atrial fibrillation prevented.

What are the characteristics of chaos? Chaotic behavior exhibits a number of characteristics that distinguish it from periodic and random behavior. The most important criteria are summarized below.

1424 *Denton et al.*

December 1990
American Heart Journal

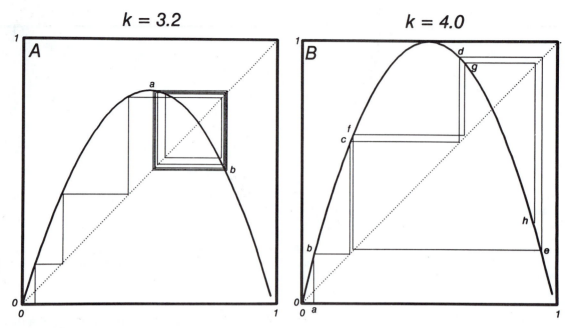

Fig. 5. Geometric solution to the logistic map. **Panel A** demonstrates a periodic solution with values oscillating between *a* and *b*. **Panel B** is a chaotic solution, with the values (*a* through *g*) falling on irregular points of the parabola. See text for explanation of the solution technique.

1. Chaos is both deterministic and aperiodic. As with Newtonian physics, there is an underlying system of mathematical equations that controls the behavior of the system. If one knows the equations (e.g., the parabola) and the initial conditions (e.g., x and k), one can predict the system's behavior accurately and precisely, no matter how complex it appears (Fig. 3, *D*). Unlike Newtonian physics, however, chaotic behavior never repeats itself exactly. There are no identifiable cycles that recur at regular intervals.

2. Chaotic systems exhibit sensitive dependence on initial conditions.[51, 58, 59] This means that very small differences in initial conditions will result in large differences in behavior at a later point in time. For example, the solid line in Fig. 6 illustrates the behavior of the logistic map if the initial value of x is 0.5, and the dotted line illustrates the behavior if the initial value of x is 0.5000001 instead. The two behaviors are almost identical at the start, but become highly divergent even with initial conditions that differ by only one part in one million. The larger the initial difference, the faster the divergence.

The so-called baker's transformation provides a material metaphor of sensitive dependence.[38, 60] Take a piece of dough and sprinkle it with raisins, taking note of their initial positions. Stretch and fold the mixture repeatedly. Now compare the final positions of the raisins to the initial positions. Even a small change in the initial position of a particular raisin will result in a very different final position if one does enough stretching and folding. In fact, any two raisins will move apart exponentially with each cycle of stretching and folding (mathematically, the logarithm of the distance separating them increases as a linear function of time).

A simple modification of the baker's transformation allows us to contrast the *exponential divergence* associated with chaos with the more commonplace *linear divergence*. Take a piece of dough and sprinkle it with raisins as before, but instead of stretching and folding the mixture, just stretch it. Two raisins will now move apart linearly rather than exponentially (mathematically, the separation itself rather than the logarithm of the separation increases linearly as a function of time). It does not take much imagination to see that the apprentice baker's stretching will not result in very good raisin bread. It is the master baker's folding of the dough that adds the nonlinear spice; no folding, no chaos, no bread.

The baker's transformation is also demonstrated on the graph of the logistic map (Fig. 5, *B*). The solution in Fig. 5, *B* starts at the initial value a. Its value is represented on the parabola by b. The value of b is "stretched" to c and c is stretched to d. Point d is stretched still farther to e, and from there e is "folded" back on itself (moves to lower values) to

Volume 120
Number 6, Part 1

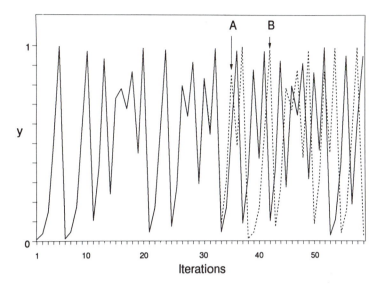

Fig. 6. Sensitive dependence on initial conditions. *The solid line* represents iterations of the logistic map (k = 3.99) with initial x = 0.5, and *the dotted line* represents the same number of iterations with initial x = 0.5000001. The two signals are exactly the same until the thirty-fifth cycle *(point A)*, when they diverge. By the forty-second cycle *(point B)*, the peaks and nadirs are completely out of phase.

point f. In essence, low values on the ascending portion of the parabola are stretched to higher values. When the new stretched value falls on the descending portion of the parabola, it is folded back on itself to low values on the ascending portion of the curve.

Although first described by Poincaré 90 years ago, sensitive dependence on initial conditions in the modern chaotic dynamic sense was rediscovered by Lorenz[2, 8] in the early 1960s. He developed a mathematical model consisting of three differential equations (now enshrined as the *Lorenz equations*) to predict the behavior of a simple microclimate over time. Initial conditions were input, and the computer generated a time series of the behavior of the three variables over many months. On one occasion, Lorenz wanted to extend a previous calculation beyond a few months. Because the calculations were time-consuming, he saved time by using data from the middle of the previous calculation as initial conditions for his longer calculation. After starting the program, he later observed that the time series did not exactly correspond to the previous calculation. The data corresponded exactly for a while, but then diverged widely from the previous behavior. Later he realized that the computer used six significant digits in its calculations, but he had only input three significant digits (there were only three on the print-out). Based on this experience, he concluded that long-term weather forecasting was impossible, and that small changes in a system at one time (the flutter of the

wings of a butterfly in Peking) could make large changes in the behavior of a system later (a weather change in New York)—the so-called "Butterfly effect."[7]

3. Chaotic behavior is constrained to a relatively narrow range. Although it appears random, the behavior of the system is *bounded,* and does not wander off to infinity. In the baker's transformation, for example, the raisins always remain embedded in the dough no matter how long or how vigorously we knead it. The behavior tends to wander because of the stretching, but always returns to a small region because it is folded back on itself. In the logistic map, the limits of the behavior are determined by the height and length of the arms of the parabola.

4. Chaotic behavior has definite form. Not only is the behavior constrained, but there is a particular pattern to the behavior. Common examples are the swirls seen as cream is mixed in coffee, the pattern of cigarette smoke as it rises in a calm room, and the pattern observed as a running stream of water is transformed into a rapid.[58] These patterns often take the form of *"bands"* (regions where behavior preferentially occurs), and *"forbidden zones"* (region where it does not). Raisin bread exhibits such a pattern. The raisins are clustered in layers; they are not randomly distributed throughout the bread. This was also seen in the logistic map, where the irregular behavior was constrained by the parabola and could not move off the curve. The extremes of behavior were limited by

1426 *Denton et al.*

December 1990
American Heart Journal

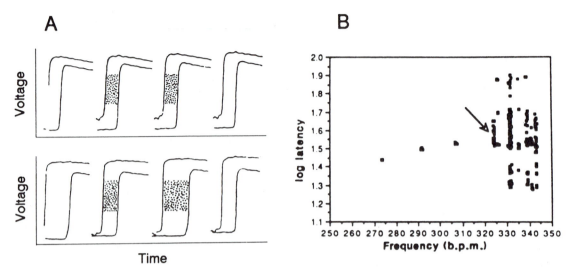

Fig. 7. A, Proximal and distal chamber action potential recordings of unstressed and stressed Purkinje fibers. The left sigmoid curve of each pair represents a depolarization in the proximal chamber and the right curve is the depolarization in the distal chamber. The time between the two curves is the conduction time between the chambers (latency). In the *top series* (no stress), all four depolarizations have the same conduction time. In the *bottom series* (stressed by compression), they oscillate; a long conduction time alternates with a short conduction time *(shading).* **B,** A bifurcation diagram of the same system. The x axis is the frequency of stimulation (the stress to the system) and the y axis represents the latency (the difference in conduction time between proximal and distal chambers). There is a constant variance in latency (just as in the logistic map bifurcation diagram) until the system is stimulated at 325 beats/min *(arrow).* At higher frequencies chaos occurs (compare this with Fig. 4) and the variance in latency increases. (Reprinted and modified by permission from Nature. 1987; 330: 751. Copyright [c] 1987 Macmillan Magazines Limited.)

the height of the parabola. As we shall see, such patterns represent presumptive—but not definitive—evidence that an underlying process is chaotic rather than random.

APPLICATION OF NONLINEAR DYNAMICS TO CARDIAC ARRHYTHMIAS

Nonlinear behavior was first identified in cardiac tissue by Guevara et al.[61-63] in 1981. They induced both periodic and aperiodic rhythms in spontaneously depolarizing chick embryonic ventricular cell aggregates by intracellular current injection, and observed a variety of phenomena *(period-doubling* and *phase locking)* similar to those that are characteristic precursors of chaos in the logistic map. Based on these data, they developed a simple nonlinear mathematical model that described the complex behavior of these heart cell aggregates. Most importantly, they found that the model could reproduce all of the behaviors seen in the heart cell aggregates, and the behavior could be predicted based on measurable parameters. This was an unequivocal demonstration of nonlinear biologic behavior. A potential clinical application of this study arises in the phase locking and period-doubling patterns observed. These patterns correspond to those associated with advanced

atrioventricular (AV) nodal disease (2:1, 3:1, 4:1 block[64-68]). The mathematical model developed by these investigators showed how these seemingly irregular conduction processes could be explained and predicted. This is an important first step in the construction of a realistic mathematical model of the AV node itself.[65]

Chialvo and Jalife[69] observed these same electrophysiologic phenomena in electrically stimulated adult sheep heart Purkinje fibers that had no pacemaker activity. By gradually increasing stimulation rate, strength of stimulation, and duration, they observed phase locking patterns similar to those reported by Guevara et al. They also subjected these Purkinje fibers to stress in a three-chamber superfusion tissue bath. The proximal and distal chambers were superfused with Tyrode's solution, and the center chamber was superfused with the electric uncoupler heptanol or was compressed mechanically. By varying stimulation rate in the proximal chamber and measuring conduction velocity to the distal chamber, bifurcations in conduction velocity similar to those in the logistic map, and aperiodic dynamics consistent with chaos were observed (Fig. 7). These observations clearly show that a biologic system is capable of exhibiting aperiodic behavior under conditions of stress, and that such behavior has many of the characteristics of chaos. Moreover, the experimental design is a reasonable model for a common clinical condition—an island of ischemic or infarcted tissue (the stressed central chamber) surrounded by normal tissue (the proximal and distal chambers), in which aperiodic behavior (extrasystoles) occurs as a result of variable conduction velocities at various heart rates.

Ritzenberg et al.[70] observed a variety of electrophysiologic and hemodynamic phenomena indicative of *prechaotic* behavior (QRS alternans, period-doubling, period-tripling, period-quadrupling, and period-quintupling) in anesthetized closed-chested dogs following intravenous noradrenaline. They also reported that hypothermia (29° C) and transient coronary artery occlusion both caused aperiodic changes in the magnitude of the QRS and T waves that followed a pattern of period-doubling similar to that for the logistic map. Whenever this characteristic precursor of chaos was observed, the ventricular fibrillation threshold was significantly decreased.[71, 72] This work extended the observation of nonlinear biologic behavior from purely electrical, in vitro systems to a mechanical, in vivo system. On the basis of these studies, these investigators developed a simple computer model of ventricular activation capable of beat-to-beat oscillations of period 2, 3, 6, and 24 during progressive increases in the rate of stimulation. This model eventually exhibited a chaotic rhythm that was considered an analog of clinical ventricular fibrillation.[73]

Goldberger et al.,[74-76] on the other hand, have questioned the hypothesis that ventricular fibrillation is chaotic. They applied a rapid train of electrical stimuli to the heart of normal, open-chested, anesthetized dogs, and analyzed the resulting ventricular fibrillation by *spectral analysis* of the hand-digitized electrocardiographic waveforms. They observed that this ventricular fibrillation was associated with a *narrow-band* frequency spectrum. Because chaos is often characterized by a *broad-band* frequency spectrum,[33] the authors concluded that ventricular fibrillation is not a chaotic process.[76]

However, recent studies by Chen et al.,[77] using a very similar model (canine ventricular fibrillation induced by a single premature stimulus), demonstrated reentrant activation at the very onset of ventricular fibrillation in a figure-of-eight pattern. This highly organized pattern of activation is analogous to sustained monomorphic ventricular tachycardia[78] and might explain the narrow-band frequency spectrum observed by Goldberger et al.[76] at the onset of ventricular fibrillation. Moreover, although investi-

gations aimed at determining if ventricular fibrillation is chaotic have so far relied exclusively on conventional spectral analysis; as we shall see, more sensitive and specific methods of detection are now available.[79, 80]

Goldberger et al.,[65, 74, 75, 81, 82] in fact, consider normal sinus rhythm rather than ventricular fibrillation to be chaotic. This counterintuitive assertion has a reasonable theoretical foundation—the sinus rhythm "system" consists of the sinoatrial (SA) node (a periodic oscillator) controlled by multiple nonlinear mechanisms (sympathetic tone, parasympathetic tone, hormones, preload, afterload), most of which have long feedback loops compared with the basic sinus cycle length—a near-perfect substrate for the generation of chaos. Recent data[83] showing a decrease in heart rate variability among patients at high risk for sudden death as a consequence of left ventricular dysfunction provide empirical support for this assertion.

Shrier et al.[84] recently demonstrated nonlinear behavior of the AV node in the intact human heart. AV nodal recovery curves were generated for seven patients undergoing routine electrophysiologic testing. The curves were constructed by plotting the time of conduction from the extrastimulus (S_2) to the His bundle spike (the S_2-H_2 interval) on the y axis, and the recovery time of the beat prior to the extrastimulus (the H_1-S_2 interval) on the x axis. Using these curves as templates, two sets of nonlinear equations were generated that described the behavior of the AV node. A variety of complex behaviors such as Wenckebach, reverse Wenckebach, alternating Wenckebach, and other advanced AV rhythms could be reproduced by these equations. This study is a logical extension of the animal models described above, and provides further support for the hypothesis that simple nonlinear mathematical models are capable of predicting—albeit only over the short-term—the complex electrodynamic behavior of the intact human heart.

Finally, Winfree[15, 85, 86] has made a remarkable series of predictions regarding the onset and form of ventricular fibrillation based on topological characteristics of biologic oscillators. He thereby predicted that a depolarization field oriented in a particular way to a repolarization field could produce an unstable state (what he called a "singular point") in the myocardium that would lead to a rotating spiral of reentry—fibrillation. The type of spiral field (circular or figure-of-eight) is a function of the orientation of the depolarizing and repolarizing fields. Various aspects of this hypothesis have been verified experimentally,[77, 87, 88] thereby demonstrating the

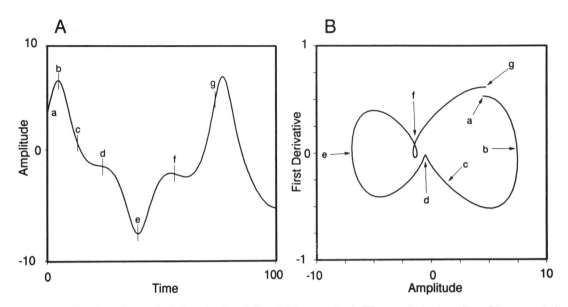

Fig. 8. A, Portion of a typical chaotic signal (Duffing's equation). The x axis is time (in arbitrary units) and the y axis is amplitude (unitless). **B,** The phase plane plot of the same chaotic signal. The x axis is amplitude and the y axis is the first derivative of the amplitude (the center of each axis is zero). The signal starts high and becomes slightly more positive for a short period of time. On the phase plane plot this is represented by starting at point *a*, moving slightly rightward (higher amplitude) and down (toward a derivative of zero). *Point b* represents an area of positive amplitude but of zero derivative. *Point c* represents a point in which the amplitude and the derivative are approaching zero. *Point d* has a slightly negative amplitude and a derivative near zero. *Point e* is the minimun with a derivative of zero. *Point f* is a small loop that represents a small suboscillation. The signal now returns toward another peak value (positive amplitude and maximally positive derivative), and the phase plane plot returns toward the starting point, *a*. The second complex in **A** does not exactly superimpose over the first, indicating that this waveform is aperiodic. Note the incidental similarity of this signal to a surface electrocardiogram (lead I in left bundle branch block).

power of applying abstract principles of mathematical analysis to the problem of cardiac arrhythmias.

ANALYTIC TECHNIQUES TO DETECT NONLINEAR DYNAMIC BEHAVIOR

Unfortunately, we usually do not know the underlying mathematical mechanisms that determine the behavior of a biologic system. We are instead presented with nothing more than a phenomenological *time series* of the behavior (the conventional electrocardiogram, or conduction properties through the AV node, for example), and must infer the mechanisms from simple measurements of that time series. The most common ways to look for nonlinear or chaotic behavior involve the study of bifurcations in *discrete* data. Other less commonly used techniques attempt to detect more complex patterns in *continuous* data (such as the electrocardiogram). We divide our discussion here into two parts; the first describing the analysis of discrete data, and the second describing the analysis of continuous data.

Discrete data. Many nonlinear systems (such as the logistic map) pass through a series of intermediate stages prior to chaotic behavior. Often, these stages are easily recognized as oscillations between two, four, eight, or more states. If a biologic system is observed to behave in this manner, then the underlying rules for the behavior might be based on a nonlinear system. Guevara et al., for example, started with observations of periodic and aperiodic behavior in their model of heart cell aggregates. By carefully stimulating the preparations, repetitive, reproducible behaviors were noted (the multiple combinations of phase-locking responses).

The next step in the analysis was the construction of a mathematical model that could reproduce the behaviors noted in vitro. This is the most difficult aspect of the problem. After developing a general theoretical model, appropriate parameters must be selected that reproduce the behavior. This step is empiric, and multiple models may need to be tried—and many parameters tested—before a successful model is found. Guevara et al. found a very simple model, the Poincaré oscillator, that described much of the behavior. It cannot be sufficiently stressed that the search for a model is an art that is not easily taught.

The final step in the process is proving that the proposed mathematical model accounts for most, if not all, of the behaviors described in the biologic model. By solving the model under many conditions analogous to those in the real biologic system, one may have the basis for studying the biology in a more systematic fashion. In addition, once a reliable model is obtained, ionic, mechanical, or biochemical mechanisms might be inferred from what we know of the biologic system.

The application of models to biologic problems has helped explain many inconsistencies in the past. An example is seen in the use of exercise stress testing. Although exercise electrocardiography has a high predictive accuracy for the diagnosis of coronary artery disease in symptomatic populations, it has a low predictive accuracy in asymptomatic populations. This paradox was resolved by showing that Bayes' theorem provided a theoretical basis for the disparate observations.[89]

Continuous data. The modeling process described above is a general framework that can be applied to many biologic behaviors. In the work of Guevara et al., the variations in behavior were relatively simple—but continuous signals present a more difficult problem. Often subtle changes in behavior are not visible in the time series; sometimes the time series appears random. In these cases, more sophisticated techniques are needed to detect the presence of underlying structure in the behavior. We now present a series of techniques commonly used in the analysis of continuous data (and sometimes of discontinuous data) that can reveal underlying structure in complicated behavior. These techniques are only the first step in providing an explanation for complex behavior. Just as in the discontinuous systems described above, once we determine there is underlying structure, we must propose a model or mechanism that fits the behavior, and demonstrate that the model applies to the biologic system. We then have a better understanding of the system, and might be able to intervene to regulate the system.

Phase plane plots. The *phase plane plot* is a representation of the behavior of a dynamic system in *state space* (the abstract mathematical area in which a behavior occurs). It typically takes the form of a graph of the position of a signal (its amplitude) on the x axis, versus the velocity of the signal (its first derivative) on the y axis. Each cycle, called a *trajectory* or orbit, represents the behavior of the system over a given period of time.[6, 13, 14, 90] Fig. 8 illustrates the phase plane plot of a typical chaotic system, and Fig. 9 is a phase plane plot based on data obtained from the experiments in Fig. 7. Graphs such as these

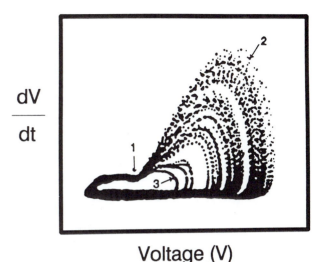

Fig. 9. A phase plane plot of the action potentials arriving at the distal chamber in the Purkinje fiber model described in Fig. 6. The pacing rate of 322 beats/min corresponds to the aperiodic region in Fig. 6, *B*. The banding and forbidden zones *(point 2)* and the sensitive dependence on initial conditions (two trajectories are very close together at *point 1,* and far apart at *point 2*) are all characteristic of chaos. (Reprinted and modified by permission from Nature 1987;330:751. Copyright [c] 1987 Macmillan Magazines Limited).

were used widely for some time to assess left ventricular function.[91] Left ventricular wall tension was plotted on the x axis against a function of its velocity of contraction on the y axis. An indirect measure of contractility (V_{max}) was determined directly from this force-velocity phase plane plot.

The two-dimensional phase plane plot is the most common representation of state space, but many others are possible. State space can also be represented in three dimensions, for example, with the axes representing the amplitude of the waveform, its first derivative (velocity), and its second derivative (accleration). In some multidimensional systems, each axis serves to represent a different variable.

Phase plane plots of periodic signals have trajectories that overlap each other precisely (Fig. 10, *B*), while those of random signals exhibit no definite pattern (Fig. 10, *J*). In contrast, although phase plane plots of chaotic signals do not have periodic trajectories, they do exhibit a definite pattern (Fig. 10, *F*). As noted earlier, two particular patterns are highly specific for chaotic behavior. Bands, similar to those in the rings of the planet Saturn, represent groups of nearby non-overlapping trajectories, while forbidden zones represent the empty space between adjacent bands.

A major disadvantage of the phase plane plot is its

1430   *Denton et al.*

December 1990
American Heart Journal

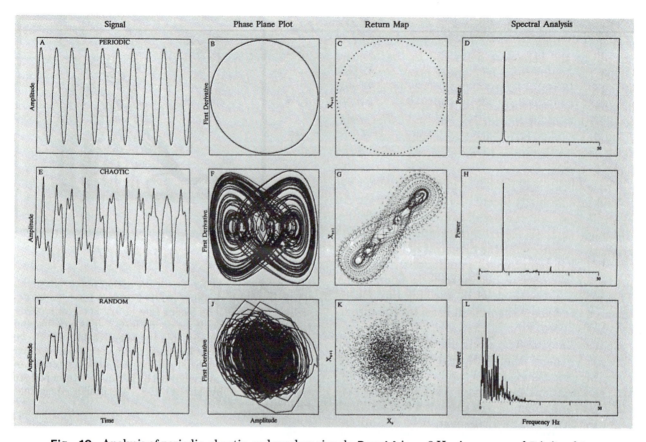

Fig. 10. Analysis of periodic, chaotic, and random signals. **Panel A** is an 8 Hz sine wave and **B** is its phase plane plot. Periodic signal trajectories all overlap; thus only a single circle is seen. Its return map **(panel C)** is very similar in structure to the phase plane plot. **Panel D** is the Fast Fourier Transform power spectrum, with one isolated spike at 8 Hz (a discrete spectrum). **Panel E** is a chaotic solution to Duffing's equation (see also Fig. 7) and **F** is its phase plane plot. Note the banding and forbidden zones, consistent with a chaotic process. **Panel G** is the return map demonstrating the same structure as the phase plane plot. The spectrum **(panel H)** has predominant spikes at 8 and 24 Hz, and very small amounts of continuous spectral power centered about 1, 16, and 19 Hz, which are the components of the signal that make it aperiodic. They are not random because Duffing's equation contains no *stochastic* components (note the similarity of Duffing's equation to polymorphous ventricular tachycardia). **Panel I** is a random, continuous, low-frequency signal generated by successive smoothing of a pseudorandom number time series. Its phase plane plot **(panel J)** and its return map **(panel K)** reflect the underlying Gaussian distribution (nonstructured) from which the data were generated. Its frequency spectrum **(panel G)** is continuous with power at all frequencies between 0 to 14 Hz.

sensitivity to noise. As little as 1% noise can severely disrupt the structure of a plot (by filling in forbidden zones, for example). Accordingly, the recording system and the data must be as noise-free as possible. Although data can be filtered to remove some of this noise, such filtering can also mask identification of an underlying chaotic structure.

Return maps. The *return map* is similar to the phase plane plot, but the analyzed data must be discrete (digital), or if not, must be converted to digital form.[55, 61] Typically, the return map represents the relation between a given point in a time series plotted on the x axis, and the next point in the time series plotted on the y axis (a next-amplitude plot). The

temporal difference between the two points is called the *lag*. The lag acts to smooth away some of the noise in the data, making the return map less sensitive to noise than the phase plane plot. This is especially useful when the data cannot be filtered. Fig. 10 illustrates examples of return maps for periodic, chaotic, and random signals. These maps are similar to phase plane plots (compare Fig. 10, *F* and 10, *G*) because the x axes are identical (amplitude), while the y axes are mathematically related (the y axis of the return map is $x + \Delta x/\Delta t$, and the y axis of the phase plane plot is dx/dt).

Shaw et al.[10, 92] have used a common water faucet as an example of a chaotic system readily analyzed by construction of a return map. The faucet is allowed to drip into a container filled with water so that one can easily hear the intervals between drops. The drip is started at a very low rate such that discrete drops fall at regular intervals. As one slowly increases the flow rate, one will note an abrupt change in the interval between the drops such that a long interval alternates with a short interval (the first bifurcation). In one continues to increase the rate of flow, one will get to a point where the intervals between drops sound random. But if one plots the relation between one interval and a subsequent interval (a next-interval plot), a remarkably ordered pattern is obtained (Fig. 11), indicating that the process is probably chaotic rather than random. With this simple graphic tool, the return map, a seemingly random pattern has been shown to have an underlying ordered structure.

A hypothetical example of the use of a return map was illustrated in the prologue of this report. The R wave amplitude time series illustrated in Fig. 1, *A* is actually the output of the logistic map with k = 3.99, and the return map in Fig. 1, *C* reveals the underlying parabolic relation. In contrast, the systolic pressure-time series illustrated in Fig. 1, *B* is really just a series of computer-generated pseudorandom numbers, and the return map in Fig. 1, *D* confirms that there is no relation between one number and a neighboring number. The return maps clearly distinguish between these chaotic and random signals. Application of this technique to the assessment of the susceptibility to ventricular fibrillation was recently awarded a United States Patent.[93]

Poincaré sections. If a phase plane plot does not have a clearly discernible pattern, this ancillary graphical technique can help reveal one.[13, 14, 50, 94] There are two kinds of *Poincaré sections*.

In the first type[50, 52, 94] a two-dimensional phase plane plot is cut by a line roughly perpendicular to the trajectories (Fig. 12, *A*). Points on that line represent where each trajectory crossed the line (Fig. 12, *B*). A graph is constructed from these points, representing the relation between adjacent trajectories (Fig. 12, *C*). Sometimes this graph reveals structure that in not apparent in the phase plane plot itself. As with the phase plane plot, this method too is sensitive to noise.

The second kind of Poincaré section[9, 13] is best explained by analogy. Imagine a common housefly in a large dark room that contains only a dresser. Over time, the fly traces a continuous path through space (its plot of state space) as it moves about the room. In one were to take a stroboscopic picture of the fly's position at regular intervals, one would generate a discrete pattern that represents where the fly has

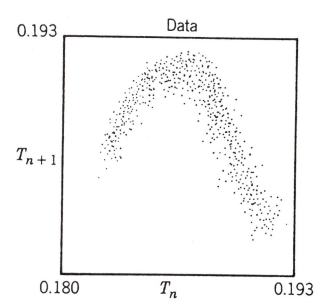

Fig. 11. Return map of the time intervals *(T)* between successive drops of water from a conventional faucet. The x axis is the duration (in milliseconds) of the index interval (n) and the y axis is the duration of the succeeding interval (n+1). Note the similarity of these empirical data to the hypothetical data in Fig. 1, *C.* The nonlinear relationship indicates that the process might be chaotic rather than random. (From Shaw R. The dripping faucet as a model chaotic system. Santa Cruz, Calif.: The Ariel Press, 1984. Reproduced with permission.)

been. In addition, one would have also amassed information about where the fly has not been. Thus because the dresser takes up space in the center of the room, our graph of where the fly has been is also a graph of a forbidden zone representing the dresser. The existence and form of the dresser is thereby detected without ever detecting the dresser itself. Just as with our analogy, this kind of Poincaré section is obtained by sampling a conventional phase plane plot at regular intervals, and replotting the data as discrete points as an amplitude versus first derivative graph.

Lyapunov exponents. The Lyapunov numerical method[13, 94-97] is used as an adjunct to the graphical analysis of state space. As noted earlier, chaotic systems characteristically exhibit sensitive dependence on initial conditions. In state space, sensitive dependence manifests itself graphically as adjacent trajectories that diverge widely from their initial close positions. The baker's transformation that was introduced as an example of sensitive dependence is also an example of exponential divergence: two raisins that are initially near each other move apart exponentially with each cycle of stretching and folding. The *Lyapunov exponent* is a quantitative measure of

1432 *Denton et al.*

December 1990
American Heart Journal

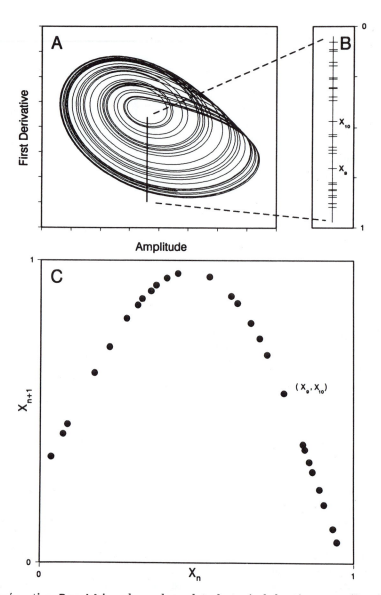

Fig. 12. Poincaré section. **Panel A** is a phase plane plot of a typical chaotic system (Rössler system). *The vertical line* intersects ("sections") a selected portion of the phase plane plot. The distribution of the points along an expansion of this line (**panel B**) reveals no apparent structure, but a return map constructed from these points shows a nonlinear pattern suggestive of a parabola **(panel C)**. Compare this with Figs. 1, *C* and 10. The phase plane plot is not a series of spirals—each trajectory crosses the line irregularly. In **panel B**, X_9 and X_{10} are the ninth and tenth trajectories—they are not adjacent. The relation between X_9 and X_{10} is shown in **graph C**.

this rate of separation. The magnitude of this exponent is related to how chaotic the system is; the larger the exponent, the more chaotic the system.[97] In three-dimensional systems, periodic signals have a Lyapunov exponent of zero; there is no divergence or convergence of trajectories because all trajectories overlap. A random signal will also have an exponent of zero because over a long period of time adjacent trajectories will converge and diverge equally. A positive Lyapunov exponent, on the other hand, indicates sensitive dependence on initial conditions and is—almost without exception[97]—diagnostic of chaos.[3, 95]

Lyapunov exponents are not easily measured.[95] The major limitation in their calculation is that currently available algorithms require large amounts of data (on the order of 1,000 to 10,000 cycles). As a result, the computing time itself can be limiting (the processing of only a few thousand points by one member of our group took 27 hours on a fast personal computer). Even then, the system being studied must remain stable over the collection period, and real biologic systems virtually never remain stable for any length of time. Clinical ventricular fibrillation serves as a good example. If one records the fibrillation over a short interval (1 to 2 seconds), there is probably little change in the underlying dynamics of the system, but this represents only 10 to 30 cycles of fibrillation—not enough for accurate computation of the exponent. With longer recording periods, adequate data can be collected, but the myocardium becomes progressively ischemic during the collection period, thereby changing the underlying dynamics of the system.

Fractal dimension. The word *fractal*, coined by Benoit Mandelbrot,[99] refers to data sets that are self-similar at all scales. Clouds are a common example; one cannot tell the distance to a large cloud because its overall form is the same at any distance, whether it be 10 miles or 10 feet. Fractal patterns cannot be thought of in conventional topological terms of three dimensions (the volume of this journal), two dimensions (the plane of this page), one dimension (this line of text), or zero dimensions (the period at the end of this sentence). Consider a ball of twine.[7, 100] At a distance of 100 yards, the ball is nothing more than a point; one dimension. As one moves closer, say 50 feet, it acquires characteristics of a plane—its spherical shape cannot be appreciated, but it takes up more space than a point; it has two dimensions. Moving closer still, it acquires all the characteristics of a sphere; three dimensions. Moving inside the ball of twine, the strands seem to be three-dimensional columns. On a still smaller scale, the individual threads of the strands are a maze of one-dimensional lines. As we magnify or shrink an object, our perception of the object's dimension will vary. A fractal has the same overall structure at all scales. The bifurcation diagram of the logistic map (Fig. 4) is a fractal pattern. Though not obvious at first, if one were to magnify the area between k = 3.5 and k = 3.6, one would see a close replica of the overall diagram; this remarkable phenomenon occurs at any scale.

This is not just an idle abstraction; *fractal dimension* can be quantified in a meaningful way.[60, 94, 99, 101-107] To do this, we observe the object (metaphorically) under many different magnifications; by varying our magnification and measuring the amount of space the object occupies, we can determine its fractal dimension. Mandelbrot uses the coast of Britain as an example. If one uses a meter stick to measure the length of the coastline, one arrives at some distance for the total length; but if one uses a millimeter stick, one will obtain a much larger

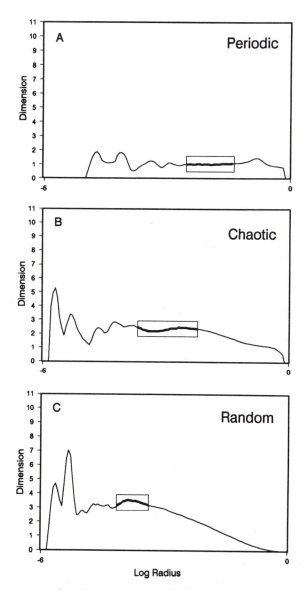

Fig. 13. Calculation of fractal dimension. For each panel, the y axis is dimension and the x axis is the "magnification" at which that dimension is calculated. The plateau portion of the curve *(boxed, thick line)* is an estimate of the dimension. **Panel A** is the dimension of an 8 Hz sine wave (Fig. 9, *A*). There is a long plateau that corresponds to a dimension close to 1. **Panel B** is a calculation using Duffing's equation (Fig. 9, *E*) and shows an approximate dimension of 2.4. **Panel C** is a random, continuous, low-frequency signal (Fig. 9, *I*) with a dimension of 3.2. Note the difficulty in selecting a plateau, and thus the limitation in accuracy and precision in the calculation. Because of this, dimensions should probably be reported semiquantitatively as high, intermediate, or low.

distance. By continuously increasing the magnification (using a smaller stick) and measuring the length of the coastline, one will observe different lengths for each magnification. Over some range, however, there

Table I. Ability of analytic methods to detect the characteristics of chaos*

	Aperiodicity	Sensitive dependence	Boundedness
Phase plane plot	Yes	Yes	Yes
Return map	Yes	Yes	Yes
Poincaré section	Yes	Yes	Yes
Lyapunov exponent	No	Yes	No
Fractal dimension	No	No	Yes
Spectral analysis	Yes	No	No

*This table is overly simplified and the investigator is referred to any of the comprehensive references for a more detailed understanding.

will be a series of magnifications for which the length of the coastline is essentially constant, and a plot of coastline length versus magnification will show a "plateau" area wherein small changes in magnification do not affect length. This plateau corresponds to the quantitative fractal dimension. The more irregular a figure, the more complex its structure, the more space it occupies, and the higher its fractal dimension. The fractal dimension of the British coastline is approximately 1.3. It is not a perfect line (dimension = 1), but neither does it fill a plane (dimension = 2).

Computation of fractal dimension is presently something of an art, and the algorithms used for analysis of unknown signals are still evolving. The most common algorithm is that developed by Grassberger and Procaccia.[104, 105] We use a particular modification of that algorithm,[106] whereby dimension is estimated by the slope of the line showing the relation between the log of the magnification factor (measuring stick length) and the log of the measured distance. As specific examples, the periodic signal in Fig. 10 has a fractal dimension of 1.1, the chaotic signal has a dimension of 2.4, and the random signal has a dimension of 3.2 (Fig. 13). Chaotic systems often exhibit low dimension because they are often simple systems, but periodic and random signals can also exhibit the same magnitude of dimension. For this reason, a diagnosis of chaos based solely on fractal dimension should be viewed with suspicion.

Spectral analysis. Spectral analysis is used as a diagnostic tool in the study of chaos because it is capable of distinguishing periodicity from the aperiodicity of randomness and chaos. There are many methods of spectral analysis, the *fast Fourier transform (FTT)* being the most common.[50, 109, 110] Spectral analysis takes a continuous signal, breaks it into component frequencies, and displays the contribution of each frequency to the total signal. A pure sine wave of 8 Hz will have an isolated spike at 8 Hz (Fig.

10, *D*), while a modulated sine wave (one that varies in a periodic manner) will have more than one spike. Spectral patterns have been classified arbitrarily into *discrete* (or narrow-band) and *continuous* (or broadband). A discrete spectrum (characteristic of periodic and some chaotic signals) contains one or more narrow spikes. The higher frequency spikes (the *harmonics*) are exact multiples of some lower frequency spike (the fundamental). A continuous spectrum (characteristic of random and some chaotic signals) exhibits curves that enclose a large number of frequencies bearing no numerical relation to each other. Often the distinction between a discrete and a continuous spectrum is qualitative rather than quantitative. Fig. 10, *L* illustrates the continuous frequency spectrum of a typical random signal.

Spectral analysis is insensitive to noise, but its application is limited to determining the presence of absence of periodic signals. It cannot distinguish between random, chaotic, or periodic signals,[50, 111] although it has been used to detect bifurcations that manifest as new harmonics.[70] Although spectral analysis alone cannot distinguish a chaotic process, some investigators believe that a particular spectral pattern (one in which the power density is inversely related to the frequency) is highly suggestive of a nonlinear or chaotic process.[67, 74, 75, 81, 112] Others, however, question the diagnostic value of this so-called 1/f pattern.[114]

Integrated analysis. Table I integrates the various graphical and numerical methods of analysis into a coherent structure that demonstrates their relative ability to detect the characteristics of chaos in an unknown signal. Because no single method is sufficient to detect all the characteristics reliably, an investigator should use combinations of these methods.[95, 115, 116] Table II demonstrates the expected results of each of the tests on periodic, chaotic, and random signals. The graphical demonstration of banding, forbidden zones, and sensitive dependence on initial conditions is highly suggestive of a chaotic process. Currently the numerical methods are all subordinate to the graphical methods, but if a reliable and rapid technique for the calculation of the Lyapunov exponent were to be developed, it would most likely be the only tool needed for the study of a stable system.

FUTURE IMPLICATIONS

Only two decades have passed since Aristotle's prophetic description of chaos (*"The least initial deviation from the truth is multiplied later a thousandfold"*) was recast with mathematical rigor. This "new math" has already helped explain a num-

Table II. Expected results of the analytic techniques on standard signals

	Periodic	*Chaotic*	*Random*
Phase plane plot	Trajectories overlap	Banding, forbidden zones, sensitive dependence	No structure
Return map	Points overlap	Banding, forbidden zones, sensitive dependence	No structure
Poincaré section	Uniform distribution of points	Non-random distribution of points	Random distribution of points
Lyapunov exponent	Zero	Positive	Zero
Fractal dimension	Usually low	Usually low	Often high, but can be low
Spectral analysis	Discrete	Discrete or continuous	Continuous

ber of heretofore puzzling phenomena in the physical sciences, and its application to biology is likely to be similarly rewarding.

Applications of nonlinear dynamics to cardiology have become common over the last few years, and a broad range of subjects is being studied by many groups. Computer models of excitable tissue have demonstrated their utility in better understanding basic cardiac physiology.[117-119] An explanation for irregular action potential dynamics seen when Purkinje fibers are repetitively stimulated may be forthcoming.[119] Mechanisms of phase-locking, and chaotic ionic mechanisms in the cell membrane are also being investigated.[120, 121] More direct clinical applications are being studied in the patterns of conduction through the AV node,[64-68] mechanisms of parasystole,[118] the nature of ventricular fibrillation, and whether chaos is normal or abnormal in physiology.[120, 121] There is some evidence that the termination of reentry may be chaotic.[122] Also of interest is the fractal nature of blood flow through the coronary tree, which may give a new insight into coronary flow dynamics and ischemia.[123] An interesting application of sensitive dependence on initial conditions, analogous to Lorenz' statement regarding the unpredictability of the weather, has been made regarding clinical prediction models[124] whereby outcome can never be reliably predicted because of initial uncertainties in a patient's condition.

SUMMARY

Nonlinear dynamics is an exciting new way of looking at peculiarities that in the past have been ignored or explained away. We have attempted to give a general introduction to the basics of the mathematics, applications to cardiology, and a brief review of the new tools needed to use the concepts of nonlinear mathematics. The careful mathematical approach to problems in cardiac electrical dynamics and blood flow is opening a window on behaviors and mechanisms previously inaccessible.

REFERENCES

1. Glass L, Mackey MC. From clocks to chaos: The rhythms of life. Princeton, N.J.: Princeton University Press, 1988.
2. Lorenz EN. Deterministic nonperiodic flow. J Atmospheric Sci 1963;20:130-41.
3. Jensen RV. Classical Chaos Am Sci 1987;75:168-81.
4. Olsen LF, Degn H. Chaos in biological systems. Q Rev Biophys 1985;18:165-225.
5. Holden AV. Chaos. Princeton, N.J.: Princeton University Press, 1986.
6. Moon FC. Chaotic vibrations. New York: John Wiley & Sons, 1987.
7. Gleick J. Chaos: making a new science. New York: Viking Penguin Inc., 1987.
8. Stewart I. Does God play dice? The mathematics of chaos. New York: Basil Blackwell Ltd, 1989.
9. Hofstadter DR. Metamagical themas. Sci Am 1981;245:22-43.
10. Crutchfield JP, Farmer JD, Packard NH, Shaw RS. Chaos. Sci Am 1986;255:46-57.
11. Kloeden PE, Mees AI. Chaotic phenomena. Bull Math Biol 1985;47:697-738.
12. Grebogi C, Ott E, Yorke JA. Chaos, strange attractors, and fractal basin boundaries in nonlinear dynamics. Science 1987;238:632-8.
13. Thompson JMT, Stewart HB. Nonlinear dynamics and chaos. New York: John Wiley & Sons, 1986.
14. Bergé P, Pomeau Y, Vidal C. Order within chaos. New York: John Wiley & Sons, 1984.
15. Winfree AT. When time breaks down: The three-dimensional dynamics of electrochemical waves and cardiac arrhythmias. Princeton, N.J.: Princeton University Press, 1987.
16. Epstein IR. Oscillations and chaos in chemical systems. Physica D 1983;7:47-56.
17. Roux JC. Experimental studies of bifurcations leading to chaos in the Belousof-Zhabotinsky reaction. Physica D 1983;7:57-68.
18. Kaplan JL, Yorke JA. The onset of chaos in a fluid flow model of Lorenz. Ann NY Acad Sci 1979;316:400-7.
19. Sussman GJ, Wisdom J. Numerical evidence that the motion of Pluto is chaotic. Science 1988;241:433-7.
20. Kurths J, Herzel H. An attractor in a solar time series. Physica D 1987;25:165-72.
21. Spiegel EA, Wolf A. Chaos and the solar cycle. Ann NY Acad Sci 1987;497:55-60.
22. Pool R. Seeing chaos in a simple system. Science 1988;241:787-8.
23. Pool R. Is something strange about the weather? Science 1989;243:1290-3.
24. Rothrock DA, Thorndike AS. Geometric properties of the underside of sea ice. J Geophys Res 1980;85:3955-63.
25. Pool R. Is it chaos, or is it just noise? Science 1989;243:25-8.
26. May RM. Biological populations with nonoverlapping generations: stable points, stable cycles, and chaos. Science 1974;186:645-7.

27. Pool R. Ecologists flirt with chaos. Science 1989;243:310-3.
28. Arneodo A, Coullet P, Peyraud J, Tresser C. Strange attractors in Volterra equations for species in competition. J Math Biol 1982;14:153-7.
29. Rogers TD, Yang ZC, Yip LW. Complete chaos in a simple epidemiological model. J Math Biol 1986;23:263-8.
30. May RM. Nonlinear phenomena in ecology and epidemiology. Ann NY Acad Sci 1980;357:267-81.
31. Decker P. Spatial, chiral, and temporal self-organization through bifurcation in "Bioids," open systems capable of a generalized Darwinian evolution. Ann NY Acad Sci 1979;316:236-50.
32. Kearney RE, Hunter IW. Nonlinear identification of stretch reflex dynamics. Ann Biomed Eng 1988;16:79-94.
33. Goldberger AL, Shabetai R, Bhargave V, West BJ, Mandell AJ. Nonlinear dynamics electrical alternans and pericardial tamponade. AM HEART J 1984;107:1297-9.
34. Goldberger AL, Findley LJ, Blackburn MR, Mandell AJ. Nonlinear dynamics in heart failure: implications of long-wavelength cardiopulmonary oscillations. AM HEART J 1984;107:612-5.
35. Glass L, Mackey MC. Pathological conditions resulting from instabilities in physiological control systems. Ann NY Acad Sci 1979;316:214-35.
36. Mackey MC, Glass L. Oscillation and chaos in physiological control systems. Science 1977;197:287-9.
37. Pyeritz RE, Murphy EA. Genetics and congenital heart disease: perspectives and prospects. J Am Coll Cardiol 1989;13:1458-68.
38. Meinhardt H. The random character of bifurcations and the reproducible processes of embryonic development. Ann NY Acad Sci 1979;316:188-202.
39. Saperstein AM. Chaos—A model for the outbreak of war. Nature 1984;309:303-5.
40. Sporns O, Roth S, Seelig F. Chaotic dynamics of two coupled biochemical oscillators. Physica D 1987;26:215-24.
41. Decroly O, Goldbeter A. Birhythmicity, chaos and other patterns of temporal self-organization in a multiply regulated biochemical system. Proc Natl Acad Sci 1982;79:6917-21.
42. Decroly O, Goldbeter A. Selection between multiple periodic regimes in a biochemical system: complex dynamic behavior resolved by use of one-dimensional maps. J Theor Biol 1985;113:649-71.
43. Babloyantz A, Destexhe A. Low-dimensional chaos in an instance of epilepsy. Proc Natl Acad Sci USA 1986;83:3513-17.
44. Watt RC, Hameroff SR. Phase space electroencephalography (EEG): a new mode of intraoperative EEG analysis. Int J Clin Monit Comput 1988;5:3-13.
45. Watt RC, Hameroff SR. Phase space analysis of human EEG during general anesthesia. Ann NY Acad Sci 1987;504:286-8.
46. Mayer-Kress G, Layne SP. Dimensionality of the human electroencephalogram. Ann NY Acad Sci 1987;504:62-87.
47. May RM. Simple mathematical models with very complicated dynamics. Nature 1976;261:459-67.
48. Feigenbaum MJ. Universal behavior in nonlinear systems. Physica D 1983;7:16-39.
49. Feigenbaum MJ. Universal behavior in nonlinear systems. Los Alamos Science 1980;1:4-27.
50. Swinney HL. Observations of order and chaos in nonlinear systems. Physica D 1983;7:3-15.
51. Procaccia I. Universal properties of dynamically complex systems: the organization of chaos. Nature 1988;333:618-23.
52. Heppenheimer TA. Routes to Chaos. Mosaic 1986;17:3-13.
53. Eckmann JP. Roads to turbulence in dissipative dynamic systems. Rev Mod Phys 1981;53:643-54.
54. Wolf A. Simplicity and universality in the transition to chaos. Nature 1983;305:182-3.
55. Manneville P, Pomeau Y. Different ways to turbulence in dissipative dynamic systems. Physica D 1980;1:219-26.
56. Beloshapkin VV, Chernikov AA, Natenzon MY, Petrovichev BA, Sagdeev RZ, Zaslavsky GM. Chaotic streamlines in preturbulent states. Nature 1989;337:133-7.

57. Devaney RL. Chaotic bursts in nonlinear dynamical systems. Science 1987;235:342-4.
58. Ruelle D. Strange attractors. Math Intelligencer 1980;2:126-37.
59. Ruelle D. Sensitive dependence on initial condition and turbulent behavior of dynamical systems. Ann NY Acad Sci 1979;316:408-16.
60. Grassberger P, Procaccia I. Dimensions and entropies of strange attractors from a fluctuating dynamics approach. Physica D 1984;13:34-54.
61. Guevara MR, Glass L, Shrier A. Phase locking, period-doubling bifurcations, and irregular dynamics in periodically stimulated cardiac cells. Science 1981;214:1350-1354
62. Glass L, Guevara MR, Shrier A. Bifurcation and chaos in a periodically stimulated cardiac oscillator. Physica D 1983;7:89-101
63. Guevara MR, Shrier A, Glass L. Phase-locked rhythms in periodically stimulated heart cell aggregates. Am J Physiol 1988;254:H1-H10
64. Glass L: Complex cardiac rhythms. Nature 1987;330:695-696
65. West BJ, Goldberger AL, Rovner G, Bhargava V. Nonlinear dynamics of the heartbeat: I. The AV junction: Passive conduit or active oscillator?. Physica D 1985;17:198-206.
66. Glass L, Goldberger AL, Courtemanche M, Shrier A. Nonlinear dynamics, chaos and complex cardiac arrhythmias. Proc R Soc Lond A 1987;413:9-26.
67. Goldberger AL, West BJ. Applications of nonlinear dynamics to clinical cardiology. Ann NY Acad Sci 1987;504:195-213.
68. Glass L, Guevara MR, Shrier A. Universal bifurcations and the classification of cardiac arrhythmias. Ann NY Acad Sci 1987;504:168-78.
69. Chialvo DR, Jalife J. Nonlinear dynamics of cardiac excitation and impulse propagation. Nature 1987;330:749-52.
70. Ritzenberg AL, Adam DR, Cohen RJ. Period multupling—evidence for nonlinear behavior of the canine heart. Nature 1984;307:159-61.
71. Adam DR, Smith JM, Akselrod S, Nyberg S, Powell AO, Cohen RJ. Fluctuations in T-wave morphology and susceptibility to ventricular fibrillation. J Electrocardiol 1984;17:209-18.
72. Smith JM, Clancy EA, Valeri CR, Ruskin JN, Cohen RJ. Electrical alternans and cardiac electrical instability. Circulation 1988;77:110-21.
73. Ritzenberg AL, Smith JM, Grumbach MP, Cohen RJ. Precursor to fibrillation in cardiac computer model. Comput Cardiol 1984;171-4.
74. Goldberger AL, West BJ. Chaos in physiology: health or disease? In: Degn H, Holden AV, Olsen LF, eds. Chaos in biological systems. New York: Plenum Publishing Corp, 1987:1-4.
75. Goldberger AL, Rigney DR. Sudden death is not chaos. In: Kelso JAS, Mandell AJ, eds. Dynamic patterns in complex systems. Singapore: World Scientific Publishers 1988:248-64.
76. Goldberger AL, Bhargava V, West BJ, Mandell AJ. Some observations on the question: is ventricular fibrillation "chaos"? Physica D 1986;19:282-9.
77. Chen PS, Wolf PD, Dixon EG, Danieley ND, Frazier DW, Smith WM, Ideker RE. Mechanism of ventricular vulnerability to single premature stimuli in open-chest dogs. Circ Res 1988;62:1191-209.
78. El-Sherif N. The figure 8 model of reentrant excitation in the canine post-infarction heart. In: Zipes DP, Jalife J, Cardiac electrophysiology and arrhythmias. New York: Grune & Stratton, Inc, 1985:363-78.
79. Garfinkel A, Karagueuzian H, Khan S, Diamond G. Is the proarrhythmic effect of quinidine a chaotic phenomenon? [Abstract] J Am Coll Cardiol 1989;13:186A.
80. Evans SJ, Khan SS, Garfinkle A, Kass RM, Albano A, Diamond GA. In ventricular fibrillation random or chaotic? [Abstract] Circulation 1989;80:II-134.
81. Goldberger AL, Rigney DR, Mietus J, Antman EM, Greenwald S. Nonlinear dynamics in sudden cardiac death syn-

drome: heart rate oscillations and bifurcations. Experientia 1987;44:983-7.

82. Goldberger AL, Bhargava V, West BJ, Mandell AJ. Nonlinear dynamics of the heartbeat. II. Subharmonic bifurcations of the cardiac interbeat interval in sinus node disease. Physica D 1985;17:207-14.

83. Myers GA, Martin GJ, Magid NM, Barnett PS, Schaad JW, Weiss JS, Lesch M, Singer DH. Power spectral analysis of heart rate variability in sudden cardiac death: comparison to other methods. IEEE Trans Biomed Eng 1986;33: 1149-56.

84. Shrier A, Dubarsky H, Rosengarten M, Guevara M, Nattel S, Glass L. Prediction of complex atrioventricular conduction rhythms in humans with use of the atrioventricular nodal recovery curve. Circulation 1987;76:1196-205.

85. Winfree AT. Sudden cardiac death: a problem in topology. Sci Am 1983;248:144-61.

86. Winfree AT. Electrical instability in cardiac muscle: phase singularities and rotors. J Theor Biol 1989;138:353-405.

87. Frazier DW, Wolf PD, Wharton JM, Tang ASL, Smith WM, Ideker RE. Stimulus-induced critical point—mechanism for electrical initiation of reentry in normal canine myocardium. J Clin Invest 1989;83:1039-52.

88. Shibata N, Peng-Sheng C, Dixon EG, Wolf PD, Danieley ND, Smith WM, Ideker RE. Influence of shock strength and timing on induction of ventricular arrhythmias in dogs. Am J Physiol 1988;255:H891-901.

89. Redwood DR, Borer JS, Epstein SE. Whither the ST segment during exercise? Circulation 1976;5:703-6.

90. Pinsker HM, Bell J. Phase plane description of endogenous neuronal oscillators in aplysia. Biol Cybern 1981;39:211-21.

91. Braunwald E, Ross J, Sonnenblick EH. Mechanisms of contraction of the normal and failing heart. N Engl J Med 1967;277:794-800, 853-63, 910-20, 962-71, 1012-22 (four parts).

92. Shaw R: The dripping faucet as a model chaotic system. Santa Cruz, Calif Ariel Press, 1984.

93. Kaplan DT, Cohen RJ. Method and apparatus for quantifying beat-to-beat variability in physiologic waveforms. United States Patent No. 4,732,157. Issued March 22, 1988. Washington, DC: U. S. Patent Office.

94. Eckmann JP, Ruelle D. Ergodic theory of chaos and strange attractors. Rev Mod Physics 1985;57:617-56.

95. Grassberger P, Procaccia I. Measuring the strangeness of strange attractors. Physica D 1983;9:189-208.

96. Benettin G, Galgani L, Giorgilli A, Strelcyn JM. Lyapunov characteristic exponents for smooth dynamical systems and for Hamiltonian systems; a method for computing all of them. Part 2. Numerical application. Meccanica 1980;15:21-30.

97. Wolf A, Swift JB, Swinney HL, Vastano JA. Determining Lyapunov exponents from a time series. Physica D 1985; 16:285-317.

98. Grebogi C, Ott E, Pelikan S, Yorke JA. Strange attractors that are not chaotic. Physica D 1984;13:261-8.

99. Mandelbrot BB. Discussion paper: fractals, attractors, and the fractal dimension. Ann NY Acad Sci 1979;316:463-4.

100. Mandelbrot B. The fractal geometry of nature. New York: W.H. Freeman, 1983.

101. Packard NH, Crutchfield JP, Farmer JD, Shaw RS. Geometry from a time series. Phys Rev Lett 1980;45:712-6.

102. Havstad JW, Ehlers CL. Attractor dimension of nonstationary dynamical systems from small data sets. Phys Rev A 1989;39:845-53.

103. Farmer JD, Ott E, Yorke JA. The dimension of chaotic attractors. Physica D 1983;7:153-80.

104. Grassberger P, Procaccia I. Characterization of strange attractors. Phys Rev Lett 1983;50:346-9.

105. Grassberger P, Procaccia I. Estimation of the Kolmogorov entropy from a chaotic signal. Phys Rev A 1983;28:2591-3.

106. Froehling H, Crutchfield JP, Farmer D, Packard NH. Shaw R. On determining the dimension of chaotic flows. Physica D 1981;3:605-17.

107. Geisel T. Chaos, randomness and dimension. Nature 1982; 298:322-3.

108. Albano AM, Mees AI, deGuzman GS, Rapp PE. Data requirements for reliable estimation of correlation dimensions. In: Holden AV, ed. Chaotic biological systems, New York: Pergamon Press, 1987.

109. McGillem CD, Cooper GR. Continuous and discrete signal and system analysis. New York: Holt, Rinehart and Winston, 1974.

110. Ramirez RW. The FFT—fundamentals and concepts. Englewood Cliffs, NJ: Prentice-Hall, 1985.

111. Farmer D, Crutchfield J, Froehling H, Packard N, Shaw R. Power spectra and mixing properties of strange attractors. Ann NY Acad Sci 1980;357:453-72.

112. Goldberger AL, Bhargava V, West BJ, Mandell AJ. On a mechanism of cardiac electrical stability, the fractal hypothesis. Biophys J 1985;48:525-8.

113. Goldberger AL, West BJ. Fractals in physiology and medicine. Yale J Biol Med 1987;60:421-35.

114. Pool R. Is it healthy to be chaotic? Science 1989;243:604-7.

115. Babloyantz A, Destexhe A. Is the normal heart a periodic oscillator? Biol Cybern 1988;58:203-11.

116. Holden AV. Chaos in complicated systems. Nature 1983; 305:183.

117. Michaels DC, Chialva DR, Matyas EP, Jalife J. Chaotic activity in a mathematical model of the vagally driven sinoatrial node. Circ Res 1989;65:1350-60.

118. Courtemanche M, Glass L, Rosengarten MD, Goldberger AL. Beyond pure parasystole: promises and problems in modelling complex arrhythmias. Am J Physiol 1989;257:H693-706.

119. Chialvo DR, Michaels DC, Jalife J. Supernormal excitability as a mechanism of chaotic dynamics of activation in cardiac Purkinje fibers. Circ Res 1990;66:525-45.

120. "Mathematical approaches to cardiac arrhythmias." Workshop sponsored by the New York Academy of Sciences, November 1989.

121. "Is cardiac chaos normal or abnormal?" Arnsdorf MF, Chairman, Postgraduate seminar. American Heart Association, 62nd Scientific Sessions, November 1989.

122. Frame LH, Rhee EK. Chaotic cycle length oscillation and bifurcation during reentry [Abstract]. Circulation 1989;80:II-96.

123. Bassingthwaighte JB, King RB, Roger SA. Fractal nature of regional myocardial blood flow heterogeneity. Circ Res 1989;65:578-90.

124. Diamond GA. Future imperfect: the limitations of clinical prediction models and the limits of clinical prediction. J Am Coll Cardiol 1989;14:12A-22A.

125. Gomes MAF. Fractal geometry in crumpled paper balls. Am J Physics 1987;55:649-50.

126. Saaty TL, Bram J. Nonlinear mathematics. New York: Dover Publications, 1964.

GLOSSARY

Aperiodic[6, 7, 8]—Irregular behavior that has no definite period. Aperiodic behavior is either *random* or *chaotic*. One exception is *quasiperiodic* behavior, which is often considered a subset of periodic.

Attractor[6, 8, 13, 14]—A geometric figure (or mathematical abstraction) in *state space* to which all *trajectories* in its vicinity (basin) are drawn. There are four types of attractors: point, limit cycle, toroidal, and strange. A point attractor will draw all trajectories to a single point, like a pendulum spiraling to rest. A limit cycle is characteristic of periodic motion and a toroid represents quasiperiodic motion. A strange attractor is associated with chaotic motion.

December 1990
American Heart Journal

The word attractor is classically associated with the solutions of *differential equations* (perfect mathematical models), but it has also been used to describe the behavior of unknown signals from physical or biologic systems. Though its use in that regard is technically inaccurate, it persists in the literature.

Autocorrelation[6, 109]—A measure of how closely a signal *(times series)* resembles a time-delayed image of itself. Periodic signals are highly autocorrelated whereas random signals are not.

Banding—Refers to bands of *trajectories* seen in plots of *state space*, inscribing zones that are not visited by the trajectories. These are analogous to the "swirls" seen in turbulent fluid. The presence of banding in state space is suggestive of chaotic behavior.

Bifurcation[6, 7, 8, 48, 49]—A point in which there is an aburpt change in behavior of a dynamic system that occurs when one of the parameters reaches a critical value.

Bifurcation diagram[1, 5, 6, 7, 8]—A graph that demonstrates the relation between the values of one parameter and the behavior of a system. An example is the bifurcation diagram for the logistic map where the x axis represented all the values of k and the y axis was all possible states of the system.

Bounded—A system's behavior is bounded if all of the behavior is in a limited region of *state space*. A bounded signal will not have any behavior that approaches infinity. "Constrained" is often used as a synonym for boundedness.

Broad-band spectrum—see *Continuous spectrum.*

Chaos—An aperiodic, seemingly *random* behavior in a *deterministic* system that exhibits *sensitive dependence on initial conditions.*

Continuous data[109]—In general terms, a *time series* that is continuous is "smooth" visually. From a mathematical viewpoint, if each point in the time series has only one derivative, the time series is continuous. An alternate mathematical definition is that if the derivatives on both sides of all points are equal, then the series is continuous.

Continuous spectrum—A spectral pattern that includes a large number of frequencies with no numerical relation to one another. Also called *broad-band;* in contrast to *discrete spectrum.*

Deterministic—A system is deterministic if its behavior is governed by known equations and initial conditions, and is therefore predictable at any past or future time. A *dynamical system* is deterministic if its evolution is completely determined by its current state and past history. There is no *stochastic* (random) component in a deterministic system.

Difference equation[1, 6, 48, 49, 109]—An equation that is solved by successive iterations, using the solution of the equation at one time as an initial condition for the next solution: of the form $x(t + 1) = f(x(t))$. The *logistic map* is an example.

Differential equation—An equation or series of coupled equations that contain(s) the derivative of one of the variables

Dimension[6, 60, 100-108]—A measure of the amount of space an object occupies. There are only four topological dimensions (point, line, surface, volume). A fractal dimension is also a measure of the "space" an object occupies, but is measured by looking at the object at different scales. The fractal dimension can be integer of non-integer and may be greater than three. Fractal dimension is also a measure a system's complexity; the more complex, the higher the dimension.

Discretely sampled data[109]—Data collected at defined intervals in time, not continuously. Digitized data are discretely sampled, whereas analog data are continuous because a value is defined at any point in time.

Discrete spectrum—A spectral pattern that consists of a series of isolated spikes, often integer multiples of a fundamental frequency *(harmonics)*. A discrete spectrum is sometimes referred to as *narrow-band* in contrast to *continuous spectrum.*

Dynamic(al) system—Any system in which the state changes with time.

Exponential divergence[6, 7, 8, 96, 97]—A property of the *trajectories* in *state space* where nearby points on adjacent trajectories diverge from each other at an exponential rate.

Fast Fourier Transform(FFT)[110]—A specific method of calculating the frequency spectrum of a signal. See *Spectral analysis.*

Forbidden zones—Areas in a graphic representation of *state space* that are never visited by the *trajectories* of the system. These are one of the two components of the "swirls" seen in turbulent systems.

Fractal[100, 125]—An object that has detailed structure at many scales. A perfect cylinder has only one structure no matter how much one reduces or magnifies it. A coastline as seen from space has an irregular structure. By magnifying the coastline (changing the scale of reference), one can see the irregularity of small inlets and sand bars. Another change in scale reveals logs and boulders that make the coastline rough. Further magnification reveals the jaggedness of grains of sand. Thus at many different scales, a coastline is "rough" and therefore fractal. The term self-similarity is also used in this setting, in that at many scales, the coastline looks like itself, rough and jagged.

Fractal dimension[100, 125]—Represents the way a set of points fills a given area of space. Defined as the slope of the function relating the numbers of points contained in a given radius ("magnification") to the radius itself. The operative dimensionality of a trajectory is defined by the flat region of the slope-radius plot.

Harmonic[109]—A frequency obtained by multiplying a fundamental frequency by an integer greater than zero.

Iteration[48, 49]—A process in which the solution to an equation is fed back into the original equation as a new initial condition.

Lag—A difference in time between one point and another. For example, a return map (also called a lag plot) plots the relation between one point in a *time series* and a subsequent point. The difference in time between the two points is called the lag. The choice of the lag is somewhat arbitrary, and is based on optimizing the amount of information in the graph.

Linear equation[126]—An equation that meets both the following criteria:

$$F(x + y) = F(x) + F(y)$$
$$F(kx) = kF(x)$$

$2^2 + 3^2 \neq (2 + 3)^2$, and $\log(2x) \neq 2 \log(x)$ are examples that do not meet the above criteria and are therefore nonlinear equations.

Linear divergence—A property of the trajectories in state space where adjacent trajectories diverge from each other at a linear rate.

Linear system[109]—A system in which the relation between input and output varies in a constant (linear) fashion. For example, if a system has a constantly increasing input, and the output increases proportionately (though perhaps at a different magnitude), the system is linear.

Logistic map[26, 48,49]—A simple nonlinear (quadratic) equation, that with special initial conditions and parameters, exhibits chaotic behavior. It is the simplest and archetypical chaotic system. The mathematical form is as follows:

$$x_{n+1} = k \cdot x_n \cdot (1 - x_n)$$

This equation states that the behavior of the system (x_{n+1}) is a function of the initial value (x_n between 0 and 1) and some parameter k (ranging between 0 and 4). From a technical standpoint, chaos occurs in this particular system when the slope of the descending arm of the parabola—as it crosses the line of identity—is less the -1. At this point, the nonlinear term in the equation is dominant.

Lorenz equations[2, 6, 14]—A series of three differential equations derived from a more complex system used in this study of fluid dynamics. The Lorenz system was used to study weather patterns, and ultimately led to the discovery of sensitive dependence on initial conditions and chaos.

Lyapunov exponent[1, 6, 96, 97]—A measure of the *exponential divergence* of a system named after the Russian mathematician Alexander Lyapunov (1857-1918). In multidimensional systems (≥ 3), an exponent of 0 indicates periodic or random systems (no net divergence of trajectories), and a positive exponent indicates a chaotic system (exponential divergence).

Mandelbrot set[100]—A simple series of two equations (containing real and imaginary components) that, when iterated and plotted on a two-dimensional graph, depict an extremely complex and classic *fractal* pattern.

Narrow band spectrum—see *Discrete spectrum*.

Nonlinear equation[126]—Any equation that does not meet the criteria for linearity (see linear equation). The logistic map contains a linear (kx) and a nonlinear (kx²) portion, but it is a nonlinear equation because a portion of it is nonlinear.

Nonlinear system[109]—Any system in which the output is disproportionate to the input. An example would be a system that has a linear input but an output that is sinusoidal.

Nonlinear dynamics—The study of nonlinear systems whose state changes with time.

Period-doubling[1, 61-64]—A system that originally had X periodic states, and now, in response to a parameter change, has 2X periodic states, is said to have undergone period doubling; one form of *bifurcation*.

Periodic behavior (periodicity)—Behavior of a system in which the output repeats itself exactly over a given time interval (the "period").

Phase locking[1, 61-64]—The behavior of a system in which a given number of input stimuli always generate a given number of output responses; the behavior of the system is "locked" to the input stimulus. For example, a system that is stimulated at one cycle per second (1 Hz) and responds at one cycle per second has 1:1 phase locking. If there are three responses for each four stimuli, there is 4:3 phase locking. A synonym is entrainment.

Phase plane plot[6, 90, 44, 45,115]—A graph of *state space* that has for its axes various combinations of the states of the system. May consist of the first, second, third, or nth derivative of the system. Each axis may also represent a different variable of the system.

Poincaré section[6, 14]—Two techniques using plots of *state space* that allow closer scrutiny of the trajecto-

1440 *Denton et al.*

December 1990
American Heart Journal

ries and their relation to each other. A *lagged section* plots points on the *phase plane plot* at defined intervals (lag). A *cross section* characterizes the relation between *trajectories* as they cross some region of interest.

Prechaotic behavior—Predictable behavior of a system before the onset of chaos. Period-doubling is one of them.

Quasiperiodic[6]—A behavior that consists of at least two frequencies in which the phases are related by an irrational number. An example would be the sum of two sine waves in which the phases are related by the square root of a prime number.

Random behavior[109]—Behavior that can never be predicted, and can only be described by summary statistics such as the mean and standard deviation. Technically, a behavior can never be reliably described as random; only organized (deterministic) behavior can be excluded.

Return map[1, 6, 13, 14]—A graphic technique that represents the relation between a point and any subsequent point in a *time series*. A lag 1 return map is a plot of an initial value on one axis and the succeeding value on the other axis. A lag 5 return map is a plot of the initial value on one axis and the fifth succeeding value on the other axis.

Sensitive dependence on initial conditions[1, 5, 6-8]—A property of chaotic systems whereby small changes in the state variables in a system at one point will make large differences in the behavior of the system at some future point.

Spectral analysis[109, 110]—A technique that breaks a signal up into its fundamental frequencies. The *Fourier transform* is the most common form of spectral analysis.

State space—That area of the universe of behavior that contains the range of values for the behavior of a particular system.

Stochastic—*Random* from a mathematical (statistical) point of view.

Subharmonic[82]—A frequency obtained by dividing a fundamental frequency by an integer greater than zero.

Time series—A series of numbers, each representative of the behavior of a system at particular points in time.

Trajectory—The representation of the behavior of a system in *state space* over a short period of time; one cycle on a *phase plane plot*.

1212

Fractal ^{15}O-Labeled Water Washout From the Heart

James B. Bassingthwaighte, Daniel A. Beard

Abstract To characterize the washout of water from the heart, we used a flow-limited (not diffusion- or permeability-limited) marker for blood-tissue exchange, namely, tracer-labeled water. Experiments were performed by injecting ^{15}O-labeled water into the inflow to isolated blood-perfused rabbit hearts and by recording the tracer content in the heart and in the outflow simultaneously for up to 5 minutes. The data exhibit a particular combination of power law forms: (1) The downslopes of the residue and outflow curves were both power law functions, with the residue diminishing as $t^{-\alpha}$ and the outflow as $t^{-\alpha-1}$, where α is interpreted to be the dimensionless exponent of a fractal power law relation characterizing the self-similarity inherent in each curve. (2) The fractional escape rate, given by the outflow curve divided by the residue curve, diminished almost exactly as t^{-1}. In 18 sets of curves, α averaged 2.21±0.27. These results lead to an improved method for extrapolating the downslopes of indicator dilution curves to estimate their areas and therefore the blood flows. The evidence also points strongly to the conclusions that myocardial water washout is a fractal process and that stirred tank models are inappropriate for the heart. (***Circ Res.*** 1995;77:1212-1221.)

Key Words • flow-limited blood-tissue exchange • power law kinetics • positron emission • oxygen-15 • capillary permeability • statistical self-similar processes

O ver the last five decades, the washout of tracers from a body or from an individual organ has been used to obtain inferential information about the processes governing the retention of the tracer within the organ. This is important for drug kinetic studies; eg, the retention of drug is usually a measure of the slowness of its dissociation from a receptor site. In other circumstances, however, when chemical binding and unbinding reactions are either very fast or not involved and when there is no limitation to tracer washout because of slow diffusion or retarded permeation of membranes, then the washout from an organ is dominated principally by the flow per unit mass of tissue. A purely intravascular marker that does not stick to or cross the endothelial barrier will be "flow-limited" in its local and global washout. Inert tracers, which distribute rapidly across the membranes of an organ so that there is effectively instantaneous local blood-tissue equilibration of each point along the capillaries, also display flow-limited washout.[1,2] Whether or not tracer washout is completely flow-limited, its mean transit time, $\bar{t}$, equals V/F, where V (in milliliters per gram) is the volume of distribution of the tracer within the organ, and F is the flow (in milliliters per gram per minute). This is simply a statement of conservation of mass and is true whether or not there are limitations to the exchange rate by membrane barriers or slow diffusion.

Organs are not normally homogeneously perfused. Regional flows in the heart are broadly heterogeneous.[3] In both the heart[4] and the lung,[5] the spatial variation appears to be fractal. This means that the spatial heterogeneity shows statistical self-similarity. The apparent variance or standard deviation of the regional flows is dependent on spatial resolution: observing smaller regions with higher resolution reveals further variation. Finding that the smaller regions are nonuniform is proof that the overall apparent heterogeneity must increase with higher resolution. In special cases, a proportional increase in resolution reveals a proportional increase in heterogeneity. This relation follows the power law function:

$$(1) \qquad \frac{RD(m)}{RD(m_0)} = \left(\frac{m}{m_0}\right)^{1-D}$$

where RD is the standard deviation divided by the mean flow for the organ at a particular resolution level defined by m, the mass of the individual pieces into which the organ has been divided (that is, piece mass) in order to make the observation; m_0 is an arbitrarily chosen reference mass, usually 1 g; and D is the fractal dimension. The spatial fractal relation holds in the hearts of awake baboons and of anesthetized sheep and rabbits over a 100-fold range of piece masses in the heart[4] and also the lung.[5]

Turn now to the temporal characteristics or kinetics of tracer exchange in the heart. These are not predictable from a knowledge of regional spatial flow distributions. For example, the spatial flow distributions are approximately gaussian: assuming that the local volume of distribution, V_i, for a tracer is the same in all regions, then the time course of tracer transit times for an intravascular tracer traveling between inflow and outflow would be directly calculable. The mean transit time for the ith path, $\bar{t}_i$, is as follows:

$$(2) \qquad \bar{t}_i = V_i/F_i$$

Received February 21, 1995; revision accepted August 2, 1995.

From the Center for Bioengineering, University of Washington, Seattle.

Correspondence to James B. Bassingthwaighte, MD, PhD, Center for Bioengineering, WD-12, University of Washington, Seattle, WA 98195. E-mail jbb@nsr.bioeng.washington.edu.

where F_i is the ith flow and V_i is the vascular volume along the ith pathway. Even if the V_is were the same everywhere, which they are not, then the distribution of the t_is would be skewed to the right in a fashion dependent on the distribution of F_is.

However, there is some heterogeneity of regional blood volumes,[6-8] so the analysis of washout times would be further confounded by the volume variation in an unpredictable fashion. The alternative is to seek a flow-limited marker with a relatively uniform distribution space, ie, one with a steady state volume of distribution that has very small regional variation. The fractional water content of the myocardium is remarkably uniform[7,9,10] at 0.78 ± 0.01 mL/g. The washout curves for water, and for the lipid-soluble substance antipyrine, have been shown to be flow-limited in the heart.[11] Therefore, these are the preferred test tracers for examining the shapes of washout curves. These washout curves will not be influenced by variation in V_i or by any diffusional retardation, nor will they be skewed by slow barrier penetration, such as that which prolongs the tails of dilution curves for potassium or sucrose or larger hydrophilic solutes. Consequently, washout curves for water will be governed by the velocities through the hundreds of thousands of vessels of the arterial and venous networks and scaled through the local equilibration via capillary-tissue exchange by the ratios of blood space to total water space. The washout time course will thus be dominated by pathway transit time distributions; the influence of the blood-tissue exchange process for water is to render all the V_is uniform, leaving the $\bar{t}_i$s reciprocal to the local F_is. The observations of Rose et al[12] suggest a small barrier limitation in the highest flow regions, which might affect the upslope and peak of the curves but would not affect the tails of the curves or our analyses.

This analysis focuses on the question of the nature of the distribution of washout times. The resultant observation that the distribution appears fractal is revealed for the first time in the present study. The result contrasts remarkably with and clearly refutes the long-held perception that washout is an exponential process. This idea was the basis of the Stewart-Hamilton method[13] for extrapolating the tails of dilution curves monoexponentially in order to measure the areas under indicator dilution curves for the estimation of organ flow or cardiac output. The results to be shown below will be used to argue that the Stewart-Hamilton method slightly but systematically underestimates the areas and so gives a minor degree of overestimation of flows.

Materials and Methods

Experiments were performed on seven isolated blood-perfused rabbit hearts (New Zealand White rabbits with hearts weighing 6 to 8 g) by using $^{15}OH_2$ water as the indicator. (^{15}O is a positron emitter with a half-life of ≈ 121 seconds.) The perfusate was Krebs-Ringer bicarbonate solution with 1% albumin, to which was added triply washed beef red blood cells to a hematocrit of 20%. The partial pressure of oxygen was 145 to 180 mm Hg. The isolated heart was mounted on a perfusion apparatus. The residual tracer activity within the heart, $R(t)$, was obtained via a pair of NaI crystal gamma detectors situated on opposite sides of the heart and used in coincidence mode to provide a measure of the two simultaneous gamma emissions resulting from positron annihilation events occurring in the heart. The

coincidence method reduces the counting of emissions from other sources, including scatter from outside the cylindrical region in which the heart was situated. The coronary sinus and right ventricular thebesian veins drained into an outflow cannula inserted through the pulmonary valve. The weight of blood in the outflow cannula, positioned below heart level, holds the pressure in the right ventricle at a negative pressure; therefore, the ventricle stays empty. ^{15}O detectors sensitive directly to the positron (positive beta) particles were set up on the inflow tubing and outflow tubing, giving the inflow, $C_{in}(t)$, and outflow concentration-time curves, $C(t)$. The structure of the detectors (made in our laboratory) was similar in design to that described by Lerch et al.[14] All three curves were corrected for the isotopic decay of ^{15}O, which has a half-life of 121 seconds.

By this experimental approach, we attempted to minimize error in the data acquisition. Because the outflow curve is a slightly dispersed and delayed measure of the derivative of the residue curve and because both outflow and residue curves must conserve mass (account for the amount of tracer in the inflow curve), analyzing the set of curves together minimizes error due to incompleteness of outflow collection because of leaks or contamination of $R(t)$ by any accumulations of tracer leaked from the heart and included in the signal because of the poor collimation.

Analytical Methods and Indicator Dilution Theory

Basic conservation theory, as summarized by Zierler,[15] maintains that after an impulse injection at $t=0$ into the entrance to an organ, the fractional residual content $R(t)$ at the next instant is 100% of the injectate. $R(t)$ remains at 1.0 until there is an appearance of tracer in the outflow. The fraction of the injectate appearing in the outflow per unit time is $h(t)$ (fraction per second). The accumulated outflow is the integral of the outflow response and is the total dose, unity, minus the fraction of dose still retained within the organ, $R(t)$:

$$(3) \qquad \int_0^t h(\lambda)d\lambda = 1.0 - R(t)$$

where λ is a dummy variable used in the integration. Further, in the ideal situation, in the absence of error in the data acquisition, the outflow fraction of the dose appearing per second is the derivative of the organ content:

$$(4) \qquad h(t) = -dR/dt$$

In practice, one records neither $R(t)$ nor $h(t)$ because injecting an impulse input is impossible. Instead, the signal recorded from the heart, $Q(t)$, is a convolution of $R(t)$ with the input:

$$(5) \qquad Q(t) = \bar{F} \cdot C_{in}(t) * R(t)$$

where $\bar{F}$ is the mean flow, and the asterisk denotes the convolution integration, more formally written as $Q(t) = \bar{F} \int_0^t C_{in}(\lambda) \cdot R(t-\lambda)d\lambda$. Likewise, the outflow concentration-time curve, $C(t)$, is as follows:

$$(6) \qquad C(t) = C_{in}(t) * h(t)$$

When the input curve, $C_{in}(t)$, is completed within a period that is short compared with the mean retention time within the organ, then the tail portion of $h(t)$ has a form influenced almost solely by the network characteristics and scarcely at all by the form of C_{in}. (For these experiments, the input was 99% complete in 18 to 22 seconds, which was short compared with washout, which took 3 to 6 minutes.) Given these conditions, a good approximation for the residue function is as follows:

1214   **Circulation Research**   *Vol 77, No 6   December 1995*

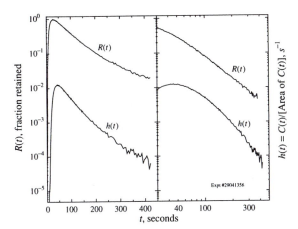

FIG 1.   Residue curves, $R(t)$, and normalized outflow concentration-time curves, $h(t)$, from a rabbit heart after injection of ^{15}O-labeled water into the coronary inflow. Both $R(t)$ and $h(t)$ have tails that are power law functions of time; ie, they are straight on log-log plots (right) and clearly not monoexponential, being concave upward on semilog plots (left).

(7)
$$R(t) \simeq \frac{Q(t)}{Q_{max}}$$

where Q_{max} is the maximum value of the curve recorded via the coincidence counters. Although the approximation is poor in the initial seconds, it is good thereafter. Likewise, the approximation for the tail of $h(t)$ is the normalized outflow concentration-time curve:

(8)
$$h(t) = \frac{C(t)}{\displaystyle\int_0^\infty C(t)dt}$$

where the denominator is the area under the curve $C(t)$. Alternatively, $h(t)$ can be calculated by using the injected dose, q_o, and the measured flow, $\bar{F}$, so that $h(t) = \bar{F}C(t)/q_o$, illustrating that $h(t)$ is the fraction of the dose reaching the outflow per unit time.

The fractional escape rate, $\eta(t)$, is defined as the fraction of residual tracer escaping per unit time, and is therefore given directly by the amount of tracer appearing in the outflow per unit time, $\bar{F}C(t)$, where $\bar{F}$ is the total flow, divided by the amount of tracer retained within the organ at each time t:

(9)
$$\eta(t) = \frac{h(t)}{R(t)} \simeq \frac{C\bar{F}(t)}{Q(t)}$$

This review of standard indicator dilution theory and of the secondary approximations sets the stage for the special approach to the analysis using fractals. Note that there are two assumptions in the normalization of Equation 9 in going from the middle to the right expression: (1) Q_{max} in Equation 7 is obtained at a time when all of the tracer is in view of the coincidence detectors, with all of the tracer having entered and none having left. (2) The area of the outflow washout is essentially complete. Assumption 1 seems reasonable in view of the fact that the input curves, C_{in}, are 99% complete by 18 to 22 seconds (not illustrated), although $R(t)$ does have a measurable plateau since the washout begins at about this time. Assumption 2 is valid within <2%, as can be seen from the final values of $R(t)$ at $t=300$ seconds in Fig 1.

A Fractal Theory To Be Tested

The fundamental feature of a fractal is self-similarity or self-affinity. A fractal washout process is therefore one for which the rate of washout decreases by some exact proportion for some chosen proportional increase in time; the self-affinity requirement is fulfilled whenever the "exact proportion" remains unchanged, independent of the moment or the segment of the data set selected to measure the proportionality constant. The length of time or the portion of the washout curve for which this relation holds is known as the "scaling region" and is necessarily finite, as is the case for all natural, nonmathematical, fractals. Fractal washout behavior can begin after the input to the organ is complete. If complete, then one would expect the late portion of $R(t)$ to have the shape of a power law relation defining the proportionality relation:

(10)
$$R(t) = At^{-\alpha}$$

where α is the power law exponent. (The observation of a power law relation is not an explanation of the phenomenon but provides an incentive for a search for an explanation.) This power law relation defines the log-log slope $d\log R/d\log t = -\alpha$. The corollary of this is that the outflow tracer concentration-time curve should also be fractal and since $h(t) = -dR/dt$, then taking the derivative of the right side of Equation 10 yields

(11)
$$h(t) = A\alpha t^{-\alpha-1}$$

and the slope on the log-log plot is $d\log h(t)/d\log t = -\alpha-1$.

According to the hypothesis, expressed in Equations 10 and 11, $\eta(t)$ should be a power law function with an exponent equal to -1:

(12)
$$\eta(t) = \frac{h(t)}{R(t)} = \frac{A\alpha t^{-\alpha-1}}{At^{-\alpha}} = \alpha t^{-1}$$

Three equations pose the tests of the fractal washout hypothesis: Over some substantial period of time late in the washout, (1) does Equation 10 provide a good fit to $R(t)$, (2) does Equation 11 provide a good fit to $h(t)$, and (3) can one value for α be used to fit Equations 10 and 11 to the data simultaneously obtained for $R(t)$ and $h(t)$? If so, then does Equation 12 provide a good fit to the data for the fractional escape rate $\eta(t)$, with the specific power law slope of -1; ie, does $\eta(t)$ decay at a rate proportional to 1/time?

Results

Eighteen sets of experimental data were recorded from seven rabbit hearts weighing 8.76 ± 0.78 g (mean$\pm$SD) with perfusate hematocrits of $20.3\pm0.01\%$. Data from inflow and outflow and from the heart itself were recorded for 140 to 440 seconds after injection. In the subsequent analysis, the figures have been chosen to give an impression of the average result rather than "best" results and to show as many different data sets as possible. Results are expressed as mean$\pm$1 SD for the 18 data sets from these seven hearts.

Fig 1 shows the type of curves obtained. Both the residue and the outflow curves are continuously concave upward on the semilogarithmic plot (left); therefore, these curves are not monoexponential. On the log-log plot, both $R(t)$ and $h(t)$ are apparently straight for times $>\approx 1$ minute. The slope of the outflow tracer concentration-time curve is steeper than that of the residue function, as was seen for all of the sets of data; this is a major point, for it denies the suitability of a stirred tank or mixing chamber model where $R(t)$ and $h(t)$ would have the same slope fitted by a single exponential.

Because the input to the system is somewhat dispersed rather than being an ideal instantaneous impulse, the values of $R(t)$ do not peak at $t=0$; the peaks of $R(t)$ occurred at 8 to 30 seconds, averaging 19 ± 8 seconds,

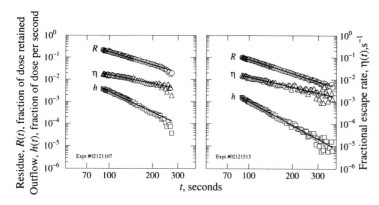

FIG 2. Fitting power law curves of general form $kt^{-\beta}$ to residue and outflow curves, $R(t)$ and $h(t)$, respectively, and to the fractional escape rate, $\eta(t)$, for two separate experiments. These are unconstrained best power law regressions fitted to the individual curves for $R(t)$, $h(t)$, and $\eta(t)$.

whereas the peaks of $h(t)$ occurred at 14 to 47 seconds, averaging 29 ± 12 seconds. The delays in the tubing from the heart to the outflow detector are on the order of 1 to 3 seconds. (The volume was 0.12 mL, and the flows were 5 to 30 mL/min.) The dispersion due to this tubing has no detectable influence on the shape or slope of the outflow curves.

The data of highest relevance to our analysis are the tails of the curves beyond the first minute, where the washout is clearly not significantly influenced by the form of the input, because all of the transit times are long compared with the duration of the input. The early parts of $R(t)$ and of $h(t)$ are therefore clearly influenced by the form of the input function, but the later portions of the curves are not, since the input was complete in 10 to 15 seconds. The subsequent analysis is performed on the data beyond, where $R(t)/R_{max}<0.2$; these are the data beyond the first 50 to 80 seconds after the injection, and the data in most runs extend to ≈300 seconds.

Unconstrained Fitting of R, h, and η

The tails of the residue $R(t)$, outflow $h(t)$, and the escape rate $\eta(t)$ for two experiments are plotted on log-log scales in Fig 2. Each curve was fit with the log-log regression to give best estimates of the power law exponent. The values from 18 experiments for α from the residue functions, fitting Equation 10, were 2.12 ± 0.33 (mean±1 SD); the values for α from the outflow curves, fitting Equation 11, were 2.13 ± 0.34. These values were obtained independently from residue and outflow data. The coefficients of variation for the fits to the $R(t)$s averaged 0.073 ± 0.042 (N=18); the coefficients of variation for the fits to the outflow curves averaged 0.074 ± 0.070 (N=18). Thus, the independently estimated values of α from residue and outflow were close to each other (2.12 and 2.13). The paired differences averaged 0.005, with a standard deviation of 0.43 for the 18 pairs. Thus, the first two tests listed below Equation 12 are satisfied and do not cause us to reject the fractal relation, since the two independent estimates of α are not statistically different, as tested by either unpaired or paired differences by Student's t test.

The curves for the fractional escape rate $\eta(t)$ are necessarily noisier than those for either $h(t)$ or $R(t)$, since $\eta(t)$ is calculated by dividing one curve by the other (Equation 9). Because of the noise, the coefficients of variation for the power law regression fitting are larger (0.21 ± 0.16, N=18). The power law exponents obtained for unconstrained fitting of the equation $\eta(t)=kt^{-\beta}$ gave

estimates of $\beta=1.12\pm0.47$ (N=18), so that the average of the unconstrained estimates of β did not differ statistically from 1.0, the value theoretically anticipated in Equation 12. Again, the fractal hypothesis cannot be rejected.

Comparing Power Law With Monoexponential Fits

Fig 3 shows optimized best fits using both the power law expressions, $\hat{R}(t)=a_1t^{-\alpha_1}$ and $\hat{h}(t)=a_2\alpha_2t^{-\alpha_2-1}$, and the exponential expressions, $\hat{R}(t)=A_1e^{-k_1t}$ and $\hat{h}(t)=A_2e^{-k_2t}$. The test was designed as a test of appropriateness of

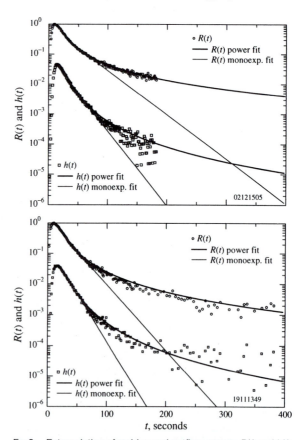

FIG 3. Extrapolation of residue and outflow curves, $R(t)$ and $h(t)$, respectively, with power law versus exponential fitting. Fitting was done over the time period where $0.2\le R(t)\le0.1$ for both $R(t)$ and $h(t)$. The power law and exponential curves beyond $R(t)=0.1$ represent the extrapolated predictions beyond 60 seconds (top) and 50 seconds (bottom).

extrapolation to predict the shape of the last parts of the tails of $R(t)$ and $h(t)$; to do this, the model functions were fit to only a limited segment of the data: for $R(t)$, from 0.2 to 0.1 only; for $h(t)$, over exactly the same time period as for $R(t)$. For this test, the power law fits were not constrained to use the same α for $R(t)$ and $h(t)$ but were best-fitting regressions, log-log for the power law and log-linear for the exponential. The rate constants for the exponential fits represent best fits over the same segments of $R(t)$ and $h(t)$ as were used for the power law fitting.

The two sets of data shown in Fig 3 on semilogarithmic, not log-log, plots are representative of the predictive capacity of the two extrapolation methods. The power law extrapolation beyond the time where $R(t)=0.1$ always lies above the exponential best fit for both $R(t)$ and $h(t)$. For 15 of 18 $R(t)$s, the power law extrapolation predicted and fit the data for $R(t)\leq0.1$ better by far than did the exponential extrapolation; in two sets, the data sets were not long enough beyond $R(t)=0.1$ to make the distinction, and in one set, $R(t)$ was better fit by the exponential, but $h(t)$ for the same set was much better fitted by the power law. For $h(t)$ the results are less secure, because the choice of the region fitted, being defined by $R(t)$ and not by $h(t)$, means that the curves are relatively noisy. For 12 curves, the power law fit was better by far; for 4 curves, the exponential fit was as good; and for 2 curves, the exponential fit was distinctly better. Of the 4 intermediate results, the data in 2 cases lay clearly in between the 2 extrapolations (power law and exponential) and did not fit either, and in 2 cases, the data points were too scattered to make the distinction.

The areas under the tail of $R(t)$ were underestimated by the monoexponential extrapolation, with the ratio to that estimated by the power law being 0.64±0.12 (N=18). For $h(t)$, the ratio of areas by exponential fit over that for power law was 0.63±0.08 (N=18).

From the point of view of estimation of total areas of curves, this difference is not great, a 3% to 4% underestimation for $R(t)$ and less than that for $h(t)$. The errors are of course greater for mean transit times, where the tails have more influence on the estimate.

Using One α for Fitting R, h, and η

The most stringent test of the hypothesis is test 3. In this approach to obtaining the best estimate of α for each experiment, the data for $R(t)$ and $h(t)$ were fitted simultaneously by using $\hat{R}(t)=a_1t^{-\alpha}$ and $\hat{h}(t)=a_2\alpha t^{-\alpha-1}$. By this approach, the hypothetical fractional escape rate must have the form $\eta(t)=a_3(a_2/a_1)\alpha t^{-1}$; the exponent is forced to be -1. The deviations of a_3 from 1.0 represent the difference in the sensitivities of the outflow detector (for positron emissions) and the residue detector (for 511-keV coincident gamma emissions). The best estimates of the a_i values and α were found by nonlinear optimization using SENSOP, a sensitivity function–based modified Levenberg-Marquardt type routine (Chan et al[16]). In this approach, the fractal hypothesis of a difference of 1.0 between the power law exponents for $R(t)$ and $h(t)$ is assumed, and with this assumption having been made, the test lies in the goodness of fit to the data for the set of three curves. Two examples are shown in Fig 4. The values of α so estimated are reported in the Table. The values of α range widely

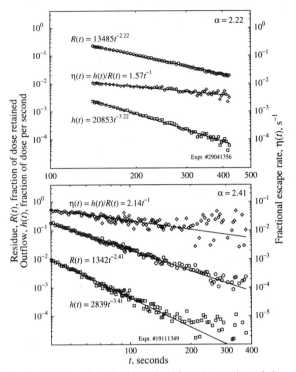

FIG 4. Optimized best fit of combined fractal power law relation for residue $R(t)=a_1t^{-\alpha}$ and outflow $h(t)=a_2\alpha t^{-\alpha-1}$ for the same value of a, forcing the fractional escape rate $\eta(t)=a_3(a_2/a_1)\alpha t^{-1}$. Top, The exponent α was 2.22, and the parameters a_1, a_2, and a_3 were 13485, 9396, and 1.01, respectively. The 95% confidence range on α was 2.22±0.01. Bottom, α was 2.41±0.03 (95% confidence limits), and a_1, a_2, and a_3 were 1342, 1178, and 1.15, respectively.

around 2.0, averaging 2.2±0.27 (mean±SD, N=18). The constrained theoretical lines appear to be close enough to the three data sets so that the hypothesis cannot be rejected. The inference from both the slopes of $R(t)$ and of $h(t)$ and of the relation between their slopes is that the tails of the transit time distributions are approximately fractal in these isolated perfused rabbit hearts.

Generally, myocardial residue curves exhibit similarity upon scaling time by dividing by mean transit time.[2] This would be the same as scaling by a flow-to-volume ratio or simply by multiplying time by F when V is constant. One might intuitively expect a higher value of α at higher flows, and this is suggested by the positive slope of α versus F in Fig 5, but it is not definitive.

In Fig 6, a more specific test is performed with respect to the question of whether α is related to flow. Three sets of curves were obtained from one heart at flows of 0.76, 1.34, and 3.44 mL·g⁻¹·min⁻¹. The three residue curves have been superimposed on each other by scaling time with respect to mean transit time (Fig 6, upper curves). The three outflow curves were treated likewise (Fig 6, lower curves). The close juxtaposition of the curves upon each other shows that their shapes are similar, meaning that their higher moments (variance and the skewness and kurtosis obtained from the third and fourth moments) are close to being the same. In Appendix A, this time scaling is applied to the function $h(t)=A\alpha t^{-\alpha-1}$, and it is shown that the exponent α is the same on the time-scaled $h(t/t)$ as on the original $h(t)$. Since scaling by flow

Fractal Exponent α for ^{15}O-Labeled Water Washout From $R(t)$, $h(t)$, and $\eta(t)$ Simultaneously

Heart	Experiment	F, mL·g^{-1}·min^{-1}	α	Confidence Limits*	CV $R(t)$	$h(t)$	$\eta(t)$
1	02121107	1.65	2.10	±0.036	0.06	0.03	0.12
1	02121112	3.32	2.59	±0.011	0.16	0.15	0.38
1	02121115	1.22	1.58	±0.050	0.04	0.03	0.11
2	02121505	3.44	2.03	±0.061	0.12	0.16	0.33
2	02121508	1.34	1.91	±0.046	0.04	0.05	0.11
2	02121513	0.76	1.82	±0.115	0.12	0.06	0.34
3	12111308	2.91	2.34	±0.034	0.06	0.05	0.17
3	12111313	2.91	2.72	±0.008	0.08	0.09	0.18
4	12111533	2.19	2.26	±0.032	0.07	0.05	0.20
4	12111545	2.19	2.29	±0.031	0.18	0.28	0.51
4	12111548	2.19	2.20	±0.074	0.20	0.30	0.62
5	19111150	1.26	2.49	±0.006	0.05	0.05	0.12
5	19111157	1.26	2.05	±0.050	0.06	0.07	0.18
6	19111342	1.10	2.33	±0.026	0.08	0.04	0.22
6	19111349	3.31	2.41	±0.035	0.09	0.10	0.19
7	29041356	0.97	2.22	±0.010	0.03	0.03	0.11
7	29041405	0.97	2.23	±0.033	0.09	0.05	0.30
7	29041411	0.97	2.14	±0.144	0.11	0.08	0.42
Mean±SD		...	2.21±0.27	...	0.09±0.05	0.09±0.08	0.26±0.15

F indicates flow; CV, coefficient of variation; $R(t)$, residual tracer activity; $h(t)$, outflow per unit time; and $\eta(t)$, fractional escape rate.

*Confidence limits for α at the 95% level for a single value of α in Equation 10 for $R(t)$, Equation 11 for $h(t)$, and Equation 12 for $\eta(t)$ a priori without any freedom.

should be equivalent to scaling by time, the theory would predict that in one heart at three different flows, the residue and outflow curves should exhibit the same power law exponent α. In this experiment (the one with the widest range of flows in the present study), the α values were 1.82, 1.91, and 2.03; ie, there is a 10% difference between the lowest and the highest. The trend for each individual heart in which there is a range of flows is like that for the whole data set in Fig 5. Thus, although the idea that α is related to flow is neither refuted nor supported by such data, there is room for suspicion despite the theory in Appendix A. Both Fig 5 and the analysis of the similarity-scaled data sets of Fig 6 leave open to further study the question of whether or not α increases with flow.

The absolute levels of myocardial blood flow influence the washout curve, $h(t)$, with higher flows giving an earlier peak and a shorter mean transit time. The fractional escape rate of tracer from the organ is higher at high flows. What is interesting about the fractional

escape rate is the exponent: the power law slope of -1 is independent of the flow and of the shapes of $R(t)$ and $h(t)$. This universality is striking: whenever the system is fractal, the relation between $R(t)$ and $h(t)$ gives rise to $\eta(t)=at^{-1}$, a power law fractal such that in all situations the escape rate diminishes as t^{-1}. This is a strong statement because $\eta(t)$ is equal to the derivative of $R(t)$ and also to $h(t)$ divided by 1.0 minus its integral. What this means is that when $\eta(t)$ has an exponent of -1, both $R(t)$ and $h(t)$ must be power law functions if either one is. The provocation provided by this observation is to find the physical explanation, as discussed below, and to ask whether it is necessarily fractal or allows some other descriptor.

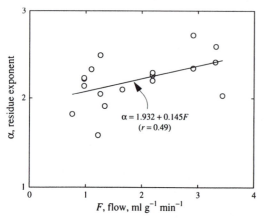

FIG 5. Fractal exponent (α) versus myocardial blood flow (F).

$$\alpha = 1.932 + 0.145F$$
$$(r = 0.49)$$

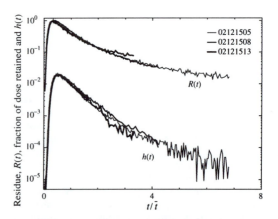

FIG 6. Residue (upper three) and outflow (lower three) curves, $R(t)$ and $h(t)$, respectively, for ^{15}O-labeled water from one heart superimposed by scaling the time axis by individual mean transit time, $\bar{t}$. There is close similarity in the shapes of the curves obtained at 0.76, 1.34, and 3.44 mL·g^{-1}·min^{-1}.

Discussion

These experiments provide data covering about two orders of magnitude in $R(t)$ and three in $h(t)$. The experiment is made particularly powerful by virtue of having data for both residue and outflow. The experimental resolution obtained here has been made possible by using radiotracers, using high time-resolution counting systems on outflow and residues simultaneously over long times, and having low background radioactivity. These conditions are only obtainable in a nonrecirculating system and are most readily obtained with short-lived positron-emitting tracers. Although the 2-minute half-life of ^{15}O has the disadvantage that the tails of the curves become rather noisy after three half-lives, correction for the decay is still adequate even when the concentrations are low, because it is practical to inject high doses of radioactivity without fear of contaminating the laboratory or risking significant radiation exposure.

It is not possible to do such experiments with standard dye dilution methods. The densitometers for indocyanine green, for example, suffer background drift of up to 2% in 1 minute with changes in blood optical density or other sources of variation, whereas with the ^{15}O-labeled water one can measure accurately down to 10^{-4} times the peak values, as is seen for the outflow curves.

The interpretation of the curves is that both the residue and outflow curves demonstrate self-similarity, in the sense that for each proportional increase in time (eg, twice as long), there is a constant proportional diminution in signal (eg, one quarter as great). In the parlance of the field of nonlinear dynamics, this is termed power law behavior. Such behavior is the hallmark of fractals—the self-similarity means that the apparent behavior (the scaling relation that says when time is twice as long, the signal is one quarter as great) is independent of the magnitude of the time unit considered.

The observation of the fractal time course of washout newly demonstrated in the present study is made secure by the simultaneous and coordinated measures of the three signals $R(t)$, $h(t)$, and $\eta(t)$. The observation that indocyanine green or ^{131}I-albumin dilution curves were not monoexponential but diminished more and more slowly as time progressed has been made when recirculation was sufficiently delayed[17] or absent.[18] When characterization of washout slopes, which were concave upward on semilog plots (as in Fig 1, left), was important, multiexponential fits were used, for example, for xenon washout from the brain by Hoedt-Rasmussen et al[19]; although this was expedient and gave good estimates of mean transit times, it also encouraged the misinterpretation that there were regions within the organ having two or three separate flows and inhibited the understanding that there was a broad heterogeneity of regional flows.

Fractal Extrapolation

For the practical purpose of measuring cardiac output, Hamilton et al[13] proposed using monoexponential extrapolation of the downslope of dilution curves to obtain an estimate of the area under the primary first-pass indicator uncontaminated with recirculated indicator. This was an excellent and powerful suggestion and

has been the method used ever since, even by those who recognized that it resulted in a minor underestimation of the area under the curve when the tails deviated (always upward) from monoexponential. Their technique is simple and allows an analytical calculation of the area under the extrapolated tail beyond the section of the downslope used to estimate the exponential rate constant. Now we propose an equally simple method of extrapolation, but we use the power law expression to exclude the recirculation while accounting for all the first-pass indicator and avoiding the systematic underestimation of the exponential extrapolation.

The method is applied to either outflow curves, $h(t)$, or to residue curves, $R(t)$. The power law exponent is the negative of the slope of the regression of $\log h(t)$ versus $\log t$ for the tail region where the relation is a straight line: $\log h(t) = \log A - \beta \log t$. (For the regression between times t_1 and t_2, an estimate of β is $\log [h(t_1)/h(t_2)]/\log [t_1/t_2]$.) The area, area 1, up to the time t_2 at which the extrapolation begins, can be obtained directly from the data. Area 2, under the extrapolated continuation of the observed data beyond t_2, is calculated analytically:

$$\text{Area 2} = \int_{t_2}^{\infty} h(t)\,dt = \int_{t_2}^{\infty} h_2 \cdot (t/t_2)^{-\beta}\, d(t/t_2)$$

(13)
$$= \frac{h_2 t_2^{1-\beta}}{\beta-1} \text{ for } \beta > 1$$

[The condition, $\beta > 1$, obviously holds for both $R(t)$ and $h(t)$ in the data of these experiments. The integral does not converge when $\beta \leq 1$, which means the area extrapolated would not be finite.] The estimate of cardiac output or flow, F, for a single path system into which a bolus of indicator of amount q_o is injected is $F = q_o/(\text{area } 1 + \text{area } 2)$.

For the residue and outflow curves in the present study, one can calculate the degree of underestimation of the areas that would result from using a monoexponential extrapolation. The calculation is based on using t_2 as the time where $R(t_2)/R_{peak} = 0.1$, and for the purpose of estimating β, the beginning of the region fitted was t_1, the time at which $R(t_1)/R_{peak} = 0.2$. The outflow $h(t)$ was fitted over the identical time period. For the 18 data sets, area 2 was calculated two ways: first as Equation 13, the fractal extrapolation, and second by monoexponential extrapolation. The monoexponential rate constant was determined from the best fitting linear regression of $\log h(t)$ or $\log R(t)$ versus t (linear). The results of the two extrapolation techniques give necessarily smaller values for the monoexponential approach: For $h(t)$, area 2 (monoexponential)/area 2 (fractal) $= 0.637 \pm 0.12$ (N=18), and for $R(t)$, area 2 (monoexponential)/area 2 (fractal) $= 0.630 \pm 0.08$ (N=18), where ± 1 SD is given. Naturally these errors in area due to the use of monoexponential extrapolation are much smaller than are errors in estimated mean transit times.

Why Is Washout Fractal?

The observed fractal washout may be explicable on the basis that regional flows per gram of tissue have fractal spatial distributions, as is well documented.[4,5] The link between the spatial and temporal events is not yet defined by any theory, but it makes sense that transit times through a network with fractal flow distributions should be fractal, since regional transit times are the local volumes of distribution divided by the local flow.

It is interesting that the observed fractal exponents are possibly dependent on flow. A theory for thinking that α and F should be independent when washout curves can be superimposed on each other by proportional time scaling[2,20] is given in Appendix A. The upward trend of α versus F in Fig 5 may be a hint that the fractal model is imperfect, which is no doubt the case, and some deviation toward multiexponential form is causing some degree of flow dependency.

The observation that washout is fractal does fit with the fractal paradigm newly recognized to apply to many aspects of biology. Self-similarity over a wide range of scales is found in time-dependent functions of many sorts. As in all physical systems, the summarizing descriptor, "fractal," applies over only a finite range. Fractals are not forever, except in the mathematics of the ideal, for every real fractal relation fails at both the large and small ends of the scale. The text of Bassingthwaighte et al[21] presents many examples of these self-similar scaling relations, all of them limited to finite ranges. Fractal power law scaling can emerge from any set of processes repeated multiple times with appropriate scaling between members of the set. See Appendix B for the general theory and an example using multiple exponentials.

It is intriguing that the coronary vascular network has so many fractal characteristics. The anatomy itself is fractal in terms of segment diameters and lengths,[22] the number of branches is a fractal function of the diameters of the vessel from which the branches derive,[23] the ratios of diameters of parent to daughter branches follow log-log scaling, and the flow distributions are spatial fractals.[4,24] The degree of heterogeneity of regional flow distributions has been approximated by those calculated from artificial fractal branching patterns by using an overly simple dichotomous branching.[25] Both Gan et al[26] and VanBavel and Spaan[8] estimate spatial distributions of flows from anatomic information; such calculations performed in our laboratory on artificial coronary systems give similar results and exhibit the same fractal correlation structure in regional flows in the heart as was observed in nature.[27] The present study adds to the story but uses the completely independent evidence on washout kinetics in vivo, as opposed to structural considerations or spatial distributions of flow at a given moment of observation. Washout kinetics, quite independently of spatial patterns or branching network structures, drive us to the same conclusion that the system is fractal.

Appendix A: Similarity of Time Scaling Means That the Fractal Exponent Should Not Be Influenced by Flow

The question of why the power law exponent α of the transport functions obtained at different flows is independent of flow can be explained mathematically on the basis of previous observations. Similarity on scaling of the time axis by the mean transit time is usually observed for the coronary system.[2,20,28] The test of "similarity" is a statistical one; namely, can the

shape of an impulse response $h_1(t)$ obtained at flow F_1 be considered similar to the response $h_2(t)$ obtained at flow F_2? Because there may be volume changes between two different physiological states, rather than scaling by F_1/F_2, one uses the more general scaling factor, the mean transit time or the ratio of mean transit times, $\bar{t}_1/\bar{t}_2$, where $\bar{t}_i=V_i/F_i$ and where the i indicates a particular state or condition or time of day when the observation of $h_i(t)$ was made. When similarity holds, then all time-normalized impulse responses have the same shape and are superimposed on each other on a plot of $\bar{t}_i h(t/\bar{t}_i)$ versus $t/\bar{t}_i$.

For the special situation where $h(t)$ is a power law function, as in Equation 11 in the text, the following equation applies:

$$(14) \qquad h(t)=A\alpha t^{-\alpha-1}$$

Then we can use $\bar{t}_i=V_i/F_i$ for clarity:

$$(15) \qquad \bar{t}_i h(t/\bar{t}_i)=\frac{V_i}{F_i}\cdot A\alpha\left(\frac{t}{V_i/F_i}\right)^{-\alpha-1}$$

$$=\frac{V_i}{F_i}\cdot A\alpha\left(\frac{F_i}{V_i}\right)^{-\alpha-1}\cdot t^{-\alpha-1}$$

$$=\left(\frac{V_i}{F_i}\right)^{-\alpha}\cdot A\alpha t^{-\alpha-1}$$

$$=(\bar{t}_i)^{-\alpha}\cdot h(t)$$

Thus, when similarity scaling holds and $h(t)$ is a fractal power law function, then the similarity scaling by mean transit time results merely in a scaling of the observed $h(t)$ by $(\bar{t})^{-\alpha}$, and the power law exponent α is unaffected by transformation. Since the scaling transformation can be performed either by using $\bar{t}_i$ generally or by using F_i when V_i is constant, then it follows that α should be unaffected by flow, as observed in Fig 5.

The same logic holds for $R(t)$ and $\eta(t)$, which have absolute values influenced by flow but have power law exponents that are not influenced by flow.

Appendix B: Sums of Scaled Functions Can Give Power Law Behavior

A power law function can be represented as the sum of a finite number of fractal-scaled basis functions. Consider approximating of the power law function of Equation 16 with the weighted sum of basis functions $f(t)$ in Equation 17:

$$(16) \qquad F=t^{-\beta}$$

$$(17) \qquad F\approx\sum_{i=1}^{N}a_i\mathrm{f}(k_it)$$

where a_i is the amplitude scalar and k_i is the time scalar for the ith member. Since the basis functions are not necessarily orthogonal, a finite sum of N scaled basis function is considered.

The minimum mean-squared error between $F(t)$ and a particular $f(k_it)$ over the interval from $t=0$ to $t=\infty$ is found by calculating a_i:

$$(18) \qquad a_i = \frac{\displaystyle\int_0^\infty f(k_i t) t^{-\beta}\, dt}{\displaystyle\int_0^\infty f^2(k_i t)\, dt}$$

From this, one can solve the relation between a_i and k_i by using a dummy variable, $\tau = k_i t$, substituted into Equation 18:

$$(19) \qquad a_i = \frac{k_i^{\beta-1} \displaystyle\int_0^\infty f(\tau)\tau^{-\beta}\, d\tau}{\dfrac{1}{k_i} \displaystyle\int_0^\infty f^2(\tau)\, d\tau} = \left(\frac{\displaystyle\int_0^\infty f(\tau)\tau^{-\beta}\, d\tau}{\displaystyle\int_0^\infty f^2(\tau)\, d\tau} \right) k_i^\beta$$

or

$$(20) \qquad a_i = C k_i^\beta$$

where C is a constant that does not depend on k_i.

A power law function can therefore be represented by a finite sum of the scaled basis functions, where the weight of each basis function is determined by the scale factor raised to the power law exponent:

$$(21) \qquad F \approx C \sum_{i=1}^{N} k_i^\beta f(k_i t)$$

In general, the k_i can be chosen on the basis of the interval over which the power law slope is fit. If the interval is defined by $t = t_a$ to $t = t_b$, then k_1 can be chosen by $k_1 = 1/t_a$ or a conveniently chosen value. In order to evenly distribute all of the k_i in the log-time domain, the rest of the k_i can be calculated over the range chosen:

$$(22) \qquad k_i = \left(\frac{k_N}{k_1} \right)^{\frac{i}{N-1}} = \left(\frac{t_a}{t_b} \right)^{\frac{i-1}{N-1}} k_1$$

An example using exponentials as the basis function is demonstrated in Fig 7. F and f are given as follows:

$$(23) \qquad F = t^{-2}$$

$$(24) \qquad f(t) = e^{-t}$$

The finite-sum approximation is shown for $N=2$, 3, and 4 exponentials. An approximate fit is achieved using only four exponentials over the interval of $t_a = 1$ to $t_b = 100$. Making t_a and t_b outside of the desired region to be fitted and increasing N allows one to approach exact power law behavior arbitrarily closely.

Acknowledgments

This study was supported by National Institutes of Health grants HL-50238 and RR-1243. The author greatly appreciates the efforts of James Ploger in analyzing these data and of Andreas Deussen (Department of Physiology, Düsseldorf), Thomas Bukowski, James Revenaugh, and James Ploger in the experimentation. FORTRAN code is available by ftp to nsr.bio-eng.washington.edu. (The linear regression program LINREG allows weighting and provides statistics: the program can be found at the ftp site in pub/NSR_linreg.tar.Z. The nonlinear optimizer is in pub/SENSOP/sensop.tar.Z.)

References

1. Bassingthwaighte JB. Blood flow and diffusion through mammalian organs. *Science*. 1970;167:1347-1353.
2. Bassingthwaighte JB. Physiology and theory of tracer washout techniques for the estimation of myocardial blood flow: flow estimation from tracer washout. *Prog Cardiovasc Dis*. 1977;20:165-189.
3. Yipintsoi T, Dobbs WA Jr, Scanlon PD, Knopp TJ, Bassingthwaighte JB. Regional distribution of diffusible tracers and carbonized microspheres in the left ventricle of isolated dog hearts. *Circ Res*. 1973;33:573-587.
4. Bassingthwaighte JB, King RB, Roger SA. Fractal nature of regional myocardial blood flow heterogeneity. *Circ Res*. 1989;65:578-590.
5. Glenny R, Robertson HT, Yamashiro S, Bassingthwaighte JB. Applications of fractal analysis to physiology. *J Appl Physiol*. 1991;70:2351-2367.
6. Tomanek RJ, Searls JC, Lachenbruch PA. Quantitative changes in the capillary bed during developing peak and stabilized hypertrophy in the spontaneously hypertensive rat. *Circ Res*. 1982;51:295-304.
7. Gonzalez F, Bassingthwaighte JB. Heterogeneities in regional volumes of distribution and flows in the rabbit heart. *Am J Physiol*. 1990;258(*Heart Circ Physiol* 27):H1012-H1024.
8. VanBavel E, Spaan JAE. Branching patterns in the porcine coronary arterial tree: estimation of flow heterogeneity. *Circ Res*. 1992;71:1200-1212.
9. Richmond DR, Yipintsoi T, Coulam CM, Titus JL, Bassingthwaighte JB. Macroaggregated albumin studies of the coronary circulation in the dog. *J Nucl Med*. 1973;14:129-134.
10. Yipintsoi T, Scanlon PD, Bassingthwaighte JB. Density and water content of dog ventricular myocardium. *Proc Soc Exp Biol Med*. 1972;141:1032-1035.
11. Yipintsoi T, Tancredi R, Richmond D, Bassingthwaighte JB. Myocardial extractions of sucrose, glucose, and potassium. In: Crone C, Lassen NA, eds. *Capillary Permeability (Alfred Benzon Symposium II)*. Copenhagen, Denmark: Munksgaard; 1970:153-156.
12. Rose CP, Goresky CA, Bach GG. The capillary and sarcolemmal barriers in the heart: an exploration of labeled water permeability. *Circ Res*. 1977;41:515-533.
13. Hamilton WF, Moore JW, Kinsman JM, Spurling RG. Studies on the circulation, IV: further analysis of the injection method, and of changes in hemodynamics under physiological and pathological conditions. *Am J Physiol*. 1932;99:534-551.
14. Lerch RA, Ambos HD, Bergmann SR, Sobel BE, Ter-Pogossian MM. Kinetics of positron emitters *in vivo* characterized with a beta probe. *Am J Physiol*. 1982;242(*Heart Circ Physiol* 11):H62-H67.
15. Zierler KL. Theoretical basis of indicator-dilution methods for measuring flow and volume. *Circ Res*. 1962;10:393-407.
16. Chan IS, Goldstein AA, Bassingthwaighte JB. SENSOP: A derivative-free solver for non-linear least squares with sensitivity scaling. *Ann Biomed Eng*. 1993;21:621-631.

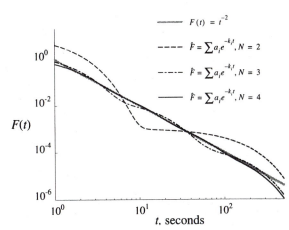

$F(t) = t^{-2}$

$\hat{F} = \sum a_i e^{-k_i t}, N = 2$

$\hat{F} = \sum a_i e^{-k_i t}, N = 3$

$\hat{F} = \sum a_i e^{-k_i t}, N = 4$

$F(t)$

t, seconds

FIG 7. Log-log plot showing multiexponential fits to $F = t^{-2}$, where F is flow and t is transit time, using two, three, and four exponentials with $t_a = 1$, $t_b = 100$, $k_2/k_1 = 100$ for $N=2$, $k_2/k_1 = 10$ for $N=3$, and $k_2/k_1 = 4.642$ for $N=4$, where k is the time scalar, and N is the number of exponentials.

17. Bassingthwaighte JB, Ackerman FH. Mathematical linearity of circulatory transport. *J Appl Physiol*. 1967;22:879-888.

18. Kuikka J, Levin M, Bassingthwaighte JB. Multiple tracer dilution estimates of D- and 2-deoxy-D-glucose uptake by the heart. *Am J Physiol*. 1986;250(*Heart Circ Physiol* 19):H29-H42.

19. Hoedt-Rasmussen K, Sveinsdottir E, Lassen NA. Regional cerebral blood flow in man determined by intra-arterial injection of radioactive inert gas. *Circ Res*. 1966;18:237-247.

20. Yipintsoi T, Bassingthwaighte JB. Circulatory transport of iodoantipyrine and water in the isolated dog heart. *Circ Res*. 1970;27:461-477.

21. Bassingthwaighte JB, Liebovitch LS, West BJ. *Fractal Physiology*. New York, NY/London, England: Oxford University Press; 1994.

22. Kassab GS, Rider CA, Tang NJ, Fung YB. Morphometry of pig coronary arterial trees. *Am J Physiol*. 1993;265(*Heart Circ Physiol* 34):H350-H365.

23. Arts T, Kruger RT, van Gerven W, Labregts JA, Reneman RS. Propagation velocity and reflection of pressure waves in the canine coronary artery. *Am J Physiol*. 1979;237:H469-H474.

24. Bassingthwaighte JB. Physiological heterogeneity: fractals link determinism and randomness in structures and functions. *News Physiol Sci*. 1988;3:5-10.

25. van Beek JHGM, Roger SA, Bassingthwaighte JB. Regional myocardial flow heterogeneity explained with fractal networks. *Am J Physiol*. 1989;257(*Heart Circ Physiol* 26):H1670-H1680.

26. Gan RZ, Tian Y, Yen RT, Kassab GS. Morphometry of the dog pulmonary venous tree. *J Appl Physiol*. 1993;75:432-440.

27. Bassingthwaighte JB, Beyer RP. Fractal correlation in heterogeneous systems. *Physica D*. 1991;53:71-84.

28. Knopp TJ, Dobbs WA, Greenleaf JF, Bassingthwaighte JB. Transcoronary intravascular transport functions obtained via a stable deconvolution technique. *Ann Biomed Eng*. 1976;4:44-59.

Is There Chaos in Cardiology?

Michiel J. Janse

*Department of Clinical and Experimental Cardiology,
Academic Medical Centre, University of Amsterdam,
Meibergdreaf 9, 1105 AZ Amsterdam Züidoost,
The Netherlands*

A recent paper stated that "the health care system in the United states is in chaos."[1] Though I am sure readers know what was meant, we have to be careful these days about the definition of chaos. Consulting a medical dictionary is unhelpful because there, chaos (*Pelomyxa carolinensis*) is an amoeba.[2] Descriptions in *Webster*[3] ("a state of things in which chance is supreme . . . nature that is subject to no law . . . a state of utter confusion completely wanting in order, sequence, organisation or predictable operation") do not quite cover the modern, mathematical redefinition of chaos.

The new chaos is characterised by deterministic behaviour, where irregular patterns obey mathematical equations and are critically dependent on initial conditions.[4] Modern chaos theory has been applied to a wide variety of biological phenomena[5] and has become quite fashionable. In certain circles you are regarded as a barbarian if your conversation is not garnished with terms such as Hopf bifurcation points, Liapunov numbers, phase locking, or fractals.

Chaos theory has been used in two areas of cardiac electrophysiology: (*a*) the behaviour of cardiac tissue, or isolated myocytes, during repetitive stimulation and (*b*) fibrillation and prefibrillatory states.

Chaos is irregular behaviour occurring in a nonlinear dynamic system. Cardiac cells may have several nonlinear, time-dependent variables (for instance supernormal excitability) and may exhibit irregular response patterns at a certain stimulation frequency.[6 7] When isolated sheep Purkinje fibres exposed to a solution containing 7 mmol/1 K^+ are repetitively stimulated at progressively faster rates, the so-called devil's staircase is seen, where 1:1 responses change into 2:1 and 3:1, with intermediate Wenckebach periodicity between the 1:1 and 2:1, and 2:1 and 3:1 responses. No irregular activity occurs. When, however, the extracellular K^+ concentration is lowered to 4 mmol/1, and the fibres exhibit a brief period of supernormal excitability during the repolarisation phase, deterministic chaotic

behaviour occurs at certain cycle lengths: either the stimulus-response pattern shows complex irregularities where no sequence is ever repeated in exactly the same way (this occurs at cycle lengths around 200 ms), or at cycle lengths of 50 ms the relation between cycle length and action potential amplitude is chaotic.[7] This example is chosen to show, on the one hand, that chaotic behaviour can indeed be induced in cardiac tissue, and that some satisfaction can be derived from the consideration that a unifying concept, chaos theory, links the stimulus-response patterns in cardiac cells with other phenomena such as growth during embryonic development[8] or the activity of phrenic nerves during mechanical ventilation of anaesthetised, paralysed cats.[9] On the other hand, the conditions in which chaotic activity arises are extreme: artificial stimulation of isolated tissue at a certain K^+ concentration at unphysiological frequencies.

Can chaotic behaviour be detected in "naturally" occurring rhythms? The obvious candidate for study is ventricular fibrillation, which traditionally has been called chaotic in the Webster sense. The identification of chaos in an existing rhythm is difficult. One technique is power spectrum analysis. A broad-band power spectrum is associated with chaos; however, ordinary random noise has a broad power spectrum as well. The power spectrum of electrocardiographic recordings during ventricular fibrillation is narrow[9 10] and Kaplan and Cohen concluded from their analysis that "there is little utility in classifying fibrillation as chaotic."[10] Would it be useful if fibrillation, or any other rhythm or conduction disorder, could be classified as chaotic? In this respect, the investigators in the chaotic domain are very enthusiastic: "A finding that ventricular fibrillation is chaos would suggest that there is a single mechanism at work in VF, and would provide guidance in the search for clinical precursors of VF";[10] ". . . such new theories may help to strengthen the ties between the basic scientist and the cardiologist by opening new research avenues which may lead to the disclosure of the fundamental mechanisms of severe cardiac arrhythmias and sudden death";[9] "The application of nonlinear systems theory to electrophysiology . . . may have clinical implications."[7] In a recent paper, describing a relation between T wave alternans in dogs with acute coronary artery occlusion and subsequent fibrillation, it was claimed that "a new approach is provided for quantification of susceptibility to malignant arrhythmia" and that "T wave alternans may represent a prechaotic state because bifurcate behaviour is the hallmark of chaos."[11]

These quotes indicate that a great deal is expected from studies applying chaos theory to cardiac rhythms: more insight into arrhythmogenic mechanisms and the identification of individuals at high risk for sudden cardiac death. It is here that I have my doubts. Certainly, new avenues should be explored, and possibly "we are sure to see dramatic advances in the field"[12] if we use nonlinear dynamics as a tool to study complex cardiac rhythms. In my view, however, cardiac arrhythmias ultimately have to be understood in terms of cardiac electrophysiology, and are due to changes in variables such as conduction velocity, excitability, automaticity, afterdepolarisations, electrotonic interactions between areas in the heart with different electrical properties, which in their turn are due to changes in properties of ionic channels, pumps, and receptors in cellular and subcellular membranes. Is my understanding that T wave alternans may be a harbinger of ventricular fibrillation in acute ischaemia improved because it is a prechaotic state (presumably leading to "chaotic" fibrillation where chaos is used in the old sense and not in the modern one) or because it marks the development of post-repolarisation refractoriness which sets the stage for unidirectional block, one of the prerequisites for re-entry?[13] [14]

In my opinion our insights into arrhythmogenesis will be advanced by the application of chaos theory only if the link between "modern" chaos theory and "old fashioned" electrophysiology is established. here, a mathematician who can model iterative non-linear systems and who understands the language of the cardiac electrophysiologist and of the practicing cardiologist may be of help.

REFERENCES

1 Young DA. Payment policy, quality of care and decision making with inadequate information. *J Am Coll Cardiol* 1989; 14(suppl A): 3A–6A.

2 *Dorland's illustrated medical dictionary*. 25th ed. Philadelphia, London, Toronto: WB Saunders, 1979.

3 *Webster's third international dictionary*. Springfield, Illinois, MA: G and C Merriam, 1971.

4 Li TY, Yorke JA. Period three implies chaos. *Am Math Monthly* 1971; 82:985–92.

5 Glass L, Mackey M.C. *From clocks to chaos. The rhythms of life.* Lawrenceville NJ: Princeton University Press, 1988.

6 Chialvo DR, Michaels D, Jalife J. Supernormal excitability as a mechanism of chaotic dynamics of activation in cardiac Purkinje fibres. *Circ Res* 1990;66:525–45.

7 Vinet A, Chialvo DR, Jalife J. Irregular Dynamics of excitation in biologic and mathematical models of cardiac cells. *Ann NY Acad Sci* 1990; 601:281–98.

8 Pyeritz RE, Murphy EA. Genetics and congenital heart disease: perspectives and prospects. *J Am Coll Cardiol* 1989;13:1458–68.

9 Goldberget AL, Uhargava V, West BJ, Mandel AJ. Some observations on the question: Is ventricular fibrillation chaos? *Physica D* 1986;19:282–9.

10 Kaplan DT, Cohen RJ. Is fibrillation chaos? *Circ Res* 1990; 67:886–92.

11 Nearing BD, Huang AH, Verrier RL. Dynamic tracking of cardiac vulnerability by complex demodulation of the T wave. *Science* 1991;252:437–40.

12 Glass L. Is cardiac chaos normal or abnormal? *J Cardiovasc Electrophysiol* 1990;1:481–2.

13 Downar E, Janse MJ, Durrer D. The effect of acute coronary artery occlusion on subepicardial transmembrane potentials in the intact porcine hart. *Circulation* 1977;56:217–24.

14 Janse MJ, Wit AL. Electrophysiological mechanism of ventricular arrhythmias resulting from myocardial ischemia and infarction. *Physiol Rev* 1989;69:1049–69.

578

Fractal Nature of Regional Myocardial Blood Flow Heterogeneity

James B. Bassingthwaighte, Richard B. King, and Stephen A. Roger

Spatial variation in regional flows within the heart, skeletal muscle, and in other organs, and temporal variations in local arteriolar velocities and flows is measurable even with low resolution techniques. A problem in the assessment of the importance of such variations has been that the observed variance increases with increasing spatial or temporal resolution in the measurements. This resolution-dependent variance is now shown to be described by the fractal dimension, D. For example, the relative dispersion (RD=SD/mean) of the spatial distribution of flows for a given spatial resolution, is given by:

$$RD(m) = RD(m_{ref}) \cdot \left[\frac{m}{m_{ref}} \right]^{1-D_s}$$

where m is the mass of the pieces of tissue in grams, and the reference level of dispersion, $RD(m_{ref})$, is taken arbitrarily to be the RD found using pieces of mass m_{ref}, which is chosen to be 1 g. Thus, the variation in regional flow within an organ can be described with two parameters, $RD(m_{ref})$ and the slope of the logarithmic relationship defined by the spatial fractal dimension D_s. In the heart, this relation has been found to hold over a wide range of piece sizes, the fractal D_s being about 1.2 and the correlation coefficient 0.99. A D_s of 1.2 suggests moderately strong correlation between local flows; a $D_s=1.0$ indicates uniform flow and a $D_s=1.5$ indicates complete randomness. (*Circulation Research* 1989;65:578–590)

It is now well established that regional myocardial blood flows show considerable spatial heterogeneity. This has been thoroughly demonstrated by those laboratories in which small tissue pieces were used and the whole of the myocardium was sampled. Probability density functions of regional flows were generated in this fashion by Yipintsoi et al[1] in the dog, by King et al[2] in the baboon, and by Bassingthwaighte et al[3] in the rabbit. Using pieces that were less than 1% of the ventricular mass, these investigators found local flows ranging from a third of the mean flow to over twice the mean flow. The relative dispersions (RDs) of the distributions (RD=SD/mean) were about 35% in these three species when observations were made by dividing the hearts into 100–250 pieces.

This large variability appeared suspect and seemed possibly attributable to inherent variation in the microsphere deposition technique, even though the results were very reproducible.[3] The spheres were recognizably large compared with the vessels in

which they were deposited, and causes of maldistribution with rheology and branching[4] are numerous. Microsphere tracer counting error exacerbates the problem. However, the studies of Bassingthwaighte et al[3] showed that in comparison to a molecular flow marker, microspheres were not seriously in error, even though a small systematic bias was observed.

The variance observed by Marcus et al[5] for regional flows in dog myocardium gave a relative dispersion of 21%, smaller than we had found. They divided the left ventricular myocardium into 96 pieces of about 1 g each; this focuses the question on sample size. In this study, we show that use of large tissue pieces underestimates the degree of observable heterogeneity and that this is not due to methodological error. An example of the dependence of the estimate of dispersion on the size of the pieces is shown in Figure 1. The finer the myocardium is cut, the broader the distributions of regional flows become. This is a fundamental property of any density function over a spatial domain.

Fractal phenomena are those that show self similarity upon scaling. In some systems, the observable degree of heterogeneity increases as resolution of the method increases. When these increases are proportional, the relation can be fractal or at least is

From the Center for Bioengineering, University of Washington, Seattle.

Supported by grants HL-19135, HL-38736, and RR-01243 from the National Institutes of Health.

Address for correspondence: James B. Bassingthwaighte, MD, PhD, University of Washington, WD-12, Seattle, WA 98195.

Received April 7, 1988; accepted February 23, 1989.

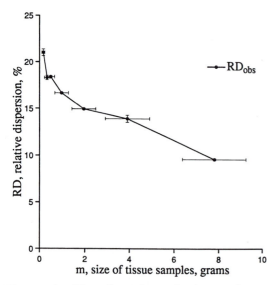

FIGURE 1. *The effect of sample size on the apparent dispersion of regional blood flow in the left ventricle of a sheep heart. Data were obtained using the "molecular microsphere" iododesmethylimipramine. The apparent relative dispersions (RD, the standard deviations divided by the mean at each level of division) are plotted against the average masses of the pieces for seven different sample sizes. Horizontal bars give the standard deviation of the piece masses, which are not uniform. Vertical bars give the standard deviations of the estimates of RD when estimates are obtained by forming aggregates of adjacent pieces in three to eight different ways.*

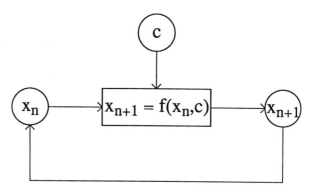

FIGURE 2. *Fractals are stochastic or deterministic recursions, giving rise to features of systems which are similar, relative to the scale of the recursion, at different scales.*

describable by a fractal relation, if it holds true over a sizable range of observation unit sizes.[6,7]

In this study, we show that a simple fractal relation provides precise descriptions of the heterogeneity of regional and myocardial blood flows over a wide range of piece sizes. The simplicity of the relation allows the variances to be described by two parameters: the variance at a particular piece size and the fractal dimension or noninteger power that relates the size of the pieces to the dispersion.

Materials and Methods

Fractal Methodology

A system having a "fractal nature" is one with one or more characteristics that remain constant when examined over a wide range of scales. A fractal boundary, for example, would be one that appears as equally invaginated or "crumpled" regardless of the magnification with which it is examined. A characteristic of such a boundary is that its apparent length increases as shorter and shorter standards are used to measure it. The change in apparent boundary length is related to the length of the measuring stick in a deterministic way. See Peitgen and Saupe[8] for a lucid explanation of fractals.

Mathematical fractals are generated by recursive expressions wherein each generation is derived

from the preceding in a specific way. The basic fractal expression is a summarizing statement describing a recursion. In a single dimension, the idea is diagrammed as in Figure 2. The recursion may be deterministic, stochastic, or some combination of both (e.g., deterministic with scatter of a specified form). The $(n+1)$th value of the recursive feature is a function of the nth value, so that even when this is a linear function the relation over two or more generations must be nonlinear.

Many of these fractal ideas and quite useful descriptions were initiated by the work of Mandelbrot,[9,10] and more practical applications are being found day by day.[7] For the Mandelbrot set, now famed for the beautiful pictures that can be produced from it, the recursion is purely deterministic and is simply $Z_{n+1} = Z_n^2 + C$, where Z and C are complex numbers.

Branching networks can be seen to be fractal, as in Mandelbrot's example of a recursion similar to the bronchial tree of the lung.[10] Branching arterial trees, bronchial trees, or mathematical analogs to real trees may be fractal in more than one dimension and have modifying features such as requirements to be space-filling. For example, ratio of parent-to-daughter branch lengths might differ from the ratio for branch diameters.

The branching network of the myocardial vascular system might be expected to have a fractal nature. If this is so, the observed heterogeneity of regional myocardial blood flow would be dependent on the size of the measuring stick, that is, on the number of pieces into which the heart is divided. This fractal relation can use either the number of pieces or the mass of the pieces. The logic is as follows: Given that a fractal relation exists between the observed RD of regional flows and N, the number of pieces into which the heart has been divided, the relation can be expressed by the equation:

$$RD(N) = RD(N=1) \cdot N^{D-1} \qquad (1)$$

where $RD(N=1)$ is the intercept obtained by extrapolating to one piece, and D is the fractal dimension, commonly a noninteger power. (The fractal relation has no meaning with respect to dispersion when there is only one piece.) A more general approach is to relate the RD to the mass of the individual pieces. Let a heart of total mass (M) be divided into N_m pieces each of mass (m) grams (i.e., $m = M/N_m$). Then, from Equation 1:

$$RD(m) \equiv RD(N_m) = RD(N=1) \cdot N_m^{D-1} \qquad (2)$$

Further, let N_{ref} be the number of pieces with individual mass m_{ref} grams and with relative dispersion $RD(m_{ref})$. Then

$$RD(m_{ref}) = RD(N=1) \cdot N_{ref}^{D-1} \qquad (2)$$

which can be rearranged to give

$$RD(N=1) = \frac{RD(m_{ref})}{N_{ref}^{D-1}} \qquad (3)$$

Substituting Equation 3 into Equation 2 gives

$$RD(m) = RD(m_{ref}) \cdot \left[\frac{N_m}{N_{ref}} \right]^{D-1} \qquad (4)$$

Since

$$\frac{N_m}{N_{ref}} = \frac{M/m}{M/m_{ref}} = \frac{m_{ref}}{m}$$

Equation 4 can be rewritten as

$$RD(m) = RD(m_{ref}) \cdot \left[\frac{m}{m_{ref}} \right]^{1-D} \qquad (5)$$

Thus, Equations 1 and 5 have the same fractal dimension. Equation 1 and Equation 5 define explicitly the hypothesis that variation in local myocardial blood flows follows fractal rules. If the equation can be well fitted to data, then we will be able to say that the fractal hypothesis cannot be rejected. Equation 5 reduces to $RD(m) = RD(m=1) \cdot m^{1-D}$, but the expression leaves out the implicit understanding that $m_{ref} = 1$ g. It is convenient to use an m_{ref} of 1 g, and the relative dispersion observed from the flows in 1-g pieces to be $RD(m_{ref})$. The logarithmic form of Equation 5 is obtained by taking the logarithm of both sides:

$$\log\left[\frac{RD(m)}{RD(m_{ref})} \right] = (1-D) \cdot \log\left[\frac{m}{m_{ref}} \right] \qquad (6)$$

or

$$D = 1 - \log[RD(m)/RD(m_{ref})]/\log[m/m_{ref}] \qquad (7)$$

Experimental Methodology

The data on deposition densities in the myocardium of baboons were obtained using standard experimental approaches for microsphere measurements of flow as outlined by Heymann et al[11] using 15-μm diameter spheres. In 10 awake baboons, injections of four to six differently labeled microspheres were made at different times in control states and during mild exercise or heat stress; in another group of three animals, differently labeled

microspheres were injected simultaneously. The methodology is outlined in detail by King et al.[3]

The methodology used in the anesthetized open-chested sheep and rabbit experiments was similar except that, in addition to microspheres, the "molecular microsphere" iododesmethylimipramine (IDMI) was also used. In five of 11 sheep and in all of the rabbits, two differently labeled IDMIs and two differently labeled 15-μm microspheres were injected simultaneously into the left atrium. In the other six sheep, only one IDMI and one microsphere type were used. The hearts were stopped 1 minute later. The methods used in rabbits are given in detail by Bassingthwaighte et al[2] and for sheep by Bassingthwaighte et al.[12]

For all of these animals, the hearts were sectioned in accord with a standard scheme similar to that used for the baboons.[3] Only the left ventricular data are used for the analysis which follows. The ventricular myocardium was studied; it was divided into four rings from apex to base, and each ring was divided into eight sectors (like sections of a pie), except that in baboons, the apical ring was only divided into four sectors. Each sector was divided into a series of slices from endocardium to epicardium (three slices in the rabbit and six in the sheep and baboons). The total number of left ventricular pieces was usually 96 in the rabbit, 168 in the baboon, and 192 in the sheep.

Data Analysis

Calculation of the observed heterogeneity of regional blood flow. From the amount of radioactivity in an LV piece, the relative deposition density (d_j) could be calculated as follows:

$$d_j = \frac{a_j/m_j}{A/M} \qquad (8)$$

where a_j is the activity measured in the piece, m_j is the mass of the piece, A is the total activity in all the LV pieces of that heart, and M is the total LV mass. From the d_js in all the LV pieces of a heart, a probability density function was constructed. Since all the d_js were in the range 0.0 to 3.0, this range was divided into 30 intervals of width 0.1. The pieces were then sorted into groups according to the interval into which d_j for the piece fell. Since each tracer gave a value for d_j in the piece, the arithmetic average of all the measurements in the piece was actually used as the sorting criterion. The probability density for a group was the ratio of the sum of the masses of the pieces in the group to the total LV mass times the interval width. Mathematically, this is expressed as

$$w_i = \qquad (9)$$

$$\frac{\Sigma m_j \text{ for all pieces for which } (d_i - \Delta d/2) < d_j < (d_i + \Delta d/2)}{\Delta d \cdot M}$$

where the subscript j refers to the pieces and the subscript i refers to the groups.

TABLE 1.   Scheme for Estimating Relative Dispersion at Different Voxel Sizes by Aggregating Pieces of Sheep LV

Number of observations	Average weight of a piece	Number of ways of calculating relative dispersion
192	0.2	1
96	0.4	3
64	0.6	3
32	1.2	6
16	2.4	8
8	4.8	8
4	9.6	8

This gives the probability density function in the form of a finite interval histogram. The area of the histogram is unity and, given a large number of observations or very narrow class widths, its mean is also unity. Because the mean of the d_js in each group is not necessarily equal to the midpoint of the interval, these relations are imperfect, but in practice the errors are less than 1%. The RD of the density function is SD/$\overline{d}$; since $\overline{d} = 1$, the RD is equal to the standard deviation, SD. It is this relative dispersion of the probability density function that is used as a measure of the heterogeneity of regional myocardial blood flow.

Calculation of the observed heterogeneity at different sample sizes. When a heart has been cut into many small locatable pieces, these pieces can be regrouped to form larger pieces composed of adjacent subpieces. The average activity of the aggregate larger piece is the mass-weighted average of the activities of the component pieces. Thus, in retrospect, the relative dispersion can be calculated from the individual pieces and then for aggregates of pairs (sets of four, eight, etc., pieces), thereby putting the heart back together again. An example of the results of this procedure is shown in Figure 1. For each grouping, a single value of RD is obtained, but adjacent pieces can be apposed in several different ways, so that for the same sizes of groups or masses of aggregated pieces, the RDs can be calculated in an increasing number of different ways as more and more pieces are put together. Table 1 lists the number of configurations of adjacent pieces to form a volume element, voxel, of each size. The table applies to the sheep studies, so that the actual masses vary from animal to animal. The number of configurations at each voxel size is less in rabbits.

Using this approach, one gets both an average dispersion at each effective piece size and an estimate of the variance of the dispersion. A complicating factor not written into our fractal expressions is that there is also variation in the piece size at each of these levels, since the aggregates were put together in a pattern fashion rather than in a fashion designed to achieve a particular mass. (If this size variation were proportionally greater at larger aggregate sizes, this would tend to underestimate the fractal slope D_s.)

Fractal Analysis

Linear least-squares regression lines were obtained for the logarithm of the relative dispersion versus the logarithm of the average mass of the aggregate pieces, at each level of division. Excluded from the regression were aggregates weighing more than 2 g. Because the correlations were high, there is no important difference between the log-log regressions and the optimized best fits of Equation 6 against the data using linear least squares, and the expedient process of using the linear least-squares fit of the logarithms was considered acceptable in this circumstance, as discussed by Berkson.[13]

When the deposition of a radioactive tracer is used to measure the relative dispersion of flows, the observed dispersion (RD_{obs}) is the composite of at least two dispersive processes which we will distinguish as spatial dispersion (RD_S) and methodological dispersion (RD_M). It is the spatial dispersion alone that is of interest, since it might be based on a fractal branching vascular network. If the variations due to the method and due to the spatial heterogeneity are independent processes, the total variance is the sum of the variances of the components. Since all the distributions are normalized to have a mean of unity, this relation can be summarized in terms of the RDs:

$$RD_{obs}^2 = RD_S^2 + RD_M^2 \qquad (10)$$

Two to six observations of activity due to IDMI or microspheres were made in each piece or aggregate. RD_M for a given spatial resolution is calculated as the average of the percent differences between two flow measurements. For example, for four observations in a piece and 192 pieces, there are six estimates of RD_M in each piece times 192 pieces, giving 1,152 estimates of RD_M, and the average of this is used. RD_M is composed of both counting error, which increases as the total number of disintegrations per minute diminishes, with the reciprocal of the number of microspheres deposited, and with weighing error. Thus, we concluded that even though the methodological error appears to follow a fractal relation very well, it is not likely to be inherently a fractal phenomenon. If RD_M is nonfractal, that is, does not follow Equation 5, then the combination of Equations 5 and 10 can still hold true for both RD_S and RD_{obs}. (Equation 10 must always be true but Equation 5 cannot be true for more than two out of RD_S, RD_M, and RD_{obs}, as can be seen by substituting.) However, since RD_{obs} contains the methodological error, the logic used in judging RD_M to be not necessarily fractal should also apply to RD_{obs}. Consequently, we consider the spatial heterogeneity as characterized by RD_S to have the best possibility of being fundamentally fractal, and observed dispersions were corrected for methodological dispersion to give RD_S before fractal analysis was applied.

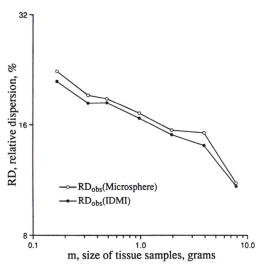

FIGURE 3. *Comparison of the observed relative dispersion (RD$_{obs}$) to piece mass (m) for iododesmethylimipramine (IDMI) and for microspheres. Data are from the left ventricle of a sheep heart. Microspheres give a larger dispersion over the range of the data but the slopes of the two lines are similar.*

Results

Data were obtained from 10 baboons, 11 sheep, and six rabbits. The physiological data in these animals are given in the publications referred to in "Materials and Methods." The baboons were awake, and the sheep were all in quite good physiological condition, as were four of six of the rabbits. However, two rabbits had low blood pressures and high heart rates at the time of the injection.

Assessment of Differences Between Microsphere and IDMI Results

The assessment of the two deposition markers for regional flow, IDMI (the "molecular microsphere")

and 16-μm diameter microspheres is the subject of two previously reported studies,[3,12] but the results are mentioned here because they provide the background methodology for the present study. The main result is that microspheres provide moderately accurate estimates of regional flow in pieces down to 0.1 g but that the methodological variation is two to four times that for the IDMI deposition technique. A secondary result is that there are small systematic biases in the deposition of particulate spheres; the larger bias is toward preferential or excessive deposition in regions of higher flow; there is also a smaller bias toward excessive deposition in subendocardial versus subepicardial regions. Both biases combine with the methodological variation in the sphere technique to produce probability density functions for sphere deposition that are slightly broader than for the deposition of the molecular marker IDMI. This is reflected in higher RDs, the standard deviations of the density functions for spheres, as is shown in Figure 3.

The data of Figure 3 are from one sheep left ventricle, cut into 186 pieces because fewer were obtained at the apex. The relative dispersions obtained for the first piecing, with an average piece mass of 0.16 g, are the largest. Grouping into larger masses gives progressively less total variation as the group mass increases. RDs from microspheres are consistently greater, as must be the case when both true regional flow variation and methodological noise contribute to the measure. What can be said is that true flow variation in samples of a given size can only be less than the values plotted. What can also be said is that larger pieces show less apparent variation, which must be true whenever there is spatial variation within the pieces. The objective is to estimate the true flow variation by accounting for these factors.

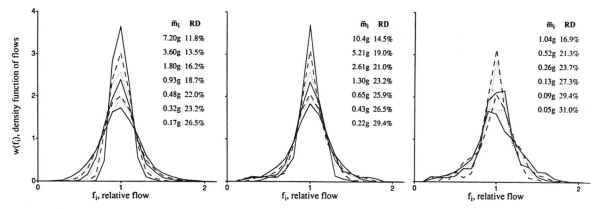

FIGURE 4. *Composite probability density functions for regional flows at differing average piece mass for three species. For each species, density functions are shown for several different piece masses. The average piece mass for each distribution is given in the details for each panel. The largest mass gives the narrowest distribution and the smallest gives the broadest.* Left panel: *Microsphere distributions in 10 baboons. Four to six microsphere measurements were made in each piece.* Center panel: *Iododesmethylimipramine distributions in 11 sheep.* Right panel: *Iododesmethylimipramine distributions in six rabbits.*

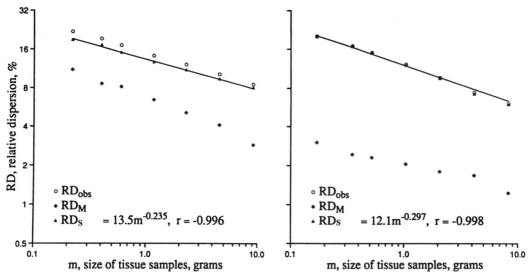

FIGURE 5. *Fractal regression for spatial flow variation in left ventricular myocardium of a baboon* (left) *and a sheep* (right). *Plotted are the relative dispersions of the observed density function (RD$_{obs}$), the methodological dispersion (RD$_M$), and the spatial dispersion (RD$_S$) at each piece mass calculated using Equation 11 for sheep and Equation 12 for baboons. RD$_{obs}$ and RD$_S$ are nearly superimposed in the sheep. Fractal analysis of the spatial dispersion on pieces up to 4 g mass showed high correlations.*

Probability Density Functions of Regional Flows

Since the LV regional flows in each animal were calculated relative to the mean flow to the entire left ventricle, the data from a group of animals could be pooled and a composite histogram constructed. Figure 4 shows composite distributions for data from the left ventricle in baboons, sheep, and rabbits. In the baboons and sheep, the distributions are shown for seven sample sizes obtained by using the number of pieces described in Table 1. Since the left ventricle of the rabbit was divided into 96 pieces, only six sample sizes are shown. Using the composite of the animals in each species provides smoother curves and illustrates that the phenomena is general. At the same time, because the shapes of the distributions in the animals do differ in whether it is skewed to the left or to the right, the composite distributions tend to be more spread than the individuals. Figure 4 emphasizes that when the heart is divided finely, the spread of the distributions is broader, and that cutting only a few large pieces per heart gives an underestimate of the underlying variation in regional flows.

Separation of Methodological, Spatial, and Temporal Components of the Observed Flow Heterogeneity

Data on five of the 11 sheep and all of the rabbits were obtained with two simultaneously injected IDMIs labeled with ^{131}I and ^{125}I. This strategy allowed an evaluation of the methodological error in the IDMI technique. Thus, the spatial dispersion in flows was calculated using a revision of Equation 10:

$$RD_S^2 = RD_{obs}^2 - RD_M^2 \qquad (11)$$

In this analysis, no assumptions are made regarding the fractal nature of the observed or methodological dispersions. At each piece mass, the observed and methodological dispersions were computed, and the resulting spatial dispersion was calculated. Fractal analysis was applied only to the spatial dispersion by fitting the values of RD$_s$ versus mass m with the regression expression of Equation 6. The relations are plotted for a single sheep in Figure 5 (right panel). The rabbit data were treated similarly since RD$_M$ was known for both spheres and IDMI.

In the baboons, one of which is shown in the left panel of Figure 5, the calculation of RD$_s$ was somewhat different because four to six temporally separated injections of different microsphere rather than a simultaneous paired control were made. Thus, the dispersions measured by the several measurements in a piece had components due to both the microsphere method and temporal dispersion:

$$RD_S^2 = RD_{obs}^2 - RD_{\tau,M}^2 \qquad (12)$$

The observed dispersions in the baboons were so corrected to yield RDs. Fractal relations between spatial dispersion and piece mass were similar to these in sheep and rabbits (see below and Table 2). We note the RD$_{\tau,M}$ is a measure of reproducibility and fails to provide a measure of the small systematic biases observed with the microsphere technique by Utley et al,[14] Yipintsoi et al,[1] and demonstrated recently in our lab where we note a small bias toward deposition of 15-μm microspheres in high flow regions compared to IDMI deposition. That there is an observed bias does not mean RD$_M$ is over

TABLE 2. **Fractal Analysis of Individual Animals**

Animal no.	Fractal Analysis		
	D_S	RD_S (m_{ref}=1 g)	r
Baboon			
01	1.16	17.9	−0.998
02	1.20	15.4	−0.993
03	1.23	15.7	−0.982
05	1.20	15.2	−0.997
06	1.14	21.8	−0.995
07	1.23	14.6	−0.999
08	1.29	11.6	−0.998
09	1.19	11.4	−0.991
10	1.23	11.8	−1.000
11	1.24	13.5	−0.996
Sheep			
230186	1.13	24.3	−0.999
010586	1.13	16.3	−0.982
220586	1.24	10.2	−0.995
290586	1.30	12.1	−0.998
050686	1.22	9.3	−0.991
190686-1	1.10	43.0	−0.998
190686-2	1.07	33.7	−0.970
080886-1	1.19	21.6	−0.989
080886-2	1.19	14.7	−0.993
300487	1.18	32.5	−0.990
060587	1.14	20.8	−0.972
Rabbit			
181185	1.22	24.0	−0.960
121285	1.18	25.6	−0.957
191285a	1.20	21.1	−0.919
090186	1.37	7.2	−0.986
160186a	1.26	7.8	−0.977
160186b	1.25	7.0	−0.995

D_S, spatial dimension; RD_S, spatial relative dispersion; m_{ref}, reference level of dispersion.

or underestimated, but it would suggest that RD_S might be overestimated slightly.

In addition to the 10 baboons discussed above, simultaneous injections of microspheres with different radioactive labels were made in a separate group of three baboons. Using the data from these three baboons to measure RD_M, corrections were applied to $RD_{\tau,M}$ to estimate the temporal dispersion RD_τ alone:

$$RD_\tau^2 = RD_{\tau,M}^2 - RD_M^2 \qquad (13)$$

The results of the analysis of the temporal data from the 10 baboons are shown in Figure 6. As for the purely spatial heterogeneity, the temporal component of the spatial variation shows a fractal regression relationship over the small, 10-fold range available to test. Since the temporal component is small compared with the spatial variation, that is, the $RD_\tau(m=1)$ of 6% is much less than the spatial $RD_S(m=1)$ of 11–21% in baboons, we conclude that

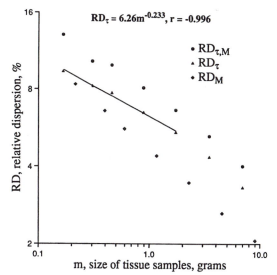

FIGURE 6. *Temporal component (RD_τ) of regional left ventricular myocardial flow variation, as a function of piece mass, from composite data in 10 baboons. Observed methodological dispersion ($RD_{\tau,M}$; ●) was measured by temporally separated injections in 10 baboons and is composed of variation due to moment-by-moment fluctuations in flow plus errors in the microsphere methodology. Microsphere method variation or dispersion (RD_M; ◆) was measured by simultaneous injections of four or six differently labeled tracer microspheres in three baboons. Temporal dispersion (RD_τ) calculated using Equation 13. Regression analysis of the temporal dispersion gave a fractal D of 1.233 (r=0.996) for RD_τ over piece sizes ranging from 0.2 to 2 g.*

the spatial distributions must be relatively stable in their spread and also that individual regions do not vary greatly in flow.

Fractal Relations for Spatial Dispersion of Regional LV Flow

The corrected RD_Ss were plotted as a function of piece mass for the composite data from the 10 baboons, 11 sheep, and six rabbits. These results are shown in Figure 7. The thin lines represent the log-log regressions for the individual animals, using pieces up to 2 g and ignoring the coarsest groups of larger aggregate mass. For the baboons, each individual line is a composite of four to six sets of microsphere observations, for a total of 1,224 observations of relative regional flow within the pieces of the smallest mass, with decreasing numbers of observations in each of the aggregated pieces of larger mass in the same animal. The composite regression, the thick line, performed on a total of 48,588 data points from the baboons, has a fractal D of 1.202 (r=0.998) while the average value of D_S from the 10 animals was 1.21±0.04. The individual values for the slope and intercept are given in Table 2.

The RD_Ss calculated from IDMI distributions determined in the sheep are shown in the center panel of

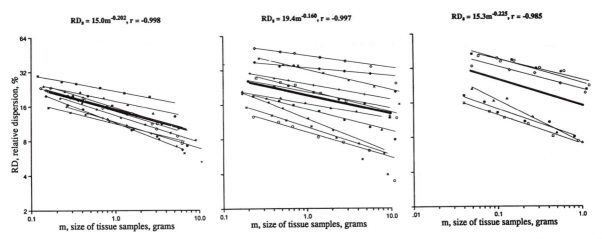

FIGURE 7. *Fractal regression lines for spatial dispersion (RD_S) in baboons, sheep, and rabbits. For each species, the calculated relative dispersions due to spatial heterogeneity of regional blood flow are shown for each level of sampling. The regression lines for the individual animals are shown by the thin lines. In each panel, the thick line is the regression obtained for all of the data points of that group of animals. The slopes, intercepts, and correlation coefficients of the regression equations for the individual animals are given in Table 2.* Left panel: *Microsphere data from 10 baboons. The composite distribution has a fractal D of 1.202 (r=0.998).* Middle panel: *Iododesmethylimipramine (IDMI) data from 11 sheep. The line for the composite data has fractal D of 1.160 (r=0.997).* Right panel: *IDMI data from six rabbits. The composite has a fractal D of 1.225 (r=0.985).*

Figure 7. The average D_s for the individual animal is 1.17±0.07 (*N*=11) and the composite D_s is 1.160 (*r*=0.997) with the total number of observations being 12,765. The IDMI data for the rabbits (Figure 7, right panel), show approximately similar slopes. The individual D_ss average 1.25±0.07 (*N*=7), and the composite is 1.225 (*r*=0.985) on 4,404 observations. Data for the individual sheep and rabbits are given in Table 2. The fractal slopes D_s for microsphere distributions in sheep and rabbits were essentially the same as for the IDMI distributions.

An unexpected finding with interesting implications is the observation that hearts with larger spatial variation at 1 g voxel size tend to have smaller fractal slopes, the fractal D, as in Figure 8. This might imply that in normal hearts there is a limit to the heterogeneity at the microvascular unit level and that hearts with RDs closer to this limit must have lower rates of increase in RD with diminishing voxel size.

Discussion

Two points are clarified by this study. First, observed variation in regional myocardial blood flow increases as the resolution is increased, and second, a two parameter fractal relation is a strikingly accurate descriptor of this change that satisfies the need for a summary of the data over the 20- to 40-fold range of sample sizes in our data. The mere fact that two parameters, the dispersion at a particular resolution RD(m_{ref}) and a noninteger slope (or fractal dimension D_s), describe the observations over a wide range of observed element sizes is a useful attribute that augments our set of descriptive statistical tools. The two-parameter description is useful for describing the variances in intensities of a characteristic over a domain that has no a priori definition of the unit size, and might augment standard statistical approaches.

The accuracy of the fractal descriptor raises the question of whether there is a true fractal phenomenon underlying the observations of regional flow. A purely deterministic branching network with a constant set of rules (e.g., a constant ratio of parent-to-child branch lengths, constant branch angles, and fixed ratios of diameter to length at each generation) will have the same resistance to flow in all the branches of a given generation and will give uniform flow per unit volume in the supplied regions.

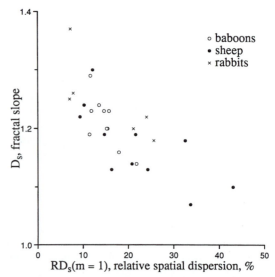

FIGURE 8. *Fractal dimension Ds for spatial variation versus RD_S(m=1), the relative dispersion of left ventricular myocardial flows at a voxel size of 1 g.*

Such deterministic rules are unlikely to lead to the situation that we observe in the myocardium: a remarkable nonuniformity of flow. On the other hand, there is no reason that the set of rules need be purely deterministic. Equally valid rules might be that each generation branches with a fixed mean angle plus or minus a prescribed random variation with branch lengths and diameter ratios also fulfilling precisely defined statistical rules. A set of stochastic rules of this type does not lead to uniformity as the different branches of the same generation will now have different resistances, and chance alone will lead to a wide range of flows in the terminal branches. The wider the individual variances prescribed by the rules, the broader will be the heterogeneity of observed regional flows.

The data of Suwa et al[15] and Suwa and Takahashi[16] show that the renal and mesenteric arteriolar trees have rather consistent log-log relations in ratios of branch lengths, diameter ratios, wall thickness to diameter ratios, radius-to-length ratios, and even intra-arterial pressures over up to a 200-fold range of lengths. These types of data are not yet available for the heart. It will be very worthwhile to undertake detailed studies of the geometry of the myocardial microvasculature and its variability in the intact state. Given sufficient information on the vascular geometry, a "fractal heart" model could be generated. This would require development of a set of rules governing the branching, lengths, diameters, etc. that adheres to the space-filling nature of the system of capillary-tissue units. The data presented in this study can serve as a test of the adequacy of any such model. Other tests would include the vascular resistances, volumes, pressures, and velocities, all of which are observable.

As the spatial resolution for cardiac flow imaging has improved, flow heterogeneity in the normal human myocardium has recently come under consideration. While the resolution of thallium imaging is so low that local variation is not seen in normal hearts, with the higher resolution positron emission tomography (PET)[17] the level of variability described in our animal studies can be recognized, but not accurately quantitated, in humans. Such recognition of the normal variation is important in defining the limits of "normality" in more precise terms than has been previously required. One wishes to avoid making diagnoses of regional underperfusion in what are actually normal people. This is especially important as it now appears that early evidence of certain cardiomyopathies may lie in an observation of flow heterogeneity.[18] The approach used in these studies to obtain the data on dispersion versus sample size could be applied to PET data. Starting with the highest resolution PET image, adjacent voxels could be combined in an ordered manner to give a set of lower resolution images that could be analyzed for flow heterogeneity. Thus, while the resolution of PET does not approach that of tissue sectioning techniques, the use of the fractal descriptor may allow extrapolation of the PET results down to the level of tissue sectioning resolution if the fractal relation holds to that level. Experiments are needed at much higher resolution to see how far one can go with this idea.

Another application of the knowledge on flow heterogeneity is in the analysis of data on solute exchange. The multiple indicator technique provides a good example. When a set of tracers are injected into the inflow of an organ and a set of outflow dilution curves is obtained by sequential sampling from the outflow, the estimation of kinetic rate constants for membrane permeation or chemical reaction are dependent on the estimates of heterogeneity of flows or transit times through the organ. For example, if the relative dispersion of regional flows is 40%, the myocardial capillary permeability-surface area products for sugars are underestimated by over 50% when the capillary flows are considered uniform instead of accounting for the flow heterogeneity.[19] This is a situation where one would like to use the fractal relationship to predict the degree of heterogeneity at the level of the functional microvascular unit size. If the fractal relationship holds down to this unit size, one would predict the heterogeneity by extrapolation and use it in the model analysis of the observed dilution curves. Our linear fractal relationships predict that, if the unit size is of the order of one cubic millimeter, the relative dispersion of flows would be more than 60%. This would give a larger estimate of capillary PS than would be obtained by assuming uniform flow, as much as 80% larger. There are two problems with simply taking the bull by the horns and applying this "fractal fix." The first is that the actual microvascular unit size is not precisely known; the second is that there is no assurance that the fractal relationship holds down to that level. Important new inferences on the unit size from the observations of Shozawa et al[20] suggest a volume of one fifth to one third of a cubic millimeter, smaller than the half to one cubic millimeter that Bassingthwaighte et al[21] conjectured. The extension of the fractal relation down to the ultimate unit size is an unlikely event. Rather, one would expect that the relative dispersion of flows would begin to plateau before this limit is reached, because one expects that flows in nearby or adjacent regions to be more similar to each other than are flows in regions distant from each other. This similarity is in keeping with our results showing a fractal dimension of about 1.2 in these hearts, whereas a purely random process would have a fractal dimension of 1.5. The association of flows in neighboring regions demands further study with techniques providing data of very high resolution.

Structures of a uniform grain size can show up as peaks in the fractal plot, as illustrated and analyzed by Wright and Karlsson.[6] They show that when there is variation in the grain sizes the peaks are less distinct. In our plots, there is no evidence of peaks deviating from a fractal line. This could conceivably mean that our sequence of steps between the piece masses used was simply so coarse that a peak was missed. If that were so, one might have expected to find a hint of a peak, a point above the fractal line, on at least one animal, but none was seen. The likely explanation is that there is no fundamental grain size or functional unit size above the size of the terminal vascular unit and which is much smaller than our crude piecing can reveal.

This study provides no insight into whether or not the regional flows are related to local metabolic needs. Certainly some variation in local metabolism is expected, as the fractions of connective tissue, myocytes, etc., must vary somewhat. The natural expectation is that metabolism drives local flow. While flow and metabolism must be fairly closely related in a functioning organ, it may also be that the branching of the vascular tree leads inevitably to flow heterogeneity that influences the growth and development of the local capacity for metabolism.

Fractal relations describe the degree of flow heterogeneity over a wide range of sample volumes in the hearts of baboons, sheep, and rabbits. Further studies are needed to elaborate the generality of these findings and to define the limits of applicability of the concept. The relation is not yet based in a secure way on the nature of the vascular tree or its dynamic behavior, although there are reasonable inferences that this may be so. How far this concept extends toward the functional microvascular units where the exchange occurs is unknown, but among the incentives to discover how far the idea can be carried is the need to account for flow heterogeneity when making estimates of transport rates, membrane permeabilities, and intracellular reaction rates in vivo, all of which are needed for both physiological studies and for the interpretation of images obtained in clinical situations by positron and single photon emission tomography.

Appendix: Fractal Dispersions of Densities

This appendix provides numerical examples of aggregates of randomly varying values. The purpose is to illustrate that the fractal dimension is lower for correlated than for random phenomena.

Begin with observations in a spatial domain of the intensities of a property. Examples are the number of stars or galaxies per unit volume in space, the number of cape buffalo per hectare in the Serengeti, or the specific gravity of a milliliter of angel cake. Even though the measurement is error free, there is variation in each concentration or density, just as there is for regional blood flows in the heart. The coefficient of variation, the RD, is an index of the variability or heterogeneity within the domain. If the variation is perfectly random, then any one set of observations at a particular size of observed unit serves to characterize it completely. The reason this can be claimed as a complete characterization is that no matter how the samples are grouped, the

standard deviation of a set of aggregates of random values is predictable from the size of the aggregate, M_{agg}, compared with any other aggregate size, M^o_{agg}; the larger the sizes of the aggregates, the smaller the variation amongst aggregates of the particular size:

$$SD(m) = SD(m_0) \cdot \left[\frac{m}{m_0}\right]^{1-D}$$

By aggregating nearest neighbors, the variance decreases. When the individual values of the smallest elements are purely random Gaussian, and no ordering of the array has been undertaken, then the fractal D is 1.5 and a doubling of the size of the aggregate reduces the variance by 30% or the SD to $1/\sqrt{2}$:

$$SD(2M_{agg}) = SD(M_{agg}) \cdot 2^{-0.5}$$

Even when the statistical basis is weak, by virtue of using only small numbers, this works pretty well, as shown in Figure A.1, and the slope gives a fractal D of nearly 1.5. Note that the observed SD at $N=4$, where the 256 values form aggregates of 64 values each, is less than the expected value of 50/8 or 6.25%; the hearts show this same tendency.

There is no law that says that log RD versus log N for the pieces of the heart or for the number of aggregates of nonrandom numbers should show self-similarity on recursion, which is what a straight line indicates. However, the grouping of neighbors must give a monotonically decreasing RD. To exemplify a couple of the possibilities of what would be the result of using the same approach on nonrandom arrays of numbers, we created ordered arrays out of random arrays. We have not yet devised a general approach to this and therefore chose to test our procedures on highly coordinated arrays created by exact rank ordering within groups. Rank ordering gives the highest degree of correlation between nearest neighbors in a group, and will serve to illustrate that such ordering creates results which are very different from the fractal relation.

Figure A.2 shows an example of the effects of rank ordering of densities or numbers from a Gaussian distribution with mean 1.0 and standard deviation 0.30. Beginning with an array of 2^{20} random Gaussian numbers, recursive twofold aggregating of neighbors gives successive reductions of RD; the result is the straight line labeled D=1.5. This is the line predicted by theory and illustrates the same phenomenon as in Figure A.1, except that now using large numbers gives a closer approximation to the theory. The straight line is in accord with self-similarity, that is, the reduction in apparent dispersion is the same with each doubling of aggregate size. Randomizing phenomena such as diffusion fit this scheme.

Three other analyses were done by aggregating nearest neighbors after rank ordering subsets of the 2^{20} random numbers. The rank ordering was done by taking N_g points (with $N_g=256$; 1,024; or 16,384 points in a group) and putting the smallest value in

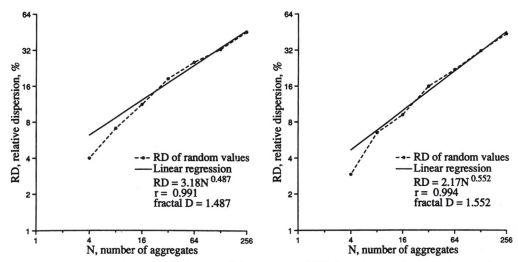

FIGURE A.1.   *Two examples of the fractal behavior of the two sets of 256 Gaussian random numbers with mean=1.0 and SD=50% grouped together by 2s to form 128 aggregates, by 4s to form 64 aggregates, etc. The theoretical fractal D is 1.5. Even with such poor statistics, especially for the large aggregates where the number of aggregates (N) is small (32, 16, and 8), the recursive grouping of nearest neighbors results in an observed log-log regression line with a fractal D close to the theoretical value of 1.5.*

the group first, the next higher value next, and so on up to the highest value in the group last. Then a plot of the 2^{20} points in order would appear as a sawtooth function with monotonic rises along each tooth and some variability in the tooth shape and height. The sequences of 2^{20} points if plotted as value versus index now forms a rough sawtooth; $N_g \times N = 2^{20}$ so that, with $N_g = 256$ there are 2^{12} teeth, each a rough ramp; with $N_g = 2^{10}$ there are 2^{10} teeth and with $N_g = 2^{14} (=16,384)$ there are 64 teeth. After this within-group rank ordering, the recursive nearest neighbor aggregation gives quite a different shape of RD

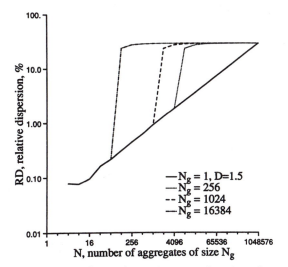

FIGURE A.2.   *Relative dispersion as a function of number of nearest-neighbor aggregates for a randomly ordered and three partially rank-ordered arrays of 2^{20} random numbers with mean 1.0 and SD=0.30. The "cuts" into the array to form the aggregates begin at the first number.*

versus group size. Because of the rank ordering, nearest neighbors in the array are closely similar, so there is very little reduction in the overall dispersion, that is, RD is reduced very little initially by the successive pairings as one progresses from the rightmost point on the graph (unpaired 2^{20} observations) to successively larger groups.

However, as the successive pairings, from right to left, increase the group size toward that of the rank ordered groups (the teeth), the RD diminishes rapidly within a few successive pairings. For Figure A.2, the successive pairings were done by starting with the first of 2^{20} numbers, so that when the number in a group exactly matched the number in a rank-ordered "tooth," the RD matches the theoretical value for a random array. This is as it should be for the content of the group of the size of the "tooth" or larger is exactly the same whether or not it had been rank-ordered internally.

Consider flows in the heart to be truly random but ordered within small regions. This approach is analogous to considering the heart to be composed of N independent regions into which flow is delivered by an artery of size A, which in turn bifurcates into 2^{20-N} or 2^N separate but ordered microvascular units. When the heart is divided into samples or groups of units smaller than that supplied by one artery of size A, then the apparent relative dispersion is close to that of a whole population of 2^{20} units. When the heart is divided exactly along borders between the 2^N groups supplied by arteries of size A or into larger groups, the RD appears as if the system were random, which it is in this case at the larger sample masses.

Next, consider the same situation as in Figure A.2, but make only a small change, namely the point in the array where the sampling is started, the

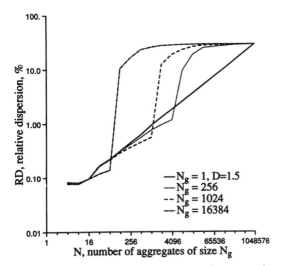

FIGURE A.3. *Relative dispersion as a function of number of nearest-neighbor aggregates for a randomly ordered and three partially rank-ordered arrays of 2^{20} random numbers with mean 1.0 and SD=0.30. The "cuts" into the array to form the aggregates begin at a random number.*

first cut made. Instead of starting with the first of the 2^{20} values, we started at a random point and cycled through the 2^{20} values (going to the last, then to first and up to the one before the starting point). The result is considerably different from that in Figure A.2, as shown by the curves in Figure A.3. Firstly, as one pairs nearest neighbors successively into larger and larger aggregates of size N_g, the diminution in RD, down from 0.3 is more rapid than in Figure A.2. This refers to the slopes near the right top end of each curve. The second difference is in the apparent RD at N=M, that is, where the number of groups equals the number of rank-ordered "teeth"; the RD is about $1/\sqrt{2}$ or less than the pure random expectation. At smaller N, larger aggregates, the RDs diminishing thereafter with a fractal slope D<1.5, about D=1.33. (The calculation for D from any pair of points on the graph is Equation 7 of the text.)

Having a random starting point for the 2^{20} points is like having an arbitrary starting point for slicing up the heart and cutting it without any specified relation to the cognate beds of the supplying arteries. For the random numbers, starting randomly within ordered groups, giving a D of 1.33 means that the RD doubles in three slicings into halves ($2\rightarrow8$ pieces) whereas purely random unordered arrays double their apparent RD with two slicings ($2\rightarrow4$ pieces). Perhaps we can extrapolate from this to suggest that if in the heart our slicing patterns fail to match the cognate beds of individual arteries, there will be some reduction in the apparent D_s compared with that obtainable with slicing at the peripheries of individual regions.

The parts of Figures A.2 and A.3 which are probably most relevant to our experimental obser-

vations are the regions with RDs greater than 10%. For each rank-ordered group size, when increasing N, as soon as N exceeds $2^{20}/N_g$, the lines of RD versus aggregate size show curves quickly reaching the plateau at 30%. These are quite unlike our data. Rank-ordering of the values within the group gives maximal local correlation; thus our local rank ordering of random values is a poor analogue to the physiological situation. The data lie in the region encompassed above by rank-ordering of large groups of random numbers (too near the plateau, too curved, flatten too fast with increasing division) and the unsorted random values (too low RDs for large samples and too steep a slope). We have no algorithm for the intermediate situation that might match the data, but we can be confident that it is very different from purely random flows and very different from groups with closely correlated rank ordered flows. From the D_ss observed in the heart we expect nearest neighbor correlations of $r=2^{3-2D}-1$ or about 0.5. We recognize that the random number string is a one-dimensional representation whereas the myocardial flows are distributed three dimensionally. Local correlation in three dimensions is to be expected, and it is probably necessary to account for the distributions in much more detail in order to understand our observations. The approach suggested by Voss[22] considering the values at partially correlated noise will certainly be useful. While we don't know its basis in vascular anatomy, rheology, and local regulation of regional flows, the fractal relations provide a fascinating new descriptive approach to sorting out the problem.

Acknowledgment

The authors are grateful for the assistance of Alice Kelly in the preparation of the manuscript.

References

1. Yipintsoi T, Dobbs WA Jr, Scanlon PD, Knopp TJ, Bassingthwaighte JB: Regional distribution of diffusible tracers and carbonized microspheres in the left ventricle of isolated dog hearts. *Circ Res* 1973;33:573–587
2. King RB, Bassingthwaighte JB, Hales JRS, Rowell LB: Stability of heterogeneity of myocardial blood flow in normal awake baboons. *Circ Res* 1985;57:285–295
3. Bassingthwaighte JB, Malone MA, Moffett TC, King RB, Little SE, Link JM, Krohn KA: Validity of microsphere depositions for regional myocardial flows. *Am J Physiol* 1987;253(*Heart Circ Physiol* 22):H184–H193
4. Yen RT, Fung YC: Effect of velocity distribution on red cell distribution in capillary blood vessels. *Am J Physiol* 1978; 235(Heart Circ Physiol 4):H251–H257
5. Marcus ML, Kerber RE, Erhardt JC, Falsetti HL, Davis DM, Abboud FM: Spatial and temporal heterogeneity of left ventricular perfusion in awake dogs. *Am Heart J* 1977; 94:748–754
6. Wright K, Karlsson B: Fractal analysis and stereological evaluation of microstructures. *J Microsc* 1983;129:185–200
7. Bassingthwaighte JB, van Beek JHGM: Lightning and the heart: Fractal behavior in cardiac function. *Proc IEEE* 1988; 76:693–699
8. Peitgen HO, Saupe D (eds): *The Science of Fractal Images.* New York. Springer-Verlag, New York, Inc, 1988

9. Mandelbrot B: *Fractals: Form, chance and dimension.* San Francisco, WH Freeman & Co, 1977

10. Mandelbrot BB: *The fractal geometry of nature.* San Francisco: WH Freeman & Co, 1983

11. Heymann MA, Payne BD, Hoffman JIE, Rudolph AM: Blood flow measurements with radionuclide-labeled particles. *Prog Cardiovasc Dis* 1977;20:55–79

12. Bassingthwaighte JB, Malone MA, Moffett TC, King RB, Chan IS, Link JM, Krohn KA: Molecular and particulate depositions for regional myocardial flows in sheep. *Circ Res* (in press)

13. Berkson J: Are there two regressions? *J Am Stat Assoc* 1950:45:164–180

14. Utley J, Carlson EL, Hoffman JIE, Martinez HM, Buckberg GD: Total and regional myocardial blood flow measurements with 25μ, 15μ, 9μ, and filtered 1–10μ diameter microspheres and antipyrine in dogs and sheep. *Circ Res* 1974;34:391–405

15. Suwa N, Niwa T, Fukasawa H, Sasaki Y: Estimation of intravascular blood pressure gradient by mathematical analysis of arterial casts. *Tohoku J Exp Med* 1963;79:168–198

16. Suwa N, Takahashi T: *Morphological and morphometrical analysis of circulation in hypertension and ischemic kidney.* Munich, Urban & Schwarzenberg, 1971

17. Budinger TF, Huesman RH: Ten precepts for quantitative data acquisition and analysis, in McMillin-Wood JB, Bassingthwaighte JB (eds): *Cardiovascular Metabolic Imaging: Physiological and Biochemical Dynamics in vivo. Circulation* 1985;72(suppl IV):53–62

18. Eng C, Cho S, Factor SM, Sonnenblick EH, Kirk ES: Myocardial micronecrosis produced by microsphere embolization: Role of an α-adrenergic tonic influence on the coronary microcirculation. *Circ Res* 1984;54:74–82

19. Bassingthwaighte JB, Goresky CA: Modeling in the analysis of solute and water exchange in the microvasculature in Renkin EM, Michel CC (eds): *Handbook of Physiology, Section 2: The Cardiovascular System, Volume IV, Microcirculation, Chapter 13.* Bethesda, Md, American Physiological Society, 1984, p 549–626

20. Shozawa T, Kawamura K, Okada E: Study of intramyocardial microangioarchitecture with respect to pathogenesis of focal myocardial necrosis. *Bibl Anat* 1981;20:511–516

21. Bassingthwaighte JB, Yipintsoi T, Harvey RB: Microvasculature of the dog left ventricular myocardium. *Microvasc Res* 1974;7:229–249

22. Voss RF: Fractals in nature: From characterization to simulation, in Peitgen HO, Saupe D: *The Science of Fractal Images.* New York, Springer-Verlag New York, Inc, 1988, pp 21–70

KEY WORDS • 2-iododesmethylimipramine • microspheres • regional myocardial blood flow • flow heterogeneity • heart • fractals • relative dispersion coefficient of variation • sheep • baboons • rabbits

Jurassic Heart: From the Heart to the Edge of Chaos

Vivian S. Rambihar, MD, FRCPC

JURASSIC PARK HAS REINTRODUCED US TO DINOSAURS and chaos. Dinosaurs died millions of years ago after a chaotic event, an unexpected meeting of a meteor and the Yucatan Peninsula. Chaos (1.2), the science not confusion, present since the origin of the universe and noted in the writings of ancient cultures and religions (2), has outlived the dinosaurs, has been revitalized since the advent of fast computers and — as shown in the editorial by Dr. R.E. Beamish (3), book by Dr. L. Glass et al (4) and review by Dr. T.A. Denton et al (5) — has relevance to cardiology. Chaos, however, is only a part of a broader paradigm shift, with potential impact on all of science (6) and on all of everything in the universe (7). This new perspective or thinking more accurately reflects the reality of the world we live in, replacing the deterministic, mechanistic, predictable universe of Newton, with a world of uncertainty, unpredictability, interrelatedness, networking, sensitivity, self-organization, etc — an open world (6).

Clinical and research cardiology is a challenge. Despite advances in modern cardiology, physicians and patients still experience the unexpected and the unexplainable . . . often. We continue to seek only a 'scientific' and deterministic explanation for these events. We cannot yet explain how or why or when a patient will develop a myocardial infarction, or which patient's isolated left anterior descending coronary artery lesion will progress to an acute coronary syndrome, which one will stabilize for years, or which 'stable' patient will suddenly deteriorate. Clinical cardiology is full of uncertainty and inexplicable phenomena. We cannot accurately predict the future course of a specific patient (8,9), even with 'diagnostic testing' (10) to avert adverse outcomes. Too often we see patients with a 'clean bill of health' or a normal exercise test succumb

to an acute event not long after. We cannot explain the nonlinearity in the clinical expression of disease, why patients with similar or only slightly different underlying pathophysiology develop completely different outcomes or why similar outcomes arise from markedly different degrees of similar pathophysiology, such as a myocardial infarction from 99% stenosis or from 30% or even from 0%. We seek increasingly finer detail and more investigations to grapple with this uncertainty and with our limitations.

Dr. Maseri (11) reflects on this "study of disease mechanisms . . . in finer and finer detail" and suggests investigation of the causes of the variable responses of individual subjects to known pathogenic mechanisms, mentioning the search for differences rather than similarities in patients with cardiac failure, hypertrophy, atherosclerosis, infarction and angina. We have all seen this variable response and seek solace in forthcoming studies or lament insufficient funding, technology, knowledge or insight. We fall back on probabilities which average out patients and events, say "things happen" or invoke Pascal — "the heart has its reasons which reason does not understand".

Jurassic Park and chaos may have reasons which reason does understand.

Chaos and complexity, the unstable area at the edge of chaos, an area of exquisite sensitivity and emergence (12,13), offer a reasonable model for understanding the variety, variability and unpredictability we see. The same laws of nature that govern the world of interplanetary motion, volcanoes, tidal waves and avalanches must, at the local level, be obeyed in the coronary artery and, at the cellular, molecular and genetic levels, affect all the areas of subspecialization we call coronary artery disease, molecular cardiology, electrophysiology, congenital disease, gene expression, etc. The principles of 'sensitive dependence' on initial conditions and interrelatedness of everything means that we are unable to collect enough information to determine precisely the outcome of any event. The laws of nonlinear dynamics that describe our world, at all levels, describe an essential and inherent unpre-

Dr VS Rambihar is a Toronto cardiologist and President of the Toronto Chaos Society

Correspondence and reprints: Dr VS Rambihar, 3302-3000

Laurence Avenue East, Scarborough, Ontario M1P 2V1. Telephone (415) 438-2100, Fax (416) 438-2106 or 438-9318

dictability in systems because as observers we have practical limitations, easily neglecting the effect of distant events, and therefore cannot contemplate all possible interrelatedness. We are thus committed to unpredictability and uncertainty. We can choose to average this out over time and list the probability for events. Chaos and complexity seem the best model we have so far to describe this variability of clinical expression of similar pathophysiology and the uncertainties we note in clinical and research medicine.

This variability and uncertainty extended outside clinical and research cardiology will have tremendous impact on the future of our patients. The self-organizing systems in health care promotion and delivery in the community, hospital and university, and in the administration and planning of cardiology would also be subject to the rules of chaos and complexity with all its ramifications (14). Slight changes in a system, strategically placed at the edge, may change the outcome tremendously and have effects that ripple throughout, creating an entirely new system. One does not need drastic or radical change to improve or to derail a system. A system touched is never the same — "you cannot step into the same river twice".

There are numerous other examples of interrelatedness and the potential for chaos on a more practical level. A patient awaiting transfer to a tertiary care bed may have that bed withdrawn because a parallel event — someone shoveling snow develops a myocardial infarction and appears by chance at the other hospital at a critical moment — determines that the bed is lost. Self-organizing systems in health prevention scattered widely across the country have a potential impact and relationship with each other even without direct communication; eg, one group may obtain a grant that limits the ability of the other to obtain funding.

The influence of one group in changing health care may change the system enough that further needs require revision. The impact of a particular study and its results may require modification of a distant study that has now become related. Medical care or traditional methods at a distant location, even years before, transcend space and time, influencing by any of numerous ways what happens today to our patients locally. It may take only a little change in lifestyle or modification of factors to cause a major change in outcome. This amplifies the value of judicious individual effort and removes the frustration of feeling that a system is insurmountable and unresponsive to the individual.

Nonlinearity exists in cardiology, as in all of medicine and science and life in general. Chaos and complexity at the edge of chaos have potential tremendous impact on cardiology, both in its technical and scien-

tific aspects, as well as in a philosophical sense. The new paradigm or thinking should lead us to a better understanding of the holistic relationship of our patient with the rest of the world at large, with unpredictability and uncertainty the rule, rather than the exception (9). Understanding the role of chaos, serendipity, and chance in clinical medicine teaches us that we may have a variable degree of impact on individual systems and on patient outcome and, used judiciously, potential tremendous impact. Our intent should be to optimize a dynamic and changing system continuously, rather than offer a simple reflex action and reaction response.

Chaos has moved from the heart to the edge of chaos (of complexity) and even further, with cautious skepticism advised "in the wake of chaos" (15).

ACKNOWLEDGEMENTS: The author thanks Debi Chaimer and Sherryn Rambihar for manuscript preparation and Dr. D. Jagdeo, Dr. T. Fox and Sherryn Rambihar for research on chaos.

REFERENCES

1. Gleick, J. Chaos — Making a new science. New York: Viking Penguin Books, 1987.
2. Briggs, J., Peat F.D. Turbulent Mirror. An Illustrated Guide to Chaos Theory and the Science of Wholeness. New York: Harper and Row, 1989.
3. Beamish, R.E. The new science of chaos — Implications for cardiology. Can J Cardiol 1993;9:607–8. (Edit)
4. Glass, L., Hunter P., McCulloch A. Theory of Heart. Biomechanics, Biophysics, and Nonlinear Dynamics of Cardiac Function. New York: Springer-Verlag, 1991.
5. Denton, T.A., Diamond GA, Helfant RH, Kahn, S., Karaguezian H. Fascinating rhythm. A primer on chaos theory, and its applications to cardiology. Am Herat J 1990;120:1419–40.
6. Davies, P., Gribbin J. The Matter Myth. Dramatic Discoveries that Challenge our Understanding of Physical Reality. New York: Simon and Schuster, 1992.
7. Lemonick, M. Life, the Universe and everything. Time Magazine, February 22, 1993.
8. Diamond, G.A. Future imperfect: The limitations of clinical prediction models and the limits of clinical prediction. J Am Coll Cardiol 1989;14:12A-22A.
9. Firth, W.J. Chaos — Predicting the unpredictable. Br Med J 1991;903:1565–9.
10. Myers, M.G., Baigrie R.S., Morgan C.D., Charlat M.L. Prediction of outcome post myocardial infarction. Can J Cardiol 1992;8:99B.
11. Maseri, A. Integration of cellular and molecular biology with clinical research in cardiology. N Engl J Med 1993;328:447. (Lett)
12. Waldrop, M.M. Complexity: The Emerging Science at the Edge of Order and Chaos. New York: Simon and Schuster, 1992.
13. Lewin, R. Complexity: Life at the Edge of Chaos. New York: MacMillan Publishing Company, 1992.
14. Ashbaugh, D.G. Chaos in Health Care. The Pharos (a publication of Alpha Omega Alpha Honor Society). Winter 1993:17–21.
15. Kellert, S.H. In the Wake of Chaos. Unpredictable Order in Dynamical Systems. Chicago: University of Chicago Press. 1993.

Application of Fractal Geometry to the Analysis of Ventricular Premature Contractions

Kenneth M. Stein, MD, and Paul Kligfield, MD

Fractals are a group of irregularly irregular geometric objects, first described by Mandelbrot.[1,2] We have previously suggested that a patient's distribution of ventricular premature contractions (VPCs) over time can be represented by a particular kind of fractal—the fractal dust.[3] This makes it possible to measure *dimension* (D), a number that quantifies the uniformity or nonuniformity of that patient's ventricular ectopy. When applied to a group of patients with severe congestive heart failure, dimension was found to have prognostic significance: Patients with nonuniform (clustered) ectopy had a higher risk of early death than those with more uniform distributions.[4] We now present some technical comments on the use of this technique.

Fractals are defined as objects whose Hausdorff-Besicovitch dimension exceeds their topologic dimension. In general they are complicated in appearance and irregular at any scale of measurement.[1,2,5] Many natural shapes have this property, among them coastlines, clouds, and the branching of Purkinje fibers in the heart or capillaries in the lung. A *fractal dust* is an object composed of topologically unconnected points. Any such object has a topologic dimension of zero. Hence, any dust with a fractal dimension greater than zero is, by definition, a fractal dust.

A set of events occurring over time can be thought of as a shape in which each event marks a point along a time axis. In this manner a set of ventricular premature contractions recorded during a defined period of ambulatory electrocardiography can be transformed into a "VPC-shape." Because any two VPCs must be separated by the time interval required for myocardial repolarization, the VPC-shape is topologically unconnected and satisfies the criterion for a dust. By extension, any VPC-shape with a Haussdorff-Besicovitch dimension greater than zero is a fractal.

Dimension is a measure of the irregularity of a shape or, more precisely, its tendency to be space-filling. One algorithm to measure the dimension from an empirically observed data set uses the correlation integral, as described by Procaccia and Grassberger.[6,7] The correlation integral is particularly well suited to measurements on dusts. In essence it expresses the probability (N) of finding a pair of data points separated by less than a given distance (r) as a function of distance. Correlation dimension is the slope of the line relating log(N) to log(r) and gives a lower limit for the object's Hausdorff-Besicovitch dimension. A review of some of the properties of this function is provided in Schaffer, et al.[8]

For a fractal dust the correlation dimension is a measure of the clustering of the points that make up the dust. A set of points that is densely clustered in space has a dimension of zero. On the other hand, for a diffuse set of points the dimension will, in the limiting case, approach the dimension of the space in which the points are embedded. In the case of points distributed along a single axis, as is the instance for the VPC-shape, the dimension that corresponds to maximum homogeneity is 1.

The uniform random distribution serves as a convenient tool for exploring the properties of the correlation integral as applied to dusts spread out along a single axis. It also provides an opportunity to discover any limitations (due to boundary effects or statistical fluctuation) that might result from applying the theory to samples of finite size. Uniform random distributions were created using a computerized ran-

From the Division of Cardiology, Department of Medicine, The New York Hospital–Cornell Medical Center, New York, New York.

Reprint requests: Paul Kligfield, MD, Division of Cardiology, Department of Medicine, The New York Hospital-Cornell Medical Center, 525 East 68th Street, New York, NY 10021.

dom number generator (GFA Basic 3.0, GFA Systemtechnik, 1988). In anticipation of applying this technique to the study of ventricular ectopy we will refer to a randomly generated point as a *complex* and to the coordinates of the line along which these complexes lie as *minutes*. In this context the points would correspond to a set of VPCs separated by random interectopic time intervals.

We analyzed a uniform random dust composed of 800 complexes spread out over 960 minutes (these values were chosen to conform with physiologic values in a population of patients with dilated cardiomyopathy and frequent ventricular ectopy). Looking at the correlation curve in the region of 1 to 10 minutes we obtain an estimated dimension of 1.02—not significantly different from the D of 1 that theory predicts for a uniform sample. (Note that it is impossible for the dimension of a linear object actually to be greater than 1!) The correlation function for this sample is plotted in Figure 1.

We used this distribution to assess the relationship between sample size and the variability of our estimate of D. The distribution of 800 complexes were subdivided into two 400-complex subintervals, four 200-complex subintervals, eight 100-complex subintervals, and sixteen 50-complex subintervals. The differences between the values for the subsamples and that for the sample as a whole and the standard deviation of this difference were calculated. We will refer to this standard deviation, expressed as a percentage of the dimension of the entire sample, as the "coefficient of difference". Details are shown in Table 1. As a result of these findings we chose to look at data in blocks of 200 complexes in all further analyses.

We have previously reported the results of applying this fractal analysis to the cases of 18 patients with dilated cardiomyopathy (either ischemic or nonischemic), looking at the correlation function in

Table 1. Variability of D as Related to Sample Size: Uniform Random Distribution

Sample Size	800	400	200	100	50
No. samples	1	2	4	8	16
	1.02	1.00	1.01	1.03	1.08
		1.03	0.97	0.99	0.94
			0.99	1.01	0.95
			1.05	0.93	1.00
				0.97	0.94
				0.99	1.06
				1.06	1.00
				1.02	0.89
					0.86
					1.01
					0.94
					1.02
					1.09
					0.97
					1.05
					0.95
Mean D	1.02	1.01	1.01	1.00	0.98
Mean difference		−0.01	−0.01	−0.02	−0.03
SD of difference		0.02	0.03	0.04	0.07
Coefficient of difference		2.1%	3.2%	3.8%	6.5%

D, dimension; SD, standard deviation

the range of 1 to 10 minutes[3,4]. Twenty-four-hour ambulatory ECGs using modified leads V_1 and V_5 were manually scanned using computer-assisted analysis (Avionics Trendsetter). Patients were selected who were predominantly in sinus rhythm and had at least 200 VPCs over the 24-hour recording period. The tapes were monitored for 200 consecutive PVCs and the time (exact to within 1 sec) of each PVC was noted. Estimated Ds for this group ranged from 0.59 to 0.99 with an average of 0.89.

To validate the choice of 200 complexes for our sample size another subsample analysis was performed. For 10 of the patients the 200-complex sample was broken down into two 100-complex subsamples and then into four 50-complex subsamples. The differences between each subsample value and the corresponding sample value were calculated and the standard deviation of these differences and coefficient of difference for the group of patients were determined, as shown in Table 2. The deviations are larger than for the random samples of similar size. This difference may reflect temporal variability in the patient data, or it may be the result of increased variability at lower dimensions.

We also determined the effect of adding "noise" to the observed patient data. Such noise might intrude from the misclassification of aberrantly conducted supraventricular complexes as PVCs. For each of the 10 sets of data referred to above we created composite data sets by adding 20 complexes assigned according to a uniform random distribution (10% noise group) or 40 uniform random complexes (20%

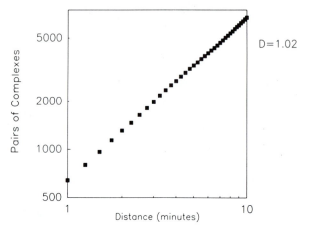

Fig. 1. Correlation function for a uniform random distribution composed of 800 complexes. D equals 1.02.

Table 2. Variability of D as Related to Sample Size: Patients With Dilated Cardiomyopathy

Patient	200 bts	100 bts	50 bts
1	0.93	0.92	0.82
		0.88	0.91
			0.79
			0.92
2	0.98	0.96	0.91
		0.98	0.98
			0.99
			0.90
3	0.97	0.99	0.99
		0.89	0.92
			0.85
			0.89
4	0.64	0.76	0.65
		0.43	0.60
			0.51
			0.37
5	0.88	0.92	0.90
		0.82	0.93
			0.87
			0.75
6	0.87	0.92	0.87
		0.86	0.96
			0.85
			0.84
7	0.89	0.77	0.77
		0.91	0.78
			0.84
			0.95
8	0.70	0.72	0.47
		0.73	0.84
			0.81
			0.46
9	0.89	0.78	0.70
		0.96	0.84
			0.91
			1.03
10	0.96	0.92	0.87
		1.17	0.75
			1.33
			1.12
Mean difference		−0.01	−0.04
SD of differences		0.09	0.12
Coefficient of difference		10.3%	14.1%

D, dimension; SD, standard deviation.

noise group) to the patient data. The mean difference ($D_{noise} - D_{real}$) was +0.02 for the 10% group and +0.03 for the 20% group. The standard deviations of the differences were 0.02 and 0.03 respectively. Thus, the addition of even relatively large amounts of nonsystematic noise led to only a minor increase in the estimate of dimension.

We have demonstrated that it is feasible, using the correlation integral, to apply a fractal approach to the measurement of clustering of ventricular ectopy. This technique yields a number called "dimension" that is near 0 in the case of highly clustered ventricular ectopy and near 1 for uniformly distributed ectopy. Even when applied to as few as 200 VPCs this measure is both reliable and robust. Ultimately it is hoped that analysis of dimension will aid clinicians in better understanding the natural history of cardiac arrhythmias and sudden death.

Although the foregoing analysis has focused on an examination of premature ventricular complexes, there is no fundamental reason to prevent the same ideas from being applied to any arrhythmia of brief duration (or, in fact, any frequent cardiac event of brief duration). Such experiments, which might identify clustering in, for example, APCs or ischemic episodes, would be of obvious interest.

References

1. Mandelbrot BB: Fractals: form, chance, and dimension. Freeman, New York, 1977
2. Mandelbrot BB: The fractal geometry of nature. Freeman, New York, 1982
3. Kligfield P, Stein K, Herrold E: Computer assisted analysis of Holter recordings. Ann NY Acad Sci, 601:353, 1990
4. Stein K, Kligfield P: Fractal clustering of ventricular ectopy in dilated cardiomyopathy. Am J Cardiol, 65:1512, 1990
5. Peitgen, H-O, Saupe D (eds): The science of fractal images. Springer-Verlag, New York, 1988
6. Grassberger P, Procaccia I: Characterization of strange attractors. Phys Rev Lett 50:346, 1983
7. Grassberger P, Procaccia I: Measuring the strangeness of strange attractors. Physica 9D:189, 1983
8. Schaffer WM, Ellner S, Kot M: Effects of noise on some dynamical models in ecology. J Math Biol 24:479, 1986

Annals of Biomedical Engineering, Vol. 21, pp. 125-134, 1993
Printed in the USA. All rights reserved.

0090-6964/93 $6.00 + .00
Copyright © 1993 Pergamon Press Ltd.

Modeling of the Heart's Ventricular Conduction System Using Fractal Geometry: Spectral Analysis of the QRS Complex

Omer Berenfeld,* Dror Sadeh,* and Shimon Abboud†

*Medical Physics Group, School of Physics, Raymond and Beverly Sackler Faculty of Exact Sciences,
Tel Aviv University, Israel, †Biomedical Engineering Program,
Faculty of Engineering, Tel Aviv University, Israel

Abstract —Many biological systems having one or more characteristics that remain constant over a wide range of scales may be considered self-similar or fractal. Geometrical and functional overview of the ventricular conduction system of the heart reveals that it shares structures common to a tree with repeatedly bifurcating "branches," decreasing in length with each generation. This system may further simplify by assuming that the bifurcating and decreasing process is the same at any generation, that is, the shortening factor and the angle of bifurcation are the same for each generation. Under these assumptions, the conduction system can be described as a fractal tree. A model of the heart's ventricles which consists of muscle cells and a fractal conduction system is described. The model is activated and the dipole potential generated by adjacent activated and resting cells is calculated to obtain a QRS complex. Analysis of the frequency spectrum of the QRS complex reveals that the simulated waveforms show an enhancement in the high frequency components as generations are added to the conduction system. It was also found that the QRS complex shows a form of an inverse power law, which was predicted by the fractal depolarization hypothesis, with a highly correlated straight line for a log-power versus log frequency plot with a slope of approximately −4. Similar results were obtained using real QRS data from healthy subjects.

Keywords —Heart modeling, Fractal geometry, ECG simulation, Spectral analysis, QRS complex.

INTRODUCTION

The use of computerized cardiac models as investigative and illustrative tools for the forward and inverse problem is widespread and many are described in the literature (2,3,10,15). Since the cardiac environment is too complex

to be considered in its full detail, models involve some degree of anatomic and physiologic simplification. This implies that models, which are oriented toward a definite object, give higher priority in description or computation to the subsystem in concern. Models usually consider conduction systems and transmission organs when the cardiac rhythmic behavior (10) or the propagation characteristics of the impulse and its spread are regarded (3). Our study investigates the conduction system function with regard to its fractal structure by the forward procedure. The concept of using fractal geometry and the formalism of self-similar structures to describe physiological systems has been known for some time (6,8,9). The His-Purkinje conduction system is an example of a physiological structure that can be described in such a manner (8,9). Scher (14) described the intraventricular conduction system as a tree, with the impulses starting near the trunk and Detweiler (5) described the transitional fibers of the Purkinje fibers as gradually diminished in size. The conduction system originates at the AV node with a single bundle and terminates at the myocardium, with numerous extremely fine fibers (5,11,14). It can generally be described by a structure of repeatedly bifurcating "branches," decreasing in length with each bifurcation. We can further simplify this description by assuming that this bifurcating and decreasing process is the same at any generation, that is, the shortening factor and the angle of bifurcation are the same for each generation. Under these assumptions, the conduction system can be described as a fractal canopy, or "tree."

The behavior of the cardiac conduction system plays an important role in the generation of a heart beat and it is this system that is responsible for the rapid and synchronized nature of cardiac muscle activity (14). The conduction system also contributes to the characteristics of the heart's electrical activity, and therefore to the form and frequency content of the ECG signal. The frequency content of the QRS complex was studied by Goldberger

Acknowledgment —This investigation was supported by the Ruth and Albert Abramson Foundation.

Address correspondence to Shimon Abboud, Biomedical Engineering Program, Faculty of Engineering, Tel Aviv University, Tel Aviv, 69978, Israel.

(Received 3/20/91; Revised 8/30/91)

O. Berenfeld, D. Sadeh, and S. Abboud

et al. (8), showing how a fractal conduction system can contribute to an inverse power law in the spectrum of the signal generated by it when a pulse propagates along the branches. In their work they analyzed the fractal hypothesis from the statistical point of view and analytically related the conduction system dimensionality to the power spectrum. They also confirmed that real QRS power spectrum indeed shows an inverse power law. However, the relation of the fractal system description to the power-law QRS spectrum has not been firmly established and the link is somewhat obscure. The conduction system dimension is obtained from the system scaling, but it is not clear how the conductive tree should be scaled and what parameters must be considered. Besides that, the question of what will be the consequences of a limited branching tree, spatially distributed sources, and surrounding myocardial cells remains open.

In our study, a finite elements computer model with a conduction system having a fractal geometry is constructed, and a high resolution simulation of the depolarization process (QRS complex) of the ventricles is obtained. The high resolution QRS complex is investigated in order to describe the results of the computer simulations according to algorithm based on fractals and to study the inverse power law of the signal generated by the model. Further development of the high resolution model, which includes repolarization process, may be used as a bridge for understanding the role of the high frequency components of QRS complex in clinical cardiology (1).

This model and its simulated results are a starting point for further research that may highlight some aspects of the conduction system role in the electric activity of the cardiac system.

DESCRIPTION OF THE MODEL

The simulation of the electrical activity in the ventricles consists of three components: (a) myocardium, (b) conduction system in the ventricles, and (c) the torso as a volume conductor.

Figure 1 shows a three-dimensional representation of the ventricles model with the fractal conduction system. This structure is realized with a three-dimensional array in which each component represents a finite element of the heart model (2). Each component stores the parameters (such as location, conduction, or myocardial cell [polarized or depolarized]) that characterizes the represented finite element. The system root is at the basal contact point of the two ventricles. The branches ramify and spread on the endocardium surface. Once the geometrical and functional parameters are established, the QRS is obtained by exciting a point at the root of the conduction system and calculating the time evolution of resulting surface potentials. The simulations are carried out on a personal computer with a 80386 processor and a 80387 mathematical coprocessor. Each simulation of a QRS complex takes to run, depending on the model configuration, between 0.5 and 2 hours.

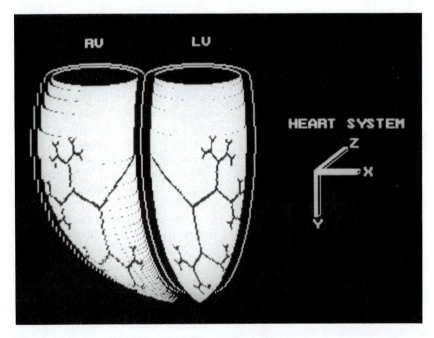

FIGURE 1. Three-dimensional representation of the model. The two ventricles with their conduction system, which is implanted in the innermost layers, can be seen. The spheres are formed by layers of building elements. The conduction system consists of bifurcating branches that gradually shorten.

The Myocardium

The ventricular wall is made mostly of muscle cells (5,14). These cells are represented in the model by abstract cubic building blocks that are joined together to form the cardiac chambers walls. The left ventricle consists of a multilayered surface of a prolate spheroid with only one apex. In the region that represents the basal ventricle wall, the apex of the spheroid is absent. The right ventricle consists of a similar chopped spheroid with a curved long axis. The wall thickness of the right ventricle is smaller than the left one. Thus, the walls of the ventricles consist of a three-dimensional lattice of cubic elements that represent the muscle cells. The geometrical size of each element is scaled by an average conduction velocity of 0.3 m/s and QRS duration of 80–100 msec. The result is a length of 0.3–0.4 mm for a single cell in each direction. This length is 3–4 times the length of the actual biological cells in the heart (12). For a ventricle length of about 5 cm, and a diameter of about 2.5 cm, the model contains about a half a million elements.

The muscle cell element can be in one of two states: resting or excited. Since our simulation considers only the depolarization process, without repolarization, the action potential of a single cell is modeled with a step function that describes the upstroke of the transmembrane potential only. When a cell is excited and one or more of its six adjacent cells are in the resting phase, a dipole moment exists and is directed toward the resting cell. The dipole of the i-th element, $\bar{D}_i$, is the potential gradient between the i and j cells:

$$\bar{D}_i = -\nabla \phi_{ij} \qquad (1)$$

and in our model each dipole is assigned with magnitude of one, namely:

$$|\bar{D}_i| = \begin{cases} 1; & \phi_i \neq \phi_j \\ 0; & \phi_i = \phi_j \end{cases} . \qquad (2)$$

The activation wavefront propagates when resting cells, with a dipole of magnitude 1 is pointing toward them, are excited. Once a cell is excited it is assumed that it is in its refractory period since it can not transmit the depolarization pulse.

In the present model the myocardial geometry is simplified to a pair of prolate spheroids, tangent to each other along a line. The walls consist of a single characteristic thickness and the individual cells are cubic. The functional characteristics are simplified, the conduction velocity is assumed to be isotropic, the same throughout the myocardium, and since only the depolarization process is considered, the transmembrane action potential is a step

function in time and space. The large number of cells assures a fine temporal resolution that is needed for the spectral analysis (up to 500 Hz).

The Conduction System

Goldberger *et al.* (8) theoretically have shown how a fractal conduction system can contribute to an inverse power law in the spectrum of the signal generated. When an electrical pulse propagates along the branches, the voltage, $V(t)$ measured at the myocardium will consist of superposition of pulses with slightly different arrival times t_j:

$$V(t) = \sum_{j=1}^{N} v(t - t_j) . \qquad (3)$$

Using the autocorrelation function of the pulses generated by a conduction system, it is shown that as the fractal structure bifurcates to infinitely fine branches, then the power spectrum can be represented as

$$S(\omega) = \frac{B_\mu}{\omega^\mu} \qquad (4)$$

where B_μ is a constant dependent on parameters characterizing the fractal system. The power spectrum of the electric signal propagating through the system should therefore be of the general form B/ω^μ and, in fact, μ is related to the averaged fractal dimension of this system. Goldberger *et al.* (8) tested the fractal hypothesis by analyzing electrocardiograms from 21 healthy men. Applying linear regression analysis to the power spectrum data in the frequency range of 7.81–249.92 Hz, a straight line $Y = 5.41 - 4.3X$ was obtained ($r = 0.99$).

The conduction system in the model refers to the fibers' network downstream the ventricular bundle branches. The Purkinje fibers system consists of specialized fibers that have an extensive ramification and gradually diminish in length until becoming continuous with myocardial muscle cells (5,11,14). In the present model, a simplification of that system is realized by certain elements, creating branches in the innermost ventricular layers, that are labeled as the conduction system fibers. The conduction system is characterized by a conduction velocity higher than the one in the muscle cells. This distinction is realized by the activation of several elements along the fibers each time step rather than only adjacent elements in the muscle propagation. The structure of the conduction system in the model is of a self-similar bifurcating tree. It is generated by repeatedly bifurcating a branch, which was previously created, into new branches. With every ramification, referred as a new generation, the branches become shorter by a certain factor r. The length of the branches at consecutive generations satisfy the following ratio:

$$L_{g-1}/L_{g-2} = L_g/L_{g-1} = \tau \quad (g = 0,1,2\ldots G) \quad (5)$$

where L_g is the length of the branches at a specific generation g and G is the final generation number. This means that the conduction system is composed of bifurcating fiber basic units. Each unit is attached to a unit of the same shape but on a different scale. The origin branch of the tree (the "trunk") contains 90 elements creating elongated fiber, and the length constant τ, was chosen to be 0.7. The number of generations is limited because the length of the branches at a progressively higher ramification stage becomes shorter, and the length of the final branches becomes the size of a fundamental building element. The angle between the splitting branches is the same throughout the system. Thus the geometry of the conduction system is controlled by only two parameters: the length factor and the angle that were both chosen.

The transitional fibers of the Purkinje system gradually diminish in size, have smaller diameter, and have lower conduction velocity (5). Since conduction velocity in the real conduction fibers shows an approximate proportionality to diameter (12), the conduction velocity along the branches of the model was decreased by a certain factor with every ramification, satisfying a relation similar to length ratio (Eq. 5). The conduction velocity at the beginning of the conduction system is 2.7 m/s and decreases to no less than 0.6 m/s at the terminals (twice the conduction velocity of the muscle cells). The implementation of the conduction system in the ventricles requires modeling the interaction between the conduction and muscle cells. It is assumed here that resting muscle cells along the conductive fibers can be excited by the conduction system elements.

The systems of the two ventricles are not interrelated. They are excited at the same time but their geometry parameters differ and their function is independent. The real right bundle branch ramifies at its end while the left one subdivides into the posterior and anterior bundles before giving rise to extensive ramification (5,14). Accounting for this bifurcation in the real left bundle branch, the modeled left system is given an additional generation throughout the simulations. This model simplifies the conduction system assuming that in each generation the conduction tree bifurcates into two branches only and that the new branches direct symmetrically to opposite directions. The value of the factors that determine the self-similar properties of the system (length, angle, and slowing of the propagation velocity) are specified deterministically without any statistical distribution function. The physiological rigidity in this model ease to isolate the basic features of the conduction system that affect the simulation results.

The Torso as a Volume Conductor

The evolution of the myocardial excitation wavefront is the source for the surface QRS complex. When the dynamics of the QRS complex are considered, the behavior of each source potential frequency component must be regarded separately. Fortunately, all field quantities arising from a given time-varying bioelectric source within the human torso, may be assumed to be in synchrony (12). This reflects the fact that the media surrounding the sources can be considered to be nondispersive in the relevant frequencies (under 1 kHz). The frequency-independent nature of the fields and the linearity of the media with respect to current and voltage, permit a formulation of the forward problem as:

$$\nabla^2 \Phi = -\frac{I_v}{\sigma} \quad (6)$$

where Φ is the potential, I_v is the source current density, and σ is the conductivity. Equation 6, subject to the boundary condition of $E_n = 0$ at the body surface, represents the basic quasi-static formulation of the electrical problem in the torso. The solution of Eq. 6 in a homogeneous media gives the potential at distance R from the source

$$\Phi = \frac{1}{4\pi\sigma} \int_V \frac{I_v}{R} \, dV \, . \quad (7)$$

As a result we obtain a multipole representation in which the dipole term alone was considered for simplicity (12).

The Limb Lead Potentials. In the case of the surface ECG obtained from the extremities, the equivalent heart vector concept and the semiempirical lead vector method are used. The use of a dipole representation of the heart in this lead configuration is supported by the study of Cuffin *et al.* (4). Using this method the electrical activity of the heart is represented by an equivalent vector $\bar{D}_{eq}$ which is the integral of all the dipole moments in the heart:

$$\bar{D}_{eq} = \sum_{elements} \bar{D}_i \, . \quad (8)$$

After the dipoles per unit volume are integrated, the result is multiplied by a lead vector $\bar{C}_l$ to yield the potential of that lead:

$$\Phi_l = \bar{D}_{eq} \cdot \bar{C}_l \, . \quad (9)$$

The lead vector method takes into consideration the location of the ventricles in the torso and the orientation of the heart within the torso must be specified. In the model, the long axis of the left ventricle is pointing downward at 70° to the left from the sagittal plane and forward at 45° to the frontal plane.

The Precordial Leads Potentials. When the ECG signal is measured at the vicinity of the heart, the equivalent vector representation does not hold because the relative distances between elements are about the same as the distance between the electrode and the heart origin. Hence, the location and orientation of each element must be considered separately. If we assume the surrounding medium to be homogeneous and infinite then the potential of the *i*-th element Φ at location *P* is

$$\Phi_i(P) = \frac{\bar{D}_i \cdot \bar{R}_i}{|R_i|^3} \qquad (10)$$

where $\bar{D}_i$ is the dipole moment of that element and $\bar{R}_i$ is the distance vector between the element *i* and the detector at *P*. This expression is calculated for all the excited elements at a given time instance and the results are summed up to give the signal at that time. In this approach a weighed contribution factor is given to each element according to its distance from the measuring point. Inhomogeneities in the torso and its finite extension are not taken into consideration. The potential calculated in this

way is actually the difference between the potential at location *P* and the potential at infinity.

The two methods involve different kinds of approximations. On the one hand, the lead vector method accounts for effects of the body inhomogeneity and boundary conditions of the potentials at its surface, that are difficult to account in an analytical approach. On the other hand, it involves the use of the equivalent vector concept which assumes a dipole distribution of the sources in the ventricles. The second method accounts for the spatial distribution of the sources within the ventricles but does not consider the effects of the inhomogeneous surrounding media and the finite size of the body.

SIMULATION RESULTS

Standard 12-Lead Electrocardiogram

Figure 2 presents the six standard limb leads and the six precordial leads resulting from the model by simulating the normal activation process of the ventricles. The normal activation refers to an artificial excitation of the two conductive systems root points and an automatic evolution of the excitation wavefront throughout the myocardium. Visually inspected, the curves obtained are similar to realistic QRS complexes. The duration of the QRS

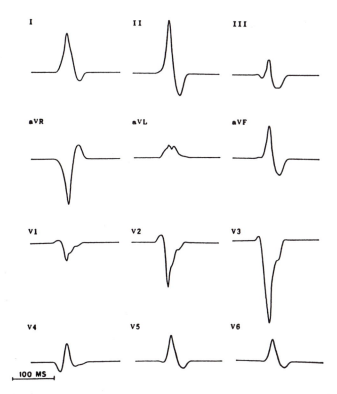

FIGURE 2. The QRS complexes from the 12 standard leads obtained by the model simulation. The model generator consists of a conduction system with 7 generations in the right ventricle and 8 generations in the left ventricle (configuration 7 in Table 1).

complexes obtained is about 80 msec. Leads I, II, and III have positive deflection, and the precordial leads signals reverse from deep negative **R** wave (at V_1, V_2, and V_3) to positive **R** wave (at V_4, V_5, and V_6). The signals obtained by the simulation have high temporal resolution of $\Delta T = 1$ msec. This resolution meets the requirements of spectral analysis with frequency components up to 500 Hz.

The Fractal Hypothesis

The number of generations in the conduction system plays an important role in the generation of the heart beat. The fractal hypothesis was tested by studying the effects of this aspect on the form and frequency content of the QRS complex generated using power spectrum analysis. The frequency content of the signal was derived using fast Fourier transform algorithms. The results obtained are summarized in Table 1. The power law scaling was tested by performing a linear regression on the plot of the Log(amplitude²) versus the Log(frequency). This analysis was applied on the frequency range between 8 Hz and 250 Hz similar to the frequency range used by Goldberger (8). This procedure was performed on signals obtained from the V_6 location by using the model with different numbers of generations in the conduction system, while other parameters are being held fixed. Figure 3 shows the QRS complex obtained in a model with 1 and 2 generations in the right (RV) and left ventricle (LV), respectively (configuration 1, Table 1). The QRS duration is 144 msec

and low level activity can be seen at the end of the simulated signal originating from late activation of muscle cells. Figure 4 shows the QRS complex and the corresponding power spectrum obtained in a model with 5 and 6 generations in the right and left ventricle, respectively (configuration 5, Table 1) and Fig. 5 in a model with 8 and 9 generations in the right and left ventricle, respectively (configuration 8, Table 1). It can be seen that as the number of generations increases, the QRS duration decreases with enhancement in the high-frequency components. Visual inspection of the power spectrum in the high frequency range clearly shows a decrease in its variance as generations are added to the tree. The linear regression analysis shows that the highest correlation coefficient ($r = 0.954$) was obtained for a model with configuration 8 with the equation $Y = 6.41 - 4.24X$. Similar analysis of a real averaged V_6 QRS complexes from 5 healthy subjects was performed (Table 1). Figure 6 shows a real QRS complex (real data 1 in Table 1) and the power spectrum obtained. The fitted linear equation for the power data was found to be $Y = 6.26 - 4.50X$ ($r = 0.927$). The intersection constant from the fitted linear equation depends on the magnification factor of the simulated QRS complex. The values in Table 1 were obtained with simulated signals scaled to an amplitude of approximately 2 mv similar to the real QRS complex analyzed. The slope constant is independent on the magnification factor and is related to the frequency content of the QRS generated.

The criteria for the most realistic conduction tree structure were obtained by calculating the normalized cross correlation coefficient between a real QRS complex (real data 1 in Table 1) and simulated signals under different conduction system configurations. Figure 7 shows the normalized cross correlation coefficient between real ECG lead of V_6 location and simulated QRS signals obtained with different configuration of the conduction system. The cross correlation analysis was performed for the low frequency region (below 100 Hz) and for the high frequency signal (100–250 Hz) separately. It can be seen that

TABLE 1. Results from simulated and real QRS complexes.

Configuration No.	Generation RV,LV	QRSD (msec)	Intersection	Slope	Correlation r Value
			Constants From Fitted Curve		
1	1,2	144	4.77	−4.29	0.938
2	2,3	129	4.78	−4.15	0.949
3	3,4	103	4.79	−4.25	0.933
4	4,5	95	5.03	−4.26	0.922
5	5,6	86	6.68	−4.93	0.938
6	6,7	83	5.56	−4.27	0.906
7	7,8	80	5.47	−4.01	0.906
8	8,9	79	6.41	−4.24	0.954
9	9,10	78	4.49	−3.19	0.911
Real Data 1	—	80	6.26	−4.50	0.927
Real Data 2	—	80	4.72	−4.12	0.938
Real Data 3	—	84	5.24	−4.67	0.958
Real Data 4	—	83	4.75	−4.72	0.942
Real Data 5	—	85	4.31	−4.24	0.924
Goldberger (8)	—	—	5.41	−4.30	0.990

RV = right ventricle.
LV = left ventricle.
QRSD = QRS duration.

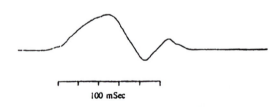

100 mSec

FIGURE 3. The QRS complex obtained in a model with 1 and 2 generations in the right and left ventricle, respectively (configuration 1, Table 1). The QRS duration is 144 msec and low level activity that originates from late activation of muscle cells can be seen at the end of the simulated signal.

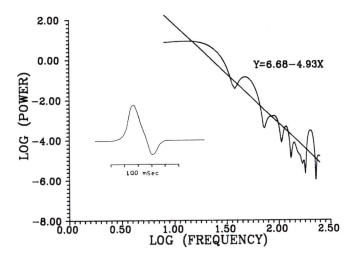

FIGURE 4. The simulated QRS complex and the corresponding spectral curve on a log-log scale obtained in a model with 5 generations in the right ventricle and 6 generations in the left ventricle (configuration 5 in Table 1). Using linear regression analysis a straight line $Y = 6.68 - 4.93X$ ($r = 0.938$) is fitted to the spectral data.

for the low frequency region (the + symbols) a maximum value (0.950) is obtained at configuration 5 which consists of 5 generations in the RV and 6 in the LV. Similar analysis with respect to the high frequency region (the $\triangle$ symbols) signals reveals that the highest correlation (0.683) is obtained for configuration 8 which consists of 8 (RV) and 9 (LV) generations.

Figure 8 shows the energy in the high frequency region

(100–250 Hz) as a function of model configuration. As can be seen, high frequency components in the QRS complex are associated with high number of generations.

DISCUSSION

The objective of the described model is to give a preliminary insight into the conduction system structure and

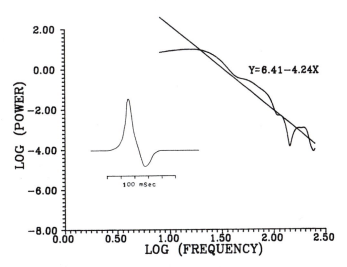

FIGURE 5. The simulated QRS complex and the corresponding spectral curve on a log-log scale obtained in a model with 8 generations in the right ventricle and 9 generations in the left ventricle (configuration 8 in table 1). Using linear regression analysis a straight line $Y = 6.41 - 4.24X$ ($r = 0.954$) is fitted to the spectral data.

O. Berenfeld, D. Sadeh, and S. Abboud

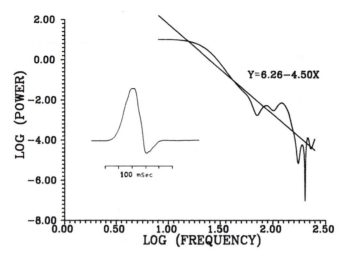

FIGURE 6. A real averaged QRS complex and the corresponding spectral curve on a log-log scale. Using linear regression analysis, a straight line $Y = 6.26 - 4.50X$ ($r = 0.927$) is fitted to the spectral data.

its relation to the QRS signal. As a narrow object-oriented model, some structural and functional simplifications were assumed while considering other relevant important factors. The model geometrical structure of the myocardium is only schematically sketched, but its large number of fundamental building elements gives a high temporal resolution. The satisfactory results of the simulated leads, which are obtained with the equivalent heart vector approximation, suggest that the model structure is acceptable as an investigative starting point.

In order to evaluate the environment effect on the results, we have performed a regression analysis on the power spectrums of the limb and precordial leads for a model whose configuration is kept the same. The six limb

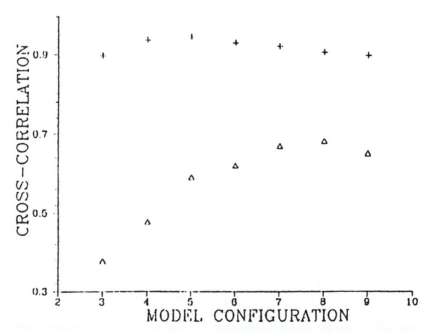

FIGURE 7. The cross correlation coefficient between a V_6 simulated signal and a real QRS (real data 1 in Table 1) as a function of the model configuration. The + symbols correspond to the low frequency region (below 100 Hz) and the $\triangle$ symbols correspond to the high frequency region (100–250 Hz).

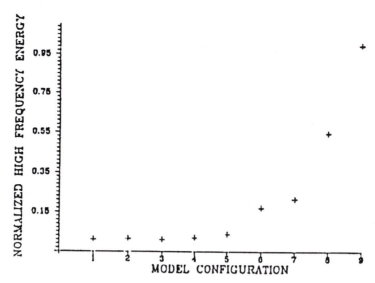

FIGURE 8. The energy in the high frequency region (100–250 Hz) as a function of model configuration. The energy is normalized to the maximum value obtained. As can be seen, high frequency components in the QRS complex are associated with high number of generations.

leads, which account for the torso medium inhomogeneity, gave an average slope of −4.42 with an average correlation coefficient of 0.958. For the six precordial leads, when inhomogeneity is ignored, we found an average slope of −4.69 with an average correlation coefficient of 0.962. Comparing the results obtained from the limb leads and the precordial leads, it seems that the volume conductor does not influence the time course of the ECG signal and the results obtained from the power spectrum are similar. Other investigators demonstrated that the geometry and nature of the volume conductor have effects on the amplitude of the potentials measured at the body surface. Rudy and Plonsey (13) have shown that the inhomogeneity aspect of the torso has large effect on the surface potentials calculation. Geselowitz (7) pointed out that the amplitude of the surface ECG is changed when the lung region is included in a spherical model. In the present study the evolution of the excitation wavefront is of concern, and priority is given to the wavefront spatial configuration over the electrical effects of the environment.

Algorithms based on fractals offer an improved approach for developing more accurate morphological descriptions of complex biological structures using mathematical models (6,8,9). The Purkinje conduction system is an example of an organ having a complex geometrical and functional structure. This system consists of a large number of fibers arranged in an inhomogeneous network. Models related to different aspects of the heart's activity are described in the literature (3,10,15) and usually either oversimplify or examine a subsample of the entire struc-

ture and determine the conduction system in such a way that the evaluated propagation sequence or activation signal is within the normal range. If essential functional roles of the system are of concern, then a governing principle rather than a detailed structure model, may be preferred. The conduction system exhibits statistical structural similarities on several different scales and this may be used to describe its organization. The purpose of the present study is to develop a model of the ventricular conduction system based upon the self-similar principle. It has been shown that the activation process of the ventricles can be controlled by including a self-similar conduction system, and simulated QRS complexes which are similar to realistic signals can be obtained. The activation wavefront propagates through the conduction system at the initial period of the QRS complex. This period does not extend 35 msec in any of the cases simulated. However, the QRS is affected by the variations in the conduction system structure even at times when the activation process travels only in the myocardium and not through conductive fibers. Thus, the configuration of the conduction tree controls the whole QRS by determining the initial conditions of the activation process. The frequency content of the QRS complex and the self-similar conduction system may be related to the fragmentation of the activation wavefront in the myocardium. As the length of the branches shortens, with increasing generation number, the wavefront fragmentation increases, contributing high frequency components to the simulated QRS complex generated. This may explain the enhancement in the high frequency components seen in the power spectrum as generations

O. BERENFELD, D. SADEH, and S. ABBOUD

are added to the system. Furthermore, the introduction of additional frequency components into the simulated signal results in a smoothing effect on the high frequency region of the power spectrum, as can be seen by comparing Figs. 4 and 5.

In our study we tried to confirm the proposed fractal depolarization hypothesis predicting that the resulting frequency spectrum of the QRS complex should take on the form of an inverse power law. In fact, one should get a nearly straight line for a healthy heart for a log-power versus log-frequency plot. The slope of this line, for data taken from 21 healthy men by Goldberger (8), was found to be -4.3 with very high correlation (0.99). Our study has shown that if a model with the fractal conduction system is used, the inverse power law can be obtained with a slope of approximately -4.3 but with lower correlation ($r = 0.954$). A similar average slope (-4.47) with an average correlation of 0.938 was obtained when an analysis of five real QRS complexes from healthy subjects was performed. Comparison between the QRS complexes obtained from the simulated signals and real data showed that the model configuration with 5 and 6 generations gave the highest correlation coefficient in the low frequency region, while the model configuration with 8 and 9 generations was in the high frequency region. It seems that the model configuration that will fit real data in both the low and high frequency regions, is the one with configuration number 7 representing 7 and 8 generations in the right and left ventricles, respectively. The simulated 12 leads presented in Fig. 2 were obtained with this configuration.

The power spectrum of the simulated QRS signal obtained by the integrated pulses generated by the branches of the conduction system, while taking into consideration the location and the direction of each dipole, shows an inverse power law. It must be stated that similar results of an inverse power law may be obtained from models with different conduction systems without having the self-similar property. The fact that the conduction fibers control the initial conditions of activation process while contributing minor energy to the QRS complex suggests that the inverse power-law should relate not only to the bifurcating branches but to the surrounding excitable media as well. It means that the relevant dimensionality depends upon the combined conduction and myocardial structure rather than the tree structure alone.

The results of these simulations may assist our understanding of cardiac conduction processes and may suggest new diagnostic measurements to detect conduction system dysfunction. It is believed (6) that the slope of the inverse power law may be a useful index of spectral reserve, and therefore healthiness, in a number of physiologic parameters. Further study is being performed in our laboratory to investigate the relations between conduction system dysfunction and the slope of the inverse power law.

REFERENCES

1. Abboud, S.; Cohen, R.J.; Selwyn, A.; Sadeh, D.; Friedman, P.L. Detection of transient myocardial ischemia by computer analysis of standard and signal averaged high frequency electrocardiogram in patients undergoing percutaneous transluminal coronary angioplasty. Circulation 76(3):585–596; 1987.
2. Abboud, S.; Berenfeld, O.; Sadeh, D. Simulation of high-resolution QRS complex using a ventricular model with a fractal conduction system—Effects of ischemia on high-frequency QRS potentials. Circ. Res. 68(6):1751–1760; 1991.
3. Aoki, M.; Okamoto, Y.; Musha, T.; Harumi, K.I. Three-dimensional simulation of the ventricular depolarization and repolarization process and body surface potentials; normal heart and bundle branch block. IEEE Trans. Biomed. Eng. BME34(6):454–462; 1987.
4. Cuffin, B.N.; Geselowitz, D.B. Studies of the electrocardiogram using realistic cardiac and torso models. IEEE Trans. Biomed. Eng. BME 24(3):242–252; 1977.
5. Detweiler, D.K. Circulation. In: Brobeck, J.R., ed. Best and Taylor's physiological basis of medical practice. 10th ed. Baltimore: The Williams and Williams Company; 1979: pp. 47–88.
6. Eberhart, R.C. Chaos theory for the biomedical engineer. IEEE Eng. Med. Biol. Mag. 8(3):41–45; 1989.
7. Geselowitz, D.B. On the theory of the electrocardiogram. Proc. of the IEEE 77(6):857–876; 1989.
8. Goldberger, A.L.; Bhargava, V.; West, B.J.; Mandell, A.J. On the mechanism of cardiac electrical stability; the fractal hypothesis. Biophys. J. 48:525–528; 1985.
9. Goldberger, A.L.; West, B.J. Fractals in physiology and medicine. The Yale Journal of Biology and Medicine 60:421–435; 1987.
10. Malik, M.; Cochrane, T.; Camm, A.J. Computer simulation of the cardiac conduction system. Comput. Biomed. Res. 16:454–468; 1983.
11. Massing, G.K.; James, T.N. Anatomical configuration of the his bundle and bundle branches in the human heart. Circulation 53(4):609–621; 1976.
12. Plonsey, R. Bioelectric phenomena. New York: McGraw Hill; 1969: pp. 1–22, 202–233, 324–332.
13. Rudy, Y.; Plonsey, R. A comparison of volume conductor and source geometry effects on body surface and epicardial potentials. Circ. Res. 46(2):283–291; 1980.
14. Scher, A.M. Electrocardiogram. In: Ruch, T.C.; Patton. H.D., eds. Physiology and biophysics II. Philadelphia: W.B. Sounders; 1974: pp. 65–101.
15. Thakor, N.V.; Eisenman, L.N. Three-dimensional computer model of the heart: Fibrillation induced by extrastimulation. Comput. Biomed. Res. 22:532–545; 1989.

Wiss. Zeitschrift der Humboldt-Universitat zu Berlin, R. Medizin 41 (1992) 4

Heart Rate, Respiration, and Baroreflex: Entrainment, Bifurcations, and Chaos

Hanspeter Herzel, Henrik Seidel, and Heinz Warzel

1. BASIC CONCEPT OF NONLINEAR DYNAMICS

In order to understand complicated patterns of physiological rhythms, such as shown in Part II [1], the concept of nonlinear dynamics (or "chaos-theory") is appropriate. In this section, we give a brief summary of the main ideas prerequisite to an understanding of the results in the next sections. More details can be found elsewhere [2–6].

Conventional time series analysis is carried out either in the time domain or the frequency domain. Nonlinear dynamics is based on an embedding of the time series in a "phase space" spanned by a set of appropriate coordinates describing the system. If only a scalar time series is available, "delay-coordinates" are often useful, i.e. subsequent measurements are taken as coordinates [4].

In this way, time-series can be considered as orbits in a phase space. If the external parameters are held constant, the orbit in phase space approaches an asymptotic regime after some initial transient.

The geometrical object in phase space corresponding to the asymptotic behaviour is termed as "attractor". Attractors can be classified as follows:

a) stable stationary states (all variables are constant)
b) limit cycles (periodic oscillations)
c) tori (superposition of two or more independent oscillations)
d) chaotic attractor (nonperiodic behaviour)

The discovery of "deterministic chaos" in nonlinear systems provides a new approach for understanding irregular observations [2–6].

Up to now we have assumed fixed external conditions. If parameters are varied, qualitative changes of the attractor might appear. Such transitions are termed "bifurcations".

For example, the transition from damped oscillations (a steady state) to self-sustained oscillations (a limit cycle) is a manifestation of a "Hopf bifurcation". The various transitions from periodic behaviour to more complicated regimes are a central issue of nonlinear dynamics theory. The most important of such bifurcations are "period-doubling" and "secondary" Hopf bifurcations. In the first case, a new limit cycle with roughly double the original period becomes stable (see Fig. 2 in Part II), i.e. in the time domain we may observe alternating large and small amplitudes. In the spectral domain one would observe the appearance of subharmonics. A secondary Hopf bifurcation is the onset of a modulation of the signal with another independent frequency, i.e. a "torus" appears in phase space.

Another frequently observed bifurcation is the sudden jump from the original limit cycle to another limit cycle with a different period and amplitude.

Attractors may coexist in nonlinear systems and, therefore, even extremely small changes of parameters may lead to abrupt jumps to other regimes (see e.g. the Figures in section 3).

The theory of nonlinear dynamics predicts that period-doubling and other bifurcations are often accompanied by deterministic chaos at adjacent parameter values.

2. BIFURCATIONS OF COUPLED OSCILLATORS

Many observations in physiology are due to the interaction of coupled oscillators. It will be argued in this section that the whole variety of dynamic behaviours discussed in section 1 can appear in the relatively simple system of two coupled nonlinear oscillators.

It is assumed in the following that the two oscillators can be characterized by their autonomous frequencies ω_1 and ω_2. We discuss now subsequently the generic behaviour for different coupling strengths:

(a) no coupling: For almost all ω_1 and ω_2 the oscillations are independent, i.e. the attractor is a torus.

(b) weak coupling: If the frequency ratio ω_1/ω_2 is close to a rational number p/q with a small denominator q (e.g. 1/1; 1/2; 2/3) the oscillators are "entrained", i.e. there is a synchronization of the oscillators due to coupling. The resulting attractor is a more or less complicated limit cycle. For the majority of ratios ω_1/ω_2 the tori persist.

(c) sufficiently strong coupling: the widths of the entrainment zones (termed "Arnold tongues") increase with the coupling. Hence, overlapping of entrainment zones appear which correspond to coexisting limit cycles. Moreover, period-doubling bifurcations and deterministic chaos occur.

The phenomena sketched above are characteristic for any system of coupled nonlinear oscillators even though the details depend on the system. Consequently, it is no surprise that entrainment zones, bifurcations and chaos are reported in a variety of systems. In the following, a few examples are listed:

(a) periodically stimulated aggregates of embryonic chick-heart cells [3]: Here the spontaneous beating of the cell and the stimulation with an intracellular microelectrode constitute the two oscillators discussed above. Arnold tongues (1/2, 3/5, 2/3, 3/4, 1/1, 3/2, 2/1, 3/1) and irregular rhythms have been observed. An empirical model based on the experimentally measured "phase response curve" was in close agreement to the observations.

(b) respiratory-locomotory coupling: 3/1, 2/1 and 3/2 entrainment of respiration and gait in a healthy human has been found [3].

(c) ventilator-respiration coupling: Experiments and model calculations show 1/2, 1/1, 3/2, 2/1 and 3/1 entrainment zones and irregular dynamics in between [3].

(d) interaction of sinus and ectopic pacemakers: Models of parasystole exhibit entrainment (3/2, 2/1, 5/2, 3/1 and 4/1) [3].

(e) vocal disorders: Normal phonation corresponds to 1/1 entrainment of all vibratory modes of vocal folds. Many observations of newborn cries [4] and rough sounding voices [6] can be interpreted in terms of irregular vibratory patterns of vocal folds. For example, localized vocal fold lesions or unilateral paralysis may lead to a de-synchronization of the left and the right vocal fold.

In the remainder of the paper we apply the concept of nonlinear dynamics to experimental findings introduced in Part II.

3. BIFURCATIONS IN HEART BEAT RECORDS

It was pointed out in Part II that the interaction of heart beat, respiration and carotid sinus nerve stimulation may induce complicated trains of heart beat intervals. In this section we present some characteristic sequences of heart beat intervals displaying bifurcations.

Under normal conditions respiratory and cardiac rhythms are usually not entrained [3]. Despite multiple feedback loops, only a slight modulation of the cardiac rhythm is observed which is termed respiratory sinus arrhythmia (RSA). In the terminology of chaos-theory the RSA is related to a torus. Fig. 1 displays a representative record without any stimulation. The RSA is superimposed by another well-known rhythm with a period of about 10 seconds [5].

Under normal physiological conditions the frequency ratio of respiratory and cardiac rhythms is about 1/4 to 1/5 (see Fig. 1). By applying stimuli a wide range of frequency ratios results. In several cases stimulation increased the respiration frequency drastically and we observed ratios of 1/2, 1/1 and even 2/1. In the latter case we have two breathing cycles per heart cycle. Just as expected from theory, in the vicinity of the 1/1 entrainment zone bifurcations and irregular rhythms (presumably "chaos") are observed.

A first example of period-doubling and subsequent irregularities was presented in Part II. Another record with several bifurcations is shown in Fig. 2. During the first 85 seconds in Fig. 2 the first R-wave during expiration triggers the stimulation. Initially, there is a 1/3 entrainment between respiration and heart. Moreover, we have 1/3 entrainment of stimulus and heart as well. At 12 and 25 seconds intermittent transitions to 1/2 entrainment occur. At around 45 seconds the system turns into 1/2 entrainment interrupted by 1/3 episodes.

After 85 seconds the stimuli are given after the fist R-peak during inhalation. This change of the external conditions leads to a nonperiodic sequence of heart beat intervals.

Wiss. Zeitschrift der Humboldt-Universitat zu Berlin, R. Medizin 41 (1992) 4

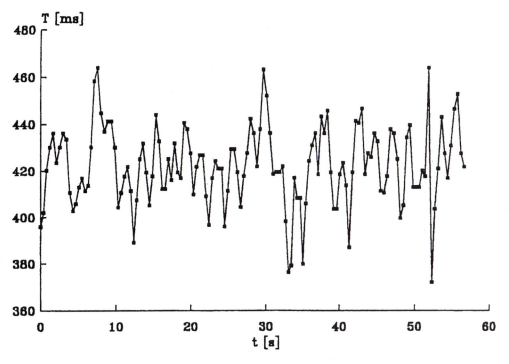

Fig. 1. Sequence of heart beat intervals displaying RSA and the 0.1 Hz rhythm. No stimulation was applied

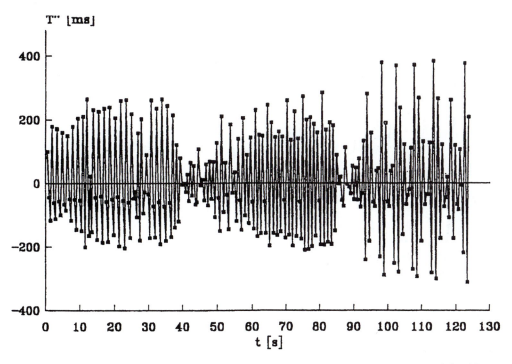

Fig. 2. Stimulation of the first R-peak during expiration (0–85 seconds) or inspiration (after 85 seconds). Different cycles of length three or two and bifurcations are visible (see text)

Wiss. Zeitschrift der Humboldt-Universitat zu Berlin, R. Medizin 41 (1992) 4

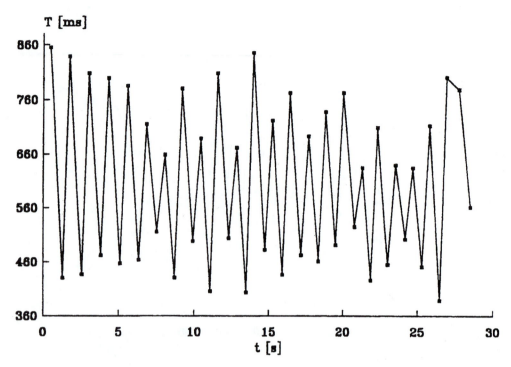

Fig. 3. Bifurcations from period two to period four to nonperiodicity (stimulation of each R-peak)

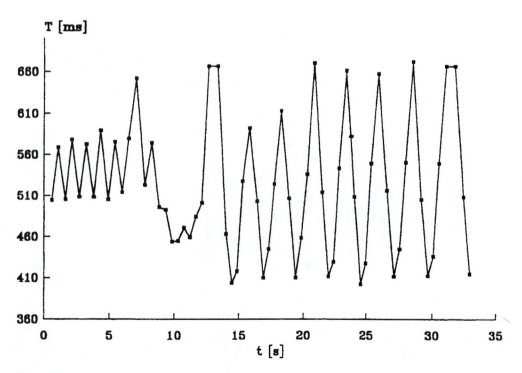

Fig. 4. Spontaneous transition from period two to period five corresponding to 1/2 and 3/5 entrainment with the respiratory rhythm (stimulation of the first R-peak during expiration)

Wiss. Zeitschrift der Humboldt-Universitat zu Berlin, R. Medizin 41 (1992) 4   55

Fig. 2 demonstrates an essential conceptional point. On one hand, bifurcations can be induced by external parameter variations (at 85 seconds) and, on the other hand, slowly drifting internal conditions may lead to sudden transitions as well. Figs. 3 and 4 display other examples of such "spontaneous bifurcations".

In Fig. 3 each R-peak triggers a stimulus without any delay. There was constantly one breath per heart cycle, i.e. the transitions depicted in Fig. 3 reflect bifurcations within the 1/1 entrainment zone. We see, therefore, a transition from a 2/2 limit cycle to 4/4 entrainment followed by nonperiodic oscillations.

Fig. 4 shows a spontaneous transition from 1/2 entrainment to 3/4 entrainment. In other words, an internal drift of certain physiological parameters induces a jump from two heart cycles per breath to five beats during three breathing cycles.

The examples above demonstrate clearly that the system respiration-heart-stimulus is capable of generating a variety of dynamic regimes. It turns out that a classification of the phenomena in terms of entrainment zones and bifurcations gives some insight into the dynamics.

The physiological reasons for the complicated dynamics are the acceleration of breathing and the relatively strong coupling between the subsystem's respiration, stimuli and heart.

4. ATTRACTOR ANALYSIS

In the preceding section bifurcations have been detected by careful inspection of the time-series. If there are relatively stationary segments of the signal a more detailed analysis of the underlying attractor is possible. Fig. 5a displays a nonperiodic sequence of heart beat intervals. For visualizing the dynamics in phase space, subsequent intervals have been plotted in Fig. 5b. Such a "next period map" is topologically equivalent to a "Poincaré section"

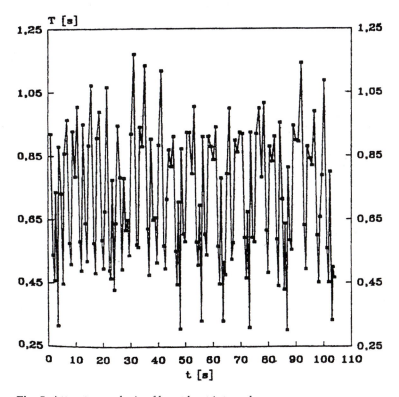

Fig. 5. Attractor analysis of heart beat intervals

(a) nonperiodic sequence

Wiss. Zeitschrift der Humboldt-Universitat zu Berlin, R. Medizin 41 (1992) 4

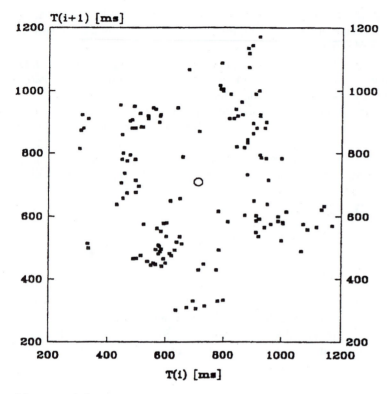

(b) next period map

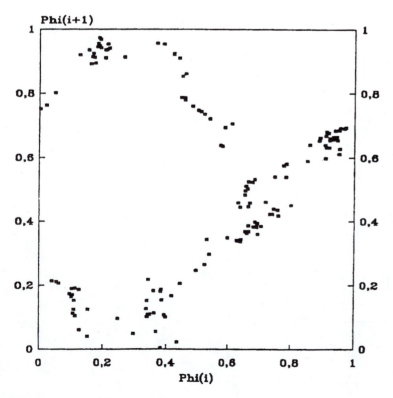

(c) return map of the rotational angle in (b)

Wiss. Zeitschrift der Humboldt-Universitat zu Berlin, R. Medizin 41 (1992) 4

of the original attractor in the ECG time series. If, for example, the original data represent a torus a section of the attractor leads to a closed curve and the dynamics is a rotational motion along the curve. The structure in Fig. 5b is more complicated, but monitoring subsequent points reveals a rotational motion around the center (denoted by 0). This observation suggests another representation of the dynamics. After introducing an angle Phi of rotation we obtain the return map in Fig. 5c. In this Figure some deterministic structure is evident. Consequently, Fig. 5c indicates that the dynamics underlying the irregular sequence in Fig. 5a is essentially deterministic. For a random sequence an unstructured cloud of points could be expected.

Beside visualizing attractors, methods have been derived to describe the attractors quantitatively with fractal dimensions and Lyapunov exponents [2, 4, 6]. However, these relatively sophisticated techniques require sufficiently stationary signals.

The observation of entrainment and low-dimensional attractors can be exploited to derive appropriate models of coupled oscillators for modelling physiological rhythms. A mathematical model based on "phase response curves' of the cardiac oscillator will be discussed in a forthcoming paper.

Address of the authors:

Dr. sc. **Hanspeter Herzel** and coll., Institute of Theoretical Physics, Humboldt University Berlin, Invalidenstraße 42, 0-1040 Berlin

REFERENCES

[1] Warzel, H.; Seidel, H.; Herzel, H.: Heart Rate, Respiration, and Baroreflex: Motivation and Experiments. — In this volume. —

[2] Holden, A. V. (Ed.): Chaos. — Manchester University Press, 1986. —

[3] Glass, L.; Mackey, M. C.: From Clocks to Chaos. — Princeton University Press, 1988. —

[4] Ebeling, W.; Engel, H.; Herzel, H.: Selbstorganisation in der Zeit. — Berlin: Akademie-Verlag, 1990. —

[5] Haken, H.; Koepchen, H. P. (Eds.): Rhythms in Physiological Systems. — Berlin: Springer, 1991. —

[6] Titze, I. (Ed.): Vocal Fold Physiology. — San Diego: Singular Publ. Group, 1992. —

Heart Rate, Respiration, and Baroreflex: Motivation and Experiments

Heinz Warzel, Henrik Seidel, and Hanspeter Herzel

The baroreceptor-heart-reflex function may be disturbed by influences like alcohol [1] and by stimulation of muscle and cutaneous afferents [2]. Heavy ethanol use causes cardiac arrhythmias [3,4] and an increased incidence of sudden cardiac death [5].

Peripheral nerve stimulation induces heart rate alterations [6], and may influence the development of arrhythmia [7] and disturbs the rhythm of the respiratory center [8]. The stimulation of the carotid sinus nerve is particularly effective if applied during expiration in prolonging the heart period [9] and increasing the amplitude of the respiratory sinus arrhythmia (RSA) [10].

The dependence of heart period on the carotid sinus nerve stimulation (CSNS) was studied at different positions of the cardiac [11] and the respiratory cycles [12].

In the present study the common effect of ethanol, sciatic nerve stimulation (SNS) and the joint function of timing of CSNS in both the cardiac and respiratory cycles is demonstrated.

The experiments were conducted on anaesthetized dogs breathing spontaneously. A respiration valve was modified to give a respiratory phase-related trigger signal. The femoral artery and vein were cannulated for measurement of arterial pressure, blood sampling and injection of ethanol (1.5g/kg) and drugs, respectively. One sciatic nerve was dissected and cut distally, and the central cut end was electrical stimulated supramaximaly (10 V, 100 Imp/s) using electrical currents. The sciatic nerve contains afferents from the skin, muscle, and joints, serving many different modalities within these structures, such as nociception, temperature, and mechanoreceptors. The impulses generated in sciatic and baroreceptor afferent fibers converge on the central components at a common cardiac vagal reflex pathway. The intact right carotid sinus nerve was stimulated with short trains of impulses (0.1–3 mA) given at various times in the cardiac cycle in either inspiration or expiration. In some cases every R-wave triggered a train of impulses. Blood pressure, instantaneous heart rate, stimulus, ECG, and breathing picked up by a thermistor were recorded simultaneously (Fig. 1). This Figure indicates that SNS increases the respiratory frequency almost to the level of the heart rate. Very complex variations were induced by the CSNS in such situations.

A variation of the delay between R-wave and CSNS results in a pattern of the heart period as shown in Fig. 2. The original time series consists of a sequence of heart period durations T_i. In order to reduce trends we have plotted the deviations from the linear trend:

$$T_i'' = \frac{T_{i-1} + T_{i+1}}{2} - T_i$$

The delay time was decreased step by step as marked in Fig. 2 (A: 500 ms, B: 450 ms, C: 400 ms, D: 300 ms, E: 200 ms, F: 100 ms).

We found a period-doubling bifurcation in the rhythm of the heart cycle. There is a period 1 for delay time 500 ms (A) and at point B a bifurcation to period 2 is induced. After switching to 400 ms delay (C) more complicated pattern appear:

At point E (200 ms delay) an initial period 1 changes into period 2. This transition without a change of the delay is presumably due to internal parameter variations. Finally we find at 100 ms delay time indications of period 4.

It is rather difficult to interpret these findings using conventional physiological methods. Therefore, in Part I the data are analyzed using techniques from nonlinear dynamics theory.

Address of the authors:
Dr. Heinz Warzel, and coll., Institute of Physiology, Medical Academy Magdeburg, Leipziger Str. 44, O-3090 Magdeburg

Wiss. Zeitschrift der Humboldt-Universität zu Berlin, R. Medizin 41 (1992) 4

59

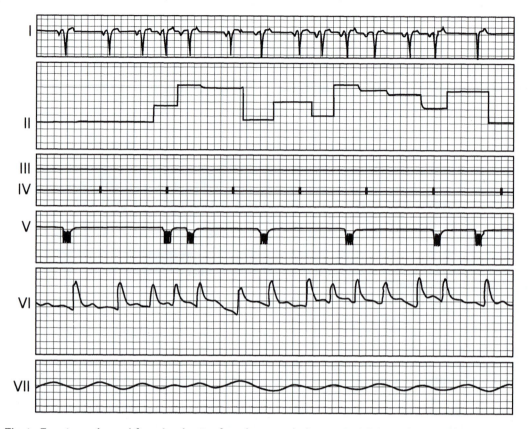

Fig. 1. Experimental record from dog showing from the top to the bottom: I. ECG, II. duration of the foregoing heart cycle, IV. one second time marker, V. (expiratory) stimulation impulses, VI. blood pressure, VII. respiration (measured by a thermistor)

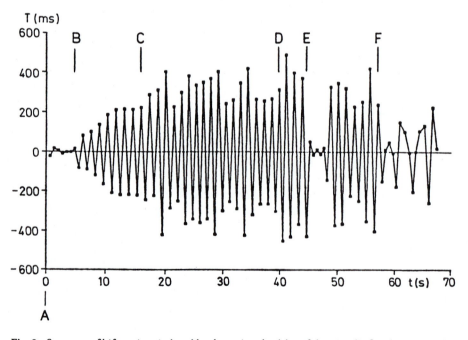

Fig. 2. Sequence of bifurcations induced by decreasing the delay of the stimuli after the R-wave (see text)

60

Wiss. Zeitschrift der Humboldt-Universität zu Berlin, R. Medizin 41 (1992) 4

References

[1] Zsoter, T. T.; Sellers, E. M.: Effect of alcohol on cardiovasvular reflexes. – In: J. Stud. Alcohol. – 38 (1977). – pp. 1–10

[2] Sato, A.; Schmidt, R. F.: The Modulation of Visceral Function by Somatic Afferent Activity. – In: Jpn. J. Physiol. – 37 (1987). – pp. 1–17

[3] Ettinger, P. O.; Wu, C. F.; De La Curuz, C.: Arrhythmias and the "holiday heart": Alcohol-associated cardiac rhythm disorders. – In: Am. Heart J. – 95 (1978). – pp. 55–62

[4] Cohen, E. J.; Klatsky, A. L.; Armstrong, M. A.: Alcohol use and supraventricular arrhythmia. – In: Am. J. Cardiol. – 62 (1988). – pp. 971–973

[5] Fraser, G. E.; Upsdell, M.: Alcohol and other discriminants between cases of sudden death and myocardial infarction. – In: Am. J. Epidemiol. – 114 (1981). – pp. 462–476

[6] Gelsema, A. J.; Bouman, L. N.; Karemaker, J. M.: Short-latency tachycardia evoked by stimulation of muscle and cutaneous afferents. – In: Am. J. Physiol. – 248 (1985). – R426–R433

[7] Maytham, J. C.; Kline, R. L.; Calaresu, F. R.: Effect of stimulation of somatic nerves on the ventricular fibrillation threshold in dogs. – In: Am. Heart J. – 94 (1977). – pp. 731–739

[8] Oliven, A.; Haxhiu, M. A.; Kelsen, St. G.: Distribution of motor activity to expiratory muscles during sciatic nerve stimulating in the dog. – In: Respir. Physiol. – 81 (1990). – pp. 165–176

[9] Koepchen, H. P.; Wagner, P.-H.; Lux, H. D.: Über die Zusammenhänge zwischen zentraler Erregbarkeit, reflektorischem Tonus und Atemrhythmus bei der nervösen Herzfrequenz. – In: Pflügers Arch. – 273 (1961). – pp. 443–465

[10] Melcher, A.: Respiratory sinus arrhythmia in man. – In: Acta Physiol. Scand., Suppl. – 435 (1976). –

[11] Levy, M. N.; Zieske, H.: Synchronization of the cardiac pacemaker with repetitive stimulation of the carotid sinus nerve in the dog. – In: Circulation Res. – 30 (1972). – pp. 634–641

[12] Warzel, H.; Eckhardt, H.-U.; Hopstock, U.: Effects of carotid sinus nerve stimulation at different times in the respiratory and cardiac cycles on variability of heart rate and blood pressure of normotensive and renal hypertensive dogs. – In: J. Autonom. Nerv. Syst. – 26 (1989). – pp. 121–127

Wiss. Zeitschrift der Humboldt-Universität zu Berlin, R. Medizin 41 (1992) 4

61

modeling in physiology

Phase dependencies of the human baroreceptor reflex

HENRIK SEIDEL,[1] HANSPETER HERZEL,[1] AND DWAIN L. ECKBERG[2]
[1]*Department of Physics, Technical University Berlin, D-10623 Berlin, Germany; and*
[2]*Departments of Medicine and Physiology, Hunter Holmes McGuire Department of*
Veterans Affairs Medical Center and Medical College of Virginia, Richmond, Virginia 23249

Seidel, Henrik, Hanspeter Herzel, and Dwain L. Eckberg. Phase dependencies of the human baroreceptor reflex. *Am. J. Physiol.* 272 (*Heart Circ. Physiol.* 41): H2040–H2053, 1997.—We studied the influence of respiratory and cardiac phase on responses of the cardiac pacemaker to brief (0.35-s) increases of carotid baroreceptor afferent traffic provoked by neck suction in seven healthy young adult subjects. Cardiac responses to neck suction were measured indirectly from electrocardiographic changes of heart period. Our results show that it is possible to separate the influences of respiratory and cardiac phases at the onset of a neck suction impulse by a product of two factors: one depending only on the respiratory phase and one depending only on the cardiac phase. This result is consistent with the hypothesis that efferent vagal activity is a function of afferent baroreceptor activity, whereas respiratory neurons modulate that medullary throughput independent of the cardiac phase. Furthermore, we have shown that stimulus broadening and stimulus cropping influence the outcome of neck suction experiments in a way that makes it virtually impossible to obtain information on the phase dependency of the cardiac pacemaker's sensitivity to vagal stimulation without accurate knowledge of the functional shape of stimulus broadening.

autonomic nervous system; neck suction; baroreflex latency; phase-response curve; modeling

ALTHOUGH SEVERAL METHODS are available for stimulating or inhibiting human baroreceptors with precisely controlled pressure changes and although methods are available for measuring the integrated efferent neural responses precisely, the simplicity of such research masks the great complexity of the underlying mechanisms.

Because the human baroreflex is a closed loop, it is difficult to distinguish between cause and effect when changes of physiological variables are provoked. Attempts have been made to overcome this problem by "opening the loop" with drugs or mechanical means. One approach has been to study responses to stimuli the duration of which is less than that of the total time delay of the baroreflex loop. This approach is quite useful in studies of fast vagal responses to baroreceptor stimulation, but it is not appropriate in studies of sympathetic responses because of the slow dynamics of sympathetic effector responses.

Another approach is to use mathematical models of the baroreflex loop (which should a priori be a closed loop) and to compare the output of the model with experimental results. Parameters of the model can be changed to give the best fit of experimental data. Using this approach, one can obtain valuable insight into the system and test hypotheses about what is cause and what is effect. Such a model should relate data that are difficult to access, such as vagal activity, to noninvasively measurable data, such as heart rate, blood pressure, and respiration. As a step in that direction, Seidel and Herzel (17) published a nonlinear model for the short-term dynamics of the baroreceptor control loop.

A serious difficulty in modeling the baroreflex loop is the limited knowledge regarding information processing in the medulla. It is well known that the magnitude of vagal responses depends on the timing of baroreceptor stimuli within the respiratory and cardiac cycles (2, 5, 6, 9, 12, 19). However, these studies investigated only the effect of stimulus timing within the respiratory or the heart cycle.

Because such data are essential for the formulation of a model, we studied the dependency of human baroreflex responses on respiratory and cardiac phases with noninvasive methods. We are aware of no earlier study in which phase-response relations were functions of both phases. Furthermore, we investigated in great detail the influence of the duration of baroreceptor stimuli on the outcome of neck suction experiments. It is well known that the sensitivity of the cardiac pacemaker with respect to short vagal stimulation depends on the cardiac phase. This was investigated by Yang et al. (19), who used electrical stimulation of vagal nerves. However, the duration of baroreceptor stimuli is much longer than the duration of these electric vagal impulses. Therefore, the response of the cardiac pacemaker is smoothed or averaged over the duration of the baroreceptor stimulus. In addition, the effect is reduced when a P peak occurs while the stimulus is active, and, therefore, only a part of the stimulus can contribute to a change of the current P-P interval.

Our results suggest that the influence of stimulus timing on the magnitude of vagal responses can be considered as the product of two independent factors, each depending only on the timing within the respiratory or the cardiac cycle. Furthermore, our analysis indicates that cropping of stimuli by P-P interval borders and smoothing of the cardiac pacemaker's responses due to the finite duration of stimuli are significant and need to be taken into account for the interpretation of data from baroreceptor stimulation.

METHODS

We used brief, moderate carotid baroreceptor stimuli to investigate the importance of stimulus timing within breathing and cardiac cycles for P-P interval responses. Mathematical modeling was used to extract some features of the results.

Subjects. We studied seven adult volunteers (5 men, 2 women) after they gave written consent to participate in the study, which was approved by the Human Research Committees of the Hunter Holmes McGuire Department of Veterans Affairs Medical Center and the Medical College of Virginia. All subjects were healthy, and none were taking medications; their ages ranged from 24 to 33 yr. We discarded data from two subjects (both men). One subject could not control his breathing adequately, and another had extremely small responses to neck suction.

Measurements. Subjects were studied supine. We recorded the following measurements with an FM tape recorder: electrocardiogram (ECG), photoplethysmographic arterial pressure (Finapres model 2300, Ohmeda, Englewood, CO), respiratory flow (ultrasonic flow measurement), and neck chamber pressure (strain gauge pressure transducer). We did not measure end-tidal carbon dioxide concentration.

Each subject was studied during three sessions on different days at the same time of the day. Each session consisted of three parts: rest periods (20 min, 10 min, 10 min), baseline periods (10 min, 5 min, 5 min), and stimulation periods (15 min, 15 min, 15 min). During each stimulation period the whole heart cycle was scanned in alternating directions (see below). Subjects maintained constant tidal volumes and breathing frequencies. The neck chamber was removed for the duration of the rest periods to avoid distortions of responses due to neck discomfort.

Neck pressure. Carotid baroreceptor afferent activity was increased briefly (0.35 s) by pressure (−70 mmHg) applied to a neck chamber (3). Stimuli were initiated after a preset delay following the upstroke of an R wave of the ECG. The delay between the R wave peak and the beginning of the stimulus was changed stepwise to scan the entire heart cycle. The respiratory cycle was scanned by chance, since stimuli were applied in intervals of ~11 s and the duration of three respiratory periods was 12 s.

Control of breathing. We measured baseline and stimulation R-R intervals during controlled breathing at 15 breaths/min and constant tidal volume, established by each subject during quiet breathing. The subjects wore headphones and were instructed to follow a computer-generated acoustic

signal for frequency control. Two horizontal lines were displayed on an oscilloscope representing current and target tidal volumes. The usual volume was established by each subject during the first rest period. Then subjects were instructed to inhale until the bottom line reached the line representing the target tidal volume.

Data analysis. Recorded data were digitized with a sampling frequency of 500 Hz. Characteristic events were marked: R-wave peak, onset of inspiration, beginning of neck chamber impulse. We calculated the timing of P waves assuming a constant P-R interval for each subject. This assumption was tested for one subject by manually marking all P-wave peaks of a 250-s data section during stimulation. The average P-R interval was 149 ± 5 (SD) ms with a maximum deviation of 11 ms, whereas changes in P-P interval due to baroreceptor stimulation were up to 200 ms. This analysis justifies the approximation of constant P-R intervals.

Inspiration onset was defined as the time when the increasing respiratory flow crossed a preset positive threshold. We chose a threshold of 5% of maximum flow. This was slightly larger than the fluctuations of flow at end expiration. The following analyses are based on the time series of these marker events.

The prolongation of heart period provoked by a neck stimulus is superimposed on slow variations of the mean P-P interval (<0.1 Hz), respiratory sinus arrhythmia (RSA), and some remaining variations considered as noise. To extract the direct effect of the baroreflex stimulus, it was necessary to subtract these other P-P interval variations from the total prolongation. Slow variations of P-P intervals were eliminated by a Gaussian filter applied in the time domain. RSA was removed by linear prediction using an autoregressive model. Noise was reduced by averaging.

Gaussian filter. A Gaussian filter has the shape of a Gaussian curve in time and frequency domains. With a center frequency of 0 Hz, it is a low-pass filter. We consider the residue of the time series of heart periods after subtraction of the filtered series. The equation for the Gaussian filter is

$$x'(t) = \frac{\sigma}{\sqrt{2\pi}} \int_{-\infty}^{\infty} e^{-\sigma^2\tau^2/2} x(t - \tau) \, d\tau \qquad (1)$$

We used 0.1 Hz for σ, the standard width of the filter. The function $x(t)$ is the spline-interpolated series of heart periods, and $x'(t)$ is the time series after filtering. We denote the residue $x(t) - x'(t)$ by $x''(t)$. Figure 1 shows some raw heart period data during baseline. The corresponding spectra before and after Gaussian filtering and linear prediction are depicted in Fig. 2. Spectra were calculated using the Lomb

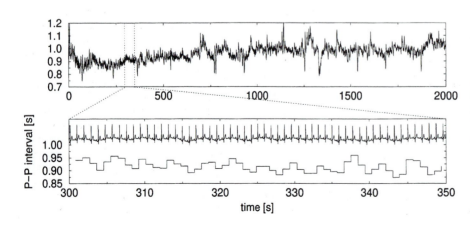

Fig. 1. Time series of P-P intervals for a baseline period (controlled breathing, no baroreceptor stimulation). ECG signal for expanded P-P interval sequence is also shown. This time series was used for demonstration of data-processing methods in Figs. 2 and 3.

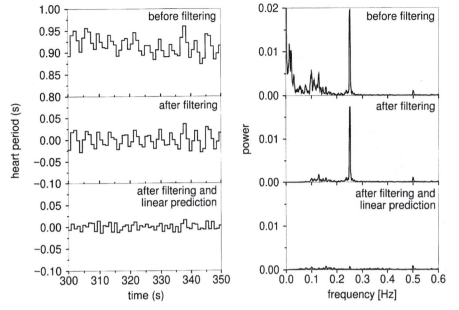

Fig. 2. Data and Fourier spectrum of time series of heart periods from Fig. 1 before filtering, after filtering, and after filtering and removal of respiratory sinus arrhythmia by linear prediction. We depict only a subsection of entire time series used for calculation of spectra to facilitate observation of effects of filtering and linear prediction on raw data.

algorithm (15), which is appropriate for unevenly sampled data, such as heart period. Low-frequency oscillations of the heart period were almost completely removed up to 0.1 Hz and were significantly reduced up to 0.15 Hz.

Linear prediction. We predict RSA to subtract its influence from the heart period of the stimulated and the subsequent heartbeat. The equations are

$$\text{RSA}(t) = \sum_{i=1}^{7} a_i x''(t - i\Delta t) \tag{2}$$

for the stimulated and

$$\text{RSA}(t) = \sum_{i=3}^{8} b_i x''(t - i\Delta t) \tag{3}$$

for the subsequent interval. We used a delay (Δt) of 1 s. It was necessary to start with $i = 3$ in *Eq. 3*, since the immediate history of this heart cycle is already influenced by the stimulus.

The coefficients a_i and b_i signify the correlations between the P-P interval we want to predict and the preceding P-P intervals. They were calculated by least-squares methods from the baseline immediately preceding the considered stimulation period. The residue $x'''(t) = x''(t) - \text{RSA}(t)$ should be the prolongation of the heart interval caused solely by neck suction, with some noise superimposed. Figure 3 shows the autocorrelation function of the Gaussian-filtered time series $x''(t)$ of P-P intervals from Fig. 1 before and after removal of RSA. The integrated power of RSA was reduced by 96.5% for a linear prediction model according to *Eq. 2*. For time series without baroreceptor stimulation, the remaining correlations can be reduced further by increasing the order of the model (see the curve for *order 15* in Fig. 3). We restricted ourselves to an order of 7, since otherwise the required history is influenced by previous stimuli for time series with stimulation.

Classes and removal of outliers. We sorted the stimuli according to their timing within respiratory and heart cycles. The respiratory period was split into five subintervals of equal length, and the heart period was split into eight subintervals. That is, we had 40 different classes with an

average of 20 points per class and subject. Stimuli were assigned to these classes according to the time of the onset of neck suction. That is, each stimulus belonged to one of the 40 classes and had a value of x''' for its prolongation of the heart interval.

Subsequently, the points in each class were averaged after the removal of outliers. There were different causes that could produce outliers. For example, subjects moved their arm or swallowed. For each class we sorted all points according to their value x''', calculated mean and standard deviation of the inner 86% of points, and removed all points that had a distance from the mean greater than three times the standard deviation. Classes with fewer than five remaining points were discarded.

Normalization of phase-response curves. There are several ways to juxtapose stimulus responses of different subjects.

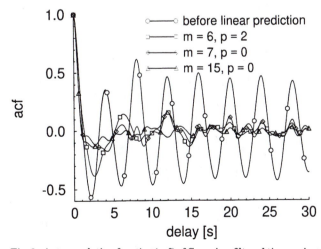

Fig. 3. Autocorrelation function (acf) of Gaussian-filtered time series of heart periods from Fig. 1 before and after removal of respiratory sinus arrhythmia by linear prediction, $\sum_{i=1+p}^{m+p} a_i x''(t - i\Delta t)$, where m is number of cardiac periods used for prediction and p is number of cardiac periods that immediately precede predicted interval but that are not used for prediction since they might already be influenced by stimulus. Symbols are added to facilitate distinguishing curves.

One can compare stimuli with the same absolute time between the first P peak of the considered heart interval and stimulus onset, or one can normalize this time by the mean P-P interval. Using the absolute time has a great disadvantage: for subjects with different resting heart rates the same absolute time can mean that for one subject the stimulus begins in midrepolarization, whereas for another subject it begins in early depolarization. Therefore, we normalize the absolute time by dividing by the resting heart period, which results in the cardiac phase. The response to a stimulus begun at a given cardiac phase means for all subjects the response to a stimulus that is initiated in the same part of the cardiac cycle. Independently of the timing of a stimulus, the magnitude of the response depends on the subject's sensitivity to neck suction and may also depend on the baseline P-P interval. To take this into account, we normalize the responses for each subject by dividing by the subject's maximum occurring prolongation.

To summarize, adding together the normalized responses of different subjects for stimuli begun at a given cardiac phase means adding together the percentages of P-P interval prolongation with respect to the subject's maximum prolongation for stimuli initiated in the same part of the cardiac cycle.

RESULTS

Raw data. Figure 4 shows a sample of raw data during stimulation for the first subject. The recorded tracks are respiratory flow, ECG, blood pressure, and neck chamber pressure. In Fig. 5 we define some of the variables we will use in the following discussion.

Influence of cardiac phase. Figure 6 shows the influence of stimulus timing within the P-P interval on the change of heart period (Δt_{pp}). Timing is represented by the phase of the cardiac pacemaker at stimulus onset (ϕ_s), i.e., the time between the opening P peak of the considered heartbeat and the beginning of baroreceptor stimulation divided by the mean P-P interval of the preceding control period ($t_{pp-mean}$). The response is averaged over all respiratory phases. We take into account that there is a substantial (with respect to the heart period) delay (ξ) between a change of carotid sinus pressure and its first effect on the cardiac pacemaker [we use $\xi = 0.35$ s, which is between the values of 0.24 s determined by Eckberg (3) and 0.55 s determined by Borst and Karemaker (1); see also discussion in APPENDIX C]. For example, if we apply a neck suction impulse exactly at the opening P peak of a heart cycle ($t_{stimulus} = t_{p-peak}$; Fig. 5), the stimulus reaches the cardiac pacemaker ~0.35 s later. That is, the phase of stimulus onset with respect to the cycle of the cardiac pacemaker is not zero but about one-third. More generally, $t'_{stimulus} = t_{stimulus} + \xi$ is approximately the time the stimulus occurs at the cardiac pacemaker, and $\phi_s = (t'_{stimulus} - t_{p-peak})/t_{pp-mean}$ is the corresponding cardiac phase. If the phase is negative, the stimulus arrives before the beginning of the considered heart interval.

We emphasize that the relations in Fig. 6 do not describe the momentary sensitivity of the cardiac pace-

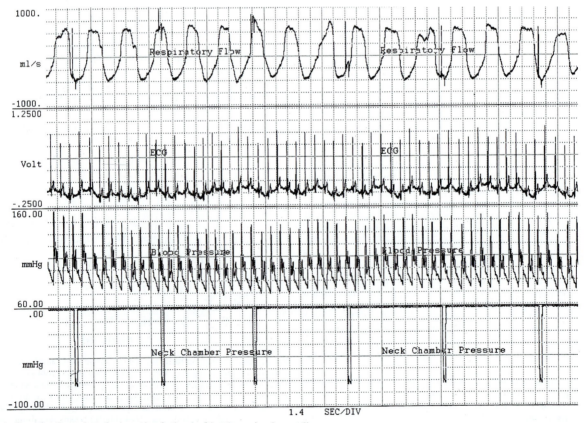

Fig. 4. Sample of raw data during stimulation (*subject 1, session 3, part 2*).

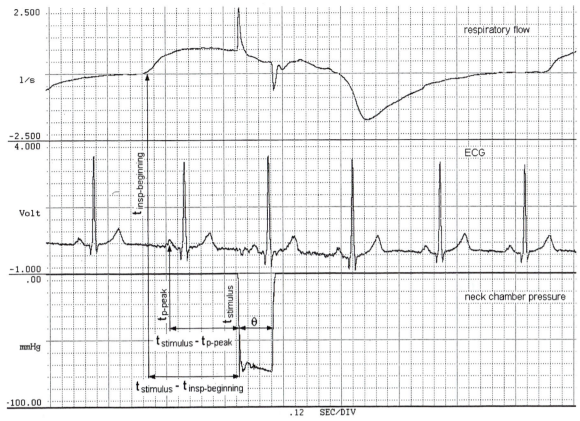

Fig. 5. Definition of variables t_{p-peak}, $t_{insp-beginning}$, $t_{stimulus}$, and stimulus duration (θ). t_{p-peak} was not measured directly but was calculated from measured timing of R peaks, assuming an average P-R interval. Data are from *subject 3*.

Fig. 6. Influence of cardiac phase (ϕ_s) on change of P-P interval (Δt_{pp}) due to carotid sinus pressure stimuli without (*A*) and with (*B*) normalization with respect to maximum of this curve [$(\Delta t_{pp})_{max}$]. *C* and *D*: corresponding curves averaged over all subjects. stddev, Standard deviation of responses.

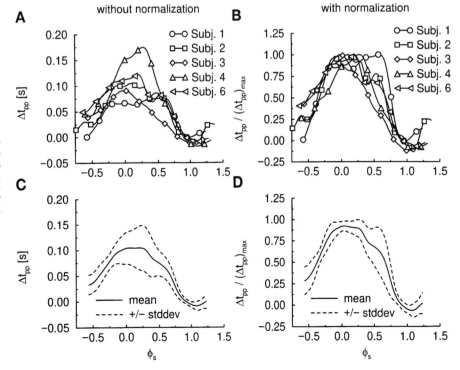

maker at the corresponding heart phase but the response to a stimulus of 0.35-s duration. As a consequence, the response shown in Fig. 6 is the sensitivity of the cardiac pacemaker at different phases integrated over the duration of the stimulus and superimposed with limitation effects that occur when only a part of the stimulus coincides with the current heart interval. Therefore, it would be desirable to use stimuli as short as possible to avoid these problems. However, neck stimuli should be of >0.25-s duration to provoke significant prolongation of heart period (4).

Figure 6A shows the response curves for all five subjects. Figure 6B shows the curves normalized by dividing by their maximum response. Because the magnitude of responses differs among subjects, this normalization allows a better comparison of the phase dependency. Figure 6, C and D, shows the response curves (mean ± SD) averaged over all subjects.

For all subjects, the heart period was prolonged maximally when the stimulus was initiated shortly after the beginning of the heart cycle. Almost no prolongation occurred near the end of the cycle. Some points for large cardiac phases seem to indicate cardiac cycle shortening. However, cycle shortening is not significant, since the smallest change of P-P interval is -15 ± 13 (SD) ms.

Influence of respiratory phase. Figure 7 depicts the influence of the timing of stimuli within the respiratory cycle on the prolongation of heart period. We averaged responses over all cardiac phases. We assumed that the respiratory influence originated from information processing in the central nervous system. Stimulation of the baroreceptor afferents by pressure stimuli occurs

nearly instantaneously (11), and the time that activity requires to travel to the central nervous system is negligible in comparison with the respiratory period (10). Therefore, for the respiratory phase-response curve, we did not shift the time axis, as for the phase-response curve of the cardiac pacemaker; i.e., the respiratory phase (ϕ_r) is defined as the time between inspiration beginning and stimulus onset normalized by the duration of the considered respiratory cycle (T_{resp}): $\phi_r = (t_{stimulus} - t_{insp-beginning})/T_{resp}$ (cf. Fig. 5).

Figure 7A shows the response curves of all subjects; Fig. 7B shows the curves normalized by dividing by their mean response (average over the respiratory cycle). Figure 7, C and D, depicts the mean response curves for all subjects. Minimum prolongation occurs when the stimulus is applied during early inspiration. Prolongation is maximal in midexpiration.

Influence of respiratory and cardiac phase. Figure 8, A and B, displays the prolongation of heart period for two subjects as a function of the cardiac phase with the respiratory phase as a curve parameter. Figure 8C depicts the averages of all subjects.

Figure 8 shows how the prolongation of P-P interval depends on stimulus timing within the cardiac and respiratory cycles. We divide the respiratory cycle into five bins corresponding to the five intervals [(0, 0.2), (0.2, 0.4), (0.4, 0.6), (0.6, 0.8), (0.8, 1)] for the respiratory phase. For each of these bins, we plot a curve that displays how the change of heart period depends on the phase of the cardiac pacemaker at stimulus onset for those stimuli that fall into the considered respiratory bin.

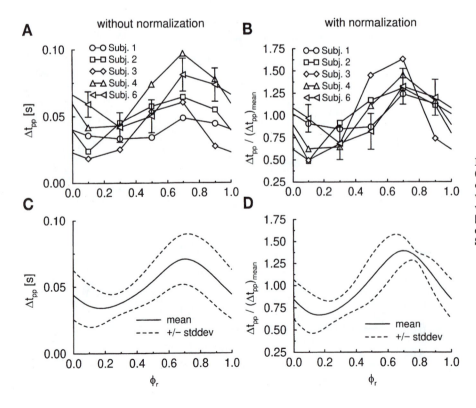

Fig. 7. Influence of respiratory phase (ϕ_r) on change of P-P interval (Δt_{pp}) due to carotid sinus pressure stimuli without (A) and with (B) normalization with respect to mean of each curve [$(\Delta t_{pp})_{mean}$]. C and D: corresponding curves averaged over all subjects. stddev, Standard deviation among subjects.

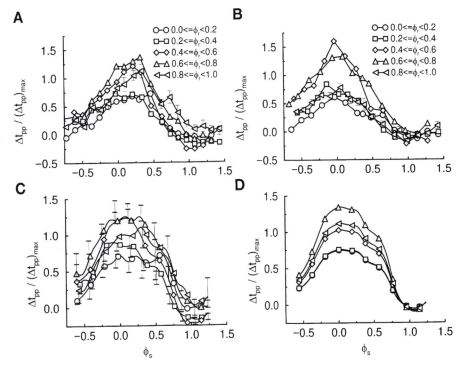

Fig. 8. Influence of respiratory phase (ϕ_r) and cardiac phase (ϕ_s) on change of P-P interval (Δt_{pp}) normalized with respect to maximum of cardiac response curve [$(\Delta t_{pp})_{max}$, average of 5 curves in each graph]. *A: subject 3.* Each point corresponds to a class. For some classes, standard errors are drawn. *B: subject 4.* *C:* mean ± SD of all subjects. *D:* calculated response curves (see text).

The graphs show very clearly the dependency of the change of P-P interval (Δt_{pp}) on the respiratory and the cardiac phase. Furthermore, the presentation of both phase dependencies in one graph allows the following analysis of the relationships between the different phase-response curves.

We have demonstrated so far how we extracted the phase dependencies from our data. In the DISCUSSION, we present some tests to show that our data handling does not distort the outcome significantly. We now use the obtained functions to obtain insight into physiological mechanisms. For this purpose, we formulate and test a functional relationship between the different phase-response curves.

In general, the response Δt_{pp} is a function of ϕ_r and ϕ_s

$$\Delta t_{pp} = f(\phi_s, \phi_r) \qquad (4)$$

If $f(\phi_s, \phi_r)$ is the product of two factors $f_1(\phi_s)$ and $f_2(\phi_r)$, each depending only on one phase, one can represent $f(\phi_s, \phi_r)$ as

$$f(\phi_s, \phi_r) = f_1(\phi_s)f_2(\phi_r) \qquad (5)$$

We want to relate $f_1(\phi_s)$ and $f_2(\phi_r)$ to our measured cardiac phase-response curve [$f_s(\phi_s)$] and to the measured respiratory phase-response curve [$f_r(\phi_r)$], which are defined by

$$f_s(\phi_s) = \langle f(\phi_s, \phi_r) \rangle_{\phi_r} \qquad (6)$$

where $\langle \rangle_{\phi_r}$ indicates averaging over the respiratory phase, with cardiac phase fixed, and

$$f_r(\phi_r) = \langle f(\phi_s, \phi_r) \rangle_{\phi_s} \qquad (7)$$

After some transformations (see APPENDIX A) we obtain

$$\frac{f(\phi_s, \phi_r)}{[\langle f(\phi_s, \phi_r) \rangle_{\phi_r}]_{max}} = \frac{f_s(\phi_s)}{[f_s(\phi_s)]_{max}} \times \frac{f_r(\phi_r)}{\langle f_r(\phi_r) \rangle_{\phi_r}} \qquad (8)$$

The left-hand side of *Eq. 8* corresponds to the normalized phase-response curves of Fig. 8C, whereas the two factors on the right-hand side correspond to the normalized cardiac phase-response curve of Fig. 6D and to the normalized respiratory phase-response curve of Fig. 7D. Thus we can use *Eq. 8* to calculate the two-dimensional response curve $f(\phi_s, \phi_r)/[\langle f(\phi_s, \phi_r) \rangle_{\phi_r}]_{max}$ from the one-dimensional response curves (Figs. 6D and 7D). If that calculated two-dimensional response curve coincides with the measured curves of Fig. 8C, our assumption (*Eq. 5*) would be justified.

In Fig. 8D we depict the theoretical response curves. They are clearly within standard deviation range of the measured curves (standard deviation among subjects). Hence, we have shown that the total prolongation of heart period by a carotid sinus pressure pulse is consistent with the hypothesis that it is the product of two factors: one depending only on the respiratory phase and one depending only on the cardiac phase. These two factors are proportional to the one-dimensional response curves of Figs. 6D and 7D.

Modeling the influence of finite stimulus duration. Earlier studies using neck suction usually did not explicitly analyze the fact that (due to the finite duration of pressure pulses) a physiological baroreceptor stimulus (an arterial pulse) does not occur at just one cardiac phase but covers a phase range. Therefore, one does not measure the sensitivity of the cardiac pacemaker at the phase of stimulus onset but, rather, a response that is the cardiac pacemaker's sensitivity smoothed over the whole phase range covered by the stimulus. Furthermore, if the considered heart cycle starts or ends while the stimulus is active, the effect of the pressure pulse on the heart period is diminished, since only a part of the stimulus can influence the current cycle. Neck suction experiments usually use stimulus durations of ≥0.25 s, i.e., one-fourth of a usual heart period. Hence, smoothing and stimulus cropping effects are significant for the interpretation of stimulus responses.

Therefore, we now address the following question: What information can be obtained from our measured phase dependencies about the baroreflex latency, stimulus broadening, and phase dependency of the cardiac pacemaker's sensitivity to vagal stimulation? Furthermore, we try to estimate how the finite stimulus duration influences the results.

Let us denote the time course of baroreceptor activity changes due to a stimulus of duration θ by $s(t)$, where t is the time since stimulus onset. The neural activity is delayed and broadened on its way to the cardiac pacemaker. We assume that this effect can be described by the convolution integral

$$s'(t) = \int_{-\infty}^{\infty} d\tau \, g(t - \tau) s(\tau) \qquad (9)$$

The function $s'(t)$ is the vagal activity that reaches the cardiac pacemaker at time t after stimulus onset and $g(t - \tau)$ models stimulus broadening and delay. The value of $g(t - \tau)$ describes how much baroreceptor activity at time τ arrives at the cardiac pacemaker at time t.

A stimulus of the considered finite duration changes the heart period by $F(\phi)$, where ϕ is the time between the first P peak of the investigated heart period and stimulus onset. We assume that the cardiac pacemaker has a phase-dependent momentary sensitivity $f(\tau)$; i.e., $f(\tau)$ is the response to a Dirac-delta impulse at time τ after the first P peak of the heart cycle. Furthermore, we assume that responses add linearly, i.e.

$$F(\phi) = \int_0^{T + F(\phi)} f(\tau) s'(\tau - \phi) \, d\tau \qquad (10)$$

where T is the undisturbed heart period.

Using Eqs. 9 and 10 in conjunction with appropriately chosen functions $s(t)$, $g(t - \tau)$, and $f(\tau)$, we can estimate the response to a finite baroreceptor stimulus. To test how the results depend on the choice of these three functions, we use two different function types (I and II) for each of them and calculate the response $F(\phi)$ for each of the eight combinations. The function types are defined in APPENDIX B. The function $s_I(t)$ describes a rectangular response of baroreceptor activity: the activity is increased by a constant value for the duration of the neck suction impulse. The function $s_{II}(t)$ describes a more differential behavior according to experimental results from Landgren (11); i.e., the baroreceptor response is not constant but decaying while the stimulus is active. The functions $g_I(t)$ and $g_{II}(t)$ are simply two

different functional shapes for the time course of stimulus broadening. Function $f_I(t)$ models a constant (i.e., phase-independent) sensitivity of the cardiac pacemaker, whereas $f_{II}(t)$ is a more realistic description according to a mathematical model of the sinus node by Reiner and Antzelevitch (16).

The essential parameters of the model are the time between the occurrence of a delta impulse and its first effect on the cardiac pacemaker (ξ), the time between first and maximum response of the cardiac pacemaker to such an impulse (η), the parameter σ, which is a measure for the width of stimulus broadening, and the amplitude of responses (A).

For all eight possible combinations of the above-defined functions, we use Powell's method (15) to determine the four parameters ξ, η, σ, and A that give the best approximation (least squares) of the measured cardiac phase-response curve by the calculated function $F(\phi)$. In this case, the measured phase-response curve is the function from Fig. 6, but without the phase shift according to the baroreflex latency. We need to use the unshifted curve here to be consistent with the modeling of the baroreflex latency by $g(t)$.

Figure 9 shows the measured cardiac phase-response curve and the fitted theoretical response $F(\phi)$ for the eight possible combinations. For each, we find parameters that give a theoretical curve that is in standard deviation range of the measured curve. However, the parameters vary considerably: the time between stimulus onset and first effect on the cardiac pacemaker (ξ) is 200 ± 130 (SD) ms, the time between first and maximum response to a delta impulse (η) is 495 ± 340 ms, the parameter σ describing the width of stimulus broadening is 280 ± 150 ms, and the time between the occurrence of a delta stimulus and its maximum effect on the cardiac pacemaker ($\xi + \eta$) is 690 ± 230 ms. Hence, the absolute values of the parameters deter-

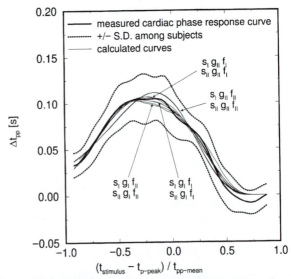

Fig. 9. Measured cardiac phase-response curve and calculated curves for mathematical model that investigates influence of finite stimulus duration. Eight calculated curves are for different combinations of s_I, s_{II}, g_I, g_{II}, f_I, and f_{II}.

mined by the fit should not be overestimated. On the other hand, their variability indicates that many different sets of parameters can approximate the measured curve $F(\phi)$.

An important result of our calculations is that not only a realistic phase-dependent sensitivity of the cardiac pacemaker $f_{II}(t)$, but also a phase-independent sensitivity $f_{I}(t)$, can reproduce the measured phase-response curve. That is, our results suggest that the measured phase-response curve does not contain enough information to determine the phase dependency $f(t)$ if no additional very accurate information on $s(t)$ and $g(t)$ is available. They rather indicate that the measured phase dependency is mainly an effect of stimulus broadening and stimulus cropping. In other words, our results suggest that it is difficult or even impossible to obtain significant information on the phase dependency of the cardiac pacemaker's sensitivity using neck suction experiments.

DISCUSSION

Phase-response curves. We investigated the influence of respiratory and cardiac phases at the beginning of short neck suction impulses on the response of P-P intervals. With a time delay of ~0.35 s between the onset of a stimulus and the first observable effect on the cardiac pacemaker taken into account, the change of P-P interval was maximal when the baroreceptor stimulus (shifted by the baroreceptor latency) was initiated near the first P peak at the beginning of the cycle and minimal shortly before the second P peak at the end of the cycle. Furthermore, the effect was maximal during midexpiration and minimal at early inspiration. These results are in accordance with those of previous studies (5, 6, 8).

As a new result, we have shown that the phase-response curve depending on both respiratory and cardiac phases can be represented by the product of two factors, each depending only on one phase. These two factors are proportional to the respiratory phase-response curve and to the cardiac phase-response curve, respectively. Such a separation of variables is consistent with the hypothesis that efferent vagal activity is a function of afferent baroreceptor activity, whereas respiratory neurons modulate medullary throughput independent of the cardiac phase.

Influence of finite stimulus duration. We investigated the influence of the finite duration of baroreceptor stimuli on the outcome of neck suction experiments. We had to make some assumptions for our calculations. The most critical of these is the assumption of a linearly accumulating change of P-P interval in *Eq. 10.* Such a linear convolution integral is only an approximation that breaks down if stimuli are strong enough to drive the trajectory of the cardiac pacemaker far from its limit cycle. For example, it was shown by Wanzhen et al. (18) in a theoretical study of the Poincaré oscillator and an experimental investigation of oscillating chick heart cell aggregates that paired stimuli may induce strong resetting of an oscillator, whereas a single stimulus of the same amplitude induces only weak

resetting. Such a topological transition of phase resetting cannot be explained by a linear approximation. However, to our knowledge, strong phase resetting has not been observed in neck suction experiments; i.e., changes of vagal activity provoked by neck suction are not strong enough to induce topological changes of the cardiac pacemaker's phase resetting. In other words, the amplitude of stimuli seems to be low enough to justify a linear approximation.

To summarize, the appropriateness of a linear convolution integral depends on how far the stimulus drives the trajectory of the cardiac pacemaker away from its limit cycle and how strong the nonlinearity in that range actually is. Without this knowledge, the best one can do is to use a linear convolution integral as a first approximation.

Nonetheless, our calculations show clearly that the finite duration of baroreceptor stimuli is of considerable importance for the interpretation of results from neck suction experiments. In particular, the measured dependency of responses on the cardiac phase seems to be caused mainly by stimulus broadening and stimulus cropping at the end of the heart cycle. The measured responses can be explained by completely different shapes for the influence of the cardiac phase on the pacemaker's sensitivity to vagal stimulation. Hence, the measured data seem to contain no significant information about this phase dependency. In other words, our results suggest that neck suction experiments alone are not suitable for the determination of the phase dependency of the cardiac pacemaker's sensitivity to vagal stimulation. An investigation of this phase dependency requires very sharp stimuli like those of Yang et al. (19), who used direct electrical stimulation of the vagal nerve.

Methods for data processing. We used several mathematical methods to extract our results from the raw data. This makes it necessary to test the appropriateness of these methods. Let us take some data of a subject during controlled breathing without baroreceptor stimulation. We change these data to simulate neck suction using the phase-response curves from Fig. 8C. Subsequently, we apply our data-processing methods to the altered data. If the resulting phase-response curves are to a reasonable degree similar to the curves used for the simulation, our data processing is appropriate.

The raw data are from an eighth subject. For this subject, we have data only during controlled breathing without baroreceptor stimulation. We generate a time series of stimulation events (i.e., the onset of neck suction) using the same stimulation regimen as in the real experiments. For each of these events, we determine its timing within the respiratory and cardiac cycles. Subsequently, we use the curves from Fig. 8C to determine the delays of the first and second subsequent heartbeats according to a stimulus with this particular timing. We shift all P peaks following and including the first heartbeat after the onset of stimulation by the just-determined delay of the first P peak. All P peaks following and including the second heartbeat after the onset of stimulation are additionally shifted by the

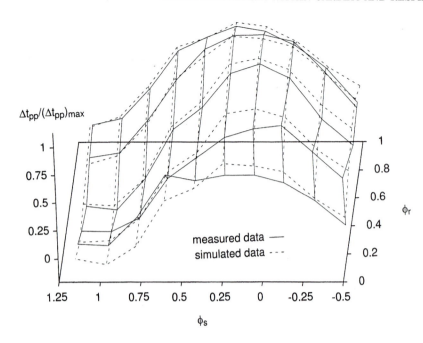

Fig. 10. Comparison of phase-response curves for real and simulated baroreceptor stimulation.

delay of the second heartbeat. In other words, we shift the right part of the time axis of the original time series to simulate a response to the stimulus. To be consistent, we also have to apply this transformation of the time axis to the respiratory data. This is necessary to keep the phase relationships between respiration and RSA.

Figure 10 shows a comparison of the phase-response curves from the real stimulation experiments (same data as in Fig. 8C) with the phase-response curves obtained from the processing of the simulated data. Both surfaces are very similar.

To test that none of the determined phase-response curves is just an effect of our data handling, we analyzed the same data without simulation of stimulus responses and calculated the corresponding phase-response curves. If our data-processing methods are appropriate, the latter should be zero. The amplitudes of the phase-response curves without baroreceptor stimulation are indeed negligible with respect to the phase-response curves with stimulation.

To summarize, our methods for data processing are able to extract the phase-response curves from the raw data without significant distortions of these curves and without the introduction of significant systematic errors.

Limitations. This study is restricted to one respiratory frequency (15 breaths/min) and one stimulus strength (70 mmHg) and duration (0.35 s). To obtain a sufficient number of points for each of the 40 classes, we had to apply ~800 stimuli to each subject. A study changing the above parameters would require a multiple of that amount. It is difficult to ensure constant conditions for an experiment extending over several weeks. For example, subjects began to feel uncomfortable after the 3rd day of neck suction.

In summary, our results show that it is possible to separate the influences of respiratory and cardiac phases at the onset of a neck suction impulse on the P-P interval prolongation by a product statement, which is consistent with the hypothesis that efferent vagal activity is a function of afferent baroreceptor activity, whereas respiratory neurons modulate that medullary throughput independent of the cardiac phase. Furthermore, we have shown that stimulus broadening and stimulus cropping influence the outcome of neck suction experiments in a way that makes it virtually impossible to obtain information on the phase dependency of the cardiac pacemaker's sensitivity to vagal stimulation without very accurate knowledge of the functional shape of stimulus broadening.

APPENDIX A

Derivation of normalization constants in Eq. 8. We substitute $f(\phi_s, \phi_r)$ in *Eqs. 6* and *7* by means of *Eq. 5* and obtain

$$f_s(\phi_s) = \langle f_1(\phi_s) f_2(\phi_r) \rangle_{\phi_r} = f_1(\phi_s) \langle f_2(\phi_r) \rangle_{\phi_r}$$

$$f_r(\phi_r) = \langle f_1(\phi_s) f_2(\phi_r) \rangle_{\phi_s} = \langle f_1(\phi_s) \rangle_{\phi_s} f_2(\phi_r) \qquad (A1)$$

Furthermore

$$\langle\langle f(\phi_s, \phi_r) \rangle_{\phi_s} \rangle_{\phi_r} = \langle\langle f_1(\phi_s) f_2(\phi_r) \rangle_{\phi_s} \rangle_{\phi_r} = \langle f_1(\phi_s) \rangle_{\phi_s} \langle f_2(\phi_r) \rangle_{\phi_r} \qquad (A2)$$

and, on the other hand

$$\langle\langle f(\phi_s, \phi_r) \rangle_{\phi_s} \rangle_{\phi_r} = \langle f_r(\phi_r) \rangle_{\phi_r} \qquad (A3)$$

Using *Eqs. 5–7* and *A1–A3* we obtain

$$f(\phi_s, \phi_r) = \frac{f_s(\phi_s) f_r(\phi_r)}{\langle f_1(\phi_s) \rangle_{\phi_s} \langle f_2(\phi_r) \rangle_{\phi_r}} = f_s(\phi_s) \frac{f_r(\phi_r)}{\langle f_r(\phi_r) \rangle_{\phi_r}} \qquad (A4)$$

Dividing *Eq. A4* by the maximum of the cardiac phase-response curve $[f_s(\phi_s)]_{max} = [\langle f(\phi_s, \phi_r)\rangle_{\phi_r}]_{max}$ yields

$$\frac{f(\phi_s, \phi_r)}{[\langle f(\phi_s, \phi_r)\rangle_{\phi_r}]_{max}} = \frac{f_s(\phi_s)}{[f_s(\phi_s)]_{max}} \times \frac{f_r(\phi_r)}{\langle f_r(\phi_r)\rangle_{\phi_r}} \quad (A5)$$

APPENDIX B

Definition of functions used for modeling the influence of finite stimulus duration. For the baroreceptor activity due to a stimulus of duration θ we use

$$s_I(t) = \begin{cases} 0 & \text{for } t \le 0 \\ 1 & \text{for } 0 < t < \theta \\ 0 & \text{for } \theta \le t \end{cases} \quad (B1)$$

(rectangular impulse) or

$$s_{II}(t) = \begin{cases} 0 & \text{for } t \le 0 \\ s_{max} & \text{for } 0 < t < t_c \\ s_{min} + \left(\dfrac{t}{b}\right)^{-a} & \text{for } t_c < t < \theta \\ 0 & \text{for } \theta \le t \end{cases} \quad (B2)$$

with $s_{min} = 0.1$, $s_{max} = 1$, $a = 0.62$, $b = 17$ ms, and $t_c = b/(s_{max} - s_{min})^{1/a}$. Function $s_{II}(t)$ simulates the differential behavior of baroreceptor responses and is a fit to data from Landgren (11). Both $s_I(t)$ and $s_{II}(t)$ are depicted in Fig. 11*A*.

Our first function type for $g(t - \tau)$ is a modified Gaussian curve

$$g_I(t - \tau) = \begin{cases} 0 & \text{for } t - \tau \le \xi \\ \dfrac{1}{\sigma}\sqrt{\dfrac{2}{\pi}} \exp\left(-\dfrac{(t - \tau - \xi - \eta)^2}{2\sigma^2}\right) & \text{for } t - \tau > \xi \end{cases} \quad (B3)$$

The parameter ξ is the mere conduction delay between baroreceptors and the cardiac pacemaker, η is the time between first and maximum response to an infinitely short impulse (delta impulse), and σ is a measure for the width of the response to a delta impulse.

Our second function type for $g(t - \tau)$ is

$$g_{II}(t - \tau) = \begin{cases} 0 & \text{for } t - \tau \le \xi \\ \chi^2_{2+\eta/\sigma}\left(\dfrac{t - \tau - \xi}{\sigma}\right) & \text{for } t - \tau > \xi \end{cases} \quad (B4)$$

where χ^2_n is the χ^2 function defined by

$$\chi^2_n(x) = \frac{x^{n/2-1}e^{-x/2}}{2^{n/2}\Gamma\left(\dfrac{n}{2}\right)} \quad (B5)$$

The meaning of the parameters is the same as above. Figure 11*B* shows $g_I(t)$ and $g_{II}(t)$ for parameters that give the best fit to the measured data.

Finally, we use

$$f_I(\tau) = A \equiv \text{const} \quad (B6)$$

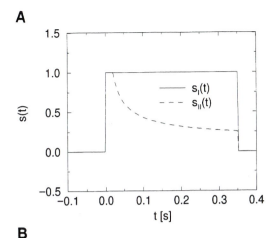

A

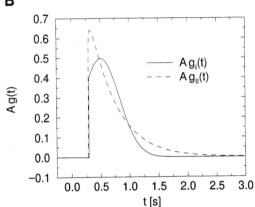

B

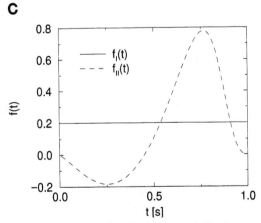

C

Fig. 11. *A*: functions $s_I(t)$ and $s_{II}(t)$ used for modeling baroreceptor activity for stimuli of 0.35-s duration. *B*: functions $g_I(t)$ and $g_{II}(t)$ used for modeling stimulus delay and broadening. $g_I(t)$ is depicted for latency (ξ) = 0.3 s, standard deviation (σ) = 0.32 s, time between first and maximum response to a Delta impulse (η) = 0.21 s, and amplitude (A) = 0.2; $g_{II}(t)$ is depicted for ξ = 0.29 s, σ = 0.21 s, η = 0.03 s, and A = 1.6. These values gave best fit of measured phase-response curve for rectangular baroreceptor activity $s_I(t)$ and for a phase-independent sensitivity of cardiac pacemaker $f_I(t)$. *C*: functions $f_I(t)$ and $f_{II}(t)$ used for modeling cardiac pacemaker's sensitivity to vagal stimulation. $f_I(t)$ is depicted for A = 0.2; $f_{II}(t)$ is depicted for A = 5.7. These values gave best fit of measured phase-response curve for rectangular baroreceptor activity $s_I(t)$ and Gaussian stimulus broadening $g_I(t)$.

or

$$f_{II}(\tau) = \begin{cases} A\tau^{1.3}(\tau - 0.45) \dfrac{(1 - \tau)^3}{(1 - 0.8)^3 + (1 - \tau)^3} & \text{for } \tau < T \\ 0 & \text{for } \tau \geq T \end{cases} \quad (B7)$$

Function $f_{II}(\tau)$ is a fit to a phase-response curve obtained from a mathematical model of the sinus node by Reiner and Antzelevitch (16). In Fig. 11C we depict $f_I(t)$ and $f_{II}(t)$ for parameters that give the best approximation of the measured data.

APPENDIX C

Baroreflex latency: critical review of Borst and Karemaker (1) and Eckberg (3). Borst and Karemaker proposed a latency of 550 ms between the onset of electrical carotid sinus nerve stimuli and the first significant effect on the P-P interval ($P < 0.01$). This is considerably longer than the delay of 0.24 s determined by Eckberg, who measured baroreceptor activity with neck suction. The discrepancy between the two values is partially due to different definitions of the term baroreflex latency. Borst and Karemaker define latency as the time between stimulus onset and first significant effect on the cardiac pacemaker, whereas Eckberg defines latency as the time between stimulus onset and the very first effect on the P-P interval, which should usually occur before the first significant effect. To determine the value for the latter definition of baroreflex latency, Eckberg uses stimuli of decreasing time between stimulus onset and subsequent P peak and extrapolates the obtained curve of P-P interval changes to obtain the delay for a prolongation of zero, which is then defined as the latency.

One should use the same definition of latency if one juxtaposes values determined by different authors. Therefore, we apply Eckberg's (3) definition of baroreflex latency to the data of Borst and Karemaker (1) to make their results comparable.

Borst and Karemaker (1) used two different methods to estimate the baroreflex latency. The first method was according to Koepchen et al. (9). Figure 12 shows the raw data adapted from Fig. 3 in Ref. 1. If the time between stimulus onset and the anticipated subsequent P peak ($t_{St \rightarrow P_a}$) is less

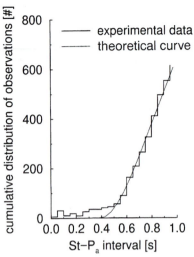

Fig. 13. Cumulative excess as a function of $t_{St \rightarrow Pa}$. Data are from Fig. 4 in Ref. 1. Theoretical curve is a fit to these data and was calculated by a model (see text).

than the baroreflex latency (ξ) [according to Eckberg (3)], there is no effect on P-P interval. However, if this time is greater than the latency, heart period prolongation should be roughly proportional to the part of the stimulus that influences the current heart cycle. Therefore, we extrapolate the steep part of the curve in Fig. 12 linearly to obtain the delay between stimulus onset and anticipated P peak for which the effect on heart period becomes zero. This yields a value of 390 ± 30 (SE) ms for Eckberg's definition of the baroreflex latency.

The second method of Borst and Karemaker (1) involves the method of cumulative sums (14). The disturbed P-P interval (I_{n+1}) was compared with the preceding undisturbed interval (I_n). Without stimulation, the probability for I_{n+1} being greater than I_n is 0.5. The excess over that probability was determined for stimulated intervals. The cumulated excess was plotted vs. the time between stimulus onset and anticipated P peak. Baroreceptor latency was determined as the time for the first significant deviation of cumulative excess from zero.

To apply Eckberg's (3) definition of latency to the method of cumulative sums, we theoretically estimate the shape of cumulative excess.

The idea is quite simple: if $t_{St \rightarrow P_a}$ is slightly larger than the baroreflex latency, the stimulus is cropped: only a part of the stimulus can contribute to the prolongation of the considered P-P interval. Hence, the excess is less than for those P-P intervals that are influenced by the entire stimulus. This causes a smaller slope of the cumulative excess for $t_{St \rightarrow P_a}$, which are only slightly larger than the latency.

To model this influence, we make the following assumptions: *1*) The P-P interval is noisy. The noise variable (ϵ) is Gaussian distributed around the mean heart period with a standard deviation σ. *2*) The average prolongation of the disturbed interval (Δt_{pp}) is proportional to the part (or duration) of the stimulus that falls within the current P-P interval. The proportionality constant (a) is the baroreflex sensitivity. To take into consideration that the impulse is delayed when it affects the cardiac pacemaker, we shift the time axis by a latency (ξ). *3*) The stimulus duration (θ) is 300 ms, as used by Borst and Karemaker (1).

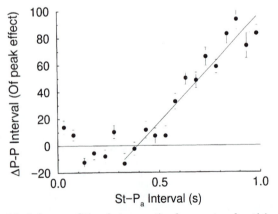

Fig. 12. Influence of time between stimulus onset and anticipated P wave ($t_{St \rightarrow P_a}$) on change of current P-P interval. Data points are from Fig. 3 in Ref. 1. We added a linear regression for steep increase of P-P interval changes for large $t_{St \rightarrow P_a}$. Linear regression intersects x-axis at $t_{St \rightarrow P_a} = 0.39 \pm 0.03$ (SE) s.

We do not take into account that the effect of 1 mmHg·s of integrated baroreceptor stimulation is not constant but depends on its timing within the cardiac cycle. An approach including this dependency is much more complicated and does not alter the general statement that the latency determined by the first significant increase in the cumulative excess is longer than the latency between stimulus onset and first effect on the cardiac pacemaker.

With the three above assumptions, we calculate the cumulative excess. The P-P interval prolongation depends on the time $\tau = t_{\mathrm{St}\to\mathrm{P_a}} + \epsilon - \xi$, which is the part of a stimulus that is within the considered P-P interval

$$\Delta\mathrm{PP} = \epsilon + \begin{cases} 0 & \text{for } \tau \leq 0 \\ a\tau & \text{for } 0 < \tau < \theta \\ a\theta & \text{for } \theta \leq \tau \end{cases} \quad (C1)$$

Using this model, one can calculate the probability that the P-P interval is prolonged [prob $(\Delta\mathrm{PP} > 0)$]

$$\mathrm{prob}\,(\Delta\mathrm{PP} > 0) = \frac{1}{\sqrt{2\pi}\sigma} \int_{-\infty}^{\infty} \Theta[\Delta\mathrm{PP}(\epsilon)] \exp\left(-\frac{\epsilon^2}{2\sigma^2}\right) d\epsilon \quad (C2)$$

$\Theta(x)$ is the Heaviside function defined by

$$\Theta(x) = \begin{cases} 0 & \text{for } x \leq 0 \\ 1 & \text{for } x > 0 \end{cases} \quad (C3)$$

The excess [$\mathrm{E}(t_{\mathrm{St}\to\mathrm{P_a}})$] is defined as the difference between the probability of P-P interval prolongation and the probability of P-P interval shortening

$$\begin{aligned} \mathrm{E}(t_{\mathrm{St}\to\mathrm{P_a}}) &= \mathrm{prob}\,(\Delta\mathrm{PP} > 0) - \mathrm{prob}\,(\Delta\mathrm{PP} \leq 0) \\ &= 2\,\mathrm{prob}\,(\Delta\mathrm{PP} > 0) - 1 \end{aligned} \quad (C4)$$

Straightforward calculations yield

$$\mathrm{E}(t_{\mathrm{St}\to\mathrm{P_a}})$$

$$= \begin{cases} 0 & \text{for } t_{\mathrm{St}\to\mathrm{P_a}} \leq 0 \\ \mathrm{erf}\left(\dfrac{a}{a+1}\dfrac{t_{\mathrm{St}\to\mathrm{P_a}} - \xi}{\sqrt{2}\sigma}\right) & \text{for } 0 < t_{\mathrm{St}\to\mathrm{P_a}} - \xi < (a+1)\theta \\ \mathrm{erf}\left(a\dfrac{\theta}{\sqrt{2}\sigma}\right) & \text{for } (a+1)\theta \leq t_{\mathrm{St}\to\mathrm{P_a}} - \xi \end{cases} \quad (C5)$$

with

$$\mathrm{erf}\,(x) = \frac{2}{\sqrt{\pi}} \int_0^x e^{-t^2}\, dt \quad (C6)$$

The cumulative excess [$\mathrm{CE}(t_{\mathrm{St}\to\mathrm{Pa}})$] is defined by

$$\mathrm{CE}(t_{\mathrm{St}\to\mathrm{Pa}}) = \int_0^{t_{\mathrm{St}\to\mathrm{Pa}}} \mathrm{E}(t)\, dt \quad (C7)$$

With *Eqs. C5–C7* we calculate the cumulative excess. These equations contain three free parameters: the standard deviation of noise σ, the baroreflex latency (ξ), and the baroreflex sensitivity (a). We use Powell's method (15) to determine the parameters that give the best fit (in the sense of least squares) to the experimental data of Borst and Karemaker (1). They are $\sigma = 51$ ms, $\xi = 406$ ms, and $a = 0.54$. Figure 13

shows the cumulative excess calculated using *Eqs. C5–C7* for this set of parameters and the cumulative excess determined experimentally by Borst and Karemaker. Borst and Karemaker did not publish the standard deviation of P-P intervals for their subjects. However, in our experiments the standard deviation ranged from 17 to 121 ms for the different subjects, with an average of 54 ms. This is well in accordance with the value of 51 ms determined by the model. The baroreflex latency of 406 ms according to Eckberg's definition (3) is considerably shorter than the value of 550 ms advanced by Borst and Karemaker. The cause for the deviation of the theoretical curve from the experimental curve for short intervals $t_{\mathrm{St}\to\mathrm{P_a}}$ is unclear.

In summary, both methods give a value of ~400 ms for Eckberg's definition (3) of baroreflex latency. Although this is 150 ms less than the latency according to Borst and Karemaker (1), it is still 160 ms longer than the value of 240 ms determined by Eckberg. A possible explanation for this discrepancy is that the authors used different groups of subjects. Eckberg studied young healthy subjects, whereas Borst and Karemaker investigated patients with coronary heart disease.

We thank Larry A. Beightol for technical assistance, and we especially thank the subjects who volunteered for the study.

This study was supported by a grant from the Department of Veterans Affairs, National Heart, Lung, and Blood Institute Grant HL-22296, National Aeronautics and Space Administration Grants NAG2-408 and NAS10-10285, and Deutsche Forschungsgemeinschaft Grant He 2168/3-1.

Address for reprint requests: H. Seidel, Technische Universität Berlin, Sekr. PN 7-1, Hardenbergstr. 36, D-10623 Berlin, Germany.

Received 5 September 1995; accepted in final form 31 October 1996.

REFERENCES

1. **Borst, C., and J. M. Karemaker.** Time delays in the human baroreceptor reflex. *J. Auton. Nerv. Syst.* 9: 399–409, 1983.
2. **Brown, G. L., and J. C. Eccles.** The action of a single vagal volley on the rhythm of the heart beat. *J. Physiol. (Lond.)* 82: 211–241, 1934.
3. **Eckberg, D. L.** Temporal response patterns of the human sinus node to brief carotid baroreceptor stimuli. *J. Physiol. (Lond.)* 258: 769–782, 1976.
4. **Eckberg, D. L., M. S. Cavanaugh, A. Mark, and F. M. Abboud.** A simplified neck suction device for activation of carotid baroreceptors. *J. Lab. Clin. Med.* 85: 167–173, 1975.
5. **Eckberg, D. L., Y. T. Kifle, and V. L. Roberts.** Phase relationship between normal human respiration and baroreflex responsiveness. *J. Physiol. (Lond.)* 304: 489–502, 1980.
6. **Eckberg, D. L., and C. R. Orshan.** Respiratory and baroreceptor reflex interactions in man. *J. Clin. Invest.* 59: 780–785, 1977.
7. **Guevara, M. R., and H. J. Jongsma.** Phase resetting in a model of sinoatrial nodal membrane: ionic and topological aspects. *Am. J. Physiol.* 258 (*Heart Circ. Physiol.* 27): H734–H747, 1990.
8. **Karemaker, J. M.** Cardiac cycle time effects: information processing and the latencies involved. In: *Psychophysiology of Cardiovascular Control*, edited by J. F. Orlebeke, G. Mulder, and L. J. O. van Dooren. New York: Plenum, 1985, p. 535–548.
9. **Koepchen, H. P., H. D. Lux, and P.-H. Wagner.** Untersuchungen über Zeitbedarf und zentrale Verarbeitung des pressoreceptorischen Herzreflexes. *Pflügers Arch.* 273: 413–430, 1961.
10. **Kunze, D. L.** Reflex discharge patterns of cardiac vagal efferent fibers. *J. Physiol. (Lond.)* 222: 1–15, 1972.
11. **Landgren, S.** On the excitation mechanism of the carotid baroreceptors. *Acta Physiol. Scand.* 26: 1–34, 1952.
12. **Levy, M. N., T. Iano, and H. Zieske.** Effects of repetitive bursts of vagal activity on heart rate. *Circ. Res.* 30: 186–195, 1972.

13. **Pickering, T. G., and J. Davies.** Estimation of the conduction time of the baroreceptor-cardiac reflex in man. *Cardiovasc. Res.* 7: 213–219, 1973.
14. **Pickering, T. G., B. Gribbin, and P. Sleight.** Comparison of the reflex heart rate response to rising and falling pressure in man. *Cardiovasc. Res.* 6: 277–283, 1972.
15. **Press, W. H., S. A. Teukolsky, W. T. Vetterling, and B. P. Flannery.** *Numerical Recipes in C.* Cambridge, UK: Cambridge University Press, 1992.
16. **Reiner, V. S., and C. Antzelevitch.** Phase resetting and annihilation in a mathematical model of sinus node. *Am. J. Physiol.* 249 (*Heart Circ. Physiol.* 18): H1143–H1153, 1985.
17. **Seidel, H., and H. Herzel.** Modelling heart rate variability due to respiration and baroreflex. In: *Modelling the Dynamics of Biological Systems,* edited by E. Mosekilde and O. G. Mouritsen. Berlin: Springer-Verlag, 1995, p. 205–229.
18. **Wanzhen, Z., L. Glass, and A. Shrier.** The topology of phase response curves induced by single and paired stimuli in spontaneously oscillating chick heart cell aggregates. *J. Biol. Rhythms* 7: 89–104, 1992.
19. **Yang, T., M. D. Jacobstein, and M. N. Levy.** Synchronization of automatic cells in S-A node during vagal stimulation in dogs. *Am. J. Physiol.* 246 (*Heart Circ. Physiol.* 15): H585–H591, 1984.

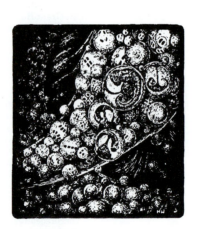

Modelling Heart Rate Variability Due to Respiration and Baroreflex

Henrik Seidel and Hanspeter Herzel

Abstract

This chapter is concerned with the interactions of heart beat, respiration, and blood pressure oscillations. We develop a nonlinear model which describes the essential parts of the baroreceptor loop: blood pressure wave, baroreceptor activity, cardio-respiratory center, and regulation of heart rate and vascular resistance via the autonomic nerves. Special attention is paid to the phase response properties of the cardiac pacemaker.

The model accounts for heart rate regulation, respiratory sinus arrhythmia (RSA), and resonant interaction of respiration and blood pressure oscillations (Mayer waves). External stimulations can induce toroidal oscillations, resonances, period-doubling, and chaotic behavior.

1 Introduction

In industrialized countries, one of the most frequent causes of death is a severe malfunction of the cardiovascular system. Yet, our present understanding of the dynamic regimes of this system and its interaction with respiration is very limited. This is partly due to the fact that many different mechanisms contribute to the control of circulation. They operate on time scales from seconds (baroreceptors, chemoreceptors) to minutes (renin-angiotensin) and even hours (renal fluid volume). Direct measurements of quantities involved in the control of the cardio-vascular system are very difficult (autonomic nervous system) or even impossible (medullary circulation centers) without serious intervention in the system. Hence, we have to deal with hidden or, at least, partially hidden variables.

For several reasons, information about the dynamics of these variables is of considerable interest. There is, for example, experimental evidence suggesting that a high sympathetic activity during myocardial infarction greatly increases the probability of a fatal cardiac arrhythmia [26]. Several diseases (e.g.

diabetes) can cause dysfunction of the autonomic nervous system. Anaesthetics may influence autonomic nerves or the vascular peripheral resistance and lead to circulation insufficiency. Failure of blood pressure control can cause hypertension and fainting or may facilitate heart arrhythmia and sudden death. Therefore, it is desirable to have a model that can relate the "hidden" variables to easily measurable data such as heart rate variability (HRV) and respiration.

The heart rate is not steady even when the level of physiological activity is constant or during deep sleep when there is no conscious psychic influence. Various rhythmic variations are observed. Coupling between the respiratory cycle and the heart beat causes oscillations of the heart rate with a frequency of approximately 0.25 Hz (4 s), referred to as respiratory sinus arrhythmia (RSA). The amplitude of RSA decreases with age. Furthermore, oscillations in heart rate appear at periods of approximately 10 s (Mayer waves) and, sometimes, 30 s. Their origin is imperfectly understood. Over a wide range, the heart rate exhibits a $1/f$ spectrum, the cause of which is also unknown [26]. Some of these rhythms are generated or, at least, influenced by circulation control mechanisms and their interaction with respiration. Their analysis by means of a model may allow conclusions about internal variables such as sympathetic and parasympathetic activity and, hence, can be used for diagnostic and prognostic purposes.

In this chapter, we attempt to establish a mathematical model which may contribute to the explanation of qualitative properties of circulation dynamics. Physiological systems are very complex, with numerous nonnegligible, interacting quantities. Only in the rarest cases it is possible to find simple mathematical expressions for these systems. Often only qualitative connections between physiological variables are known, and many parameters have to be guessed. Therefore, detailed modelling is nearly impossible, and we have to look for a compromise: the model must be complex enough to reconstruct essential features of the system. On the other hand, it must be simple enough to be useful for conceptualization.

The system treated in this chapter contains elements, where even qualitative properties are still disputed. This is particularly true for medullary interactions. For that reason, our model cannot and does not claim quantitative agreement with the physiological experiments. We want to investigate the qualitative behavior of the model and to compare it with experimental results. We hope that it can be a help in answering some as yet open physiological questions.

2 Heart, Respiration, and Baroreflex: Basic Dynamical Features

Before we present our model, we want to discuss some of its basic mechanisms. This discussion is very introductory, and the reader is referred to standard physiological literature [40, 3] for further information.

2.1 Heart

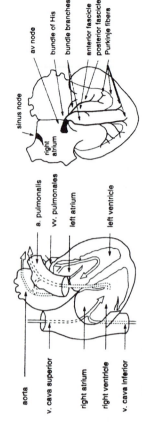

Fig. 1. The heart and its stimulus conducting system (adapted from [39])

The heart can be considered a complex oscillator. It contains several elements of specialized myocardial tissue forming a stimulus conducting system (Fig. 1). The sinus node, the atrio-ventricular node, and the Purkinje system are capable of oscillating independently. There is a hierarchy among these pacemakers with respect to their firing rates. If the heart is normal, the sinus node determines the heart rate (ca. 70 min^{-1} at rest). After the excitation has passed the AV-node, it quickly spreads along the bundle of His, to the Purkinje fibers, and then over the whole heart, resulting in a contraction. The frequency of the atrio-ventricular node is somewhat less (40–60 min^{-1}). Normally, the AV-node gets entrained by the sinus node. Only if the conduction from the sinus node towards the AV-node fails or is weakened (AV-block), the AV-node becomes the active pacemaker of the heart. If neither impulses from the sino-atrial nor from the atrio-ventricular node can reach the ventricles, the Purkinje system takes over rhythm generation (ca. 20 min^{-1}).

The myocardial tissue shows a post-systolic refractory behavior, i.e. each heart beat is followed by a certain time span characterized by the inexcitability of the cells. Hence, usually one impulse cannot excite a myocardial cell twice after an infarction, the impulse may reenter a previously excited area after the end of the refractory period, leading to an extra-systolic heart beat or, even worse, to circulating waves or fibrillation.

Another cause of arrhythmia are *ectopic pacemakers*. They consist of degenerated self-oscillating cardiac muscle tissue. Sinus node and ectopic pacemakers interact and influence each other. Hence, they form a system of two coupled oscillators which is capable of evoking complex rhythms as entrainment, period doubling, and chaos [31, 4, 25, 20, 22, 5, 33, 19]

The heart is influenced by the autonomic nervous system in order to react to different stress situations. Three main effects are distinguished. High sympathetic activity increases, and high parasympathetic activity decreases the frequency of the sinus node (chronotropic effect), the contractility of the heart (inotropic effect), and the velocity of atrio-ventricular conduction (dromotropic effect).

2.2 Respiration

In the respiratory system, the rhythm generating pacemaker and the executing organ are spatially separated. Usually a central pattern generator is assumed to be situated in the *medulla oblangata*. Numerous physiological experiments have been performed in order to localize exactly the source of the respiratory rhythm. Until now, however, only preliminary concepts about the rhythm generation exist. A number of mathematical models have been established. These models are based on several groups of neurons mutually inhibiting or exciting [15, 14, 18, 50, 28, 44, 43, 16, 36] and are still rather speculative.

The impulses generated in the medulla oblangata are carried by the *phrenic nerve* to the diaphragm. Feedback is given by thoracic stress receptors and chemoreceptors sensitive to the blood concentrations of CO_2, H^+, and O_2. Numerous authors have tried to model these feedback loops. Some of the models include metabolic changes during muscular activity and contain more than one hundred equations [32].

2.3 Baroreceptors

Baroreceptors, sometimes also called *pressure receptors*, are neuronal cells wound around blood vessels. They respond with a change in their firing frequency to a strain in their cell membrane. The vascular walls expand at high pressures, enabling the baroreceptors to sense the blood pressure.

Upon closer examination, it turns out that the firing frequency of the baroreceptors depends both on the pressure and on its time derivative. Fig. 2 shows typical responses of baroreceptors to pressure waves. A review of baroreceptor models is given in [41].

Baroreceptors are located along the aorta. The most important of them are situated in the *aortic arch* directly at the heart and at the *sinus caroticus* in the neck. Their impulses are led by the *aortic nerve* and the *carotid sinus nerve* towards the brain. Both nerves cause a decrease in blood pressure when

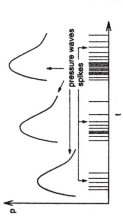

Fig. 2. Responses of baroreceptors to blood pressure waves of different strengths (schematic).

stimulated. Thus, it it possible to understand how the baroreceptors manage their task of regulating the blood pressure: when the pressure increases, the vascular walls expand, the firing rates of the baroreceptors and, consequently, of the aortic and the carotid sinus nerve rise, causing a drop in blood pressure. Without any time delay in that control loop, the blood pressure would approach a constant value. However, as a consequence of the finite conduction times and further time delays, complicated rhythms can occur.

3 The Baroreceptor Loop

In figure 3, the structure of the baroreceptor loop is depicted. In this section we introduce the remaining parts of that loop.

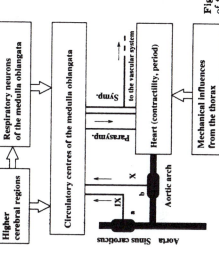

Fig. 3. Schematic representation of the baroreceptor control loop

3.1 Medullary Circulation Centers

The *medullary circulation centers* mix several inputs. Afferents from the baro- and chemoreceptors, impulses from higher cerebral regions, and from respiratory neurons are combined. The result of this process is led by the *sympathetic* and the *parasympathetic nerves* to the effector organs.

The knowledge about information processing in the medulla is very limited. The following points are generally accepted:

1. The sympathetic activity is reduced by an increased activity of the aortic nerve or the carotid sinus nerve.
2. The parasympathetic activity is enhanced by an increased activity of the aortic nerve or the carotid sinus nerve.
3. The phase of the respiratory cycle determines the strength of the influences mentioned above.

Statements going beyond this are hard to defend. In the physiological literature, one often finds contradicting opinions [29, 23, 42, 11, 13, 9, 17, 6, 36, 37]. A commonly accepted quantitative transfer function from the efferent to the afferent activities does not exist.

For these reasons, it is very difficult to model the medulla. Hence, it seems reasonable to limit our description to a minimal set of plausible equations representing the medulla at least qualitatively.

3.2 Sympathetic and Parasympathetic Nerves, Heart and Vascular System

In addition to voluntary movements and to the hormonal system, the autonomic nervous system controls the reaction of an organism to a change of its environmental or internal state. The autonomic system's afferent parts are the antagonistic *sympathetic* and *parasympathetic* nerves. Feedback is given by *visceral afferents*. Usually, the sympathetic nerves have an activating effect, whereas the parasympathetic nerves are inhibiting.

Large parts of the parasympathetic system are located in the left or right *vagus*. The common vagal synaptic transmitter is *acetylcholine*, the sympathetic nerves usually use *noradrenaline*. In consequence of their mythelization, the vagal axons have a very high impulse velocity (up to 100 m/s) in comparison with sympathetic neurons (ca. 1 m/s). Furthermore, the effect of acetylcholine is faster than that of noradrenaline. Acetylcholine is decomposed by *cholinesterases* in the synaptic gap. Noradrenaline needs to be removed from the synaptic gap and broken down at another location. This process takes much longer than the decomposition of acetylcholine. Hence, sympathetic dynamics are slower than their parasympathetic counterpart, and we will treat the two influences as mathematically distinct.

Now we want to turn to the actions of the autonomic nerves on several elements of the baroreceptor control loop. The blood vessels are influenced

nearly exclusively by the sympathetic system. An elevated sympathetic activity decreases the elasticity of the vascular walls and thereby produces an increase in blood pressure.

The heart is supplied both by the sympathetic and the parasympathetic system. The sympathetic nerves innervate the whole heart. A high sympathetic activity increases the contractility and the heart rate by opening calcium channels. The vagus innervates mainly the sinus node and the atria. Its left part is responsible for the AV-node, the right one for the sinus node and the right atrium. The parasympathetic effect on the contractility is restricted to the atria. Since the main work of the heart is done by the ventricles, we shall neglect the vagal influence on the contractility in order not to complicate the model. The parasympathetic effect on the heart rate is based on the activity of potassium channels.

As a consequence of the slow sympathetic dynamics, the distribution of sympathetic impulses over a heart cycle is not very important. The noradrenaline concentration acts like a buffer.

This is completely different for the parasympathetic influence on the heart. The acetylcholine concentration follows the vagal activity nearly immediately. The effect of acetylcholine on the time course of the sino-atrial action potential strongly depends on the phase of the heart cycle. We shall use a *phase-response curve* to describe this behavior.

The respiration acts on the other elements of the baroreceptor loop by medullary respiratory neurons and by mechanical influences of the thorax on the heart. According to [9], the latter causes only approximately ten percent of the overall interaction between heart and respiration. In a first approach to modelling the system, we shall neglect mechanical influences.

4 The Model

Let us now try to formulate a nonlinear model of the baroreceptor control loop that accounts for processes within a heart cycle. A popular beat-to-beat-model was published some years ago by De Boer and Karemaker [7] (another one is given, e.g., by Baselli et al. [2]). However, their model has a number of severe disadvantages:

1. Respiration is taken into account only through its mechanical influence. As mentioned above, according to [9], the nervous influence by respiratory neurons is much stronger than the mechanical one.
2. Contrary to experimental evidence, a direct sympathetic influence on the contractility of the heart does not exist in that model.
3. In the physiological system several time delays occur. These are accounted for by considering the preceding six heart beats. This implies that there is no absolute time scale in the model – the duration of the heart period being used as the time step. Consequently, the simulated time delays

decrease to the same extent as the heart rate increases. This may distort the dynamics.

4. The effect of a vagal stimulation of the sinus node depends on the phase of the heart cycle [51]. Since the smallest time scale used by de Boer and Karemaker is the heart period, this essential effect cannot be taken into account in the model.
5. The model has been examined only in its linearized form.

We shall attempt to develop a model that overcomes these problems.

4.1 Modelling Neuronal Activity

In order to model neuronal activity on time scales of milliseconds, several complications have to be overcome. Typical firing rates of the fibers of the autonomic nervous system are in the order of 4–5 s⁻¹. Consequently, it seems not to be possible to describe neuronal activity only by firing rates. On the other hand, with current physiological knowledge, it is not possible to model such a complex system as circulation control on the basis of single spikes, especially given the lack of knowledge concerning the medullary processes.

To find a way out of this situation, one could try to use firing rates (particularly for the medullary transfer function) and to switch to single spikes for elements that are highly sensitive to the exact moment of occurrence of an impulse. A probability distribution for the occurrence of a spike at a given firing frequency could be used to determine the moment of the next spike.

In our model we adopt another formulation. Usually, a nerve consists of numerous axons. We assume that these fibers correlate in their firing frequency on greater time scales, but not in the occurrence of single spikes. Then it is possible to define an activity ν of single fibers for the transition to an infinite number N of axons by

$$\nu = \lim_{\delta t \to 0} \frac{1}{\delta t} \lim_{N \to \infty} \frac{N(\delta t)}{N} \qquad (1)$$

where $N(\delta t)$ is the number of fibers firing in the time interval δt. Let τ be the duration of an impulse and f the mean firing frequency of a fiber. Then the limit is well approximated for $N \gg 1/(\tau f)$. With $\tau \approx 1$ ms and $f \approx 5$ s⁻¹, this means $N \gg 200$. In the following we assume that the number of fibers is high enough for this approximation to be valid.

4.2 Modelling Baroreceptors

In order to describe the response of the baroreceptor's activity to the blood pressure wave, we use the simple equation

$$\nu_b = k_1 \left(p - p^{(0)} \right) + k_2 \frac{dp}{dt}, \qquad (2)$$

originally proposed by Warner [47]. More complicated models are available (see the review given by Taher et al. [41]). However, it is not a good idea to put much effort into the modelling of one particular element of the system, when this accuracy may be lost because of insufficient knowledge in other parts. By applying (2) we neglect that

1. baroreceptors run into saturation at high pressures,
2. baroreceptors show adaption to a changed mean pressure,
3. there is a slight asymmetry in k_2 in dependence on the direction of the pressure change,
4. different baroreceptors have different inputs (the wave form changes along the aorta) and outputs (the coefficients k_1 and k_2 may vary for different baroreceptors),
5. the conduction times towards the medulla depend on the location of the baroreceptors.

Some of these phenomena may be included as the physiology of the medulla becomes known in more detail.

4.3 Modelling Sympathetic and Parasympathetic Activity

The description of the response of sympathetic and parasympathetic activity to the afferents from the baroreceptors and to respiratory influences is the most critical point of the model. As already mentioned, very little is known about medullary processes. For that reason, we shall keep the equations as simple as possible and assume a linear dependence of the sympathetic and parasympathetic activity on the activity of the baroreceptors.

One can find different, often contradictory opinions about the influence of respiratory neurons on the autonomic nerves. Eckberg [11, 10, 9, 12] found augmented sympathetic and vagal activities during expiration, though he points to the fact that other authors draw opposite conclusions.

Fortunately, concerning our model, it is not important during which phase in the respiratory cycle autonomic activity is augmented or reduced so long as we restrict the interaction between the respiration and baroreceptor loops to a single location only. Since we shall consider only medullary neuronal influences of respiration, this holds true in our case. An incorrectly chosen activating phase of the respiratory cycle corresponds to a shift of respiration relative to circulatory rhythms. Their dynamics remains unchanged, however. If we wanted to include mechanical interaction, we would have to use exact phase relations of gating.

In accordance with the above considerations, we shall describe the activities of the sympathetic and vagal activities, respectively, by the equations

$$\nu_s = \max\left(0, \nu_s^{(0)} - k_s^b \nu_b + k_s^r \sin\left(\pi f_r t + \Delta \phi_s^r\right)\right) \qquad (3)$$

214   Henrik Seidel and Hanspeter Herzel

$$\nu_p = \max\left(0, \nu_p^{(0)} + k_p^b \nu_b + k_p^r \left|\sin\left(\pi f_r t + \Delta\phi_p^r\right)\right|\right)$$ (4)

where superscripts of the proportionality constants k are mere labels. The sympathetic activity ν_s is composed of a resting-tone $\nu_s^{(0)}$, an inhibitory influence $k_s^b \nu_b$ from the baroreceptors, and an additional modulation by respiratory neurons. These three components are assumed to be linearly integrated by neurons of the circulation centers. When the inhibition is very strong, this integration can give a negative result, implying a complete suppression of sympathetic activity. We take this into account by means of the maximum function.

The description of the parasympathetic activity is performed analogously, with an activating effect of the baroreceptors.

4.4 Modelling the Heart

Our representation of the heart includes a variety of different phenomena:

4.4.1 Dromotropic Effect

The contractility of the heart is externally influenced by the sympathetic nerves. We neglect parasympatheticly induced contractility changes of the atria. Because of the slow dynamics of noradrenaline, it is necessary to introduce a cardiac noradrenaline concentration c_{cNa}:

$$\frac{dc_{cNa}}{dt} = -\frac{c_{cNa}}{\tau_{cNa}} + k_{cNa}^s \nu_s(t - \theta_{cNa}),$$ (5)

where $\nu_s(t)$ is the sympathetic activity at the medulla at time t. A time delay is taken into account by θ_{cNa}. This delay is caused by finite conduction velocity and the time that noradrenaline needs to produce an effect on the heart.

Furthermore, at high heart rates fatigue may occur and decrease the contractility. In addition, the potassium conductivity does not return to its resting-value. This has an accelerating effect on the next repolarisation and thereby decreases the contractility S_i. For these reasons, we use the equations

$$S_i' = S^{(0)} + k_S^c c_{cNa} + k_S^t T_{i-1}$$ (6)

$$S_i = S_i' + (\hat{S} - S_i')\frac{S_i'^{n_S}}{S_i'^{n_S} + \hat{S}^{n_S}}$$ (7)

to describe the contractility S_i of the ith heart beat. T_{i-1} denotes the duration of the heart beat immediately preceding the systole. By equation (7), at high values the contractility is saturated. The fraction in the second term of that equation is a threshold function. Figure 4 shows this function for some exponents n_S.

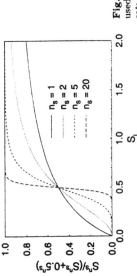

Fig. 4. Threshold function used for the description of saturation.

4.4.2 Chronotropic Effect

We want to model the heart on time scales less than the heart period. With this purpose we introduce a phase φ of the sinus node, satisfying the equation

$$\frac{d\varphi}{dt} = \frac{1}{T^{(0)}} f_s f_p.$$ (8)

The factors f_s and f_p represent the sympathetic and parasympathetic influence on the phase velocity. They are given by

$$f_s = 1 + k_\varphi^{cNa}\left(c_{cNa} + (\hat{c}_{cNa} - c_{cNa})\frac{c_{cNa}^{n_{cNa}}}{\hat{c}_{cNa}^{n_{cNa}} + c_{cNa}^{n_{cNa}}}\right)$$ (9)

$$f_p = 1 - k_\varphi^p\left(\nu_{p,\theta_p} + (\hat{\nu}_p - \nu_{p,\theta_p})\frac{\nu_{p,\theta_p}^{n_p}}{\hat{\nu}_p^{n_p} + \nu_{p,\theta_p}^{n_p}}\right)F(\varphi)$$ (10)

where $\nu_{p,\theta_p} \equiv \nu_p(t - \theta_p)$. Saturation is achieved analogously to equation (7). When the phase φ reaches the value 1, a new heart beat is stimulated (integrate-and-fire-model). The phase is reset to 0 and the contractility S_i is added to the diastolic pressure to give the new systolic pressure.

The function F in equation (10) requires some explanation. We already mentioned that the effect of vagal impulses on the sinus node depends on the phase at which they occur during the heart cycle. For single stimuli, this can be described by a phase-response curve [30, 24, 5, 19, 45, 46]. The theory of phase-response curves usually assumes instantaneous relaxation to a limit cycle after a perturbation. This is approximately attained if the relaxation time is negligible in comparison with the time interval between spikes. However, since we use vagal activities instead of single spikes, there are no longer discrete parasympathetic events, and the phase-response concept is not applicable in its original form. Nevertheless, we want to take into account that an increase of vagal activity has another effect at the beginning of a heart cycle than at the end. Therefore, we introduce a *phase-effectiveness curve*. In order to explain the meaning of that curve, let us first assume the activity

216   Henrik Seidel and Hanspeter Herzel

to be a single rectangular impulse starting at t_s, having a duration of θ and an amplitude a with $\theta a = b \equiv$ const. Let T be the undisturbed period of the system and t_0 the time of the last point of intersection of the trajectory with the ($\phi = 0$)-plane. Then, the effect of an impulse can be calculated using the phase-effectiveness curve by

$$\Delta\phi = \int_{t_s}^{t_s+\theta} aF\left(\frac{t-t_0}{T}\right) dt. \quad (11)$$

For continuous F, this can be written as

$$\Delta\phi = bF\left(\frac{t_\xi}{T}\right), \quad (12)$$

where $t_\xi \in [t_0+t_s, t_0+t_s+\theta]$. Hence, for $\theta \to 0$ the phase-effectiveness should approach the phase-response curve

$$\Delta\phi = f_b(\phi) \quad (13)$$

except for a proportionality constant. In other words, if one knows the phase-response curve of a system, it is reasonable to set the phase-effectiveness curve proportional to that curve.

Of course, even the phase-effectiveness curve is only an approximation of the real processes. Each perturbation causes a deviation from the attractor. Consequently, the distance between the system's phase space position and the attractor depends on the stimulation history. Therefore, to be exact, F should be a function of the whole history of the system. Unfortunately, this would destroy our hope of getting a simple description of the system by means of phase-response concepts.

For that reason, we have to accept the inaccuracies resulting from the use of a phase-effectiveness curve. In order to estimate the error, one must know the complete high-dimensional system, as it is described, e.g., for the sinus node by the DiFrancesco-Noble-equations [8, 34]. Such an analysis is difficult and would require much time and effort. Presently, we restrict ourselves to the investigation of the capabilities of the model and try to compare its output with experimental results.

The phase-effectiveness curve that we have chosen is of the form

$$F(\varphi) = \varphi^{1.3}(\varphi - 0.45)\frac{(1-\varphi)^3}{(1-0.8)^3 + (1-\varphi)^3}, \quad (14)$$

approximating a phase-response curve derived numerically from a mathematical model of the sinus node by Reiner et al. [35] (fig. 5).

The functional form of equation (8) is similar to a model of Rosenblueth and Simeone [38]. They proposed that the dependence of the heart rate on autonomic activity can be expressed by

---

Modelling Heart Rate Variability Due to Respiration and Baroreflex   217

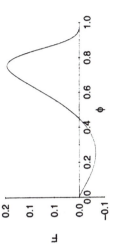

Fig. 5. Graph of the phase-effectiveness curve used in the model, see equation (14).

$$R = R^{(0)}f_s f_p = R^{(0)}\left[1 + \frac{\nu_s}{R^{(0)}(k_1 + k_2\nu_s)}\right]\left[1 - \frac{\nu_p}{R^{(0)}(k_3 + k_4\nu_p)}\right]. \quad (15)$$

Katona et al. [27] have shown the compatibility of this equation with another model proposed by Warner and Russel [48]. In both models, the total effect of vagal and sympathetic activity on the heart rate can be represented by a product of two factors, each depending only on the activity of one of the nerves.

4.4.3 Modelling the Vascular System

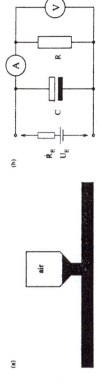

Fig. 6. (a) Origin of the *Windkessel* model, (b) Electric analogue

We use a *windkessel* model (fig. 6) to represent the vascular system. An elevated sympathetic activity causes a constriction of the blood vessels and, consequently, leads to an augmented peripheral resistance or, in other words, to an increased time constant τ of the *windkessel* model. Similarly to (5), we introduce another noradrenaline concentration at the blood vessels

$$\frac{dc_{vNa}}{dt} = -\frac{c_{vNa}}{\tau_{vNa}} + k^s_{c,vNa}\nu_s(t - \theta_{vNa}). \quad (16)$$

Then, the *windkessel* time constant is given by

$$\tau_v = \tau_v^{(0)} + \bar{\tau}_v\left(c_{vNa} + (\hat{c}_{vNa} - c_{vNa})\frac{c_{vNa}^{n_{vNa}}}{\hat{c}_{vNa}^{n_{vNa}} + c_{vNa}^{n_{vNa}}}\right), \quad (17)$$

where $\tau_v^{(0)}$ and $\bar\tau_v$ are constants.

Finally, we need a representation for the blood pressure itself. We divide each pulse wave into two parts. During the systolic increase of pressure, we use

$$p_I = d_{i-1} + S_i \frac{t - t_i}{\tau_{sys}} \exp\left\{1 - \frac{t - t_i}{\tau_{sys}}\right\}, \quad (18)$$

where d_{i-1} is the diastolic pressure immediately preceding the onset of systole at time t_i. Phase I has the constant duration τ_{sys}. For the diastolic part of the pulse wave we write

$$\frac{dp_{II}}{dt} = -\frac{p_{II}}{\tau_v(t)} \quad (19)$$

according to the *windkessel* model.

5 Simulations

Let us hereafter present some of the results obtained from simulations with the model proposed in the preceding section.

5.1 Interaction of Mayer Waves and RSA

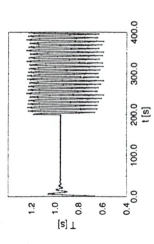

Fig. 7. Time series of the heart period. The first 200 seconds show a damped oscillation towards a constant period. The transition to a large amplitude cycle after the onset of stimulation can be seen (see 5.3.).

Mayer waves are blood pressure fluctuations with periods in the range of six to twenty seconds with a mean of ten seconds. They are quite common; their period and stability, however, can vary widely among individuals.

Our simulations show that the sympathetic part of the blood pressure control loop represents an oscillator with frequencies in the range mentioned above. Usually these oscillations are damped; for strong feedback or long time

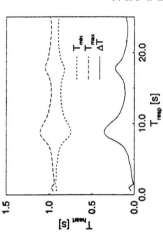

Fig. 8. Resonance between respiration and blood pressure control loop. T_{resp} and T_{heart} are the respiratory and the heart period, respectively.

delays, however, sustained oscillations are also possible. In figure 7 one can see a damped rhythm with a period of about nine seconds at the beginning of the record before the onset of stimulation.

The influence of respiratory neurons on the sympathetic and parasympathetic activity causes variations in blood pressure and heart period, called *respiratory sinus arrhythmia* (RSA, see fig. 9). If the respiratory frequency is approximately equal to the frequency of the sympathetic control loop, resonance effects occur. Figure 8 shows the maximum and minimum heart period during RSA, as well as the RSA's amplitude for varying breathing periods.

5.2 Response to Vagal Stimulation by Single Impulses

In some calculations, we have simulated the behavior of the system which is stimulated vagally both by single and repeated impulses. First we shall consider the system's response to single stimuli given near the medulla. We increase the parasympathetic activity ν_p for a stimulus duration τ_{stim} by a stimulus amplitude A_{stim}.

Figure 11 shows the period changes of the disturbed heart cycle T_i and the two following cycles T_{i+1} and T_{i+2} for several stimulus strengths, where θ is the time delay between the onset of systole of cycle i and the application of the stimulus, and T_0 is the heart period without additional stimulation. The phase-response curves of figure 11 are similar to those obtained experimentally by Yang et al. [51]. Both in our simulation and in Yang's experiments, the influence of respiration was suppressed.

5.3 Response to Repeated Vagal Stimulation

Finally, we would like to investigate the system's response to repeated vagal stimulation. Each heart cycle is stimulated after a time delay θ following the beginning of systole (see fig. 10). Some *return maps* for several time delays

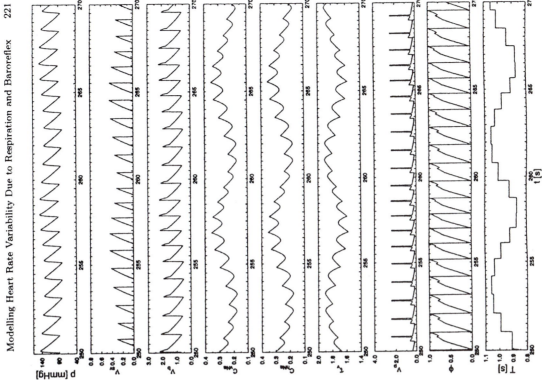

Fig. 10. Repeated stimulation (constant time delay $\theta = 0.2$ between systolic onset and stimulus), no respiratory influence

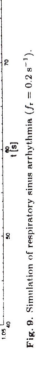

Fig. 9. Simulation of respiratory sinus arrhythmia ($f_r = 0.2\ \mathrm{s}^{-1}$).

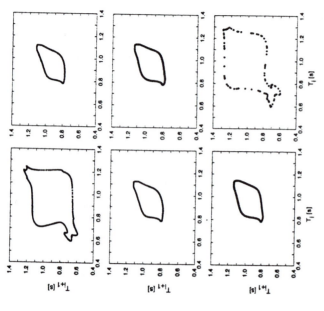

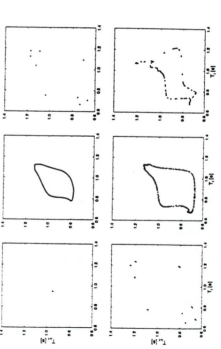

Fig. 13. Some tori for several time delays (θ = 0.20, 0.23, 0.24, 0.25, 0.26, 0.28 s) A_{stim} = 5.0, τ_{stim} = 0.05.

are depicted in figure 12. θ turns out to be an essential bifurcation parameter. Changes in the time delay can result in stable nodes, periodic attractors, and tori, the latter sometimes being quite wrinkled.

Periodicity is observed only when the total period is in the range of the period of the baroreceptor loop or of one of its multiples. We found periods of 9–12, 18, and 35. Period doubling was also observed (transition from period 9 to period 18, see fig 12). The complicated shapes of some of the tori indicate chaotic dynamics for certain time delays. In figure 13 and 14 some of these tori and the corresponding Fourier spectra are depicted. The first of these spectra shows an augmented background, indicative of chaos. A comprehensive bifurcation analysis of the model will be left for further investigations.

A strong influence of the time delay on circulation rhythms has also been found in stimulation experiments on anaesthetized dogs [49]. This emphasizes that phase-response concepts are required for adequate modelling.

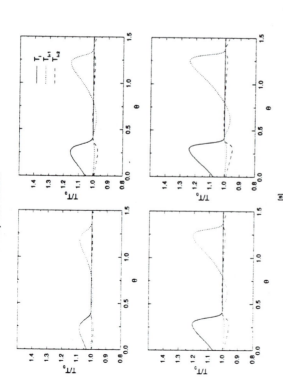

Fig. 11. Phase-response curves for several stimulus strengths (1.0, 2.0, 3.0, and 4.0), see text. The influence of respiration is not taken into account here.

Fig. 12. Return map $T_{i+1}(T_i)$ for several time delays (θ, A_{stim}, τ_{stim}) = (0.1, 2.0, 0.1) (0.23, 5.0, 0.05) (0.2, 2.0, 0.1) (0.25, 2.0, 0.1) (0.15, 2.0, 0.1) (1.0, 2.0, 0.1).

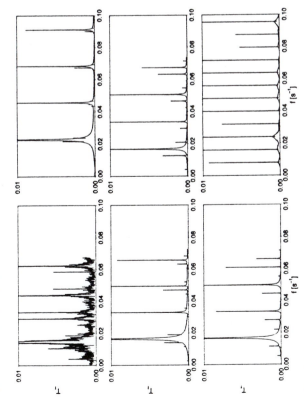

Fig. 14. Fourier spectra for the tori of fig. 13.

6 Discussion

We have introduced a model for the dynamics of the blood pressure control loop. It was designed to explain basic dynamical features of the system on time scales from milliseconds to minutes. Changes of the concentrations of CO_2, O_2, and H^+ are not included; neither are metabolic impacts on the system and influences from higher cerebral regions. The respiratory pattern generator is assumed to have a constant period. Mechanical interactions between respiration and heart beat are neglected.

In spite of these simplifications we are able to reproduce a number of experimental findings as such Mayer waves, respiratory sinus arrhythmia, resonance effects between respiration and Mayer waves, phase dependence of the impact of vagal activity on the heart, and the occurrence of complex dynamics at repeated vagal stimulation.

Appendices

A.1 Simplified Delay Model of Blood Pressure Control

In section 5.1 we saw that the circulation control exhibits a resonance around 0.1 s^{-1}. We shall now show that this rhythm can also be obtained by a strongly simplified model. This model includes only the sympathetic part of blood pressure control, synonymous with cut vagi. The influence of respiration is neglected as well, and we are going to use an averaged blood pressure without the wave form induced by heart beats.

Let us assume that an augmented cardiac noradrenaline concentration leads to a blood pressure increase by way of a strengthened contractility

$$\frac{d\bar{p}}{dt} = \alpha(\bar{c} - c_0).$$ (20)

On the pre-condition that the sympathetic activity never vanishes completely, so that we can delete the maximum function, one can derive the equation

$$\frac{d\bar{c}}{dt} = -\beta\bar{c} + \gamma - \sigma(\bar{p}(t-\theta) - p_0)$$ (21)

from our model. The substitution $(\bar{c} - c_0) \to c$ and $(\bar{p} - p_0) \to p$ yields the two-dimensional linear differential delay equation system

$$\frac{dp}{dt} = \alpha c$$ (22)

$$\frac{dc}{dt} = -\beta c + \gamma - \sigma p(t-\theta)$$ (23)

or

$$\ddot{c}(t) + \beta\dot{c}(t) + \alpha\sigma c(t-\theta) = 0.$$ (24)

Equation (24) exhibits a Hopf bifurcation for increasing time delay (see, e.g., [1]). In order to calculate the bifurcation point, we use $c = \hat{c}\exp(i\omega t)$. The conditions for a vanishing imaginary part of ω are

$$\omega^4 + \omega^2\beta^2 - \alpha^2\sigma^2 = 0$$ (25)

$$\tan(\omega\theta) = \frac{\beta}{\omega}.$$ (26)

The frequency of the system is determined by $\alpha\sigma$ and β according to

$$\omega = \frac{\beta}{\sqrt{2}}\sqrt{\sqrt{1 + \left(\frac{2\alpha\sigma}{\beta^2}\right)^2} - 1}.$$ (27)

With $\alpha = 30$, $\beta = 0.5$, and $\sigma = 0.2$, approximating our global model, the period of the blood pressure variations is in the order of ten seconds. The linear model allows, however, no analysis of the resulting limit cycle.

If the damping β is small or the feedback $\alpha\sigma$ is strong ($\alpha\sigma/\beta^2 \gg 1$), equation (26) can be expanded to yield

$$\theta \approx \frac{\beta}{\omega^2} = \frac{\beta T^2}{4\pi^2}. \tag{28}$$

For a strong damping or a weak feedback ($\alpha\sigma/\beta^2 \ll 1$) equation (27) gives

$$\frac{\beta}{\omega} \approx \frac{\beta^2}{\alpha\sigma} \gg 1. \tag{29}$$

According to equation (26) the lowest frequency of the system is given by $\omega\theta \lesssim \pi/2$ or, in other words,

$$\theta \lesssim \frac{T}{4}. \tag{30}$$

Hence, for strong damping or weak feedback we get sustained oscillations if the time delay is greater than a quarter period of the system's smallest frequency.

According to figure 15, for a period of ten seconds one can expect stable sustained oscillations at time delays $\theta \gtrsim 1.5$ s.

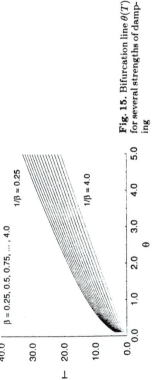

Fig. 15. Bifurcation line $\theta(T)$ for several strengths of damping

To sum up, one can say that even the extremely simplified approximation introduced in this section can account for the occurrence of sustained oscillations and resonance phenomena at periods around ten seconds. We want to emphasize that this result does not exclude the generation of these rhythms at other locations (e.g. in the *formatio recticularis*).

A.2 Sample Parameter Set

$p^{(0)}$	50.0 mmHg	θ_p	0.5 s
k_1	0.02 1/mmHg	$S^{(0)}$	25 mmHg
k_2	0.00125 s/mmHg	k_S^c	40 mmHg
$\nu_s^{(0)}$	0.8	k_S^t	10 mmHg/s
k_s^b	0.7	n_S	2.5
k_s^r	0.1	$\hat{S}$	70.0 mmHg
f_r	0.2 1/s	$T^{(0)}$	1.1 s
$\Delta\phi_s^r$	0.0	k_φ^{cNa}	1.6
$\nu_p^{(0)}$	0.0	$\hat{c}_{cNa}$	2.0
k_p^b	0.3	n_{cNa}	2.0
k_p^r	0.1	k_φ^p	5.8
$\Delta\phi_p^r$	0.0	$\hat{\nu}_p$	2.5
τ_{cNa}	2.0 s	n_p	2.0
k_{cNa}^s	1.2	$\tau_v^{(0)}$	2.2 s
θ_{cNa}	1.65 s	$\bar{\tau}_v$	1.5 s
τ_{vNa}	2.0 s	$\hat{c}_{vNa}$	10.0
k_{cvNa}^s	1.2	n_{vNa}	1.5
θ_{vNa}	1.65 s	τ_{syn}	0.125 s

References

1. U. an der Heiden, A. Longtin, M. C. Mackey, J. G. Milton, and R. Scholl: Oscillatory modes in a nonlinear second-order differential equation with delay. Journal of Dynamics and Differential Equations **2**, 423–449 (1990)

2. G. Baselli, S. Cerutti, S. Civardi, A. Malliani, and M. Pagani: Cardiovascular variability signals: Towards the identification of a closed-loop model of the neural control mechanisms. IEEE Trans. Biomed. Eng. **35**, 1033–1046 (1988)

3. R. M. Berne, N. Sperelakis, and S. R. Geiger, editors: Handbook of Physiology, volume I. American Physiological Society 1979

4. T. R. Chay and Y. S. Lee: Phase resetting and bifurcation in the ventricular myocardium. J. Physiol. **47**, 641–651 (1985)

5. M. Courtmanche, L. Glass, M. Rosengarten, and A. L. Goldberger: Beyond pure parasystole: promises and problems in modelling complex arrhythmias. Am. J. Physiol. **257**, H693–H706 (1989)

6. M. R. Cowie and J. M. Rawles: A modified method of quantifying the carotid baroreceptor–heart rate reflex in man: the effect of age and blood pressure. Clin. Sci. **77**, 223–228 (1989)

7. R. W. de Boer, J. M. Karemaker, and J. Strackee: Hemodynamic fluctuations and baroreflex sensitivity in humans: a beat-to-beat model. Am. J. Physiol. **253**, 680–689 (1987)

8. D. DiFrancesco and D. Noble: A model of cardiac electrical activity incorporating ionic pumps and concentration changes. Phil. Trans. R. Soc. Lond. B **307**, 353–398 (1985)

9. D. L. Eckberg: Human sinus arrhythmia as an index of vagal cardiac outflow. J. Appl. Physiol. **54**, 961–966 (1983)

228   Henrik Seidel and Hanspeter Herzel

10. D. L. Eckberg, Y. T. Kifle, and V. L. Roberts: Phase relationship between normal human respiration and baroreflex responsiveness. J. Physiol. **304**, 489–502 (1980).
11. D. L. Eckberg and C. R. Orshan: Respiratory and baroreflex interactions in man. J. Clin. Inv. **59**, 780–785 (1977).
12. D. L. Eckberg, R. F. Rea, O. K. Andersson, T. Hedner, J. Pernow, J. M. Lundberg, and B. G. Wallin: Baroreflex modulation of sympathetic activity and sympathetic neurotransmitters in humans. Acta Physiol. Scand. **133**, 221–231 (1988).
13. R. B. Felder and M. D. Thames: Interaction between cardiac receptors and sinoaortic baroreceptors in the control of efferent cardiac sympathetic nerve activity during myocardial ischemia in dogs. Circ. Res. **45**, 728–736 (1979).
14. J. L. Feldman and J. D. Cowan: Large-scale activity in neuronal nets I: A model for the brainstem respiratory oscillator. Biol. Cybern. **17**, 29–38 (1975).
15. J. L. Feldman and J. D. Cowan: Large-scale activity in neuronal nets II: A model for the brainstem respiratory oscillator. Biol. Cybern. **17**, 39–51 (1975).
16. J. L. Feldman et al.: Neurogenesis of respiratory rhythm and pattern: emerging concepts. Am. J. Physiol. **259**, R879–R886 (1990).
17. F. M. Fouad, R. C. Tarazi, C. M. Ferrario, S. Fighaly, and C. Alicandri: Assessment of parasympathetic control of heart rate by a noninvasive method. Am. J. Physiol. **246**, H838–H842 (1984).
18. S. Geman and M. Miller: Computer simulation of brainstem respiratory activity. J. Appl. Physiol. **41**, 931–938 (1976).
19. L. Glass: Cardiac arrhythmias and circle maps – a classical problem. Chaos **1**, 13–19 (1991).
20. L. Glass, A. L. Goldberger, and J. Bélair: Dynamics of pure parasystole. Am. J. Physiol. **251**, H841–H847 (1986).
21. L. Glass and M. C. Mackey: From Clocks to Chaos. Princeton University 1988.
22. A. L. Goldberger, D. R. Rigney, J. Meitus, E. M. Antman, and S. Greenwald: Nonlinear dynamics in sudden cardiac death syndrome: heartrate oscillations and bifurcations. Experientia **44**, 983–987 (1988).
23. N. M. Greene and R. G. Bachand: Vagal component of the chronotropic response to baroreceptor stimulation in man. Am. Heart J. **82**, 22–27 (1971).
24. M. R. Guevara, A. Shrier, and L. Glass: Phase-locked rhythms in periodically stimulated heart cell aggregates. Am. J. Physiol. **254**, H1–H10 (1988).
25. N. Ikeda, S. Yoshizawa, and T. Sato: Difference equation model of ventricular parasystole as an interaction between cardiac pacemakers based on the phase response curve. J. theor. Biol. **103**, 439–465 (1983).
26. Danial T. Kaplan and Mario Talajic: Dynamics of heart rate. Chaos **1**, 251–256 (1991).
27. P. G. Katona, P. J. Martin, and J. Felix: Neuronal control of heart rate: A conciliation of models. IEEE Trans. Biomed. Eng. **23**, 164–166 (1976).
28. T. Kawahara: Coupled Van der Pol oscillators - a model of excitatory and inhibitory neuronal interactions. Biol. Cybern. **39**, 37–43 (1980).
29. P. Lindgren and J. Manning: Decrease in cardiac activity by carotid sinus baroreceptor reflex. Acta physiol. scand. **63**, 401–408 (1965).
30. L. G. Michael, R. Guevara and A. Shrier: Phase locking, period-doubling bifurcations, and irregular dynamics in periodically stimulated cardiac cells. Science **214**, 1350–1353 (1981).
31. G. K. Moe, J. Jalife, W. J. Mueller, and B. Moe: A mathematical model of parasystole and its application to clinical arrhythmias. Circulation **56**, 968–979 (1977).

Modelling Heart Rate Variability Due to Respiration and Baroreflex   229

32. E. Mosekilde and J. I. Jensen: Dynamic simulation of human ventilatory regulation. System Dynamics Conf. Albany, New York 1981.
33. L. Glass, P. Hunter and A. McCulloch, editors: The Theory of Heart. Springer-Verlag New York 1991.
34. D. Noble and S. J. Noble: A model of sino-atrial node electrical activity based on a modification of the DiFrancesco-Noble (1984) equations. Proc. R. Soc. Lond. B **222**, 295–304 (1984).
35. V. S. Reiner and C. Antzelevitch: Phase resetting and annihilation in a mathemetical model of sinus node. Am. J. Physiol. **249**, H1143–H1153 (1985).
36. D. W. Richter and K. M. Spyer: Cardiorespiratory control. In A. D. Loewy and K. M. Spyer, editors: Central Regulation of Autonomic Functions. Oxford University Press 1990, pp. 189–207.
37. D. W. Richter, K. M. Spyer, M. P. Gilbey, E. E. Lawson, C. R. Bainton, and Z. Wilhelm: On the existence of a common cardiorespiratory network. In H.-P. Koepchen and T. Huopaniemi, editors: Cardiorespiratory and Motor Coordination. Springer-Verlag Berlin, 1991, pp. 118–130.
38. A. Rosenblueth and F. A. Simeone: The interrelations of vagal and accelerator effects on the cardiac rate. Am. J. Physiol. **110**, 42–55 (1934).
39. R. F. Schmidt and G. Thews, editors: Physiologie des Menschen. Springer-Verlag Berlin, 22nd edition, 1985.
40. R. F. Schmidt and G. Thews, editors: Human Physiology. Springer-Verlag Berlin, 3rd edition, 1989.
41. M. F. Taher et al.: Baroreceptor responses derived from a fundamental concept. Ann. Biom. Eng. **16**, 429–443 (1988).
42. S. F. Vatner, C. B. Higgens, D. Franklin, and E. Braunwald: Extent of carotid sinus regulation of the myocardial contractile state in conscious dogs. J. Clin. Inv. **51**, 995–1008 (1972).
43. C. von Euler: On the central pattern generator for the basic breathing rhythmicity. J. Appl. Physiol. **55**, 1647–1659 (1983).
44. C. von Euler: On the origin and pattern control of breathing rhythmicity in mammals. In A. Roberts and B. Roberts, editors: Neuronal origin of rhythmic movements. Society for Experimental Biology, Society for Experimental Biology 1983, pp. 469–485.
45. Z. Wanzhen, L. Glass, and A. Shrier: Evolution of rhythms during periodic stimulation of embryonic chick heart cell aggregates. Circ. Res. **69**, 1022–1033 (1991).
46. Z. Wanzhen, L. Glass, and A. Shrier: The topology of phase response curves induced by single and paired stimuli in spontaneously oscillating chick heart cell aggregates. J. Biol. Rhythms **7**, 89–104 (1992).
47. H. R. Warner: The frequency-dependent nature of blood pressure regulation by the carotid sinus studied with an electric analog. Circ. Res. **6**, 35–40 (1958).
48. H. R. Warner and R. O. Russel: Effect of combined sympathetic and vagal stimulation on heart rate in the dog. Circ. Res. **24**, 567–573 (1969).
49. H. Warzel, H.-U. Eckhardt, and U. Hopstock: Effects of carotid sinus nerve stimulation at different times in the respiratory and cardiac cycles on variability of heart rate and blood pressure of normotensive and renal hypertensive dogs. J. Auton. Nerv. Syst. **26**, 121–127 (1989).
50. R. J. Wyman: Neuronal generation of the breathing rhythm. Ann. Rev. Physiol. **39**, 417–448 (1977).
51. T. Yang, M. D. Jacobstein, and M. N. Levy: Synchronisation of automatic cells in S-A node during vagal stimulation in dogs. Am. J. Physiol. **246**, H585–H591 (1984).

Fractal analysis of role of smooth muscle Ca^{2+} fluxes in genesis of chaotic arterial pressure oscillations

T. M. GRIFFITH AND D. H. EDWARDS

Departments of Diagnostic Radiology and Cardiology, Cardiovascular Sciences Research Group, University of Wales College of Medicine, Heath Park, Cardiff CF4 4XN, United Kingdom

Griffith, T. M., and D. H. Edwards. Fractal analysis of role of smooth muscle Ca^{2+} fluxes in genesis of chaotic arterial pressure oscillations. *Am. J. Physiol.* 266 (*Heart Circ. Physiol.* 35): H1801–H1811, 1994.—We have investigated the role of vascular smooth muscle Ca^{2+} fluxes in the genesis of chaotic pressure oscillations induced by histamine in isolated resistance arteries from the rabbit ear. The responses exhibited distinct "fast" and "slow" components, with periods of 5–20 s and 1–5 min, respectively, which could be dissociated pharmacologically. The fast subsystem involved ion movements at the cell membrane and was inhibited by both low (<2 mM) and high (>5 mM) extracellular Ca^{2+} concentration ($[Ca^{2+}]_o$) by verapamil (which inhibits voltage-dependent Ca^{2+} influx) and by charybdotoxin (ChTX) and apamin (which block Ca^{2+}-activated K^+ channels). In contrast, the slow subsystem was intracellular and was selectively attenuated by ryanodine, which inhibits Ca^{2+}-induced Ca^{2+} release from sarcoplasmic reticulum. The effects of these interventions on the complexity of the responses were quantified by calculating their fractal dimension, a parameter that estimates the minimum number of independent variables contributing to an irregular time series. Its mean value was generally >2 under control conditions but decreased to <2 in a concentration-dependent fashion in the presence of verapamil, ChTX, apamin, or ryanodine and when $[Ca^{2+}]_o$ was outside the range of 2–3 mM. Each intervention thus removed one dimension of complexity from the mechanisms generating the rhythmic activity. We conclude that the interaction of a fast membrane oscillator, which involves Ca^{2+} influx, Ca^{2+}-activated K^+ efflux, and therefore presumably changes in membrane potential, and a slow intracellular oscillator involving Ca^{2+} sequestration and release from stores is responsible for vascular chaos in our model. The coupling between these subsystems is likely to be mediated by cytosolic $[Ca^{2+}]$.

nonlinear dynamics; strange attractor; fractal dimension; endothelium-derived relaxing factor; ryanodine; verapamil; charybdotoxin; apamin; glibenclamide

WE HAVE PREVIOUSLY PROVIDED evidence that irregular fluctuations in perfusion pressure, induced by histamine in isolated rabbit ear resistance arteries, are generated by nonlinear interactions between distinct fast and slow oscillatory mechanisms within the vascular smooth muscle cell (13). The responses were analyzed by calculating their fractal dimension, a parameter that estimates the minimum number of control variables involved in an irregular time series, and was shown to be at least 3 (12, 13). A value >2 is necessary to classify irregular signals as chaotic, because it is theoretically impossible to generate the complex patterns of behavior that characterize chaos with just two variables (13). The endogeneous nitrovasodilator endothelium-derived relaxing factor (EDRF) and the concentration of histamine used to induce rhythmic activity

were both shown to influence the superficial form of oscillations, but not their intrinsic complexity, as assessed by fractal dimension. EDRF and histamine may thus be regarded as modulatory and permissive factors, respectively, rather than essential determinants of the overall responses (13).

In the present study we have employed pharmacological probes to elucidate the biological determinants of excitation-contraction coupling involved in the genesis of the irregular histamine-induced responses by analyzing their effects on the fractal dimension of experimental data. We have studied the effects of altered extracellular calcium ($[Ca^{2+}]_o$), inhibition of Ca^{2+} influx through voltage-dependent membrane channels (with verapamil) (29), inhibition of Ca^{2+}-activated and ATP-sensitive K^+ channels [with charybdotoxin (ChTX), apamin, and glibenclamide] (7), and inhibition of intracellular Ca^{2+}-induced Ca^{2+} release from intracellular stores (with ryanodine) (1, 8, 16, 19, 21). The findings demonstrate how nonlinear analysis of the consequences of pharmacological interventions can identify key vasomotor control variables and interactions, and thereby provide a means of differentiating the mechanisms that determine the nature of the responses from those that simply modulate their superficial appearance, such as altered EDRF activity and histamine concentration.

METHODS

The preparation and technique for studying single resistance arteries in the isolated rabbit ear has been described in detail elsewhere (13). Briefly, first-generation arteries (1–1.5 cm long and ~150 μm in diam) arising from the central ear artery were perfused in situ at 0.5 ml/min with oxygenated (95%O_2-5%CO_2) Holman's buffer (composition in mM: 120 NaCl, 5 KCl, 2.5 $CaCl_2$, 1.3 NaH_2PO_4, 25 $NaHCO_3$, 11 glucose, and 10 sucrose, pH 7.2–8.4) at 35°C, via a cannula secured in the central ear artery, which was itself ligated distally to divert all flow into the branch vessel under study. In one group of experiments the concentration of extracellular Ca^{2+} present in the buffer was varied (0–5 mM). Perfusion pressure was monitored continuously via a sidearm connected to the perfusion circuit.

Ryanodine was obtained from Novabiochem, ChTX from Alomome Laboratories (Jerusalem, Israel), and glibenclamide from Hoechst. All other reagents were obtained from Sigma (Poole, Dorset, UK). Stock solutions were freshly prepared on the day of the experiment, with all reagents being dissolved in saline except glibenclamide and verapamil hydrochloride, which were dissolved in absolute ethanol. All experiments were conducted in the presence of nitric oxide synthase blockade with 50 μM N^G-nitro-L-arginine methyl ester (L-NAME) to exclude secondary effects on EDRF production, which is dependent on extracellular $[Ca^{2+}]$ influx in rabbit arteries (14). In experiments characterizing the concentration-dependent effects of the various drugs on fractal dimension, 2.5 μM histamine was employed in all cases. Spectral analysis of the responses was performed on segments of data at least 5 min long (range 5–15 min) digitized as 4,096 points, the power ordinate being given in arbitrary units. Considerations of space have not allowed the complete sections of data used to calculate the fractal dimension of the responses and derive the corresponding power spectra to be illustrated in all instances. The effects of the various pharmacological interventions on perfusion pressure, fractal dimension, and the frequencies of the principal slow and fast components of the oscillations were compared by the Student's t-test or analysis of variance as appropriate, with $P < 0.05$ being considered as significant.

Theoretical Analysis

The method of analysis involves calculating the correlation dimension (D_c) of the responses by the method of Grassberger and Procaccia (12), which provides one measure of their fractal dimension. Briefly, time-varying fluctuations in perfusion pressure, P(t), were digitized as a series of temporally equidistant points to generate a vector set $\mathbf{P}_i = \{P_i(t), P_i(t + \tau), ...$ $P_i[t + (m - 1)\tau]\}$, where τ is a suitably chosen time delay, and m is an integer known as the embedding dimension (D_E). These vectors were then used to calculate the Grassberger and Procaccia correlation integral

$$C(l) = \lim_{N \to \infty} \frac{1}{N^2}$$

$$\times \left[\begin{array}{l} \text{number of pairs } (i, j) \text{ whose distance} \\ \text{from each other } (|\mathbf{P}_j - \mathbf{P}_i|) \text{ is less than } l \end{array} \right] \quad (1)$$

where l is an arbitrarily chosen distance in the m-dimensional phase space created by the analysis. For a deterministic data set

$$C(l) \propto l^v \quad (2)$$

where v is a measure of the fractal dimension (D_c) of the time series for sufficiently large m. When rounded up to the nearest integer, D_c provides an estimate of the minimum number of independent control variables contributing to an irregular time series. In the present analysis a single value of embedding dimension ($D_E = 10$) was employed to estimate the D_c of the responses, because a value that is too high can produce inadvertent errors (13). The τ was selected as $0.2 \times$ average oscillatory period. Validation of these parameter choices in the context of histamine-induced pressure oscillations has been presented elsewhere (13).

RESULTS

A total of 62 arteries was studied, 49 of which exhibited oscillatory responses when perfused with 1 or 2.5 µM histamine. In 34 preparations full concentration-response curves were constructed for the pharmacological interventions.

Effects of Changes in Extracellular [Ca²⁺]

Preparations perfused by 2.5 µM histamine and 50 µM L-NAME generally exhibited slow pressure oscillations (period 1–5 min) lacking a detectable fast component following brief equilibration (for 5–20 min) in nominally Ca²⁺-free buffer (Fig. 1). Such slow oscillations were observed in 7 of 10 vessels thus challenged. Subsequent introduction of Ca²⁺ into the perfusate unmasked superimposed fast oscillations of period 5–20 s {mean frequency 0.053 ± 0.009 Hz at 2 mM extracellu-

lar Ca²⁺ concentration ([Ca²⁺]$_o$), $n = 7$}. When [Ca²⁺]$_o$ was in the intermediate range (2 mM), the mean value of D_c was indicative of chaotic dynamics ($D_c > 2$), otherwise falling to a value $1 < D_c < 2$ at both low and high [Ca²⁺]$_o$ (Figs. 1 and 2A). There was, however, considerable variation in the responses of the individual preparations in this respect (Fig. 2A). With [Ca²⁺]$_o \geq 5$ mM, both slow and fast fluctuations in pressure were either markedly diminished in amplitude or abolished altogether (Fig. 1).

Spectral analysis indicated that the activity of the slow oscillatory subsystem was relatively insensitive to [Ca²⁺]$_o$. Mean values of the principal slow frequency peak in the power spectra were 0.004 ± 0.0004, 0.004 ± 0.0003, and 0.005 ± 0.0009 Hz for [Ca²⁺]$_o$ = 0, 2, and 4 mM, respectively, and not significantly different from each other. The rise in perfusion pressure induced by histamine and L-NAME after brief exposure to nominally Ca²⁺-free buffer was generally greater, and that in the presence of 5 mM [Ca²⁺]$_o$ lower, than that observed when [Ca²⁺]$_o$ was within the "physiological" range of 2–3 mM (Fig. 2A).

Effects of Ca²⁺ Antagonism

Verapamil caused a selective, concentration-dependent decrease in the amplitude of the fast component of the pressure oscillations induced by 2.5 µM histamine and 50 µM L-NAME without inhibiting the slow component when this was present (Fig 3A). Indeed, in three of eight preparations tested, varapamil actually promoted the appearance of slow, large-amplitude relaxation oscillations (Fig. 3B). Both patterns of response were nevertheless associated with a concentration-dependent fall in D_c. Although there were individual variations in the initial value of D_c, the mean value ultimately attained in the present of 1 µM verapamil fell from a control between 2 and 3 to a value <2 ($n = 7$) (Fig. 2B). The average values of the principal slow frequency peak in the power spectra for the control situation and 1 µM verapamil were 0.009 ± 0.003 and 0.012 ± 0.004 Hz, respectively, and not significantly different from each other ($n = 7$). Verapamil generally induced a concentration-dependent fall in mean perfusion pressure (control 97 ± 13 vs. 53 ± 7 mmHg with 1 µM; $P < 0.05$, $n = 7$).

Role of Ca²⁺-Sensitive Outward K⁺ Channels

Apamin induced a concentration-dependent fall in the amplitude of the fast, but not the slow, component of the responses induced by 2.5 µM histamine and 50 µM L-NAME, in association with a significant reduction in average D_c from a mean value between 2 and 3 to <2 ($n = 9$, Figs. 4A and 5A), although in some preparations there was an initial increase (Fig. 4B). Mean values of the principal slow frequency peak in the power spectra for the control situation and 100 nM apamin were 0.010 ± 0.002 and 0.009 ± 0.002 Hz, respectively, and were not significantly different from each other. Apamin did not significantly affect mean perfusion pressure.

In contrast to apamin, ChTX elevated perfusion pressure in arteries constricted by 2.5 µM histamine and 50

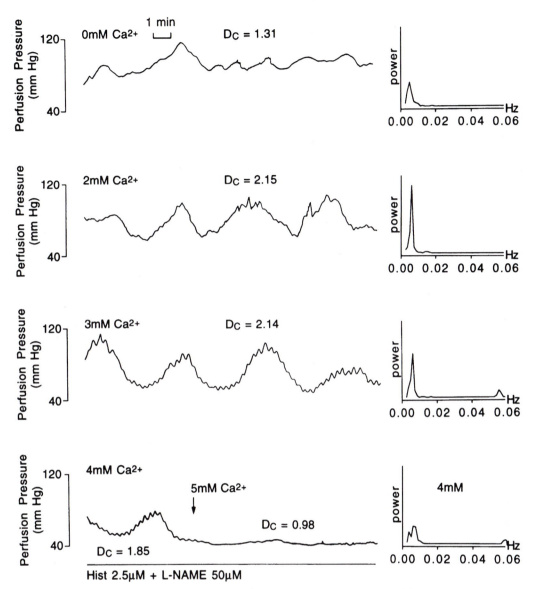

Fig. 1. Effects of increasing extracellular Ca²⁺ concentration ($[Ca^{2+}]_o$) in an artery initially perfused for ∼10 min with nominally Ca²⁺-free buffer in the presence of 2.5 µM histamine (Hist) and 50 µM N^G-nitro-L-arginine methyl ester (L-NAME). Slow oscillations were present at all concentrations <5 µM. Superimposed fast oscillations also became conspicuous with $[Ca^{2+}]_o$ in the range of 2–4 mM. Spectral analysis demonstrated that the predominant frequency of either component was only minimally influenced by $[Ca^{2+}]_o$. Oscillatory activity was virtually abolished by 5 mM $[Ca^{2+}]_o$ in this preparation. D_c, fractal dimension.

µM L-NAME (control 88 ± 17 vs. 137 ± 15 mmHg with 10 nM; $P < 0.05$, $n = 6$). Nevertheless, there was a similar concentration-dependent decrease in mean D_c from a control value between 2 and 3 ($n = 6$, Fig. 5B, Fig. 6, A and B), although in occasional preparations an initial increase in complexity was observed, as in the case of apamin (e.g., Fig. 6A). ChTX selectively decreased the amplitude of the fast component of the oscillations, which was usually abolished at a concentration of 100 nM, but did not suppress the activity of the slow oscillatory subsystem (Fig. 6). Mean value of the principal slow frequency peak in the power spectra for the control situation and 10 nM ChTX were 0.004 ±

0.001 and 0.003 ± 0.001 Hz, respectively, and were not significantly different from each other.

Blockade of ATP-sensitive K⁺ channels did not influence mean perfusion pressure or the appearance and complexity of the pressure fluctuations, D_c being 2.60 ± 0.23 in the absence and 2.65 ± 0.13 in the presence of 10 µM glibenclamide ($n = 5$, not significant).

Role of Intracellular Ca²⁺ Movements

Ryanodine selectively diminished the amplitude of the slow oscillatory component of the responses induced by 2.5 µM histamine and 50 µM L-NAME, in association

264 • Chapter 27

H1804

ANALYSIS OF ROLE OF SMOOTH MUSCLE CA^{2+} FLUXES

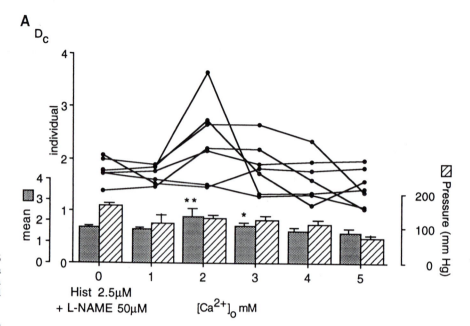

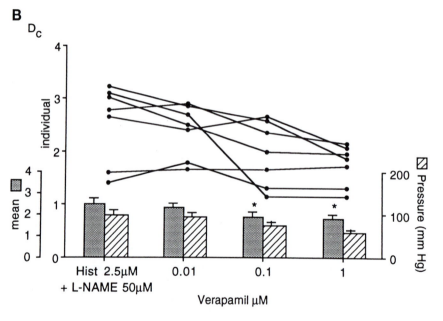

Fig. 2. D_c of oscillations induced by 2.5 μM Hist and 50 μM L-NAME as a function of $[Ca^{2+}]_o$ and verapamil (with $[Ca^{2+}]_o$ = 2.5 mM). *A*: dynamics could generally be classified as chaotic ($D_c >$ 2) only at values of $[Ca^{2+}]_o$ ~ 2 mM ($n =$ 7, **$P <$ 0.01, *$P <$ 0.05 vs. $[Ca^{2+}]_o$ = 0 mM). *B*: verapamil induced a significant decrease in overall D_c from between 2 and 3 to a value <2 ($n =$ 7, *$P <$ 0.05 vs. control) and a decline in mean perfusion pressure.

with a concentration-dependent decrease in average D_c from between 2 and 3 to a value <2 at a concentration of 30 μM ($n =$ 5, Figs. 7 and 8). Indeed, in preparations in which a fast component was undetectable, slow pressure oscillations could be completely abolished by ryanodine (Fig. 7*B*). Although there was sometimes a small decrease in the amplitude of the fast oscillatory component, when initially present it was always still conspicuous at concentrations as high as 30 μM, and there was no significant effect on its frequency. Mean values for the main high-frequency component in the control situation and with 30 μM ryanodine were 0.10 ± 0.02 and 0.11 ± 0.02 Hz, respectively ($n =$ 5, not significant). Ryanodine generally exerted no significant effect on mean perfusion pressure (Fig. 8).

DISCUSSION

We have shown that nonlinear analysis of the effects of pharmacological manipulation of vascular smooth muscle Ca^{2+} and K$^+$ fluxes permits differentiation of the key control mechanisms responsible for chaotic pressure oscillations in an isolated rabbit ear resistance artery. As in a previous study (13), the fractal dimension of the irregular responses induced by histamine, estimated as the D_c of Grassberger and Proccacia (12), generally averaged between 2 and 3, but in a relatively small number of cases it took a value between 3 and 4. D_c is a measure of the intrinsic complexity of a chaotic time series and provides an estimate of the minimum number of independent control variables involved, which in the

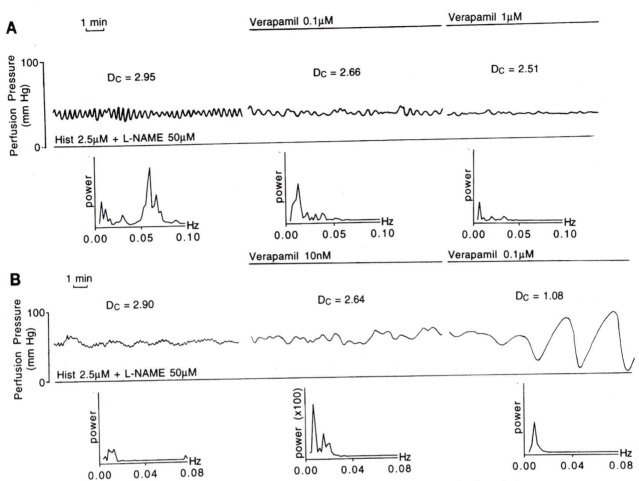

Fig. 3. Effects of verapamil on responses to 2.5 μM Hist in presence of 50 μM L-NAME. *A*: concentration-dependent inhibition of irregular fast oscillations lacking a major slow component by a low concentration of verapamil. *B*: trace exhibiting superimposed fast and slow oscillations. Verapamil inhibited fast but enhanced slow subsystem, unmasking sustained large-amplitude relaxation oscillations. Note that similar relaxation oscillations also occurred in absence of verapamil (see Fig. 7*B*). Spectral analysis confirmed loss of a high frequency component in both examples (note change in scale). Markedly contrasting effects of verapamil in these two preparations may be an illustration of inherently unpredictable behavior of nonlinear dynamical systems.

present model of "vasomotion" is therefore 3. We have previously shown that distinct fast and slow mechanisms contribute to the rhythmic vasomotor activity induced by histamine in these rabbit ear vessels (13). The present findings are consistent with the hypothesis that the fast subsystem involves Ca^{2+} and K^+ movements at the vascular smooth muscle cell membrane and the slow subsystem an interaction between free cytosolic Ca^{2+} and intracellular stores of Ca^{2+}; i.e., Ca^{2+}-induced Ca^{2+} release (CICR). Furthermore, spectral analysis of the data indicated that the frequencies of these two oscillatory mechanisms were effectively independent of each other.

The fast component of the pressure oscillations was usually evident only with $[Ca^{2+}]_o$ in the range of 2–3 mM, whereas slow changes in pressure were not suppressed by brief exposure to nominally Ca^{2+}-free buffer, the overall dynamics being chaotic ($D_c > 2$) only when $[Ca^{2+}]_o$ was in an intermediate range. High concentrations of extracellular Ca^{2+} (>5 mM) decreased mean

perfusion pressure and inhibited both fast and slow oscillations, presumably in part by stimulating Na^+-K^+-adenosinetriphosphatase activity and thus inducing membrane hyperpolarization (41). Previous workers have similarly reported that rhythmic fluctuations in tone in other artery types are abolished by both low and high $[Ca^{2+}]_o$ (20, 32). In the present study, the rise in perfusion pressure induced by the combination of histamine and L-NAME was enhanced by brief exposure to Ca^{2+}-free buffer compared with that obtained with $[Ca^{2+}]_o$ within the normally accepted physiological range. The explanation for this is not clear, but it is unlikely that the duration of the exposure of Ca^{2+}-free buffer was sufficient to deplete intracellular Ca^{2+} stores to a level that ultimately depressed contraction. Possible contributory factors are that low $[Ca^{2+}]_o$ enhances depolarization of vascular smooth muscle by inhibiting endothelium-derived hyperpolarizing factor activity (3) and that force development in low $[Ca^{2+}]_o$ is enhanced by Mg^{2+}-free buffer such as was used experimentally (19).

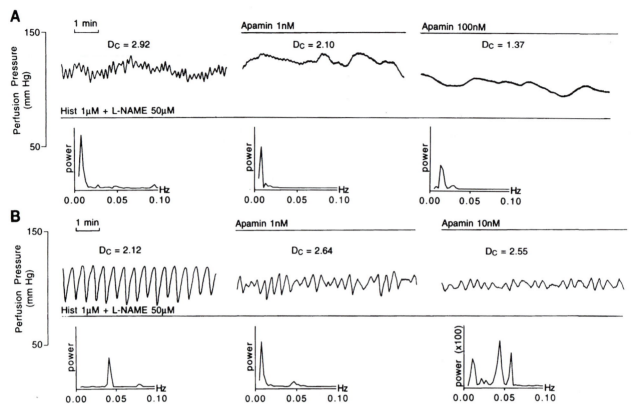

Fig. 4. Effects of apamin on responses to 1 μM Hist in presence of 50 μM L-NAME. *A*: selective inhibition of fast pressure oscillations, confirmed by spectral analysis as loss of a high frequency peak near 0.10 Hz with little effect on frequency of predominant slow component, which was still evident in presence of 100 nM apamin. There was an associated concentration-dependent fall in D_c to a value <2. *B*: concentration-dependent decrease in amplitude of a predominantly fast oscillation with an initial increase in D_c and thus complexity. Fast component was subsequently abolished by 100 nM apamin in association with a fall in D_c to a value <2, as in *A*.

The role of extracellular Ca²⁺ influx was also investigated by inhibition of membrane-bound, voltage-dependent Ca²⁺ channels with verapamil (29), which selectively suppressed the fast component of the pressure oscillations and induced a concentration-dependent fall in mean D_c to a value <2, without inhibiting expression of the slow control subsystem. Indeed, in ~40% of all preparations thus studied, verapamil actually promoted the appearance of slow, large-amplitude relaxation oscillations, whereas in others it suppressed virtually all rhythmic activity. These observations may reflect the inherently unpredictable and often surprising responses of chaotic systems to perturbation ("sensitivity to initial conditions"). The distal microcirculation can, analagously, respond unpredictably to administration of Ca²⁺ antagonists in vivo. Thus nifedipine is capable of inducing large-amplitude diameter oscillations in rat cremaster muscle (23), whereas in a hamster skinfold model, verapamil suppresses all rhythmic activity (4).

The role of K⁺ efflux through channels activated by intracellular Ca²⁺, which mediate membrane hyperpolarization, was investigated with the peptides ChTX and apamin, which are generally accepted to block a spectrum of medium/high and specific low-conductance, Ca²⁺-dependent K⁺ channels, respectively (7). It should nevertheless be noted that ChTX has also been reported

to inhibit voltage-dependent K⁺ channel subtypes in certain nonvascular cells, and apamin has been reported to block voltage-dependent L-type Ca²⁺ channels in cardiac myocytes (2, 7). A spectrum of different K_{Ca} channels has been described in blood vessels of the rabbit and other species (18, 29), but apamin is reportedly without effect on the steady contractile responses of the rabbit aorta (6). In analogous fashion, apamin did not significantly affect mean perfusion pressure in the present experiments with rabbit ear arteries; its action being apparently selective for the oscillatory component of their responses. Functional blockade of voltage-dependent Ca²⁺ channels by apamin in these vessels seems unlikely given that there was no fall in perfusion pressure, as in the case of verapamil. Conversely, ChTX caused a significant increase, as would be expected of an agent likely to promote membrane depolarization.

The effects of both peptides were similar in that they selectively abolished the fast component of the pressure oscillations, with an associated concentration-dependent decrease in mean D_c to a value <2, and, in contrast to the findings with verapamil, did not enhance the activity of the slow subsystem. This is consistent with observations that pinacidil, which hyperpolarizes vascular smooth muscle by opening ATP-sensitive outward K⁺ channels (and whose action is therefore mechanisti-

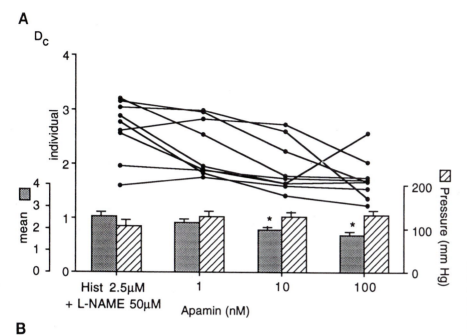

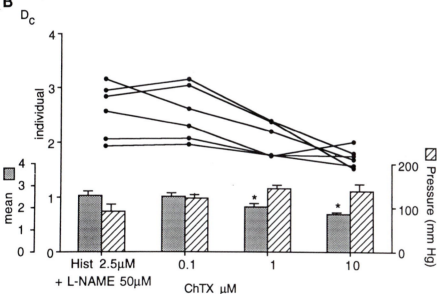

Fig. 5. D_c and mean perfusion pressure of oscillations induced by 2.5 μM Hist and 50 μM L-NAME as a function of the concentration of apamin (A, $n = 9$) and ChTX (B, $n = 6$). Both agents caused a significant concentration-dependent decrease in average D_c from a value >2 to <2 (*$P < 0.05$ vs. control). ChTX significantly increased mean perfusion pressure, but apamin did not.

cally the converse of ChTX and apamin), induces rhythmic oscillations in tone in pharmacologically constricted rat arteries (15). The specific involvement of ATP-sensitive K⁺ channels in the genesis of rhythmic activity in rabbit ear vessels was excluded by the lack of effect of glibenclamide (7).

The role of intracellular Ca²⁺ release was examined with the alkaloid ryanodine, which also induced a concentration-dependent fall in mean D_c to a value <2, without significantly affecting the frequency or abolishing the expression of the fast subsystem. Its action was therefore selective for the slow component of the pressure oscillations. Present evidence suggests that there are two major intracellular pools of stored Ca²⁺ in vascular smooth muscle: 1) type Sα, which possesses

both Ca²⁺-induced and inositol 1,4,5-trisphosphate [Ins(1,4,5)P₃]-induced Ca²⁺ release mechanisms (CICR and IICR); and 2) type Sβ, which possesses only IICR (16). Ryanodine does not influence depolarization-dependent Ca²⁺ influx, but at nanomolar concentrations it locks the channels that mediate CICR in an open state, causing a leak of Ca²⁺ from the Sα store, which becomes unresponsive to both Ca²⁺ and Ins(1,4,5)P₃. At micromolar concentrations ryanodine actually closes the channels (1, 16, 21). Ryanodine thus abolishes CICR, whereas Ins(1,4,5)P₃ can still evoke Ca²⁺ release from the Sβ store. An interaction between CICR and membrane ion fluxes has previously been demonstrated in hog carotid artery in which histamine stimulates periodic ryanodine-sensitive Ca²⁺ release from sarcoplas-

268 • Chapter 27

H1808   ANALYSIS OF ROLE OF SMOOTH MUSCLE CA²⁺ FLUXES

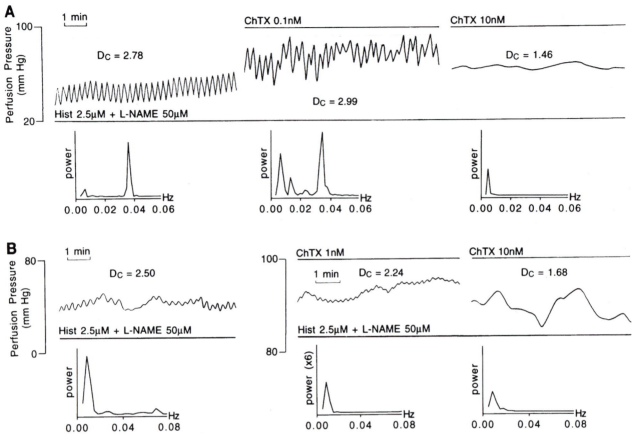

Fig. 6. Effects of charybdotoxin (ChTX) on responses to 2.5 μM Hist in presence of 50 μM L-NAME. *A*: initial increase in D_c and thus complexity of predominantly fast chaotic oscillations followed by a reduction in both overall amplitude and D_c to a value <2. *B*: selective abolition of fast, but not slow, pressure oscillations by ChTX, again with an associated concentration-dependent fall in D_c confirmed by spectral analysis. Note change of pressure scale in center and left panels. In both experiments spectral analysis confirmed loss of high frequency but preservation of a low-frequency component, and ChTX elevated mean perfusion pressure (note change of scale in center panel).

mic reticulum, thereby inducing oscillations in Ca²⁺-activated K⁺ currents at the cell membrane (8).

The above interventions manipulating Ca²⁺ movements generally reduced D_c of the responses to a value <2 when >2 but did not substantially affect its value when initially <2. This is in marked contrast to the effects of stimulating EDRF activity in these rabbit ear arteries with acetylcholine, which suppresses oscillatory activity in a concentration-dependent fashion without affecting the intrinsic complexity of the responses; i.e., the mean value of D_c remains >2 until the oscillations disappear (13). This observation is perhaps surprising because nitrovasodilators exert multiple effects on Ca²⁺-dependent mechanisms in vascular smooth muscle, mediating relaxation by decreasing both intracellular Ca²⁺concentration ([Ca²⁺]ᵢ) and the Ca²⁺ sensitivity of contractile proteins. These effects follow activation of soluble guanylyl cyclase, and thus elevation of guanosine 3′,5′-cyclic monophosphate (cGMP) levels and phosphorylation of multiple target (including contractile) proteins by cGMP-dependent protein kinase (10, 30). There is an associated increase in Ca²⁺ extrusion and Ca²⁺ sequestration within sarcoplasmic reticulum (33,

39), inhibition of extracellular Ca²⁺ influx (5), and membrane hyperpolarization (37). The lack of effect of EDRF on D_c is potentially explained by the competing effects of the various maneuvers affecting ion fluxes employed in the present study. Thus blockade of Ca²⁺ influx by verapamil and CICR by ryanodine, which both caused a decrease in D_c, may be respectively considered as functionally equivalent to the limitation of extracellular Ca²⁺ influx and increased intracellular sequestration of Ca²⁺ promoted by EDRF. The expected fall in D_c could, however, be offset by EDRF-induced membrane hyperpolarization, which may directly involve activation of Ca²⁺-activated K⁺ channels, and should theoretically increase D_c, given that ChTX and apamin both cause a fall (38).

Mathematical models have shown how a two-variable nonlinear interaction between free cytosolic and stored intracellular pools of Ca²⁺ can generate oscillations in [Ca²⁺]ᵢ but also require a constant supply of Ca²⁺ to the cytosol, either from an Ins(1,4,5)P₃-sensitive store or steady influx of extracellular Ca²⁺ through the cell membrane (9, 11, 35). Oscillations in [Ca²⁺]ᵢ then result from cycling of Ca²⁺ between the cytosol and an

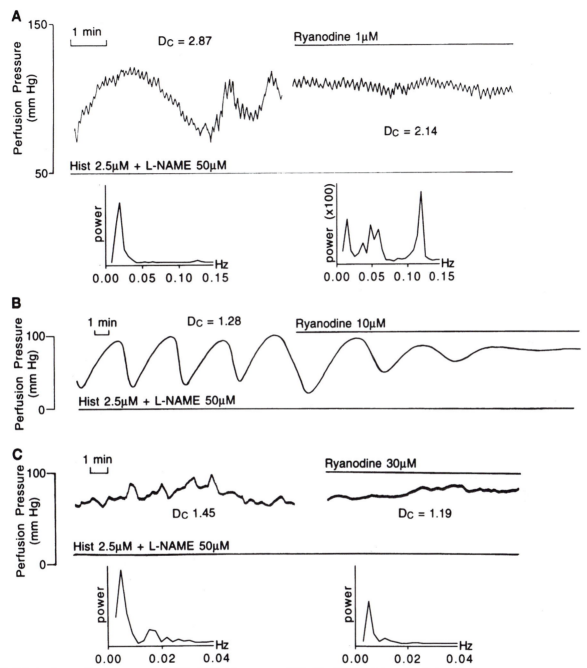

Fig. 7. Effects of ryanodine on responses to 2.5 μM Hist in presence of 50 μM L-NAME. *A*: irregular fast oscillations superimposed on a slow component. A low concentration of ryanodine minimally affected frequency of fast component but markedly attenuated the slow component, as confirmed by spectral analysis (note change of scale on right panel). *B*: unusually large sustained relaxation oscillations completely abolished by 10 μM ryanodine, final steady-state perfusion pressure being close to that at peak of oscillations. *C*: attenuation of irregular slow pressure oscillations lacking an obvious fast component by 30 μM ryanodine, with minimal effect on their frequency or mean perfusion pressure.

Ins(1,4,5)P_3-insensitive store through CICR, rather than periodic changes in Ins(1,4,5)P_3 concentration. They can be triggered by increases in $[Ca^{2+}]_o$ but are paradoxically suppressed when $[Ca^{2+}]_o$ is elevated above a critical level because the resulting high $[Ca^{2+}]_i$ then overrides the CICR mechanism (9, 11, 35). These models predict

qualitatively certain properties of the slow oscillatory subsystem investigated in the present study in that *1*) slow pressure oscillations were inhibited by ryanodine, which abolishes CICR; *2*) $[Ca^{2+}]_o > 5$ mM suppressed slow oscillatory activity; and *3*) verapamil sometimes induced slow, large-amplitude oscillations, possibly by

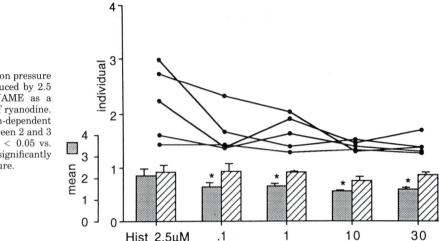

Fig. 8. D_c and mean perfusion pressure of pressure oscillations induced by 2.5 μM Hist and 50 μM L-NAME as a function of concentration of ryanodine. There was a concentration-dependent fall in average D_c from between 2 and 3 to a value <2 ($n = 5$; *$P < 0.05$ vs. control). Ryanodine did not significantly affect mean perfusion pressure.

limiting excessive Ca^{2+} influx. Spectral analysis indicated that neither altered [Ca^{2+}]$_o$ nor verapamil significantly affected the frequency of the slow subsystem, suggesting that the steady supply of Ca^{2+} necessary for oscillations derives preferentially from intracellular Ca^{2+} release by Ins(1,4,5)P$_3$, rather than influx. Experimentally, such a scenario is supported by observations that acetylcholine can evoke oscillatory Ca^{2+} release from an internal store that is triggered by a constant small Ins(1,4,5)P$_3$-evoked Ca^{2+} flow (40).

A two-variable model cannot, however, explain the chaotic nature of the experimental responses induced by histamine, because such dynamics require the participation of at least three independent control variables (12, 13). The findings with altered [Ca^{2+}]$_o$, verapamil, ChTX, and apamin suggest that two additional contributory mechanisms could be vascular smooth muscle cell membrane potential and the open-state probability of plasmalemmal Ca^{2+}-sensitive K$^+$ channels. Although electrical and mechanical events may correspond very closely in some vessel types, depolarizing action potentials being accompanied by synchronous increases in force development, in others they cannot be equated absolutely as oscillations in potential may also be functionally "integrated" over time to produce a tonic rise in force (20, 28, 32, 34, 37).

More complex biochemical pathways could also play a role in the genesis of the responses, and it has been proposed that oscillations in Ins(1,4,5)P$_3$ (and therefore [Ca^{2+}]$_i$ and tone) could arise through positive feedback between an Ins(1,4,5)P$_3$-gated intracellular channel and phospholipase C via [Ca^{2+}]$_i$ (25). Furthermore, sequentially positive then negative feedback by [Ca^{2+}]$_i$ on the opening of IICR Ca^{2+} channels by Ins(1,4,5)P$_3$ may promote oscillatory Ca^{2+} release, a mechanism functionally equivalent to CICR from ryanodine-sensitive stores (1, 17). Other possibilities include: 1) spontaneous discharge of the Ins(1,4,5)P$_3$-sensitive store when overloaded with Ca^{2+} (26), 2) activation of a sustained Ca^{2+}-activated K$^+$ current dependent on external Ca^{2+}

as a consequence of a synergistic interaction between Ins(1,4,5)P$_3$ and inositol 1,3,4,5-tetrakisphosphate (27), 3) inhibition of Ca^{2+} influx through voltage-operated Ca^{2+} channels by elevated [Ca^{2+}]$_i$ (31), 4) enhancement of Ca^{2+} influx through voltage-operated channels by calmodulin-dependent protein kinase II (24), and 5) diminished buffering of [Ca^{2+}]$_i$ by internal stores in response to vasoconstrictor agonists (36). Further experiments are necessary to evaluate the participation of these mechanisms.

In conclusion, we have shown how nonlinear analysis can provide insights into the dynamics of the mechanisms regulating vasomotor tone. "Conventional" approaches such as pharmacological and/or biochemical "isolation" and characterization of the component mechanisms may in comparison provide relatively limited insights into their overall functional integration. Given the multiplicity of the possible interactions among Ca^{2+} and K$^+$ fluxes, membrane potential, and inositol phosphates (among others), it is perhaps surprising that the fractal dimension and complexity of the vascular chaos induced by histamine are so low.

The authors thank Mike Stanton, David Harvey, and Roger Marshall for assistance with software development, Ros Maylin for secretarial assistance, and Professor Geraint Roberts for support and encouragement during the study (all at Univ. of Wales College of Medicine). We are also grateful to Professor Robert May and Alun Lloyd, Dept. of Zoology, University of Oxford, for helpful comments during the preparation of the manuscript.

This work was supported by the British Heart Foundation.

Address for reprint requests: T. M. Griffith, Dept. of Diagnostic Radiology, UWCM, Heath Park, Cardiff CF4 4XN, UK.

Received 6 July 1992; accepted in final form 22 September 1993.

REFERENCES

1. **Berridge, M. J.** Inositol phosphate and calcium signalling. *Nature Lond.* 361: 315–325, 1993.
2. **Bkaily, G., A. Sculptoreanu, D. Jacques, D. Economos, and D. Menard.** Apamin, a highly potent fetal L-type Ca^{2+} current blocker in single heart cells. *Am. J. Physiol.* 262 (*Heart Circ. Physiol.* 31): H463–H471, 1992.

3. **Chen, G., and H. Suzuki.** Calcium dependency of the endothelium-dependent hyperpolarization in smooth muscle cells of the rabbit carotid artery. *J. Physiol. Lond.* 421: 521–534, 1990.

4. **Colantuoni, S., A. Bertuglia, and M. Intaglietta.** The effects of α- or β-adrenergic receptor agonists and antagonists and calcium entry blockers on the spontaneous vasomotion. *Microvasc. Res.* 28: 143–158, 1984.

5. **Collins, P., T. M. Griffith, A. H. Henderson, and M. J. Lewis.** Endothelium-derived relaxing factor alters calcium fluxes in rabbit aorta: a cyclic guanosine monophosphate-mediated effect. *J. Physiol. Lond.* 381: 427–437, 1986.

6. **Cook, N. S.** Effect of some potassium channel blockers on contractile responses of the rabbit aorta. *J. Cardiovasc. Pharmacol.* 13: 299–306, 1989.

7. **Cook, N. S., and U. Quast.** Potassium channel pharmacology. In: *Potassium Channel Structure Classification, Function and Therapeutic Potential*, edited by N. S. Cook. Chichester, UK: Harwood, 1990, p. 181–255.

8. **Desilets, M., S. P. Driska, and C. M. Baumgarten.** Current fluctuations and oscillations in smooth muscle cells from hog carotid artery. *Circ. Res.* 65: 708–722, 1989.

9. **Ferrier, J., A. Kesthely, E. Lagan, and C. Richter.** An experimental model for repeated Ca²⁺ spikes in osteoblastic cells. *Biochem. Cell Biol.* 69: 433–441, 1990.

10. **Fiscus, R. R., R. M. Rapoport, and F. Murad.** Endothelium-dependent and nitrovasodilator-induced activation of cyclic GMP-dependent protein kinase in rat aorta. *J. Cycl. Nucleotide Protein Phosphorylation Res.* 9: 415–425, 1984.

11. **Goldbeter, A., G. Dupont, and M. J. Berridge.** Minimal model for signal-induced Ca²⁺ oscillations and for their frequency encoding through protein phosphorylation. *Proc. Natl. Acad. Sci. USA* 87: 1461–1465, 1990.

12. **Grassberger, P., and I. Procaccia.** Measuring the strangeness of strange attractors. *Physica D* 9: 189–208, 1983.

13. **Griffith, T. M., and D. H. Edwards.** EDRF suppresses chaotic pressure oscillations in an isolated resistance artery but does not influence their intrinsic complexity. *Am. J. Physiol.* 266 (*Heart Circ. Physiol.* 35): H1786–H1800, 1994.

14. **Griffith, T. M., D. H. Edwards, A. C. Newby, M. J. Lewis, and A. H. Henderson.** Production of endothelium-derived relaxant factor is dependent on oxidative phosphorylation and extracellular calcium. *Cardiovasc. Res.* 20: 7–12, 1986.

15. **Hermsmeyer, K., and H. Akbarali.** Cellular pacemaker mechanism in vascular muscle. *Prog. Appl. Microcirc.* 15: 32–40, 1989.

16. **Iino, M.** Calcium release mechanisms in smooth muscle. *Jpn. J. Pharmacol.* 54: 345–354, 1990.

17. **Iino, M., and M. Endo.** Calcium-dependent immediate feedback control of inositol 1,4,5-trisphosphate-induced Ca²⁺ release. *Nature Lond.* 360: 76–78, 1992.

18. **Inoue, R., M. Kitamura, and H. Kuriyama.** Two Ca-dependent K-channels classified by the application of tetraethylammonium distribute to smooth muscle membranes of the rabbit portal vein. *Pfluegers Arch.* 405: 173–179, 1985.

19. **Ito, K., T. Ikemoto, and S. Takakura.** Involvement of Ca²⁺ influx-induced Ca²⁺ release in contractions of intact vascular smooth muscle. *Am. J. Physiol.* 261 (*Heart Circ. Physiol.* 30): H1464–H1470, 1991.

20. **Johansson, B., and D. F. Bohr.** Rhythmic activity in smooth muscle from small subcutaneous arteries. *Am. J. Physiol.* 210: 801–806, 1966.

21. **Kanmura, Y., L. Missiaen, L. Raeymaekers, and R. Casteels.** Ryanodine reduces the amount of calcium in intracellular stores of smooth-muscle cells of the rabbit ear artery. *Pfluegers Arch.* 413: 153–159, 1988.

22. **Lamb, F. S., and R. C. Webb.** Potassium conductance and oscillatory contractions in tail arteries from genetically hypertensive rats. *J. Hypertens.* 7: 457–463, 1989.

23. **Magers, S., and J. E. Faber.** Real time measurements of microvascular dimensions using digital cross-correlation image processing. *J. Vasc. Res.* 29: 241–247, 1992.

24. **McCarron, J. G., J. H. McGeown, S. Reardon, M. Ikebe, F. S. Fay, and J. V. Walsh.** Calcium-dependent enhancement of calcium current in smooth muscle by calmodulin-dependent protein kinase II. *Nature Lond.* 357: 74–77, 1992.

25. **Meyer, T., and L. Stryer.** Molecular model for receptor-stimulated calcium spiking. *Proc. Natl. Acad. Sci. USA* 85: 5051–5055, 1988.

26. **Missiaen, L., C. W. Taylor, and M. J. Berridge.** Spontaneous calcium release from inositol trisphosphate-sensitive calcium stores. *Nature Lond.* 352: 241–244, 1991.

27. **Morris, A. P., D. V. Gallacher, R. F. Irvine, and O. H. Petersen.** Synergism of trisphosphate and tetrakisphosphate in activating Ca²⁺-dependent K⁺ channels. *Nature Lond.* 330: 653–655, 1987.

28. **Myers, J. H., F. S. Lamb, and R. C. Webb.** Norepinephrine-induced phasic activity in tail arteries from genetically hypertensive rats. *Am. J. Physiol.* 248 (*Heart Circ. Physiol.* 17): H419–H423, 1985.

29. **Nelson, M. T., J. B. Patlak, J. F. Worley, and N. B. Standen.** Calcium channels, potassium channels, and voltage dependence of arterial smooth muscle tone. *Am. J. Physiol.* 259 (*Cell Physiol.* 28): C3–C18, 1990.

30. **Nishikawa, M., P. De Lanerolle, T. H. M. Lincoln, and R. S. Adelstein.** Phosphorylation of mammalian myosin light chain kinase by the catalytic subunit of cyclic AMP-dependent protein kinase and by cyclic GMP-dependent protein kinase. *J. Biol. Chem.* 259: 8429–8436, 1984.

31. **Ohya, Y., K. Kitamura, and H. Kuriyama.** Regulation of calcium current by intracellular calcium in smooth muscle cells of rabbit portal vein. *Circ. Res.* 62: 375–383, 1988.

32. **Osol, G., and W. Halpern.** Spontaneous vasomotion in pressurized cerebral arteries from genetically hypertensive rats. *Am. J. Physiol.* 254 (*Heart Circ. Physiol.* 23): H28–H33, 1988.

33. **Popescu, L. M., C. Panoiu, M. Hinescu, and O. Nutu.** The mechanism of cGMP-induced relaxation in vascular smooth muscle. *Eur. J. Pharmacol.* 107: 393–394, 1985.

34. **Smeda, J. S., and E. E. Daniel.** Elevations in arterial pressure induce the formation of spontaneous action potentials and alter neurotransmission in canine ileum arteries. *Circ. Res.* 62: 1104–1110, 1988.

35. **Somogyi, R., and J. W. Strucki.** Hormone-induced calcium oscillations in liver cells can be explained by a simple one pool model. *J. Biol. Chem.* 266: 11068–11077, 1991.

36. **Sturek, M., K. Kunda, and Q. Hu.** Sarcoplasmic reticulum buffering of myoplasmic calcium in bovine coronary artery smooth muscle. *J. Physiol. Lond.* 451: 25–28, 1992.

37. **Tare, M., H. C. Parkington, H. A. Coleman, T. O. Neild, and G. J. Dusting.** Hyperpolarization and relaxation of arterial smooth muscle caused by nitric oxide derived from the endothelium. *Nature Lond.* 346: 69–71, 1990.

38. **Thornbury, K. D., S. M. Ward, H. H. Dalziel, A. Carl, D. P. Westfall, and K. M. Saunders.** Nitric oxide and nitrocysteine mimic nonadrenergic, noncholinergic hyperplarization in canine proximal colon. *Am. J. Physiol.* 261 (*Gastrointest. Liver Physiol.* 24): G553–G557, 1991.

39. **Twort, C. H. C., and C. Van Breemen.** Cyclic guanosine monophosphate-enhanced sequestration of Ca²⁺ by sarcoplasmic reticulum in vascular smooth muscle. *Circ. Res.* 62: 961–964, 1988.

40. **Wakui, M., Y. V. Osipchuk, and O. H. Petersen.** Receptor-activated cytoplasmic Ca²⁺ spiking mediated by inositol trisphosphate is due to Ca²⁺-induced Ca²⁺ release. *Cell* 63: 1025–1032, 1990.

41. **Wu, C.-C., and D. F. Bohr.** Mechanisms of calcium relaxation of vascular smooth muscle. *Am. J. Physiol.* 261 (*Heart Circ. Physiol.* 30): H1411–H1416, 1991.

Physiol. Meas. **14** (1993) 309–315. Printed in the UK

Fractal analysis of foetal heart rate variability

Nigel A J Gough

Department of Obstetrics and Gynaecology, University of Wales College of Medicine, Heath Park, Cardiff CF4 4XN, UK

Received 5 February 1993, in final form 10 May 1993

Abstract. Current methods for analysing foetal heart rate (FHR) patterns have yet to meet their full potential in the recognition of hypoxia in the foetus. Following the recent suggestion that fractal analysis can be applied to FHR recordings, the current paper describes a method for distinguishing two simultaneous fractal dimensions in FHR variation.

An irregular line was plotted from 2500 consecutive foetal heart beat to beat intervals derived from an ultrasound source. A window of 500 intervals was moved along the line in steps of 20 intervals. At each step the Richardson technique was used to make estimates of the length of the line within the window using 40 different ruler lengths. When the estimates were plotted against the ruler lengths on log–log axes the resulting curve exhibited two distinct linear regions, each demonstrating an inverse power relationship. From the two slopes the fractal dimensions were derived for unspecified low- and high-frequency FHR variation in the current window. The values of both fractal dimensions were plotted simultaneously with the irregular FHR line and were found to accord with perceived changes in FHR variation. The method described is simply a measure of the irregularity in a series of foetal heart beat to beat intervals: the existence of fractal properties in the irregular line does not of itself imply underlying deterministic dynamics (e.g. chaos).

This new method of observing FHR variability requires no preprocessing of the measured data, which are all taken into account. Not only does it represent a method for studying normal foetal behaviour but also has potential as a sensitive indicator of impending foetal compromise.

1. Introduction

Antenatal foetal heart rate (FHR) measurement has been ubiquitous in the West for the past 20 years and is often used as an indicator of foetal well-being in combination with other obstetric factors. The measurement is made continuously using an electronic FHR monitor which produces a chart of rate against time. When a recording is long enough, the FHR patterns are analysed. The common method of analysis is visual and subjective, the accuracy depending on the experience of the observer. A study carried out by Trimbos and Keirse (1978) showed how it was possible for obstetricians not only to disagree with each other when assessing equivocal FHR traces, but also to disagree with themselves when shown the same traces some months later. While gross patterns of heart rate variability such as accelerations, decelerations or reductions of short-term variability are easily recognized by eye, they are not reliable indicators of foetal status. The promise of this conventional FHR monitoring has yet to be realized (Neilson 1991).

In the absence of any alternatives, FHR monitoring is likely to remain in use for the foreseeable future. Therefore, efforts must be made to achieve more objective methods for the analysis of FHR variation. The first prerequisite is to improve the understanding of the behaviour of FHR variability. Much work has been carried out on statistical analysis (Visser *et al* 1981, Dawes *et al* 1981), complex demodulation (Orr and Hoffman 1974, Dalton *et al*

310   *N A J Gough*

1986) and spectral analysis (Ferrazzi *et al* 1989, Breborowicz *et al* 1988, Abboud and Sadeh 1990) with varying degrees of success. Of these methods only that of the Dawes group has been adopted as an analytical tool in clinical practice. It has been suggested that the normal sinus rhythm of the developed adult heart may be chaotic (Babloyantz and Destexhe 1988), in which case the phase space plot of the attractor will possess fractal properties (Eberhart 1989). Techniques have been developed for determining the fractal dimension of such attractors (Grassberger and Procaccia 1983, Kroll and Fulton 1991). However, Albert (1991) has questioned the validity of using established signatures of chaos in the analysis of adult heart rate. The method described in this paper treats the FHR line as a fractal line similar to a one-dimensional Brownian line (Peitgen *et al* 1992). That fractal properties can be demonstrated does not necessarily imply the presence of chaotic dynamics.

Richardson (1961) demonstrated the ambiguity in measuring the length of the border between neighbouring countries. He showed how estimates of the lengths of international borders were inversely related to the length of the ruler used to make the measurement. Plotting these estimates against ruler length produced a straight line on log–log paper. Mandelbrot (1967) took the slope of this line to be a measure of the geometric dimensionality D of the boundary ($1 \leqslant D \leqslant 2$). This value is fractional and Mandelbrot later coined the term *fractal dimension*. Using the *ruler* method described by Richardson (1961), Kaye (1989) has described how fine particles may be classified by the fractal dimension of their rugged boundaries. Kaye also showed how natural boundaries can possess two fractal scalings giving rise to two simultaneous fractal dimensions. These are manifested as two distinct straight portions on the log–log plot of length estimate against ruler length. Kaye related the fractal dimension associated with short and long rulers to *texture* and *structure* respectively.

The justification for applying fractal measurement techniques to FHR variation is illustrated in figure 1. When fractal objects are magnified they reveal more *self-similar* detail. The top trace (a) in figure 1 shows a plot of 2500 sequential beat to beat intervals (approximately 20 min). A window of 500 intervals is enlarged both vertically and horizontally and plotted beneath (b). This window has been taken from a portion of the upper trace which would conventionally be considered as a pattern reflecting a quiet foetal state with all the variability being attributable to inter-beat variation. Yet it has many similarities to the longer trace plotted above which has both high- and low-frequency variation. Much of the information that can be seen in the lower trace is usually smoothed out in conventional FHR recordings, yet given the appropriate tools, this short-term data could be rich in physiological information.

The author has recently shown that the irregular line formed by plotting sequential FHR beat to beat intervals does possess measurable fractal properties (Gough 1992). The current paper describes the method for studying these fractal properties and demonstrates the existence of two fractal scalings which appear to be related to higher- and lower-frequency variation (yet to be defined in terms of fractal dimension). However, it must be remembered that these fractal measures are not suggestive of any underlying deterministic law (*chaos*, see Gleick 1987, Denton *et al* 1990), but are simply a measure of the geometric irregularity of a line plotted from a series of numbers and having a fractal dimension, D ($1 \leqslant D \leqslant 2$). The underlying cause of this irregularity could be random or chaotic.

2. Method

FHR recordings were made using the ultrasound channel of a Hewlett Packard 8040 FHR monitor. A tape recorder was attached to the audio output of the foetal monitor and

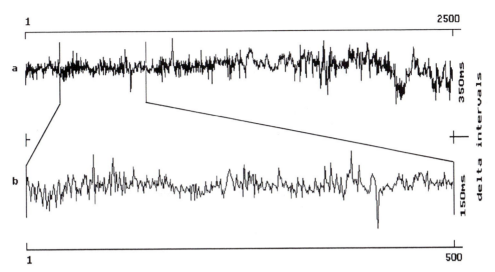

Figure 1. (*a*) 2500 FHR beat to beat intervals plotted sequentially (vertical range of interval differences = 350 ms); (*b*) 500 samples taken from a low-variability portion of (*a*) and expanded both vertically (vertical range of interval differences = 150 ms) and horizontally. Qualitatively similar detail can be seen in both traces, suggesting the existence of fractal properties.

recordings of 20 min were made. The audio signal was then played back through a system that has been described elsewhere (Gough *et al* 1986). The system measured the intervals between each heart sound complex by identifying a trigger point on the Doppler ultrasound envelope. The interval between this and the next trigger point was measured by a 1 kHz clock to a resolution of 1 ms. For statistical FHR analysis the error in ultrasonically derived interval measurements has been shown to be negligible (Dawes *et al* 1981). The values of the intervals were passed to a Toshiba T3200SX lap top computer for analysis. Each record was trimmed to 2500 consecutive beat to beat intervals. These values were then used to plot a continuous line of intervals on the vertical axis against evolution number on the horizontal axis (figure 1(*a*)). It must be noted that the horizontal axis is *not* a time axis but simply represents the relative positions of the intervals within the epoch under scrutiny. This permits consideration of the data set as a continuous non-time-sampled space filling line rather than a series of irregularly placed intervals.

A window $N = 500$ samples long ($x_0, x_1, \ldots, x_{N-1}$) was moved along the line in jumps of 20 samples. 40 estimates of the length of the line were made within the current window using a different ruler length λ for each estimate ($\lambda = 1$ to 40); the ruler was moved horizontally end to end. A Pythagorean technique was used to make an estimate of the length of each segment of line, λ samples long on the horizontal. The horizontal ruler length between $x_{i\lambda}$ and $x_{(i+1)\lambda}$ formed one side of a right angled triangle and the difference between $x_{i\lambda}$ and $x_{(i+1)\lambda}$ formed the adjacent side ($i = 0$ to $(k-1)$, and is the ruler counter, see the equation below). The hypotenuse then gave the length estimate for each segment (figure 2). The estimate $e(\lambda)$ of the length of the line within the current window for each ruler length λ was the sum of the hypotenuses and was derived from the following equation:

$$e(\lambda) = \frac{1}{N-1}\left\{ \sum_{i=0}^{k-1} \sqrt{\lambda^2 + (x_{i\lambda} - x_{(i+1)\lambda})^2} + \sqrt{(N - \lambda k - 1)^2 + (x_{\lambda k} - x_{N-1})^2} \right\}$$

$$k \doteq \mathrm{TRUNC}[(N-1)/\lambda] \qquad \lambda = 1, 2 \ldots, 40 \qquad N = 500.$$

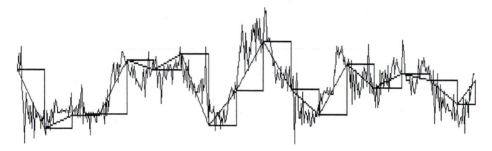

Figure 2. 500-sample-long window. The hypotenuse of each triangle gives an estimate of the length of each λ-sample-long segment of line (for this demonstration $\lambda = 30$). The estimate for the length of the whole window, $e(30)$, is the sum of the hypotenuses. A set of length estimates $e(\lambda)$ are made for each window using $\lambda = 1, 2, \ldots, 40$ (see figure 3).

The last square rooted term is included so that the length estimate can be made to the end of the data series when λ is not a factor of $N - 1$ and is equal to 0 when λ is a factor of $N - 1$. Dividing by $N - 1$ normalizes the estimates $e(\lambda)$ to the shortest length of the data series. The TRUNC function gives the integer part of $(N - 1)/\lambda$ rounded toward zero, e.g. $\frac{3}{2} = 1.5$, TRUNC $(\frac{3}{2}) = 1$. i is the ruler counter. k gives the number of whole ruler lengths that may be laid end to end along the window.

The estimates $e(\lambda)$ became shorter as the ruler length increased and conformed to an inverse power relationship, i.e. $e(\lambda) \propto \lambda^{-d}$. When $e(\lambda)$ was plotted against λ on log–log scales, a straight line with negative slope was produced. The fractal dimension D was determined from the slope $-d$ as follows (Mandelbrot 1982):

$$D = 1 - (-d).$$

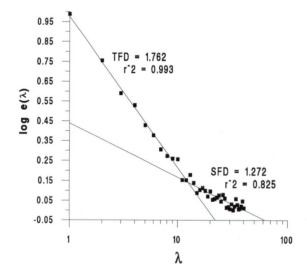

Figure 3. $\log e(\lambda)$ against $\log \lambda$ for an $N = 500$ window. The slopes of the regression lines give TFD and SFD from $D = 1 - (-d)$ (see text).

3. Results

Figure 3 shows a log–log plot of $e(\lambda)$ against λ for a window of $N = 500$ samples. It can be seen that there are two straight portions to the curve with different slopes. The first portion of the slope is related to the short ruler lengths (1 to 10) while the second is related to long ruler lengths (11 to 40). When using this technique to characterize fine-particle profiles, Kaye (1989) related these portions of the curve to texture and structure. Since the relationship between fractal dimension and the current definitions of long- and short-term variability of FHR is as yet unknown, the terms texture and structure are used here for descriptive purposes. For FHR variability, texture relates to the perceived high-frequency variation, and structure to lower-frequency variation. Automatic separation of the two straight portions of the curve was achieved by subtracting the entire data set from a least-squares fit. The point at which the maximum positive difference occurred identified the join separating the two subsets. A least-squares fit was then made to each subset and the corresponding fractal dimensions determined as described above. Figure 4 shows the textural (TFD) and structural (SFD) fractal dimensions plotted against the FHR trace.

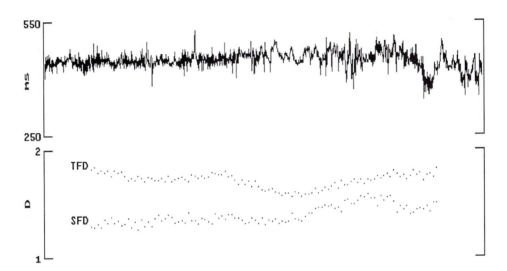

Figure 4. Evolution of beat to beat interval variation for 2500 intervals plotted with TFD and SFD. It can be seen that both TFD and SFD are sensitive to changes in high- and low-frequency variation (texture and structure).

Figure 4 shows how the TFD and SFD are affected by perceived high-and low-frequency variation respectively. The first portion of the trace has little low-frequency variation while the beat to beat variability is very apparent. This is reflected by low SFD and a high TFD. As the evolution of the trace progresses, so the low-frequency variation increases, and this is reflected in the increasing SFD. Throughout the trace high-frequency variation fluctuates and is readily identified from the TFD although it is not always apparent by observation.

4. Discussion

The fractal technique described here has shown there to be two distinct fractal structures within the FHR variation curve yielding two simultaneous fractal dimensions. These fractal dimensions are related to the high-frequency variation which gives the appearance of texture (TFD), and low-frequency variation giving the appearance of structure (SFD). The more complex spectral analysis using filtering and Fourier transforms described by Abboud and Sadeh (1990) identified two significant regions in the power spectrum relating to long- and short-term variability and categorized these regions with a long- and short-term index. It seems likely that the indices are equivalent to, or at least related to, SFD and TFD. The method described here, however, requires no preconditioning of the data such as filtering: it is possible that the characteristics of a filter could influence the resulting measures.

Dawes *et al* (1981) demonstrated how foetal breathing has the effect of slightly increasing short-term variability ($\sim$ 1 ms). This increase in short-term variability will increase the value of TFD. Abboud and Sadeh (1990) did not associate the short-term variability peak they found in the power spectrum with foetal breathing. However, this peak does coincide with the foetal breathing peaks in the power spectra of Cerutti *et al* (1989) and Ferrazzi *et al* (1989). In the absence of foetal breathing the latter two groups showed no peaks at this point in the power spectrum. This raises the question as to whether the peak disappears as foetal breathing abates or whether it is necessary to adjust the data to allow the information to be observed. It cannot be assumed that short-term variability ceases in the absence of foetal breathing and therefore power spectral techniques are possibly too insensitive to be useful.

Fractal analysis together with chaos theory is now stimulating interest in several branches of medical science (West 1990). Although a significant departure from the traditional methods of FHR analysis, the method described here has shown that the irregularity in foetal beat to beat interval values conforms to the fractal definitions of Mandelbrot (1982). The current investigation was intended to determine the presence of fractal structures in patterns of FHR obtained using a conventional source—Doppler ultrasound. Whilst fractal structures have been demonstrated, if the analysis is to be developed further, it will be helpful to determine any systematic error in interval measurement which could affect TFD. However, for detailed statistical analysis, Dawes *et al* (1981) have shown the acceptability of ultrasound for signal derivation when compared with the direct foetal ECG in labour.

The technique described here is relatively simple and natural compared with other methods. All the measured data are taken into account and require no preprocessing: what is traditionally dismissed as noise may now be treated as a legitimate component of the observed data set. The analysis is simply a geometric measure of the irregularity in a set of FHR interval values and does not imply the presence of deterministic, chaotic dynamics. It remains to explore the usefulness and applicability of fractal measurement of FHR in clinical practice, but the limited predictive value of current methods would seem to make further investigation worthwhile.

References

Abboud S and Sadeh D 1990 Power spectrum analysis of foetal heart rate variability using the abdominal maternal electrocardiogram *J. Biomed. Eng.* **12** 161–4

Albert D E 1991 Chaos and the ECG: fact and fiction *J. Electrocardiol.* **24** Supplement 102–6

Babloyantz A and Destexhe A 1988 Is the normal heart a periodic oscillator? *Biol. Cybern.* **58** 203–11

Breborowicz G, Moczko J and Gadzinowski J 1988 Quantification of the fetal heart rate variability by spectral analysis in growth-retarded fetuses. *Gynecol. Obstet. Invest.* **25** 186–91

Cerutti S, Civardi S, Bianchi A, Signorini M G, Ferrazzi E and Pardi G 1989 Spectral analysis of antepartum heart rate variability *Clin. Phys. Physiol. Meas.* **10** Supplement B 27–31

Dalton K J, Denman D W, Dawson A J and Hoffman H J 1986 Ultradian rhythms in human fetal heart rate: a computerised time series analysis *Int. J. Biomed. Comput.* **18** 45–60

Ultrasonic Imaging 15, 304–323 (1993)

Potential of Fractal Analysis for Lesion Detection in Echographic Images

J.T.M. Verhoeven and J.M. Thijssen

Biophysics Laboratory, Institute of Ophthalmology
University Hospital Nijmegen
6500 HB Nijmegen, The Netherlands

The application of fractal analysis to parametric imaging of B-mode echograms and to differentation of echographic speckle textures was investigated. Echograms were obtained from realistic simulations and from a clinical study on diffuse liver disease. The simulations comprised tissue models with randomly positioned scatterers in a 3-D volume in which the number density was varied over a range from 0.5 to 25 mm^{-3}. The clinical echograms comprised both normals and patients with liver cirrhosis. Three methods of estimating the fractal dimension were investigated, two in the spatial image domain and one in the spatial frequency domain. The results of these methods are compared and the applicability and the limitations of texture differentiation using fractal analysis is discussed. The main conclusion is that fractal analysis offers no obvious advantage over statistical analysis of the texture of echographic images. Its use for parametric imaging is further limited by the need to use relatively large windows for local estimation of the fractal dimension.   © 1993 Academic Press, Inc.

Key words: B-mode images, echographic image processing, fractal analysis, parametric imaging, texture differentiation, ultrasonic speckle.

1. INTRODUCTION

Analysis of echographic image texture has been applied in many clinical pilot studies. The analysis was based either on tissue-ultrasound interaction models of image formation [1–7], or on purely (first and second order) statistical approaches [8,9]. The quantitative parameters involved were to some extent dependent on the employed equipment. Moreover, the retrospectively performed studies involved a limited number of clinical cases. Therefore, it is still not possible to indicate with certainty the clinical impact of echographic image analysis.

It has become clear from physical modelling of the ultrasound propagation and image formation, that image texture contains information about the physical characteristics [10] and the spatial distribution [3,4,11–13] of the scattering structures within the tissue. Echographic image texture is dominated by speckle formation, which is due to the interference at reception of a great number of partially coherent backscattered echoes [14–17]. It has been shown in theoretical studies [18,19] and simulation experiments [10,20] that the moments of the grey level statistics are systematically dependent on the number density of the scatterers. Moreover, structural patterns of the spatial distribution of scatterers are revealed by spatial and grey level modulations of the speckle pattern, i.e., yielding a particular image texture [21–23].

The scattering of ultrasound by parenchymal tissue is dominated by collagen-rich histological structures. Experimental studies of the backscattering by liver tissue indicated that possibly three dimensional levels are involved: cells, portal triads, and the (arterial) vasculature [24]. These are discrete dimensions of the order of 10 μm, 100 μm and 1 mm or larger, respectively. From these characteristics, mainly, the vascular tree is present in a large

305

Ultrasonic Imaging 15, 304–323 (1993)

range of dimensions. The range of the imaging dimensions is two orders of magnitude: from 1 to 100 mm. The lower value corresponds to the resolution limit of a 3.5 MHz transducer, whereas the upper limit is induced by the practical size of the region of interest (ROI). The aforementioned lower resolution limit applies to the axial direction. In the lateral direction the speckle dimension is up to five times larger. Therefore, any image analysis has to be performed in the two directions separately. The conditions are further complicated by the change of — mainly the lateral — speckle dimension with depth [10]. Therefore, any analysis of the lateral texture characteristics should be adapted to the depth range involved.

Recently, some papers have been published on fractal analysis of echographic images. The approaches used were based on the concept of fractional Brownian motion (fBm), either in the spatial domain [25,26], or in the frequency domain [27]. The analysis yields an estimate of the so-called Hurst coefficient (H), from which the fractal dimension can be calculated. Another approach of fractal analysis is based on the estimation of the Minkowski index (M) from a scale-space approach of image analysis [28–30]. The fractal dimension can be related to the Minkowski index. The application of the analysis methods to medical echograms comprise very limited sets of patients in these papers.

In this paper, a comparison is made of these three approaches of fractal analysis. In addition, the results are compared to those obtained by more conventional methods of image analysis. The material analyzed consists of computer stimulated one- and two-dimensional echograms, as well as liver echograms of normal subjects and of patients with a proven liver disease taken from a clinical pilot study [4–6].

2. FRACTALS

2.1 Geometric model

The basic concept of fractal models can be most easily explained by the "coastline of Britain" measurement as described by Mandelbrot [31]. The length, L, of the coarse coastline is measured by a one-dimensional yardstick of length λ_1. The length is now the number of times we can place this yardstick along the coastline, $N_1(\lambda_1)$, multiplied by the length of the yardstick

$$L = N_1(\lambda_1)\lambda_1 \tag{1}$$

When we take a shorter yardstick of length λ_2, we find a different number $N_2(\lambda_2)$.

However,

$$N_1(\lambda_1)\lambda_1 \neq N_2(\lambda_2)\lambda_2 \tag{2}$$

This is because any yardstick skips bays and peninsulas that are smaller than the yardstick itself. In general, the length will increase with decreasing length of the applied yardstick because smaller details are taken into account.

The apparent length of the coastline is therefore dependent on the length of the applied yardstick, or, more in general, dependent on the applied resolution. We may demand the length L to be independent of λ by introducing a new dimension, D_F. Now we demand:

$$L = N_1(\lambda_1)\lambda_1^{D_F} = N_2(\lambda_2)\lambda_2^{D_F} = \text{constant} \tag{3}$$

where D_F = Hausdorff-Besicovitch dimension.

As a result:

$$D_F = \frac{\ln\left(\dfrac{N_1(\lambda_1)}{N_2(\lambda_2)}\right)}{\ln\left(\dfrac{\lambda_2}{\lambda_1}\right)} \tag{4.1}$$

Ultrasonic Imaging 15, 304–323 (1993)

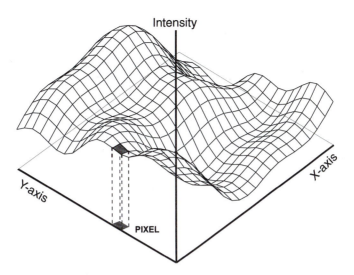

Fig. 1 Examples of the intensity surface of a small region in a B-mode image. The intensity of a pixel located in the XY-plane, is displayed along the vertical intensity axis.

In general, D_F differs from the topological dimension, T, (i.e., $D_F>1$ for the one-dimensional problem considered here) and does not have an integer but rather a fractional value; hence the more generally used term fractional, or fractal, dimension. This fractal dimension is not a fixed value but depends on the measurement problem, i.e., it is dependent on the roughness of the coastline in the problem considered here. In general, D_F can be used to describe the roughness of a curve in a plane.

This one-dimensional case can easily be extended from curves to surfaces and volumes. Now, the area of a surface is measured by a two-dimensional unity surface (with area λ^2) instead of the one-dimensional yardstick. Again, we demand the area of the surface to be independent of the size of the unity surface. The fractal dimension for which this condition holds, is found from:

$$D_F = \frac{\ln\left(\dfrac{N_1\left(\lambda_1^2\right)}{N_2\left(\lambda_2^2\right)}\right)}{\ln\left(\dfrac{\lambda_2^2}{\lambda_1^2}\right)} \qquad (4.2)$$

When we regard the pixel intensities of an image as heights above a plane (Fig. 1), then the intensity surface of this image can be viewed as a rugged surface. The fractal dimension can now be used to quantify the roughness, i.e., the texture, of the image. In this way, it provides a scale invariant description of complex image textures. Therefore, it may possess potential for image segmentation purposes and for lesion detection methods based on the detection of abnormal texture regions.

2.2 Selfsimilarity

An interesting aspect of fractals is that they posses the property of selfsimilarity. This means that every part of a curve (or surface) is similar to the curve (or surface) as a whole, except for a scaling factor. A curve defined by a

307

Ultrasonic Imaging 15, 304–323 (1993)

function $f(r)$ is said to be selfsimilar with parameter H if for any $h>0$:

$$f(r+\Delta r) = \frac{f(r+h\Delta r)-f(r)}{h^H} \tag{5}$$

where r = distance,
       H = Hurst coefficient ($H \in (0,1)$).

When we try to describe a real object as a fractal, this object is, in general, only selfsimilar in a certain range of scales (i.e., an object with finite size), whereas the fractal is selfsimilar on all scales. So we can expect the fractal dimension of a real object to be constant over a limited range only.

2.3 Statistical fractals

Natural fractal surfaces do not, in general, possess this geometric selfsimilarity described above. Instead however, they exhibit *statistical* selfsimilarity; that is, they are composed of distinct subsets each of which is scaled down from the original and is identical in all statistical respects to the scaled original. This statistical selfsimilarity is often referred to as selfaffinity. An important, and well known, class of statistically selfaffine fractals are the fractional Brownian functions [40,33].

2.4 Fractal images

Pentland [32] has presented evidence that most natural surfaces are spatially isotropic fractals and that intensity images of these surfaces are also fractals. Mandelbrot has demonstrated [31] that such fractal surfaces are generalizations of random walks and Brownian motion; that is, they result as a limit of processes that randomly modify local shape at each scale. This generalization, which is an expansion of the ordinary Brownian motion, is called a fractional Brownian function (fBf) and its properties are extensively described in [33].

Medical images typically have a degree of randomness associated with the characteristics of the underlying structures. The intensity surface of such an image is often viewed as resulting from a random walk in 2D space [26]. Therefore, in our fractal model, the texture of the intensity images, $I(\vec{r})$, is considered to be modeled by a fractional Brownian function. In this case for all $\vec{r}$ and $\Delta\vec{r}$ the following relation holds:

$$Pr\left(\frac{I(\vec{r}+\Delta\vec{r})-I(\vec{r})}{\|\Delta\vec{r}\|^H} < y\right) \doteq F(y) \tag{6}$$

where $\vec{r}$ = (x,y), position in 2-dimensional space,
      I = intensity of pixel at position $\vec{r}$,
     $F(y)$ = a cumulative distribution function (typically a zero-mean Gaussian with
             unit variance), and
     H = Hurst coefficient as defined above.

For $H = \frac{1}{2}$ we obtain the classical nonfractional Brownian motion [27,33].

For fractal images (i.e., physical fractals), it is required that [27]:
1. each segment of the image is statistically similar to all other segments, and
2. the properties of these segments are invariant to scale transformation.

Ultrasonic Imaging 15, 304–323 (1993)

3. FRACTAL ANALYSIS

The three methods for estimation of the fractal dimension studied in this paper are described below. Two of these methods, one estimating the Hurst coefficient (*method 1*) and one estimating the Minkowski dimension (*method 2*), are carried out in the spatial image domain. The *third method*, also estimating the Hurst coefficient, is carried out in the spatial frequency domain. The relation between the two parameters resulting from these analysis methods, and the fractal dimension is defined.

3.1 Spatial domain

Method 1: From Eq. (6) we can derive the following expression [27]:

$$E\left\{\left[I(\vec{r}+\Delta\vec{r})-I(\vec{r})\right]^2\right\} = \left\|\Delta\vec{r}\right\|^{2H} s^2 \tag{7}$$

where E = expectation,
H = Hurst coefficient, and
s^2 = the variance of the distribution $F(y)$.

Taking the logarithm, we obtain:

$$\ln E\left\{\left[I(\vec{r}+\Delta\vec{r})-I(\vec{r})\right]^2\right\} = 2H\ln\left\|\Delta\vec{r}\right\| + 2\ln s \tag{8}$$

The texture of an echographic image (i.e., the roughness of the surface of a fBf) can now be described by the parameter H while keeping the variance s^2 constant. When we define $\Delta I_{\Delta\vec{r}} = \left|I(\vec{r}+\Delta\vec{r})-I(\vec{r})\right|$ then:

$$\ln E\left\{\Delta I_{\Delta\vec{r}}^2\right\} = 2H\ln\left\|\Delta\vec{r}\right\| + \text{ constant} \tag{9}$$

(It should be noted that $\ln E\left\{\Delta I_{\Delta\vec{r}}^2\right\}$ cannot be simplified to $2\ln E\left\{\Delta I_{\Delta\vec{r}}\right\}$ as is done in [26]).

From Eq. (9), the Hurst coefficient, H, can now be estimated using the following procedure [32]. First, from the intensity image, the mean squared intensity difference, $E\left\{\Delta I_{\Delta\vec{r}}^2\right\}$, is calculated for various distances between two pixels, $\Delta\vec{r}$. Second, the logarithm of $E\left\{\Delta I_{\Delta r}^2\right\}$ is plotted versus the logarithm of $\left\|\Delta\vec{r}\right\|$. An example of the resulting curve is shown in figure 3. Finally, the slope of this curve, which corresponds to H, is estimated by applying a linear least-squares method [34].

For practical reasons, the range of $\Delta\vec{r}$ has to be limited between a minimum and a maximum value. The smallest "information grain" in an echographic image is the speckle cell [15]. Therefore, the lower limit is set to the size of the speckle cell as expressed by the Full-Width-at-Half-Maximum of its autocovariance function [10]. It should be noted that this size is different in the axial and lateral direction. Therefore, the lower limit is dependent on the direction of the analysis. In general, the upper limit is determined by the size of the organs or structures being examined. However, our test images, both the computer simulated images and the clinical echograms, are entirely of one homogeneous structure. Therefore, the upper limit is determined by the size of the image. To ensure sufficient data for the estimating of $E\left\{\Delta I_{\Delta\vec{r}}^2\right\}$, the upper limit was set at half the length of an image line.

Method 2: A somewhat different approach is based on the "scale-space" filtering concept [35,36]. Scale-space filtering implies the convolution of an image with a kernel over a certain range of resolutions. It can be proven that a Gaussian kernel is optimal in preserving spatial signal characteristics [37] and for this reason the Gaussian kernel is used in this study. The width of the Gaussian kernel is expressed by its standard deviation value σ_s, and the convolution is written as:

$$V(x,y;\sigma_s) = I(x,y) \otimes G(x,y;\sigma_s)$$
$$= \iint I(\zeta,\eta)G\big((\zeta-x),(\eta-y);\sigma_s\big)d\zeta d\eta \tag{10}$$

309

Ultrasonic Imaging 15, 304–323 (1993)

where $I(x,y)$ is the original echographic image and

$$G(x,y;\sigma_s) = \frac{1}{2\pi\sigma_s}\exp\left(-\frac{x^2+y^2}{2\sigma_s^2}\right)$$ (11)

is the Gaussian kernel. σ_s is used to vary the width of the kernel (i.e., vary the resolution) and is, therefore, referred to as "scale parameter".

As quoted in [28], Minkowski developed a method for defining the area, A, of a (not necessarily smooth) surface in $\mathbf{R}^3$. For a smooth surface, and applying the scale-space filtering concept described above, the following formula estimating the so-called Minkowski dimension, M, which is related to the fractal dimension, was obtained:

$$M = T - \frac{\ln(A(\sigma_s))}{\ln(\sigma_s)}$$ (12)

where $A(\sigma_s)$ = area of the intensity surface of the image after convolution with a kernel (i.e., of $V(x,y;\sigma_s)$ in Eq. (10)),
$\quad\sigma_s\quad$ = standard deviation of the Gaussian.

This relation is supposed to hold over a certain range of σ_s-values [28], although Minkowski described a rigorous proof for the limit case of $\sigma_s \to 0$ only.

The Minkowski dimension can now be estimated by using the following procedure. First, the image is filtered (as expressed in Eq. (10)) applying Gaussian kernels over a certain range of the scale parameter σ_s (figure 2 shows an example of the resulting intensity surfaces for three values of σ_s). Second, the areas, $A(\sigma s)$, of the surfaces spanned by the grey-levels of the filtered images are computed. For a two-dimensional image, the area of the surface spanned by the grey-levels in the image follows from:

$$A(\sigma_s) = \iint_{xy} \sqrt{1+V_x^2(x,y;\sigma_s)+V_y^2(x,y;\sigma_s)}\,dxdy$$ (13)

where $V_x(x,y;\sigma_s) = \dfrac{\partial V(x,y;\sigma_s)}{\partial x}$, i.e., the first derivative with respect to x, and $V_y(x,y;\sigma_s)$ is defined accordingly.

Next, the logarithm of $A(\sigma_s)$ is plotted versus the logarithm of the scale parameter, σ_s, and the slope of the resulting curve is estimated by a linear least-squares fit [34]. Finally, M is found by subtracting the result of this fit from the topological dimension, T. Since the curve generally has a negative slope (the area, $A(\sigma_s)$, increases with decreasing scale parameter because smaller details are taken into account), the Minkowski dimension will be found to be larger than the topological dimension.

Because for real images the selfsimilarity property only holds over a certain range of scales (section 2.2), the curve is not a straight line (see figure 6). Both for small values of the scale parameter ($\sigma_s \to 0$), where the filtered image approaches the original image, and for large values of the scale parameter ($\sigma_s \to \infty$), where the filtered image ap-

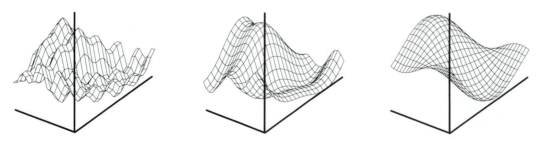

Fig. 2 Example of the smoothing effect of *method* 2. From left to right, normalized intensity surfaces of a region in a B-mode image after convolution with a Gaussian kernel with increasing scale parameter.

Ultrasonic Imaging 15, 304–323 (1993)   310

proaches the mean value of the original image, the curve approaches a fixed value. Therefore, the fit of a straight line can only be performed over a limited range of the scale parameters. This range is centered around the bending point of the curve.

3.2   Frequency domain

Method 3: A third possibility to estimate the fractal dimension is to consider the power spectrum of a fBf [32,38]. Given a fBf, B(r), a frequency representation was obtained by Hunt [33,39]:

$$B(r_2) - B(r_1) = C \int_0^\infty \left(e^{2\pi i f r_2} - e^{2\pi i f r_1} \right) f^{-H-1/2} dB(f) \tag{14}$$

with frequency f and C a constant. Although it is difficult to exactly determine the power spectrum of nonstationary random functions, like fBf's, it is suggested [33] from Eq. (14) that fBf's have a power spectrum proportional to f^β with $\beta = 2H + 1$.

Now, taking the Fourier transform of an echographic intensity image, the following relation applies:

$$\mathcal{F}\{I(r)\} \propto f_s^{-\beta} \tag{15}$$

with

$$\beta = 2H + 1 \tag{16}$$

and $\mathcal{F}$ = spatial Fourier transform,
      f_s = spatial frequency, and
      r = either the x or the y direction (for one-dimensional analysis in axial and lateral direction separately).

Like before, the Hurst coefficient can now be estimated via regression in the logarithmic domain of $\mathcal{F}\{I(r)\}$ over the spatial frequency, f_s. However, Gårding [27] showed with simulated fractal images that the linear relation in Eq. (16) only holds over a limited range of the values of H ($H \in (0.1, 0.8)$).

3.3   Relation between derived parameters, M and H, and the fractal dimension, D_F

Hurst coefficient: The fractal dimension can be found from the Hurst coefficient by [27,40]:

$$D_F = T + 1 - H \tag{17}$$

where D_F = the fractal dimension, and
        T = the topological dimension.

Therefore, in case of a one-dimensional analysis of a 2-D image (i.e., analysis in the axial and lateral directions separately), the fractal dimension can be estimated from the Hurst coefficient by:

$$D_F = 2 - H \tag{18}$$

while in case of a full two-dimensional analysis the fractal dimension is given by:

$$D_F = 3 - H \tag{19}$$

Minkowski dimension: Zähle [28] defined a general relation between the Minkowski dimension, the Hausdorff-Besicovitch dimension and the topological dimension:

$$0 \le D_F \le M \le T + 1 \tag{20}$$

311

Ultrasonic Imaging 15, 304–323 (1993)

Applying Eq. (17) and $H \in (0,1)$ we find:

$$T \leq D_F \leq M \leq T + 1 \tag{21}$$

4. TEST IMAGES

The fractal analysis methods were applied to computer simulated echographic images and to clinical B-mode images of the liver. Both one-dimensional simulations, i.e., echolines rather than echo-images, and full 3-D simulations [41], yielding realistic 2-D (B-mode) images, were used.

The one-dimensional images consisted of 64 lines of 1024 data points. Each line was divided in two, and each half represented different tissue. The left 512 samples were made by using a tissue model containing 50 scatterers/cm and the right 512 samples by using a model containing 500 scatterers/cm. The mean amplitude level in both sides was made equal.

The medium in the 3-D simulations consisted of a volume of nonattenuating tissue placed in the focal zone of a 3 MHz transducer (–6 dB bandwidth of 1.55 MHz). The tissue consisted of randomly distributed point scatterers. The number density of scatterers was 100, 200, 500, 5000 and 25000 scatters/cm³, resulting in images with different speckle textures [10]. The B-mode image was derived by a linear scan around the focus and covered a 4×4 cm² area. These simulated images were visualized and processed using a 512×512 pixel, 256 gray level image memory. The second order statistics of the one-dimensional simulated images using 50 and 500 scatters/cm corresponded to that of the axial direction of the 3-D simulated images using 500 and 5000 scatterers/cm³, respectively.

The fractal dimension was also extracted from images of six healthy and seven cirrhotic livers. For each liver, five images were used. Each image consisted of approximately 72 scan lines of 65 mm of tissue. These images were obtained by scanning different (independent) cross-sections of the same liver and were taken shortly after each other in one diagnostic session. The transducer geometry of the echoscanner (Sonoline 3000, Siemens, Inc.) corresponded to that of the transducer in the computer simulations.

5. RESULTS

5.1 Spatial domain

The *first method* was applied to computer simulated test images and to clinical echograms of the liver. The simulations were of tissues containing various number densities of scatterers. For each number density, six independent images were simulated. The clinical images were of patients with a normal or a cirrhotic livers. For each patient, five images of different cross-sections of the liver were used. The fractal dimension of these images was estimated using a one-dimensional analysis in the axial direction. The mean Hurst coefficient resulting from the analysis of the simulated images together with its computed standard deviation (s.d.) is shown in table I. In figure 3, an example of a graph of the logarithm of $E\{\Delta I_{\Delta r}^2\}$ plotted versus the logarithm of Δr is shown. Table II shows the results of the analy-

Table I Mean Hurst coefficient, H, resulting from the analysis of simulated echograms of tissues with various scatterer densities (*method 1*). For each density, six independent images were analyzed (n=6).

scatterer density cm⁻³	H ($\cdot 10^{-3}$)	s.d. ($\cdot 10^{-3}$)
100	82	12
200	70	9
500	64	8
5000	69	6
25000	72	10

Ultrasonic Imaging 15, 304–323 (1993)

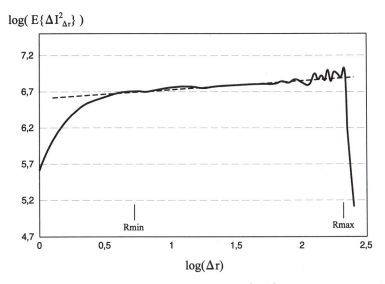

Fig. 3 Example of *method 1*. The logarithm of $E\{\Delta I^2_{\Delta r}\}$ plotted versus the logarithm of Δr for computer simulated images containing 500 scatterers/cm^3 (solid curve) and the fitted line (dashed curve). The fit procedure was performed over the indicated range (R_{min}, R_{max}).

sis of the clinical images. The mean Hurst coefficient for each patient (mean of the different cross-sections of one liver) and for each class (mean of all images within a class) is presented.

The *second method*, based on the scale-space filtering concept, was applied to one-dimensional simulations of tissue models containing 50 and 500 scatterers/cm. A one-dimensional analysis in the axial direction was performed. In this case, the surface $A(\sigma_s)$ in Eq. (12) is the simple line integral over the samples. The resulting Minkowski dimensions (for each half of the simulation separately) are shown in table III. The Minkowski dimension resulting from each analysis window individually was plotted versus its axial postion. A window size of 64×64 samples was used and they were 32 samples apart, resulting in an overlap of 50%. Only the central window (number 16) was present both in tissue containing 50 and in tissue containing 500 scatterers/cm. The result is shown in figure 4.

Table II Hurst coefficient, H, of normal and cirrhotic livers calculated for each patient separately (5 images/patient) and for the normal and cirrhotic class as a whole (*method 1*).

healthy livers			cirrhotic livers		
patient index	H ($\cdot 10^{-3}$)	s.d. ($\cdot 10^{-3}$)	patient index	H ($\cdot 10^{-3}$)	s.d. ($\cdot 10^{-3}$)
1	60	6	7	71	12
2	88	10	8	64	7
3	87	7	9	67	6
4	70	8	10	73	7
5	75	6	11	56	6
6	67	8	12	87	13
			13	74	9
total	75	13	total	70	14

313   Ultrasonic Imaging 15, 304–323 (1993)

Table III Minkowski dimension, M, minus the topological dimension ($T = 1$) for the one-dimensional simulated echograms (*method 2*).

scatterer density cm^{-1}	M-T (·10^{-3})	s.d. (·10^{-3})
50	14.5	0.43
500	11.6	0.50

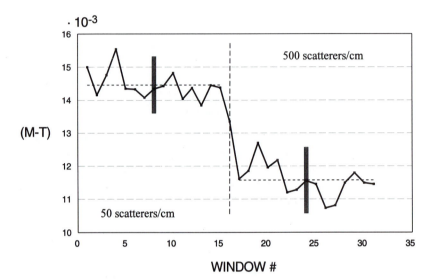

Fig. 4 (M-T) versus position, #, of analysis window ($T = 1$). The vertical dashed line indicates the transition between the two tissues. The horizontal dotted lines indicate the mean values, the vertical bars specify the ±2s.d. ranges.

This method was also applied to the computer simulated test images of tissues with various number densities of scatterers. A full two-dimensional analysis was performed. Now, the function $A(\sigma_s)$ is the area as computed numerically from Eq. (13). The results are shown in table IV and in figure 5. In figure 6, examples of the graphs of the logarithm of A plotted versus the logarithm of σ_s are shown for two different scatterer densities.

Finally, the clinical images were analyzed. Again, a one-dimensional analysis in the axial direction was carried out. The results of this analysis are shown in table V.

Table IV Minkowski dimension, M, minus the topological dimension ($T = 2$) for the computer simulated test images (*method 2*).

scatterer density cm^{-3}	M-T (·10^{-3})	s.d. (·10^{-3})
100	160	10
200	139	6
500	121	7
5000	104	3
25000	103	4

Ultrasonic Imaging 15, 304–323 (1993)

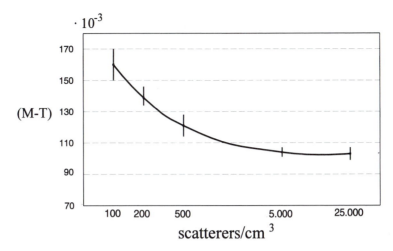

Fig. 5 (*M-T*) versus scatterer density (*T* = 2). The vertical bars indicate the ±s.d. range (see table IV).

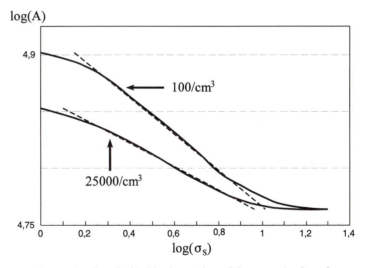

Fig. 6 Example of *method 2*. The logarithm of the area, *A*, plotted versus the logarithm of σ_s for computer simulated images containing 100 and 25000 scatterers/cm³ (solid curves) and the fitted lines (dashed curves).

Table V Minkowski dimension, *M*, minus the topological dimension (*T* = 1) of normal and cirrhotic livers (*method 2*).

healthy livers			cirrhotic livers		
patient index	*M-T* ($\cdot 10^{-3}$)	s.d. ($\cdot 10^{-3}$)	patient index	*M-T* ($\cdot 10^{-3}$)	s.d. ($\cdot 10^{-3}$)
1	12.8	0.8	7	14.3	1.3
2	10.9	0.9	8	13.7	1.0
3	11.5	1.1	9	15.3	1.1
4	13.1	1.0	10	12.8	1.2
5	12.3	0.9	11	15.9	1.2
6	10.4	1.0	12	13.9	0.8
			13	13.5	0.9
total	11.8	1.3	total	14.2	1.5

315   Ultrasonic Imaging 15, 304–323 (1993)

Table VI Hurst coefficient, H, resulting from the analysis of simulated echograms of tissues which various scatterer densities using *method 3* (frequency domain).

scatterer density cm^{-3}	H ($\cdot 10^{-3}$)	s.d. ($\cdot 10^{-3}$)
100	34	15
200	45	13
500	50	20
5000	72	19
25000	65	21

Table VII Hurst coefficient, H, of normal and cirrhotic livers, calculated for each patient separately and for the normal and cirrhotic class as a whole, using *method 3* (frequency domain).

healthy livers			cirrhotic livers		
patient index	H ($\cdot 10^{-3}$)	s.d. ($\cdot 10^{-3}$)	patient index	H ($\cdot 10^{-3}$)	s.d. ($\cdot 10^{-3}$)
1	56	27	7	66	21
2	37	24	8	39	28
3	73	18	9	80	20
4	−9	27	10	52	16
5	24	26	11	−11	23
6	12	21	12	17	18
			13	74	14
total	32	31	total	45	34

5.2 Frequency domain

Method 3: The method in the frequency domain was applied to the computer simulated test images and to the clinical echograms. To determine the frequency spectrum a discrete fast Fourier transform (DFT) was used. The results of the, one-dimensional, analysis are shown in table VI and VII.

6. DISCUSSION

Comparing the results of the three investigated methods, only the second method in the time domain, based on the scale-space filtering concept, shows potential for texture differentiation purposes in echographic images.

Method 1: Our study, both using computer simulated images and clinical liver images, produces no evidence that this method is applicable, although Chen [26] presented promising results based on a limited set of clinical echographic images. In this method, it is assumed that the image texture can be fully described by the fractal dimension while keeping the variance in Eq. (7) constant. However, the converse is also applicable: describing the image texture by the variance while keeping the fractal dimension constant. Gårding [27] suggested that both parameters are needed to fully describe image texture modeled by a fBf.

Method 2: This method showed potential for classifying clinical liver images (normal versus cirrhotic) and for distinguishing between echographic image textures. To further assess its potential, we applied this method to a computer simulated image of an isoechoic lesion (Fig. 7). This image consisted of background tissue containing 5000

Ultrasonic Imaging 15, 304–323 (1993)

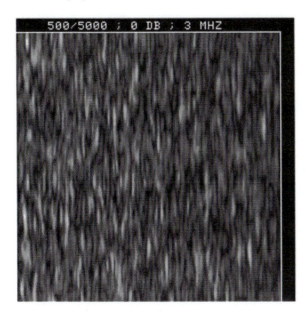

Fig. 7 Simulated echographic image of an isoechoic lesion (background: 5000/cm³, lesion: 500/cm³).

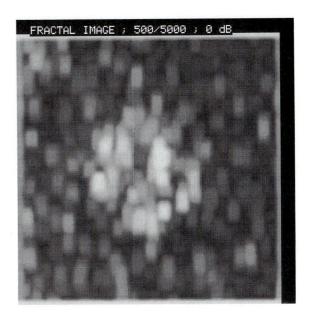

Fig. 8 Parametric image showing the Minkowski dimension minus the topological dimension $(M - T)$. White corresponds to $(M - T) = 140 \ 10^{-3}$, black to $(M - T) = 80 \ 10^{-3}$.

scatterers/cm³ with circulair lesion tissue containing 500 scatterers/cm³ located in the center. A two-dimensional analysis was performed using 32×32 pixel windows. The results are displayed in a two-dimensional fashion, thus creating a new parametric image (Fig. 8) where black represents a $(M\text{-}T)$ value of $80 \ 10^{-3}$ and white of $140 \ 10^{-3}$. This image clearly reveals the presence of a deviant image texture in the center of the original image.

Method 3: Although some dependency of the fractal dimension on the investigated image texture is apparent, differentiation is not feasible because of the large spread in the results. This method requires a very accurate estimation of the power spectrum. Even using the computer simulated images (which consist of a regular speckle pattern), we were not able to achieve the required precision when applying DFT's for the estimation of the frequency spectrum. A drawback of DFT's is that, for an accurate estimation of the spectrum, many samples are needed. Therefore, this method could only be used to analyze complete images. Using an Auto-Regressive (AR) spectral estimation algorithm [42,43], which requires fewer samples, did not solve this problem. Even when using higher order models, no reliable fit could be made because of the dependency of the spectral peaks on the AR-model.

It is assumed that the fractal dimension of a scene dictates the fractal dimension in its echographic image. Pentland has shown [32] that this assumption only applies under restricted conditions. In this paper, we do not study this imaging problem. However, because we do not intend to exactly classify image regions but only try to segment regions with different textures, this should not be a major problem.

In this paper, the fractal dimension is used to quantify changes of the texture pattern in an echographic B-mode image that result from changes in the number density of scatterers in the tissue being investigated. However, the first (Signal-to-Noise Ratio (SNR) [44]) and second (width of the autocovariance function (ACFV) [10]) order statistical parameters can also be used, which require less computational effort. These parameters appeared to change by a factor of the order of 1.2 (ACFV) to 1.5 (SNR) over the range of scatterer number densities used in the present paper. The maximum result for the fractal analysis (*method 2*), as given in table IV, is similar to the result of the SNR analysis. However, the algorithm for calculating the SNR is more simple and more precise. Therefore, smaller windows can be used and SNR imaging is to be preferred rather than imaging the fractal dimension (Fig. 8). If it would show that the fractal dimension is statistically independent of the other texture measures, it could still be employed in a multiparameter approach to tissue characterization.

ACKNOWLEDGMENTS

This work was supported by a grant from the Technical Science Branch (STW) of the Netherland's Organization for Scientific Research (NWO). The authors would also like to thank P. Kniest and M. Wijshoff for their contributions.

REFERENCES

1 Insana, M.F., Wagner, R.F., Garra, B.S., Brown, D.G. and Shawker, T.H., Analysis of ultrasound image texture via generalized Rician statistics, *Opt. Eng. 25*, 743–748 (1986).

2 Garra, B.S., Insana, M.F., Shawker, T.H. and Russell, M.A., Quantitative estimation of liver estimation and echogenicity: normal state versus diffuse liver disease, *Radiology 162*, 61–67 (1987).

3 Fellingham, L.L. and Sommer, F.G., Ultrasonic characterization of tissue structure in the in vivo human liver and spleen, *IEEE Trans. Sonics Ultrason. SU-31*, 418–428 (1984).

4 Hartman, P.C., Oosterveld, B.J., Thijssen, J.M., Rosenbusch, G.J.E., and van den Berg, J., Detection and differentiation of diffuse liver disease by quantitative echography: a retrospective assessment, *Invest. Radiol. 28*, 1–6 (1993).

5 Oosterveld, B.J., Thijssen, J.M., Hartman, P.C. and Rosenbusch, G.J.E., Detection of diffuse liver disease by quantitative echography: dependence on a priori choice of parameters, *Ultrasound Med. Biol. 19*, 21–25 (1993).

6 Romijn, R.L., Thijssen, J.M., Oosterveld, B.J. and Verbeek, A.M., Ultrasonic differentiation of intraocular melanomas: parameters and estimation methods, *Ultrasonic Imaging 13*, 27–55 (1991).

7 Thijssen, J.M., Oosterveld, B.J., Hartman, P.C. and Rosenbusch G.J.E., Correlations between acoustic and texture parameters from RF and B-mode liver echograms, *Ultrasound Med. Biol. 19*, 13–20 (1993).

8 Nicholas, D., Nassiri, D.K., Garbutt, P. and Hill, C.R., Tissue characterization from ultrasound B-scan data, *Ultrasound Med. Biol. 12*, 135–143 (1986).

9 Schlaps, D., Zuna, I., Walz, M., Volk, J. and Raeth, U., Ultrasonic tissue characterization by texture analysis: Estimation of tissue independent factors, in *Proc. SPIE Congress, Vol. 768*, Ferrari, L.A., ed., pp. 128–134 (SPIE, Bellingham, 1987).

10 Oosterveld, B.J., Thijssen, J.M. and Verhoef, W.A., Texture of B-mode echograms: 3-D simulations and experiments of the effects of diffraction and scatterer density, *Ultrasonic Imaging 7*, 142–160 (1985).

11 Wagner, R.F., Insana, M.F. and Brown, D.G., Unified approach to the detection and classification of speckle texture in diagnostic ultrasound, *Opt. Eng. 25*, 738–742 (1986).

12 Wagner, R.F., Insana, M.F. and Brown, D.G., Statistical properties of radio-frequency and envelope-detected signals with applications to medical ultrasound, *J. Optical Soc. Am. 4*, 910–922 (1987).

13 Insana, M.F., Wagner, R.F., Garra, B.S. and Brown, D.G., Analysis of ultrasound image texture via generalized Rician statistics, *J. Opt. Eng. 25*, 732–748 (1986).

14 Abbott, J.G. and Thurstone, F.L., Acoustic speckle: theory and experimental analysis, *Ultrasonic Imaging 1*, 303–324 (1979).

15 Burckhardt, C.B., Speckle in Ultrasound B-mode scans, *IEEE Trans. Sonics Ultrasonics SU-25*, 1–6 (1978).

16 Bamber, J.C. and Dickinson, R.J., Ultrasonic B-scanning: A computer simulation, *Phys. Med. Biol. 25*, 463–479 (1980).

17 Wagner, R.F., Smith, S.W., Sandrik, J.M. and Lopez, H., Statistics of speckle in ultrasound B-scans, *IEEE Trans. Sonics Ultrasonics 30*, 156–163 (1983).

18 Jakeman, E., Speckle statistics with small number of scatterers, *Opt. Eng. 23*, 453–461 (1984).

19 Cardoso, J.-F., 3-D Ultrasonic speckle modeling: Below the Rayleigh limit, in *Proc. SPIE Int. Symp. on Pattern Recognition and Acoustical Imaging*, L.A. Ferrari, ed., pp. 207–214 (SPIE, Bellingham, 1987).

20 Foster, D.E., Arditi, M, Foster, F.S., Patterson, M.S. and Hunt, J.W., Computer simulations of speckle in B-mode images, *Ultrasonic Imaging 5*, 308–330 (1983).

21 Nicholas, D., Time-frequency-domain analysis: one-dimensional phantom studies, *Phys. Med. Biol. 27*, 665–682 (1982).

22 Mesdag, P.R., *Estimation of Medium Parameters by Acoustic Echo Measurements*, (Thesis, Delft University of Technology, 1985).

23 Jacobs, E.M.G. and Thijssen, J.M., A simulation study of echographic imaging of diffuse and structurally scattering media, *Ultrasonic Imaging 13*, 316–333 (1991).

24 Nicholas, D., Evaluation of backscattering coefficients for excised human tissues: results, interpretation and associated measurements, *Ultrasound in Med. Biol. 8*, 17–28 (1982).

25 Keller, J.M., Chen, S. and Crownover, R.M., Texture description and segmentation through fractal geometry, *Comp. Vision Graphics Image Process. 45*, 150–166 (1989).

26 Chen, C.C., Daponte, J.S. and Fox, M.D., Fractal features analysis and classification in medical imaging, *IEEE Trans. Medical Imaging 8*, 133–143 (1989).

27 Gårding, J., Properties of fractal intensity surfaces, *Pattern Recognition Letters 8*, 319–324 (1988).

28 Zähle, U., Sets and measures of fractional dimension, *Journ. of Inform. Process. and Cybernetics 20*, 261–269 (1984).

29 Mussigmann, U., Texture analysis, fractals and scale space filtering, in *Proc. 6th Scandinavian Conf. on Image Analysis*, Oulo, pp. 987–994 (1989).

30 Mussigman, U., Homogeneous Fractals and their Application in Texture Analysis, in *Proceedings of the 1st IFIP Conf. on Fractals*, H.O. Peitgen, J.M. Henriques and L.F. Penedo, eds. (Elsevier, Amsterdam, 1990).

31 Mandelbrot, B.B., *The Fractal Geometry of Nature* (W.H. Freeman and company, New York, 1963).

32 Pentland, A.P., Fractal based description of natural scenes, *IEEE Trans. Pattern Analys. and Mach. Intell. PAMI-6*, 661–674 (1984).

33 Mandelbrot, B.B. and van Ness, J.W., Fractional Brownian motions, fractal noises and applications, *SIAM review 10*, (1968).

34 Bevington, P.R., *Data Reduction and Error Analysis for the Physical Sciences* (McGraw-Hill, New York, 1969).

35 Witkin, A.P., Scale-space filtering, in *Proc. Joint Conference on Artificial Intelligence*, Karlsruhe, pp. 329–332 (1983).

Ultrasonic Imaging 15, 304–323 (1993)

36 Rueff, M., Scale space filtering and the scaling regions of fractals, in *From Pixels to Features*, Simon, J.C., ed., pp. 49–60 (Elsevier, Amsterdam, 1989).

37 Baband, J., Witkin, A.O., Baudin, M. and Duda, R.O., Uniqueness Gaussian kernel for scale-space filtering, *IEEE Trans. Patt. Anal. Mach. Intell. PAMI-8*, 26–33 (1986).

38 Kube, P. and Pentland, A., On the imaging of fractal surfaces, *IEEE Trans. pattern Anal. Mach. Intelligence 10*, 704–707 (1988).

39 Hunt, G.A., Random Fourier transforms, *Trans. Amer. Math. Soc. 71*, 38–69 (1951).

40 Adler, R.J., *The Geometry of Random Fields* (Wiley, New York, 1981).

41 Jacobs, E.M.G.P. and Thijssen, J.M., A simulation study of echographic imaging of diffuse and structurally scattering media, *Ultrasonic Imaging 13*, 316–333 (1991).

42 Kay, S.M. and Marple, S.L., Spectrum analysis — a modern perspective, *Proc. IEEE 69*, 1380–1419 (1981).

43 Makhoul, J., Linear prediction: a tutorial review, *Proc. IEEE 63*, 561–580 (1975).

44 Verhoeven, J.T.M., Thijssen, J.M. and Theeuwes, A.G.M., Improvement of lesion detection by echographic image processing: signal-to-noise-ratio imaging, *Ultrasonic Imaging 13*, 238–251 (1991).

A New Technique for Fractal Analysis Applied to Human, Intracerebrally Recorded, Ictal Electroencephalographic Signals

Edward Bullmore, Michael Brammer, Gonzalo Alarcon and Colin Binnie

Departments of Neuroscience and Clinical Neurophysiology, Maudsley Hospital and Institute of Psychiatry, London (UK)

(Received 29 June 1992; Revised version received 18 August 1992; Accepted 24 August 1992)

Key words: Fractal; Epilepsy; Quantitative EEG analysis; Synoptic visualisation

Application of a new method of fractal analysis to human, intracerebrally recorded, ictal electroencephalographic (EEG) signals is reported. 'Frameshift-Richardson' (FR) analysis involves estimation of fractal dimension (1<FD<2) of consecutive, overlapping 10-s epochs of digitised EEG data; it is suggested that this technique offers significant operational advantages over use of algorithms for FD estimation requiring preliminary reconstruction of EEG data in phase space. FR analysis was found to reduce substantially the volume of EEG data, without loss of diagnostically important information concerning onset, propagation and evolution of ictal EEG discharges. Arrhythmic EEG events were correlated with relatively important information concerning onset, propagation and evolution of ictal EEG discharges. Arrhythmic EEG events were correlated with relatively increased FD; rhythmic EEG events with relatively decreased FD. It is proposed that development of this method may lead to: (i) enhanced definition and localisation of initial ictal changes in the EEG presumed due to multi-unit activity; and (ii) synoptic visualisation of long periods of EEG data.

Fractal analysis of electroencephalographic (EEG) data has been computationally feasible since the mid-1980s [3]; reconstruction of the EEG signal as a strange attractor in multidimensional phase space has since been repeatedly accomplished [8]; and the geometric or dynamic characteristics of various such strange attractors, derived from EEG data recorded from patients in various neuropsychological states, have been quantitatively compared in terms of their relative fractal (correlation) dimensions [11], or Lyapunov exponents [6]. It has been reported that higher dimensional EEG attractors tend to have more positive Lyapunov exponents, to be more dissipative and unpredictable, and to be associated with behavioural states such as relaxed wakefulness with alpha rhythm [5] and performance of mental arithmetic [9]; whereas lower dimensional EEG attractors tend to have fewer positive Lyapunov exponents, to be more constrained and repetitive, and to be associated with states such as absence seizures [2],

coma and stage IV sleep [5], and meditation [12]. These findings have suggested that fractal dimensions of the EEG may generally be related to concomitant level of consciousness or cognitive state; and that fractal dimension might therefore have considerable pragmatic value in the development of improved software for computerised diagnosis of EEG data [7]. However, it has also been widely realised that estimation of fractal dimension by some algorithms requires large numbers of data points input (dpi). For example, Mayer-Kress and Layne [8] have shown that the Grassberger-Procaccia algorithm for estimation of fractal (correlation) dimension does not yield an asymptotic value for EEG dimension even as dpi exceeds 15,000 (equivalent to 75 s of EEG signal digitised at 200 Hz); and Gallez and Babloyantz [5] found that Eckmann's algorithm for estimation of Lyapunov exponent demanded up to 10^6 dpi (equivalent to 5,000 s of EEG signal digitised at 200 Hz), depending on the fractal (correlation) dimension of the underlying attractor. Data requirements of this order have constituted a major impediment to adequate temporal resolution by fractal analysis of the non-stationary EEG signal.

Correspondence: E. Bullmore, Departments of Neuroscience and Clinical Neurophysiology, Maudsley Hospital and Institute of Psychiatry, Denmark Hill, London SE5 8AZ, UK.

We report here a novel method of fractal analysis (comparable in some respects to the method reported by Arle and Simon [1]) which we believe offers significant operational advantages over previously published techniques; and application of this method to the quantification and representation of ictal EEG changes.

An algorithm for the estimation of fractal dimension was written, based on Richardson's technique [10] for calculating fractal dimension of coastlines. This algorithm was validated by testing its estimation performance against a range of artificially generated curves. Each test curve had been generated by interpolation of a line of known fractal dimension between 2000 data points [4] (the same number of data points as a 10-s epoch of EEG digitised at 200 Hz). High dimensional test curves appeared relatively convoluted and space-occupying, increasingly so as fractal dimension approached a maximum of 2; whereas low dimensional test curves appeared relatively smooth and linear, increasingly so as fractal dimension approached a minimum of 1. It was shown that the algorithm was able accurately to estimate fractal dimension of a range of test curves without preliminary reconstruction of data in phase space, and on the basis of fewer data points input than algorithms previously used to estimate fractal (correlation) dimension, or Lyapunov exponents.

All EEG signals were obtained with 15 intracerebral electrodes, stereotactically implanted in bilateral temporal lobe structures (amygdala, anterior and posterior hippocampus), from a patient with complex partial seizures, refractory to medical treatment, who was being assessed for neurosurgery. The EEG was recorded using a 32-channel cable telemetry system (Telefactor Beehive); band pass filtered, time constant 0.3 s, low pass cutoff frequency 70 Hz; and digitalised at 200 Hz with a 12 bit analog-to-digital converter and 2 mV input range. Four complex partial seizures with secondarily generalised tonic-clonic convulsions were recorded over a 6-day period; 3 of these seizure recordings (S1, S2, S3) were submitted to analysis.

Digitised EEG signal was input to the algorithm as a consecutive series of overlapping 10-s epochs, the time 0.5 s Fractal dimension of each epoch was estimated, the dimensions of consecutive epochs plotted as a time series, and smoothed using a Savitzky-Golay smoothing algorithm (single pass: 99 point window). This process of 'frameshift-Richardson' (FR) fractal analysis was demanding of CPU time (15 s of 486-PC processing time required per second of single channel EEG data), but promised fine temporal resolution of brain electrical change as well as a substantial contraction of the somewhat voluminous raw EEG data (the ratio between dpi input:output is 99:1). FR analysis was individually undertaken for each recording channel. The resulting time series of EEG dimension seemed sensitively to summarise diagnostically significant events in the raw EEG waveform.

Thus, onset of a burst of spiking at seizure onset was correlated with decrease in dimension relative to baseline; while termination of spiking was correlated with a return to baseline dimension (Fig. 1A). Periods of low

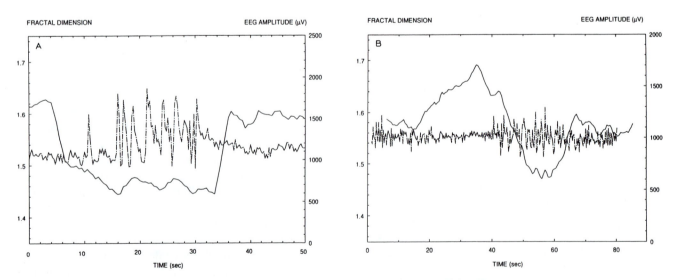

Fig. 1. A: burst of spiking at seizure onset. Broken line, 50 s of EEG signal, recorded from left anterior hippocampus (LAH) 50 s prior to onset of S3; solid line, 50-s time series of fractal dimension derived by Frameshift-Richardson (FR) analysis of same EEG data. B: early ictal rhythmic transformation. Broken line, 80 s of EEG signal recorded from left posterior hippocampus (LPH) 140 s prior to onset of S2; solid line, 80-s time series of fractal dimension of same EEG data, derived as in A.

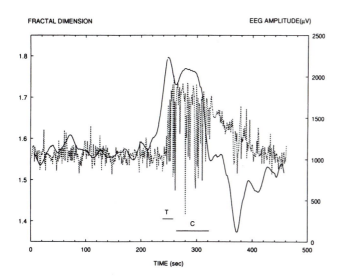

Fig. 2. Secondarily generalised seizure (S2): single channel. Broken line, 450 s of EEG signal, recorded from LAH before, during and after seizure; solid line, 450-s time series of fractal dimension derived by FR analysis of same EEG data. T, duration of tonic convulsions; C, duration of clonic convulsions.

amplitude, arrhythmic EEG waveform, which preceded periods of ictal rhythmic transformation on visual inspection, were correlated with a phase of relative increase in dimension, followed by a phase of relative decrease in dimension (Fig. 1B). In general, perceptible increases in rhythmicity of the EEG, which could be relatively easily detected by visual inspection of the raw data, were correlated with a decrease in dimension; whereas episodes of 'white', arrhythmic, or de-synchronised EEG activity, which had been relatively difficult to detect on visual inspection of the raw data, were correlated with an increase in dimension.

Secondarily generalised seizures were also associated with biphasic changes in fractal dimension (Fig. 2). Seizure onset was preceded by a period of increasing dimension of the EEG, presumably due to multi-unit activity. Fractal dimension remained relatively increased throughout the first phase of the seizure, before decreasing rapidly in the second phase. Such ictal changes in fractal dimension were most extreme in data recorded from electrodes which showed the earliest EEG signs of seizure onset. Post-ictal dimensions were decreased in all channels relative to their pre-ictal dimensions. The pattern of biphasic dimensional change occurring in all channels during generalised seizures was notably similar to the biphasic pattern associated with the early episode of ictal rhythmic transformation, which occurred 140 s prior to onset of secondarily generalised seizure, but

only in the left posterior hippocampus (compare Figs. 1B and 2).

In order to facilitate comparison between channels of these pathophysiologically relevant changes in dimension, the mean fractal dimension of each time series was subtracted from all constituent data points, generating time series of deviations from mean fractal dimension. As shown in Fig. 3, propagation of ictal activity between anatomically related structures was reflected by relatively delayed increase in fractal dimension of EEG data recorded from anatomically related electrodes; and there was greatest coherence between channels at the moment of transition between relatively high and low dimensional phases.

Temporal evolution of these ictal perturbations of fractal dimension could be compactly represented by colour-coded, or grey-scaled, displays of time series of deviations from mean fractal dimension in data recorded from all electrodes. A grey-scaled version of this display format is shown in Fig. 4. This image represents 460 s of 15-channel EEG data. Diagnostically important features, such as seizure onset, focal episodes of early ictal rhythmic transformation, and global post-ictal decrease in dimension are preserved even at small image sizes. Application of this technique might consequently prove useful in the synoptic visualisation of long periods of EEG data (e.g. several hours of sleep or telemetric recording) recorded for clinical

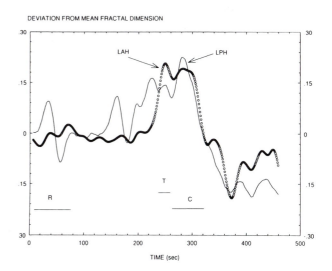

Fig. 3. Secondarily generalised seizure (S2): two channels. Broken line, 450-s time series of deviations from mean fractal dimension derived by FR analysis of EEG data recorded from LAH; solid line, 450-s time series of deviations from mean fractal dimension derived by FR analysis of EEG data recorded from LPH. R, early ictal rhythmic transformation in LPH (see Fig. 1B); T, duration of tonic convulsions; C, duration of clonic convulsions.

230

Intracerebral locus

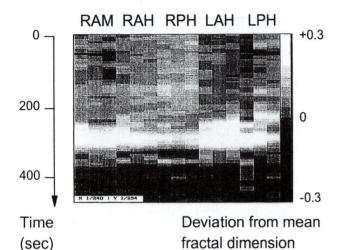

RAM RAH RPH LAH LPH

Time (sec)

Deviation from mean fractal dimension

Fig. 4. Secondarily generalised seizure (S2): 15 channels, 450-s time series of deviations from mean fractal dimension derived by FR analysis of EEG data recorded from all electrodes. X-axis: RAM, right amygdala (electrodes 1–3); RAH, right anterior hippocampus (4–6); RPH, right posterior hippocampus (7–9); LAH, left anterior hippocampus (10–12); LPH, left posterior hippocampus (13–15). Y-axis: time (s). Grey scale codes, as shown by bar on the right side of the image, for deviation from mean fractal dimension in each channel (range: –0.3 to +0.3). Ictal onset with desynchronisation in LPH at 160 s and spread of desynchronised activity throughout left hippocampus at 250 s, correlated with increased fractal dimension; secondarily generalised seizure 250–320 s, correlated with coherent biphasic dimensional change in all channels; generalised slow wave activity postictally 320–450 s, correlated with fractal dimensions decreased relative to pre-ictal baseline in all channels.

purposes of spatial and temporal localisation of epileptic seizure onset.

REFERENCES

1 Arle, J.E. and Simon, R.H., An application of fractal dimension to the detection of transients in the electroencephalogram, Electroencephalogr. Clin. Neurophysiol., 75 (1990) 296–305.
2 Babloyantz, A. and Destexhe, A., Low dimensional chaos in an instance of epilepsy, Proc. Natl. Acad. Sci. USA, 83 (1986) 3513–3517.
3 Babloyantz, A., Nicolis, C. and Salazar, J.M., Evidence for chaotic dynamics of brain activity during the sleep cycle, Phys. Lett., 111 (1985) 152–156.
4 Barnsley, M.F., Fractal functions and interpolation, Constr. Approx., 2 (1986) 303–329.
5 Gallez, D. and Babloyantz, A., Predictability of human EEG: a dynamic approach, Biol. Cybern., 64 (1991) 381–391.
6 Iasemedis, L.D., Sackellares, J.C., Zaveri, H.P. and Williams, W.J., Phase space topography and the Lyapunov exponent of electrocorticograms in partial seizures, Brain Topogr., 2 (1990) 187–201.
7 Jansen, B.H., Quantitative analysis of electroencephalograms: is there chaos in the future?, Int. J. Biomed. Comput., 27 (1991) 95–123.
8 Mayer-Kress, G. and Layne, S.P., Dimensionality of the human electroencephalogram, Ann. N.Y. Acad. Sci., 504 (1986) 3513–3517.
9 Rapp, P.E., Bashore, T.R., Martinerie, J.M., Albano, A.M., Zimmerman, I.D. and Mees, A.I., Dynamics of brain electrical activity, Brain Topogr., 2 (1989) 99–118.
10 Voss, R.F., Fractals in nature: from characterisation to simulation. In H.O. Peitgen and D. Saupe (Eds.), The Science of Fractal Images, 1st ed., Springer, New York, 1988, pp 21–76.
11 Watt, R.C. and Hameroff, S.R., Phase space electrocorticography: a new mode of intraoperative EEG analysis, Int. J. Clin. Monit. Comput., 5 (1988) 3–13.
12 Xu, N. and Xu, J., The fractal dimension of EEG as a physical measure of conscious human brain activities. Bull. Math. Biol., 50 (1988) 559–565.

112

Neuroscience Letters, 130 (1991) 112–116
© 1991 Elsevier Scientific Publishers Ireland Ltd. 0304-3940/91/$ 03.50
ADONIS 0304394091004923

NSL 08008

A fractal analysis of pyramidal neurons in mammalian motor cortex

R. Porter, S. Ghosh*, G. David Lange** and T.G. Smith Jr.***

Faculty of Medicine, Monash University, Clayton, Vic. (Australia)

(Received 18 April 1991; Revised version received 31 May 1991; Accepted 3 June 1991)

Key words: Motor cortex; Pyramidal neuron; Fractal dimension

Pyramidal neurons in the mammalian cerebral cortex can be described by a fractal dimension (Mandelbrot, 1982), which is an objective, quantitative measure of the complexity of their soma/dendritic borders. In the cat, the fractal dimensions of lamina V cells, which include pyramidal tract neurons (PTN), indicate that these cells are more complex than other pyramidal neurons (PN) in the same region of motor cortex. The lamina V cells of the cat are also more complex than those in motor cortex of the monkey. Moreover, lamina III neurons in the monkey are more complex than monkey lamina V neurons. The fractal dimension of the intracortical axon collateral arborizations of the same pyramidal neurons indicated, in all cases, that the branching of these terminals is less complex than the branching of the dendrites of the same cells. In line with the observation that the fractal dimensions of some homologous cellular populations are different in different species, it is suggested that the fractal dimension and the degree of morphological complexity may relate to the requirement for the number of separable functions to be accommodated within one neuron. For example, as the size of the cortex and the number of neurons in a region increase, the opportunity exists within a given cortical zone, for individual functions to be segregated and for functional specialization to be accommodated with less morphological complexity of the individual neurons performing each of these functions.

The morphological classification of neurons in the vertebrate nervous system has been examined at a number of levels. Perhaps the most common definition is according to gross anatomical location, (dorsal root ganglion neurons). Other classifications are based on the connectivity of the neurons, (spino-thalamic tract neurons). Some are related to a characteristic shape of the neuron's soma, (pyramidal neurons). The names may indicate physiological function, (spinal motoneurons). The distinctive shapes or locations of the neurons may be used and are often eponymous, e.g. Purkinje neurons of the cerebellum. More general schemes have been proposed on the basis of the overall structural characteristics or gestalt of soma-dendritic branching patterns [12].

Most quantitative analyses of individual neurons have involved measurements of the number, diameters and lengths of branches of dendritic trees. Such measurements have been useful in relating certain physiological functions, e.g. the spread of membrane potential changes through dendritic trees, to morphological structure [6, 13]. There are, however, certain morphological characteristics of individual neurons that are generally recognised as important but are characterised with a relative 'more' or 'less' of the attribute. One such attribute is a cell's morphological complexity, with, for example, a Purkinje cell being recognised as 'more complex' than, say, a retinal ganglion cell.

Recently, however, the concepts of Mandelbrot's fractal geometry have afforded a means of quantitatively measuring the complexity of the borders or geometrical outlines of neurons and glia in a completely objective and unbiased manner [9, 16, 17]. The 'measure' is the fractal dimension (D) of the cell's border, which increases in value with increase in complexity. Here we report on such measurements made on camera lucida reconstructions of cat and monkey cortical pyramidal neurons in area 4 (motor cortex), some identified as pyramidal tract neurons (PTN) by sending axons into the basis pedunculi or the pyramidal tract. We find statistically significant differences among the fractal dimensions of several different neuronal types, which conceivably may have relevance to their physiological function.

As to the interpretation of D as a measure of complexity, it is the fractional part of D that is relevant for comparison purposes. The integer (1.) denotes a dimensiona-

*Present address: Department of Physiology and Pharmacology, University of Queensland, Qld. 4072, Australia.
**Present address: Instrumentation and Computer Section NINDS, National Institutes of Health, Bethesda, MD 20892, U.S.A.
***Present address: Laboratory of Neurophysiology, National Institutes of Health, Bldg. 36, Room 2C 02, Bethesda, MD 20892, U.S.A.
Correspondence: R. Porter, Faculty of Medicine, Monash University, Clayton, Vic. 3168, Australia.

lity for the object that lies between a straight line and a flat plane (2. means a dimensionality between a plane and a volume). The fractional part is obtained from the slope of a line in a log-log plot and is a unitless ratio of two log values (Fig. 1). It is this ratio that expresses the relative complexity of two objects. An increase in the fractional part of D from 0.1 to 0.2 represents a doubling in complexity, and the range of 1.39 to 1.63 found in cat motor cortex cells in this study represents an approximately 1.5 to 2-fold difference in complexity.

The experimental procedures for the initial experiments on the live animals have been reported completely elsewhere [3–5]. Basically, anaesthetized cats and monkeys were studied, intracellular records were made from motor cortex neurons and these cells were then injected with horseradish peroxidase. Subsequently, camera lucida drawings of the completely filled cells were made from superimposed serial sections of fixed tissue on microscope slides. This generated two dimensional illustrations of the outlines of the total branched surface of these cells. Even in the reconstructions there is little 'loss' of definition caused by the superimposition of dendritic profiles. The method of calculating the fractal dimension from an image of a cell's border or outline has also been reported extensively elsewhere [2, 16, 17].

Thirty-one cells from area 4 of the cat, and thirteen cells from area 4 of the monkey were analysed for their fractal dimensions. Thirteen cells from the cat and three from the monkey were identified as pyramidal tract neurons (PTN); the others were classified as pyramidal neurons (PN) by the shape of their somata, the arrangement and distribution of their apical dendrites and the exit of their axon from the cortex. They were assigned to the cortical laminae (II–VI) occupied by their somata. All PTN neurons were from lamina V. The fractal dimension results of individual cells or parts of cells of each cell group were analysed for statistically significant differences between them by employing analysis of variance and the Scheffe post hoc test (SuperAnova, Abacus Concepts, Inc., Berkeley, CA, U.S.A.). We have chosen a 95% confidence level ($P < 0.05$) as our criterion for significant difference.

Fig. 1. illustrates both the camera lucida projection of the most complex fast PTN in the cat (C20) and the graphical representation of its fractal dimension (1.63). As can be seen in Tables I and II the fractal dimensions (D) for the entire soma-dendritic arbor of individual cat pyramidal neurons ranged from 1.39 to 1.63, while those for cells from the monkey were from 1.34 to 1.56. Taken as a whole, and using a Student's t-test, for example, the cat and monkey data are not significantly different. However, when an analysis of variance allowing for classification according to species and lamina (two-way

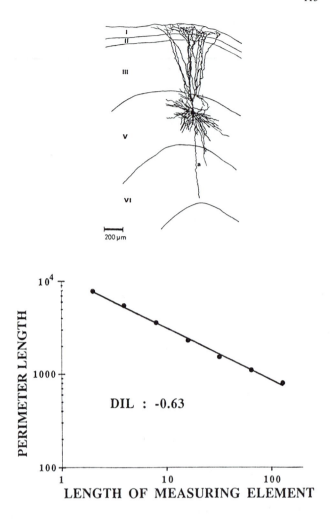

Fig. 1. Upper panel: silhouette from camera lucida projection drawing of a cat motor cortex PTN neuron (C20), with cortical laminae indicated (I–VI). Lower panel: Richardson plot of the log of the perimeter of the cell's border vs. the log of the length of the measuring element (e.g., ruler, caliper), using the DILATION method [2, 17]. The fractal dimension is calculated from the measured slope (S; Dil: -0.63), $$D = 1 - S = 1 - (-0.63) = 1.63$$

ANOVA) is employed, then significant differences are revealed. Post hoc analysis shows differences between homologous laminae in the two species. There are also differences among the various categories of cat neurons. The most interesting results are obtained when the fast and slow PTNs, which are not themselves significantly different, are lumped and are included with the other lamina V cells, rather than being considered in separate categories. All lamina V neurons project to relatively distant targets and, in this sense, may have some common characteristics. Post hoc analysis indicates that the neurons of the various laminae fall into overlapping groups along a continuum of decreasing complexity. Although the laminar groups were not completely separable statistically in the cat, the rank order of the means of each group with decreasing complexity was: lamina V >

114

lamina III > lamina II > lamina VI. It should be noted, however, that there were fewer than five cells in the samples of laminae III and VI. However, in the monkey, D was statistically significantly greater in lamina III (mean 1.53) than in lamina V (mean 1.46). These results are indicated in Table I for cats and Table II for monkeys.

A correlation matrix examined the relationship between D and thirteen conventional physiological and anatomical parameters, e.g. conduction velocity of the axon, somatic diameters, number of apical dendrites, dendritic extent and orientation, density of dendritic spines and spread of intracortical axon collaterals. (These measures are reported in Ghosh et al. [3] and reconstructions of many of the cells are illustrated in this and associated publications.) No correlations greater than 0.65 were found. This would indicate that no more than 42% of the variance in any of these measures can be explained by D. Such analyses do not rule out a possible non-monotonic or other nonlinear relationship of D with these other measures.

In order to test for the presence of the defining property of a fractal object, namely, self-similarity, the fractal dimension of a portion, say a quarter to a half, of the dendritic tree, was calculated for each of the cat neurons (Table I). Self-similarity means that the object looks qualitatively the same, irrespective of scale or magnification. The average D of the entire cell was 1.52, while the average D of the part-cell images was 1.54 and the means were not significantly different ($P < 0.24$). On the other hand, the D of the intracortical collateral arborization of the axon of each cell in the cat (mean of 1.39), when available (8 cells), was statistically different from its corresponding whole cell – soma and dendrites ($P < 0.0001$). Moreover, as is indicated in both Table I and Table II, in each cell's case, for both the lamina III and the lamina V neurons of the monkey as well as the cat, the D of the intracortical axonal arborization was lower (less complex) than that of the soma-dendritic tree.

Perhaps the most interesting result came from a comparison of the cells in laminae III and V of the cat and monkey. Somewhat surprisingly, the cat laminar V cells had a significantly larger D (mean of 1.55) than those of lamina V of the monkey (mean of 1.48). Moreover, the lamina III neurons of the monkey (mean 1.53) were significantly more complex than those of monkey lamina V (mean 1.48).

The fractal dimension of an object is generally taken to measure, quantitatively, the complexity of whatever aspect of the object is being measured. Here the borders of the branched profiles of cat and monkey motor cortex

TABLE I

FRACTAL DIMENSIONS OF CAT PYRAMIDAL NEURONS AREA 4

S.D., soma dendritic boundary; PART, fractal dimension for part of cell; I.A.C., intracortical axonal arborizations; C.V., conduction velocity of axon.

Neuron type[1]	D				Neuron type	D		
	S.D.	Part	I.A.C.	C.V. m/s		S.D.	Part	I.A.C.
Fast PTN	1.60	1.66	–	35.7	Lamina II	1.48	1.48	
Fast PTN[a]	1.63	1.66	1.59	27.0	Lamina II	1.49	1.52	
Fast PTN[b]	1.54	1.56	1.36	27.5	Lamina II[e]	1.48	1.50	
Slow PTN	1.55	1.62	–	5.7	Lamina II[f]	1.41	1.45	
Slow PTN	1.49	1.53	–	11.0	Lamina II	1.57	1.51	
Slow PTN[c]	1.60	1.64	1.49	11.0	Lamina II[g]	1.47	1.43	
Slow PTN	1.60	1.66	–	8.8	Lamina III[h]	1.52	1.58	
Slow PTN	1.53	1.55	–	5.0	Lamina III	1.48	1.49	
Slow PTN	1.51	1.59	1.29	11.4	Lamina III	1.55	1.50	
Slow PTN	1.49	1.43	1.37	19.2	Lamina III	1.50	1.50	
Slow PTN	1.54	1.51	–	8.3	Lamina VI[i]	1.47	1.49	
Slow PTN	1.53	1.56	–	19.2	Lamina VI[j]	1.41	1.50	
Slow PTN[d]	1.57	1.60	1.44	19.2	Lamina VI[k]	1.39	1.47	
Lamina V	1.55	1.63	–					
Lamina V	1.59	1.53	1.33					
Lamina V	1.52	1.51	–					
Lamina V	1.44	1.48	1.26					
Lamina V	1.52	1.48	–					

[1]A number of these neurons have been illustrated in a previous paper [3] and may be identified in that paper as follows: (a) Fig. 9B; (b) Fig. 9A; (c) Fig. 7B; (d) Fig. 11; (e) Fig. 3B; (f) Fig. 3C; (g) Fig. 3E; (h) Fig. 5A; (i) Fig. 16A; (j) Fig. 16B; (k) Fig. 16C.

115

TABLE II

FRACTAL DIMENSIONS (*D*) OF MONKEY PYRAMIDAL NEURONS AREA 4

S.D., soma/dendritic complex; I.A.C., intracortical axon collateral arborization.

Lamina III	*D*		Lamina V	*D*	
	S.D.	I.A.C.		S.D.	I.A.C.
1	1.52	1.32	1 (Fast)	1.49	1.39
2	1.54	1.51	2 (Fast)	1.51	1.27
3	1.53	1.46	3 (Slow)	1.46	1.30
4	1.51		4	1.48	1.42
5	1.56		5	1.34	
6	1.49		6	1.47	
			7	1.45	
Mean	1.53	1.43		1.46	1.34
S.D.	0.02	0.09		0.06	0.07

neurons were examined. For these outlines, as for the edge traces of other complex geometric forms, the higher the *D*, the more complex the object.

With respect to what aspects of cellular morphology the *D* measures, we have found three characteristics to be important [16, 17]. The first is the degree of branching of the dendritic tree, with the greater branching giving a higher *D*. Second, is the ruggedness of the border of the cell, with a more rugged, jagged or uneven border leading to a higher *D*. And, third, is the degree to which the border fills the plane of the projection of the two-dimensional image. These categories are not independent. The distinction between branching and ruggedness is, to some extent, a question of scale, with increases in either, being more space filling [16, 17]. In the neurons studied here, the first aspect, the degree of branching, appeared to be the most important.

The importance of dendritic branching to the functioning of neurons is likely to arise because the number and modes of interaction of the inputs to a cell are critical to the cell's output behaviour. It seems quite likely that degree of branching and the number and distribution of inputs are correlated and that dendritic branching affords a medium for complex interactions among these inputs. Specialisations, such as dendritic spines which accommodate synaptic inputs, would be expected further to increase the measure of complexity of the cell's border and also the degree of input/output interactions. Separation of different inputs on different dendritic branches may provide for different input/output characteristics for separate aspects of a neuron's functions. A high *D* in cat lamina V neurons, which includes the pyramidal tract neurons (PTNs), may therefore signify a high degree of computational complexity in these cells. This level of complexity is revealed in other studies of such cells by Deschenes et al. [1]. Here, a more complex geometry may be required for computationally greater requirements of neurons that control many other elements far removed from the somatic location of the cell, than for the cells that have only local intracortical connections or synapses with relatively localised nearby targets in the thalamus or basal ganglia. The opposite may be true of monkey lamina III neurons, which must be presumed to be ipsilateral cortico-cortical or cortico-callosal neurons [7], and which are more complex than the lamina V neurons, including fast and slow pyramidal tract neurons, whose axons innervate distant targets, including spinal motoneurons. We still need to understand the extent and functional implications of the territory innervated by an individual pyramidal neuron in either lamina III or lamina V. For PTN in the cat and the monkey, it may be relevant that, in general, the more complex cells of the cat appear to have a wider spread of their spinal terminal arborizations than those of the monkey [8, 14, 15]. However, for individual cells, direct correlations between complexity of soma/dendritic morphology and extent of terminal arborization cannot be made.

The findings that cat and monkey have reciprocal degrees of the complexity in laminae III and V are interesting and challenge explanation. In another study, of Bergman glial cells of the cerebellum of rodents, monkeys and man (A. Reichenbach et al., personal communication), it was found that *D*'s were significantly different in the three species, in the order rodent > monkey > man. If it were known, for example, that *D*'s for cerebellar glial cells were inversely related to the motor repertoire of the various species, it might be an important development. We do not, however, have a well-defined measure of motor repertoire.

116

The fact that no large correlations were found between D and conventional physiological and anatomical measures indicates that measuring the D of a cell cannot substitute for measuring other aspects of function and form directly. For example, Spain et al. [18] have recently identified different membrane channel properties in different pyramidal cells of lamina V of in vitro slices of cat's motor cortex.

The demonstration of self-similarity in motor cortex neurons is consistent with our findings in other neuronal and glial studies [16, 17] and indicates that the borders of these neurons may be considered to be fractal objects. Here, as elsewhere [16, 17], the borders were fractal over a range of scale of from 1.5 to 2 decades, a range common for biological objects [11]. While the entire soma-dendritic complex demonstrated self-similarity, the same was not true of the intracortical axon terminals of their parent cells, where the terminals were considerably less complex. While 'true' fractals are self-similar everywhere in their structure [10] it is common in 'natural' fractal objects to find that D changes with either a large change of scale [11] or with different parts of the same object, e.g., in the leaves of a tree compared to the branches of the same tree.

One can raise the legitimate question as to the validity of measuring D from two-dimensional projections of what are, in fact, three-dimensional structures. In the field of fractal geometry, where the rules are still being developed, this is a matter of some controversy. Mandelbrot, the father of fractal geometry, says that such estimates of D can be considered a rough approximation of the 'true' complexity and are more likely to underestimate the latter [9]. The methods of reconstruction of the images of the cells from serial histological sections will certainly result in distortions of the length of processes which traverse the plane of the sections. However, the demonstration, provided here, of self-similarity, revealed by the same measure of the fractal dimension for parts of the dendritic arbor as for the whole cell, indicates that such non-uniform representations of lengths of dendrites in different planes have had little influence on D. Methods for estimating D in higher dimensions are under development, but until we have those methods and the data in the proper format, we are limited to what we have done here. Such measures as we have performed may, nonetheless, be useful quantifiers of cellular morphology which could illuminate relationships between cellular structure and function which are not revealed by other measures of cellular geometry and tell us something about the importance and function of homologous cells across species.

1 Deschênes, M., Labelle, A. and Landry, P., Morphological characterization of slow and fast pyramidal tract cells in the cat, Brain Res., 178 (1979) 251–274.

2 Flook, A.G., The use of dilation logic on the quantimet to achieve fractal dimension characterisation of textured and structured profiles. Powder Technol. 21 (1978) 295–298.

3 Ghosh, S., Fyffe, R.E.W. and Porter, R., Morphology of neurons in area 4 γ of the cat's cortex studied with intracellular injection of HRP, J. Comp. Neurol., 269 (1988) 290–312.

4 Ghosh, S. and Porter, R., Morphology of pyramidal neurones in monkey motor cortex and the synaptic actions of their intracortical axon collaterals, J. Physiol., 400 (1988) 593–615.

5 Ghosh, S. and Porter, R., Corticocortical synaptic influences on morphologically identified pyramidal neurones in the motor cortex of the monkey, J. Physiol., 400 (1988) 617–629.

6 Jack, J.J.B. and Redman, S.J., An electrical description of the motoneurone, and its application to the analysis of synaptic potentials, J. Physiol., 215 (1971) 321–352.

7 Jones, E.G. and Wise, S.P., Size, laminar and columnar distribution of efferent cells in the sensory-motor cortex of monkeys, J. Comp. Neurol., 175 (1977) 391–438.

8 Lawrence, D.G., Porter, R., Redman, S.J., Cortico-motoneuronal synapses in the monkey: light microscopic localization upon motoneurons of intrinsic muscles of the hand, J. Comp. Neurol., 232 (1985) 499–510.

9 Mandelbrot, B., The Fractal Geometry of Nature, W.H. Freeman, New York, 1982.

10 Mandelbrot, B., Fractals – a geometry of nature, New Scientist, 127, No. 1734 (1990) 23–29.

11 Peitgen, H.-O. and Richter, P.H., The Beauty of Fractals, Springer, New York, 1986.

12 Ramon Molinar, E., An attempt at classifying nerve cells on the basis of their dendritic patterns, J. Comp. Neurol., 119 (1962) 211–227.

13 Rall, W., Electrophysiology of a dendritic neuron model, Biophys. J., 2 (1962) 145–169.

14 Shinoda, Y., Yamaguchi, T. and Futami, T., Multiple axon collaterals of single corticospinal axons in the cat spinal cord, J. Neurophysiol., 55 (1986) 425–448.

15 Shinoda, Y., Yokota, J. and Futami, T., Divergent projection of individual corticospinal axons to motoneurons of multiple muscles in the monkey, Neurosci. Lett., 23 (1981) 7–12.

16 Smith, T.G. Jnr., Behar, T.N., Lange, G.D., Marks, W.B. and Sheriff, W.H., A fractal analysis of cultured rat optic nerve glial growth, Neuroscience, 41 (1991) 159–169.

17 Smith, T.G. Jnr., Marks, W.B., Lange, G.D., Sheriff, W.H. and Neale, E.A., A fractal analysis of cell images, J. Neurosci. Methods, 27 (1989) 173–180.

18 Spain, W.J., Schwindt, P.C. and Crill, W.E., Two transient potassium currents in layer V pyramidal neurones from cat sensorimotor cortex, J. Physiol., 434 (1991) 591–607.

Journal of Pathology, vol. **170**: 479–484 (1993)

Quantitation of the Renal Arterial Tree by Fractal Analysis

Simon S. Cross*, Roger D. Start*, Paul B. Silcocks†, Andrew D. Bull‡, Dennis W. K. Cotton* and James C. E. Underwood*

Departments of *Pathology and †Public Health Medicine, University of Sheffield Medical School, P.O. Box 596, Beech Hill Road, Sheffield S10 2UL, U.K.: ‡Department of Histopathology, Northern General Hospital, Herries Road, Sheffield, S5 7AU, U.K.

Received 15 January 1993
Accepted 4 March 1993

SUMMARY

To determine whether the renal arterial system has a fractal structure, the fractal dimension of renal angiograms from 52 necropsy cases was measured using an implementation of the box-counting method of an image analysis system. The method was validated using objects with known fractal dimensions. The method was accurate with errors of less than 1·5 per cent and reproducible with initial values with 1·2 per cent of the mean of ten sets of measurements (reliability coefficient 0·968, 95 per cent confidence limits 0·911–0·984). In the 36 satisfactory angiograms the mean fractal dimension was 1·61 (SD 0·06), which was significantly greater than the topological dimension of 1 ($P<0.0001$), indicating that the renal arterial tree has a fractal structure. There was no significant relationship between age ($P=0.494$), sex ($P=0.136$), or systolic ($P=0.069$) or diastolic ($P=0.990$) blood pressure, but two congenitally abnormal kidneys (hypoplastic dysplasia and renal artery stenosis) had fractal dimensions at the lower end of the normal range (third percentile). Since the renal arterial tree has a fractal structure. Euclidean geometric measurements, such as area and boundary length, are invalid outside precisely defined conditions of magnification and resolution.

Key words: Fractals, fractal dimension, morphometry, renal artery.

INTRODUCTION

Branching structures in the body such as the coronary arterial, pulmonary arterial, and bronchial trees have been shown to have a fractal structure.[1-5] A fractal structure retains a similar level of complexity through a wide range of magnifications; conventional Euclidean measurements, such as perimeter length and area, do not adequately describe this property.[6] The fractal dimension gives an index of the degree to which a fractal structure fills the metric space in which it is embedded[7]

and it has been shown that a three-dimensional fractal structure retains its fractal properties when projected onto a two-dimensional plane.[8] The definition of a fractal structure is an object with a fractal dimension which is greater than its topological dimension.[7] Subjective examination of an object for self-similarity at different scales of magnification can suggest that the object has a fractal structure but empirical measurement is required to fulfill the strict definition. The renal arterial tree is a branching structure in which small peripheral branches have a similar appearance to large central divisions—subjective self-similarity. This study uses fractal geometric analysis to determine whether the renal arterial tree has a fractal structure and to investigate the utility of the fractal dimension as a measure of abnormalities in this structure.

Addressee for correspondence: Dr S. S. Cross, Department of Pathology, University of Sheffield Medical School, P.O. Box 596, Beech Hill Road, Sheffield S10 2UL. U.K.

0022-3417/080479-06 $08

METHODS

Renal arteriography

The study population consisted of 52 hospital necropsy cases (22 female, 30 male, age range 21–89 years, median age 72 years). At necropsy the aorta was opened posteriorly and the renal arteries were identified. A 340 g in 65 ml aqueous suspension of barium sulphate ('E-Z'HD', Henley Medical Supplies Ltd., Welwyn Garden City, U.K.) was injected down each artery using a cannula and syringe until firm resistance was felt. The arteries were ligated and the kidneys dissected from surrounding tissue. Radiographs of each kidney were made by placing the kidneys on radiograph film (Kodak MIN-R) in a cabinet X-ray system (Faxitron, Hewlett Packard, McMinniville, Oregon, U.S.A.) using a constant exposure of 60 s at 55 kV. A radiograph was defined as satisfactory if the visualized vessels extended to within 2 mm of the border of the soft tissue shadow of the kidney and if air bubbles were absent from the vessels. Histological samples were taken from each kidney and haematoxylin and eosin-stained paraffin sections were examined. The age, sex, systolic and diastolic blood pressure (before any agonal change), and macroscopic appearance of the kidneys were recorded for each case.

Fractal analysis

The fractal dimension of the radiographic image of the renal arterial tree was measured using an implementation of the box-counting method[9–11] (Seescan plc. Cambridge, U.K.). Radiographs were placed on a light box and an area of 30 × 25 mm of the renal periphery opposite the hilum was digitized to a resolution of 512 × 512 pixels using a video camera (Panasonic WV-71. Matsushita Communications Industrial Co. Ltd., Japan) and an image analysis system (Seescan Salandra, Seescan plc, Cambridge, U.K.). The light box gave a constant level of illumination and the settings of focus, zoom, and aperture on the video camera were kept constant, giving a total magnification of 8, a single pixel representing 0·095 mm. The images were processed to threshold the renal arterial tree without background interference; there was no processing of the edges (by functions such as binary noise reduction) of the image included in the analysis. The fractal analysis software converted the solid thresholded image to an outline of single pixels and then applied grids of squares with side lengths from 1 to 200 pixels to this image, counting the number of squares which contained the outline.

Log-log graphs were plotted of the reciprocal of the side length of the square against the number of outline-containing squares. The gradient of linear segments of these graphs was calculated using the least-squares method of regression. Images of a circle, a square, and a quadric Koch island (with known fractal dimensions of 1·00, 1·00, and 1·61, respectively) were also analysed to test the accuracy of the method. Ten sets of measurements were made on these shapes and on 20 renal angiograms; reliability coefficients were calculated for these using estimation of variance components by a restricted maximum likelihood method[12] with confidence limits found by application of Fieller's theorem.[13] The Shapiro-Wilk test was used to determine whether the values for the measurement of fractal dimension were normally distributed; a single sample t-test was used to determine whether the mean fractal dimensions differed from the topological dimension (=1). A two-sample Kolmogorov-Smirnov test was used to compare the distributions of fractal dimension for satisfactory and incompletely filled angiograms. Analysis of covariance was used to investigate the relationships between fractal dimension and age, sex, and systolic and diastolic blood pressure.

To determine the size of the barium sulphate particles, and thus the size of vessels into which they would penetrate, a sample was examined microscopically and the diameters of 100 particles were measured using the image analysis system.

RESULTS

Seventy-two normal kidneys were radiographed; 36 produced satisfactory angiograms, the others were incompletely filled or contained air bubbles. The log–log graph for the renal angiograms produced a line of points which had a linear segment for the box sizes from 2 to 19 pixels side length (Fig. 1) but curved and then scattered distribution for larger box sizes. The fractal dimension was calculated from the gradient of the line for boxes with side lengths of 2–19 pixels; all correlation coefficients were greater than 0·995 for this segment. Plots for the objects with known fractal dimensions gave errors of less than 1·5 per cent (circle +0·5 per cent, square +0·1 per cent, Koch island –1·2 per cent). A cumulative mean graph of ten sets of measurements on these objects and 20 satisfactory angiograms showed that the initial value was within 1·2 per cent of the mean of ten sets (Fig. 2). For a single measurement taking a subject at random, the reliability coefficient was 0·968 (1·000=perfect agreement) with 95 per cent confidence limits of 0·911–0·984. The single t-test showed that the population mean of the satisfactory angiograms was significantly greater than the theoretical topological dimension of 1 ($P<0.0001$). Comparison of the 36 satisfactory angiograms with the

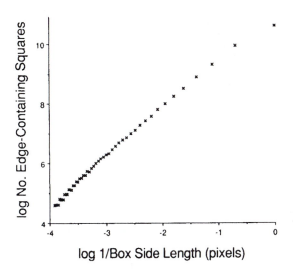

Fig. 1—Log–log graph of the reciprocal of the box side length (pixels) against the number of edge-containing squares showing a linear segment at boxes with side lengths of 2–19 pixels but a curved and progressively scattered set of points at larger box sizes

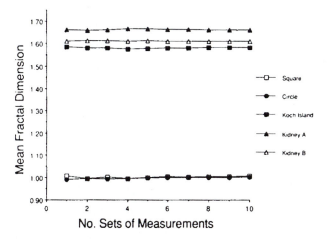

Fig. 2—Cumulative mean plot for the calculated fractal dimensions of a circle, a square, a Koch island, and two sample renal angiograms showing little difference between the initial value and the mean of ten sets of measurements.

36 unsatisfactory angiograms showed that their distributions differed significantly (Kolmogorov–Smirnov test $P<0.001$). In particular, the fractal dimensions of the 36 satisfactory angiograms of normal kidneys had a mean of 1.61 (standard deviation 0.06) and were normally distributed (correlation coefficient of normal probability plot=0.989, critical value to reject normality by Shapiro–Wilk test <0.97 at $P=0.05$). On the other hand, the fractal dimensions of the 36 unsatisfactory

angiograms had a mean of 1.47 (significantly lower than the satisfactory angiograms) and were positively skewed (correlation coefficient of normal probability plot=0.957, critical value to reject normality by Shapiro–Wilk test <0.97 at $P=0.05$).

In the satisfactory preparations, there was no significant association between fractal dimension and age ($P=0.494$), sex ($P=0.136$), or systolic ($P=0.069$) or diastolic ($P=0.990$) blood pressure.

Four abnormal kidneys were radiographed (Fig. 3): a congenitally dysplastic kidney (fractal dimension 1.50) from a case of bilateral hypoplastic renal dysplasia,[14] a kidney with congenital renal artery stenosis (fractal dimension 1.50), a kidney from a case of chronic renal failure due to recurrent thromboembolism (fractal dimension 1.57), and a small granular kidney from a case of end-stage renal failure due to hypertension (fractal dimension 1.62).

The mean diameter of the barium sulphate particles was 0.0090 mm (range 0.0054–0.0114).

DISCUSSION

The results for objects with known fractal dimension show that this implementation of the box-counting method is accurate (errors less than 1.5 per cent) and reproducible with very small differences between the initial and final mean values of ten sets of measurements (less than 1.2 per cent) and high reliability coefficients. The main methodological problem in this study was assessing the filling of the vessels; if the results are to be valid, then all the vessels that could have been analysed should have been visualized in the radiographs. The box-counting method used detects the presence of an outline of an object in boxes with side lengths from 1 to 200 pixels; in this study, 1 pixel represented 0.095 mm on the radiograph. The particles of barium sulphate in the contrast medium had a mean diameter one-tenth of this pixel size (0.009 mm), so would have penetrated smaller vessels if sufficient medium had been injected. Arterioles are usually as vessels less than 100 μm in diameter,[15] so in this method arterioles would be at the limits of the resolution of the image analysis system but the barium sulphate particles should have penetrated small arterioles and some capillaries. The amount of contrast medium injected was deemed to be sufficient if the visualized vessels extended to within 2 mm of the soft tissue outline on the radiograph at all three renal poles, since this is as far as vessels in the kidney would be expected to extend. It therefore seems reasonable to assume that all vessels detectable by the image analysis system were visualized in the radiographs defined as

482

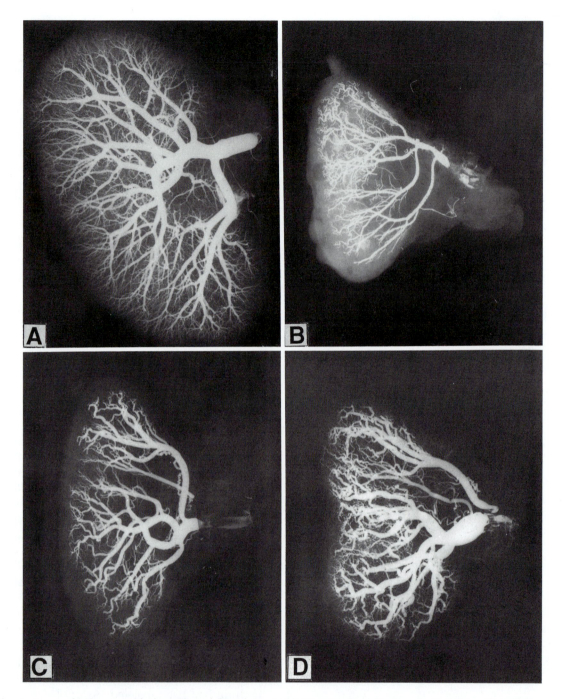

Fig. 3—Angiograms of (a) a normal kidney (fractal dimension 1·60), (b) a congenitally dysplastic kidney (fractal dimension 1·50), (c) a kidney with renal artery stenosis (fractal dimension 1·50), and (d) a kidney with recurrent thromboembolic lesions (fractal dimension 1·57). All pictures at same magnification

satisfactory unless there were focal blockages in the arterial tree within individual renal poles, a phenomenon which was not seen on subjective examination of the radiographs.

The results for the satisfactory angiograms show that the renal arterial tree has a fractal structure since the fractal dimension exceeded the topological dimension in all cases. This fractal property of the renal arterial tree invalidates any Euclidean measurement that is not performed under precisely defined conditions of magnification and measuring instrument resolution; even then, the fractal dimension is likely to be a more useful descriptor.[6]

In a two-dimensional system, a fractal dimension of 2 would indicate that all the embedding space was filled by the object and a value of 1 would indicate that effectively no space was occupied (the idealized mathematical line with no measurable width). These results show that the renal arterial tree fills a considerable amount of the space in which it is embedded, a property which produces a large surface area for plasma filtration in a compact organ and is illustrated by the relatively small size of the kidneys in relation to the fraction of cardiac output that they receive (about 25 per cent). The fractal dimension of the retinal vasculature has been measured by other investigators with mean values of 1·63[16] and 1·64[17] for the arterial tree. These values are very similar to our value (1·61) for the renal arterial tree and all these values are within the range that can be found in artificial fractal structures generated by diffusion-limited aggregation processes,[18–21] so it is possible that such processes are present in blood vessel formation and growth. There was no significant relationship between fractal dimension and age, or systolic or diastolic blood pressure. This suggests that the structure of the renal arterial tree is not greatly altered by factors after its formation and this was confirmed by the results on the four abnormal kidneys. The congenitally dysplastic kidney had a fractal dimension at the third percentile of the distribution of the satisfactory angiograms and the specimen with renal artery stenosis was also at this percentile, but the specimens in cases of end-stage hypertension and recurrent embolic disease were within the main body of the normal distribution (38th and 28th percentiles, respectively). In hypertension, there are changes in the walls of the smaller arteries which may eventually occlude the lumen but the vessels remain patent (and thus counted in the measurement of the fractal dimension) until advanced disease. The main changes in hypertension are in arteriolar walls, which lie at the limits of the resolution of this system.

The fractal dimension in the box-counting method is taken as the gradient of a log–log graph of the reciprocal of the box side length against the number of edge-containing squares. Mathematical fractal objects exhibit boundaries with a similar level of complexity at all box sizes but natural objects are constrained by the materials that they are constructed from and have a fractal structure over a more limited range of magnification.[7] Some natural objects, such as coral reefs,[22,23] have different fractal dimensions at different scales of magnification related to the processes which determine their shape at these different scales. It is possible that the renal arterial tree may have fractal dimensions of differing values to those calculated in this study if it is examined at widely differing magnifications but only one linear segment was seen on the graph of 200 box sizes at this magnification ($\times$ 8).

This methodology could be applied to other vascular trees in the body, particularly the coronary arterial tree where 'small vessel' disease is thought to play an important role in some deaths due to myocardial ischaemia but is difficult to quantitate.[24]

ACKNOWLEDGEMENTS

Simon Cross is a Medical Research Council Training Fellow. We thank Janet Brammer for her assistance with radiography, Liz Crook of Seescan plc for her advice on the fractal analysis software, and Dr L. J. R. Brown for a helpful comment on our methodology. We also thank Drs Channer, Holt, Kennedy, O'Neil, Rogers, Shortland, Smith, and Warren for providing material for this study.

REFERENCES

1. Lefevre J. Teleonomical optimization of a fractal model of the pulmonary arterial bed. *J Theor Biol* 1983; **102**: 225–248.
2. Bassingthwaite JB, Van Beek JHGM, King RB. Fractal branchings: the basis of myocardial flow heterogeneities? *Ann NY Acad Sci* 1990; **591**: 392–401.
3. Glenny RW, Robertson HT. Fractal properties of pulmonary blood flow: characterization of spatial heterogeneity. *J Appl Physiol* 1990; **69**: 532–545.
4. Horsfield K. Diameters, generations, and orders of branches in the bronchial tree. *J Appl Physiol* 1990; **68**: 457–461.
5. West BJ. Fractal Physiology and Chaos in Medicine. Singapore: World Scientific, 1990.
6. Cross SS, Cotton DWK. The fractal dimension may be a useful morphometric discriminant in histopathology. *J Pathol* 1992; **166**: 409–411.
7. Mandelbrot BB. The Fractal Geometry of Nature. New York: Freeman, 1983.
8. Falconer K. Fractal Geometry: Mathematical Foundations and Applications. Chichester: John Wiley, 1990; 83–85.
9. Morse DR, Lawton JH, Dodson MM, Williamson MH. Fractal dimension of vegetation and the distribution of arthropod body lengths. *Nature* 1985; **314**: 731–733.
10. Peitgen H-O, Jurgens H, Saupe D. Fractals in the Classroom: Part One—Introduction to Fractals and Chaos. New York: Springer-Verlag, 1992; 240–244.
11. Gulick D. Encounters with Chaos. New York: McGraw-Hill, 1992; 190–191.
12. Dunn G. Design and Analysis of Reliability Studies. London: Edward Arnold, 1989; 114–136.
13. Lloyd E. Handbook of Applicable Mathematics. Volume VI, Part A. Chichester: John Wiley, 1984; 161–162.
14. Darmady EM, MacIver AG. Renal Pathology. London: Butterworths, 1989, 69.
15. Gallagher PJ. Blood vessels. In: Sternberg SS, ed. Histology for Pathologists. New York: Raven Press, 1992; 198.
16. Mainster MA. The fractal properties of retinal vessels: embryological and clinical implications. *Eye* 1990; **4**: 235–241.

484

17. Mission GP, Landini G, Murray PI. Fractals and ophthalmology. *Lancet* 1992; **339**: 872.

18. Witten TA, Sander LM. Diffusion-limited aggregation: a kinetic critical phenomenon. *Phys Rev Lett* 1981; **47**: 1400–1403.

19. Witten TA, Meakin P. Diffusion-limited aggregation at multiple growth sites. *Phys Rev B* 1983; **28**: 5632–5642.

20. Witten TA, Sander LM. Diffusion-limited aggregation. *Phys Rev B* 1983; **27**: 5686–5697.

21. Meakin P. A new model for biological pattern formation. *J Theor Biol* 1986; **118**: 101–113.

22. Bradbury RH, Reichelt RE. Fractal dimension of a coral reef at ecological scales. *Mar Ecol Prog Ser* 1983; **10**: 169–171.

23. Bradbury RH, Reichelt RE, Green DG. Fractals in ecology: methods and interpretation. *Mar Ecol Prog Ser* 1985; **14**: 295–296.

24. James TN, Bruschke AVG. The spectrum of diseases of small coronary arteries and their physiologic consequences. *J Am Coll Cardiol* 1990; **15**: 763–774.

Ultrasound in Med. & Biol. Vol. 19, No. 8, pp. 661–666, 1993
Printed in the USA

0301–5629/93 $6.00 + .00
© 1993 Pergamon Press Ltd.

●*Original Contribution*

FRACTAL CONCEPT AND ITS ANALYSIS METHOD FOR DOPPLER ULTRASOUND SIGNALS

Yuan-Yuan Wang and Wei-Qi Wang

Department of Electronic Engineering, Fudan University, Shanghai 200433, China

(*Received 25 September* 1992; *in final form 25 March* 1993)

Abstract—A method to obtain the fractal dimension of Doppler ultrasound signals is described, and its application to the analysis of simulated and real Doppler signals is demonstrated.

Key Words: Ultrasound Doppler, Fractal dimension, Simulated Doppler signal, Least-squares method.

INTRODUCTION

Fractals, a new concept of the last 10 years, of which B. B. Mandelbrot (1982) gave a detailed description in his works in the 1980s, has been successfully applied in many areas. Now, some scientists have begun to pay attention to its application in the area of medical ultrasound (Javanaud 1989). As a further exploration of its worthiness in this area, we have used the fractal concept to analyze Doppler ultrasound flow signals. This paper introduces the method of fractal analysis and describes the results of preliminary studies in which the method is used to analyze simulated Doppler signals and clinically recorded Doppler signals.

Points are zero-dimensional, lines are one-dimensional and space is three-dimensional. Higher dimension, even infinite dimension, is used in some research areas where the variable "time" is regarded as one dimension or degrees of freedom are regarded as dimensions. These are all integer dimensions. However, many objects in nature such as coast-lines, clouds, blood vessels and the trachea of mammals are of fractal dimension, which are characterized by the properties of self-similarity, no characteristic length and no differential. A simple and typical example of a fractal graph is the Koch curve. The graph in Fig. 1a consists of four straight lines. When we reduce four replicates of this graph to $\frac{1}{3}$ of their old sizes, then rotate them and put them together, a graph shown in

Fig. 1b is obtained. As the process continuously repeats, a Koch curve is formed.

It is well known that doubling the length of a one-dimensional line results in the equivalent two of the old lines, doubling the length of each side of a two-dimensional square makes four of the old squares, while doubling the length of each side of a three-dimensional cube brings about eight of the old cubes. Therefore, $\log_a p$ is the dimension of the object if enlarging this object "a" times along one of its dimensions leads to "p" of the old objects. When $\log_a p$ is a fraction, the object is said to be of fractal dimension. The dimension of the Koch curve is therefore $\log_3 4 \approx 1.26$, which is a fractal dimension.

Doppler ultrasound technique has been widely used in the clinical noninvasive assessment of cardiac and vascular disease, where one often considers the mean frequency waveform and/or maximum frequency waveform only. The Doppler ultrasound flow signal is a random process. Now, we want to explore the worthiness of the fractal dimension of the Doppler ultrasound signal in clinical diagnosis. A method to calculate the fractal dimension of Doppler signals, and its results from simulated data and recorded data are described in the following sections. The results of clinical application will be reported in another paper.

PRINCIPLE AND METHOD

According to Mo and Cobbold (1986), Doppler ultrasound flow signals can be regarded as a quasi-wide-sense stationary (quasi-WSS) random process during a short enough time period (generally $T \leq 10$ ms). The fractal dimension of Doppler signal wave-

Address correspondence to: Prof. Wei-Qi Wang, Department of Electronic Engineering, Fudan University, Shanghai 200433, China.

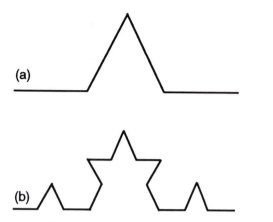

Fig. 1. Formation of Koch curve: (a) original graph, (b) modified graph.

forms will therefore be analyzed in this interval. Doppler signals can be written: $y(t) = f(t)$, in which $0 \leq t \leq T$ and amplitude, y is the function of variable, time t. In order to calculate the fractal dimension of waveforms easily and provide a distinct physical concept, we first rewrite the above formula. If the maximum amplitude of the waveforms in this interval is A, we define: $Y = y/A$ and $\tau = t/T$. So, the corresponding expression becomes: $Y(\tau) = g(\tau)$ where $0 \leq \tau \leq 1$. As the $Y - \tau$ curve has the same shape as the $y - t$ curve, the fractal dimension of the $Y - \tau$ curve in fact reflects that of the $y - t$ curve, which is a characteristic value in the time domain of Doppler ultrasound flow signals.

Here, we use the scale-changing method (Mandelbrot 1982) to calculate the fractal dimension of the waveforms for Y and τ. The main principle of the scale-changing method to calculate the fractal dimen-

sion of the graph is: when n steps are needed if we measure the length of a graph with single step length l, the total length of this graph is $L = nl$. As the single step length l changes, the step number n changes correspondingly. If n and l have the following relation: $n = kl^{-D}$ (k is constant), the total length of the graph can be expressed:

$$L = nl = kl^{1-D} = kl^{-\alpha}. \tag{1}$$

So, the fractal dimension D of the graph is obtained:

$$D = 1 + \alpha. \tag{2}$$

In our method, Doppler signal waveforms $Y(\tau) = g(\tau)$ have been already normalized, so the region of τ is $[0, 1]$ and the total length L of Doppler signal waveform is the sum of n segments of single length l_i which is the length of the straight line connecting the two neighboring points when we divide $\tau \in [0, 1]$ into m segments and the step length is $\Delta\tau$. Then, there are m points in the graph and $m = 1/\Delta\tau$. Figure 2 demonstrates the above process.

Total length is:

$$L = \sum_{i=1}^{m} l_i \tag{3}$$

where

$$l_i = \sqrt{(Y_i - Y_{i-1})^2 + (\tau_i - \tau_{i-1})^2}$$
$$= \sqrt{[Y(i\Delta\tau) - Y(i\Delta\tau - \Delta\tau)]^2 + \Delta\tau^2}. \tag{4}$$

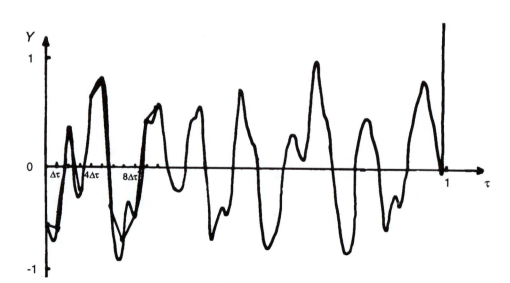

Fig. 2. Method to measure the length of waveforms.

Altering the single step length $\Delta\tau$ will cause a corresponding variation of the total length L. Changing eqn (1), we get the following:

$$\ln L = k_o - \alpha \ln \Delta\tau \qquad (5)$$

where $k_o = \ln k$. From eqn (5), it is known that the relation between $\ln L$ and $\ln \Delta\tau$ is a line with the slope $-\alpha$, shown in Fig. 3. Therefore, the procedure is to first calculate the total length L under the different single step length $\Delta\tau$ and then to obtain the fractal dimension by using the least-squares method to work out the slope $-\alpha$ of the best fit straight line between $\ln L$ and $\ln \Delta\tau$ (see Appendix).

RESULTS

Simulated Doppler flow signals with $T \leq 10$ ms

The Doppler frequency shift is greatly less than the emitting frequency of ultrasound, so the Doppler ultrasound flow signal is a narrow band signal. According to communication theory, Doppler ultrasound flow signals can be approximated (Mo and Cobbold 1986):

$$X(t) \approx \sum_{m=1}^{M} a_m \cos(2\pi f_m t + \varphi_m) \qquad (6)$$

where

$$f_m = (m - \tfrac{1}{2})\Delta f,$$
$$a_m = \sqrt{2 S_x(f_m)\Delta f y_m}, \quad \Delta f = f_{max}/M. \qquad (7)$$

y_m is an independent χ^2 random variable with two degrees of freedom, φ_m is an independent random variable uniformly distributed on the region $[0, 2\pi]$ and $S_x(f_m)$ is the power spectral density function of the Doppler signal. If the resolution of the spectrum is $1/T$, M should be chosen:

$$f_{max}/M \ll 1/T, \quad i.e., \quad M \gg f_{max}T. \qquad (8)$$

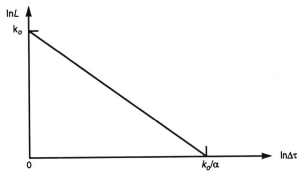

Fig. 3. The relation between $\ln L$ and $\ln \Delta\tau$.

Table 1. Fractal dimension of simulated Doppler signals with different velocity profiles.

Velocity profile index p	Fractal dimension	
	Equation (10)	Equation (11)
2.0	1.6366	1.6479
2.5	1.6566	1.6644
3.0	1.6668	1.6747
3.5	1.6750	1.6830
5.0	1.6919	1.6997
10	1.7123	1.7191
30	1.7266	1.7317
100	1.7319	1.7350

So, simulated Doppler flow signals can be generated when the power spectral density functions of the desired signals are known. Here, we assume the flow velocity profile $V(r)$ of a vessel is axis-symmetric, its form is:

$$V(r) = V_{max}[1 - (r/R)^p] \qquad (9)$$

where R is the radius of the vessel, p is an index of velocity profile, V_{max} is the velocity at the vessel center, and r is a variable coordinate originated from the vessel center. Different flow velocity profiles will cause different signal power spectral density functions. The relation between the velocity profile and signal power spectral density function is complicated. Here, we only pay attention to two simple formulae:

(a) Assuming the vessel in the infinitely wide plane wave ultrasound field, we have derived (Wang et al. 1992):

$$S(f) = k(1 - f/f_{max})^{2/p-1} \qquad (10)$$

where f_{max} is the maximum frequency shift of Doppler signal, and k is a constant.

(b) According to Bascom et al. (1986), the following formula is for the power spectral density of Doppler signals received by a circular transducer whose radius is equal to that of the vessel being insonated:

$$S(f) = [4r^3[\{4\rho(1-\rho) - r^2\}/\{3\rho(1-\rho^2)^2\}]$$
$$- 16r/3 + (2r/3\rho)(3r^2 - 2)(3\pi - 4) + 4r$$
$$\times \{r^2 - \rho(1-\rho)\}/\{\rho(1-\rho)^2\} + 2[(\pi - 2\sin^{-1}\rho)/$$
$$\{\rho(1-\rho^2)\}] \times \{\rho^2(1-\rho) - r^2(1-\rho) - r^2\rho\}]$$
$$\times \{-(1 - f/f_{max})^{1/p-1}\}(3p/16) \qquad (11)$$

where $r = (1 - f/f_{max})^{1/p}$, and $\rho = (1 - r^2)^{1/2}$.

According to Mo and Cobbold (1986), within

664   Ultrasound in Medicine and Biology   Volume 19, Number 8, 1993

the interval for which the Doppler flow signal is a quasi-WSS process, the signal power spectral density does not change and is only a function of frequency, f. We have simulated Doppler signals with two kinds of power spectral density (eqns 10 and 11). All calculations were under the same conditions: emitting ultrasound frequency, 5 MHz; radius of the vessel, 2 mm; angle between ultrasound beam and flow, 60°; distance between the center of the transducer face and the flow axis, 3 cm; maximum velocity, 80 cm/s; f_{max} = 3 kHz; T = 10 ms; M = 500. Table 1 shows the fractal dimension of these simulated signals.

From Table 1 we find that the fractal dimension of Doppler signals is different for different velocity profiles (different p).

Simulated Doppler signals over one or more cardiac cycles

According to the simulation model of Doppler flow signals (eqns 6 and 7), we can generate Doppler flow signals over one or more cardiac cycles when the function between the power spectral density and variable, time, is known. Mo and Cobbold (1989) obtained the relation between the power spectral density of Doppler ultrasound flow signal in normal carotid artery and its maximum frequency $f_{max}(t)$ from experimental statistics:

$$S(f, t) = A_1(f_{max}(t) - f)^2 \exp[-B_1(f_{max}(t) - f)^2] + A_2(f_{max}(t) - f)\exp[-B_2(f_{max}(t) - f)^2] \quad (12)$$

where

$$B_1 = 1/(0.215 f_{max}(t) - 0.094),$$
$$B_2 = B_1/10,$$
$$A_1 = (0.47 f_{max}(t) + 2.18)/[\pi/4 B_1^{3/2} + 0.125(1 - \exp(-B_1 f_{max}^2(t)/10)/B_1]$$
$$A_2 = 0.025 A_1. \quad (13)$$

So, the relevant power spectral density can be calculated if the maximum frequency $f_{max}(t)$ is known. Thus, Doppler signals over long periods can be simulated.

To obtain a practical maximum frequency curve, the Doppler signals in normal carotid artery over two cardiac cycles were acquired by a computer. The maximum frequency curve was then obtained with maximum frequency estimation algorithm (Mo et al. 1988). Figure 4a is the sonogram of recorded Doppler signals. Figure 4b is the maximum frequency curve, which was used to simulate long-period Doppler signals.

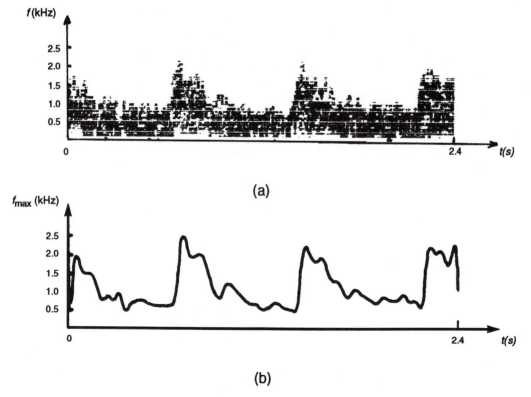

Fig. 4. Sonogram of Doppler signals in normal carotid artery (a) and maximum frequency curve (b).

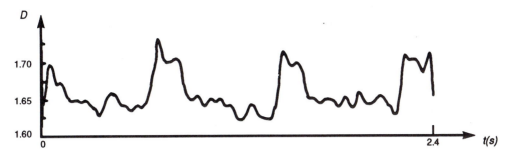

Fig. 5. Fractal dimension curve of simulation Doppler signal waveforms.

Calculate the power spectral density over the same period. This in turn was used to simulate the corresponding Doppler flow signals. Figure 5 shows the fractal dimension D curve which resulted from applying fractal analysis to the Doppler signal simulated from the maximum frequency curve in Fig. 4.

It can be seen from Fig. 5 that the fractal dimension curve and the maximum frequency curve are very similar. On the algorithm and software, the calculation of fractal dimension is simpler and easier than that of frequency spectrum analysis.

Real Doppler signals over one or more cardiac cycles

We can analyze the fractal dimension of recorded Doppler ultrasound signal waveforms of human normal carotid artery. The results of a fractal dimension analysis of Doppler signal from which Fig. 4 was obtained are shown in Fig. 6.

The cardiac rhythm can be easily seen from the fractal dimension curve, which is also very similar to the Doppler mean velocity waveform.

DISCUSSION AND CONCLUSION

Fractal geometry is a new branch of mathematics. Some graphs are characterized by their fractal dimension, and signal waveforms can be regarded as one kind of graph. According to this point, signal waveforms have the characteristics of the fractal dimension. Therefore, the fractal dimension is an index

which reflects the essence of signal waveforms, not just a mathematic tool such as Fourier Transform.

Doppler signals are time-domain signals whose horizontal coordinate and vertical coordinate have different dimensions. Therefore, in our method, we first normalize time and amplitude of signal waveforms. In this way, the method of calculating the fractal dimension of graphs can be used to analyze the fractal dimension of time-domain signals.

The maximum frequency of Doppler signals is an important index for diagnosing vessel diseases such as stenosis. The fractal dimension curve of Doppler signals corresponds with the maximum frequency curve of Doppler signals, so it is expected that the fractal dimension curve of Doppler signals can be applied in the clinical diagnosis. However, on the algorithm and software structure, fractal dimension calculation is simpler than maximum frequency analysis which can lead to simplicity and cheapness of instrument hardware and/or software. The clinical application of the fractal dimension of Doppler signals still needs further research work.

The velocity profile is an important index of blood hydrodynamics. In our method, we only use the simple model: axis-symmetric velocity profile. We have discussed the corresponding relation between velocity profile index p and fractal dimension, but velocity profile is actually not axis-symmetric. It is rather complicated. Our further work will focus on analyzing the sonogram of recorded Doppler signals to ob-

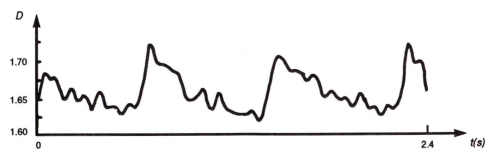

Fig. 6. Fractal dimension curve of recorded Doppler signal.

tain the fractal dimension of the sonogram. The spectrum of Doppler signals reflects the velocity distribution of red cells in the blood. Fractal dimension in the frequency domain should have a more clear physical concept of velocity profile than time-domain signals.

REFERENCES

Bascom, P. A. J.; Cobbold, R. S. C.; Roelofs, B. H. M. Influence of spectral broadening on continuous wave Doppler ultrasound spectra: A geometric approach. Ultrasound Med. Biol. 12:387–395; 1986.

Javanaud, C. The application of a fractal model to the scattering of ultrasound in biological media. J. Acoust. Soc. Am. 86:493–496; 1989.

Mandelbrot, B. B. The fractal geometry of nature. San Francisco: Freeman; 1982.

Mo, L. Y. L.; Cobbold, R. S. C. "Speckle" in CW Doppler ultrasound spectra: A simulation study. IEEE Trans. Ultrason. Ferroelectr. Freq. Contr. UFFC-33:747–752; 1986.

Mo, L. Y. L.; Cobbold, R. S. C. A nonstationary signal simulation model for CW and PW Doppler ultrasound. IEEE Trans. Ultrason. Ferroelectr. Freq. Contr. UFFC-36:522–530; 1989.

Mo, L. Y. L.; Yun, L. C. M.; Cobbold, R. S. C. Comparison of four digital maximum frequency estimators for Doppler ultrasound. Ultrasound Med. Biol. 14:355–363; 1988.

Wang, Y. Y.; Wang, W. Q.; Shao, Q. M. Computer simulation of Doppler ultrasound signal. J. Fudan Univ. 31:461–470; 1992.

APPENDIX

If m different total lengths $L_1, L_2, \ldots$, have been calculated respectively under m different single step lengths $\Delta\tau_1, \Delta\tau_2, \ldots, \Delta\tau_m$, a function $y_i = \ln L_i - k_o + \alpha \ln \Delta\tau_i$ can be constructed. For different $\Delta\tau_i$, we want $\sum y_i^2 \to 0$, i.e., make $\sum\limits_{i=1}^{m} y_i^2 = \sum\limits_{i=1}^{m} (\ln L_i - k_o + \alpha \ln \Delta\tau_i)^2$ reaching minimum.

According to the least-squares method, we have:

$$\begin{cases} \partial(\sum\limits_{i=1}^{m} y_i^2)/\partial k_o = 0 \\[2mm] \partial(\sum\limits_{i=1}^{m} y_i^2)/\partial \alpha = 0 \end{cases} \quad (A1)$$

i.e.,

$$\begin{cases} -2 \sum\limits_{i=1}^{m} (\ln L_i - k_o + \alpha \ln \Delta\tau_i) = 0 \\[2mm] 2 \sum\limits_{i=1}^{m} [\ln \Delta\tau_i (\ln L_i - k_o + \alpha \ln \Delta\tau_i)] = 0. \end{cases} \quad (A2)$$

With α value worked out form eqn (A2) replacing its value in eqn (2), we get the fractal dimension of the waveforms:

$$D = 1 + \{ n \sum\limits_{i=1}^{m} [(\ln \Delta\tau_i)\ln L_i] - \sum\limits_{i=1}^{m} \ln \Delta\tau_i \sum\limits_{i=1}^{m} \ln L_i \}$$

$$/[(\sum\limits_{i=1}^{m} \ln \Delta\tau_i)^2 - n \sum\limits_{i=1}^{m} (\ln \Delta\tau_i)^2]. \quad (A3)$$

Neuroscience Research, Suppl. 10 (1989) S131–S140
Elsevier Scientific Publishers Ireland Ltd.

S131

FRACTAL ANALYSIS OF GANGLION CELL DENDRITIC BRANCHING PATTERNS OF THE RAT AND CAT RETINAE

KATSUKO MORIGIWA*, MASAKI TAUCHI** AND YUTAKA FUKUDA*
*Department of Neurophysiology, Biomedical Research Center, Osaka University Medical School, Kita-ku, Osaka 530 and **Department of Sensory Impairments, Research Institute, National Rehabilitation Center for the Disabled, Tokorozawa 359 (Japan)

INTRODUCTION

Despite the body of information on ganglion cell morphology in the mammalian retina, to date there exist no established methods to objectively quantify its dendritic complexity. By intracellularly injecting Lucifer Yellow (LY) into prelabeled cells[1,2] and thereby completely staining the terminal dendrites, we have applied fractal analysis to quantify the complexity of the dendritic branching patterns.

Fractal analysis has already become one of the most widely used measures of complexity and randomness in such seemingly unrelated studies as: diffusion-limited aggregations[3], electrodeposition[4], dielectric breakdown (such as lightning)[5], earthquake prediction[6], cloud sizes and shapes[7], or cardiac rhythms and His-Purkinje network[8]. They all involve "random" patterns that traditional Euclidean geometry has been unable to quantify. The analysis reveals "regular irregularities," e.g., an organizing structure or pattern that lies hidden within the apparent randomness or complexity of a system. This measure, originally suggested by the German mathematician Felix Hausdorff, was revived by Benoit Mandelbrot to seek patterns in the random fluctuations of noise in electrical transmission, (temporally distributed as a Cantor set,) or of cotton prices in the United States of America.

The fractal dimension of a set is a number that expresses how densely this set occupies the metric space in which it exists. Fractals are structures in which this fractal dimension (D) is distinctly smaller than the Euclidean dimension (d) of the space[9]. The underlying regularity of fractal structures is due to their quality of self-similarity, i.e., they are scale invariant and look the same under different magnifications; they are also recursive, containing pattern inside of pattern. Hausdorff suggested one way to define the dimension of these self-similar figures where we can reduce the scale by some ratio $1/\underline{a}$ and obtain a reduced figure that is of the same form as the original one. Suppose that in this way we subdivide the original figure into $\underline{b}$ similar parts, then the exponent D in the equation $b=a^D$ expresses a dimension that is solved by taking their logarithms: $D=\log b/\log a$*. Generally, the higher this fractal dimension (D) the more complex the pattern.

---

*To give an example, the frequently cited Koch's snowflake curve is generated by recursively reducing the scale by 1/3, and obtaining 4 similar parts to that of the original one. Thus after n steps, the original length of a unit line has increased by a factor of $(3/4)^n$, giving us the fractal dimension $(D)=\log 4/\log 3 =1.26$. In contrast, a conventional straight line reduced by 1/3 has 3 identical segments, and its length is unchanged after recursive $\underline{n}$ steps; that is, $D=\log 3/\log 3 =1$, an integer. Similarly, in the case of a unit square, if one side is reduced by 1/3 we obtain $3^2=9$ identical squares; thus $D=\log 3^2/\log 3 =2$.

Presented at the 11th Taniguchi International Symposium on Visual Science, November 28–December 2, 1988
0168-0102/89/$03.50 © 1989 Elsevier Scientific Publishers Ireland Ltd.

In the present study, we have redefined the morphological properties of rat alpha ganglion cells, particularly of the ON and OFF cell subclasses having different dendritic stratifications in the inner plexiform layer (IPL)[10,11]. We not only show distinct morphological differences between ON and OFF alpha ganglion cells at defined eccentricities from the optic disk, but also demonstrate that their dendritic branching patterns have fractal structures. Furthermore, our results show that the fractal dimensions of ON and OFF alpha cells appear to differ with eccentricity, indicating that a particular fractal dimension does not serve to define and to catergorize ON and OFF subclasses. The dimensions do seem to reflect different branching rules, however, possibly due to differing promoting principles or dendritic competition during growth, or both. To examine how fractal dimensions vary in cells undergoing developmental changes, we have tentatively subjected to fractal analysis developmental data of three types of retinal ganglion cells of the rat described by Masilm et al.[12] and two types of ganglion cells of the cat described by Dann et al.[13] and Ramoa et al[14].

MATERIAL AND METHODS
Intracellular injection of Lucifer Yellow

Twenty-five albino rats (Wistar) were anesthetized with 4% chloral hydrate (i.p., 1 cc/ 100 g) for craniotomy; all surgical wounds were infiltrated with 2% Xylocaine. Using a microsyringe or a piece of gelatinized sponge, 4.5-6 μl of 5% granular blue (GB) in 5% DMSO was stereotaxically injected into the lateral geniculate nucleus or the superior colliculus. After a 48-72 h postinjection survival, animals were perfused with saline under deep anesthesia, and the eyes were enucleated. The retinae were then dissected into eye cups, and wholemounts were prepared in warm oxygenated Ames' solution. The wholemounts (n=42) were placed vitreous side up in a small chamber superfused with Ames' solution, and observed under a Nikon fluorescence microscope. Using a BV excitation filter (400-450 nm), we aimed a glass micropipette filled with 3% LY at GB-prelabeled cells with a soma diameter of over 20 μm. Negative currents of 2 to 5 nA were passed through the tip for 5 to 10 min so as to allow for the filling with LY of the cell's terminal dendrites. The cells identified as alpha cells (n=185), which had thick axons and 3 to 6 thick primary dendrites, were then subclassified into ON (n=75) or OFF types (n=84) based on the depths of their dendritic stratification in the IPL. ON types extended their dendrites within the inner sublamina, and OFF types within the outer. Those cells that did not meet the morphological criteria of alpha cells (n=21), and those that could not be subclassified into ON or OFF types, or that had incompletely filled dendrites (n=26), were excluded from the data. Individual LY-filled cells were drawn for detailed analysis.

Fractal analysis

We used the box-counting method[7] to analyze the fractal dimensions of the dendritic branchings of 8 ON and 8 OFF type alpha cells found at different eccentricities from the optic disk. The drawings of the 16 alpha cells were each placed under grids of different unit sizes (see Fig. 2). These grids of different scales were constructed by successively dissecting the largest grid covering the whole alpha cell. The grids thus made had $2^1, 2^2, ..., 2^6$ boxes on one side (the minimum grid was

10 x 10 μm). For each scale grid, the number of boxes entered by the dendritic branches (N(r)) were counted (the soma and axon excluded) and plotted as a function of the number of boxes on one side of the grid (r) on a logarithmic scale. To obtain estimates of the fractal dimension D, straight lines were least square fitted to the coordinates (log N(r), log (r)) and further divided by a correction factor of log 2 to yield estimates at base 10. Mean correlation coefficients were checked to ensure goodness of fit.

We tentatively analyzed the fractal dimensions of the dendrites of class I, II and III ganglion cells of rat peripheral retina at different developmental stages (postnatal day P6, P14 and adult), based on the representative drawings depicted by Maslim et al[12]. We also subjected to fractal analysis representative drawings of alpha and beta ganglion cells of cat peripheral retina (from fetal day E45 to postnatal day P31) as described by Ramoa et al.[14] and those (P0 and adult) by Dann et al[13]. Drawings of the different morphological types of retinal ganglion cells of the rat and cat at varying developmental stages were photocopied. They were enlarged and subjected to fractal analysis at the same magnification (1 μm = 5 mm) as our original drawings of ON and OFF alpha ganglion cells of the rat.

RESULTS
Morphological differences between ON and OFF alpha cells of the albino rat

A total of 75 ON cells and 84 OFF cells were sampled from all four quadrants of the retina at eccentricities of 0 to 5 mm from the optic disk. Table I summarizes the morphological differences between the ON and OFF types.

TABLE I

MORPHOLOGICAL PROPERTIES OF ON AND OFF ALPHA CELLS OF THE ALBINO RAT RETINA

	ON-type		OFF-type
Dendritic termination in IPL	sublamina b		sublamina a
Soma diameter (μm)	32.0 ± 6.45	>	27.1 ± 4.82
Dendritic field diameter (μm)	607 ± 120	>	499 ± 76.7
Number of primary dendrites	5.58 ± 0.92	>	4.33 ± 1.66
Fractal dimension	1.38 ± 0.12	>	1.53 ± 0.05
Dendritic branching	distal		proximal
	sparse		profuse

Besides the depth of their dendritic stratifications, the dimensions of soma diameter as well as dendritic field diameter differed between the two cell types. They differed also in the number of primary dendrites and their soma shape: ON cell had 4 to 7 primary dendrites with triangular or

S134

cubic shaped soma, whereas OFF cells had 3 to 6 primary dendrites and oval or spherical soma. The difference between the two types was particularly evident in their dendritic branching patterns as can be appreciated from Fig. 1. At a similar eccentricity from the optic disk (ON cell, 2.9 mm; OFF cell, 3.0 mm), not only was the dendritic field of the OFF cell smaller, but its proximal dendrites were denser and appeared to branch more regularly and successively than those of the ON type. This difference between the dendritic patterns of the two cell types became more prominent as the dendritic field dimensions of both ON and OFF types increased with eccentricity (correlation

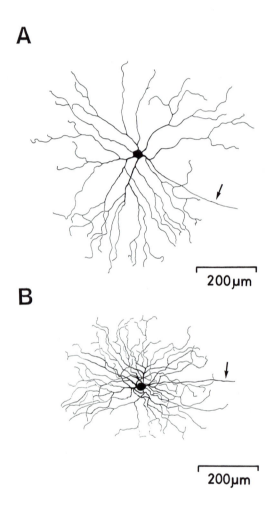

Fig. 1. Drawings of LY-injected alpha ganglion cells of the albino rat retina. A: ON type cell at 2.9 mm from the optic disk. B: OFF type cell at 3.0 mm from the optic disk. Axons are indicated by arrows. Note the difference in soma diameter and dendritic branching patterns between ON and OFF types at similar eccentricity.

coefficients of 0.65 and 0.64 respectively, P<0.01). There was relatively little correlation between eccentricity and the dimensions of their soma diameter.

Fractal analysis of ON and OFF alpha cells of the albino rat

To quantify the differences in the dendritic complexity noted above, drawings of 8 pairs of ON and OFF cells at different eccentricities from the optic disk were subjected to fractal analysis (Fig. 2A). In all cells subjected to analysis we found that the number of boxes of the dendrite region (N(r)) aligned linearly to the number of boxes on one side of grid (r) with high correlation (mean correlation coefficient 0.9989 ± 0.0004) (Fig. 2B). This finding implies that the dendritic arborizations of rat alpha ganglion cells have fractal structures, and that they do not branch out randomly but follow certain rules.

The fractal dimensions of 8 ON cells varied with eccentricity from 1.2 to 1.6 with a mean of 1.38 ± 0.12 (TableI). Those of the 8 OFF types ranged from 1.43 to 1.58 with a mean of 1.53 ± 0.05 (Table I). As depicted in Fig. 3, not only were the fractal dimensions of OFF cells relatively higher than those of the ON cells, but they remained relatively constant irrespective of eccentricity.

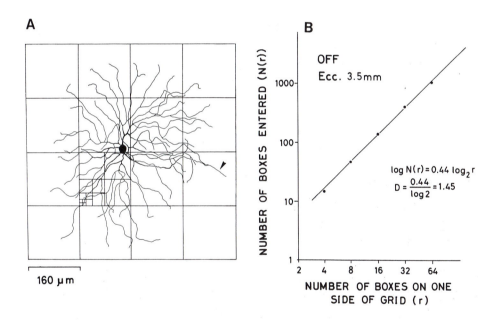

Fig. 2. Fractal analysis (box-counting method) of dendritic branching patterns. A: a grid of unit size covering the dendritic field of an alpha cell is successively dissected into smaller and smaller grids, the smallest, 10 x 10 μm, having 2^6 boxes on one side. B: logarithmic plots of the number of boxes entered by dendritic branches (N(r)) as a function of the number of boxes on one side (r) (2^1, 2^2, 2^3, 2^4, 2^5, and 2^6 boxes). The axon indicated by an arrowhead in A was excluded. Note the logarithmic straight line which implies fractal structure with D = 1.45.

S136

In contrast, there was a marked decrease in the dimensions of the ON types with eccentricity. These results support our impression that OFF types indeed have relatively complex dendritic arborizations branching uniformly throughout the retina (see Figs. 1, 2). ON cells were found to have less complex branching, which is manifested more clearly in cells with large dendritic fields at increasing eccentricities. In other words, the dendrites of OFF alpha cells originate from few primary dendrites that branch elaborately, while ON cells have more primary dendrites that extend distally without being subjected to repeated bifurcations.

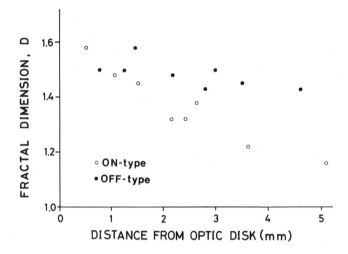

Fig. 3. Fractal dimensions of ON (open circles) and OFF (filled circles) alpha cells of the albino rat retina plotted as a function of distance from the optic disk. Note that the dimensions of ON alpha cells decrease with eccentricity while those of the OFF cells are relatively high and constant.

Fractal analysis of dendritic development of rat and cat retinal ganglion cells

Of the representative drawings of Maslim et al.[12], we subjected to fractal analysis only the data classifiable into the three ganglion cell classes of the rat retina: those at postnatal day 6 (P6), day 14 (P14) and adult stage. The mean fractal dimensions were 1.49 ± 0.03, 1.54 ± 0.04 and 1.36 ± 0.02 for class I, II and III cells (corresponding to cat alpha, beta and gamma cells), respectively, with an overall correlation coefficient of 0.9965 ± 0.004. As illustrated in Fig. 4, the dimensions of all three cell classes rise in parallel at P14 and drop again at the adult stage. It appears also from this limited data that class II cells have the highest dimensions and class III cells the lowest ones, which supports our impressions of their dendritic arborizations.

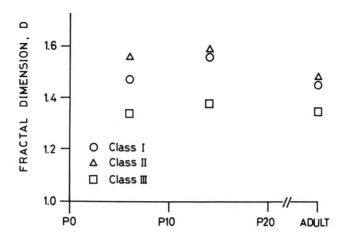

Fig. 4. Developmental changes in the fractal dimensions of Class I (circles), Class II(triangles), and Class III (squares) cells of the rat retina at P6, P14 and adult stage, derived from representative drawings in Maslim et al[12]. Note that, although the dimensions of the three different morphological types rise and fall in parallel with age, Class II cells have the highest dimensions, and Class III the lowest ones.

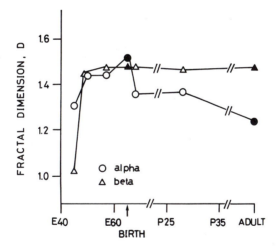

Fig. 5. Developmental changes in the fractal dimensions of alpha (circles) and beta (triangles) of the cat retina. Filled symbols: dimensions derived from the data reported by Dann et al.[13]; P0 and adult. Open symbols: dimensions derived from those reported by Ramoa et al.[14]; E45, E50/52, E57, P3 and P31; arrow indicates the time of birth. Note that the dimensions of beta cells are relatively high and constant, whereas those of alpha cells are high in the prenatal stage but drop in the postnatal stage.

S138

Figure 5 shows developmental changes in the fractal dimensions of alpha (circles) and beta (triangles) cells of peripheral cat retina. The filled symbols represent data of alpha and beta cells from Dann et al.[13], and the open symbols data from Ramoa et al[14]. Although there are limitations in directly comparing dimensions analyzed from two different sources (their overall correlation coefficient was 0.9985 ± 0.0005), the results suggest that, excluding the initial stage (E45), the fractal dimensions of beta cells are relatively constant throughout the developmental stages with a mean of 1.47 ± 0.01. On the other hand, the dimensions of alpha cells (mean 1.40 ± 0.09) appear to be as high as beta cells in prenatal stage, but gradually decline postnatally towards a minimum value at the adult stage.

DISCUSSION

The technique of relabeling the prelabeled neurons with intracellular injection of the fluorescent dye LY has made it possible to apply fractal analysis to the dendritic branching patterns of retinal ganglion cells. It should also be noted that the two-dimensional growth of the ganglion cell dendrites and the use of wholemount preparations have all made it relatively simple to subject the ganglion cells to such an analysis. The most significant result of our study is the fact that ganglion cell branching patterns have fractal structures. We believe that the fact that fractal analysis can be applied to the dendritic branching patterns of retinal ganglion cells in itself opens the door to exciting possibilities in studying function as well as cell structure.

Our morphological study on the ON and OFF alpha cells is only the first step in this direction. We have shown that OFF cells have more complex, but smaller dendritic fields than those of ON cells, particularly in the periphery. The results of our fractal analysis of the two cell types further indicates that their dendritic arborizations follow certain branching rules expressed by the fractal dimensions: OFF cells have relatively high and constant fractal dimensions at all eccentricities (mean 1.53 ± 0.05), whereas the dimensions of ON cells vary and decrease with eccentricity (mean 1.38 ± 0.12). The difference may be genetically encoded; but they may also be modified by varying nearest neighbor conditions within the inner and outer halves of the IPL.

To see how the dendritic branchings of ganglion cells undergo changes during growth, we analyzed developmental data for the cat[13,14] as well as for the rat[12]. The fractal dimensions obtained from these data are tentative; nevertheless, they suggest certain trends in the development of the ganglion cells. The result of the rat data shown in Fig.4 suggests that there might be definite differences in the genetically encoded rules governing the different ganglion cell types (Class I, II and III). Results from the cat data depicted in Fig. 5 further support this possibility: The fractal dimensions of alpha cells increase and decline with age, whereas those of beta cells appear to be relatively constant. Indeed, morphological types of ganglion cells appear to be identifiable by E50 in the cat and by P6 in the rat during development[12].

Figure 5 also reflects the fact that small spine-like processes, abundant in developing cells, peak around P0 to P5 in the cat[13,14] and that alpha cells subsequently undergo more extensive remodelling than do beta cells[14]. Ramoa et al.[14] have noted that the proliferation of dendritic spines observed in developing cat ganglion cells coincides with the period of conventional synapse

S139

formation with amacrine cells in the IPL[15] and that the disappearance of spines, and declining dendritic complexity coincides with the formation period of ribbon synapses[14]. The difference in the constancy of fractal dimensions between alpha and beta cells during development may reflect their differing synaptic connectivity within the IPL.

Maslim et al.[12] also note that the segregation of rat ganglion cell dendrites to the IPL occurs between P6 and P14, corresponding to the period during which amacrine-like processes make synapses in the IPL[16]; dendritic competition also begins to affect dendritic field size at this stage when dendritic processes cease to extend by means of growth cones[12]. It is therefore plausible that the dimensions of ON and OFF alpha cells may reflect further diversification of synaptic connectivity as well as dendritic competition in the two halves of the IPL during this stage. A thorough LY-study on the morphological variations with eccentricity of the ON and OFF subclasses of the different ganglion cell types is necessary to examine this possibility.

ACKNOWLEDGEMENTS

We should like to thank Dr. Mitsugu Matsushita for his helpful comments and discussions on fractal analysis, and Drs. Y. Ogata and Y. Tamura of the Institute of Statistical Mathematics for their useful advice.

REFERENCES

1. Tauchi M, Masland RH (1984) Proc R Soc Lond B **223**:101-119
2. Vaney DI (1984) Proc R Soc Lond B **220**:501-508
3. Witten TA, Sander LM (1981) Phys Rev Lett **47**:1400-1403
4. Matsushita M, Sano N, Hayakawa H, Honjo H, Sawada Y (1984) Phys Rev Lett **53**:286-289
5. Takayasu H (1985) Phys Rev Lett **54**:1099-1101
6. Scholz CH (1982) Bull Seism Soc Ame **72**:1-14
7. Lovejoy S (1982) Science **216**:185-187
8. Goldberger AL, Bhargava V, West BJ, Mandell AJ (1985) Biophys J **48**:525
9. Mandelbrot BB (1982) The Fractal Geometry of Nature. Freeman, San Francisco
10. Boycott BB, Wässle H (1974) J Physiol **240**:397-419
11. Peichl L, Ott H, Boycott BB (1987) Proc R Soc Lond B **231**:169-197
12. Maslim J, Webster M, Stone J (1986) J Comp Neurol **254**:382-402
13. Dann JF, Buhl EH, Peichl L (1988) J Neurosci **8**:1485-1499
14. Ramoa AS, Campbell G, Schatz CJ (1988) J Neurosci **8**:4239-4261
15. Maslim J, Stone J (1986) Brain Res **373**:35-48
16. Wiedman T, Kuwabara T (1986) Arch Ophthalmol **79**:970-984

ELSEVIER

Brain Research 634 (1994) 181–190

BRAIN RESEARCH

Research Report

Comparative fractal analysis of cultured glia derived from optic nerve and brain demonstrate different rates of morphological differentiation

T.G. Smith Jr. *, T.N. Behar

Laboratory of Neurophysiology, NINDS, NIH, Bethesda, MD 20892, USA

(Accepted 17 August 1993)

Abstract

O-2A progenitor cells derived from neonatal rat cerebral hemispheres or optic nerves, were induced to differentiate in culture into either oligodendrocytes or type 2 astrocytes. The fractal dimensions, a measure of morphological complexity, of the differentiating glial cells were measured over time. Analysis of the changes in fractal dimension (D) with respect to time revealed specific rates of growth for each glial phenotype and a specific final D. The time course of these changes is well fit by a simple mathematical model. While brain-derived oligodendrocytes matured faster than the astrocytes, they ultimately attained comparable levels of complexity, with similar maximum fractal dimensions. Oligodendrocytes from nerve also matured faster than nerve derived astrocytes, in contrast, however, they attained a greater morphological complexity than nerve astrocytes. While the brain-derived oligodendrocytes showed a faster rate of maturation than their optic nerve counterparts, astrocytes from both regions had similar rates of morphological differentiation. Self-similarity, a defining property of fractal objects was investigated, by determining the fractal dimension of cells over a range of magnifications. The calculated fractal dimension remained constant over a 10-fold range in optical magnification, illustrating that cultured glial cells exhibit this important characteristic of fractal objects. In addition, we analyzed the branching patterns of glial processes by the Sholl method and found that the results were not as interpretable or meaningful as those of fractal analysis.

Key words: Glia; Differentiation; Fractal dimension

1. Introduction

Oligodendrocytes and type 2 astrocytes, the two cells that cooperate in myelinating axons in the adult CNS, arise from a common precursor cell, the O-2A progenitor [22]. In vivo, signals from both neurons and type 1 astrocytes probably influence the induction of the precursor's maturation, however, the cellular and molecular signals underlying the glial cells' differentiation have yet to be elucidated. Tissue culture provides an opportunity to study the factors and mechanisms involved in glial cell growth and differentiation.

By manipulating the culture conditions, enriched populations of precursor cells can be selectively induced to differentiate into either oligodendrocytes or type 2 astrocytes ahead of their in vivo time table. Cells cultured in chemically defined media differentiate into oligodendrocytes, while progenitors grown in the presence of fetal calf serum (FCS) become type 2 astrocytes [22].

Traditionally, the appearance of specific antigenic markers have served as 'milestones' for assessing the stages of glial differentiation. For example, the appearance of galactocerebroside (GC) defines oligodendrocytes, while the combination of glial fibrillary acidic protein (GFAP) and A2B5-ganglioside is a marker specific for type 2 astrocytes. Emergence of a sulfatide recognized by the monoclonal antibody O4 [5] designates one stage along the developing pathway. These qualitative descriptions do not address the broad spectrum of cellular, molecular and morphological changes which take place during the course of differentiation of each phenotype. As the progenitor differentiates it undergoes striking morphological changes. Initially bipolar, the cell develops an extensive network of branches as it matures.

We have previously reported that cultured differentiating O-2A progenitor cells derived from rat optic

---

* Corresponding author. Fax: (1) (301) 402-1565.

Elsevier Science B.V.
SSDI 0006-8993(93)E1192-6

nerve can be *quantitatively* described on the basis of their morphological complexity, by measuring the fractal dimension (*D*) of the cells. The fractal dimension is a calculation of the measure of the rate of addition of detail with increasing magnification. Few natural objects are well described or modeled by Euclidian measures (e.g., circles, squares, etc.), where the measures are given in units raised to integer powers; however, many such objects are well described by measures raised to non-integer or fractional powers and are called fractals [10,19]. Increases in measured *D* correlate with perceived increases in morphological complexity [26,28]. Furthermore, specific *D*'s correlate with specific degrees of maturation. Thus, cells can be described quantitatively and objectively, at any given stage of differentiation, by their *D* value, which we think is better than the aforementioned, qualitative antigenic markers.

D has become a useful quantitative measure of the complexity of cellular forms. For example, one study examined how the measured *D* compared with the observed complexity of cultured neurons [28]. Another study examined changes in *D* among cultured optic nerve derived glial cells that were differentiating in vitro [26]. In addition, the complexity of liver cells [18], motor cortex cells [21], cerebellar glial cells [24], Purkinje cells [29] and retinal ganglion cells [1,13–15] grown in vivo have been measured. More recently, rodent spinal cord neurons have been classified and their morphological differentiation followed by measuring *D* [16,17]. In all studies, *D* appeared to correlate with perceived complexity, as previously observed [4]. In the optic nerve glial cell [26] and spinal neuronal [17] studies, however, there was a surprisingly good fit of the data with a simple, one parameter model's description of how the fractal dimension changed with growth. That model predicted that the rate of increase in the fractal dimension with growth and differentiation decreased over time in a manner described by a single time constant (τ) [26,17].

In this study we have cultured O-2A progenitor cells derived from two different regions of the CNS, the optic nerve and cortex, in an effort to quantify all cultures simultaneously and compare their relative values. Oligodendrocytes were identified by immunocytochemical detection of GC. Type 2 astrocytes were identified by A2B5 immunoreactivity. *D* was calculated and compared for samples from each culture condition over a 10-day period. In addition, the rate of morphological differentiation was determined by analyzing the changes in *D* of each phenotype from each region over time.

An important and defining property of fractal objects is called 'self similarity', which means that objects look qualitatively the same at all magnifications. This means that extra detail appears in the object at quanti-

tatively the same rate over many changes in scale or magnification. 'True', theoretical or deterministic fractals are self-similar over an infinite range of scales and they exist only in computers. In the real world, fractal objects are self-similar over ranges of 2–4 orders of magnitude [19].

In the present study we have examined whether the borders of cultured cells are, in fact, self-similar, i.e., do they really look qualitatively the same and have essentially the same *D* when viewed under different magnifications? Thus, does the *D* of a homogeneous population of cells, viewed under low magnification have the same *D* as individual cells or even parts of individual cells within the same population when viewed under higher magnifications? The answers to these questions have important implications about how *D* is actually measured, the limitations that need to be imposed in undertaking the measurement and the meaning that is imparted to the values of *D*. We show that, within certain limits, the *D* value of a group of cells is essentially the same over all magnifications examined, thus within that range of magnification, the borders of the cells are self-similar.

In addition, we find that the branching pattern of glial processes can also be characterized quantitatively by a single parameter, the Sholl coefficient, which is a measure of the difference in the rate at which branches are forming minus branch termination as a function of distance from the cell soma. Sholl [25] found that some cerebral cortical cells were best fit by a straight line on a semi-log plot, while others were best fit on a log–log plot. We found that nerve-derived glial cells were best fit on a semi-log plot, while brain-derived cells fit a log–log plot better. This method, however, does not appear to be as useful in yielding meaningful results as the fractal dimension analysis.

2. Materials and methods

Cell cultures

Brain derived O-2A progenitor cells were isolated by a modified panning technique as described elsewhere [2]. Briefly, cerebral hemispheres from neonatal Sprague–Dawley rats were dissected, mechanically dissociated and cultured for 7 days prior to seeding onto coverslips. Flasks of primary mixed cultures were shaken overnight on a rotary shaker at 37°C and precursor cells were harvested from the supernatant. Progenitors were further purified by a panning technique, as reported [2]. Optic nerve progenitors were isolated from 7-day-old rat pups, as described previously [2]. 50 μl (1×10^4) of cells were seeded onto poly-D-lysine coated coverslips and allowed to adhere for 2 h at 37°C, then the cultures were fed with defined medium or medium containing FCS as described [2]. At the time of the first feeding, enriched cultures contained 90–95% pure O-2A progenitors. Cultures were maintained at 37°C in a humidified incubator containing 95% air/5% CO_2. Two coverslips from each culture condition were collected for processing and *D* analysis after 2 h (Day 0) and thereafter every 24 h from day 1 to day 5. Samples were also collected on days 7 and 10 for brain derived cells.

T.G. Smith, T.N. Behar / Brain Research 634 (1994) 181–190 183

Immunocytochemistry and preparation of cells for fractal analysis

Cells were fixed in 2% paraformaldehyde in phosphate buffered saline (PBS), pH 7.2 for 10 min at room temperature. Cultures maintained in defined medium were incubated 20 min in anti-GC ascites (1:300, PBS), washed and incubated 20 min in rhodamine (RITC)-conjugated rat anti-mouse IgG. Cells grown in serum-containing media were incubated 15 min in A2B5 ascites (1:300, PBS), washed, and incubated 15 min in fluorescine (FITC)-conjugated goat anti-mouse IgM. Following three washes in PBS, coverslips were mounted onto slides in 80% glycerol/20% PBS, then sealed with nail polish.

Immunoreactive cells were visualized on a Zeiss photomicroscope equipped with epifluorescence and appropriate filters for the visualization of fluorescine and rhodamine, using a 63× Planapochromatic objective. For the comparison of self-similarity, cells were also examined with 10–100× Planapochromatic objectives.

Six–ten cells from each coverslip were photographed using T-MAX, ASA 400 film (KODAK) pushed to 1600 and developed in D19 (KODAK). Black and white negatives were illuminated on a light box, the images were captured with a video camera fitted with a telephoto lens, digitized and analyzed with an image processor as described elsewhere [27] and below.

Calculation and analysis of fractal dimensions

The borders of binary silhouettes of the cells were generated from grey-scale images (Fig. 1) with a modified Marr-Hildreth filtering-convolution algorithm and a Laplacian convolution operation [27]. Fractal dimensions were calculated with Flook's border-dilation method [6,7]. This method was previously calibrated against images of known fractal dimensions [28]. This procedure measures the length of the equivalent perimeter of the borders with different magnitude measuring elements. D is calculated from the slope (S) of the plot of the log of the equivalent perimeter versus the log of the measuring element (Richardson plot) and $D = 1 - S$. Examples of single cells for each of the four cell types are shown in Figs. 2A,B–5A,B.

Sholl analysis of morphology was determined as described elsewhere [17,25]. The Sholl coefficient was obtained as follows. First, a 'stick' or skeletonized image was obtained from its binary silhouette of the cell (Figs. 2–5C). Then, a series of circles of increasing diameter was superimposed on the stick image with the center of the circle located at the center of the soma (Fig. 6). The number of intersections of the branches with each circle was counted (a Boolean AND operation) and then divided by the length of perimeter of the circle (number of intersections per unit length). This latter number

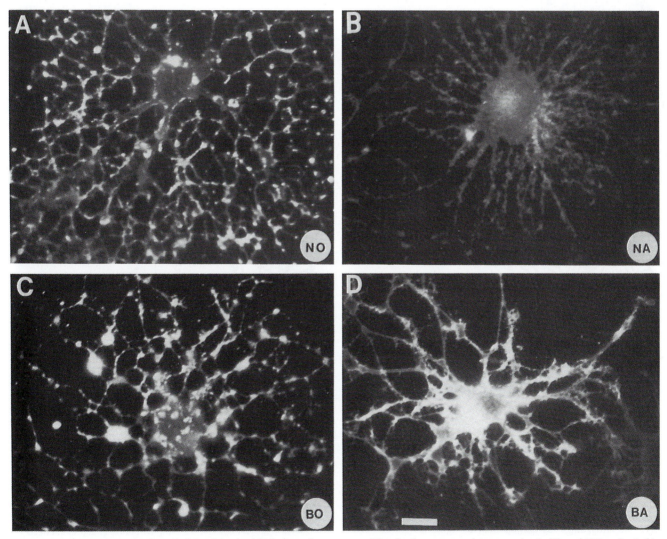

Fig. 1. Photomicrographs of cultured glial cells stained by immunofluorescence. Oligodendrocytes were immunostained with anti-GC antibody (A and C); type-2 astrocytes (B and D) were immunostained with monoclonal A2B5 ascites (see Materials and Methods). A: optic nerve-derived oligodendrocyte (NO) maintained in culture for 5 days; B: optic nerve-derived astrocyte (NA) cultured for 4 days. C: brain-derived oligodendrocyte (BO) cultured for 10 days; D: a brain-derived type-2 astrocyte (BA) cultured for 10 days. Bar = 20 μm.

184   *T.G. Smith, T.N. Behar / Brain Research 634 (1994) 181–190*

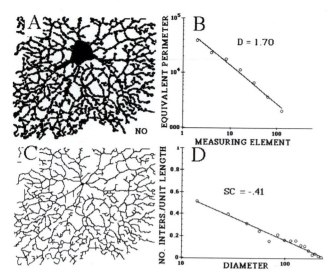

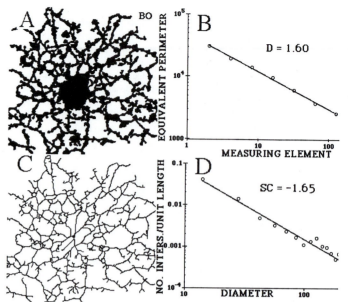

Fig. 2. The binary image (A) and the Richardson plot (B), used to determine the fractal dimension ($D = 1.70$) of a cultured oligodendrocyte (from Fig. 1A) derived from the optic nerve (NO) and maintained in vitro for 5 days (see Materials and Methods). The Sholl coefficient (SC) of the same cell is determined by generating a stick figure of the cell (C) and calculating the coefficient (D, $SC = -0.41$) as described in Materials and Methods.

Fig. 4. The binary image (A) and the Richardson plot (B), used to determine the fractal dimension ($D = 1.60$) of a cultured oligodendrocyte (from Fig. 1C) derived from the cortex (BO) and maintained in vitro for 10 days (see Materials and Methods). The Sholl coefficient (SC) of the same cell is determined by generating a stick figure of the cell (C) and calculating the coefficient (D, $SC = -1.65$) as described in Materials and Methods.

was plotted against the diameter of the circles on a semi-log or log-log scales and the slope of the best straight line fit was taken as the Sholl coefficient (SC). Examples of single cells for each of the four cell types are show in Figs. 2C,D–5C,D.

When the number of branches intersecting with each circle are determined automatically with image processing software, as here, there are potential errors that might not be present if the counting were done manually. These are illustrated by the letters (A, B and C) in Fig. 6. The intersections are done by a Boolean AND operation

between the stick processes and the circles. Then the resultant pixels are counted by determining the zero values (black pixels) from a histogram of the AND result. Fig. 6A illustrates a case when the process extends beyond the largest circle; 6B shows a situation where the process bends back on itself and is counted twice; and C-arrow illustrates a process that turns and traverses along a circle and thus is

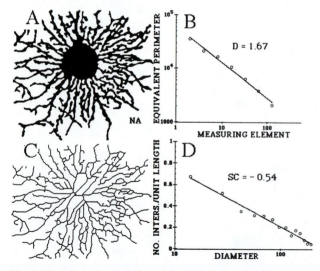

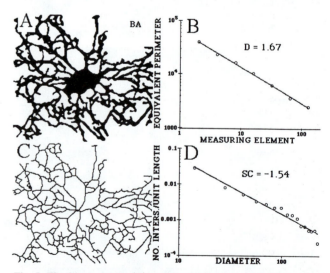

Fig. 3. The binary image (A) and the Richardson plot (B), used to determine the fractal dimension ($D = 1.67$) of a cultured type-2 astrocyte (from Fig.. 1B) derived from the optic nerve (NA) and maintained in vitro for 4 days (see Materials and Methods). The Sholl coefficient (SC) of the same cell is determined by generating a stick figure of the cell (C) and calculating the coefficient (D, $SC = -0.54$) as described in Materials and Methods.

Fig. 5. The binary image (A) and the Richardson plot (B), used to determine the fractal dimension ($D = 1.67$) of a cultured type-2 astrocyte (Fig. 1D) derived from the cortex (BA) and maintained in vitro for 10 days (see Materials and Methods). The Sholl coefficient (SC) of the same cell is determined by generating a stick figure of the cell (C) and calculating the coefficient (D, $SC = -1.54$) as described in Materials and Methods.

T.G. Smith, T.N. Behar / Brain Research 634 (1994) 181–190   185

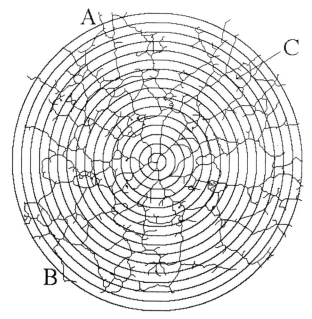

Fig. 6. Illustration depicting the skeletonized image of an oligodendrocyte and the concentric circles which are used to determine Sholl coefficient (see text). The branching pattern presents problems in determining the number of processes that cross each circle. A: branches which extend beyond the outer-most circle; B: a branch that bends back on itself and is counted twice; C: a process that aligns with one circle and is counted several times (see Materials and Methods).

counted multiply. While these potential error-creating situations are not common, neither are they rare and this may account, in part, for the lack of utility we find with the Sholl method.

The D and SC for every cell of each cell type were calculated each day for up to 10 days, with day 0 taken as the time the cells were plated. For each day, six or more typical cells were selected for analysis. The time course of changes in D were fitted to a simple dynamic model, which has the form:

$$D = A + B \cdot e^{t/\tau} \tag{1}$$

where D is the fractal dimension, A and B are variables, t is time grown in culture and τ is a time-constant. No meaningful or easily interpretive quantitative curve fits were found for the Sholl plots. This may reflect the fact that the individual Sholl plots did not fit a straight line as well as the D plots did (cf. Figs. 2–5 B vs. D).

3. Results

Typical nerve-derived and brain-derived glia are illustrated in Figs. 1–5. Included are the fluorescently labeled cells (Fig. 1), the binary silhouette images derived from each of the photograph negatives (Figs. 2–5): (A), their skeletonized forms (C), each cell's Richardson plot (B), where D = the calculated fractal dimension of the cell and its Sholl plot (D), where SC = the Sholl coefficient (Figs. 2–5). (The borders of the cells, not the silhouettes shown in Fig. 2–5A, were used to perform the fractal measurements. The border was obtained by a Laplacian convolution operation on

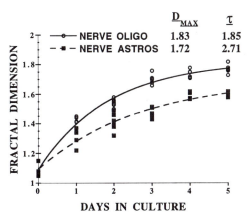

Fig. 7. Plots of the formula: $D(t) = A + B \cdot e^{-t/\tau}$ for the nerve-derived glial phenotypes, where the numbers represent the mean $D_{\max}$ for each phenotype and τ is the time constant for each phenotype. The nerve-derived glia reached their maximum D value within 5 days in vitro.

the silhouettes; see Materials and Methods.) Fig. 7 illustrates the changes in D for each nerve-derived cell type over time, while Fig. 8 illustrates similar changes in D for brain glia.

Nerve glia had larger D's than their brain counterparts (Figs. 7,8). Nerve oligodendrocyte (oligo) D ranged from 1.1 to 1.85, with a mean maximum D ($D_{\max}$) of 1.83. Nerve astrocyte (astro) D ranged from 1.1 at time 0 to a $D_{\max}$ of 1.73. The mean $D_{\max}$ of astros was 1.72. In contrast, the average $D_{\max}$ of the two phenotypes from brain were similar. Brain oligos had a $D_{\max}$ of 1.51, while astros were 1.52. Thus by this measure, the two glia from brain reached comparable levels of complexity, but they were both less complex than their optic nerve counterparts.

Analysis of changes in the fractal dimension of all phenotypes over time revealed that the differentiation of complex morphology occurred at an exponentially

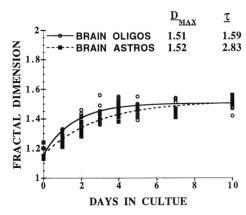

Fig. 8. Plots of the formula: $D(t) = A + B \cdot e^{-t/\tau}$ for the brain-derived glial phenotypes, where the numbers represent the mean $D_{\max}$ for each phenotype and τ is the time constant for each phenotype. The brain-derived glia reached their maximum D value within 10 days in vitro.

186   *T.G. Smith, T.N. Behar / Brain Research 634 (1994) 181–190*

A   D = 1.86

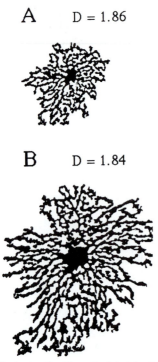

B   D = 1.84

A   **D = 1.68**

B   **D = 1.65**

C   **D = 1.65**

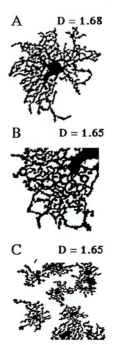

Fig. 9. Self-similarity in glia. The calculated fractal dimensions (*D*) of a single cell viewed under low (A) and high (B) magnifications are similar

Fig. 10. Self-similarity in glia. The fractal dimensions (*D*) calculated from the binary images of a group of cells (C), a single cell on the same coverslip (A), or a portion of the single cell (B) are remarkably similar.

declining rate (Figs. 7,8). Brain oligos differentiated faster (τ = 1.59) than nerve oligos (τ = 1.85) and oligos from both regions increased in complexity faster than their corresponding astrocytes (τ = 2.83 and τ = 2.71, respectively). The time constant for brain oligos (1.59) is approximately 56% of that for the astros (2.83), indicating the oligos differentiated faster than the astros.

Self-similarity is a defining characteristic of fractal objects [10,19], thus we analyzed the phenomenon of self-similarity by calculating the fractal dimension of oligodendrocytes under different magnifications. A sin-

gle oligodendrocyte was photographed under two magnification conditions, and the resultant *D*'s were calculated and compared. Fig. 9 illustrates the binary silhouette of such a cell, where B is twice the magnification of A. The calculated *D*'s of both binary images were nearly identical, with *D*'s of 1.86 and 1.84, respectively. Fig. 10 shows the silhouettes of cultured oligodendrocytes from a single coverslip viewed over a 10-fold change in magnification. The silhouette of a single cell is illustrated in Fig. 10A. (*D* = 1.68). Part of the lower left hand quadrant of the same cell is illustrated in Fig. 10B (*D* = 1.65). Fig. 10C is a composit low power view of a cluster of cells from the coverslip. Although the

Table 1
Culture numbers
An analysis of self-similarity of glial cells of all types. Within each culture, the fractal dimensions calculated from images taken at different magnifications are similar. Note the similarity of *D* in each individual culture and the small values of standard deviation. The images were collected with 10–100× objectives through the cine port of the microscope onto the face of a CCD video camera. The camera was mounted on an optical bench such that the camera could be moved along the optical axis of the light beam. This allowed for optimum magnification adjustment to achieve maximum resolution for image processing. In practice, this means filling about 3/4 of a TV-frame, although this prevents a precise knowledge of the magnification of any given image. A 'composite' magnification is illustrated in Fig. 10C. (See text.)

Magnificiation:	1	2	3	4	5	6	7	8	9	10
Composite	1.88	1.87	1.80	1.54	1.67	1.75	1.80	1.65	1.48	1.37
Low		1.86	1.81							
Medium	1.84	1.84	1.78		1.60	1.76	1.76	1.68	1.55	1.42
High	1.78	1.86	1.77	1.53	1.66	1.76	1.75	1.65	1.55	1.42
Very high	1.75	1.86	1.77			1.72	1.72	1.65		1.42
Mean	1.81	1.86	1.79	1.54	1.64	1.75	1.76	1.66	1.51	1.41
Standard deviation	0.06	0.01	0.02	0.01	0.04	0.02	0.03	0.01	0.04	0.02

T.G. Smith, T.N. Behar / Brain Research 634 (1994) 181–190

cluster contains 10 cells, the D of the entire border of congruent silhouetted cells has a D of 1.65. Table I shows the results of ten similar experiments on oligodendrocytes. The fractal dimension is consistent over a wide range of magnifications in each individual experiment (note small standard deviations), thus these cultured oligodendrocytes display self-similarity.

In Sholl's original work on pyramidal cells of the mammalian cortex of the brain [25], he found that the branching pattern of basilar dendrites were best fitted with a semilog function, while the apical dendrites were best described by a power or log–log function. We find nerve glial cells best fit by a semi-log function, while the brain derived glia best fit by a log–log function (Figs. 2D–5D), although the fits were not as good as the fractal curves (cf. Figs. 2–5B with 2–5D).

While the various glial cells did show changes in their SC's over time, unlike the fractal dimension, the SC's could not be fit by any meaningful or interesting mathematical function. There was, however, some linear correlation between the D's and SC's when each cell type was compared separately in a pair-wise manner for the total cell population (not shown; correlation coefficient of approximately 0.5).

4. Discussion

Measuring the fractal dimension

O-2A progenitor cells undergo visually striking changes in morphology as they differentiate in vitro. Simple spherical to bipolar cells develop into mature, differentiated cells that exhibit very complex morphology. Under controlled culture conditions, the O-2A progenitor can be induced to develop into either an oligodendrocyte (Fig. 1A,C), with luxurious multiple branches, or a type-2 astrocyte which contains fine spindle-like branches and often flat membrane sheets (Fig. 1B,D). Morphological complexity of any given cell can be measured, quantified and assigned a numerical value expressed as the fractal dimension (D). Increases in D correlate with increases in complexity. As the progenitor undergoes the process of differentiation, the D can be measured at any given stage in time. Analysis of changes in the D with respect to time illustrate the rate of cellular development and growth as the cells mature. This change in the rate is described by a time constant, τ.

The fractal dimensions of cultured O-2A progenitor cells derived from optic nerves and cerebral hemispheres of neonatal rats, selectively differentiating into either oligodendrocytes or type 2 astrocytes, were analyzed and compared. Cells differentiating along the oligodendrocyte pathway had smaller time constants than cells induced to become astrocytes. Thus, oligodendroctyes reached their maximum level of complex-

ity earlier than the astrocytes. While O-2A progenitor cells are capable of proliferation, when cultured in defined medium, mitotic activity ceases and the cells are induced to differentiate at an accelerated pace [23]. In the presence of FCS, however, the O-2A progenitor may undergo cell division, thus delaying differentiation and commitment to the astrocyte phenotype. Alternatively, these differences in rates of maturation between the two cell types may reflect genetic, pre-programmed differences involving various stages along each pathway. Interestingly, studies of precursors differentiating in situ in the rat optic nerve demonstrate that oligodendrocytes appear during the first postnatal week, while type 2 astrocytes do not emerge until the second week postnatally [23].

Although the two types of glial cells from brain demonstrated different time constants, their maximum fractal dimensions were remarkably similar. While each phenotype has a unique characteristic morphology, the fractal dimension reflects the degree of complexity of that morphology, but not the form of that morphology or cell size, to which D is insensitive [10,19]. Both the ruggedness of a cell's border as well as the branching of its processes contribute to the D [17,26,28]. In any given cell, one characteristic may dominate or both may play a role. Thus, two cells with morphologies that differ considerably can have the same fractal dimension [17,26,28]. Thus, there is a clear need to develop other measures to distinguish between such cells.

In general, both the nerve-derived oligodendrocytes as well as the nerve-derived type 2 astrocytes attained greater levels of morphological complexity than their age-matched, brain-derived counterparts cultured under identical conditions. Differences in the D of cells of the same phenotype, derived from various locations within the CNS, may reflect unique characteristic differences among regional subpopulations of glial cells. These differences may be related to function. For example, an oligodendrocyte in the optic nerve may myelinate more axons than an oligodendrocyte in the cerebral cortex, thus the cells from nerve elaborate more complex processes.

The nerve and brain-derived oligos exhibited different rates of growth. These differences suggest that the O-2A progenitors originally isolated from the two sources could be at different stages of development when initially put into culture. As is well known, within the CNS, regional patterns of gliogenesis vary. O-2A cells migrate from the subventricular zones adjacent to the lateral ventricles into the formative white matter. Evidence suggests that the precursor cells, influenced by platelet-derived growth factor (PDGF), undergo a limited number of mitoses before they stop dividing and differentiate into oligodendrocytes [23]. During the first postnatal week, when brain progenitors are cultured, there are still substantial germinal zones within

T.G. Smith, T.N. Behar / Brain Research 634 (1994) 181–190

the subventricular zones [8]. At this time, however, no residual germinal plate remains in the optic nerve. Thus the progenitors migrating into the nerve and isolated for culture at day 7, may be further along in their natural course of differentiation than the precursors isolated from the brain, which include the more immature precursors associated with germinal centers of the subventricular zone. The nerve and brain derived precursor cells may have different capacities of responding to growth factors that modulate their differentiation.

Evidence suggests this may be the case. Brain-derived O2A progenitors have a greater mitogenic response to PDGF than nerve-derived precursors [2]. However, that same study indicates that brain-derived cells may respond to factors signalling oligodendrocyte differentiation more readily than precursors isolated from nerve. In contrast, progenitors from brain and nerve show similar rates of response to factors that induce astrocyte differentiation. Insulin, a constituent of chemically defined medium, and ciliary neurotrophic factor [9] which is present in fetal calf serum, influence glial maturation. Insulin and Insulin-like growth factor I have been shown to induce oligodendrocyte differentiation [11,12], whereas ciliary neurotrophic factor stimulates progenitors into the astrocyte pathway [9].

Methodology

In the present study, we have enhanced the method of capturing images of the cells and converting them to binary silhouettes. In previous studies [26], cells were immunostained using peroxidase-conjugated second antibodies and video images of the cells were captured directly from the microscope. Binary images were generated from grey-scale images. Here, we have stained the cells by immunofluorescence, photographed the cells under higher magnification and captured the video images from the developed negatives. Immunofluorescence illuminates fine processes of the cells and the black and white negatives afford greater contrast, thus finer detail of cellular morphology can be visualized. Enhanced resolution of detail could result in more accurate calculated fractal dimensions. Higher magnification alone, however, would not likely be a contributing factor to the fractal dimension, since D is not a function of size (see below) [10].

It should be noted that in this study, the values calculated for the nerve-derived fractal dimension and τ are similar, but differ from the values reported previously [26]. In the present study, the mean D_{max} and τ's for the oligos and astros were 1.83 and 1.85, 1.72 and 2.71, respectively, while our previous measurements were 1.75 and 1.25, 1.62 and 2.19. This may reflect the different histological stains used in the two studies (see Materials and Methods and above). On the

other hand, for a given cell type, D and τ may vary slightly from one study to another; calculated D's and τ's from one experiment may not be compared directly with D's and τ's calculated in previous studies. Comparative studies of the effects of given factors may require simultaneously run controls to measure D in every experiment, unless it is found, with identical techniques, that D and τ are stable for each phenotype over a number of experiments.

Significance of D

It may be helpful to examine the significance of the numerical values or change in the values of D. It is the fractional part of D, the slope (S), that is important in assessing significance and it is the ratio of two logarithmic numbers. Thus, a change from 1.1 to 1.2 in D indicates a (0.2/0.1) doubling in complexity and a change from 1.1 to 1.5 indicates a 5-fold increase in complexity. These observations may help put into context the comparative value of the fractal dimension. For example the nerve oligos are 1.63 times more complex as the brain derived oligos and the nerve astros show a 1.38-fold increase in complexity over the brain astros. The time constant data indicate, for example, that the brain astros take about 1.53 times longer to mature than the nerve oligodendrocytes. Thus, a major conclusion of this study is that processes, like changes in complexity during morphological differentiation, which could only be described previously in a qualitative way, can now be analyzed in a *objective and quantitative* manner.

Self-similarity

Self-similarity, an important and defining characteristic of fractal objects, means that extra detail appears at quantitatively the same rate over changes in scale, or magnification [10]. The fractal dimension of a composite field of oligodendrocytes viewed under low magnification was the same as one individual cell from the same culture. Furthermore, the fractal dimension of only a portion of the cell viewed under higher magnification was the same as the fractal dimension of the entire cell. Thus over an approximately 10-fold range of magnification, the calculated fractal dimensions were similar. Similar findings were found in motor cortex pyramidal cells in monkey and cat [21]. This suggests if small parts of a cell are not captured in the image to be analyzed, it is of no great consequence in determining D. We should point out that such optical experiments would give similar results only on certain types of cells, for example only with radially symmetrical structures like oligodendrocytes or cells that have prominent, uniform dendrites like motor cortex pyramidal cells. Thus, the optical method is of restricted use in showing self-similarity.

T.G. Smith, T.N. Behar / Brain Research 634 (1994) 181–190   189

Fractal growth

It should be noted that Casserta, et al. [3] and Pellinoisz [20] have suggested that if a cell border has a fractal dimension, the object became fractal by 'fractal growth'. Fractal growth usually means that the fractal dimension of the object remains constant as it grows in other ways (size, area, etc.) [10]. All of the cells we analyzed possess fractal dimensions at each stage of their growth, but the dimensions change as differentiation proceeds. These results indicate that these cells do not exhibit fractal growth during the period studied. This raises questions about the influences and mechanisms involved in producing fractal objects whose dimensions change during differentiation.

Sholl method

The utility of the Sholl coefficient (SC) is less clear as a quantifier of cellular morphology. The SC is a measure of the rate in the difference in which branches are forming minus branch termination as a function of distance from the soma. What this implies in terms of cellular growth and differentiation is uncertain. The observation that there was some correlation between pair-wise measurements of individual cells in D and SC among glial cell types is not surprising, since both are a measure of cellular branching. However, D also measures the ruggedness of the cellular border, to which the SC is insensitive [17]. We feel, therefore, that D is the better measure of morphological complexity and differentiation. Similar conclusions were reached in a comparable study of differentiation of spinal cord neurons [17].

Significance

These results demonstrate that large changes in cellular morphological complexity (up to 8-fold) take place over relatively short periods of time and that such changes can be described by a simple model. It is noteworthy that such dramatic changes in morphology can be described by a simple mathematical model. These results suggest that morphological complexity is an important component of cellular differentiation. We have proposed that the fractal dimension, which is recognized as a good measure of complexity, may also be a good quantitative measure of the degree of morphological differentiation [26]. This is consistent with the Webster's New College Dictionary definition of differentiation, namely, '(the) development from … the simple to the complex …' [30]. As such, the fractal dimension can be used to quantify changing states of differentiation in a completely unbiased and objective manner. It also appears to be a useful measure for comparative studies across and among species, as they relate to cellular evolution [29]. Finally, we mentioned earlier in this discussion certain known factors that can change morphological differentiation of the cell types

studied here. But they are known only in a qualitative or semi-quantitative manner. Now we have a baseline that can analyze such changes in a *quantitative* manner.

Conclusion

Analysis of changes in fractal dimension of two populations of glial cells differentiating in vitro, revealed that each phenotype had a specific final D and a specific developmental rate. Dissimilarities in the rate of differentiation for each phenotype suggests that the mechanisms which underlie maturation of the lineage may be more complex for one cell type versus the other. The fractal dimension of an object provides insight into how elaborate the process that generated the object may be; since the larger the dimension, the larger the number of degrees of freedom likely to be involved in that process.

Within the context of molecular biology and traditional histological and immunocytochemical techniques, fractal dimension analysis could provide a new strategy for studying cellular differentiation. Specifically, strategies similar to the one we have employed may be used to see if other cellular types change their fractal dimensions as they differentiate and, if so, can they be described by the simple model we have developed.

References

[1] Amthor, F.R., Quantitative fractal analysis of dendritic trees of identified rabbit retinal ganglion cells, *Soc. Neurosci. Abstr.*, 14 (1988) 603.

[2] Behar, T., McMorris, F.A., Novotny, E.A., Barker, J.L., and Dubois-Dalcq, M., Growth and differentiation properties of O-2A progenitors purified from rat cerebral hemispheres., *J. Neurosci. Res.*, 21 (1988) 168–180.

[3] Caserta, F., Stanley, H.E., Eldred, W.D., Daccord, G., Hausman, R.E. and Nittmann, J., Physical mechanisms underlying neurite outgrowth: a quantitative analysis of neuronal shape, *Phys. Rev. Lett.*, 64 (1990) 95–98.

[4] Cutting, J.E. and Garvin, J.J., Fractal curves and complexity, *Percep. Psychophys.*, 42 (1987) 365–370.

[5] Dubois-Dalcq, M., Characterization of a slowly proliferative cell along the oligodendrocyte differentiation pathway, *Eur. Mol. Biol. Org. J.*, 6 (1987) 2587–2597.

[6] Flook, A.G., The use of dilation logic on the Quantimet to achieve fractal dimension characterization of textured and structured profiles, *Powder Technol.*, 21 (1978) 295–298.

[7] Flook, A.G., Fractal dimensions: their evaluation and significance in stereological measurements, *Acta Stereol.*, 1 (1982) 79.

[8] LeVine, S.M. and Goldman, J.E., Embryonic divergence of oligodendrocyte and astrocyte lineages in developing rat cerebrum, *J. Neurosci.*, 11 (1988) 3992–4006.

[9] Lillien, L.E., Sendtner, M., Rohrer, H., Hughes, S.M. and Raff, M.C., Type-2 astrocyte development in rat brain cultures is initiated by a CNTF-like protein produced by type-1 astrocytes, *Neuron*, 1 (1988) 485–494.

[10] Mandelbrot, B.B., *The Fractal Geometry of Nature*, W.H. Freeman, New York, 1982.

190   *T.G. Smith, T.N. Behar / Brain Research 634 (1994) 181–190*

[11] McMorris, F.A. and Dubois-Dalcq, M., Insulin-like growth factor I promotes cell proliferation and oligodendroglial commitment in rat glial progenitor cells developing in vitro, *J. Neurosci. Res.*, 21 (1988) 199–209.

[12] McMorris, F.A., Smith, T.M., DeSalvo, S. and Furlanetto, R.W., Insulin-like growth factor I/somatomedin C: a potent inducer of oligodendrocyte development, *Proc. Natl. Acad. Sci. USA*, 83 (1986) 822–826.

[13] Montague, P.R. and Friedlander, M.J., Expression of an intrinsic growth strategy by mammalian retinal neurons, *Proc. Natl. Acad. Sci. USA*, 86 (1989) 7223–7227.

[14] Montague, P.R. and Friedlander, M.J., Morphogenesis and territorial coverage by isolated mammalian retinal ganglion cells, *J. Neurosci.*, 11 (1991) 1440–1457.

[15] Morigiwa, K., Tauchi, M. and Fukuda, Y., Fractal analysis of ganglion cell dendritic branching patterns of the rat and cat retinae, *Neurosci. Res. Suppl.*, 10 (1989) S131–S140.

[16] Neale, E.A., Bowers, L.M. and Smith Jr., T.G., Early dendrite development described by fractal dimension, *Soc. Neurosci. Abstr.*, 17 (1991) 36.

[17] Neale, E.A., Bowers, L.M. and Smith Jr., T.G., Early dendritic development in spinal cord cell cultures: a quantitative study, *J. Neurosci. Res.*, 34 (1993) 54–66.

[18] Ng, Y.-K. and Iannaccone, Fractal beometry of mosaic pattern demonstrates liver regeneration is a self-similar process, *Dev. Biol.*, 151 (1992) 419–430.

[19] Peitgen, H.-O. and Richter, P.H., *The Beauty of Fractals*, 1986, Springer, New York.

[20] Pellionisz, A.J., Neural geometry: towards a fractal model of neurons. In R.M.J. Cotterill (Ed.), *Models of Brain Function*, Cambridge University Press, Cambridge, 1989, pp. 453–464.

[21] Porter, R., Ghosh, S., Lange, G.D. and Smith Jr., T.G., A fractal analysis of pyramidal neurons in mammalian motor cortex, *Neurosci. Lett.*, 130 (1991) 112–116.

[22] Raff, M., Miller, R.H. and Noble, M., A glial progenitor cell that develops in vitro into an astrocyte or an oligodendrocyte depending on culture medium, *Nature*, 303 (1983) 390–396.

[23] Raff, M.C., Lillien, L.E., Richardson, W.D., Burne, J.F., and Noble, M.D., Platelet-derived growth factor from astrocytes drives the clock that times oligodendrocyte development in culture, *Nature*, 333 (1988) 562–565.

[24] Reichenbach, A., Siegel, A., Senitz, D. and Smith Jr., T.G., A comparative fractal analysis of various mammalian astroglial cell types, *Neuroimage*, 1 (1992) 66–77.

[25] Sholl, D.A.D., Dendritic organization in the neurons of the visual and motor cortices of the cat, *J. Anat.*, 87 (1953) 387–406.

[26] Smith Jr., T.G., Behar, T.N., Lange, G.D., Marks, B., W. and Sheriff Jr., W.H., A fractal analysis of cultured rat optic nerve glial growth and differentiation, *Neuroscience*, 41 (1991) 159–169.

[27] Smith Jr., T.G., Marks, W.B., Lange, G.D., Sheriff Jr., W.H. and Neale, E.A., Edge detection in images using Marr-Hildreth filtering techniques, *J. Neurosci. Methods*, 26 (1988) 75–82.

[28] Smith Jr., T.G., Marks, W.B., Lange, G.D., Sheriff Jr., W.H. and Neale, E.A., A fractal analysis of cell images, *J. Neurosci. Methods*, 27 (1989) 173–180.

[29] Smith, T.G., J., Brauer, K. and Reichenbach, A., Quantitative Phylogenetic Constancy of Cerebellar Purkinje Morphological Complexity, *J. Comp. Neurol.*, 331 (1993) 402–406.

[30] Woolf, H.B., *Webster's New Collegiate Dictionary*, 1976, G & C Merriam, Springfield, MA, USA.

Neuroscience Vol. 41, No. 1, pp. 159–166, 1991
Printed in Great Britain

0306-4522/91 $3.00 + 0.00
Pergamon Press plc
IBRO

A FRACTAL ANALYSIS OF CULTURED RAT OPTIC NERVE GLIAL GROWTH AND DIFFERENTIATION

T. G. Smith Jr,*† T. N. Behar,* G. D. Lange,‡ W. B. Marks§
and W. H. Sheriff Jr‡

*Laboratory of Neurophysiology, NINDS, National Institutes of Health, Bethesda, MD 20892, U.S.A.
‡Instrumentation and Computer Section, NINDS, NIH, Bethesda, MD 20892, U.S.A.
§Laboratory of Neural Control, NINDS, National Institutes of Health, Bethesda, MD 20892, U.S.A.

Abstract—Fractal dimension can be used as a quantitative measure of morphological complexity. Separate, enriched populations of oligodendrocytes or type 2 astrocytes derived from neonatal rat optic nerves were allowed to differentiate *in vitro*. Fractal dimensions of differentiating glial cells were measured over time. The fractal dimension correlated with perceived complexity and increased in value as the glial cells matured.

Analysis of the changes in fractal dimension with time revealed unique rates of growth and differentiation for each glial phenotype.

Most natural structures are too complex to be readily described as collections of Euclidian points, straight lines, rectangles, etc. On the other hand, many natural shapes look qualitatively the same over a wide range of magnifications. This "self-similar" property, an important and defining characteristic of fractal objects, means that extra detail appears at quantitatively the same rate over many changes in scale or magnification. Mandelbrot's[19] geometry of fractal objects includes the calculation of a quantity (fractal dimension: D) which is a measure of the rate of addition of detail with increasing magnification. We have shown[30] that as cells increase in morphological complexity, the fractal dimension increases. The function relating D to time then becomes a quantitative description of the growth and differentiation of the cell to the extent that these are expressed in morphology. Amthor[1] distinguished several classes of retinal ganglion cells in the rabbit by means of their fractal dimension and Caserta *et al.*[7] have shown that such cells have different fractal dimensions when grown *in vivo* or *in vitro*. Pellionisz[22] demonstrates the approximate qualitative similarity of a guinea-pig cerebellar Purkinje cell to a model of it generated by iteratively scaling down and substituting a simple tree structure for the model branches. He suggests that "The growth of cellular (neural) elements reveals a fractal geometry that is a direct manifestation of a process based on repeated access to the genetic code during growth."[22]

Cultured O-2A progenitor cells derived from newborn rat optic nerve provide a model in which one can control the differentiation of two cell types, oligodendrocytes and type 2 astrocytes. Recent studies of the developing optic nerve in the neonatal rat have provided evidence that the oligodendrocyte and type 2 astrocyte, the two glial cells that cooperate in myelinating axons in the CNS, arise from a common, bipotential progenitor cell.[13,23,25] When the progenitor cell is grown *in vitro*, it develops into an astrocyte or oligodendrocyte depending on the culture medium in which it is maintained. The simple bipolar precursor undergoes striking morphological changes as it develops either the stellate morphology of the type 2 astrocyte or the intricate branched processes of the multipolar oligodendrocyte. Precursors differentiate *in vitro* in a synchronized manner, ahead of their *in vivo* schedule.[24] Differentiation of these optic nerve progenitors has been studied extensively.[8,13,23,25,27]

Oligodendrocytes, type 2 astrocytes and the O-2A progenitors can be identified by specific surface and cytoskeletal molecules which serve as markers. The progenitor stains with the monoclonal antibody designated A2B5, which is directed against gangliosides on the cell's surface.[5,11] It also has vimentin-containing intermediate filaments. The type 2 astrocyte can also be surface labeled with the A2B5 antibody. This astrocyte also contains vimentin but in addition has filaments containing glial fibrillary acidic protein (GFAP), a marker for astrocytes. The oligodendrocyte loses A2B5 surface reactivity soon after it begins to express galacto-cerebroside (a glycolipid of myelin) on its surface. The presence of galactocerebroside is considered a marker for differentiated oligodendrocytes.[26] Oligodendrocytes do not contain any of the known classes of intermediate filaments.[16]

---

†To whom correspondence should be addressed at: Building 36, Room 2C02, National Institutes of Health, Bethesda, MD 20892, U.S.A.
Abbreviations: DMEM, Dulbecco's modified Eagle's medium; FCS, fetal calf serum; GFAP, glial fibrillary acidic protein; MEM, minimum essential medium; PBS, phosphate-buffered saline.

During a 5 day period both cell types differentiate morphologically from very simple spherical shapes into cells with considerable morphological complexity. Until now, however, such changes in complexity could only be described qualitatively since there was no readily available way to quantify them. The fractal dimension provides a quantitative measure of the complexity of these glial cell types at several stages in their morphological differentiation. The borders of less complex glial cells have a small D while more complex cells have a large D. For both cell types, D increases during growth at an exponentially declining rate. The rates are specific for each cell type.

EXPERIMENTAL PROCEDURES

Tissue culture

Optic nerve glial cultures were generated by a modified method of Raff *et al.*[23] Briefly, littermates of 7-day-old Sprague–Dawley rats were decapitated and their optic nerves removed. The nerves were immersed in minimum essential medium (MEM; Gibco, Grand Island, NY) buffered with 25 mM HEPES, then cleaned of meninges. Cleaned nerves were pooled and incubated for 30 min at 37°C in Ca- and Mg-free Hanks balanced salt solution (Gibco) containing 0.25% trypsin (Sigma Chemical Corp., St Louis, MO) and 0.04% collagenase (Worthington Biochemcials, Freehold, NJ). The initial enzyme solution was aspirated, and the nerves were incubated at 37°C for 30 min in a solution of 0.05% trypsin in Versene (Whittaker M.A. Bioproducts, Walkersville, MD). The enzyme solution was removed and replaced with 1 ml of Dulbecco's modified Eagle's medium (DMEM; Gibco) containing 5% fetal calf serum (FCS) (Whittaker M.A. Bioproducts), 1.7 mg/ml bovine serum albumin, 0.04 mg/ml DNase, and 0.5 mg/ml soybean trypsin inhibitor (all from Sigma Chemical Co., St Louis, MO). The tissue was dissociated by trituration through a 25-gauge needle. Dispersed cells were seeded in drops onto poly-D-lysine-coated, 12 mm glass coverslips at a density of 10,000–20,000 cells per drop. For coating coverslips, poly-D-lysine (50,000 mol. wt, Sigma Chemical Co.) was diluted to 5 μg/ml in sterile water, applied to the coverslips for 60 min, then air dried. Cells were allowed to adhere to the polylysine-coated coverslips for 1–2 h at 37°C before being covered with additional growth medium. Cultures were maintained at 37°C in a humidified atmosphere of 90% air and 10% CO_2. The medium was renewed every 48 h.

Growth and differentiation media

Two types of culture medium were used for experiments on cell growth and differentiation: (1) DMEM (Gibco) supplemented with 10% FCS, which is known to induce the development of astrocytes from optic nerve O-2A progenitors;[23] and (2) defined medium[6,10] consisting of DMEM supplemented with 50 μg/ml of transferrin, 30 nM of selenium, 30 nM of tri-iodothyronine, and 5 μg/ml of bovine insulin (all from Sigma Chemical Co, St Louis, MO) and to which 0.5% FCS was added. In defined medium, the O-2A progenitors differentiate into oligodendrocytes.[8,23]

Immunolabeling

Cells were fixed at 12 or 24 h intervals for 10 min in 2% formaldehyde in phosphate-buffered saline (PBS) (prepared freshly from paraformaldehyde) prior to immunolabeling.

The following antibodies used for immunolabeling have been described in previous publications:[8,23,26] the IgM mouse monoclonal antibody in ascites fluid from A2B5 cells (American Type Culture Collection, Rockville, MD) and the IgG3 mouse monoclonal anti-galactocerebroside.

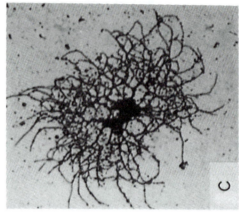

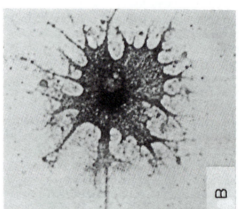

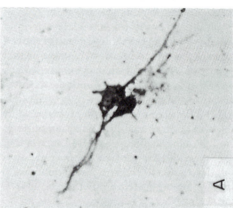

Fig. 1. Optic nerve-derived glial cells grown in the presence or absence of FCS and maintained in culture for different periods of time were fixed and identified by immunolabeling with specific antibodies as described in Experimental Procedures. (A) Bipolar O-2A progenitor cell cultured for 24 h and stained with A2B5 antibody. (B) Type 2 astrocyte grown for 4 days in the presence of FCS, stained with A2B5 antibody. (C) Oligodendrocyte grown for 5 days without serum, stained with anti-galactocerebroside antibody.

Immunoperoxidase staining

A minimal modification of the peroxidase–antiperoxidase method of Sternberger[32] was employed. Formaldehyde-fixed cells on coverslips were incubated for 60 min in a 1:300 dilution of primary antibody (ascites fluid) in PBS (cultures grown in DMEM with 10% FCS were labeled with A2B5 antibodies, while cells maintained in the defined media were labeled with the anti-galactocerebroside antibody). Coverslips were then washed in PBS (this wash and all subsequent washes were done with three changes of buffer for 5 min each). The cells were overlaid with a 1:30 dilution of rabbit anti-mouse IgGs in PBS (Accurate Chemical and Scientific Corp, Westbury, NY), incubated at room temperature for 60 min and washed. The last overlay was incubated on the cells for 24 h at 4°C with a solution of horseradish peroxidase mouse anti-peroxidase (Accurate) diluted 1:80 in PBS; this was followed by a wash. Finally, the coverslips were incubated for 8 min in a solution containing 0.5 mg/ml of 3,3'-diaminobenzidine·4 HCl (Polysciences) and 0.01% H_2O_2 v/v in saline Tris–HCl buffer, pH 7.6, then washed. The peroxidase staining was enhanced by exposing the coverslips to a 0.1% solution of osmium tetroxide in PBS for 2 min. Following extensive washes in buffer, the coverslips were mounted onto slides with 80% glycerol in PBS, and sealed with nail polish. Photographs of typical cells are shown in Fig. 1.

Image processing methods

The details of our image processing and analysis techniques are given elsewhere.[29,30] Briefly, images of the cells were captured from a light microscope with a video camera, then digitized and analysed with an image processor. Binary silhouettes of the cells were generated from a gray-scale image with a modified Marr–Hildreth filtering-convolution algorithm.[20,29] A typical result is shown in Fig. 2. The original gray-scale image is shown in (A) and its binary silhouette in (B). From these solid silhouettes, border silhouettes could be generated when needed.

Fractal dimensions were calculated with a border dilation method (DILATE) and a tile-covering procedure (GRID). These methods were previously calibrated against images of known fractal dimensions.[30] The amount of detail in the border of a two-dimensional object is directly related to its length. The length of a border (L) can be measured by counting caliper spans each of length E. Another method which seems less straightforward but is easier to implement in an image processing computer consists of widening the border to a width E, measuring the area, then dividing by E. In either case details of the border that are small compared with E are lost. If E is decreased, more detail is resolved and L increases. If the border is self-similar, each successive reduction of E by a constant factor produces an increase in L by a different constant factor. This implies that L, the measured length, is proportional to E, the caliper span, raised to a constant power (S); i.e. $L = L_0 E^S$, where L_0 is the length with a unitary measuring scale. S is negative since decreases in E lead to increases in L. If the border is a smooth Euclidean line of length L_0, the measured length L will be L_0 for all E, i.e. $S = 0$. For a family of self-similar borders of increasing roughness, borders that are smooth will have an S near 0 and those so rough as to be almost space-filling will have an S near -1 (see p. 62 of Mandelbrot's book[19]). If one sets $D = 1 - S$, then for a smooth line of Euclidean dimension 1, the "fractal dimension" D will also be 1. For natural lines of increasing roughness on a plane, D ranges through non-integral fractal dimensions from just above 1 to just below 2.

The quantity S is measured using a Richardson plot, which is a graph of the logarithm of the length of the border vs the logarithm of the length of the measuring element (e.g. caliper span, border width, or grid spacing). Over the range where such a plot is a straight line, with slope S, the object is "fractal".

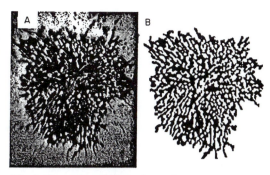

Fig. 2. Generation of binary image from gray-scale image. (A) Gray-scale image of oligodendrocyte grown in tissue culture. (B) Binary image generated by application of Marr–Hildreth convolution algorithm.

Analysis of growth and differentiation

D values were calculated at eight time periods over 5 days following plating of the progenitor cells. Zero time was taken to be the moment when the cells were placed in differentiating medium. Time is expressed in days in all the figures. At each time period, six typical cells were selected from each culture group. Each cell was acquired as a gray-scale image (Fig. 2A) from the microscope stage to the image processor. It was converted to a binary image and the border was isolated (Fig. 2B).[29] D values were calculated for each cell along with appropriate statistics.[30] Finally, functions of D were fitted to a simple dynamic model.

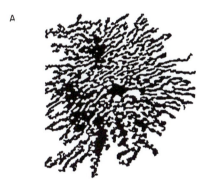

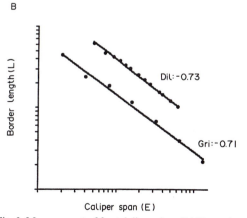

Fig. 3. Measurement of fractal dimension. (A) Binary image of oligodendrocyte. (B) Richardson plots of log of the length of cell border against the log of the length of the measuring variable ("caliper span") by the dilation (DIL) and grid (GRI) methods. The numbers are the slopes (S) of the plots. The fractal dimension (D) is $1 - S$.

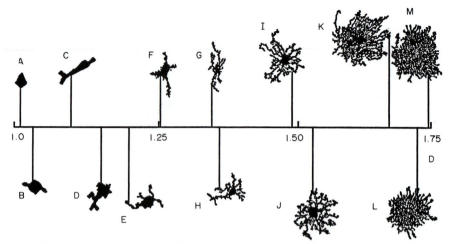

Fig. 4. Glial cells vary in their fractal dimensions. Composite of typical silhouettes (A–H) of glial cells studied. A line connects the silhouettes to their value on the *D* axis.

RESULTS

The two fractal dimension measuring methods (DILATE and GRID) gave results that closely agreed for each cell. The fractal dimensions of the total (0–5 days) population ranged from 1.02 to 1.81. All the youngest cells had a fractal dimension near 1. Astrocyte mean *D* increased to a final value of about 1.62, while oligodendrocyte mean *D* increased to about 1.75. Thus, oligodendrocytes become, by this measure, morphologically more complex than astrocytes. This is consistent with one's perception, under microscopical viewing, of the two cell types.

A typical result is illustrated in Fig. 3, which shows a silhouette of a 5 day oligodendrocyte and its Richardson plots. As can be seen, the slope, *S*, is about −0.72, and is invariant over 1.5–2 decades. The two methods give essentially identical results (*D* = 1.71 for GRID and *D* = 1.73 for DILATE).[1]* Similarly good fits to lines were obtained with the other cells with slopes from −0.02 to −0.81.

Examples of silhouettes of glial cells ordered by their fractal dimensions are illustrated in Fig. 4. It is apparent that as the cells go from relatively simple shapes and borders (A–F) to more complex (G–M), their *D* values increase. Furthermore, while cells with similar *D* values (Fig. 4C, D) may appear similar in structure, this may not always be so. This is because both the ruggedness of the cell's border and the branching of its processes contribute to *D*. For any particular cell it is not always clear which characteristic contributes predominantly to *D*. In some cells, one characteristic appears to dominate. For example,

the two cells shown in Fig. 5 have similar *D* values, while their morphologies differ considerably. In (A), the border ruggedness contributes most to *D*; while in (B) luxurious branching appears to dominate.

Fractal dimension as a function of time for cells differentiating along the astrocyte or oligodendrocyte pathways are shown in Figs 6 and 7, respectively. Binary silhouettes of representative cells from each population are also shown at various stages of differentiation. A line connects each cell to its *D*-time point on the graph. As can be seen in Figs 6 and 7, there is an increase in *D* and in perceived complexity of the cellular borders as growth proceeds. *D* increases rapidly at first and then more slowly at the end of the growth period.

A

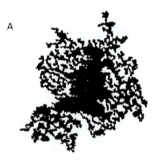

B

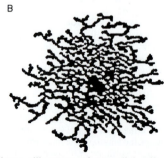

Fig. 5. Binary silhouettes of two glial cells with similar fractal dimensions, but with clearly different shapes.

---

*The images may, in fact, be fractal over a wider scale span for longer rulers; however, practical considerations prevented that determination. For example, for a 512 × 512 pixel image our software did not allow the use of discs larger than 61 pixels in diameter in the dilation program, DILATE. It is also not useful to employ tiles larger than 128 pixels on edge in the program GRID since all images would likely give the same values for such large tiles.

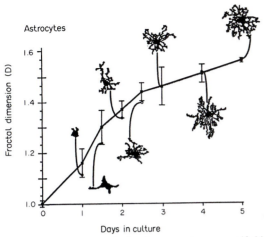

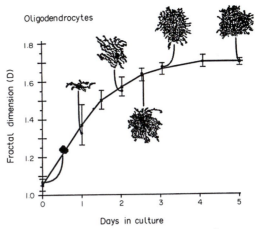

Fig. 6. Astrocyte complexity increases in a quantifiable manner. Plot of the mean ± S.D. of the fractal dimension (D) of astrocytes vs the number of days grown in culture. Silhouettes of typical cells with solid lines joined to their value of D and to their time in culture.

Fig. 7. Oligodendrocyte complexity increases in a quantifiable manner. Plot of the mean ± S.D. of the fractal dimension (D) of oligodendrocytes vs the number of days grown in culture. Silhouettes of typical cells with solid line joined to their value of D and to their time in culture.

We find that morphological complexity expressed as $D(t)$ of both glial phenotypes progresses according to the equation:

$$D(t) = D_{max} - (D_{max} - D_0)\exp(-t/\tau),$$

where D_{max} is the maximum, plateau value of D, D_0 is the value of D at the beginning of the experiment; t is time; and τ is the time constant of approach to D_{max}. The differentiation of complex morphology of both phenotypes occurs at an exponentially declining rate, as illustrated in Fig. 8. The curves in the figure were drawn using the equation. The time constant (τ) for the oligodendrocytes (1.25 days) is approximately

75% that for astrocytes (2.19 days), which is consistent with the observation that the oligodendrocytes differentiate faster. Also, at all times the oligodendrocytes are more complex than the astrocytes.

DISCUSSION

We have demonstrated previously[30] that the principles of Mandelbrot's fractal geometry can be applied to quantify cell morphology, as has been done fruitfully in other areas of biology.[4,33] Increases in fractal dimensions correlate with increases in perceived morphological complexity. Both astrocytes

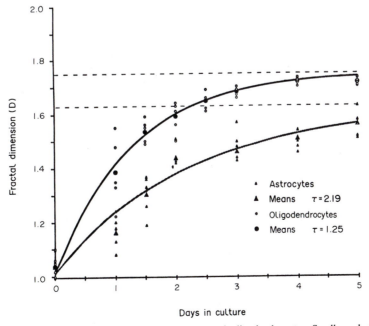

Fig. 8. Comparison of the changes in D of astrocytes and oligodendrocytes. Small symbols represent individual cells; large symbols represent means. Dashed horizontal lines represent asymptotic values. τ = time constant in days.

and oligodendrocytes increase in D as they undergo differentiation. Analysis of the changes in fractal dimension in the two maturing populations studied in this research demonstrates differing rates of differentiation. Oligodendrocytes have a smaller time constant; i.e. they differentiate faster than type 2 astrocytes.

Some attention should be paid to the interpretation of changes in D and their relationship to our common sense perception of complexity. It is the magnitude of the quantity S that is most easily related to complexity. Recall that S is the slope of the line in a Richardson plot and is, therefore, the ratio of two logarithmic physical measurements. Its magnitude is the fractional part of the fractal dimension D. Therefore, a change in D from 1.1 to 1.2 represents a doubling of complexity. Likewise, a change from 1.1 to 1.7 would represent a seven-fold increase in complexity. Though a useful way of trying to relate D to psychophysical reality, this line of reasoning breaks down as D approaches 2, which is the point where the border entirely fills the image plane.

One might also ask what aspect of the cell's "complexity" is the fractal dimension actually measuring. In experiments on computer constructed test images, it was found that two important properties are the ruggedness of the border and the profusion of branching. D increases as either of these characteristics increases.[30] These two characteristics can be considered to be part of a continuum with no precise dividing line between them. That is, a rugged border might appear as profuse branching at higher magnification and branches might appear to be the textural elements of borders at lower magnification. These may, in fact, be manifestations of self-similarity.

Since fixation and staining are essential elements of this research and can surely affect the appearance of cells, it is rational to inquire as to the verity of our claims to be studying genuine changes in morphology. There are many instances in the literature where given glial cells have been microscopically studied both live and fixed.[3,12,14,17,21] Under these conditions no striking differences were seen. Most immunochemical and biochemical work on glial cells has been done using fixed material. We are primarily interested at this stage in our work to be able to begin to compare our results to those results. However, as physiologists, our primary interest is in cell function–morphology relations and, therefore, in future work we hope to follow quantitative morphological changes in individual live cells.

We could not stain our presumed astrocyte cultures for the definitive marker, GFAP, because the fixation methods that are required cause cell shrinkage and, thereby, alter the relevant morphology. However, with the trained eye, it is always possible to identify type 2 astrocytes based on morphological criteria.[5] We estimate that the contamination with other cell types (predominantly type 1 astrocytes) would be less than 2% initially and less than 10% by the fifth day.

As the bipotential progenitor differentiates along the oligodendrocyte pathway, biologists have described three stages of differentiation by using conventional qualitative means. The initial A2B5 +, vimentin + cell is bipolar, capable of migration and proliferates in response to specific growth factors including Platelet-Derived Growth Factor and Insulin-like Growth Factor 1. Along this pathway, an intermediate progenitor cell, considered to be slightly more differentiated, has been described. This multipolar cell has short processes, continues to label with A2B5, and acquires a sulfatide on its surface that is detected by the monoclonal antibody designated O4. The intermediate progenitor is capable of proliferation, but like the oligodendrocyte it is devoid of intermediate filaments. Insulin or insulin-like growth factors stimulate this cell to differentiate further.[8] The differentiated oligodendrocyte, which continues to express the O4 marker, expresses galactocerebroside on its surface and ordinarily does not proliferate. Along the astrocyte pathway, a multipolar intermediate precursor may transiently express O4 and GFAP simultaneously.

Descriptions of "intermediate progenitors" along the two glial cell pathways can be viewed as "milestones" which one can identify and define by available technologies. During the 72 h in which the bipolar progenitor differentiates into the multipolar oligodendrocyte, the cell undergoes many changes that reflect the various stages of differentiation, which up to now have not been quantifiable. Analysis of a homogeneous population of progenitor cells, differentiating in a synchronized manner, reveals that the calculated fractal dimensions of the cells within that population at a given time are similar, and thus D reflects the mean morphological complexity of the population at that time. Thus, the fractal dimension may be considered as a quantitative description of the stage of morphological differentiation of the population. As the population undergoes differentiation along the oligodendrocyte pathway, the mean fractal dimension increases rapidly between time 0 and 72 h, when 95% of the cells express galactocerebroside. Once the cells are committed oligodendrocytes that are expressing galactocerebroside, the D of the population plateaus, although the oligodendrocytes do not yet express other myelin proteins such as myelin basic protein or proteolipid protein.[9] The period of rapid increase in fractal dimension of the population correlates with the period when most of the cellular changes associated with differentiation occur. Analysis of the mean D of the differentiating astrocyte population reveals that the fastest period of increasing D is between 12 and 60 h. This may indicate the period in which the precursor is undergoing most of the changes associated with differentiation, and by 60 h it may be committed to the astrocyte pathway.

Progenitor cells express a complex spectrum of ionic conductances in the rat that disappear during oligodendrocytic differentiation and are followed by the singular appearance of anomalous rectification potassium conductance.[3,31] It may be possible to relate the developmental transformation of cytoplasmic and surface antigens in the cells to both membrane conductance expression and fractal dimension. If, for example, the early appearance of ion conductances play a role in oligodendrocyte differentiation, then alterations in those conductances may have recognizable effects on the development of morphological complexity and/or on cellular differentiation. Various growth factors are known to induce differentiation of progenitor elements and their associated second messenger signal transduction mechanisms can be studied to compare, quantitatively and objectively, the development of morphological complexity. Thus, it may be possible to characterize the genomic and cytoplasmic mechanisms that drive the progenitor cells into their characteristic, complex morphologies. Naturally, similar types of studies can also be performed with neuronal and other cellular phenotypes differentiating in culture.

Quantitative analysis of the increase in morphological complexity during the process of differentiation may provide a new strategy for studying morphology. The complex genomic and cytoplasmic mechanisms that generate the differences in glial morphology can now be probed in an entirely objective and quantitative manner. Analysis of changes in fractal dimension can be used to complement both conventional histological techniques and immunocytochemical demonstrations of surface and cytoplasmic antigens. The fractal dimension of an object places significant constraints on the morphological possibilities of the processes that generated the object and the magnitude of D provides some insight into how elaborate the process may be, since the larger the D, the larger the number of degrees of freedom likely to be involved in the process.

Moreover, the appearance of the various markers for differentiation and various other physiological and functional milestones could be expressed with respect to a D axis rather than to a time axis. This could be useful in making comparisons of development between regions of the CNS or across species where "characteristic times" might differ but the ordering of stages and the relationships to cell morphology might be invariant.

Fractal dimension may also be a useful classification variable. It will be of interest to see how classification of cells based on fractal dimension relates to current classification schemes. The fact that large changes in morphological complexity (measured as D) can be well described by a simple mathematical model having no more than three parameters suggests that perhaps the dynamics of the mechanisms underlying the phenomenon are themselves quite simple. Only by devising experiments where the model is tested at the extremes of its applicability will we be able to decide whether this apparent simplicity is due to an averaging of many mechanisms or to some inherently simple determinant of morphological differentiation.

CONCLUSION

The reader should be cautioned that our results do not imply, rather they rule out, mechanisms that are characterized as "fractal growth". For example, Mandelbrot[19] gives a number of examples of objects which grow by a rule where size increases and the fractal dimension is invariant: i.e. fractal growth. Typically, the range of scale over which the object is fractal also increases. The object grows in a way analogous to a steady increase in optical magnification. Clearly we have established that in our glial cultures the fractal dimension itself increases as well as the size and, therefore, cannot be considered as fractal growth. Other authors have examined growth rules which produce botanical shapes ("L-systems"),[15,18,28] and various textures ("iterated transforms").[2] Often these do not have straight Richardson plots during differentiation, in which cases they are not pure fractals. Mandelbrot calls these "sub-fractals". Their range is vast, and seems capable of producing glia-like shapes. Could there be growth rules in this class with Richardson plots straight enough at each stage of growth to define a value of D, but which increases during growth? Our results suggest the need to search for such rules.

REFERENCES

1. Amthor F. R. (1988) Quantitative/fractal analysis of dendritic trees of identified rabbit retinal ganglion cells. *Soc. Neurosci. Abstr.* **14,** 603.
2. Barnsley M. F. (1988) *Fractals Everywhere.* Academic Press, New York.
3. Barres B. A., Chun L. L. and Corey D. P. (1988) Ion channel expression by white matter glia: I. Type 2 astrocytes and oligodendrocytes. *Glia* **1,** 10–30.
4. Bassingthwaighte J. B. (1988) Physiological heterogeneity: fractals link determinism and randomness in structures and functions. *News physiol. Sci.* **3,** 5–10.
5. Behar T., McMorris F. A., Novotny E. A., Barker J. L. and Dubois-Dalcq M. (1988) Growth and differentiation properties of O-2A progenitors purified from rat cerebral hemispheres. *J. Neurosci. Res.* **21,** 168–180.
6. Bottenstein J. E. (1986) Growth requirements *in vitro* of oligodendrocyte cell lines and neuronatal rat brain oligodendrocytes. *Proc. natn. Acad. Sci. U.S.A.* **83,** 1955–1959.
7. Caserta F., Stanley H. E., Eldred W. D., Daccord G., Hausman R. E. and Nittman J. (1990) Physical mechanism underlies neurite outgrowth: a quantitative analysis of neuronal shape. *Phys. Rev. Lett.* **64,** 95–98.

166   T. G. SMITH JR *et al.*

8. Dubois-Dalcq M. (1987) Characterization of a slowly proliferative cell along the oligodendrocyte differentiation pathway. *Eur. molec. Biol. Org. J.* **6**, 2587–2597.

9. Dubois-Dalcq M., Behar T., Hudson L. and Lazzarini R. A. (1986) Emergence of three myelin proteins in oligodendrocytes cultured without neurons. *J. Cell Biol.* **102**, 384–392.

10. Eccelston P. A. and Silberberg D. H. (1984) The differentiation of oligodendrocytes in a serum-free, hormone supplemented medium. *Devl Brain Res.* **16**, 1–9.

11. Eisenbarth G., Walsh F. S. and Nirenberg M. (1979) Monoclonal antibody to a plasma membrane of neurons. *Proc. natn. Acad. Sci. U.S.A.* **76**, 4913–4917.

12. Espinosa de los Monteros A., Roussel G., Gensburger C., Nussbaum J. L. and Labourdetti G. (1985) Precursor cells of oligodendrocytes in rat primary cultures. *Devl Biol.* **108**, 474–480.

13. Ffrench-Constant C. and Raff M. C. (1986) The oligodendrocyte–type-2 astrocyte cell lineage is specialized for myelination. *Nature* **323**, 335–338.

14. Gilbert P., Kettenmann H. and Schachner M. (1984) Gamma-aminobutyric acid directly depolarizes cultured oligodendrocytes. *J. Neurosci.* **4**, 561–569.

15. Jurgensen H. and Lindenmayer A. (1987) Inference algorithms for developmental systems with cell lineages. *Bull. Math. Biol.* **49**, 93–123.

16. Kachar B., Behar T. and Dubois-Dalcq M. (1986) Cell shape and motility of oligodendrocytes cultured without neurons. *Cell Tiss. Res.* **244**, 27–38.

17. Kettenmann H., Sonnhof U. and Schachner M. (1983) Exclusive potassium dependence of the membrane potential in cultured mouse oligodendrocytes. *J. Neurosci.* **3**, 500–505.

18. Lindenmayer A. (1984) Positional and temporal control mechanisms in inflorescence development. In *Developmental Order: Its Origin and Regulation* (eds Subtelny S. S. and Green P. B.), pp. 461–486. Cambridge University Press.

19. Mandelbrot B. B. (1982) *The Fractal Geometry of Nature.* W. H. Freeman, New York.

20. Marr D. and Hildreth E. (1980) Theory of edge detection. *Proc. R. Soc. Lond. B* **207**, 187–217.

21. Noble M., Murray K., Stroobant P., Waterfield M. D. and Riddle P. (1988) Platelet-derived growth factor promotes division and motility and inhibits premature differentiation of the oligodendrocyte/type-2 astrocyte progenitor cell. *Nature* **333**, 560–562.

22. Pellionisz A. (1991) Neural geometry: towards a fractal model of neurons. In *Models of Brain Function* (ed. Cotterill R. M.). Cambridge University Press (in press).

23. Raff M., Miller R. H. and Noble M. (1983) A glial progenitor cell that develops *in vitro* in to an astrocyte or an oligodendrocyte depending on culture medium. *Nature* **303**, 390–396.

24. Raff M. C. (1989) Glial cell diversification in the rat optic nerve. *Science* **243**, 1450–1455.

25. Raff M. C., Williams B. P. and Miller R. H. (1984) The *in vitro* differentiation of a bipolar glial progenitor cell. *Eur. molec. Biol. Org. J.* **3**, 857–864.

26. Ranscht B., Clapshaw P. A., Price J., Noble M. and Seifert W. (1982) Development of oligodendrocytes and Schwann cells studied with a monoclonal antibody against galactocerebroside. *Proc. natn. Acad. Sci. U.S.A.* **79**, 2709–2713.

27. Small R. K., Riddle P. and Noble M. (1987) Evidence for migration of oligodendrocyte–type 2 astrocyte progenitor cells into the developing optic nerve. *Nature* **328**, 155–157.

28. Smith A. R. (1984) Plants, fractals and formal languages. *Comput. Graphics* **18**, 1–10.

29. Smith T. G. Jr, Marks W. B., Lange G. D., Sheriff W. H. Jr and Neale E. A. (1988) Edge detection in images using Marr–Hildreth filtering techniques. *J. Neurosci. Meth.* **26**, 75–82.

30. Smith T. G. Jr, Marks W. B., Lange G. D., Sheriff W. H. Jr and Neale E. A. (1989) A fractal analysis of cell images. *J. Neurosci. Meth.* **27**, 173–180.

31. Sontheimer H., Trotter J., Schachner M. and Ketterman H. (1988) Developmental regulation of channel expression in oligodendrocytes. *Soc. Neurosci. Abstr.* **14**, 787.

32. Sternberger L. A. (1986) *Immunocytochemistry*, pp. 90–210. John Wiley, New York.

33. West B. J. and Goldberger A. L. (1987) Physiology in fractal dimensions. *Am. Scient.* **75**, 354–365.

(*Accepted* 18 *July* 1990)

Lucifer Yellow, Retrograde Tracers, and Fractal Analysis Characterise Adult Ferret Retinal Ganglion Cells

Richard J.T. Wingate, Tom Fitzgibbon, and Ian D. Thompson

Oxford University, University Laboratory of Physiology, Parks Road, Oxford OX1 3PT, United Kingdom

ABSTRACT

The dendritic morphology of retinal ganglion cells in the ferret was studied by the intracellular injection of lucifer yellow in fixed tissue. Ganglion cells were identified by the retrograde transport of red or green fluorescent microspheres that had been injected into different target nuclei, usually the lateral geniculate nucleus or superior colliculus. This approach allows the comparison of dendritic morphologies of ganglion cells in the same retina with different central projections and also identifies cells with branching axons. The digitised images of dendritic arbors were analysed quantitatively by a variety of measures. Dendritic complexity was assessed by calculating the fractal dimension of each arbor. The ferret has distinct alpha, beta, and gamma morphological classes of cells similar to those found in the cat. The gamma cell class was morphologically diverse and could be subdivided into "sparse," "loose," and "tight" groups, reflecting increasing dendritic complexity. Whereas the beta cell projection was limited to the lateral geniculate nucleus alone, alpha and gamma cells could project to either or both nuclei. Retinal ganglion cells labelled from the pretectal nuclei formed a morphologically distinct class of retinal ganglion cells. The ipsilateral projection lacked alpha cells and the most complex, "tight" gamma cells. However, ipsilaterally projecting "loose" gamma cells overlapped alpha cells in both soma and dendritic dimensions. Different morphological classes of retinal ganglion cells hence show characteristic axon behaviour both in their decussation at the chiasm and in which targets they innervate. Fractal measures were used to contrast variation within and between these identified classes.

Key words: dendritic arbors, intracellular dye, morphometry, lateral geniculate nucleus, superior colliculus

Mammalian retinae are characterised by the great morphological diversity of retinal ganglion cells (Cajal, 1893), which send axons along the optic nerve to a variety of central nuclei. Classification of these cells, by anatomical and physiological approaches, has greatly increased the understanding of how visual information is coded. Such studies have revealed that different functional classes have distinct dendritic morphologies, cover the retina in independent mosaics, and vary in their subcortical targets (Wässle and Boycott, '91). Most recently, in vivo tract tracing and in vitro intracellular techniques have been combined to determine the detailed dendritic characteristics of retinal ganglion cells with a projection to a single identified nucleus (Buhl and Peichl, '96; Dann and Buhl, '87; Ramoa et al., '87, '88, '89; Buhl and Dann, '88; Pu and Amthor, '90a,b). We have extended these techniques in the adult ferret (*Mustela putorius furo*), to compare retinal ganglion cells within a single retina that have been identified by their projection to one or more central targets.

In this study, we used latex microspheres conjugated with two different fluorochromes as contrasting retrograde tracers (Katz et al., '84; Katz and Larovici, '90). The dendritic morphology of labelled cells was revealed by intracellular injection of a compatible,

Accepted May 22, 1992.

Address reprint requests to Dr. R.J.T. Wingate, University Laboratory of Physiology, Parks Road, Oxford OX1 3PT, United Kingdom.

T. FitzGibbon is now at the Department of Clinical Ophthalmology (C09), Sydney University, Sydney, New South Wales 2006, Australia.

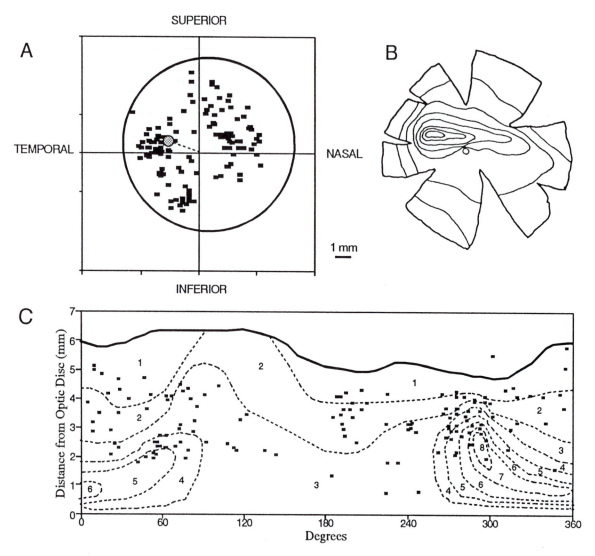

Fig. 1. Construction of equivalent density zones. **A:** Polar plot of intracellularly filled and analysed cell bodies, relative to the optic disc (origin), on a standard right retina. The shaded circle denotes the area centralis, from which the dotted line traces the axis to the optic disc. The ellipse represents the line of best fit through the superimposed perimeters of each retina. **B:** Isodensity contours on an equivalent right retina (Henderson, '85). **C:** Isodensity contours (dotted lines) and retinal circumference (solid line) from B mapped onto a rectilinear projection of the polar plot in A (0° is superior). This allowed us to assign cells to one of eight equivalent density zones: 1, <500 mm^{-2}; 2, 500–1,000 mm^{-2}; 3, 1,000–1,500 mm^{-2}; 4, 1,500–2,000 mm^{-2}; 5, 2,000–2,500 mm^{-2}; 6, 2,000–3,000 mm^{-2}; 7, 3,000–3,500 mm^{-2}; 8, >3,500 mm^{-2}. One very peripheral cell in A fell outside the reconstructed polar borders of the retina shown in B. Scale bar = 1 mm.

fluorescent dye, lucifer yellow, in lightly fixed retinae (Tauchi and Masland, '84; Teranishi and Negishi, '86; Dann and Buhl, '87; Dann et al., '87; Peichl et al., '87a). In this way, we have been able to compare populations of retinal ganglion cells whose somas have been retrogradely labelled from two different target nuclei and also identify those cells with bifurcating axons. Finally, by using image-analysis techniques to estimate the fractal dimension of individual dendritic arbors (Montague and Friedlander, '89, '91; Morigiwa et al., '89; Smith et al., '89; Caserta et al., '90; Wingate et al.,

'90), the branching characteristics of dendrites in identified populations of retinal ganglion cells have been contrasted by using a scale-independent measure of complexity.

Our approach combines methods that have been used in numerous studies to investigate the relationship of morphological class to the retinofugal projection of mammalian retinal ganglion cells. In the cat, retrograde tracing with horseradish peroxidase (HRP) has been used widely to demonstrate the various different projections of ganglion cells, where at least three

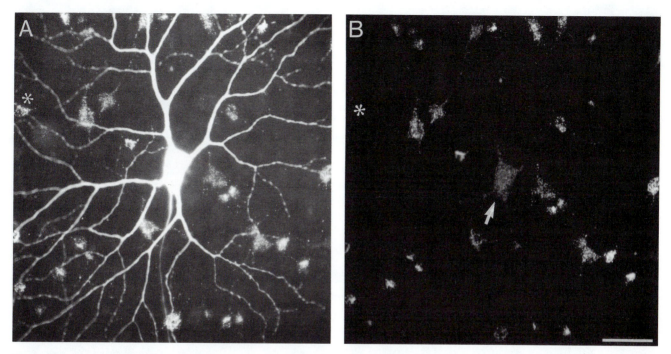

Fig. 2. The different labelling characteristics of retrograde and intracellular tracers. **A:** Photomicrograph of a peripheral alpha cell (arrow, cell body) filled intracellularly with the fluorescent dye lucifer yellow. This cell has also taken up green beads and red beads retrogradely from different terminal nuclei. The somatic green bead label is obscured by the intense lucifer yellow fluorescence, which shares similar excitation and emission spectra. Beta cells in this particular field of view were not heavily labelled by either retrograde tracer. The cell soma labelled by an asterisk (*) is labelled with only green beads transported from the superior colliculus **B:** The lucifer yellow filled cell is co-labelled with red beads retrogradely taken up from the lateral geniculate nucleus, which are revealed when the cell body (arrow) is photographed with the appropriate UV excitation and interference filters for rhodamine. The soma labelled with green beads alone (asterisk, *) is no longer visible. There is very little fluorescence "leakage" between filters. In general, our protocol was to fill only cells labelled with green beads and determine the presence of red beads subsequently, during photography. Alpha cells could be recognised prior to impalement by the characteristically even retrograde label. Scale bar = 50 μm.

basic cell classes have been distinguishable on the basis of soma size and dendritic morphology (Boycott and Wässle, '74; Kelly and Gilbert, '75; Leventhal et al., '80, '85; Wässle and Illing, '80; Illing and Wässle, '81; Leventhal, '82; Koontz et al., '85). Double retrograde labelling studies have been carried out to directly assess axonal branching within soma size classes (Illing, '80). Otherwise, the degree of axonal branching for a group of retinal ganglion cells has been deduced from the numbers and types of cells labelled by retrograde HRP transport from different nuclei (Wässle and Illing, '80; Illing and Wässle, '81). However, the degree to which discrete dendritic classes are revealed by retrograde transport of HRP is variable and, in general, not as good as intracellular injection of fluorescent dyes (Dann et al., '87; Ramoa et al., '87; Dann et al., '88; Ramoa et al., '88, '89) or Golgi impregnation (Boycott and Wässle, '74; Stone and Clarke, '80).

In the ferret, HRP studies have shown a range of cell classes based on soma sizes and dendritic profiles similar to those in the cat (Vitek et al., '85; Morgan et al., '87; Thompson et al., '91). Unlike the cat there is no

clear evidence of a trimodal distribution of soma sizes, nor are central to peripheral size gradients so marked (Fukuda and Stone, '74; Henderson, '85; Leventhal et al., '85). However, cells projecting to the superior colliculus (SC) differ in soma size distribution from those projecting to the lateral geniculate nucleus (LGN), suggesting differential targeting of retinal ganglion cell types (Morgan et al., '87). In addition, both the range of cell classes contributing to ipsilateral and contralateral projections and the course of fibre diameters through the optic chiasm suggest that different types of retinal ganglion cells display different decussation patterns (Vitek et al., '85; Reese and Baker, '90). In this study, we investigated how variations in axonal projection correlate with the detailed dendritic morphology of retinal ganglion cells. We also examined how different quantitative parameters of dendritic morphology vary within and between different ganglion cell classes. The purpose of this comparison was twofold: to investigate to what extent an objective classification of retinal ganglion cell classes is possible and to provide a framework for subsequent studies of ganglion cell development and

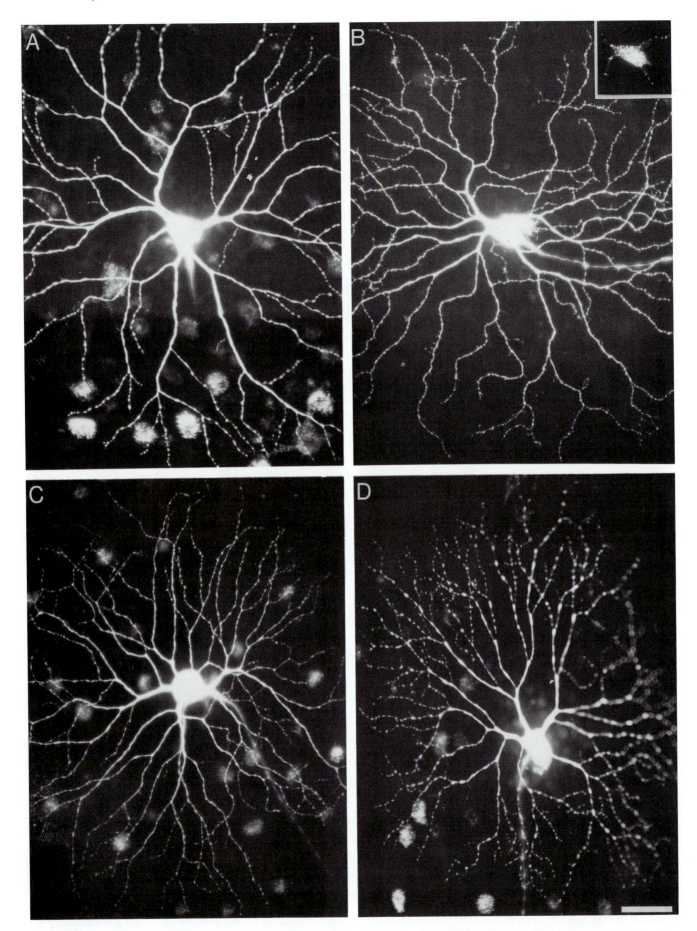

Figure 3

plasticity. The ferret is relatively immature at birth and so provides an excellent model for developmental studies of the visual system (Jackson and Hickey, '85).

MATERIALS AND METHODS

Thirteen adult pigmented ferrets provided data for this study.

Surgery

Anaesthesia was induced by the administration of Alphaxalone 0.9% and Alphadolone acetate 0.3% (Saffan; Pitman-Moore, Uxbridge, U.K., 2 ml/kg i.m.) and maintained with additional doses (0.5 ml) as necessary. Atropine sulphate (0.1 ml, i.p.) was administered to reduce respiratory secretions. The animal was placed in a stereotaxic headholder (Eldridge et al., '85). A craniotomy was made lateral to the midline and anterior to the sagittal sinus, the dura mater removed, and the cortex overlying the SC and LGN aspirated. Fine borosilicate tubing pipettes (Plowden and Thompson, Stourbridge, U.K., 0.7–0.8 mm outer diameter, 0.4 mm inner diameter, volume @ 125 nl/mm) were pulled on a horizontal pipette puller and calibrated. The tips were broken back to a diameter of 20–30 μm. These were backfilled with a dilution (1:10 in sterile saline) of either green or red fluorescent latex microspheres (Lumafluor, New York). In most animals, one tracer was injected by pressure into the SC and the other into the LGN. Multiple injections (total volume 5.0–6.0 μl) were made unilaterally into each nucleus to produce an even application of tracer with minimal spillage. In two animals, red bead injections were made unilaterally into the pretectal nuclei (PT) and green beads into the SC. In one animal, small, nonoverlapping injections of red beads (500 nl) and green beads (1 μl) were made unilaterally into the rostral and caudal poles of the SC, respectively. The region above the exposed midbrain and thalamus was then packed with Sterispon (Allen and Hanburys Ltd., London, U.K.), the bone flap re-

placed, and the wound sutured. A local anaesthetic, Xylocaine (Astra Chemicals, King's Langley, U.K.), was applied to the wound. After a minimum of 4 days survival time, an overdose of pentobarbitone sodium (Sagattal; RMB Animal Health Ltd., Dagenham, U.K.) was administered (120 mg/kg, i.p.). While under deep anaesthesia, the animal was perfused with phosphate buffered saline and then approximately 30 ml of filtered 1% paraformaldehyde in 0.1 M phosphate buffer (pH 7.4). The dorsal pole of the cornea was incised with a fine scalpel blade to mark the orientation of the eye. The eyes were removed and placed in 0.1 M phosphate buffer (pH 7.4). The animal was then perfused with 4% paraformaldehyde in 0.1 M phosphate buffer (pH 7.4). The brain was removed and sunk in 30% sucrose in 0.1 M phosphate buffer prior to sectioning at 50 μm on a freezing microtome.

Intracellular dye filling

The lightly fixed eyecup was opened up by making four to six radial incisions through the sclera and retina. The neural retina was dissected away from the eyecup and the vitreous humor teased away from its surface with paintbrushes and forceps. The retina was then placed in a tissue chamber in filtered 2 mM ascorbic acid in 0.1 M phosphate buffer (pH 7.4; Dann et al., '87; Peichl et al., '87a) with the ganglion cell layer uppermost. The fluid-air interface was regulated at approximately 0.5 mm above the retinal surface, and the tissue held in place by tungsten pins mounted on moveable, magnetic strips. The tissue chamber was positioned under a fixed stage compound microscope (M2 Micromanipulation Microscope; Oxford Microinstruments, Oxford, U.K.) with UV epifluorescence (HBO-50 W high pressure mercury vapour lamp) and the appropriate excitation and interference filters (green/yellow: Zeiss BP .450–490 FT 510 BP 515–560; red: Zeiss BP 510–560 FT 580 LP 590). Retrogradely labelled cells were identified through long working distance objectives (Zeiss Neofluar ×10/0.30 and Nikon Plan ×40/0.55 ELWD). Micropipettes were pulled from filament containing capillary glass (Clark Electromedical Instruments, Reading, U.K.; GC120–F10) and were backfilled with 15% lucifer yellow CH (LY; Sigma) in 0.1 M lithium chloride (Ramoa et al., '87) producing a typical DC resistance of 30–80 MΩ in 0.1 M phosphate buffer. The micropipette was advanced at an angle of 35° to the retinal surface and cell bodies were impaled under direct visual control and filled with lucifer yellow by applying small steady or oscillating hyperpolarising currents across the electrode tip (1–2 nA, 500 milliseconds, 1 Hz). Our standard protocol was to impale cells identified by green beads that had been retrogradely transported from the SC or LGN; the presence of red beads in the soma was assessed

Fig. 3. Photomicrographs of alpha cells retrogradely labelled with green beads from the lateral geniculate nucleus (LGN) and intracellularly filled with lucifer yellow. Cells **A, B,** and **D** have inner stratifying arbors while **C** shows an outer stratifying dendritic tree. The density zones of the four cells in A–D, respectively, are: 4, 3, 4, and 2. The cell in B is an example of a triple labelled alpha cell retrogradely labelled with green beads from the LGN, red beads from the superior colliculus (SC, inset) and subsequently with lucifer yellow. The patchy background fluorescence is due to retrogradely labelled somas of adjacent retinal ganglion cells that lie outside the focal plane. Scale bar = 50 μm.

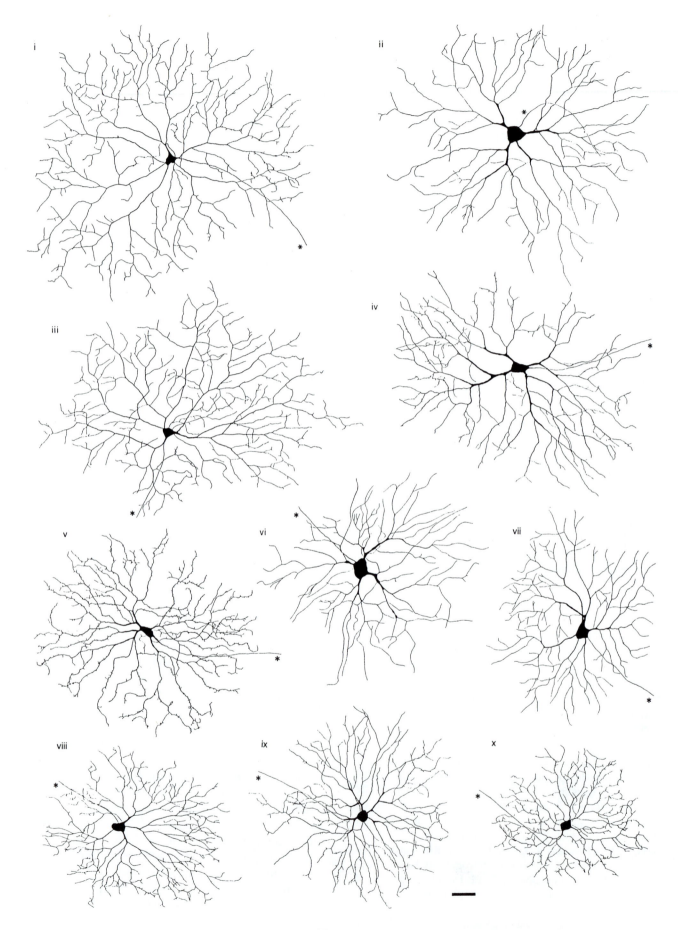

Figure 4

subsequently. Cells were judged to be well labelled with lucifer yellow when a sufficient extent of axon and the finest dendritic processes were clearly visible. When a number of cells had been filled, the retina was postfixed for at least 1 hour in filtered 4% paraformaldehyde in 0.1 M phosphate buffer (pH 7.4) at 0–4°C, while flattened under a glass coverslip, and then washed in three changes of 0.1 M phosphate buffer (pH 7.4). The retina was dried onto a subbed slide to minimise shrinkage, further dehydrated through a series of alcohols (95%, 100%, 100%; 30 seconds each) to xylene (30 seconds), and mounted in Fluoremount GURR (Sigma).

Morphometric analysis

Only cells clearly labelled by transport and showing complete intracellular dendritic staining were photographed. A total of 131 dendritic arbors were reconstructed by tracing the projected negatives of 3–15 serial photographs (Kodak T-MAX 400 ASA), taken at high power through the depth of the inner plexiform layer. The retinal location of each photographed, double or triple labelled cell was reconstructed by means of a camera lucida and a computer aided morphometric programme (Halasz and Martin, '84). Given the pronounced visual streak and dorsal-ventral asymmetries in cell density across the ferret retina (Henderson, '85; Vitek et al., '85; Peichl et al., '87b), local cell density was believed to represent a better value by which to compare changes in arbor size than distance from the area centralis (Watanabe and Rodieck, '89). The location of each lucifer yellow filled cell was plotted relative to the optic disc onto a schematic right retina (Fig. 1A).

Cells close to the optic disc are underrepresented because of the technical difficulty of impaling cells through the thickness of the fibre layer in this region. When published isodensity contours (Fig. 1B, drawn from Henderson, '85) were superimposed onto a rectilinear projection of these data (Fig. 1C), the retina could be subdivided according to ganglion cell density. Each filled cell was hence assigned to one of 8 zones of increasing equivalent density.

The stratification of dendritic arbors was assessed from the microscope fine focus calibration at high magnification (Zeiss Neofluar ×40/0.9) and classified as simply inner or outer depending on their proximity to the ganglion cell layer or amacrine cell layer, respectively. The sizes of the soma and dendritic arbor were estimated by tracing their perimeters onto a digitising tablet (Summagraphics, Fairfield, CT) by means of a morphometric analysis computer programme (Sigmascan V3.0, © Jandel Scientific, Sausolito, CA, '87); area values are given as μm^2.

The branching complexity of a retinal ganglion cell was assessed by its Hausdorff-Besicovitch or fractal dimension (*Df*; Mandelbrot, '77). This value can be seen as a measure of the space-filling characteristics of a particular branching form independent of its topology or size. Its application depends upon the assumption that retinal ganglion cells are essentially planar and have an intrinsic fractal structure (Caserta et al., '90). Drawings of the dendritic arbors were digitised onto a 256 × 256 pixel array by means of a video camera attached to a parallel microprocessor (Seescan Imaging Ltd., Cambridge, U.K.). The images were skeletised to one pixel width, reducing the soma to a point and the axons "painted" out to leave only a representation of the dendritic structure. The fractal dimension was calculated by a pixel dilation protocol (Flook, '78; Smith et al., '89; Wingate et al., '90), whereby the rate of areal expansion of the image for the addition of successive layers of pixels to the skeletised arbor was used to derive a value of *Df* (Seescan Analytical Services, Cambridge, U.K.). This method was chosen for reasons of processing efficiency that relate to the choice of image analysis hardware. Alternative strategies were assessed; both "caliper" methods (Nittman et al., '85; Smith et al., '89) and box-counting methods (Smith et al., '89; Montague and Friedlander, '89, '91; Caserta et al., '90) gave similar values of *Df*.[1]

To assess the degree of displacement of the soma from the geometric centre of the dendritic arbor, the centres of gravity of the soma and of the dilated pixel

---

Fig. 4. Alpha cells of differing morphologies. Drawings were made by tracing serial photomicrograph negatives. The more peripheral cells, top left; more central, bottom right. Cells **i–x** represent the variety of dendritic form and soma size found at various retinal locations. Note that cells of a similar arbor size can vary greatly in soma dimensions, such as cells i and ii. Similarly, dendritic processes can be either spiny or smooth regardless of arbor size (compare cells v and vi). The density zone (1–8) for each cell and whether its arbor is inner (*i*) or outer (*o*) stratifying are as follows: i, 2*i*; ii, 5*o*; iii, 2*i*; iv, 3*o*; v, 3*i*; vi, 5*i*; vii, 1*o*; viii, 2*i*; ix, 4*o*; x, 3*i*. Asterisk (*) denotes axons. Scale bar = 50 μm.

---

[1]The former method relies on the assumption that when measured with a "caliper" of increasing length, *r*, the resolvable perimeter of a fractal structure becomes smaller at a rate that relates to its complexity (×r^{1-Df}; Mandelbrot, '77). For box-counting methods, the fractal image is superimposed onto a sampling mesh of boxes of length *d*. The number of boxes (*K(d)*) intersected by the image decreases as the mesh becomes coarser (i.e., as the individual box sizes increase), such that:

$$\log(K(d)) \times -Df \cdot (\log(d)).$$

Hence, a double log plot of the size of the fractal structure, either in terms of perimeter length in units of *r*, or of boxes intersected *k(d)*, against the length of *r* or *d* as both increase, yields a slope of 1 – *Df* or –*Df*, respectively.

image of the arbor were calculated. The distance between these two points was expressed as a percentage of the average (Feret) radius of the dilated image.

RESULTS

The results are presented in three sections. In the first section, the types of retinal ganglion cell found in the ferret that project to the superior colliculus and lateral geniculate nucleus are described following the conventions of previous studies. In the second section, the details of the relation between these classes and different retinofugal projections are discussed. In the third section, quantitative classification of retinal ganglion cell arbor types, in combination with projection pattern, is used to investigate the possibility of a natural classification system for ferret retinal ganglion cells (Rodieck and Brening, '83).

A note on nomenclature

Ferret retinal ganglion cells projecting to the LGN and SC were found to fall into a variety of classes based on their distinctive dendritic branching styles, soma sizes, and arbor sizes at a particular retinal location. We found that the major classes agreed well with the previous descriptions of mammalian alpha and beta cells (Boycott and Wässle, '74; Wässle et al., '81a,b; Wilson and Condo, '85; Peichl et al., '87a,b; Peichl, '89, '91; Dann and Buhl, '90; for review see Wässle and Boycott, '91). This confirms previous HRP studies on the ferret (Henderson, '85; Vitek et al., '85) and hence we feel able to adopt this nomenclature. A third heterogeneous, "gamma" class of cells is here used to describe a variety of types. These non-alpha, non-beta cells embrace the various gamma morphologies described for the cat in Golgi studies (Boycott and Wässle, '74; Stone and Clarke, '80) and various retrograde HRP studies (Leventhal et al., '80, '85; Leventhal, '82; Koontz et al., '85) but also more delicate arbor types as demonstrated by Ramoa et al. ('88). It is clear that the pooling of morphologies into a single gamma class is an oversimplification. For instance, Kolb et al. ('81) have described 21 different types of ganglion cell in the cat. For the purpose of simply categorising the more distinct variants, we have used "loose," "tight," and "sparse" to describe the differing gamma morphs. While not suggesting a homology, these can be seen to correspond to the types I, II, and III morphologies encountered in the rodent (Perry, '79). In the cat, the gamma class has been subdivided into g1 (group 1) and g2 (Leventhal, '82) and, in addition, delta (Boycott and Wässle, '74; Wässle and Boycott, '91) and epsilon cells (Leventhal et al., '80, '85; Leventhal, '82; Vitek et al., '85) have been described. The relationship of ferret "gamma" cells to these vari-

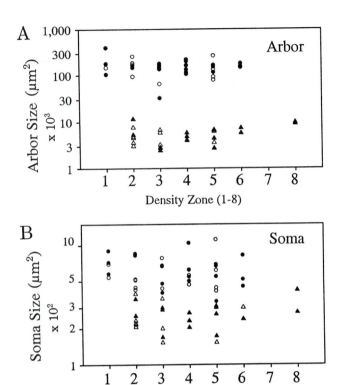

Fig. 5. Variation in cell dimensions with local cell density for the alpha (circles) and beta (triangles) retinal ganglion cell classes. Local density was assessed by plotting individual cell locations onto local density zones mapped out in Figure 1. Zones range, in steps of 500 mm^{-2}, from <500 mm^{-2} (zone 1) to >3,500 mm^{-2} (zone 8). **A:** Log arbor size with equivalent density zone (1–8). **B:** Log soma size with equivalent density zone (1–8). Inner and outer stratifying arbors are represented by empty and solid symbols, respectively. While the variation within each zone is clearly high, a sampling bias away from the highest density zones may account for the lack of a clear gradient in size with changing eccentricity.

ous classes is discussed. No bistratified cells were found in our sample.

Alpha Cells. The alpha class have the largest somas at a given retinal eccentricity, and can be easily distinguished prior to lucifer yellow injection on the basis of their size. In addition, fluorescent microspheres had a distinctly even distribution through the cell body that characteristically spread into the proximal primary dendrites. Figure 2A shows an intracellularly filled alpha cell photographed under UV epifluorescence, with filters passing green/yellow fluorescence. The same field is shown in Figure 2B, photographed with the appropriate filter set for rhodamine. The lucifer yellow filled dendrites are no longer revealed; however, the even distribution of diffuse, punctate fluorescence of rhodamine beads in the cell soma and proximal dendrites becomes visible. Although most cells in this retinal field are double la-

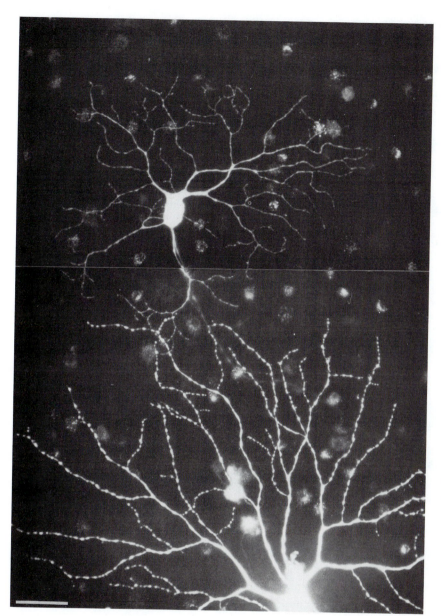

Fig. 6. Montage of photomicrographs showing the relationship of a "small" alpha cell (top) to an adjacent alpha cell (bottom) of normal dimensions. The former is distinguished by dendrites ramifying in the same layer of the inner plexiform layer (IPL) as the ganglion cell soma. The arbor of the "small" alpha cell resembles that of more central alpha cells (See Fig. 3D). While the soma and dendrites of the small alpha cell (above) are in the same focal plane, the soma of the alpha cell (below) is out of the focal plane. Scale bar = 50 μm.

belled, the cell body labelled with an asterisk in Figure 2A is labelled only with green beads and does not fluoresce in Figure 2B. Figure 3A–D shows photomicrographs of alpha cells of different sizes and detailed morphology. All cells were labelled with green beads whose fluorescence is obscured by the much brighter intracellular dye. Green beads are clearly visible in neighbouring soma that have not been filled with lucifer yellow. The cells in Figure 3B was retrogradely co-labelled with green beads from the LGN and red beads from the SC. A photomicrograph of the red bead label is shown in the inset.

In general, there appears to be no systematic variation in alpha cell dendritic morphology with retrograde label, or with cell size. Processes can be spiny or smooth regardless of dendritic branching pattern (con-

trast Fig. 3A with the relatively more twiggy Fig. 3B). Axons arise either from the perikaryon or from the largest of four to seven primary dendrites (12 out of 40 cases). Intraretinal axon calibers appear greater than in other cell classes. Axon trajectories are relatively undeviating, any corrections being consistent with the organisation of the raphe. Dendrites branch regularly and taper to form characteristically uniform dendritic fields. Alpha cells show the least mean displacement of soma relative to the centre of gravity of the arbor (11% ∓ 7.9). Both soma size (657–1,875 μm²) and arbor size (32,000–147,000 μm²) were found to be quite variable for any given density zone.

Figure 4 shows drawings from photomicrograph negatives of a variety of complete alpha cells. Cells with relatively smaller somas (Fig. 4i, iii, and v) are

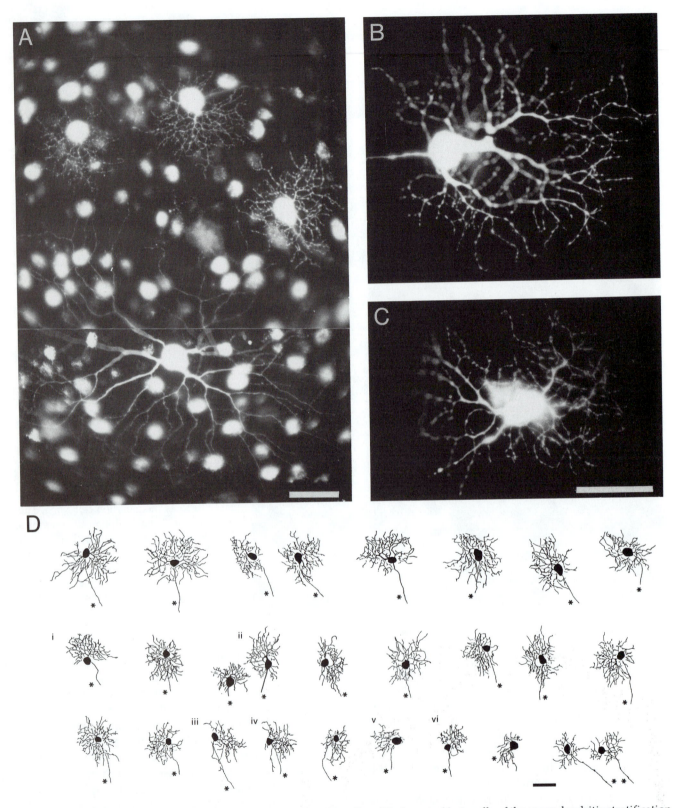

Fig. 7. Beta cells. **A:** Photomicrograph montage of three lucifer yellow filled, central beta cells of the same dendritic stratification in the IPL and adjacent to a morphologically distinct alpha cell. **B, C:** Photomicrographs of individual beta cells filled intracellularly with lucifer yellow in regions where background retrograde labelling was at a low density. **D:** Beta cell drawings chosen to represent a variety of sizes and morphologies. These are shown to the same scale as Figure 4 for comparison. Cells indicated (**i–vi**) are examples in which the centre of the dendritic arbor is considerably displaced relative to the soma. In i, ii, and vi, the direction of this displacement is away from the axon initial segment. Asterisk (*) denotes axons. Scale bars = 50 μm.

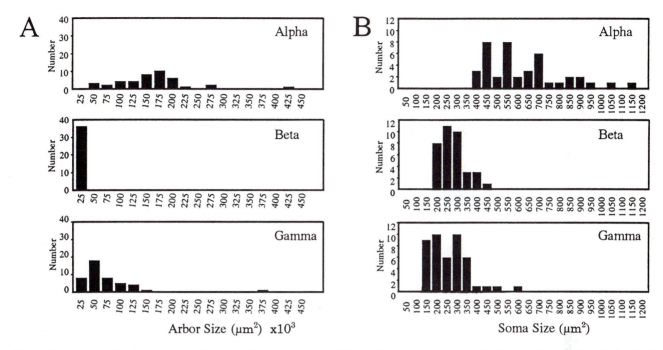

Fig. 8. Frequency distributions of arbor size (**A**) and soma size (**B**), pooled across all eccentricities, for three subjectively identified classes of ganglion cells: alpha, beta, and gamma. Within classes, there is no clear tendency for either arbor sizes or soma sizes to fall into clear size classes. Given the lack of clear central-peripheral size gradients, it seems unlikely that by comparing cells from across the extent of the retina we are obscuring any strong class differences. Unlike in the cat, alpha and beta arbor dimensions do not overlap. Gamma cell arbor sizes overlap both alpha and beta cells. Alpha cells show a generally larger cell body whilst gamma and beta soma sizes show highly overlapped distributions. The smallest soma sizes were found in the gamma population.

displayed next to cells with relatively larger cell bodies but similar dendritic extent (Fig. 4ii, iv, and vi) for comparison. A plot of arbor size against density zone reveals a shallow gradient of increasing arbor sizes with eccentricity (Fig. 5A) towards the periphery (zone 1), where both the largest arbors and range of arbor sizes are found. The variation in soma size with local cell density (Fig. 5B) reflects the morphological heterogeneity seen in Figure 4. This diversity of form does not seem to relate to which sublamina of the inner plexiform layer (IPL) a particular cell ramifies. Alpha cells clearly stratify in either outer or inner sublaminae of the inner plexiform layer but we found no systematic difference in the size of form of inner and outer arbors. Occasionally, the dendritic arbor of a particular alpha cell might be significantly smaller than those of its neighbours. Figure 6 shows one such cell in which axon, cell body, and dendrites are in focus. Part of the arbor of an adjacent alpha cell is also shown whose soma and axon lie out of the focal plane. These rare, small alpha cells are characterised by dendritic trees and cell bodies that lie in the same plane.

Beta cells. Beta cells have small densely branching arbors arising from one to four primary dendrites. The axons are of a smaller calibre than alpha cells and arise directly from the perikaryon (152–417 μm^2). The den-

dritic arbor (2,420–18,700 μm^2) arises from one to four primary dendrites and is relatively complex. Figure 7A shows a photomicrograph of a central retinal field in which one alpha and three adjacent beta cells have been filled with lucifer yellow. Figure 7B and C shows higher power photomicrographs of typical beta cells from a retinal region where the background retrograde label was low.

Although the morphology of beta cells is quite distinct from that of alpha cells at any given retinal location (compare Figs. 4 and 7D, which are to the same scale), Figure 7D does show variability within the population. Beta cells can ramify in either the inner or outer sublaminae of the inner plexiform layer but this does not correlate with any heterogeneities in dendritic morphology. At any particular eccentricity, sizes can be variable and the soma considerably displaced from the geometric centre of the arbor (33% ∓ 19). In Figure 7D, the tracings of serial photomicrographs of beta cells labelled i–vi represent cases where the arbor and soma have very different centres of gravity. Note that the arbor tends to be displaced away from the origin of the axon initial segment (also Fig. 7B and Di, ii, and vi). We found little variation with eccentricity in the distribution of beta soma sizes or dendritic arbors (Fig. 5A,B). When the sizes of alpha and beta cells are compared

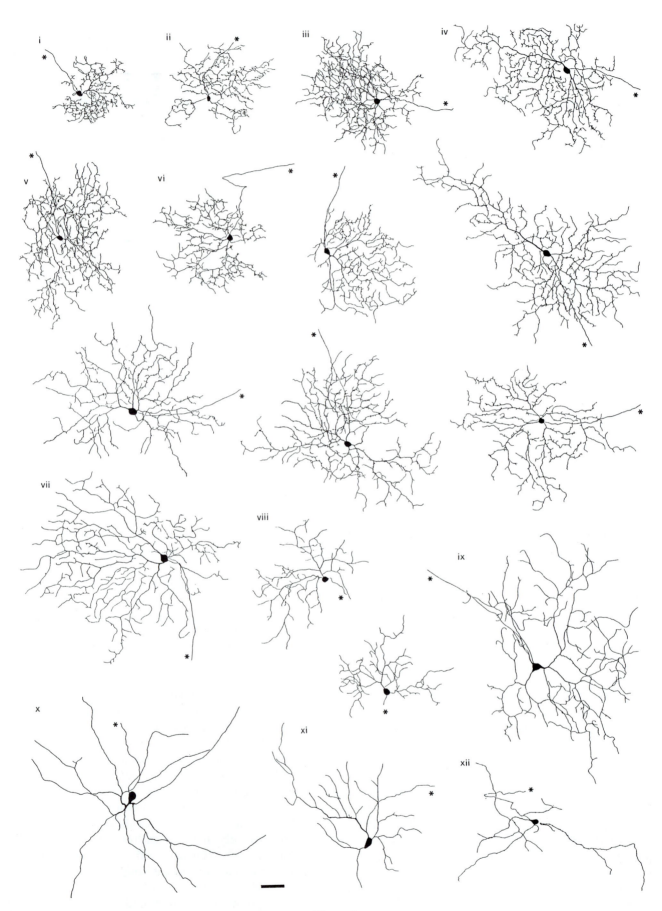

Figure 9

(Fig. 8), there is no overlap in arbor size distribution and only a small overlap in the distribution of soma sizes, although within any one density zone this overlap is minimal (Fig. 5B).

Gamma cells. The third major class of cells consists of a heterogeneous distribution of morphologies that are clearly neither alpha nor beta (Figs. 9–11). For the smallest cells of beta cell arbor dimensions, cell bodies tend to be relatively smaller, and dendritic processes thinner and spinier. For the largest gamma cells, overlapping alpha soma and arbor dimensions, dendritic branching is less orderly and processes more curved. The range of cell body sizes (115–569 μm^2) is coincident with the beta class (Fig. 8A) whilst arbor sizes (63,000–368,000 μm^2) are intermediate between beta and alpha ranges (Fig. 8B). Axons arise from the perikaryon or occasionally the initial segment of one of 2–8 primary dendrites. Axon calibers tend to be relatively smaller and more erratic in their initial trajectories than alpha cells. Given the heterogeneity of this class, a plot of size measurements with equivalent cell density yields no information. Figure 9 shows drawings of the range of dendritic arbors that are characteristically encountered, ranging from the most complex (top left) to the sparsest (bottom right).

The most densely branched, "tight" gamma cell arbors (Figs. 9i–vi, 10A–D) have very fine, spiny processes, resembling the rodent type II morphology as described by Perry ('79). Figure 10 shows photomicrographs of four cells classed as tight. Despite the density of branching, their fine processes and relatively small somas distinguish these from beta cells. Less highly branching "loose" morphologies (Figs. 9vii–ix, 11A) show complexities similar to those of alpha cells. These resemble rodent type I cells (Perry, '79) and, to a certain extent, the delta cells of the cat (Boycott and Wässle, '74). Loose and tight forms stratify in either the inner or outer IPL. Where "loose" gamma cells overlap alpha cells in size, alpha cells remain distinct on the basis of their retrograde label pattern, axon caliber and straightness, and characteristic regular dendritic branching style. This region of morphological overlap is described more fully below.

There is a range of intermediate forms of gamma cell, so that the labels "tight" and "loose" apply to quite distinct extremes of an apparently continuous distribution. Additionally, a number of gamma cells show sparsely branching dendritic trees (Figs. 9x-xii, 11B,C), reminiscent of the rodent type III morphology (Perry, '79) and cat gamma and epsilon cells. Again this "sparse" subclass is subjectively continuous with "loose" forms. Given the nature of this variation, we will use the labels as an aid to description rather than as definitions of rigid subtypes. However, cells subjectively classified as tight or loose do tend to differ parametrically (Fig. 12). Tight cells tend to have relatively smaller somas for a given arbor size when compared to loose cells.

Although there is some degree of overlap in soma and arbor dimensions between alpha, beta, and gamma cells, these groups can be contrasted by using only these measures and regardless of dendritic complexity. By plotting log arbor area versus the log of the cross-sectional area of the cell body, the three major classes can be seen to cluster differently in the plane of morphological space (Fig. 13). A region of overlap between gamma and alpha cells represents morphologies that differ in only branching characteristics and is described fully below. Semi-schematic outlines of the territories occupied by each cell class were superimposed onto each cluster after Leventhal et al. ('80). This mapping of a subjective classification onto a quantitative space provides a descriptive template by which populations of cells characterised by their projection patterns can be compared.

Cell types and axonal targets

Injections of retrograde tracer into the projection nuclei of the optic pathway allowed us to correlate axonal projections and branching patterns in terms of dendritic morphology. The combination of direct visualisation of the midbrain and thalamus during injection and the limited diffusion properties of the latex microspheres allowed accurate labelling of target nuclei. Reconstruction of injection sites revealed that placement of retrograde tracer outside the boundaries of the intended target nuclei was very limited. Figure 14 shows photomicrographs of typical injection sites in the lateral geniculate nucleus (Fig. 14A,D), pretectum (Fig. 14B,E), and superior colliculus (Fig. 14C,F), contrasting Nissl stained sections (above) with the fluorescence image of the adjacent section (below). The possibility of uptake by fibres of passage was investigated in one animal, illustrated in Figure 15, by making rostral versus caudal placements of red and green fluorescent microspheres into the superior colliculus. Discrete patches of the temporal/central and nasal retina were labelled, respectively, with no double labelled cells in the former (Fig. 15C), despite the fact that the rostral injection site passes through the stratum

Fig. 9. Gamma cell drawings showing a representative sample of different morphologies. Morphologies show a continuous gradation of form, from "tight" (top let **i–vi**), to "loose" (**vii–ix**), to "sparse" (bottom right, **x–xii**). The density zone (1–8) for each labelled cell and for i–x, whether its arbor is inner (*i*) or outer (*o*) to stratifying are as follows: i, 3*o*; ii, 5*o*; iii, 5*o*; iv, 3*o*; v, 3*o*; vi, 3*i*; vii, 5*o*; viii, 2*o*; ix, 1*i*; x, 5*o*; xi, 2; xii, 2. Asterisk (*) denotes axons. Scale bar = 50 μm.

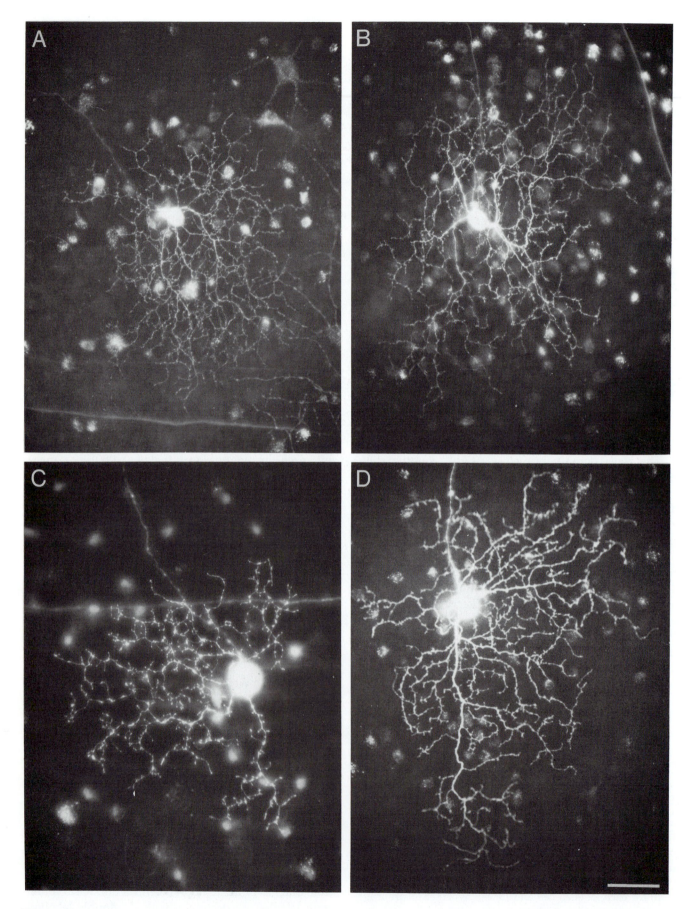

Fig. 10. Photomicrographs of four lucifer yellow filled gamma cells (**A–D**), classified as tight. Dendritic processes are thin and display numerous large spines or twigs. Scale bar = 50 μm.

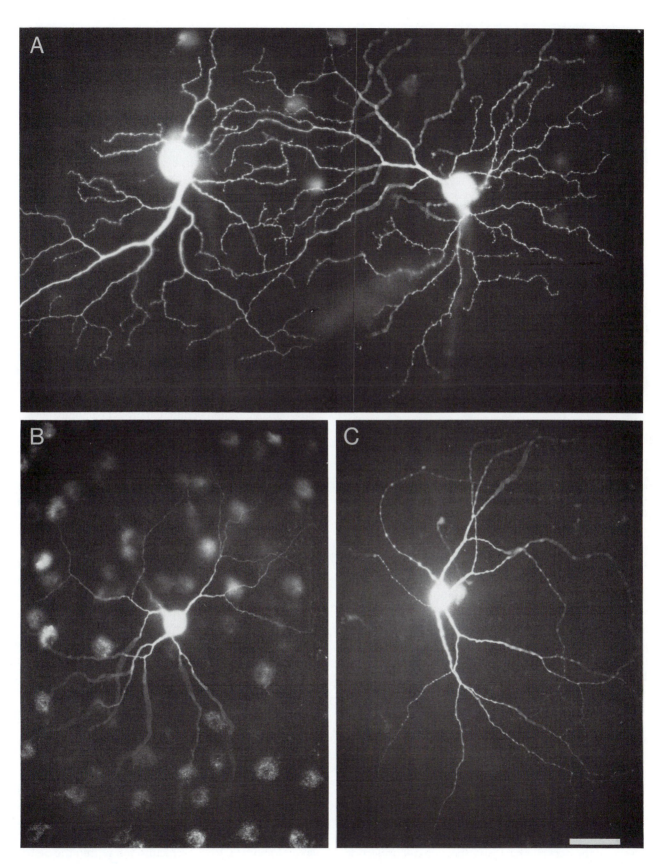

Fig. 11. Photomicrographs of loose and sparse gamma cells. **A:** Montage of adjacent lucifer yellow filled cells from the ipsilateral projection in the temporal crescent. Both of these cells have been classified as loose, on the basis of an intermediate dendritic complexity. Notice that both dendritic arbors are spiny. **B, C:** Sparse retinal ganglion cells with smooth, infrequently branching processes. Scale bar = 50 μm.

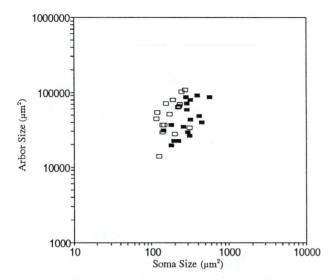

Fig. 12. The relationship between subjectively classified loose (filled square, ■) and tight (empty square, □) gamma cells on a double log plot of arbor size vs. soma size (both μm²).

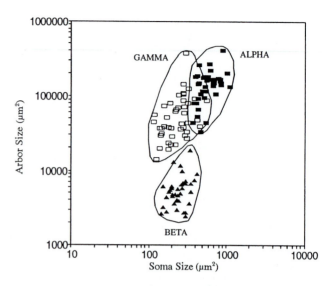

Fig. 13. Comparison of arbor and soma dimensions between classes. Different morphological classes—alpha (filled square, ■), beta (filled triangle, ▲), and gamma (empty square, □)—are segregated on the basis of a double log plot of arbor size vs. soma size (both μm²). Semi-schematic outlines of the territories occupied by each cell class are drawn around the clusters. These outlines are used as a template by which to assess the composition of different projection populations.

opticum containing fibres of passage running to the caudal pole.

Whilst the limited spread of tracer within the injection site allows a confident identification of target for each labelled retinal ganglion cell body, it also can result in a patchy overall pattern of labelling. This means that while cells containing the two tracers can be identified unambiguously as having bifurcating axons, the presence of only one tracer does not rule out the possibility of branching axons. Although we attempted to sample regions of the retina that were well labelled with both tracers, we have not used the absence of double labelling by retrograde tracers to discriminate otherwise identical sets of cells.

In the following section, cell soma sizes are plotted against dendritic arbor sizes for different populations that have been characterised on the basis of their projection patterns.

Lateral geniculate nucleus versus superior colliculus. Retrograde label from the SC and LGN labels populations across the entire extent of the retina. Plotting dendritic area as a function of soma size reveals the heterogeneity of lucifer yellow filled cells with respect to the projections (Fig. 16A). Cells labelled from the LGN (solid squares) are found across all morphological types. Cells that project to the SC are distributed only through the alpha and gamma classes; none can be seen in the beta cluster. Thus, the beta cell projection is to LGN but not SC. Of the cells projecting to the SC, 67% were also labelled retrogradely from the LGN. However, gamma or alpha cells labelled with both retrograde tracers were not restricted to any observed

morphological subtypes. The number of lucifer yellow injected cells projecting to these nuclei are summarised in Table 1.

Pretectum versus superior colliculus. An injection of tracer into the pretectum labelled a population of retinal ganglion cells scattered at a low density across the extent of the retina. A discrete injection of contrasting tracer into the caudal SC produced a focus of uniform labelling in nasal retina. In this region, cells co-labelled from both nuclei were encountered. The dendritic morphologies of cells projecting to the pretectum all fell into the gamma category. Cells that had no observable projection to the SC (i.e., cell bodies within the focus of retrograde label from the SC but only labelled with tracer injected into the pretectum) had "tight" dendritic arbors composed of very fine processes (Fig. 17) and small somas (41–252 μm2). The overall distribution of arbor and soma sizes of cells projecting to the pretectum overlaps with the rest of the gamma population (Fig. 18). When log dendritic arbor size was plotted as a function of log soma area (Fig. 16B), these cells partially overlapped the gamma cluster defined in Figure 13. Cells with a branching axon to both SC and pretectum fell within the distribution already observed for loose and sparse cells with an SC projection.

The ipsilateral projection. Ganglion cells projecting ipsilaterally to the midbrain and thalamus are prin-

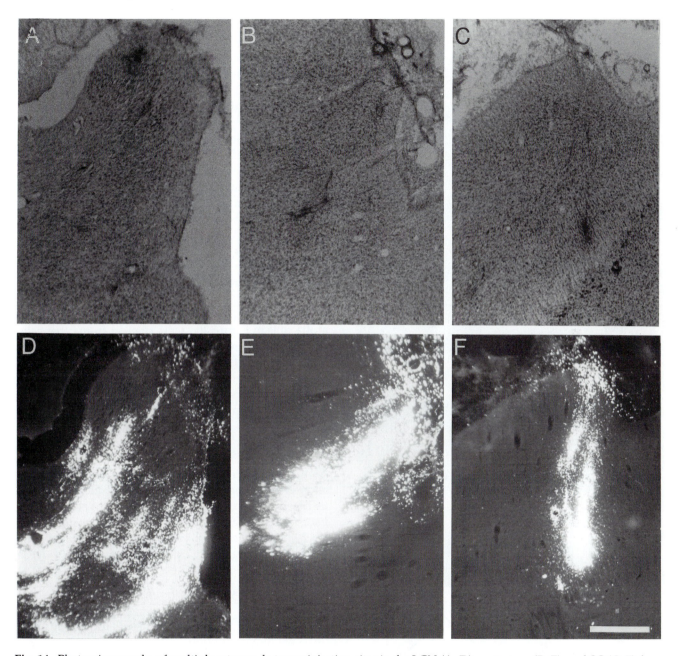

Fig. 14. Photomicrographs of multiple retrograde tracer injection sites in the LGN (**A, D**), pretectum (**B, E**), and SC (**C, F**) from different animals. Parasagittal sections were cut at 50 μm thickness. Nissl stained sections are shown above, with the fluorescence image of an adjacent, unstained section below. In F, only one of several injection sites is visible. Adjacent sections show both more rostral and more caudal sites. The rostral-caudal axis is left to right; superior–inferior, top to bottom. Tracer was delivered by multiple punctate deliveries of beads into the nuclei. The spread of tracer by diffusion within the injection site was very limited. Scale bar = 500 μm.

cipally found in a distinct temporal crescent. Outside this region, only a very small population of scattered cells projects to the ipsilateral LGN and/or SC. This latter population is aberrant in that a correct binocular topography cannot be present at their axonal targets. In terms of arbor size and soma size, aberrant ipsilateral (ABIPSI) retinal ganglion cells show a range of arbor and soma sizes similar to gamma cells (Fig. 18A,B).

The ipsilateral projection does not display the full complement of cell types (summarised in Table 2). Figure 19 shows a representative selection of dendritic morphologies. Most notably, we found no alpha cells with an uncrossed projection in the temporal crescent. In addition, there are no gamma cells with tightly branching, spiny dendritic arbors. Our impression was that the loose gamma cells formed a regular matrix

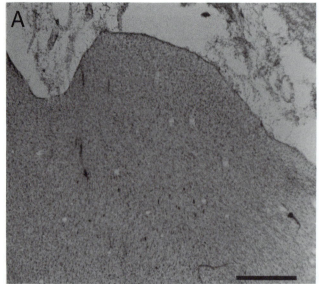

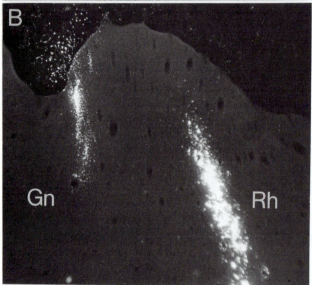

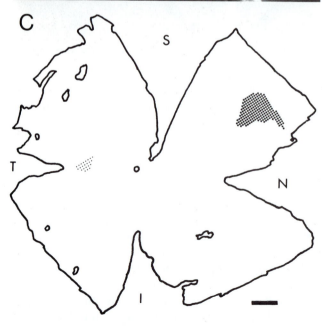

(see, for example, the adjacent cells in Fig. 11A) and in general branched to both the SC and LGN. This matrix is independent of the beta cell matrix in which the arbors are smaller and the cells only project to the LGN.

In Figure 20, the clusterings of alpha, beta, and gamma cells within contralateral and ipsilateral projections are compared. The region of overlap between alpha and gamma cells in terms of arbor and soma size is examined in detail. In the contralateral projection (Fig. 20A), all the cells in the region of overlap between the alpha and gamma templates in Figure 13 have an alpha morphology. Drawings of examples of these alpha cells (Fig. 20α) are contrasted with cells from the same "space" in the arbor size—soma size distribution that project ipsilaterally (Fig. 20γ). Though of similar dimensions (Fig. 20B), these cells were indistinguishable from surrounding retrogradely labelled beta cells on the basis of some size prior to injection of lucifer yellow. By comparison, the corresponding alpha cells in Figure 20α were distinct from other cells on the basis of retrograde label alone. Their dendritic branching patterns are different from the gamma cells in Figure 20γ, with more regular branching and fewer internodal twigs. A comparison of the overall contralateral and ipsilateral gamma cell has a generally smaller arbor as a function of soma size. This corresponds to the observation that tight morphologies are lacking from the ipsilateral projection (see Fig. 12 for a comparison of the soma and arbor dimensions of loose and tight morphologies). The small sample of aberrant ipsilateral cells shows a range of soma and arbor dimensions in both the gamma and beta size range (Figs. 17, 20), but the cells all have a uniformly sparse dendritic morphology (Fig. 20C).

Quantifying morphological diversity

The distribution of fractal dimensions in various identified ganglion cell populations is shown in Figure 21.

Fig. 15. Localised dual injection of tracer into the SC. **A:** Nissl stained parasagittal section through both injection sites. The rostral-caudal axis runs right to left. **B:** Double-exposure photomicrograph of an adjacent section with UV epi-illumination and appropriate filters for green and red fluorescence wavelengths. A single injection of green beads (Gn) was made into the caudal SC while a larger and deeper injection of red beads (rhodamine, Rh) was made into the rostral SC. Adjacent sections show rhodamine fluorescence in superficial, rostral SC. Scale bar = 500 μm. **C:** A camera lucida drawing of the pattern of labelling in the right retina 1 week after injection shows two foci of retrograde label. Green beads accumulate in cell bodies in the nasal periphery (heavy shading), while red beads are taken up by a much more restricted area of ganglion cells in the temporal retina (light shading). Scale bar = 1 mm.

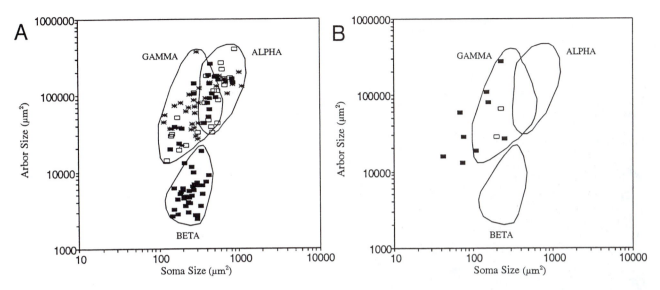

Fig. 16. The morphology of cells with different central projections as assessed by a double log plot of arbor vs. soma size (both μm²). Superimposed is the template of cell classes derived from Figure 13. **A:** Cells projecting to the LGN only (filled squares, ■), to the SC only (empty squares, □), and to both SC and LGN (asterisks, *). **B:** Cells with a projection to the pretectum (filled squares, ■) and with a projection to both SC and pretectum (empty squares, □).

Table 1. Summary of the Number of Lucifer Yellow Filled Cells and Their Projections, for Animals in Which Contrasting Retrograde Tracers Were Injected Into the Lateral Geniculate Nucleus (LGN) and Superior Colliculus (SC)

	SC	SC and LGN	LGN	Total
Alpha	11	11	16	38
Beta	—	—	34	34
Gamma	6	24	6	36

Although the range of alpha fractal dimensions overlaps that of beta and gamma cells, it has significantly different distribution characteristics from both (Mann–Whitney U test: alpha vs. beta, $z = 2.89$, $P = 0.0036$; and alpha vs. gamma, $z = 2.23$ $P = 0.0258$, respectively, for a two-tailed test). The broader range of gamma cell complexity matches the observed diversity of form, with no clear peak in the distribution. The range of beta cell complexities falls within that of the gamma distribution, but is shifted to lower values. Similarly, cells that branch to the pretectum show a broad range of complexities that are coincident with the gamma distribution. The population of aberrant cells has a highly significantly reduced space-filling capacity when compared to the other classes ($z = 4.28$, $P < 0.00006$, for a two-tailed test).

While the fractal dimension describes the space-filling characteristics of an arbor, the branching complexity of dendritic structure can also be examined semi-topologically. The total length of processes con-

tributing to the dendritic tree can be divided by the number of terminal segments in the arbor to give a rough approximation of how often dendrites branch in each arbor. Since this value is proportional to the extent of the dendritic tree, it has been scaled by dividing by the Feret radius of the expanded pixel cell image. This produces a dimensionless value, T, that is independent of the arbor size (Fig. 22A). The larger this value, the greater the mean relative length of dendrite contributing to each terminal segment for the particular cell. The frequency distribution of these values is plotted for each of the different cell classes in Figure 22B.

Alpha and beta cells show similarly unimodal distributions with similar modal values of T, while the range of values of T displayed in the gamma class is much greater and skewed towards the lower values. Our sample beta distribution extends higher than that of alpha cells and is significantly different from that of the gamma cell sample (Mann–Whitney U test: gamma vs. beta, $z = 2.15$, $P = 0.011$, for a two-tailed test). By comparison, aberrant ipsilateral cells show far less branching (large T) than any of these three groups and have a highly significant different range of T values ($z = 4.74$, $P = 0.00006$, for a two-tailed test). As with values of Df, the spread of values for cells with a projection to the pretectum is coincident with the gamma distribution.

When the log of T is plotted against fractal dimension, the various cell types as defined by their sizes maintain integral clusters in nonparametric space (Fig. 23). However, their distribution is no longer discrete. Alpha and beta cells converge onto the same cluster,

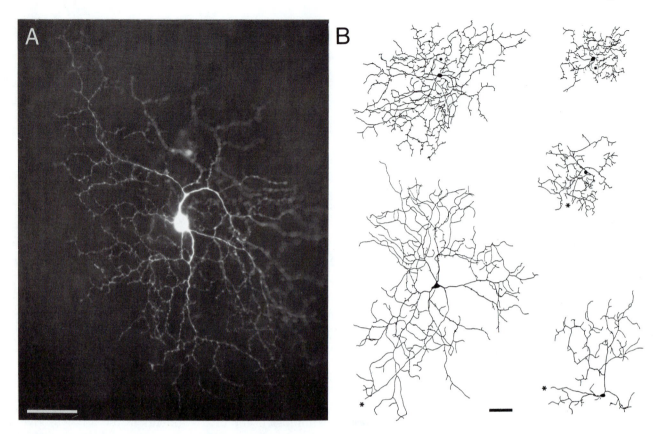

Fig. 17. Retinal ganglion cells with a projection to the pretectum. **A:** Photomicrograph showing the comparatively delicate dendritic processes that typify such cells. **B:** Drawings of a selection of retinal ganglion cells with a projection to the pretectum but with no observed axonal branching to the SC within the region of double retrograde label from pretectum and SC. Asterisk (*) denotes axons. Scale bars = 50 μm.

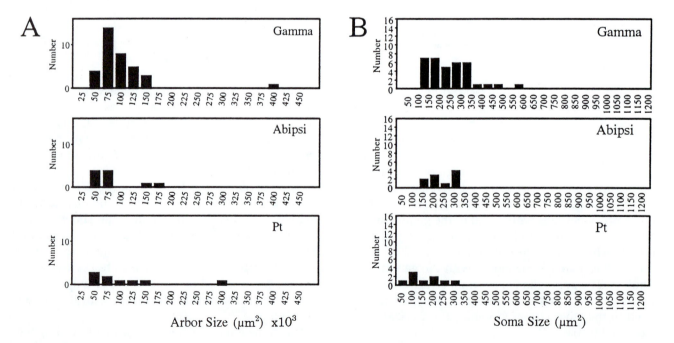

Fig. 18. Frequency distributions within non-alpha and non-beta cells. **A:** Arbor sizes. **B:** Soma sizes. The gamma population has been subdivided so that aberrant nasal ganglion cells with an ipsilateral projection (Abipsi, middle) can be compared to the rest of the gamma population (above). Both are contrasted with the population of ganglion cells with a pretectal projection that contains cells with the smallest cell bodies (Pt, below).

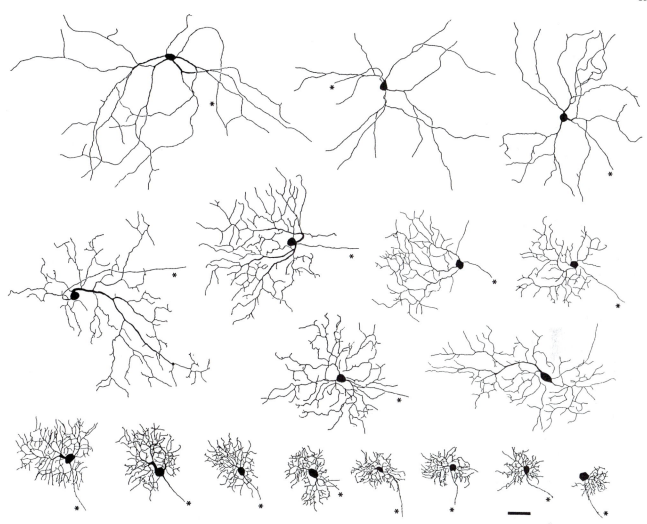

Fig. 19. Cells with an ipsilateral projection to the midbrain. The projection from the temporal crescent includes sparse and loose gamma cells (top and middle) and beta cells (bottom). Beta cells only project to the LGN; gamma cells may send axons to the LGN and/or SC. Asterisk (*) denotes axons. Scale bar = 50 μm.

indicating that their complexity is achieved by similar relative branching characteristics (Fig. 23A). Gamma cells of the same fractal complexity have a lower value of T, but overlap the alpha and beta cluster as their fractal complexity decreases (Fig. 23B). Gamma cells with an equivalent or lower branching "rate" than alpha and beta cells, in terms of a large T value, achieve a lower fractal complexity. Hence the cluster of gamma cell types is essentially a continuous distribution of complexities where space-filling capacity (as Df) increases as the frequency of branching increases. This is in distinct contrast to alpha and beta cells, which show no marked relationship of Df with T. This difference in behaviour is demonstrated explicitly in Figure 23C. The sparsest (aberrant ipsilateral) gamma cells (low Df) have the lowest branching rate. The medium complex,

"loose" gamma cells overlap the alpha/beta distribution. The most complex, "tight" gamma cells branch relatively more often than alpha/beta cells of a similar fractal dimension.

DISCUSSION

In this study we have used intracellular injection of lucifer yellow to extend previous descriptions of ferret retinal ganglion cells that were based on retrograde HRP transport studies (Vitek et al., '85; Morgan et al., '87). The intracellular fills have confirmed their basic categorisation of ferret retinal ganglion cells into alpha, beta, and gamma classes whose morphologies closely resemble those found in the cat (Boycott and Wässle,

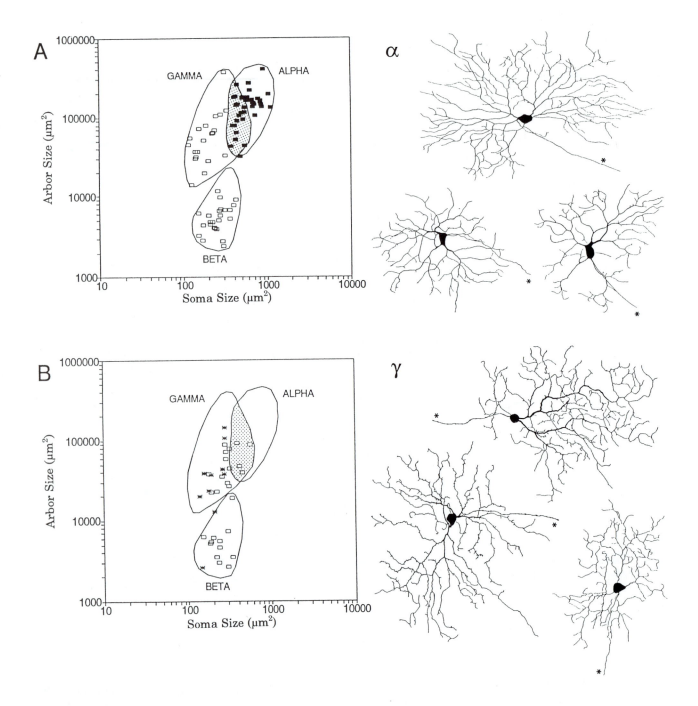

C: Aberrant

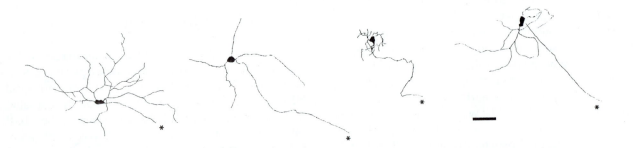

Figure 20

'74; Wässle and Boycott, '91), where they have been shown to correspond to separate Y, X, and W physiological types (Enroth–Cugell and Robson, '66; Peichl and Wässle, '81, '83; Saíto, '83; Stanford, '87). Quantitative description of soma and arbor dimensions and a fractal analysis of complexity have revealed varying degrees of diversity within and between these ganglion cell classes. By employing retrograde tracers in conjunction with morphometric techniques, we have been able to examine whether this diversity relates to the organisation of retinofugal projections.

Our approach has shown that there is indeed a systematic variation in both decussation pattern and target nuclei with different types of dendritic morphology. This is true for the alpha and beta cells and, notably, within the variable gamma population. It has also enabled us to quantitatively describe the nature of alpha, beta, and gamma categories, which should prove useful in understanding the generation of retinal ganglion cell diversity during development.

Table 2. Composition of Ipsilateral (IPSI), Aberrant Ipsilateral (ABIPSI), and Contralateral (CONTRA) Projections in Terms of the presence (Y) or Absence (—) of Identified Morphological Classes

	IPSI	**ABIPSI**	**CONTRA**
Alpha	—	—	Y
Beta	Y	—	Y
Gamma (sparse)	Y	Y	Y
Gamma (loose)	Y	—	Y
Gamma (tight)	—	—	Y

Fig. 20. Comparison of the contralateral (**A**) and ipsilateral (**B**) projections in terms of the dendritic arbor vs. soma dimensions of their constituents. Cells identified as alpha are shown as solid squares (■). In B, cells projecting ipsilaterally from the nasal retina are shown as asterisks (*). Superimposed on each is the template of identified cell types derived from Figure 7. The region where alpha cell and gamma cell clusters overlap is stippled, and the representative cells from this region of morphological space from each projection are shown to the right. In the contralateral projection, only alpha cells are found in this region (α). In the ipsilateral projection, the region of overlap defines loose gamma cells (γ). Despite similar dimensions, the dendritic branching of the gamma cells is less regular. Individual gamma cell dendrites meander more and produce shorter collaterals than in an equivalent alpha cell. Aberrant ipsilateral retinal ganglion cells fall into both gamma and beta clusters in B. **C:** Drawings of aberrant ipsilateral cells showing their distinctly sparse dendritic morphology. In α, γ, and C, asterisk (*) denotes axons. Scale bars = 50 μm.

In considering these results there are certain technical limitations that place constraints on the interpretation and analysis of our data. By combining the use of three tracers, our sample rates are necessarily low. In addition, the complete dendritic fills required for fractal measures required that poor intracellular fills were rejected. While the choice of retrograde tracer ensured

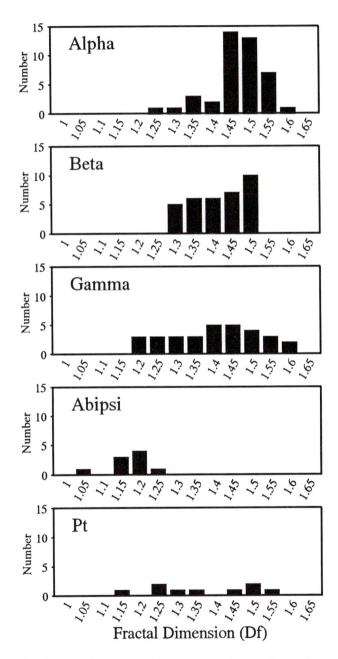

Fig. 21. The frequency distributions of fractal dimensions (*Df*) within four identified populations of retinal ganglion cells: alpha, beta, gamma, and aberrant cells (Abipsi). The alpha distribution is significantly different from the gamma and beta distributions. Aberrant ipsilateral ganglion cells have a significantly different distribution from alpha, beta, and gamma cells. See text for details. Pt, cells that branch to the pretectum.

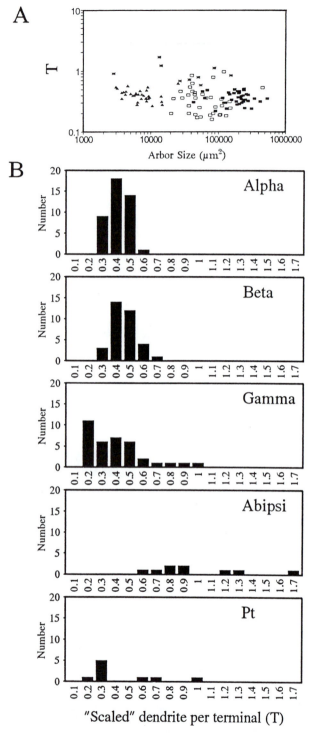

Fig. 22. A: The relationship of T, a scaled measure of branching, with dendritic area, demonstrating its invariance with size for alpha (solid square, ■), beta (solid triangle, ▲), gamma (empty square, □), and aberrant (asterisk, *) classes. **B:** The frequency distributions of the scaled branching "rates" (T) within five identified populations of alpha, beta, gamma, aberrant cells (Abipsi), and cells that branch to the pretectum (Pt). The gamma distribution is significantly different from the beta distribution. Aberrant ipsilateral retinal ganglion cells have a significantly different distribution from alpha, beta, and gamma cells. See text for details.

unambiguous labelling and compatibility with in vitro intracellular dye injection, the limited spread of beads from their punctate injection sites meant that the distribution of labelled cells was patchy. This has two consequences. Firstly, an absence of label is not always diagnostic of absence of a projection. Secondly, the local density of retrograde label could not be used to assess retinal ganglion cell numbers reliably. Since the usual Nissl counterstains are incompatible with fluorescence, ganglion cell density gradients had to be derived from previously published data, as opposed to calculating the exact local density for any particular filled cell.

Alpha and beta cells

Ferret alpha and beta cells are strikingly similar to those of the cat. Both display inner and outer stratifying subtypes and we can presume that this gives rise to Y_{ON} Y_{OFF} X_{ON} X_{OFF} units found in the ferret LGN (Stryker and Zahs, '83; Price and Morgan, '87; Roe et al., '89). Peichl et al. ('87b) reported arbor coverage differences between inner and outer mosaics in the ferret. We were unable to measure differences in the dimensions of arbors stratifying in different sublaminae of the IPL. The only exception was a group of very small alpha cells characterised by arbors that stratified next to the ganglion cell layer and that may represent developmental anomalies. However, alpha heterogeneity has been reported in the cat on the basis of, for example, selective immunoreactivity to somatostatin (White and Chalupa, '91) and subdivisions of ferret alpha class cannot be ruled out.

Two features of cat alpha and beta cells that we did not observe in the ferret are a consistently oriented displacement of dendritic fields relative to their cell bodies and the shaping of the arbors into oriented ellipses. In the cat, Schall and Leventhal ('87) argue that while the displacement of dendritic fields relative to their cell bodies follows the local ganglion cell density gradient, the elliptical shape and orientation of these fields relates to the geometry of retinal maturation, which is centred on the area centralized (Walsh and Polley, '85). In the ferret, there is a far shallower ganglion cell density gradient in the adult and much more uniform expansion of the retina during development (Henderson, '85; Henderson et al., '88). Spatial distribution of retinal ganglion cell somas and, moreover, the actual extent of their dendritic arbors can be strongly influenced by competitive dendritic interactions (Linden and Perry, '82; Perry and Linden, '82; Eysel et al., '85; Kirby and Chalupa, '86; Leventhal et al., '88). In the ferret, where the local gradients of ganglion cell density are far lower than in the cat, the differential dendritic competition across an array of arbors that could lead to a consistently oriented displacement of dendritic fields relative

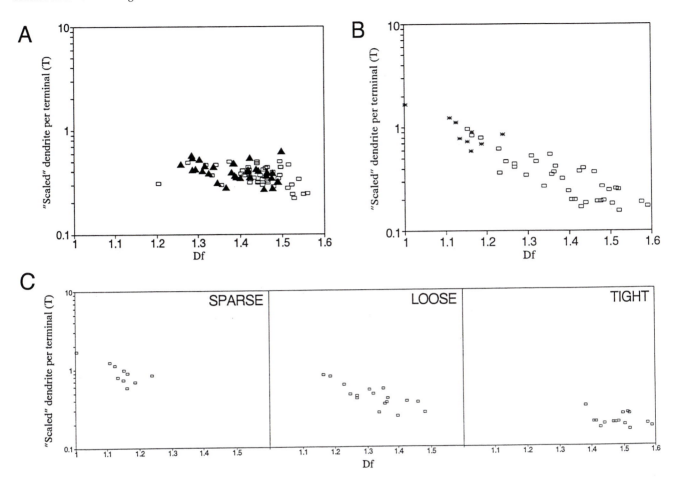

Fig. 23. Segregation of morphological classes on the basis of branching characteristics shown by plotting log T vs. Df. **A:** Alpha (empty square, □) and beta (filled triangle, ▲) populations. **B:** Gamma (empty square, □) and aberrant ipsilateral (asterisk, *) populations. **C:** Subdivisions of the gamma cell class. Subjective classification of gamma cells into three types on the basis of dendritic complexity can be seen to cluster together, quantitatively, on the basis of T and Df.

to cell bodies would be lacking. In addition, a less specialised area centralis, reflecting shallower gradients of retinal maturation, might account for our inability to detect oriented elliptical dendritic fields. The lack of such arbors in either alpha or beta cells may not be too surprising, as they are not a general feature of mammalian retinae (see Watanabe and Rodieck, '89).

However, dendritic competition is not necessarily reduced in the ferret retina. Class related variation in the general degree of displacement of cell bodies relative to their arbors may point to underlying stochastic variations in the characteristic mosaics of each cell class. Local dendritic competition (Perry and Maffei, '88) might be expected to compensate for irregularities in the packing of cell somas to produce a nevertheless even coverage of dendritic arbors. A more irregular array of somas will consequently have a higher general soma/arbor displacement. The higher value of this displacement that we measure in the beta cell population may hence reflect a less regular overall packing of beta

cell bodies. The lower gradient of change of packing density in both alpha and beta cells may similarly determine the relatively weak increase in both soma and arbor size with increasing eccentricity, which is a marked feature of cat and primate (Leventhal and Schall, '89).

The lack of a beta cell projection to the SC agrees with previous studies of decussation patterns in the ferret (Morgan et al., '87). The X-pathway carries the qualitative, "fine-grain," linear component of the visual image. The SC is conventionally seen as an attentional centre regulating eye movement and orientation, whereas the LGN provides the major afferent pathways for higher visual processing. The lack of a detectable alpha component in the ipsilateral projection has been observed before (Vitek et al., '85; Reese and Baker, '90; Thompson et al., '91). The implication is that the relatively "coarse," movement sensitive, Y-cell input does not contribute directly to binocular spatial analysis in the ferret.

Subdivisions of the gamma cell class

The considerable diversity of cells classified as non-alpha and non-beta is in agreement with previous studies on the ferret and cat; however, the general complexity of their dendritic form is not. Complex dendritic forms in the gamma cell class have rarely been described in carnivores (see, however, Fig. 2 of Stone and Clarke, '80) and yet are common in lucifer yellow material (see Fig. 8 of Ramoa et al., '88). It is possible that the fineness of gamma dendritic processes prejudices their labelling in retrogradely labelled HRP material. The sparse morphologies of gamma (g1 and g2), delta, and epsilon cells described in such studies may well be poorly filled examples of the cells described here. It hence seems appropriate to try to relate our own classifications to the standard morphological classes in the cat.

Gamma cells in the ferret are best described in terms of three archetypal forms within a continuous distribution. Loose gamma cells correspond approximately to the description of delta cells in rat (Peichl, '89) and cat (Boycott and Wässle, '74; Wässle and Boycott, '91). The most complex forms overlap the "tight" gamma morph. The presence of inner and outer forms of both these archetypes suggests that they contribute to ON- and OFF- pathways. The lack of the "tight" gamma morphology from the ipsilateral projection suggests that this type is discrete from the loose gamma cell. Disregarding their branching density, smaller cell bodies as a function of arbor size (Fig. 12) would label "tight" gamma cells as epsilon cells by previous schema (Leventhal et al., '80, '85). The remaining "sparse" forms correspond to the gamma cells as originally described in the cat (Boycott and Wässle, '74).

While our subjective subgroups did not correlate to specific projections to either the LGN or the SC, they demonstrate different decussation patterns at the optic chiasm. Tight gamma cells are restricted to the contralateral projection while the ipsilateral projection from the temporal crescent contains only loose and sparse gamma cells. In the cat, this ipsilateral, W-cell projection has a mainly tonic physiological response while the contralateral W-cell population is mainly phasic (Stone and Fukuda, '74). This implies that both the "fine" (beta/X-cell) and "coarse-grain" (gamma/W-cell) components of the ferret ipsilateral retinal output are broadly tonic.

The variation in decussation pattern that is seen between different retinal ganglion cell classes in the cat (Stone and Fukuda, '74; Wässle and Illing, '80; Illing and Wässle, '81) has been correlated with different relative birth dates (Walsh et al., '83). The pattern of fibre reordering in the retinal pathways of both cat and ferret also implies a relationship between decussation and the time of axon arrival at the chiasm (Walsh, '86;

Baker, '90; Reese and Baker, '90; Reese et al., '91). This relationship has been made explicit in cell birth-dating studies in the rodent (Dräger, '85), which showed that contralaterally projecting cells in the temporal retina are born after ipsilaterally projecting cells. Extending these arguments to gamma cells in the ferret predicts that "loose" gamma (delta-like) ganglion cells that project ipsilaterally from the temporal crescent are born earlier than the exclusively uncrossed, "tight" variant. The presence of discontinuous decussation patterns within the gamma cell grouping, which may relate to neuronal birth dates, strengthens the argument for a greater diversity of function for these cell types.

The aberrant ipsilaterally projecting cells outside the temporal crescent were uniformly sparse and of a significantly lower mean fractal dimension. Although the sample was admittedly small, a particularly sparse morphology is believed to be associated with anomalous development in both the hamster (Wingate and Thompson, '89a,b; Wingate, '90) and the rat (Yamasaki and Ramoa, '90).

The specialised input to the pretectum, which includes very small cells, is consistent with findings in the cat by HRP studies (Koontz et al., '85). The absence of such small retinal ganglion cells from the projection to the lateral geniculate nucleus is another indication that uptake by fibres of passage was not a problem in our preparation. The pretectal region contains a number of nuclei, which makes functional interpretation of a specialised input difficult to interpret. However, in the ferret the nucleus of the optic tract receives a binocular input and may compare the consistency of image movement across the retinae of both eyes (Klauer et al., '90).

Quantitative taxonomy of retinal ganglion cells

The use of fractal measures to describe the complexity of essentially planar neurons has been justified in various studies of cultured and in vitro retinal ganglion cells (Montague and Friedlander, '89, '91; Morigiwa et al., '89; Smith et al., '89; Caserta et al., '90; Wingate et al., '90). However, as a tool for categorising neurons it has been of little use. While correlating well with perceived complexity (Cutting and Garvin, '87) and, indeed, our subjective divisions of the gamma class (Fig. 23C), fractal dimension is insensitive to a variety of features that subjectively unite classes of neurons. However, when topological parameters (reflecting the number of branches) are contrasted with fractal dimension (measuring "space-filling capacity"), we have been able to approach a numerical basis for defining patterns of branching. While a statistical description of morphology is not only taxonomically advantageous (Rowe and Stone, '80; Rodieck and Brening, '82, '83), it would also be of considerable use for defining morphological changes in identified populations during normal and perturbed development.

In this study, we have shown that the clustering of alpha, beta, and gamma cells is distinct in terms of soma size and dendritic arbor size. A numerical analysis of branching styles reveals different relationships. Our measure of branching, T, indicates that alpha and beta cells achieve a similar adult range of complexity (as fractal dimension, Df) with a similar relationship of branching to overall dendritic length. This suggests that the morphological "plan" of alpha and beta cells is similar in spite of the difference in the size of their arbors. The absence of a relationship between T and Df implies that increased space-filling in alpha and beta cells is achieved through relatively symmetrical branching, which will tend to keep T constant. By comparison, gamma cells show a relation between T and Df (Fig. 23C), implying that increased space-filling is achieved by the asymmetric elaboration of dendritic branches. This would tend to increase the relative number of dendritic terminals in gamma arbors, which are consequently more "twiggy" than alpha and beta cells of an equivalent fractal dimension. Twiggy arbors are generally a feature of immature retinal ganglion cells (Dann et al., '88; Ramoa et al., '88).

Journal of Thoracic Imaging, Vol. 9. No. 1, 1994

8

Fractal Analysis of Pulmonary Arteries: The Fractal Dimension Is Lower in Pulmonary Hypertension

Lawrence M. Boxt, M.D., Jose Katz, M.D., Larry S. Liebovitch, Ph.D., Rosemary Jones, M.D., Peter D. Esser, Ph.D., and Lynne Reid, M.D.

Summary: We analyzed the spatial structure of contact radiographs of barium-filled pulmonary arteries of rats raised in room air and in two environments that induce pulmonary arterial hypertension (PAH)—hypoxia and hyperoxia. We found that the spatial structure of the pulmonary arteries was fractal in both the control and the hypertensive lungs. The fractal dimension of the pulmonary arteries of the control lungs was 1.62 ± 0.01 (mean ± SEM), which is greater than that of both the hypoxic lungs 1.50 ± 0.03 ($p < 0.01$) and the hyperoxic lungs 1.44 ± 0.01 ($p < 0.01$). There was no significant difference between the hypoxic and hyperoxic lungs. The fractal dimension may be a useful clinical index to quantify pathologic changes in the pulmonary arterial tree.

Key Words: Fractal—Pulmonary artery—Hypertension, pulmonary arterial.

Pulmonary arterial hypertension (PAH) may complicate a variety of diseases that are associated with increased pulmonary vascular resistance or pulmonary blood flow (1,2). In a smaller population of patients, a primary form of PAH may occur in which no apparent etiology is demonstrated (3–5). Regardless of its etiology, once PAH occurs, it may continue to worsen (6). Although longitudinal studies describing the natural history of secondary PAH are lacking (7), the prognosis in patients diagnosed with primary PAH is grim (8).

Certain structural changes are common to most forms of PAH. In virtually all cases there is an increase in the thickness of the muscular and adventitial coats of the pulmonary arteries and a decrease in the luminal area of the affected arteries (9–11). Morphometric studies have demonstrated specific differences among the

various types of PAH (12–14). Pulmonary arteriograms of hypertensive lungs show both altered tapering of segmental and subsegmental pulmonary arteries (11) and fewer arterial branches ("pruning") than in the normotensive lungs (15). From results of quantitative analysis of pulmonary arteriograms, it is possible to predict both pulmonary arterial resistance and the degree of abnormality that will be seen from open biopsy results in children with PAH secondary to congenital heart disease. Furthermore, in patients with primary PAH, computation of segmental pulmonary artery taper correlated strongly with pulmonary arterial pressure (16,17). Pulmonary arteriograms in patients with PAH may be characterized by a loss of side branches that results from the occlusion and narrowing of the lumina of the affected vessels. This leads to a decrease in total cross-sectional area of the pulmonary arterial bed, and hence to a further increase in pulmonary arterial resistance. The ability to quantify this morphologic observation would be useful in the investigation of pulmonary hypertension because it would provide a means of estimating the current status of the pulmonary vascular bed; this information cannot be obtained by direct pressure measurements. Furthermore, it would provide quantitative information concerning serial changes in the bed, as might be found in pro-

From the Departments of Radiology (L.M.B., J.K., P.D.E.), Medicine (J.K.), and Ophthalmology (L.S.L.), Columbia University, College of Physicians and Surgeons, New York, New York; and Department of Pathology (R.J., L.R.), Harvard Medical School and The Children's Hospital Medical Center, Boston, Massachusetts, U.S.A.

Address correspondence and reprint requests to Dr. L. M. Boxt at Department of Radiology, College of Physicians and Surgeons of Columbia University, 177 Fort Washington Avenue, New York, NY 10032, U.S.A.

L. M. Box et al.

gressive disease or in regression of disease secondary to medical intervention. This type of information currently can only be obtained by means of serial open lung biopsies. In addition, serial quantitative analyses would provide a means of studying the mechanisms responsible for these changes.

Experimental chronic PAH has been produced by exposing animals to hypobaric hypoxia (10,18) or to normobaric hyperoxia (19,20). In addition to vasoconstriction, hypoxic exposure (air at one-half atmosphere of pressure) leads to development of severe PAH on the basis of structural remodeling of the peripheral pulmonary vasculature; this remodeling includes the appearance of smooth muscle in smaller and more peripheral pulmonary arteries than is normal. Hyperoxic exposure (87% oxygen at atmospheric pressure) produces obliterative changes in those pulmonary arteries that survive, and reduction in luminal diameter of both muscular and nonmuscular pulmonary arteries. In this model muscle also is found in previously nonmuscular pulmonary arteries. On barium-filled contact radiographs of the pulmonary arteries in both the hypoxia-induced and hyperoxia-induced models of PAH, the background haze and the number of arteries detected as individual lines are reduced. This is because of narrowing of arterial lumina in hypoxia and arterial occlusion in hyperoxia. The loss of peripheral branches has been quantitated by microscopic examination; however, the corresponding changes described on pulmonary arteriograms previously has not been quantitated. Fractal analysis has been found to be useful for studying and characterizing branching structures. We investigated the use of fractal analysis to quantify morphologic changes in the pulmonary arteries of rats with hypoxia- and hyperoxia-induced PAH.

A fractal can be defined as an object that is self-similar (21–23) and has a non-integer scaling dimension. Self-similarity means that, the properties of each piece of the fractal are similar to those of the whole object. Thus, for example, the branching of twigs from a tree limb has the general appearance of the larger limbs branching from the trunk. The noninteger scaling dimension of a fractal is referred to as the fractal dimension (21–23). The mathematical equations of the scaling dimension are given in the Materials and Methods section. We note here that the significance of the scaling dimension is that it tells us how many new elements are revealed when the object is examined at higher resolution. For example, consider a straight line in a two-dimensional plane. As we magnify pieces of the line, no new details appear. Such a line has a scaling dimension equal to 1. Now consider the contact pulmonary arteriogram of a normotensive rat as illustrated in Fig. 1. It consists of an arterial trunk that divides into shorter narrower trunks, which branch

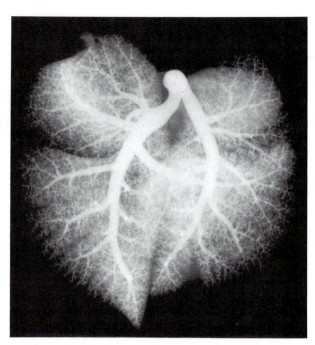

FIG. 1. Barium-gelatin contact pulmonary arteriogram of the lungs of a normal control rat maintained in room air at one atmosphere of pressure.

into shorter trunks and so forth. As we magnify pieces of this object, we discover even more of its finer branches. Such an object has a fractal dimension between 1 and 2. The fractal dimension is higher when a greater number of smaller branches are found as the magnification is increased. Conversely, when there is a disproportionate loss of smaller vessels, then the fractal dimension is decreased. If there are so many branches that the object fills the two-dimension plane, then the fractal dimension approaches 2. Thus, the fractal dimension quantifies the space filling or branching characteristics of an object. The larger the fractal dimension of an object, the more its branches fill the space that it occupies.

Many different anatomic and physiologic systems have been shown to possess fractal features that have been described and quantitated by fractal analysis. Fractals have been used to characterize the shapes of neurons (24,25). Plots of the relative dispersion of the velocity of coronary blood flow have fractal properties (26). The power spectrum of the QRS complex in normal individuals has fractal properties that may be due to fractal branching of the HIS-Purkinje system (27). The branching pattern of the bronchial tree is fractal (28). The retinal arteries of the eye are fractal (29,30). Furthermore, the fractal dimension of the retinal arteries is decreased in patients with vasculitis and angioid streaks suggesting that this form of analysis might be useful for ophthalmologic diagnosis (29).

In this study, we analyzed the contact radiographs of the barium-injected pulmonary arteries of three populations of rats; these included animals with normal pulmonary artery pressure, with hypoxia-induced PAH, and with hyperoxia-induced PAH. We determined whether the pulmonary arterial tree in each of these populations is fractal and whether determination of the fractal dimension could distinguish these populations from each other.

MATERIALS AND METHODS

Animal preparation

We analyzed the contact radiographs of the lungs of 12 adult male rats (weighing between 175 and 225 gm) from two previously reported experiments (10,19). Four control adult Sprague-Dawley rats had been maintained in room air. In four, hypoxic PAH was experimentally induced by exposure to air at $\frac{1}{2}$ atm pressure for 10 days. In four, hyperoxic PAH was produced by exposure to 87% oxygen at 1 atm of pressure for 28 days. All groups had received ad lib food and water. The animals were sacrificed by an overdose of sodium pentobarbital. The thoracic block (heart, lungs, thymus, trachea, and esophagus) was quickly excised from each animal. The thymus and esophagus were then removed.

Contact pulmonary arteriograms were prepared in the following manner. The pulmonary arteries of each animal were injected with a gelatin-barium sulfate suspension at 60°C and 100 cm of water pressure (19). This technique of injection recruits and distends all pulmonary arteries > 15 μm in diameter. The capillaries and pulmonary veins are not filled. The bronchial tree of each specimen was then distended at 23 cm of water pressure, and contact radiographs of the lungs were obtained (40 kV, 30 mAs). These radiographs were digitized with an Apple scanner attached to a Macintosh SE computer and were thresholded to produce binary (black on white background) images.

Scaling dimension

The scaling dimension was determined from the binary images by using a fast box-counting algorithm (31). In this method, the image is divided into square boxes of side r, and the number of boxes $N(r)$ that contain at least one pixel of the image is determined. This procedure is then repeated for different box sizes. The scaling dimension d can then be found from the relationship $N(r) \propto 1/r^d$. This is done by determining the absolute value of the slope of the least squares fit of the

plot of log $N(r)$ vs. log (r). As mentioned in the introduction, the scaling dimension d is also referred to as the fractal dimension when d is not an integer. The fractal dimension of each radiograph was determined using this procedure.

Statistical analysis

A Wilcoxon's rank sum test (32) was used to test the statistical significance of the difference in the fractal dimension between the control group and the experimental groups.

RESULTS

Examples of contact radiographs of barium-injected pulmonary arteries of control rats and those with hypoxia-induced and hyperoxia-induced PAH are shown in Figs. 1 to 3.

For each image, a plot of $N(r)$, the number of boxes that contain at least one pixel of the image versus the box size r, was determined. A typical plot of log $N(r)$ versus r obtained from the analysis of the contact radiograph of the lungs of a normal rat is shown in Fig. 4. The plots of log $N(r)$ versus log r from all the images could be well fit by straight lines having correlation coefficients >0.99. The fact that the data is well described

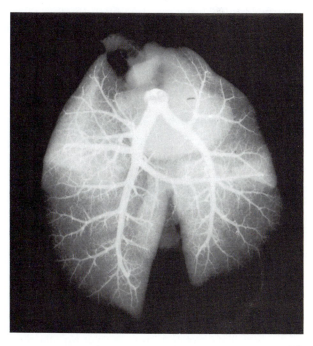

FIG. 2. Barium-gelatin contact pulmonary arteriogram of the lungs of a rat with hypoxia-induced pulmonary arterial hypertension (PAH). Note the significant loss of arborization and the background haze typical of PAH compared to Fig. 1.

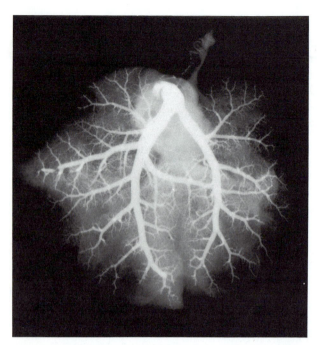

FIG. 3. Barium-gelatin contact pulmonary arteriogram of the lungs of a rat with hyperoxia-induced pulmonary arterial hypertension (PAH). Note the similarity to Fig. 2 and the different appearance from Fig. 1.

TABLE 1. Fractal dimension of control and hypertensive pulmonary arteries

Population	Specimen	Fractal dimension
Control	1	1.60
	2	1.59
	3	1.63
	4	1.65
	Mean (±SEM)	1.62 ± 0.01
Hypoxia-induced hypertension	1	1.41
	2	1.53
	3	1.53
	4	1.55
	Mean (±SEM)	1.51 ± 0.03[a]
Hyperoxia-induced hypertension	1	1.44
	2	1.43
	3	1.45
	4	1.43
	mean (±SEM)	1.44 ± 0.01[a]

SEM, standard error of the mean.
[a]Indicates significant difference from control value ($p < 0.01$).

by this relationship indicates that the images are fractal. The fractal dimensions measured for the 12 animals are reported in Table 1. The mean fractal dimension of the normal control lungs was 1.62 ± 0.01 (mean ± SEM). The mean fractal dimension of the hypoxia-induced hypertensive lungs was 1.50 ± 0.03, and the mean fractal dimension of the hyperoxia-induced hypertensive lungs was 1.44 ± 0.01. The difference of the fractal dimension between the control group and both the hypoxic group and the hyperoxic group were found to be significant ($p < 0.01$, Wilcoxon's rank sum test). The difference between the hypoxic group and the hyperoxic group was not statistically significant ($p < 0.17$, Wilcoxon's rank sum test).

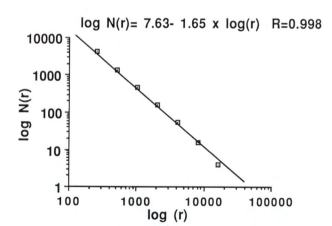

log N(r)= 7.63- 1.65 x log(r)   R=0.998

FIG. 4. Logarithmic plot of the regression of $N(r)$, the number of boxes of size r that contain at least one pixel of the image, versus r, the size of each box. The strong correlation coefficient ($R = .998$) indicates that the pulmonary artery is fractal. The absolute value of the slope of the regression line, 1.65, is the fractal dimension of the pulmonary artery.

DISCUSSION

We found that the pulmonary arterial trees of normal control rats and rats with hypoxia-induced and hyperoxia-induced PAH are fractal. Thus, pulmonary artery tree structures can be characterized by its fractal dimension. We also found that the fractal dimension of the pulmonary arteries of normal control lungs was higher than that of PAH. The fractal dimension of the pulmonary arteries of the hypoxic and hyperoxic lungs was not significantly different.

The existence of a fractal pattern is indicated by the significant linear correlation between log $N(r)$ and log r. The fractal character of the pulmonary arteries may be related to the mechanism of their formation. During the fourth week of gestation, the lung arises as a diverticulum of the foregut. By the 16th week, the major airways have developed from dichotomous branching of this diverticulum (that is, buds form and become tubes, then smaller buds branch from these tubes, and so on).

Thus, the observed self-similar branching of the pulmonary airways (28) may result from its self-similar pattern of morphogenesis. The pulmonary arterial bed and proximal pulmonary arterial branches develop in a similar way. That is, endothelialized intraparenchymal lacunae may bud to form branches that form smaller buds and smaller branches, and so on, thus producing a self-similar fractal structure. There are, however, many more arterial branches than airway branches.

The fractal dimension found in other arterial beds such as the retina suggests certain properties of their morphogenesis. The retinal arteries are self-similar with a fractal dimension of ~1.7; this fractal dimension is seen in structures produced by a mechanism known as diffusion-limited aggregation (29,30). In the diffusion-limited aggregation model, the growth of an object depends on the interaction between the object itself and its local chemical, electrical, or hydrostatic environment. As the object grows, the local changes in its structure alter the manner in which the environment affects its further growth. It has not been shown, however, that this is the only mechanism that produces structures with fractal dimensions of ~1.7.

The quantitative value of the fractal dimension of the pulmonary arteries was found to be related to the pruned tree appearance of the pulmonary arteries seen on radiographs of patients with PAH. Previous studies also have found that the qualitative appearance of cells and organs is correlated with their fractal dimension (24,25,33).

We found that the fractal dimension can differentiate normal from pathologic pulmonary arteries. The man fractal dimension of the pulmonary arteries in the normal control lungs was 1.62 ± 0.01. This was significantly greater than the fractal dimension of 1.44 ± 0.03 ($p < 0.01$) found in the lungs with hyperoxia-induced PAH. Thus, the fractal dimension may be used to differentiate normal populations from those with PAH and may be able to quantitate the degree of abnormality. Clinical use of the word "complex" to characterize the qualitative appearance of normal pulmonary arteries compared to the pruned-tree appearance of the hypertensive lung may be quantified by the numerical value of the fractal dimension.

The lower mean fractal dimension of the lungs with PAH indicates that the arteries in these lungs have proportionately fewer fine branches, at least as seen with the spatial resolution of the contact radiographs. The detailed mechanism that would account for this change is not yet understood. It may, however, reflect remodeling of the smaller vessels (34) caused by pathologic processes in the pulmonary arteries or lung parenchyma.

Artery taper and other indices also have been used to characterize changes in the pulmonary arteries in patients with PAH (11,16). These indices characterize the properties of individual arteries. The fractal dimension, in contrast, is affected by any structural change that affects space filling such as narrowing of artery lumen and pruning of side branches at all levels. Because of these global characteristics, the fractal dimension is not specific to a particular structural change. Other measures of structure may be needed to differentiate exactly what these changes are. Future studies will be needed to determine the complete range of capabilities and limitations of the fractal dimension as a clinical tool to quantify pathologic changes in the pulmonary arterial tree and in other vascular beds.

Acknowledgment: This work was done during the tenure of an established investigatorship from the American Heart Association (L.S.L.) and also supported by grants from the Whitaker Foundation and the National Institutes of Health RO1 EY6234 and RO1 HL34552.

REFERENCES

1. Grossman W, Braunwald E. Pulmonary hypertension. In Braunwald E, ed. Heart disease. Philadelphia: Saunders, 1988:793–818.
2. Anderson G, Reid L, Simon G. The radiographic appearances in primary and in thromboembolic pulmonary hypertension. *Clin Radiol* 1973;24:113–20.
3. Voelkel NF, Reeves RJ. Primary pulmonary hypertension. In: Moser KM, ed. Pulmonary vascular disease. New York: Dekker, 1979:573–628.
4. Wagenvoort CA, Wagenvoort N. Primary pulmonary hypertension. A pathologic study of the lung vessels in 156 clinically diagnosed cases. *Circulation* 1970;42:1163–84.
5. Edwards WD, Edwards JE. Clinical primary pulmonary hypertension: three pathological types. *Circulation* 1977;56:884–8.
6. Meyrick B, Reid L. Pulmonary hypertension: anatomic and physiologic correlates. *Clin Chest Med* 1983;4:199–217.
7. Robin ED. Some basic and clinical challenges in the pulmonary circulation. *Chest* 1982;81:357–63.
8. Fuster V, Steele PM, Edwards WD, Gersh BJ, McGoon MD, Frye RL. Primary pulmonary hypertension: natural history and the importance of thrombosis. *Circulation* 1984;70:580–7.
9. Hislop A, Reid L. Changes in the pulmonary arteries of the

Fractal and Morphometric Analysis of Lung Structures After Canine Adenovirus-Induced Bronchiolitis in Beagle Puppies

Mark L. Witten, PhD,[1,2,6] **Joseph L. McKee,**[1] **R. Clark Lantz, PhD,**[3,6] **Allison M. Hays,**[1] **Stuart F. Quan, MD,**[4,6] **Richard E. Sobonya, MD,**[5,6] **and Richard J. Lemen, MD**[1,2,6]

Summary: Acute viral respiratory infections are commonly associated with alteration in lung growth and with chronic obstructive disease. However, it is difficult to quantify these changes in lung function. We determined that the recently described techniques of fractal analysis gave additional information about the changes in lung function after viral illness compared to standard morphometric techniques. Fractal and morphometric parameters change with lung growth after acute infection with canine adenovirus type 2 (CAV2, n = 5) or no infection (controls, n = 6) in beagle puppies. Lung pathological studies showed areas of obliterative bronchiolitis and chronic small airways inflammation but no emphysema in the CAV2-infected puppies. Morphometric studies at ~236 days of age demonstrated accelerated lung growth in the CAV2-infected dogs as evidenced by significant increases in lung volume (V_L) and internal surface area (ISA). Fractal analysis showed an increased fractal dimension (D_f) of the alveolar perimeter length in the CAV2 group associated with increased growth that was similar to the percentage change in V_L and ISA. These data suggest that a single infection with CAV2 in beagle puppies accelerates lung growth and increases the complexity (D_f) of the alveolar structure. **Pediatr Pulmonol. 1993; 16:62–68.**

Key words: Lung growth; fractal dimension; percent change of lung volume; internal surface area; pathological histology.

INTRODUCTION

Viral respiratory infections are major causes of morbidity and mortality in infants and children,[1,2] and are frequent precipitants of acute asthmatic exacerbations[3] in patients of all ages. Furthermore, childhood viral respiratory infections may play a major role in the development of chronic lung disease and altered lung growth.[4,5]

We have developed a beagle puppy using canine adenovirus-2 (CAV2) to induce lung injury. An acute

From the Critical Care Medicine Section of the Department of Pediatrics and Steele Memorial Children's Research Center,[1] Departments of Physiology,[2] Anatomy,[3] Internal Medicine,[4] Pathology,[5] and the Respiratory Sciences Center,[6] University of Arizona College of Medicine, Tucson, Arizona.

Received February 20, 1992; (revision) accepted February 25, 1993.

Address correspondence and reprint requests to Dr. M. L. Witten, Department of Pediatrics, Arizona Health Sciences Center, 1501 N. Campbell Avenue, Tucson, AZ 85724-0001.

This research was supported by grants HL 14136 and 07249, and USAFOSR 91-0199.

infection with CAV2 in 80-day-old beagle puppies produces transient airway hyperresponsiveness to aerosolized histamine[6,7] and mild-to-moderate inflammation of bronchi and bronchioles.[6–8] Pulmonary function abnormalities suggestive of delayed growth occurred between 12 and 14 days after infection with CAV2.[4]

Recently, fractal analysis of lung structure and function has demonstrated the complex nature of the lung. Glenny and Robertson have shown that fractal branching models relate structure and function of the pulmonary vascular tree and provide a mechanism to describe the spatially correlated distribution of blood flow and the gravity-independent heterogeneity of blood flow.[9] Other investigators have demonstrated fractal components for the lung's bronchial tree[10] and pulmonary microvasculature.[11] Thus, fractal analysis of the lungs may give new insight into the pathological processes caused by infection or disease. The purpose of the current study was to determine by morphometric and fractal analysis whether CAV2-induced bronchiolitis in specific pathogen-free beagle puppies altered lung growth using morphometric and fractal analysis. We also compared the sensitivity of fractal analysis and standard morphometrics to detect changes in lung function after a single respiratory illness.

MATERIALS AND METHODS

Study Animals

Pregnant beagles were purchased from a single outbred colony (Laboratory Research Enterprises, Kalamazoo, MI) and transported to Tucson 2–3 weeks before anticipated parturition. Pregnant females were immunized for parainfluenza, adenovirus, parvovirus, and distemper only at 4 weeks of age to minimize maternal antibodies in their offspring. Puppies were delivered vaginally and weaned at 4 weeks of age. Bitches and their puppies were raised in strict isolation and remain pathogen free. The puppies were immunized for distemper, rabies, and hepatitis at 5 weeks of age and were negative for maternal antibody to CAV2 by 8 weeks of age. All protocols were approved by the Laboratory Animal Care Committee of the University of Arizona College of Medicine in accordance with guidelines for the humane care of laboratory animals established by the National Institutes of Health.

Experimental Protocol

The source of the CAV2 virus and the methods used for preparation of inocula, measuring antibody titers, and culturing CAV2 have been described elsewhere.[6–8] Between 9 and 12 weeks of age, 11 puppies were assigned to two groups: controls (n = 6) and those inoculated with CAV2 (n = 5). Some of the physiologic and morphometric data for the CAV2 and control groups have appeared in a prior publication.[4] Each litter was allocated to a single experimental group because of the high infectivity rates of CAV2. Random assignment of littermates to different experimental groups was not possible without the risk of inadvertent infection.

Lung Pathology

Lung fractal and morphometric studies were performed in six control dogs (C, mean ages of 238 ± 2 days) and five CAV2 dogs (mean ages of 235 ± 2 days). The dogs were killed by exsanguination, and their lungs were removed rapidly and weighed. The lungs were inflated to 30 cm H_2O pressure with 10% neutral buffered formalin solution for 24–72 hours. After gross inspection, the lungs were sliced parasagittally and randomized sections were processed for light microscopy. These consisted of four sections from each apical-cardiac lobe, four sections from each diaphrag-

matic lobe, and two sections from the intermediate lobe for each lung.

Morphometric measurements, including lung volume by water displacement (V_L) and internal surface area (ISA), were performed, as has been described elsewhere.[8,12,13] The diameter of 100 small airways (<1 mm) were calculated by projecting the light microscopic sections onto a screen and measuring the size of the airways. For determination of ISA, tissue blocks for light microscopy sections were taken suing a 2 × 1.5-cm template. For each section, intercepts with a pattern of three intersecting lines were counted in contiguous fields covering each slide (usually 10–15 fields/slide). Data for all fields in a slide were averaged, and then data for all slides were averaged for each dog. To quantify the amount of bronchiolar inflammation, a scoring system, bronchiolar inflammation score (BIS), was used which graded each nonalveolated small airway on a scale of 0–3, compared with a panel of photomicrographs of small airways inflammation of varying severity.[14] The BIS was expressed as the ratio of the observed score to the maximum possible score.

Fractal Analysis

In general, fractal objects are complex irregular objects that are characterized by detail nested within detail. Closer observation of fractal objects reveals more detail than is predicted on the basis of scale correction. Thus, the absolute area, length, or volume of a fractal object cannot be determined; these measures depend on the scale of observation. The concept of the fractal nature of the lung can be seen in Figure 1, which is an example of a Minkowski figure.

Fractal analysis of light microscopy alveolar sections was performed according to the method of Iannaccone.[15] Twenty-five alveoli from each dog were selected randomly and viewed with four different objectives (4, 10, 20, and 40). The corresponding magnifications for the four different objectives are 208×, 520×, 1040×, and 2080×, respectively.

Alveolar perimeter length was determined at the four different levels of magnification by using a Bioquant measurement system (R and M Biometrics, Inc., Nashville, TN). The logs of the 25 alveolar perimeter lengths for each dog at the four different magnifications were then averaged to obtain a mean log value at each magnification for each animal. This mean log value for each animal at the four different magnifications was then averaged to obtain the mean log for the control and CAV2 groups. The mean log of the alveolar perimeter length was plotted vs. the absolute value of the log of the reciprocal of the magnification for the control and CAV2 groups (Fig. 2). The slope of the line was determined by the least squares method.

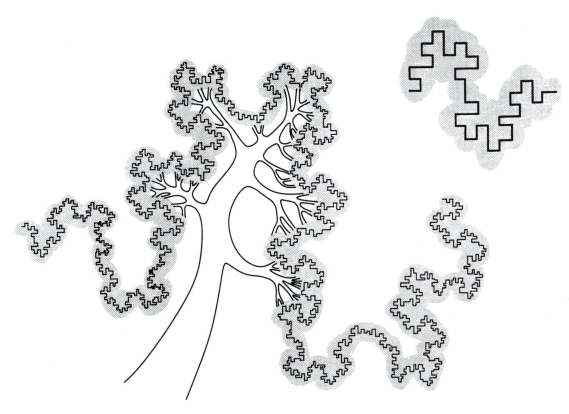

Fig. 1. Conceptual drawing of an alveolar septal area that demonstrates the fractal nature of the lung. The enlarged alveolar septal area is an example of a Minkowski fractal figure.[18]

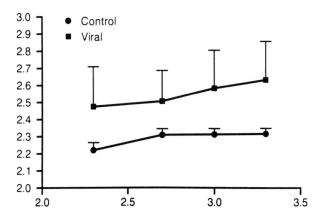

Fig. 2. A log–log plot of mean alveolar perimeter length (microns) (y-axis) vs the mean absolute value of the reciprocal of the magnification (x-axis) for the control and CAV2 groups. The small SEM (bars) of the control group vs the larger SEM in the CAV2 group demonstrates the uniformity of the alveolar perimeter length in the control group.

This resultant slope estimates the Hausdorff-Besicovitch dimension, which has been identified with the fractal dimension (D_f). If the object has a fractal geometry, then the resultant slope of the log–log trans-formed data of the alveolar perimeter length plotted against the scale of magnification will not be zero. If we find that a nonzero slope for alveolar perimeter length exists, then we conclude that the alveolar perimeter has a D_f equal to 1 minus the slope, since the topological dimension of a nonfractal length, such as a straight line is 1.[16] The value for D_f must exceed the topological dimension (D_t), which is 1 for nonfractal lines. For present purposes, a fractal object is one in which $D_t < D_f$. The D_f values were corrected by 0.02 after 10 trials at each magnification with a square figure which demonstrated a D_f of 1.02.

Analysis of morphometric data was performed using a nonparametric one-way analysis of variance.[17] The fractal data analysis was performed using Student's t test. All statistical tests considered a P value < 0.05 as significant. The data are shown as mean ± SEM.

RESULTS

On light microscopy, chronic inflammation in the walls of small airways was noted consistently in the lungs of dogs in the CAV2 group (Fig. 3). Focal fibrosis was

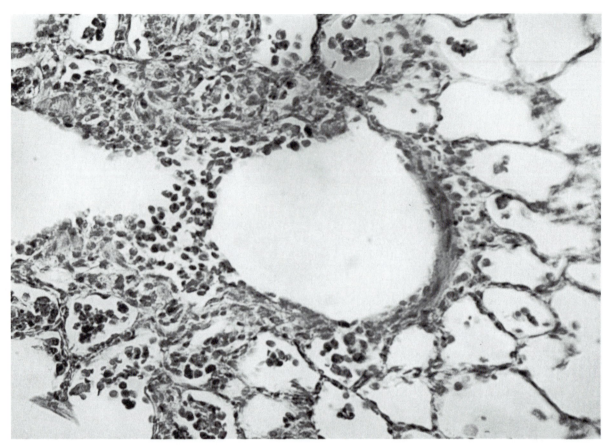

Fig. 3. Bronchiolitis obliterans in a dog exposed to CAV2. Small airway lumen is filled with fibrous tissue and inflammatory cells. (Hematoxylin and eosin; ×200.)

Table 1—Fractal Dimension (D$_f$) of Alveolar Perimeter Length

	D$_f$ of alveolar perimeter length
CAV2 dogs	
#1	1.144
#2	1.162
#3	1.087
#4	1.127
#5	1.128
	(1.130 ± 0.012)*
Control dogs	
#1	0.993
#2	1.046
#3	1.096
#4	1.119
#5	1.000
#6	1.115
	(1.062 ± 0.023)

D$_f$ is the fractal dimension as defined in the text. D$_f$ was determined by obtaining the slope of the line describing the relationship between the log of the alveolar perimeter length and the log of the reciprocal of magnification (see Materials and Methods). Mean ± SEM in parentheses.

*$P < 0.05$ compared to control dogs.

sometimes seen near these lesions, but no emphysema was present.

The log–log plot of alveolar perimeter length vs. the absolute value of the reciprocal of the magnification (Fig. 2) demonstrates the fractal geometry for both the control and CAV2 groups, since the resultant slopes of the regression lines are not equal to zero. The D$_f$s for alveolar perimeter length in the CAV2 and control groups are shown in Table 1. The mean D$_f$ for alveolar perimeter length in the CAV2 group was 1.130 (±0.012), which was significantly increased over the control value of 1.062 (±0.023; Figs. 4 and 5).

Morphometric data for the CAV2 and control groups supports qualitative evaluation on light microscopy. An increase in the BIS and a decrease in small airways diameter indicated a significant small airways inflammation in the CAV2 group. In this group the BIS was larger, 0.41 ± 0.05 vs. 0.09 ± 0.01 for controls ($P < 0.01$), and the diameter of small airways was narrower; CAV2, 0.50 ± 0.05 mm vs. 0.59 ± 0.01 mm for controls ($P < 0.05$). Furthermore, the percentage of small airways less than 0.35 mm was significantly increased in the CAV2 group, 26 ± 6, compared to the control percentage of 11 ± 3 ($P < 0.01$). The V$_L$ and ISA were sig-

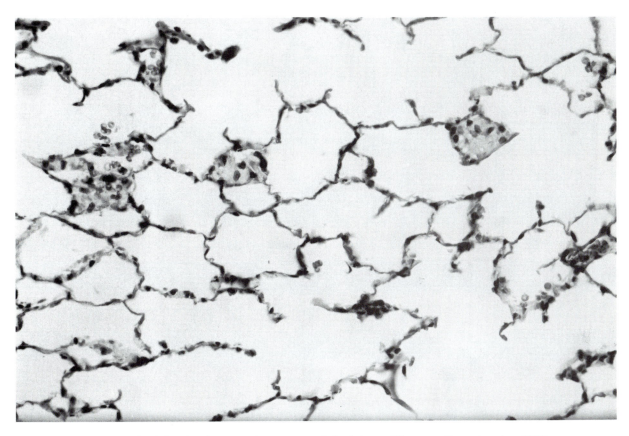

Fig. 4. Light micrograph of the alveolar septa from a control dog's lung. (Hematoxylin and eosin; ×305.)

nificantly increased in the CAV2 dogs by 71.5% and 93.2%, respectively, over control values (Table 2).

DISCUSSION

Many patterns of nature are irregular and fragmented, i.e., clouds, a coastline, or a tree. Mandelbrot developed a new geometry of nature that describes many of the irregular patterns by identifying a family of shapes called fractals.[18] These shapes tend to be scaling, which implies that the degree of irregularity is similar at all scales. We have utilized this fractal technique to analyze alveolar structures after a single infection with CAV2. There were significant changes in lung structure, V_L, ISA, and the diameter of small airways. Furthermore, these changes were accompanied by an increase of D_f for alveolar perimeter length. We interpret these changes to suggest that an acute viral respiratory infection may be a sufficient stress to alter lung growth.

In humans, lung volume after birth increases by addition of alveolar number until approximately 8 years of age (proliferative stage). Thereafter, an increase in lung volume occurs through an enlargement of exist-

ing alveoli (equilibrative stage). The puppies in the present study were infected with CAV2 at 80 days of age and subsequently killed at 232–256 days of age. According to Le Beau,[19] the corresponding age span in humans is 4.5–14.2 years of age, a time when both proliferative and equilibrative growth occur.[20]

The proliferative stage of lung growth is dominated by increased alveolarization. Previous studies have demonstrated that hypoxia,[21] cold exposure,[22] resection of lung,[23] and atelectasis[23] in young animals can produce more rapid lung growth. Furthermore, chronic exercise in rats during the second month of postnatal growth can increase alveolar proliferation, as indicated by greater alveolar densities and surface area to volume ratios.[24] Inasmuch as puppies in this study were infected with a virus at a time when there was alveolar proliferation, retardation or chronic impairment of lung development was expected. However, the opposite appears to have occurred. CAV2 infection in puppies appears to accelerate lung alveolarization.

An increased oxygen demand and/or pulmonary blood flow have been proposed to be important variables in affecting lung growth. Moreover, Castleman[25] has demonstrated that postmortem lung volume in

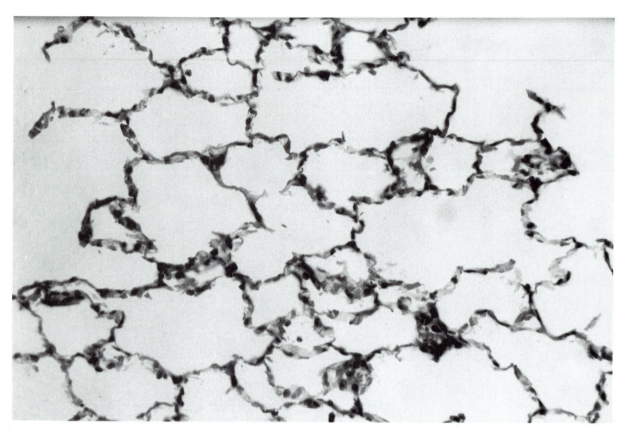

Fig. 5. A light micrograph of the alveolar septa of a CAV2 dog's lung. The alveolar perimeters are more irregular and complex than the control dog's alveolar perimeters in Figure 4. (Hematoxylin and eosin; ×305.)

Table 2—Morphometric Data (Mean ± SEM)

Group	V_L	ISA
CAV2	1091 ± 60*	31.1 ± 3.7*
Control	636 ± 77	16.1 ± 1.2

V_L, lung volume (mL); ISA, internal surface area (m²).

*$P < 0.01$ compared to control values.

Sendai virus-infected weanling rats was greater 30 and 60 days after inoculation. Thus, our data and those of Castleman[25] support the possibility that virus infection can accelerate alveolarization.

The pre- and postnatal development of saccules/ alveoli by septation is closely related to the elastic tissue network in the lung parenchyma.[26] The septal fiber system is a network of short, extremely fine fibers that are found in the alveolar walls themselves. Alveoli are formed in the meshes of this delicate connective tissue latticework so that these fibers form, in their terminal boundaries, the reinforced entrance rings of individual alveoli. Each new septum begins as a crest that has an elastic fiber as its base. The fishnet-like network of elastic fibers in the developing lung are the foundation upon which alveolar formation is centered. This occurs by creating boundaries of the lattice through which new alveoli emerge. Murray proposes that there is an interdependence of structure and function in the alveolarization process based upon an optimum design for functional requirements.[26] Thus, if a viral infection alters the functional metabolic requirements of the lung, i.e., oxygen demand and/or pulmonary blood flow, then according to Murray's postulate, one would expect an altered structure of the lung to result.

There is evidence that viral infection can alter alveolar structure. Castleman and co-workers have demonstrated that infection with Sendai virus in neonatal rats resulted in delayed or impaired growth of secondary septa into alveolar saccules. The impaired septal ingrowth was multifocal and predominantly centriacinar in distribution and was associated with alveolar enlargement and significant decreases in alveolar surface density.[27] Furthermore, in Sendai virus-infected weanling rats, at an age more closely corresponding to the age of the CAV2 infected puppies in this study, postmortem lung volume and specific alveolar surface area were increased 60 days post virus inoculation.[25] These latter observations are similar to the changes in V_L and ISA found in our current canine study.

In contrast to the evidence that viral infection accelerated alveolarization of the lung, our findings of chronic bronchiolar inflammation and a reduction in small airways diameters indicates that there was an inhibition in bronchiolar enlargement in virus-infected puppies. This observation differs somewhat from the findings of Castleman[25] in weanling rats that did not have a change in terminal bronchiolar cross-sectional area 30–60 days after Sendai virus infection. However, Sendai virus infection reduced bronchiolar diameter in neonatal rats.[27] This discrepancy may be related to differences in the regulation of airway enlargement with maturation among species. Nevertheless, our data and those of Castleman and co-workers demonstrate that viral lower respiratory tract infection can inhibit small airway growth.

We have demonstrated that changes in V_L, ISA, and D_f for alveolar perimeter all increase in CAV2-infected puppies' lungs compared to control values. It is interesting to note that the mean slope of the linear relationship between the alveolar perimeter length and the scale of magnification was increased 82.9% over the control slope. The V_L and ISA were increased 71.5% and 93.2%, respectively, over control values. The increases in V_L and ISA suggest that more alveoli are developed in the CAV2 dogs; while an increased D_f for alveolar perimeter demonstrates a more complex alveolar structure. However, this finding implies that some unknown physiological process(es) altered by viral infection cause increases of the same order of magnitude in V_L, ISA, and the slope for alveolar perimeter.

We hypothesize that viral infection alters the growth-regulatory process of the fishnet of elastic fibers that are the foundation and latticework for the alveolarization process. Bruce and co-workers demonstrated that prolonged hyperoxic exposure is associated with alterations in both total length and structure of lung elastic fibers.[28] Furthermore, there is evidence that diabetes and undernourishment have different effects on connective tissue synthesis in the lung that affect lung growth and structure.[29]

In conclusion, we have determined that a single infection of CAV2 can alter lung growth as measured by V_L and ISA. Furthermore, the alveolar perimeter in CAV2-infected lungs acquires a significant fractal dimension compared to controls. We hypothesize that the virus may stimulate the release of growth factors that alter the latticework of elastic fibers that govern the formation of new alveoli in the lung.

REFERENCES

1. Denney FW, Collier AM, Henderson FW, Clyde WA, Jr. Infectious agents of importance in airways and parenchymal diseases in infants and children with particular emphasis on bronchiolitis.

2. Smith JJ, Lemen RJ, Taussig LM. Mechanisms of viral-induced lower airway obstruction. Pediatr Inf Dis. 1987; 6:837–842.

3. Hudgel DW, Langston, L, Jr., Selner JC, McIntosh K. Viral and bacterial infections in adults with chronic asthma. Am Rev Respir Dis. 1979; 120:393–397.

4. Quan SF, Lemen RJ, Witten ML, Sherrill DL, Grad R, Sobonya RE, Ray CG. Changes in lung mechanics and reactivity with age after viral bronchiolitis in beagle puppies. J Appl Physiol. 1990; 69:2034–2042.

5. Samet JM, Tager IB, Speizer FE. The relationship between respiratory illness in childhood and chronic airflow obstruction in adulthood. Am Rev Respir Dis. 1983; 127:508–523.

6. Lemen RJ, Quan SF, Witten ML, Sobonya RE, Ray CG, Grad R. Canine parainfluenza type 2 bronchiolitis increases histamine responsiveness in beagle puppies. Am Rev Respir Dis. 1990; 141:199–207.

7. Quan SF, Witten ML, Grad R. Sobony RE, Ray CG, Dambro NN, Lemen RJ. Acute canine adenovirus 2 infection increases histamine reactivity in beagle puppies. Am Rev Respir Dis. 1990; 141:414–420.

8. Wagner JS, Minnich L, Sobonya R, Taussig LM, Ray CG, Fulginiti V. Parainfluenza type II infection in dogs: A model for lower viral respiratory tract infection in humans. Am Rev Respir Dis. 1983; 127:771–775.

9. Glenny RW, Robertson HT. Fractal modeling of pulmonary blood flow heterogeneity. J Appl Physiol 1991; 70:1024–1030.

10. Nelson TR, West BJ, Goldberger AL. The fractal lung: Universal and species-related scaling patterns. Experientia. 1990; 46:251–254.

11. McNamee JE. Fractal character of pulmonary microvascular permeability. Ann Biomed Eng. 1990; 18:123–133.

12. Butler C. Lung surface area in various morphologic forms of human emphysema. Am Rev Respir Dis. 1974; 11:347–352.

13. Thurlbeck WM. The internal surface area of nonemphysematous lungs. AM Rev Respir Dis. 1967; 96:765–773.

14. Cosio M, Ghezzo H, Hogg JC, Corbin R, Loveland M, Dosman J, Macklem PT. The relations between structural changes in small airways and pulmonary function tests. N Engl J Med 1977; 298:1277–1281.

15. Iannaccone PM. Fractal geometry in mosaic organs: A new interpretation of mosaic pattern. FASEB J. 1990; 4:1508–1512.

16. Glenny RW, Robertson HT, Yamashiro S, Bassingthwaighte JB. Applications of fractal analysis to physiology. J Appl Physiol. 1991; 70:2351–2367.

17. Zar JH. Biostatistical Analysis. Englewood Cliffs, NJ: Prentice-Hall, 1974:130–150.

18. Mandelbrot BB. The Fractal Geometry of Nature. New York: W.H. Freeman and Co., 1983:1–3.

19. LeBeau A. L'age du chien et celui de l'homme—essai de statisque sur la mortalite canine. Bull Acad Vet Fr. 1953; 26:229–232.

20. Reid L. Influence of the pattern of structural growth of lung on susceptibility to specific infectious diseases in infants and children. Pediatr Res. 1977; 11:210–215.

21. Lechner AJ, Banchero N. Lung morphometry in guinea pig acclimated to hypoxia during growth. Respir Physiol. 1980; 42:155–169.

22. Lechner AJ, Banchero N. Lung morphometry in guinea pigs acclimated to cold during growth. J Appl Physiol. 1980; 48:886–891.

23. Tartter PI, Gross RJ. Compensatory pulmonary hypertrophy after incapacitation of one lung in the rat. J Thorac Cardiovasc Surg. 1973; 66:147–152.

24. Fu FH. The effects of physical training on the lung growth of infant rats. Med Sci Sports. 1976; 8:226–229.

25. Castleman WL. Alterations in pulmonary ultrastructure and morphometric parameters induced by parainfluenza (Sendai)

virus in rats during postnatal growth. Am J Pathol. 1984; 114:322–335.

26. Murray, JF. The Normal Lung. Philadelphia: W. B. Saunders, 1986:43–59.

27. Castleman WL, Sorkness RL, Lemanske RF, Grasee G, Suyemoto MM. Neonatal viral bronchiolitis and pneumonia induces bronchiolar hypoplasia and alveolar dysplasia in rats. Lab Invest. 1988; 59:387–396.

28. Bruce MC, Pawlowski R, Tomashefski JF, Jr. Changes in lung elastic fiber structure and concentration associated with hyperoxic exposure in the developing rat lung. Am Rev Respir Dis. 1989; 140:1067–1074.

29. Ofulue AF, Kida K, Thurlbeck WM. Experimental diabetes and the lung. I. Changes in growth, morphometry, and biochemistry. Am Rev Respir Dis. 1988; 137:162–166.

Current Eye Research

Volume 12 number 1 1993, 23—27

Fractal analysis of the normal human retinal fluorescein angiogram

Gabriel Landini, Gary P.Misson and Philip I.Murray

Academic Unit of Ophthalmology, University of Birmingham, Birmingham and Midland Eye Hospital,
Church Street, Birmingham B3 2NS, UK

ABSTRACT
The fractal dimension of the retinal vasculature and isolated venous and arterial trees down to a caliber of 40 μm was estimated in 23 routine fluorescein angiograms of normal retinas. Fractal dimension was determined with a method based on the box counting theorem. This method is less susceptible to the radial architecture of the retinal vascular tree than those previously reported (mass-radius relation and density-density correlation function). Two scale ranges with different fractal dimension were consistently present. The estimated fractal dimensions showed no significant difference between isolated arterial and venous trees which is not supported by previous reports. This method was designed for simple application in a clinical setting.

INTRODUCTION

Many natural structures are statistically self-similar, a geometrical quality of possessing increasing detail under magnification (1). Such objects are termed 'fractal' and may be assigned a fractional dimension rather than the integer dimension of classical Euclidean geometry. The degree of complexity and self-similarity of a fractal object may be expressed by a single (and usually fractional) number, the fractal dimension (D).
Blood vessel trees have fractal properties: there is a relationship of the number of branches to the branch generation (1). In simple terms, the self-similarity of blood vessels means that as scale decreases the number of branches increase in a statistically predictable way.

Retinal blood vessels are good candidates for fractal analysis as they develop predominantly on a surface (the retina) which can be regarded as two-dimensional, they are relatively easy to access with noninvasive methods and they undergo structural changes in different pathological conditions.

Previous investigations on small numbers of cases using mass-radius relation and the density-density correlation function showed that the retinal vasculature is fractal (2-5), findings which have led to speculation concerning their development (6,7). Moreover, D could be used as an objective parameter for characterizing the complexity of the retinal blood tree in normality and disease. The previously reported methodology assessed the fractal dimension of the entire photographically accesible retina which requires exhaustive photographic survey and subsequent reconstruction by a 'collage' of angiograms. However, the routine 60° angiograms include principally areas of special interest such as the optic disc and macula in which the quantification by the fractal dimension could be of clinical significance. With the aim of validating a method for the estimation of D, the area surveyed was reduced to single shot from routine 60° angiograms including the disc and macular areas. Additionally the procedure for estimating the fractal dimension in this study was based in the box counting theorem, which lacks a systematic error present in the mass-radius and density-density correlation function used in early reports (3-7).

MATERIALS AND METHODS

The methodology was implemented using a personal computer by one of us (G.L.) to achieve a semi-automatized procedure and involved the following stages: image collection, digitization and estimation of fractal dimension.

Image collection

The study material consisted of 23 routine fluorescein angiograms from patients with no ophthalmic disease taken with a 60° Topcon TRC 50VT fundus camera. The angiograms were projected onto paper and hand traced at high magnification and constant thickness down to vessels of 40 μm diameter (the size limit to which the vessels throughout the fundus could be accurately and consistely traced in our photographs). As this investigation is concerned with the spatial distribution of vessels, their diameters were not considered. Studies on the fractal dimension of retinal ganglion cells showed that D is insensitive to the branch width thus supporting this approach (8).

Received on June 24, 1992; accepted on November 24, 1992

Current
Eye
Research

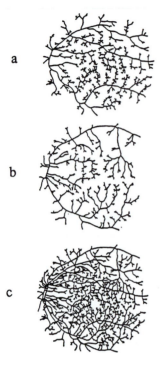

a

b

c

Figure 1. A digitized fluorescein angiogram as used in the fractal analysis a) arterial, b)venous, c) arterio-venous trace.

Table 1. Calculated and mean estimated fractal dimension of known objects.

Object	Calculated D	Estimated D ± SD
Line	1.0000	0.994 ± 0.004
Circle	1.0000	1.004 ± 0.013
Square (perimeter)	1.0000	1.000 ± 0.000
Square (filled)	2.0000	1.972 ± 0.013
Koch triadic island perimeter	1.2618	1.264 ± 0.018
Koch quadric island perimeter	1.5000	1.496 ± 0.018
Vicsek fractal	1.4649	1.468 ± 0.014

The mean values were obtained from 5 measurements starting at random initial positions of the grid.
SD: standard deviation.

Table 2. Estimated fractal dimension of arteries and veins combined in two test cases.

Case	Sex	Age	Mean fractal dimension (± SD)		
			D0	D1	D2
A	M	63	1.63 ± 0.020	1.31 ± 0.008	1.76 ± 0.021
B	M	56	1.62 ± 0.004	1.29 ± 0.013	1.76 ± 0.008

The mean values were obtained from 5 different traced angiograms. SD: standard deviation.
D0: 50 to 3200 μm, D1: 50 to 250 μm, D2: 250 to 3200 μm

The arterial and venous trees were traced separately and in combination.

Digitization

Tracings were digitized into a personal computer as binary images with an image scanner (OMRON, Japan). The scanned image was represented on a graphic window of 400 x 400 pixels. Resolution was 1 pixel equal to 25 μm (Fig. 1).

Estimation of fractal dimension

Binary images were analyzed by the GRID method for estimation of fractal dimension (9) which is based on the box counting theorem (10). This method consists of overlapping the figure with a grid of increasing unit size r, and counting the number of 'tiles' or 'boxes' N(r) of size r that contain the image. A maximum of 58 different grid sizes ranging from 1 to 128 pixels were used. If the subsequent log-log plot and linear regression of r versus N(r) tends to a straight line with a high correlation coefficient (always above 0.98 in this study) within a range of r, the object is considered fractal. Best fit estimation of the line was performed interactively. The fractal dimension D was calculated as:

D = -S

where S is the slope of the regression line.

For validating the method, a series of computer generated Euclidean and fractal shapes of mathematically determined fractal dimension was analyzed. An average value of D was obtained from 5 random initial positions of the grid (Table 1).

The reproducibility of the method as applied to traced angiograms was assessed by analyzing 5 angiograms (combined veins and arteries) of the same eye taken on different occasions in two further patients.

RESULTS

The results are summarized in Tables 3-5. The log-log plots of the analyzed angiograms in their three versions (arterial, venous and combined) had a tendency to a 'double slope' line. One of them ranging from 50 to 250μm (D1) and the other from 250 to 3200 μm (D2) (Fig. 2). Because this effect was always present, we fitted curves for the two slopes separately as well as for the general plot (D0) (Tables 3 & 4). At high resolutions (50 to 250 μm) the fractal dimension values obtained (D1) were smaller than at low resolutions (D2).

Analysis of the two cases in which repeated measurements were taken shows the results to be highly reproducible (Table 2).

Duncan's multiple range test for differences of means was

Current
Eye
Research

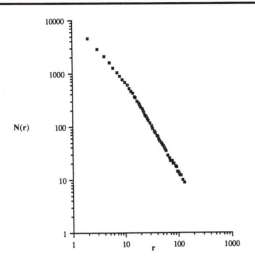

Figure 2. Log-log plot of the number of boxes N(r) of side size r necessary to cover the digitized angiogram. Note the two slopes of the plot: D1 between r = 2 and r + 10 and D2 between r = 10 and r = 100. 1 pixel = 25µm.

Table 3. Summary of experimental data.

No.	Sex	Age	Arteries			Veins			Arteries and veins		
			D0	D1	D2	D0	D1	D2	D0	D1	D2
1	F	14	1.62	1.20	1.65	1.55	1.23	1.72	1.66	1.28	1.80
2	F	27	1.48	1.23	1.62	1.52	1.23	1.69	1.60	1.29	1.71
3	F	28	1.41	1.09	1.59	1.45	1.13	1.63	1.61	1.27	1.76
4	F	34	1.54	1.20	1.71	1.53	1.22	1.68	1.67	1.32	1.77
5	F	43	1.54	1.17	1.72	1.53	1.15	1.71	1.68	1.27	1.81
6	F	45	1.48	1.23	1.63	1.49	1.21	1.65	1.64	1.30	1.76
7	F	55	1.53	1.23	1.68	1.53	1.22	1.69	1.67	1.34	1.79
8	F	70	1.50	1.20	1.68	1.48	1.21	1.64	1.64	1.30	1.77
9	M	15	1.55	1.25	1.75	1.57	1.25	1.75	1.72	1.36	1.80
10	M	18	1.45	1.12	1.63	1.43	1.15	1.60	1.62	1.29	1.74
11	M	20	1.45	1.12	1.64	1.43	1.09	1.63	1.62	1.22	1.76
12	M	22	1.47	1.17	1.63	1.46	1.17	1.61	1.62	1.29	1.73
13	M	25	1.47	1.25	1.61	1.40	1.25	1.53	1.60	1.31	1.72
14	M	29	1.53	1.23	1.69	1.52	1.20	1.70	1.67	1.30	1.81
15	M	34	1.49	1.21	1.66	1.52	1.22	1.68	1.67	1.30	1.80
16	M	40	1.49	1.23	1.64	1.56	1.24	1.70	1.66	1.32	1.78
17	M	45	1.48	1.16	1.65	1.48	1.22	1.63	1.60	1.24	1.74
18	M	55	1.47	1.16	1.64	1.50	1.17	1.66	1.64	1.27	1.77
19	M	63	1.40	1.14	1.58	1.43	1.17	1.66	1.58	1.29	1.72
20	M	63	1.45	1.29	1.59	1.53	1.30	1.67	1.63	1.30	1.77
21	M	65	1.44	1.21	1.60	1.45	1.19	1.62	1.59	1.28	1.74
22	M	72	1.48	1.20	1.69	1.48	1.19	1.66	1.64	1.28	1.78
23	M	73	1.49	1.15	1.67	1.51	1.15	1.69	1.64	1.25	1.75

D0: 50 to 3200 µm, D1: 50 to 250 µm, D2: 250 to 3200 µm

applied to evaluate the differences between values of D in the 3 ranges of the arterial, venous and arterio-venous groups.

No correlation was found between age or sex of the patients and the arterial, venous or arterio-venous fractal dimensions or the

Table 4. Mean values of the fractal dimension D and standard deviation of the retinal vascular tree in 23 patients.

	All data D0	Slope 1 D1	Slope 2 D2
Arteries			
Females	1.51 ± 0.05	1.19 ± 0.04	1.66 ± 0.04
Males	1.47 ± 0.03	1.19 ± 0.04	1.64 ± 0.03
All	1.48 ± 0.04	1.19 ± 0.04	1.64 ± 0.04
Veins			
Females	1.51 ± 0.03	1.20 ± 0.03	1.67 ± 0.03
Males	1.48 ± 0.04	1.19 ± 0.04	1.65 ± 0.05
All	1.49 ± 0.04	1.19 ± 0.04	1.66 ± 0.04
Arteries & veins			
Females	1.64 ± 0.02	1.29 ± 0.02	1.77 ± 0.02
Males	1.63 ± 0.03	1.28 ± 0.03	1.76 ± 0.02
All	1.63 ± 0.03	1.29 ± 0.02	1.76 ± 0.02

D0: 50 to 3200 µm, D1: 50 to 250 µm, D2: 250 to 3200 µm
SD: standard deviation

Table 5. Duncan's multiple range test for the difference of means between the different fractal dimensions in the arterial, venous and arterio-venous angiograms.

		D0		D1			D2		
		V	AV	A	V	AV	A	V	AV
D0	A	NS	S	S	S	S	S	S	S
	V		S	S	S	S	S	S	S
	AV			S	S	S	NS	NS	S
D1	A				NS	S	S	S	S
	V					S	S	S	S
	AV						S	S	S
D2	A							NS	S
	V								S

D0: 50 to 3200µm, D1: 50 to 250 µm, D2: 250 to 3200 µm
A:arterial, V: venous, AV: arteries and veins combined
S: statistically significant (p< =.01)
NS: non significant (p>.05)

ratios D(vein)/D(artery) for any of the 3 estimated values of D. The results of Duncan's test are expressed in Table 5. No statistically significant difference was found between arterial and venous fractal dimensions in any of the 3 slopes considered.

DISCUSSION

Two hypotheses concerning retinal angiogenesis have been proposed on the basis of estimated fractal dimension of the retinal vasculature. Our determination of the fractal dimension of the posterior retinal vasculature, including the macula and optic

Current
Eye
Research

disc areas, are comparable to previous reports (3-6) in which the similarity of the retinal vascular fractal dimension and that of physical model of diffusion limited aggregation (D = 1.66 - 1.67) (11) was noted. A recent study of fundus photographs of 12 normal subjects (24 eyes), using the grid method estimated D at 1.7 ± 0.01 (12). Although the amount of neural tissue within the retina is well defined but not uniformly distributed, it is possible that the developing nerve tissue dictates the patterns of angiogenesis. However, the similar values of D to difussion limited aggregation led to the suggestion that a similar non-equilibrium Laplacian processes could be involved in retinal angiogenensis (3-6). Our results support this view.

A substantially higher estimate of D = 1.875 has been determined by the density-density correlation function method (13) and used as evidence for an alternative hypothesis of angiogenesis similar to the "invasion percolation model" which explains drainage networks (D = 1.896)(14). Subject data and details of measurement of the density-density correlation function study are not reported so the validity of the higher fractal dimension cannot be assessed. This higher value does not agree with our estimate or those of other authors.

In previous studies, D was obtained by the relation mass-radius or the density-density correlation function (2,3). The GRID method was considered more appropiate as routine angiograms are not necessarily centered at the optic disk whereas the other procedures are sensitive to the statistical radial symmetry of the shape under study i.e. the measurements, in general, start from the optic disc and expand centrifugally.

A tendency to two regression lines of the log-log plot in the range form 50 to 3200 μm was also found, a feature which has not been previously documented. There are several possible explanations for this: (a) the result of arbitrarily analyzing a fraction of the entire retina including the disc and macular areas, the latter being avascular. This fact may be of clinical significance and its value could be revealed with comparative measurements in normal and pathological conditions, (b) it may be related to the concept of 'asymptotic fractal' (fractal tendency at low resolutions and asymptotic tendency to a single value at high ones) (15). Although mathematical deterministic fractals are self similar *ad infinitum*, natural fractals have upper and lower limits, the upper ones, usually asymptotic to a specific value. For the retinal vascular tree, the lower limit is the branching of the main retinal arteries and veins and the upper limit is the capillary bed. This fact limits the meaning of "scale independence" to a finite range as seen in Fig. 2. Our plots show an inverse power law in a range between one and two decades (orders of magnitude).

The limitations of the type of graphic analyses as presented here relate to object size and to pixel resolution. For achieving ranges of resolution of several decades, then large graphic arrays have to be used. As an example, if we keep 1 pixel as the smallest box size (25 μm), adding further decades of data points to the plot implies a box size of 1000 pixels (2.5 cm) for a third decade, or size 10000 pixels (25 cm) for a fourth. Clearly these ranges are far larger than the eye itself and therefore meaningless. Conversely, with addition of boxes at the low end of the range (with magnification of the image prior to tracing), unit pixel size would be, for example 2.5 μm or 0.25 μm, depending on addition of one or two decades. For these sizes, even the capillary bed is reached in theory (although not resolved by manually traced fluorescein angiograms), but at this magnification vessels are unlikely to be self-similar.

In the asymptotic fractal concept (15), one should look for the asymptotic value of the upper part of the log-log plot, but we preferred to approach the same problem with 2 regression lines because they revealed high correlation coefficients and the upper limit at 40μm (limit of accurate resolution of the angiogram) is arbitrarily imposed. Therefore, the behaviour beyond this resolution up to the capillary bed is unknown and consequently the asymptotic values would not be valid.

No difference could be found with age or sex in the patients over the resolution range observed. This is not surprising as there is no documented age-related change in the form or branching of the vascular tree. In previous reports (4,5) based on small numbers of cases, the fractal dimension of the venous tree was reported to be higher than the arterial one, but no statistically significant difference could be found in this study.

The similarity of fractal dimension of retinal vasculature to computer generated fractals based on diffusion precesses has been used to support the involvement of such processes in normal (2,4) and pathological angiogenesis (16). If correct, then similar factors may influence development of both retinal arteries and veins resulting in comparable fractal dimensions.

It is possible that small discrepancies in the estimation of dimension values by various authors are related to the image adquisition technique (all the reports use manual tracings) or the ranges of estimation rather than differences in the fractal dimension itself. With improvements in image processing, computerized analysis will aid interpretation of such clinical investigations as fundus photography and fluorescein angiography. Fractal analysis is a method which can be easily applied to images of branching structures. It may be expected that diseases which alter the distribution of retinal vasculature, such as proliferative retinopathies, would also change their fractal dimensions.

CORRESPONDING AUTHOR

Dr. G. Landini. Oral Pathology Unit, The Dental School, University of Birmingham. St Chad's Queensway, Birmingham B4 6NN, UK

REFERENCES

1. Mandelbrot, B.B. (1982) The Fractal Geometry of Nature. Freeman, San Francisco.
2. Masters, B.R. (1990) Fractal analysis of human retinal blood vessels patterns: developmental and diagnostic aspects. In "Noninvasive Diagnostic Techniques in Ophthalmology", (Ed. Masters, B.R.) pp.515-527, Springer-Verlag, N.Y.
3. Family, F., Masters, B.R. and Platt, D.E. (1989) Fractal pattern formation in human retinal vessels. Physica D , 38, 98-103.
4. Mainster, M.A. (1990) The factal properties of retinal vessels: Embryological and clinical implications. Eye, 4, 235-241.
5. Kinoshita, M. and Honda, Y. (1991) The fractal property of retinal vascular pattern. Invest. Ophthalmol. Vis. Sci., 32 (suppl), 1082.
6. Masters, B.R. and Platt, D.E. (1989) Development of human retinal vessels: a fractal analysis. Invest. Ophthalmol. Vis. Sci., 30 (suppl), 391.
7. Masters, B.R., Family, F. and Platt, D.E. (1989) Fractal analysis of human retinal vessels. Biophys. J., 55 (suppl), 575a.
8. Caserta, F., Stanley, H.E., Eldred, W.D., Daccord, G., Hausman, R.E. and Nittmann, J. (1990) Physical mechanisms underlying neurite outgrowth: a quantitative analysis of nuronal shape. Phys. Rev. Lett., 64, 95-98.
9. Voss, R.F. (1986) Characterization and measurement of random fractals. Physica Scripta, T13, 27-32.
10. Barnsley, M. (1988) Fractals Everywhere. Academic Press, San Diego.
11. Witten, T.A., and Sanders, L.M. (1983) Diffusion-limited aggregation. Phys. Rev. B, 27, 5686-5697.
12. Masters, B.R., Sernetz, M. and Wlczek, P. (1992) Image analysis of human retinal blood vessels and their characterization as fractals. Acta Stereol., 11(suppl 1), 355-360.
13. Daxer, A. (1992) Fractals and retinal vessels. Lancet, 339, 618.
14. Stark, C.P. (1991) An invasion percolation model of drainage network evolution. Nature, 352, 423-425.
15. Rigaut, J.P. (1984) An empirical formulation relating boundary lengths to resolution in specimens showing 'non-ideally fractal' dimensions. J. Microsc., 133 Pt1, 41-54.
16. Landini, G. and Misson, G. (1993) Simulation of corneal neo-vascularization by inverted difussion limited aggregation. Invest. Ophthalmol. Vis. Sci. (in press).

Cancer Letters 77 (1994) 183–189

183

The Application of Fractal Analysis to Mammographic Tissue Classification

Carey E. Priebe*[a], Jeffrey L. Solka[a], Richard A. Lorey[a], George W. Rogers[a], Wendy L. Poston[a], Maria Kallergi[b], Wei Qian[b], Laurence P. Clarke[b], Robert A. Clark[b]

[a]Naval Surface Warfare Center, Dahlgren Division, Advanced Computation Technology Group, Code B10, Dahlgren, VA 22448, USA

[b]H. Lee Moffitt Cancer and Research Center, University of South Florida, Tampa, FL 33612, USA

(Received 19 September 1993; revision received 25 October 1993; accepted 29 October 1993)

Abstract: As a first step in determining the efficacy of using computers to assist in diagnosis of medical images, an investigation has been conducted which utilizes the patterns, or textures, in the images. To be of value, any computer scheme must be able to recognize and differentiate the various patterns. An obvious example of this in mammography is the recognition of tumorous tissue and non-malignant abnormal tissue from normal parenchymal tissue. We have developed a pattern recognition technique which uses features derived from the fractal nature of the image. Further, we are able to develop mathematical models which can be used to differentiate and classify the many tissue types. Based on a limited number of cases of digitized mammograms, our computer algorithms have been able to distinguish tumorous from healthy tissue and to distinguish among various parenchymal tissue patterns. The preliminary results indicate that discrimination based on the fractal nature of images may well represent a viable approach to utilizing computers to assist in diagnosis.

Key words: Computational statistics; Computer assisted diagnosis; Wolfe patterns; Feature extraction; Pattern recognition; Fractals; Probability density function

1. INTRODUCTION

The development of computer assisted diagnosis (CAD) as a physician's tool is widely recognized as a desirable goal [4]. The application of CAD to mammography could well lead to broader based screening without increased medical costs. Additionally, a successful CAD system could aid radiologists in evaluating the myriad normal mammograms and segregate the questionable ones for further diagnosis. Any successful CAD system applied to medical imagery must necessarily be concerned with such issues as image segmentation, feature extraction, and pattern recognition. This paper addresses one method of feature extraction and pattern recognition based on image texture. The feature extraction technique is derived from the theory of frac-

tals [2]. Related work in fractal analysis of mammographic images can be found in references [3,7,9]. The pattern recognition system we have developed is based on a branch of statistics known as Computational Statistics [19].

Computational Statistics is most useful in dealing with extremely large data sets and data sets that cannot be represented by usual statistical models such as normal (or other closed form) distributions. The texture information in a digitized medical image such as a mammogram easily represents a data set of 100 000 local observations. Additionally, our observations indicate this data is not well represented by a normal (or gaussian) distribution. With the advent of current computer technology, manipulation of data sets of this size or lager is quite feasible. Hence, the application of Computational Statistics to medical imagery and CAD represents a quite natural blend of technologies.

*Corresponding author.

C.E. Priebe et al. / Cancer Lett. 77 (1994) 183–189

In dealing with the issues raised above we need to address and define several mathematical terms. The first is a probability density function or pdf. The pdf is analogous to a mass density which is described with respect to some variable (e.g., the mass density of the earth as a function of distance from the center). Here, the probability density will be a function of the image data. To estimate the pdf, we use a technique such as adaptive mixtures [12,13]. Adaptive mixtures is a means of calculating the pdf without making strict assumptions about the actual statistical distribution of the data and is a hybrid approach designed to maintain the best features of both kernel estimation [16] and finite mixture models [18]. That is, we do not assume that the data is normally distributed.

In order to compute the pdf estimate, we need to extract image features. For this work we have used features based on the concept of fractals which can be used to represent various textures [11]. Fractals have been used to describe many common images such as coastlines, clouds, and fern leaves [8]. In other words, fractals are geometric objects which have a non-Euclidean (nonman-made) character which can be described in part by a property called the fractal dimension which is different than the normal Euclidean dimension.

The science of fractals was first pioneered by Mandelbrot [8]. Barnsley, et al. [1] showed that many biological systems could be described using fractal geometry. This quantity (fractal dimension f_d) has been shown to correlate with subjective human texture classification and is defined by Pentland [10] as

$$E\{|\Delta I(\Delta x)|\} = E\{|\Delta I(1)|\} \|\Delta x\|^H$$

Here H is the difference between the normal Euclidean dimension (e_d) and the fractal dimension ($H = e_d - f_d$). The Euclidean dimension for an image is, of course, two. $E\{...\}$ is the expected value of the quantity in brackets. $E\{|\Delta I(1)|\}$ is the expected change in the intensity one unit away from a given point $E\{\Delta I(\Delta x)\}$ is the expected change in the intensity Δx units away. The symbol $\|...\|$ is the standard Euclidean norm or distance. For the case of a Euclidean object where the fractal and Euclidean dimensions are the same (i.e., a non-fractal object) the expected change in the image intensity at a distance × units from some point is the same as the expected change one unit away. This result is in keeping with our intuition since the grayscale value is constant for such an object. Previous work of Caldwell et al. [3] has shown a correlation between fractal dimension and the subjective human classification of parenchymal patterns.

Many of the methods for estimating f_d are based on Richardson's Law [8]

$$M(\varepsilon) = K\varepsilon^{(e_d - f_d)},$$

where $M(\varepsilon)$ is the measured property of a fractal at a scale of ε and K is a constant of proportionality. The measured quantity at a given point is the change in image intensity as a function of scale. Using this equation, and the technique described in Solka et al. [17], we extract three features that describe the texture. The first is directly related to the fractal dimension, the second is a measure of how well the fractal model fits the data, and the third is related to the local degree of contrast in the image. As will be seen below, the use of all three features gives improved results over the use of any single feature.

The process of extracting fractal features and computing a pdf must be done for each class of data represented in the image. Once we have the estimates of the class pdfs our job is to discriminate each class from the other classes. If we plot the various pdfs and show that they are distinct from one another, we can calculate discrimination boundaries and the task of discriminating the various classes is a relatively straightforward application of Bayes' rule [5]. Once we have good estimates of the pdfs based on data from a number of images (i.e., from training data) and have determined appropriate discrimination boundaries, we can, in effect, turn the process around and use these boundaries to classify regions in new images.

As stated above, when we extract fractal features for a given class we determine three features for each observation. We can think of these three features as being the coordinates of a vector in three dimensional space. While more information is often contained in higher dimensional feature space, the difficulty associated with pdf estimation increases dramatically with any increase in the dimensionality of the observations [15]. To simplify our computations we can use the Fisher linear discriminant (FLD) [5] which allows us to project these three dimensions to the one dimension that is in some sense best for discrimination and thus decreases the computational complexity. Additionally, this projection eases the problem of illustration since we are able to plot the results.

For each class of training data we have some number of observations that we label as X_i which represents the observations from class i (where $i = 1,2$ for two classes). Using the fractal features as components we can represent each observation vector as $\underline{x} = [x_1, x_2, x_3]^T$, where each observation vector $\underline{x}$ is contained in the set X_i. The FLD yields a projection vector whose use results in a projected one dimensional observation y for each vector $\underline{x}$. Thus we obtain a set of observations Y_i for each class i. Then we employ a normalization transformation which yields Y'_1 with a mean of 0 and variance of 1. This same transformation is applied to class

Cancer Letters 77 (1994) 183–189

2 of the projected observations yielding Y'_2 from Y_2. Next we estimate the pdfs for Y'_1 and Y'_2 using the adaptive mixtures technique and determine the discriminant boundary.

For a different image, which we label as testing data, we apply the FLD projection vector and the normalization transformation which were determined from the training data. We then estimate the pdfs for the two classes of data from the testing image using the projected and transformed data. This allows us to obtain performance estimates of this overall procedure and to judge its utility to CAD.

2. METHODS

Images used in this study were provided courtesy of the H. Lee Moffitt Cancer Center and Research Institute and the Department of Radiology at the University of South Florida. The acquisition of the mammograms was accomplished under the breast screening program of the Center. The selected cases represent a variety of cancers of different subtlety. All tumorous regions were biopsy proven. The mammograms were digitized at ~220 mm/pixel and 8 bit/pixel by the Mindax Corporation of Minneapolis, MN using DuPont FD-2000 scanner.

Using the techniques described by Solka et al. [17], features for tumorous and healthy tissues are extracted (10 000 healthy tissue observations and 500 tumorous tissue observations) from mammogram A shown in Fig. 1. This represents the training data. We develop the FLD projection vector and the normalization transformation from this image (which contains a malignant stellate mass ~10 mm).

A second mammogram not pictured here (mammogram B) was used for testing (10 000 healthy tissue observations and 300 tumorous tissue observations). The mammogram contains a malignant stellate mass (~6 mm). We apply the FLD projection and transformation developed from mammogram A to the data from mammogram B. We next reverse the order of training and testing data. That is, we use mammogram B as training data and mammogram A as testing data.

At this point, one might well ask if the process of projection from three dimensions to one dimension results in any degradation in discriminant capabilities. For the small number of images we are using in our work we can of course calculate the estimated pdfs using the full three dimensional vectors. We can also calculate the correlation matrices which show numbers which are a measure of how well any given feature correlates to the class variable for the two mammograms in this study.

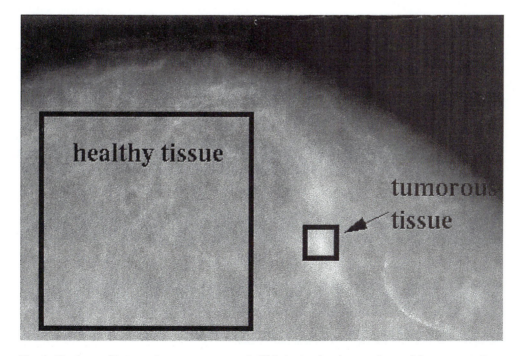

Fig. 1. Regions of interest in mammogram. A. This image has been enhanced for presentation.

186

C.E. Priebe et al. / Cancer Lett. 77 (1994) 183–189

The last part of our analysis utilized the four tissue patterns (labeled as N1, P1, P2, DY) which have been distinguished by Wolfe [20] and correspond to increasing breast tissue density and different morphology. The relationship of these patterns with breast cancer risk is the subject of much discussion. See, for instance, Saftlas and Szklo [14]. To determine the applicability of this technique to the discrimination of Wolfe patterns, we analyzed an additional eight mammograms. Our method consisted of determining pdfs for two Wolfe patterns, using this as training data, and using two other Wolfe patterns as testing data.

3. RESULTS

3.1. Two class data discrimination

Fig. 2 is a plot of the pdfs of the projected data showing the separation of the healthy and tumorous classes. This figure indicates that for this image, the fractal dimension features can be used to distinguish healthy tissue from tumorous tissue.

We apply the FLD projection and transformation developed from mammogram A to the data from mammogram B. The estimated pdfs from this testing data are shown in Fig. 3. The discrimination boundary is clearly evident. Furthermore, this boundary appears to be invariant. That is, the boundaries in Figs. 2 and 3 are in the same place.

When the roles of mammograms A and B are reversed, the plots obtained exhibit the same behavior but with a different discriminant boundary. However, the results indicate that once a projection is chosen the discriminant boundary is invariant from training to testing data. This indicates that the discriminant boundary obtained from training images can be successfully applied to new test images. We hasten to add

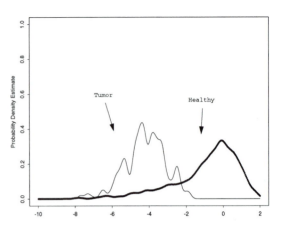

Fig. 3. Fisher linear discriminant pdfs for mammogram B using the independent projection.

that since this is based on just two mammograms this represents an indication of what might be possible.

To examine the feature correlation we can consider the correlation against class obtained from the mammogram A data. The correlation number for the single projected dimension is −0.749. The correlation numbers for the three original features are 0.128, 0.367, and 0.094. Comparing absolute values, we find in each case that the number associated with the projected single dimension correlates better with class than any of the three original features. For the data from mammogram A, the FLD projection correlation of −0.749 is significantly higher than any of the class correlations for the original features. Although the magnitude of the correlations are smaller for the data from mammogram B, this same pattern still holds. This result is the motivation for using all three features with the FLD rather than any single feature such as the fractal dimension by itself. We can also compute correlations based on one image used as a training set and the other image used as a testing set. Comparing the correlations of the projected data, there is no serious degradation in the correlation when the projection is obtained independently. For example, we obtain a correlation of −0.749 for the projected mammogram A data when the projection is obtained using this same data. When the projection used is obtained from the mammogram B data this correlation is nearly unchanged (−0.724). The numbers obtained for the mammogram B data follow this same pattern for the correlation. This gives further credence to the generalization property, i.e., the projection obtained from one image can be used on data extracted from a separate image.

3.2. Wolfe's pattern analysis

The pdfs for the Wolfe patterns N1 and DY are shown in Fig. 4. This figure, along with Fig. 5 and Fig. 6, indicates the ability to discriminate among the various

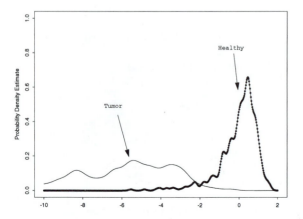

Fig. 2. Fisher linear discriminant pdfs for mammogram A.

Cancer Letters 77 (1994) 183–189

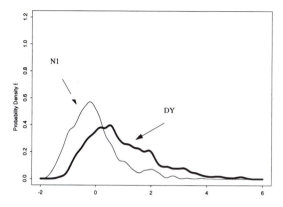

187

Fig. 4. FLD pdfs for mammogram N1 vs. mammogram DY.

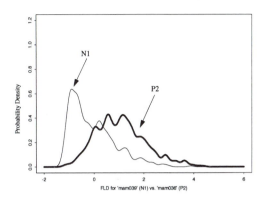

Fig. 6. FLD pdfs for mammogram N1 vs. mammogram P2.

Wolfe patterns. These particular combinations of patterns were chosen simply for illustration and are not meant to be exhaustive. To demonstrate the same kind of generalization shown above, FLD projection vectors were determined using the data drawn from these new mammograms and were used in producing the pdfs for the combinations N1–DY, N1–P1, and N1–P2 represented by Figs. 4, 5, and 6. In all cases, the patterns could be discriminated from one another and the discriminant boundaries generalize from training to testing image.

The pdfs here have a greater overlap than those discussed previously and certainly this overlap represents a measure of the amount of error, or probability of error, of incorrect classification of a single observation associated with a testing set. However, in the case of spatial data for which multiple observations can be assumed to be from a single class, this probability of error is drastically reduced by considering the joint pdfs as a product of the (independent) individual pdfs. In fact, as few as 10 observations, which is certainly a reasonable number for this application, could reduce the probability of error significantly.

4. CONCLUSIONS

Based on the limited number of cases studied, the preliminary indications are that the extraction of features based on the fractal nature of images, the reduction of dimensionality employing the Fisher Linear Discriminant projection vector, and the estimation of probability density functions using adaptive mixtures, represents a viable approach to pattern recognition that may be useful in the application of Computer Assisted Diagnosis to mammography. If the results of the efforts involving the Wolfe patterns can be extended to include non-malignant abnormal tissue this technique may aid in distinguishing these tissue types.

Research is continuing in this area and we have begun the digitization of a larger number of mammograms. Our plans are to develop an FLD projection vector based on training data from healthy tissue and tumorous tissue extracted from a substantial quantity of mammograms. The normalization transformation will be calculated and the pdfs of these two classes will be estimated. This model will then be tested on a sizable number of distinct mammograms to determine its utility. We will continue our research and testing until there exists sufficient evidence to support the viability of the approach. Additionally, we will extend our efforts to include non-malignant abnormal tissue.

For any system to be of practical value, the model must be formed from a sufficiently large pool of mammograms to instil confidence in the method. The pdfs formed from this large pool will form the baseline system and will be stored for archiving and reference purposes. The adaptive mixtures approach to pdf estimation will give the system the capability to update the pdfs with each new mammogram that is tested. Finally, our previous work indicates that the performance of our system can be improved through the use of wavelet transformations to enhance the areas of interest in the images [6].

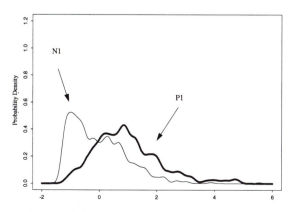

Fig. 5. FLD pdfs for mammogram N1 vs. mammogram P1.

5. ACKNOWLEDGMENTS

The authors would like to thank an anonymous reviewer for helpful comments.

REFERENCES

1 Barnsley, M.F., Massopust, P., Strickland, H. and Sloan, A.D. (1987) Fractal modeling of biological structures. Ann. NY Acad. Sci., 504, 179–194.

2 Barnsley, M.F. (1988) Fractals Everywhere. Academic Press, San Diego, CA.

3 Caldwell, C.B., Stapleton, S.J., Holdsworth, D.W., Jong, R.A., Weiser, W.J., Cooke, G. and Yaffe, M.J. (1990) Characteristics of mammographic parenchymal pattern by fractal dimension. Phys. Med. Biol., 35, 235–247.

4 Chan, H.P., Doi, K. Vyborny, C.J., Schmidt, R.A., Metz, C.E., Lam, K.L., Ogura, T. Wu, Y. and MacMahon, H. (1990) Improvements in radiologists' detection of clustered microcalcifications on mammograms. Invest. Radiol., 25, 1102–1110.

5 Duda, R.O. and Hart, P.E. (1973) Pattern Classification and Scene Analysis. John Wiley and Sons, New York, NY.

6 Li, H.D., Qian W., Clarke, L.P., Kallergi, M. and Clark, R.A. (1993) Mammographic image features extraction and enhancement by wavelet transform. Proceedings of the 35th Annual Meeting of the AAPM (Abs), Washington DC, August 8–12.

7 Magnin, I.E., Cluzeau, F., Odet, C.L. and Bremond, A. (1986) Mammographic texture analysis: an evaluation of risk for developing breast cancer. Opt. Eng., 25, 780–784.

8 Mandelbrot, B. (1977) The Fractal Geometry of Nature. W.H. Freeman and Company, New York, NY.

9 Miller, P. and Astley, S. (1992) Classification of breast tissue by texture analysis. Image Vision Comput., 10, 277–282.

10 Pentland, A.P. (1986) From Pixels to Predicates. Ablex Publishing Corporation, Norwood, NJ.

11 Pietgen, H. and Saupe, D. (Eds.) (1988) The Science of Fractal Images. Springer-Verlag, New York, NY.

12 Priebe, C.E. and Marchette, D.J. (1991) Adaptive mixtures: recursive nonparametric pattern recognition. Pattern Recognition, 24, 1197–1209.

13 Priebe, C.E. and Marchette, D.J. (1993) Adaptive mixture density estimation. Pattern Recognition, 26, 771–785.

14 Saftlas, A.F. and Szklo, M. (1987) Mammographic parenchymal patterns and breast cancer risk. Epidemiol. Rev., 9, 146–174.

15 Scott, D.W. (1992) Multvariate Density Estimation. John Wiley and Sons, New York, NY.

16. Silverman, B.W. (1986) Density Estimation. Chapman and Hall. New York, NY.

17 Solka, J.L., Priebe, C.E. and Rogers, G.W. (1992) An initial assessment of discriminant surface complexity for power law feature. Simulation, 58, 311–318.

18 Titterington, D.M., Smith A.F.M. and Makov, U.E. (1985) Statistical Analysis of Finite Mixture Distributions. John Wiley and Sons, New York, NY.

19 Wegman, E.J. (1988) Computational Statistics: a new agenda for statistical theory and practice. J. Wash. Acad. Sci., 78, 310–322.

20 Wolfe, J.N. (1976) Breast patterns as an index of risk for developing breast cancer. Am J. Radiol., 126, 1130–1139.

Bio-Medical Materials and Engineering, Vol. 3, No. 3, pp. 117–126, 1993

117

Fractal Dimension Analysis of Aluminum Oxide Particle for Sandblasting Dental Use

Yoshiki Oshida*, Carlos A. Munoz**, Mark M. Winkler*, Azza Hashem*, and Michio Itoh†

*Department of Dental Materials, Indiana University School of Dentistry, Indianapolis, IN 46202-5186

**Department of Prosthodontics, Indiana University School of Dentistry, Indianapolis, IN 46202-5186

†Institute for Dental Science, Matsumoto Dental College, Shiojiri Nagano, 399-07 Japan

Abstract—Aluminum oxide particles are commonly used as a sandblasting media, particularly in dentistry, for multiple purposes including divesting the casting investment materials and increasing effective surface area for enhancing the mechanical retention strengths of succeedingly applied fired porcelain or luting cements. Usually fine aluminum oxide particles are recycled within the sandblasting machine. Ceramics such as aluminum oxides are brittle, therefore, some portions of recycling aluminum oxide particles might be brittle fractured. If fractured sandblasting particles are involved in the recycling media, it might result in irregularity metallic materials surface as well as the recycling sandblasting media itself be contaminated. Hence, it is necessary from both clinical and practical reasons to monitor the particle conditions in terms of size/shape and effectiveness of sandblasting, so that sandblasting dental prostheses can be fabricated in optimum and acceptable conditions. In the present study, the effect of recycling aluminum oxide particles on the surface texture of metallic materials was evaluated by Fractal Dimension Analysis (FDA). Every week the alumina powder was sampled and analyzed for weight fraction and contaminants. Surface texture of sandblasted standard samples was also characterized by FDA. Results indicate very little change in particle size, while the fractal dimension increased. Fractal dimension analysis showed that the aluminum oxide particle as a sandblasting media should be replaced after 30 or 40 min of total accumulated operation time.

Key Words—fractal dimension analysis, sandblasting, aluminum oxide particle, contamination, X-ray diffraction

INTRODUCTION

DENTAL MANUFACTURERS of sandblasting or an airborne particle abrasive (ABPA) machines provide an array of systems. Some systems can vary the operating pressure or provide recycling and non-recycling capability or vary the nozzle size.

Many commercial dental laboratories used ABPA systems that recycle the aluminum oxide and will have units with a dedicated purpose, such as one for divesting castings, another for preparation of the metal prior to porcelain application, or the use of different blasting media such as glass beads, aluminum oxide, or walnut shells.

In prosthodontics, one of the many steps in the preparation of the metal substrate prior to the application of porcelain is the creation of microscopic irregularities. These irregularities serve to enhance mechanical retention and increases the surface area of the substructure. This is accomplished by the use of stones and burs, airborne particle abrasion or a combination of the two. The preferred method is to prepare the surface with burs and stone and then to air abrade the metal by injecting 50 μm alumina under pressure into the metal's surface to form a plurality of small indentation.

Research has shown that the rough texture generated by airborne particle abrasion increases the surface area of the metal and thus enhances the interfacial bond strength of porcelain fused to metal (1–15). The increased surface area caused by ABPA can be roughly estimated. Suppose a rectangular-shaped unair-abraded metal coupon has a surface area of S_o (= L_o^2, where L_o is length), after air abrading, L_o will be increased by $L_i = (2\pi r_i/B_i) \times (L_o/r_i) \times C_i$, where r_i is the radius of used alumina-abrading media, B_i is cross-sectional contact fraction of each media, and C_i is the total coverage of air abrading in percentage. B_i normally ranges from 12.5% to 50%; i.e., $8 > 1/B_i > 2$ (12). The size of the air-abrading media, r_i, (usually varying from 25 μm to 200 μm) is cancelled out in the above equation. The term C_i is normally 200%, meaning that the entire surface will be air abraded twice under the same blasting condition. Hence, if we assume that 20% of the spherical surface of individual blast media particle is impinged into the substrate (i.e., $B_i = 1/5$), L_i yields $L_i = (2\pi/5) \times L_o \times 2 \approx 2.5L_o$ or $Si = (2.5L_o)^2 = 6.25S_o$. Therefore, it can be suggested that at least the surface area will increase by factor of 6.25 than the unair-abraded surface area.

Usually dental technicians will air abrade a framework for 5 s under a pressure of 20 psi by using 50 μm alumina (α–Al_2O_3) powder and keeping a distance between the tip of the nozzle and the framework of approximately 30 mm. If a system that recycles the Al_2O_3 is used, the alumina, being a brittle material, will fracture into smaller particles. Also during the blasting process, the impingement reaction with sharp-edged fractured alumina over the metal will cause metal to be abraded away into small fractured metal elements, thus causing possible contamination on both alumina powder and metal surfaces.

The aim, therefore, of this study is to (a) investigate the altering characteristics of alumina powder as a function of time, (b) to evaluate the microstructure and element analysis of 50 μm Al_2O_3 media, and (c) to recommend the optimum condition for replacement time of the alumina powder in the ABPA machines in order to maintain a reliable mechanical retention strength at an interface between the metal and porcelain. The characterization of the ever-changing alumina morphology was conducted by the new statistical concept—Fractal Dimension Analysis—which has been used widely in various sectors in science and engineering fields.

Fractal Dimension Analysis

Since this research project deals with the fractal dimension analysis, it will be discussed in detail below. We are accustomed to the Euclidian dimension (d) of 0, 1, 2, and 3, which respectively corresponds to a dot, a line, a surface, and a three-dimensional object. In reality however, many geometrical shapes do not quite fit into one of these categories. Fractals are a new geometric concept whose primary object is to describe the great variety of natural structures that are irregular, rough, or fragmented, have irregularities of various sizes that bear a special "scaling" relationship to one another (16). Namely, the structure is "self-similar" over a wide range of scales (17). To accommodate such geometries, Mandelbrot introduced the idea of intermediate fractal dimension, D_f (>d) such that $2 \leq D_f \leq 3$; higher value for the D_f value, the rougher surfaces; while for a line, $1 \leq D_f \leq 2$ (16,17). Rough surfaces are also known to exhibit the feature of geometric self-similarity and self-affinity (16,18–21), by which similar appearances of the surfaces are seen under various degrees of magnification (22). Since increasing amounts of detail in the roughness are observed at decreasing length scales the concept of slope and curvature, which inherently assume the smoothness of a surface, cannot be defined. Hence, it is necessary to characterize rough surfaces by intrinsic parameters that are independent of all scales of roughness (22). This suggests that the fractal dimension, which is invariant with length scales and is closely linked to the concept of geometric self-similarity, is an intrinsic property and should be used for surface characterization 922). The D_f satisfies the properties of continuity, nondifferentiability, and self-affinity (22,23).

There are several ways to define the fractal dimension, e.g., slit island method (17), vertical section method (24), or box counting method (25). It was reported that the D_f obtained by the slit island method provided the same value as the D_f obtained by the vertical section method after the Fourier analysis (24). In this study, the box counting method was employed because this method has an easy assess to a computerized data acquisition and processing.

One can find various applications of the fractal analysis in surface science and engineering fields. Surface sciences on a surface adsorption phenomena (26), sandstone porosity (27), fine particle profiles (28), or wettability (29) utilized the fractal dimension. Fracture surface of ductile materials were extensively characterized by the D_f (17,24,30,31,32) as an application to practical fractography. Surface fracture topology of brittle materials was also studied by the fractal dimension (33). Application of the fractal analysis to the tribological phenomena can be found in various articles (34,35,36). Fractal concept has been successfully employed to characterize metallographic features (37,38,39). One of the present authors (Y. Oshida) had employed the Richardson plot method to characterize the surface roughness of shot-peened steel surfaces and concluded that the D_f can serve as a measure for determining and monitoring the optimum surface coverage percentage in shot-peening industry (12).

The rough surface and surface texture of various materials were analyzed by the fractal dimension (18,22,40). Majumdar and Tien, studying the machined stainless steel surface, found that the $D_f = 1.5$, and the power spectra indicated the power law of $1/\omega^2$, which corresponds to a Brownian process (22). Furthermore, Chesters, Wen, Lundin, and Kasper, using a contact diamond stylus profilometer to characterize the surface of stainless steel with various surface finishes, reported that $D_f = 1.3 - 1.9$ for as-machined condition, $1.1 - 1.2$ for electropolished surface and $1.2 - 1.7$ for chemically polished surfaces. It was also found that the higher R_a (arithmetic average roughness) and R_m (its largest single deviation), the higher D_f (18).

MATERIALS AND METHODS

Equipment Setup

An airborne particle abrasion machine (Ticonium, Model 5102A1, Albany, NY) was set up in the graduate prosthodontic laboratory. Aluminum oxide powder (Sterngold, Attleboro, MA) was used. Nominal particle size of unused alumina was 50 μm.

It was requested that all residents use this system prior to porcelain application. Every time it was used, the user filled out a record sheet regarding date, approximate blasting duration and type of alloy used. The machine was set up at a constant 20 psi and checked periodically to ascertain that the pressure was constant. Weekly, a sample was collected from the upper compartment and used for measuring weight fraction of the different particle size. A reference steel sample coupon (15 × 15 × 3 mm) was air abraded under 20 psi, of 5 s, with a distance from nozzle tip to metal sample of 30 mm. The air-abraded metal coupon was further characterized by the fractal dimension analysis, as described below.

Aluminum Oxide Particle Analysis: Particle Size

Approximately 50 g of alumina powder was sampled each week from the upper compartment. Using two mesh-sized (61 μm and 44 μm), sampled powder was separated into three groups: (a) coarse size alumina powder, not passing through the 61 μm mesh (i.e., +61 μm); (b) medium size alumina powder, passing through the 61 μm mesh, but not passing through the 44 μm mesh (i.e., –61 μm > particle size >+44 μm); and (c) fine size alumina powder, passing through the 44 μm mesh (i.e., –44 μm). Each grouped powder was weighed, and the weight fraction, W_f, was calculated in percentage for each group. After obtaining W_f, all sampled powder was returned to the upper recycling compartment of the ABPA machine.

Fractal Dimension Analysis

As explained before, a steel coupon (15 × 15 × 3 mm) was air abraded for 5 s under 20 psi of pressurized air. The surface of the steel coupon was subjected to a surface texture analysis before and after air abrasion using a profilometer (Surtronic 3P, Rank Taylor-Hobson, Leicster, England) with a diamond stylus (tip radius: 5 μm); a printed readout of each reading was obtained. The printed surface profile was then subjected to the Fractal Dimension Analysis. For this study, the box counting method (a Richardson plot) was employed. Referring to Fig. 1, the box size, r, can be related to the box number, $N(r)$, in a formula of $N(r) \propto 1/r^D$. The negative slope of a log–log plot of r and $N(r)$ is the fractal dimension, D_f, of the profile. In this study, three scales (r) were prepared; 3 × 3 mm, 5 × 5 mm, and 10 × 10 mm. Each scale was superimposed over the surface roughness profile chart and total number of boxes containing the profile, $N(r)$, was counted, as illustrated in Fig. 1.

Microstructure and Element Analysis of Alumina Powder

Both unused and used alumina powder (which was sampled at total accumulated time of 2,400 seconds) were observed under the scanning electron microscope (SEM) and element analyzed with the Energy-Dispersive X-Ray Spectroscopy (EDXS) (Kevex-Ray®).

X-ray Diffraction of Alumina Powder

Both unused and used alumina powder after 2,400 s were subjected to x-ray diffraction (XRD) to identify the crystalline structures as well as to further investigate the diffracted line broadening, if any, XRD was conducted using $CuK_{\alpha 1}$ radiation with a Ni filter, under 50kV and 40mA, with scanning speed of 4 deg/min.

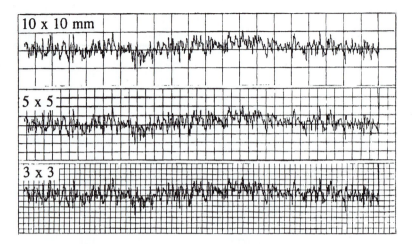

FIG. 1. Surface roughness profile superimposed with three different sizes of fractal scale (10×10, 5×5, and 3×3 mm).

RESULTS AND DISCUSSION

Operation Record

The accumulated total time was 4,310 s (72 min over a 6 month period). The material types that were air abraded during this period included high gold content metal ceramic alloys, base metal alloys, Ni-Cr alloys, pure Ti, stainless steel, and Fe-based alloys. The time fraction was as follows; 44% of 4,310 total times were utilized for air-abrading base metal alloys, 28% for Ti-based alloys, 18% for Fe-based alloys, and 10% for Ni-Cr alloys.

Fractal Dimension, D_f

Figure 2 shows the changes in D_f (fractal dimension) as a function of time. After new α-Al$_2$O$_3$ powder was filled into the ABPA machine, an Fe-C coupon was air abraded for 5 s at 20 psi with a 30 mm distance between the nozzle tip and the sample. The D_f was calculated to be 1.2. It increased to 1.5 even after total time of less than 3 min. The D_f

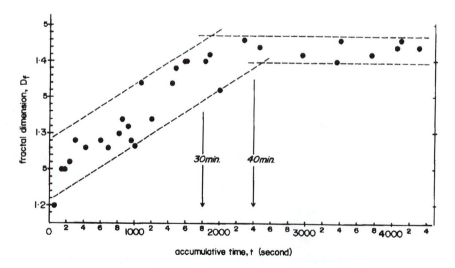

FIG. 2. Changes in fractal dimension, D_f, as a function of time, showing remarkable breaking point at about 30–40 minutes.

changed from 1.26 to 1.30 between 200 to 1,000 s, which is very close to a famous Koch's ideal fractal dimension; 1,2619 (= log4/log3) (41). D_f appears to increase within a scattered band until 30–40 total minutes had elapsed, when the D_f started to be fairly constant with slight scattering between 1.35 and 1.43. When the D_f reached 1.39 ± 0.4, it seems not to alter significantly up to 4,310 total s when this research project was completed. It is obvious that, from Fig. 2, the D_f behavior exhibits a remarkable breaking point at about 30–40 total minutes.

Weight Fraction of Powder, W_f

Sampled alumina powder was subjected to sieving-separation by using 61 μm and 44 μm mesh sieves. As indicated previously, sampled powder was categorized into three groups, coarse, medium, and fine size alumina powder. After separation, each group was weighed, and weight fraction, W_f, was calculated in percentage. The result on un-used powder indicated that coarse size alumina had W_f of 30 weight%, while W_f of the medium size powder was 55%, and W_f of the fine size powder was 15%. These data confirms that the nominal particle size of unused alumina powder was 50 μm (namely, –60 μm > 50 μm > +44 μm).

Changes in W_f for each size group as a function of accumulated time are presented in Fig. 3. Although it was anticipated that W_f for coarse size powder will decrease while W_f for fine size alumina powder will increase as a function of time, all particle size groups appeared not to change significantly during this research period up to 4,310 s (72 min).

Microanalytical Studies

Figure 4 shows scanning electron micrographs (SEMs) of unused and used alumina powder. Used powder was collected from the upper recycling compartment of the ABPA machine at the total time of 2,400 s. It was found that a used particle was fractured in a cleavage manner. Even though the number of broken particles increased as time went on, it did not reshape into a uniform spherical size of fine size particle, so that W_f in fine size particle remained unchanged.

Both unused and used powder were further investigated with energy-dispersive X-ray spectroscopy attached to the SEM (Kevex-ray) under 20kV. Total elapsed time for the element analyses was 100 s. The unused alumina powder showed 100 weight % of Al; while used powder (sampled at 2,400 s) indicated that it contained various elements; namely, Al(83.32 weight%), Ti(5.48%), Ca(1.68%), Ni(1.36%), Mo(1.31%), S(1.02%), Si(0.65%), P(0.55%), Mn(0.49%), K(0.29%), Cl(0.26%), and V(0.08%). It is speculated that these contaminants were partially from metallic materials that were air abraded and partially from trace amounts of investment materials that were used for casting these alloys.

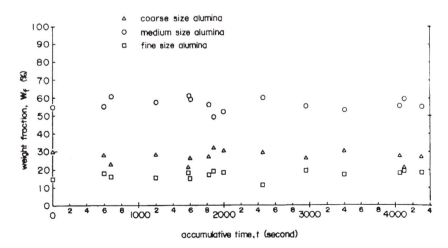

FIG. 3. Changes in weight fraction, W_f, of separated three different sizes of alphas-alumina powder as a function of time.

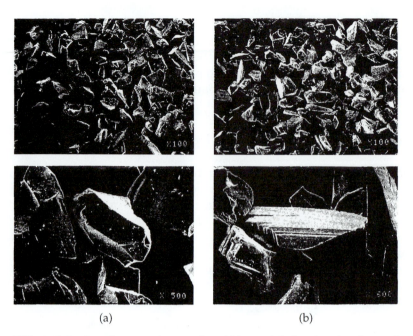

(a)   (b)

FIG. 4. Scanning electron micrographs of (a) unused alumina powder, and (b) used powder after 2,400 total seconds.

X-Ray Diffraction on Alumina Powder

Figures 5 and 6 show X-ray diffractograms of unused alumina (Fig. 5) and used powder (Fig. 6), at 2,400 s. Although main diffracted lines were identified as α-Al$_2$O$_3$ (hkℓ) as marked in both figures, there found three significant differences between two XRDs. Namely, for used alumina powder it was found that (a) integrated intensities of all diffracted lines decreased, (b) abnormality in relative intensity was noticed, and (c) background level increased. Although these phenomena are interacting each other, they will be discussed individually. First, decreased integrated intensity indicates that amount of crystalline particle contributing to the diffraction decreases. Assuming that both unused and used alumina powder were diffracted with same density, if alumina powder were fractured upon collision with each other and/or with a metal piece, to refine its particle size, it should reflect to the diffracted line broadening, not to integrated intensity. However, no remarkable line broadening in lines diffracted from used

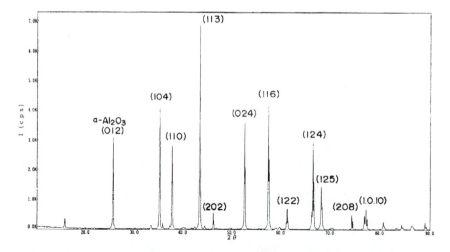

FIG. 5. X-ray diffractogram of un-used alumina powder by CuK$_\alpha$ (Ni filter).

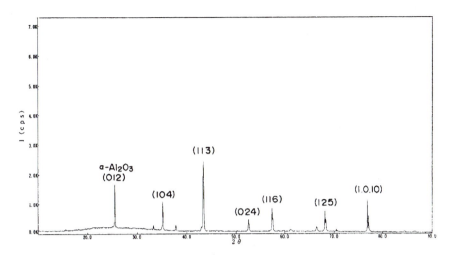

FIG. 6. X-ray diffractogram of powder used for total 2,400 seconds.

powder was found (see Fig. 6), so that it suggested that the majority of sampled used powder still maintained the original shape. This confirmed the results on W_f analysis (see Fig. 3). Secondly, the abnormality in relative intensity is usually recognized when the sample exhibits crystallographic heterogeneity. Crystal structure of α-Al_2O_3 is hexagonal, and its closed packed planes are (00ℓ), on which most of alumina will be fractured in a cleavage manner. Hence, it might cause a directional orientation on the XRDs. According to ASTM X-Ray Powder Data File No. 10-173 (α-Al_2O_3), there is only one diffraction line on 006) at d - 2.165Å. The I/I_1 is less than 1, indicating that the relative intensity is very weak. Although, because of this reason, both Figs. 5 and 6 did not show any diffraction lines from (006) basal plane, it can be speculated that the diffraction planes that are close to (00ℓ) might be intensified. These could be (012) and (104) planes in this case. For example, if diffraction intensities on (012) and (104) planes from unused and those from used powder are compared, it is noticed that their relative intensities are reversed. Therefore, this suggests that the α-Al_2O_3 crystals were selectively cleavage-fractured on planes that were close to the basal (00ℓ) plane. Thirdly, the background level will be caused by fluorescent X-ray, continuous X-ray, non-coherency scattering, or crystalline defects. Since a monochromator was utilized, any other X-rays than $CuK_{\alpha 1}$ line should not be involved in the background increment. The only possibilities left to explain the increased background detected in used powder might be either (a) fluorescent X-ray from element (such as Fe) having a larger mass absorption coefficient for $CuK_{\alpha 1}$ energy level, or (b) non-coherency scattering X-ray from light elements (such as Si), or (c) both. As discussed previously, since used powder contains various heavier and lighter elements than $CuK_{\alpha 1}$, it can be said that these secondary X-ray caused increased background level.

Shot Energy and Deterioration of Metals/Alloys

The velocity of sandblasting (or shot-peening) media, V, can be defined as: $V = b \times \rho^{-1/2} \times D^{-1/3} \times p^{3/4}$, where ρ is density of used show media, b is a constant, depending mainly upon nozzle geometry, D is mean size of shot media, and p is the applied pressure (42). The jet energy of blasting media, E, can also be defined as $E = \pi/12 \times \rho \times D^3 \times V^2$, where ρ is mass volume of total shot, D is shot diameter, and V is velocity (43). Substituting V into this equation yields that $E = \pi/12 \times D^{1/3} \times p^{6/4}$.

The energy, E, defined above is for a case in which individual media is impinged perpendicular to the work piece surface. If the blasting media is impinged with a certain angle, it is anticipated that E will be decreased as a function of $\tan\theta$, where the angle θ is a declining angle. Felton, Bayne, Kanoy, and White studying the effects of air abrasives used for air abrading (25 μm Al_2O_3 under 80 psi) on various marginal configurations of metal ceramic casting alloys, found that the smaller the margin angle, the greater was the loss of alloy after air abrasion (6).

Furthermore, Tiller, Magnus, Gobel, Musil, and Garscke measured the amount of wear volume due to air-abrasive action during the air abrading using 250 μm Al_2O_3 under 20 psi, and observed that the amount of wear was dependent upon the distance between the nozzle tip and the work piece, and 0.5–0.7 μm/second was recorded when the distance was 30 mm. It was also concluded that the worn amount increased in materials with a lower hardness and a lower melting point (44).

According to the equation described above, if D (particle size) decreases, the jet energy will increase under a constant pressure. In the present study, the changes in D were not significant, rather it was indicated that the irregularity in shape and the degree of the contamination increased. This might cause the fractal dimension, D_f, increase after the accumulated total time of 30 to 40 min was reached.

Effects of morphological changes in alumina powder (in terms of fractal dimension) on succeeding bonding strength after the porcelain is applied are under progress.

CONCLUSIONS

In order to determine the effects of air-particle abrasion on metal when the Al_2O_3 is recycled, an air-particle abrasion with recycling capabilities was set up for this project for approximately 6 months. During this project period, alumina powder was sampled weekly to analyze the weight fraction in terms of changes in particle size. A steel coupon was abraded for 5 s under 20 psi and the surface was further subjected to the fractal dimension analysis to characterize the surface topological changes. The accumulated total time for this project was 4,310 s.

The main conclusions drawn from this project are as follows;

1. Even after 2,400 s (40 min), the alumina that had been recycled in the upper compartment of the ABPA machine was contaminated with various elements from the metals/alloys air abraded as well as investment materials for casting.
2. Weight fraction, W_f, for coarse, medium, and fine size alumina does not appear to change significantly, although the scanning electron microscopy reveals a cleavage-fracture of alumina.
3. The X-ray diffraction patterns for both unused and used powder indicated that (a) cleavage fracture took place on planes close to the basal (00ℓ) plane and (b) secondary X-rays caused by contaminants increase the background level.
4. Fractal Dimension Analysis was successfully introduced in the dentistry to characterize the surface texture. Specifically, if it was applied to the ever-changing alumina powder used for the ABPA machine, it can be concluded that alumina media (50 μm nominal particle size) should be replaced entirely from the blaster every 30 to 40 min of total operation time.

Acknowledgements—The authors are grateful to all graduate students from the Departments of Prosthodontics and Operative Dentistry who participated in this project by filling out the record sheet with the important data on which this project relied. The authors would also like to thank Miss Lesley Wilson (Summer Research Program, National Institutes of Health, 1992) for her contribution at an early phase of this project. The project was partially funded by the IUPUI (Indiana University Purdue University at Indianapolis) Faculty Development Grant (No. 22-761-63).

REFERENCES

1. Carpenter, M. A.; Goodbind, M. S. Effect of varying surface texture on bond strength of one semi-precious and one non-precious ceramo alloy. J. Prosthet. Dent. 42:86–95; 1979.
2. Newitter, D. A.; Schlissel, E. R.; Wolff, M. S. An evaluation of adjustment and postadjustment finishing techniques on the surface of porcelain-bonded-to-metal crowns. J. Prosthet. Dent. 48:388–395; 1982.
3. McInnes, P. M.; Wendt, S. L.; Retief, D. H.; Weinberg, R. Effect of dentin surface roughness on shear bond strength. Dent. Mater. 6:204–207; 1990.
4. Schäffer, H.; Differ, A. Evaluation of the electrolytic etching depth of a nickel-chromium base alloy used in resin-bonded cast restorations. J. Prosthet. Dent. 64:680–683; 1990.
5. Eliades, G. C.; Tzoutzas, J. G.; Vougiousklakis, G. J. Surface alternations on dental restorative materials subjected to air-powder abrasive instrument. J. Prosthet. Dent. 65:27–33; 1991.
6. Felton, D. A.; Bayne, S. C.; Kanoy, B. E.; White, J. T. Effect of air abrasive on marginal configurations of porcelain-fused-to-metal alloys: An SEM analysis. J. Prosthet. Dent. 65:38–43, 1991.
7. Toth, P.; Varsanyi, M.; Kovacs, J. Electrochemical or mechanical preparation of metal surfaces of fixed dentures or splints. Fogow-Sz. 83:90–93; 1990.
8. Trifunovic, D. M.; Gligic, M.; Todorovic, A. B. Study of Co-Cr-Mo alloys in metal-ceramics. Stomatol. Glas. Srb. 37:369–374; 1991.
9. Susz, C. P.; Meyer, J. M.; Orosz, P. F. Thermal expansion of precious metal alloys for porcelain-metal use. Metallurgie Dentaire, 124–134; 1981.
10. Kononen, M.; Kivilaht, J. testing of metal-ceramic joint using scanning acoustic microscopy. Dent. Mater. 7:211–214; 1991.
11. Murakami, I.; Vaidyanathan, J.; Vaidyanathan, T. K.; Schulman, A. Interactive effects of etching and preoxidation on porcelain adherence to non-precious alloys: A guided planar shear test study. Dent. Mater 6:217–222; 1990.

12. Sohida, Y.; Seno, T.; Nishihara, T.; Itoh, A. Fractal characterization of shot-peened surfaces. In Niku-Lari A. ed. Shot Peening. Institute for Industrial Technology Transfer; 1992:253–260.
13. Thompson, V. P.; del Castillo, E.; Livaditis, G. J. Resin-bonded retainers. Part I: Resin bond to electrolytically etched nonprecious alloys. J. Prosthet. Dent. 50:771–779; 1983.
14. Isidor, F.; Hassna, N. M.; Josephsen, K.; Kaaber, S. Tensile bond strength of resin-bonded non-precious alloys with chemically and mechanically roughed surfaces. Dent. Mater. 7:225–229; 1991.
15. Verziden, C. W. G. J. M.; Feilzer, A. J.; Creugers, N. H. J.; Davison, C. L. The influence of polymerization shrinkage of resin cements on bonding to metal. J. Dent. Res. 71:410–413; 1992.
16. Mandelbrot, B. B. The fractal geometry of nature. New York: Freeman; 1983:34.
17. Mandelbrot, B. B.; Passoja, D. E.; Paullay, A. J. Fractal character of fracture surfaces of metals. Nature 308:721–722; 1987.
18. Chesters, S.; Wen, H. Y.; Lundin, M.; Kasper, G. Fractal-based characterization of surface texture. Appl. Surf. Sci. 40:185–182; 1989.
19. Nayak, P. R. Random process model of rough surfaces. J. Lubr. Tech. 93:398–407; 1971.
20. Sayles, R. S.; Thomas, T. R. Surface topography as a non-stationary random process. Nature 271:431–434; 1978.
21. Peitgen, H. O.; Saupe, D. The science of fractal images. New York: Springer; 1988:152.
22. Majumdar, A.; Tien, CL. Fractal characterization and simulation of rough surfaces. Wear 136:313–327; 1990.
23. Berry, M. V.; Lewis, Z. V. On the Weierstress-Mandelbrot fractal function. Proc. Roy. Soc. Lond. [A] 370:459–484; 1980.
24. Pande, C. S.; Richards, L. E.; Louat, N.; Dempsey, B. D.; Schwoeble, A. J. Fractal characterization of fractures surfaces. Acta Metall. 35:1633–1637; 1987.
25. Richardson, L. F. General systems yearbook 6:139–145; 1961.
26. Pfeifer, P.; Anvir, D. Chemistry in noninteger dimensions between two and three. I. Fractal theory of heterogeneous surfaces. Surf. Sci. 79:3558–3565; 1983.
27. Katz, A. J.; Thompson, A. H. Fractal sandstone pores: Implications for conductivity and pore formation. Phys. Rev. Lett. 54:1325–1328; 1985.
28. Kaye, B. H. Fractal geometry and the characterization of rock fragments. Isr. Phys. Soc. 21:1; 1978.
29. Hazlett, R. D. Fractal application: Wettability and contact angle. J. Colloid Interface Sci. 137:527–533; 1990.
30. Coster, M.; Chermant, J. L. Recent development in quantitative fractography. Int. Metals Rev. 28:228–250; 1983.
31. Underwood, E. E.; Benerji, K. Fractal analysis of fracture surfaces. Fractography 12:193–198; 1987.
32. Dauskardt, R. H.; Hanbensak, F.; Ritche, R. O. On the interpretation of the fractal character of fracture surfaces. Acta Metall. 38:143–159; 1986.
33. Mecholsky, J. J.; Passoja. D. E.; Fenberg-Ringel, K. S. Quantitative analysis of brittle fracture surfaces using fractal geometry. J. Am. Ceram. Soc. 72:60–65; 1989.
34. Ling, F. F. The possible role of fractal geometry in tribology. Tribology Trans. 32:497–505; 1989.
35. Stupak, P. R.; Donovan, J. A. Fractal analysis of rubber wear surfaces and debris. J. Mater Sci. 23:2230–2242; 1988.
36. Majumdar, A.; Bhushan, B. Role of fractal geometry in roughness characterization and contact mechanics of surfaces. J. Tribology 112:205–216; 1990.
37. Nishihara, T. Characterization of metals using fractal theory. Heat Treat. 29:99–102; 1989.
38. Hornbogen, E. Fractal analysis of grain boundaries in hot-worked poly-crystals. Zeit Matllk. 78:622–625; 1987.
39. Hornbogen, E. Fractals in microstructure of metals. Int. Mater. Rev. 34:277–296; 1989.
40. Keller, J. M.; Chen, S.; Crownover. Texture description and segmentation through fractal geometry. Comp. Vis. Graph. Image Proc. 34:150–166; 1989.
41. Lauwerier, H. Fractals: Images of chaos. New York: Penguin Books; 1991:32–37.
42. Mueller, P. P.; Urffer, D. Peening with ceramic beads. In Wohlfahrt et al., eds. Shot Peening: Science, technology, application. Informationsgesellschaft Verlag; 1987:49–54.
43. Lieurade, H. P. Fundamental aspects of the effect of shot peening on the fatigue strength of metallic parts and structures. In Wohlfahrt et al., Shot peening: Science, technology, application. Informationsgesselschaft Verlag; 1987;343–359.
44. Tiller, H. J.; Magnus, B.; Gobel, R.; Musil, R.; Garscke, A. Der Sandstrahprozess und seine Einwirkung auf den Oberflaschenzustand von Dentallegierungen. Quintessenz. 36:1927–1934; 1985.

(*Received 7 July* 1993)

Epilogue: Into a Chaotic Future

R. J. Baken, Ph.D.

Director of Laryngology Research
New York Eye and Ear Infirmary

Despite very significant efforts by many of our best researchers over a significant period of time, there remain large gaps in our understanding of laryngeal behavior, and in particular in our ability to explain many anomalies of vocal function. The "pitch breaks" of the adolescent, for example, lack a coherent explanatory model. So does the normal frequency and amplitude perturbation of the healthy voice, and even more so the increased jitter and shimmer that are characteristic of vocal disorder. In short, we have developed a fairly clear picture of the mechanisms of the phonationally regular, but we have not done nearly as well in explaining the vocally erratic.

On the whole, that is not very surprising, for the truth is that we have done no worse in our small territory than the larger sciences of which we are a part have done in their much broader domains. The explanation for this state of affairs was mostly to be found in a lack of optimal scientific tools for characterizing the irregular, in an absence of adequate models of instability, and in a want of a paradigm of the capricious.

The situation has recently changed very much for the better with the recognition of the pivotal importance, near-ubiquitous applicability, and enormous explanatory power of a very different way of looking at natural phenomena. A young science is in the throes of explosive development, and it has already begun to revolutionize our understanding of much of the seemingly-random in the natural, and more relevant to our interests, in the biomedical, world. Cochlear function (1, 2), abnormal motor behavior (3), cardiac electrical instability (4, 5, 6, 7, 8), Cheyne-Stokes respiration (9), cerebral electrophysiology (10) even menopausal hot flashes (11) have been explored quite profitably with the new tools—quantitative as well as qualitative—that this science is providing. The new discipline is formally known as the theory of nonlinear dynamics. Its more popular name is the theory of chaos[1]. It is the science of the unpredictable and the erratic, and it provides an underpinning for a very wide expanse of physiological modelling (24, 25, 26). Chaos theory is probably coming soon to a research lab near you because it holds the promise of powerful breakthroughs in understanding just those erratic phenomena of voice, normal and disordered, that have proven so intractable.

The very term "chaos" has achieved the status of a buzzword, and so before going on it is important to specify precisely what chaos means. Basically, behavior can be called chaotic if and only if

1. It is the product of a deterministic nonlinear system. That is, the behavior must be governed by some nonlinear rule. It is obviously not a requirement that we know what the rule is, only that it exists. In other words, chaos is NOT randomness.
2. Despite the determinism of the generating system, the output must nonetheless be unpredictable. This requirement needs to be understood carefully. It does, of course, imply that the behavior may be random looking. But it also allows, for example, that the system produce a number of different *patterns* of response, within each of which a succession of output states is completely predictable. If one is not able to predict which pattern will be produced at any given time, the system may validly be described as chaotic (provided, of course, that the other requirements are met).

---

1. There is a voluminous literature in the area of nonlinear dynamics. Good introductory sources include (12, 13, 14, 15, 16, 17, 18, 19, 20, 21, 22). An overview of the basic principles of chaos theory as they might relate to voice production is available in (23).

3. Finally,—and this requirement is crucial—**the behavior must be "exquisitely sensitive to initial conditions."** That is, infinitesimal differences in some controlling parameter can have dramatically large effects on system behavior. Note that "infinitesimal" is used here in its literal, mathematical sense, and thus the implication of this requirement is that we can never have enough decimal places in our quantification of the controlling variable to be able to specify the resultant behavior to any arbitrary degree of certainty.

An example will be useful in demonstrating what a chaotic system is and how it functions. It will also serve to show how chaos might clarify some puzzling aspects of laryngeal function. For the present purposes we choose a classic example of a very simple chaotic system, represented by what is called the "logistic equation." Originally derived to model changes in insect populations (27, 28), with some imagination and some gross simplification (together, perhaps, with apologies to laryngeal physiologists) we can adapt it to our didactic needs.

Imagine that, by virtue of some analytical sleight of hand and mathematical legerdemain, we can summarize in a single coefficient, all of the factors (longitudinal tension of the vocal fold cover, stiffness of the body, driving pressure, acoustic load, and so on) that determine the duration of a vocal period. We can call this coefficient a (for $a$djustment!). Then we could say that the period, P, of a vocal cycle is proportional to a. However, it is clear that every glottal cycle is influenced by the cycle that came before it. The force of the immediately-preceding collision of the vocal folds, for instance, strongly affects the rate of rebound of the folds and the extent to which they are likely to separate, thereby altering the duration of the post-collisional cycle. Therefore, to predict the period of a given cycle, P_n, we need to include not only the adjustment coefficient, a, but also some factor that accounts for the period of the previous cycle, P_{n-1}. Let us assume that that factor is $P_{n-1}(1-P_{n-1})$. We can therefore state that the relative period of a given vocal cycle is

$$Pn = aP_{n-1}(1-P_{n-1}).$$

Note that the equation is recursive (the answer to one application, P_n, is plugged into the next calculation as P_{n-1}) and that it is nonlinear, since it contains the term P_{n-1}^2.

Suppose that the vocal fold adjustment, a, is 1.5. To apply our predictive equation we need some starting value, P_{n-1}—say 0.75. Then repeated application of the equation gives us P_n = 0.281, 0.303, 0.317, 0.325, 0.329, 0.331, 0.333, 0.333, 0.333. . . . By way of validating the equation, we can begin the calculation with a different starting value—perhaps 0.65. Then successive P_ns are 0.341, 0.335, 0.334, 0.334, 0.334, 0.333, 0.333, 0.333, 0.333. . . . One more test: starting with a value of 0.9 (but keeping a = 1.5) gives the series 0.135, 0.175, 0.217, 0.255, 0.285, 0.306, 0.318, 0.325, 0.329, 0.331, 0.333, 0.333, 0.333, 0.333. . . . If vocal fold adjustment, a, is changed to 2.5 then (starting with 0.45) the P_n series is 0.618, 0.590, 0.605, 0.597, 0.601, 0.600, 0.600, 0.600 . . . For the same a, starting with 0.75 gives P_n = 0.469, 0.622, 0.587, 0.606, 0.597, 0.601, 0.600, 0.600, 0.600. . . . The predictive equation appears to be quite reliable: irrespective of the starting point, the vocal period seems to converge to a value that depends on the vocal fold adjustment parameter, a.

But the behavior of the predictive equation is not as neat as these examples might lead us to believe. Look at what happens if a is raised to 3.25: the P_n output series is 0.500, 0.812, 0.495, 0.812, 0.495, 0.812, 0.495, 0.812 . . . When a is 3.25 the series of vocal periods converges to *two* alternating values: the equation generates *diplophonia*.

The outputs of the predictive equation across a broad range of a values is summarized in Figure 1. (To generate the plot the equation was given a value of a, allowed to run for 150 iterations—which permitted transient start-up behavior to die away—and then the next 75 output values were plotted as separate points on the P_n axis. A new value of a was then assigned and the process repeated.) There is a richness of behavior which is surprising, given the extreme simplicity of the generating equation. At first, as we have already seen, the model produces a single fundamental period for each setting of the adjustment coefficient. But quite suddenly, when a exceeds about 3.05, two different pe-

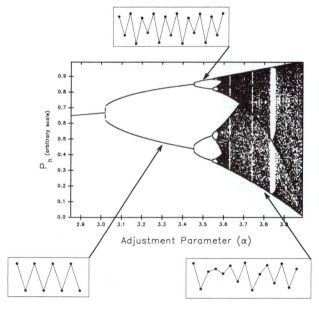

Figure 1. Behavior of the predictive equation as a function of the adjustment parameter a. Insets show sequential outputs at $a \approx 3.3$, 3.5, and 3.8.

riods are alternately generated. (The successive period values at about $a = 3.3$ are plotted in the lower-left inset.) In the technical jargon this is referred to as a period-2 output of the system. The sudden change in behavior is called a *bifurcation*, and it is typical of chaotic systems. In the region of $a = 3.45$ a second bifurcation occurs, and the model produces four successive output periods for each value of a. (A sample of successive periods at $a \approx 3.5$ is shown in the upper inset.) Another bifurcation occurs between $a = 3.5$ and 3.6, as a result of which we get a period-8 output. Beyond $a \approx 3.6$, however, order disappears. The model produces an infinitely-long string of different period values at most settings of a, and hence, for each locus on the a-axis, the plot shows scattered points within a restricted range along the P_n axis. (A sample of the output at $a \approx 3.8$ is plotted in the lower-right inset.)

Three more details of the behavior of the predictive equation, all demonstrated in Figure 1, are instructive and relevant to consideration of the utility of a chaotic model for explaining phonatory phenomena.

First, the period-doubling bifurcations (from period-1 to period-2 or period-2 to period-4, for example) occur with infinite suddenness as a increases. That is, the magnitude of the change in a that is needed to produce a bifurcation from one state to another is infinitesimal. Therefore, we can never have enough decimal places of a to allow us to specify exactly where a bifurcation occurs. The behavior of the system, like that of all chaotic systems, is exquisitely sensitive to the value of its governing parameter[2].

Second, even in the area of $a > 3.6$, where successive outputs of the equation are completely erratic, there are small islands of stability in which the system's behavior is a period-n output. One such relatively-large region is at $a \approx 3.84$, where the output is period-3. (Smaller stable regions are visible at lower values of a.) An enlargement of the zone between $a = 3.75$ and $a = 3.8$ (Figure 2A) shows one of these stable regions (it is also visible in Figure 1) of period-7. But the greater resolution of Figure 2A just barely reveals another area of stability at about $a = 3.765$. Further enlargement (Figure 2B) shows it to be period-9. In fact, it can be mathematically demonstrated that ever-grater enlargements of Figure 1 will reveal ever-smaller islands of period-n stability, each separated from a neighboring region of completely unpredictable output by an infinitesimal difference of a.

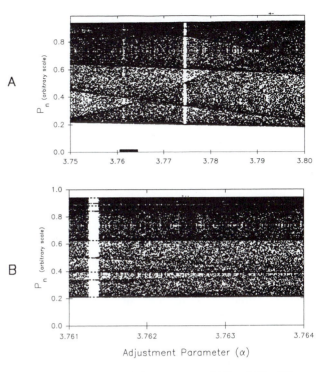

Figure 2. Enlargement of the region $a = 3.75$ to 3.80 of Figure 1. B. Detail of a small region of A (marked by a heavy bar on the a axis of A) demonstrating finer detail.

Finally, it turns out that the outputs in the regions of total unpredictability are not quite as disorganized as they first seem. If, for a given a, one plots each output, P_n, against the following output, P_{n+1}, we find that the points describe a simple geometric structure (Figure 3). It is as if the results of recursive application of our predictive equation are drawn to this parabolic line in the P_n–P_{n+1} plane. It is therefore called an *attractor*.[3]

Consideration of the properties of the predictive equation in light of the defining characteristics of chaos enumerated on page 2 clearly demonstrates that our simple model is truly chaotic. We have borrowed this equation from May (28) and adapted it to our own illustrative purposes only to show what chaotic systems are like, to demonstrate that they can be quite simple, and that they are characterized by some very strange behavior. If we can now show that the real phonating larynx is likely to be chaotic, then we will have laid a foundation for novel hypotheses that might explain strange aspects of phonatory function.

---

2. It is worthwhile to note, if only as a matter of intellectual interest, that the bifurcations occur at an ever-diminishing distance along the a axis. There is a lawfulness to this spacing that is characteristic of all chaotic mappings of this sort. The phenomenon has been studied extensively by Feigenbaum (29), who has derived a constant that characterizes it. The Feigenbaum constant may well turn out to be one of the foundational descriptors of the natural world as are, for example, π and e.

3. Non-chaotic dynamic systems also have attractors, of course. The attractor of a chaotic system shares certain of their characteristics. But there is also a very important difference: a chaotic attractor is fractal. This means that its geometry departs in some significant ways from the rules of the geometry of Euclid. Most importantly, the dimension of the geometric structure that is the chaotic attractor is not an integral number, but rather is fractional. The attractor is therefore one example of a *fractal* shape.

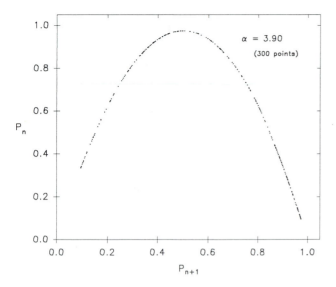

Figure 3. Outputs (P_n) of the predictive equation at $a = 3.90$ plotted against the following output, P_{n+1}. All of the points fall on a parabolic "attractor," demonstrating that the output is not as disordered as it might appear from Figure 1.

The strongest available evidence for the chaotic nature of voice production lies in the finding—by several researchers working independently—of obvious bifurcations in vocal behavior. Bifurcation behavior has been observed in three different contexts: mathematical models of phonatory function, normal infant cry, and the abnormal phonation of adults with demonstrable laryngeal disorder.

The difficulty of conducting physiologic experiments on the phonating larynx (both in vivo and in vitro) has led researchers to turn to mathematical models of laryngeal function. To the extent that a given model is a valid representation of actual physiological processes the presence of chaotic characteristics in its behavior is particularly instructive, because we can be certain that any chaotic output is not the result of stochastic influences that inescapably plague experiments with real organs. Awrejcewicz (34) has shown that an important class of laryngeal models is indeed chaotic, producing through bifurcations all of the behaviors that have been considered in the case of our simple "predictive equation." Wong, Ito, et al. (35) have demonstrated that a hybrid of the Ishizaka-Flanagan (36) and Tize (37, 38) models is also inherently chaotic and produces outputs that mimic important characteristics of the voices of pathologic larynges. What these studies demonstrate is that we should expect the real larynx to be chaotic.

The infant's cry has been recognized for some time as a rich source of vocal characteristics rare or unknown in the adult voice. Among the most salient and puzzling are the phenomena labeled "subharmonic breaks," and "turbulence" in a classic series of studies by Scandinavian investigators (39, 40). Essentially, these involve period doubling and aperiodicity, respectively, during the cry. The sound spectrograms in these studies clearly demonstrate the extreme rapidity with which these "aberrant" vocal modes may appear and disappear. More recent evaluation of these behaviors using the techniques of nonlinear dynamics theory clearly reveals them to be bifurcations of a chaotic system (41, 42).

In an unpublished study undertaken at the Health Sciences Center of the University of Texas at Dallas, Baken, Watson, and Dembowski observed bifurcations in the voices of patients with demonstrable laryngeal disorder. They were qualitatively similar to the bifurcations seen in the output of mathematical models and in the voices of infants.

Three sustained phonations from that study are shown in Figure 4. In each case the period of every glottal cycle was determined, and the periods were plotted sequentially. The resulting traces have something of the appearance of acoustic waves, but it is important to keep in mind that they are not: each trace is the record of vocal period (or equivalently, of F_o) over time.

The phonation represented in A shows quasi-normal period variability (A_1) that is intermittently in-

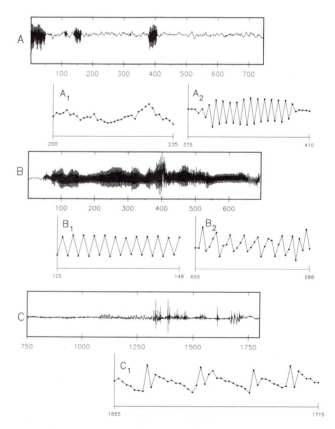

Figure 4. Sustained phonations by three dysphonic patients. The traces represent the period of each cycle (y axis) plotted against the sequential period number in the sample (x axis). Insets below each sample show sequential period values of selected regions at greater resolution.

terrupted by intervals of diplophonic phonation, as shown in A_2. That is, the phonatory system of this patient shows bifurcations to period-2 output. Sample B, on the other hand, begins as normally-variable voicing, but it quickly bifurcates to diplophonic (period-2) phonation (B_1), which continues for most of the sample. Near the end, however, another bifurcation occurs and the vocal behavior changes for a while to a period-4 output, which is unstable and thus bifurcates back to period-2 (B_2). Sample C shows the most complex behavior consisting of intermittent repetition of a complex pattern of period values on the order of 10 to 14 periods long (C_1).

So, mathematical models predict very strange vocal behaviors, and those behaviors are observable in the function of both the normal immature (infantile) larynx and in the abnormal adult. None of the widely-accepted theories of vocal physiology can explain these behaviors. Given that the phonatory system is highly nonlinear, however, the theory of nonlinear dynamics would predict the appearance of exactly these—and other—strange vocal attributes.

At this stage, it seems indisputable that the vocal system is chaotic. That is very good news, because it means that we finally have a model that includes the unpredictable events and the bizarre products that are frequently characteristics of vocal disorder. Even better, the theory of nonlinear dynamics offers tools for evaluating and quantifying the specific characteristics of the dynamical system that produces chaotic outputs. Those methods offer the potential of accurate differential diagnosis based on acoustic and physiologic measurement—a goal that has until now been very highly elusive. Best of all, very recent work (43–46) suggests that chaos can be controlled, providing hope for much more effective rehabilitation of the heretofore more intractable categories of dysphonia.

The future of vocal research seems very chaotic indeed.

REFERENCES

1. Teich MC, Keilson SE, Khanna SM, et al: Chaos in the cochlea. In Lim DJ (ed): Abstracts of the 14th Midwinter Meeting: Association for Research in Otolaryngology, 1991, p. 50.

2. Teich MC, Lowen SB, Turcott RG: On possible peripheral origins of the fractal auditory neural spike train. In Lim DJ (ed): Abstracts of the Fourteenth Midwinter Meeting: Association for Research in Otolaryngology, 1991, p. 50.

3. Beuter A, Labrie C. Vasilakos K: Transient dynamics in motor control of patients with Parkinson's disease. Chaos 1:279–286, 1991.

4. Goldberger AL, Bhargava V, West BJ, et al: On a mechanism of cardiac electrical stability. Biophys J 48:525–528, 1985.

5. Sheldon R, Riff K: Changes in heart rate variability during fainting. Chaos 1:257–264, 1991.

6. Kaplan DT. Talajic M: Dynamics of heart rate. Chaos 1:251–256, 1991.

7. Coumel P, Maison-Blanche P. Complex dynamics of cardiac arrhythmias. Chaos 1:335–342, 1991.

8. Skinner JE. Goldberger AL, Mayer-Kress G, et al: Chaos in the heart: Implications for clinical cardiology. Biotechnology 8:1018–1024, 1990.

9. Kryger MH, Millar T: Cheyne-Stokes respiration: Stability of interacting systems in heart failure. Chaos 1:265–269, 1991.

10. Rapp PE, Bashore TR, Martinerie JM, et al: Dynamics of brain electrical activity. Brain Topogr 2:99–118, 1989.

11. Kronenberg F: Menopausal hot flashes: randomness or rhythmicity. Chaos 1: 271–278, 1991.

12. Crutchfield, JP, Farmer JD, Packard NH, Shaw RS: Chaos. Sci Amer 254 no. 12: 46–57, 1986.

13. Cvitanovic P (Ed.): Universality in Chaos. New York, Adam Hilger, 1989.

14. Eubank S, Farmer D: An introduction to chaos and randomness. Jen E (Ed.): 1989 Lectures in Complex Systems (SFI Studies in the Sciences of Complexity), Lecture volume II. Addison-Wesley, 1990, p 75.

15. Glass L, Mackey MC: From Clocks to Chaos: The Rhythms of Life. Princeton, NJ, Princeton, 1988.

16. Gleick J: Chaos: Making a New Science. New York, Viking, 1987.

17. Holden AV (Ed.): Chaos. Princeton NJ, Princeton, 1986.

18. Moon FC: Chaotic Vibrations: An Introduction for Applied Scientists and Engineers. New York, Wiley, 1987.

19. Stewart I: Does God Play Dice: The Mathematics of Chaos. Cambridge, MA, Blackwell, 1989.

20. Thompson JMT, Stewart HB: Nonlinear Dynamics and Chaos: Geometrical Methods for Engineers and Scientists. New York, Wiley, 1986.

21. West BJ: Fractal Physiology and Chaos in Medicine. Teaneck, NJ, World Scientific, 1990.

22. Hall N (Ed.): Exploring Chaos. New York, Norton, 1991.

23. Titze IR, Baken RJ, Herzel H: Evidence of chaos in vocal fold vibration. In Titze IR (Ed.): Vocal Fold Physiology: Frontiers in Basic Science. San Diego, CA, Singular, 1993, p 143.

24. Glass L: Nonlinear dynamics of physiological function and control. Chaos 1: 247–250, 1991.

25. Goldberger AL, Rigney DR, West BJ: Chaos and fractals in human physiology. Sci Amer 262 no. 2: 43–49, 1990.

26. Pool R: Is it healthy to be chaotic? Science 243: 604–607, 1989.

27. May RM: Stability and Complexity in Model Ecosystems. Princeton, NJ, Princeton, 1973.

28. May RM: Biological populations with nonoverlapping generations: Stable points, stable cycles, and chaos. Science 186: 645–647, 1974.

29. Feigenbaum MJ: Quantitative universality for a class of nonlinear transformations. J Stat Phys 19: 25–52, 1978.

30. Barnsley M: Fractals Everywhere. New York, Academic, 1988.

31. Jurgens H, Peitgen H-O, Saupe D: The language of fractals. Sci Amer 263 no. 2: 60–67, 1990.

32. Le Méhauté A: Fractal Geometries: Theory and Applications. Boca Raton, FL, CRC, 1991.

33. Baken RJ: Irregularity of vocal period and amplitude: A first approach to the fractal analysis of voice. J Voice 4: 185–197,1990.

34. Awrejcewicz J: Bifurcation portrait of the human vocal cord oscillations. J Sound Vib 136: 151–156, 1990.

35. Wong D, Ito MR, Cox NB, Titze IR: Observation of perturbations in a lumped-element model of the vocal folds with application to some pathological cases. J Acous Soc Amer 89: 383–391, 1991.

36. Ishizaka K, Flanagan JL: Synthesis of voiced sounds from a two-mass model of the vocal cords. Bell Syst Tech J 51: 1233–1268, 1972.

37. Titze IR: The human vocal cords: A mathematical model. Part I. Phonetica 28: 129–170, 1973.

38. Titze IR: The human vocal cords: A mathematical model. Part II. Phonetica 29: 1–21, 1974.

39. Truby HM, Lind J: Cry sounds of the newborn infant. In Lind J (Ed.): Newborn Infant Cry. Uppsala, Almqvist and Wiksells, 1965, p 8.

40. Wasz-Höckert O, Lind J, Vuorenkoski V, Partanen T, Valanné E: *The Infant Cry: A Spectrographic and Auditory Analysis. (Clinics in Developmental Medicine*, no. 29). London, Spastics International Medical Publications, 1968.

41. Mende W, Herzel H, Wermke K: Bifurcations and chaos in newborn infant cries. *Phys Let A* 145: 418–424, 1990.

42. Herzel H, Steinecke I, Mende W, Wermke K. Chaos and bifurcations during voiced speech. In Mosekilde E (Ed.): *Complexity, Chaos and Biological Evolution*. New York, Plenum, 1991, p 41.

43. Ditto WL, Pecora LM: Mastering chaos. *Sci. Amer* 269 no. 2: 78–84, 1993.

44. Pecora LM, Carroll TL: Synchronization in chaotic systems. *Phys Rev Let* 64: 821–824, 1990.

45. Ditto WL, Rauseo SN, Spano ML: Experimental control of chaos. *Phys Rev Let* 65: 3211–3214, 1990.

46. Garfinkel ML, Spano ML, Ditto WL, Weiss JN: Controlling cardiac chaos. *Science* 257: 1230–1235, 1992.

Journal of Voice
Vol. 4, No. 3, pp. 185–197
© 1990 Raven Press, Ltd., New York

Irregularity of Vocal Period and Amplitude: A First Approach to the Fractal Analysis of Voice

R. J. Baken

Speech Research Laboratory, Columbia University, New York, New York, U.S.A.

Summary: Fractal geometry, a relatively young branch of mathematics, offers new ways of evaluating the irregularity of the physiologic and acoustic aspects of speech. The validity and reliability of a box-counting method for estimating the fractal dimension (D_F) of the period and amplitude of vocal signals were demonstrated, and the method was applied to sustained vowels produced by four men and four women. Mean D_F of the fundamental period was 1.46; D_F of the amplitude records averaged a slightly, but significantly, higher 1.54. The potential of D_F as a research and clinical tool is considered. **Key Words:** Fundamental frequency (F_0)—Amplitude—Fractal dimension (D_F)—Chaos—Perturbation—Jitter—Shimmer.

Irregularity is an important characteristic of all components of the speech signal, but perhaps in no area has its measurement been the focus of more interest, or the object of more research, than in the study of voice production and voice disorders. In the domain of voice, irregularity is generally referred to as "perturbation." Numerous indices of both frequency and amplitude perturbation ("jitter" and "shimmer," respectively) have been devised to characterize both normal and disordered voices (1–11).

Two aspirations have motivated research on vocal perturbation. First, understanding the irregularity of the vocal signal may provide important insights about laryngeal or vocal tract mechanisms (5,12–21). Second, because perturbation is likely to increase in the presence of laryngeal pathology, jitter and shimmer might prove to be useful metrics of the severity—and perhaps even the type—of voice disorder (2,9,22–33). Progress in this latter area, however, has been disappointing (34).

Dedicated to the memory of Edward D. Mysak, Ph.D.
Address correspondence and reprint requests to Dr. R. J. Baken at Box 3, Columbia University, 525 West 120 Street, New York, NY 10027, U.S.A.

It is implicit in the concepts of jitter and shimmer that they represent essentially *random* variations. Yet, with the exception of the directional perturbation factor proposed by Hecker and Kreul (3), perturbation measures represent some sort of average of the difference between the periods (or amplitudes) of successive vocal cycles (35). As such, perturbation indices quantify vocal *variability* rather than vocal *irregularity*.

The distinction is not a trivial one. Consider the case of the two records of 300 consecutive vocal periods shown in Fig. 1. The upper record is of phonation at a comfortable pitch by a middle-aged man. The lower plot is synthetic and was created to match the perturbation characteristics (as normally measured) of the natural record. Both records have a mean period of 8.65 ms. Both have a period SD of 0.05 ms and a mean absolute jitter of 27 μs. In short, they have the same variability. But they are very different in what one might choose to call their shape or *geometry*. Clearly, the lower plot is much less irregular and less disorganized than the upper one. The usual measures of *variability* have masked an important difference in the *irregularity* of the two sets of data.

There is a way to describe irregularity, or disor-

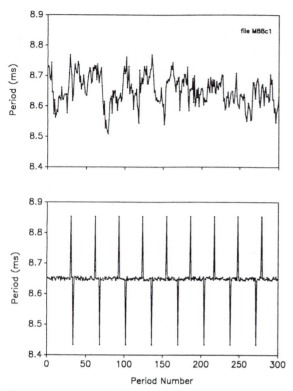

FIG. 1. Two records of 300 sequential fundamental periods. The upper represents phonation of /a/ by a normal male. The lower record is synthetic. Both have the same variability.

derliness, independent of variability. That method lies in the use of a relatively new branch of mathematics known as *fractal geometry*. Although an attempt has been made to characterize the fractal dimension of speech waveforms (36), fractal analytic procedures have not previously been applied to the records of vocal signals. Because the rationales and methods involved are, therefore, likely to be unfamiliar to voice specialists, a brief overview and nontechnical explanation of basic principles may prove useful.[1]

FRACTAL GEOMETRY AND THE CONCEPT OF FRACTAL DIMENSION

Initially created by Mandelbrot (37,38), the field of fractal geometry has experienced almost explosive growth and refinement in the past several years. At the most fundamental level, it is a system for describing the shapes of objects of the real world, rather than the abstract or ideal structures that are the focus of the more traditional Euclidean geometry. Given this difference, it is not surprising that fractal and Euclidean geometries differ at their most basic levels. In general, a common educational background leads one to consider natural structures in Euclidean terms. Understanding fractal geometry, therefore, requires significant reconceptualization of the way the world is.

A small demonstration will help. Tear the corner off a sheet of paper. (Do not crease it beforehand—just tear it.) A roughly triangular piece of paper results. Two of its edges—the untorn ones—represent straight lines. The torn edge, however, is likely to be very irregular. It is an easy matter to describe the straight segments, either in words or by very simple equations. But how can the erratic, disorderly shape of the torn edge be characterized? Traditional mathematics attempted to solve the problem by making the assumption that if the irregular edge were magnified sufficiently it would appear as a series of (extremely short but perfectly straight) simple line segments, each of which could be easily described by traditional geometry. Since a straight line is a one-dimensional shape, the implication of this method is that a complex, irregular, disorderly line can be described as a string of very much shorter (but individually orderly) one-dimensional structures.

Looking at the torn edge with ever-stronger magnifying glasses quickly shows the problem with this assumption: Every time the irregular line is magnified, more irregularity appears. In fact, no matter how much it is enlarged, the torn edge of a real piece of paper can *never* be reduced to a set of perfectly straight lines. (In the formal language of fractal geometry, the edge is said to be "self-similar" at all scalings.) This implies that it cannot be a one-dimensional shape. On the other hand, the irregular edge obviously cannot have a dimension of as much as two, which is the dimension of a plane surface. However counterintuitive it may seem at first, logic demands that the irregular edge must have a dimension that is between one and two. That is, its dimension must be *fract*(ion)*al*.

ESTIMATING THE FRACTAL DIMENSION

There are many methods by which one can estimate the fractal dimension of any geometric shape,

---

[1] More mathematically rigorous treatments of this subject are readily available in a number of sources. Among the best for the beginner, however, are to be found in Mandelbrot (38) and Barnsley (40).

including, of course, the shape of a graph of vocal period or amplitude values. The simplest, in terms of conceptualization and implementation, is the "box-counting method." Although perhaps not applicable in the case of complex structures in higher-dimensional spaces (39), this method has several virtues that recommend it strongly for the purposes at hand. The following discussion will present an intuitive approach to box-counting estimation of fractal dimension. For those who need them, the mathematical formalisms are available in a number of sources (37,40–42).

Imagine a filled rectangle (a two-dimensional structure) that completely fills a plane. Let the plane be divided into five divisions on a side, as in Fig. 2A. The gray rectangle fills all 25 boxes into which the plane has been divided. (Call these boxes "occupied.") Now let the plane be divided to make 10 divisions horizontally and 10 divisions vertically, as in Fig. 2B. This time the rectangle occupies 100 boxes. Finally, let the horizontal and vertical dimensions of the plane each be divided into 15 equal

segments (Fig. 2C). Now the rectangle fills 225 boxes. In short, the number of boxes increases as the *square* of the number of divisions of each dimension.

Now draw a straight line on an otherwise empty plane. Proceed in the same manner as with the rectangle, dividing the vertical and horizontal dimensions of the plane into 5, 10, and 15 segments each (Fig. 3). Count the number of boxes that are "occupied" by having the line pass through them. We find that with a 5-by-5 division the line occupies 5 boxes, a 10-by-10 division has 10 boxes occupied, and a 15-by-15 division causes 15 boxes to be occupied. In the case of a line, the number of boxes that are occupied increases in direct proportion to the number of divisions of each dimension.

These two sets of results can be summarized by saying that the number of boxes occupied by a one-dimensional structure increases directly with the linear divisions of the plane, whereas the number occupied by a two-dimensional structure increases as the square of the linear divisions of the plane. Stated in mathematical terms, if N = the number of

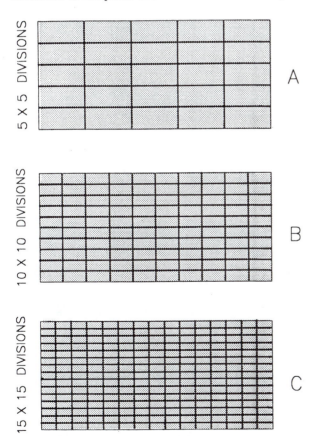

FIG. 2. Subdivision of a plane that is completely occupied by a rectangle (shaded) into 5 × 5, 10 × 10, and 15 × 15 segments.

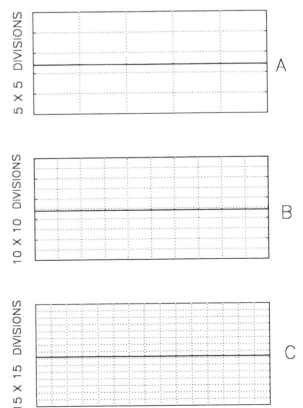

FIG. 3. Subdivision of a plane on which a line has been drawn into 5 × 5, 10 × 10, and 15 × 15 segments.

188

R. J. BAKEN

divisions of each side of the plane, then for a one-dimensional structure, occupied boxes $\propto N^1$; and for a two-dimensional structure, occupied boxes $\propto N^2$.

In fact, the dimensionality of the shape that has been placed on the plane is specified by the exponent in the proportionality between the number of divisions and the number of boxes occupied. With a very small trick, this relationship can be recast into a more convenient form. Raising a number to a power is equivalent to multiplying the *logarithm* of that number by the power. Thus, it is possible to say that for a one-dimensional shape, ln(occupied boxes) $\propto 1 \cdot \ln(N)$; and for a two-dimensional shape, ln(occupied boxes) $\propto 2 \cdot \ln(N)$. In this form, the dimension of a shape is specified by the *coefficient* in the equation.

Finally, place a graph of fundamental period values over time on the plane, as in Fig. 4. Consider this graph to be not a set of numerical data, but just a shape—perhaps a very ragged line. At least to a useful approximation, this shape can be considered similar to the torn edge of a piece of paper. That is, it may be assumed that, up to a finite limit, increasing magnification will demonstrate increasing irregularity. This implies that its dimension must be greater than one. But its dimension must also be less than two, since it is clear that it does not fill the plane completely. So, this record of vocal fundamental periods must have a dimension that is fractional: It is a *fractal* shape. And its dimension can be determined by the same box-counting method, as shown in Fig. 5.

Note that estimating the fractal dimension is a problem in *geometry* and that the data are considered to constitute a *shape,* not a set of numbers. Since the actual numerical values are of no importance, the graph can be expanded to fill the plane in which the measurement is to be done.

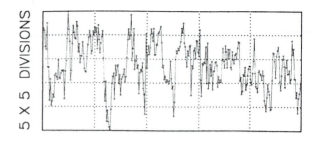

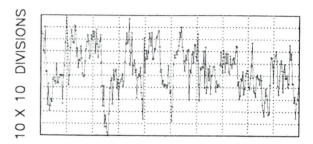

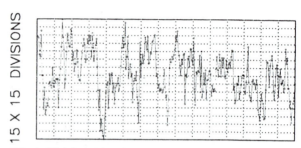

FIG. 5. Division of the plane on which the period values of Fig. 5 have been plotted.

Counting boxes for the three sets of divisions of the plane shown in Fig. 5 results in the following data:

Divisor	ln(Divisor)	Occupied boxes	ln(Occupied boxes)
5	1.609	23	3.135
10	2.303	74	4.304
15	2.708	148	4.997

If these data are plotted, as in Fig. 6, it is easy to see how they can be used to derive an equation of the form ln(occupied boxes) = A · ln(divisor), in which the coefficient A represents the (fractal) dimension of the data shape. The line through the three data points on the graph is the regression line, whose calculation will be familiar from basic statistics. Its slope is the coefficient A in the equation. That is, its slope is the fractal dimension (D_F) of the original data record. For the tabled data, the regres-

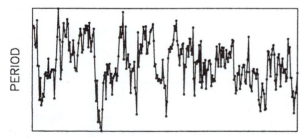

FIG. 4. Graph of sequential period values during a sustained vowel by a normal male speaker.

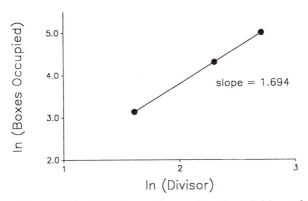

FIG. 6. Relationship between the number of subdivisions of each side of the plane and the number of boxes occupied by the data curve. The data points are connected by a regression line, whose slope is the best estimate of the D_F of the data record.

sion equation is ln(occupied boxes) = 1.694 · ln(divisor) + a remainder. The fractal dimension of the data record of Fig. 4 is therefore $D_F = 1.694$.

The box-counting method of estimating a fractal dimension is thus quite simple. It could, in fact, be performed by hand. But it is obviously very well suited to implementation on any microcomputer with a graphics terminal, a fact that greatly enhances its attractiveness for both research and, ultimately, clinical applications.

PRELIMINARY VALIDATION STUDIES

Before undertaking estimation of the D_F of vocal signals using the box-counting algorithm, it seemed prudent to assess the adequacy of its performance when implemented on commonly available microcomputers and to verify experimentally that the fractal dimension does indeed quantify disorder and not variability. In addition, explorations of the fractal characteristics of data sets provided an opportunity to develop a sense of what fractal dimension means in the everyday world of real data and of how fractal values relate to the more traditional measures of data variability.

To these ends, software was developed to derive box-counting estimates of D_F on an IBM-PC/XT, which was considered representative of the minimal level of computer sophistication that would be expected in research and clinical settings. The computer's IBM CGA graphics adapter provided a resolution of only 640 (horizontal) by 200 (vertical) pixels.

Validity and robustness of the algorithm in the IBM-PC environment

Effect of screen resolution

Because the box-counting algorithm is a graphics-dependent method, it was important to assess the degree to which limited screen resolution might influence the resulting estimate of D_F. To do this, a sample record of vocal periods was repeatedly evaluated (using screen divisions from 10 to 50 in 5-division steps) when plotted on increasingly smaller proportions of the computer screen's maximal horizontal and vertical size. The results of this analysis are shown in Fig. 7.

Shrinkage of the plotting area, with an attendant loss of graphics resolution, clearly causes overestimation of D_F, but the effect is marginal until reduction of either vertical or horizontal size approaches 50%. It seemed reasonable to conclude that the box-counting method is compatible with commonly available computer graphics hardware.

The other side of the resolution coin concerns the size of the maximal divisor that is required for a reliable estimate of D_F. In theory, one should continue to divide the measurement plane until the divisions are infinitesimal. (In mathematical terminology, one actually needs to ascertain the *limit* of the number of occupied boxes as the divisor approaches infinity.) But the issue of screen resolution clearly circumscribes one's ability to do this: Boxes cannot get smaller than 1 pixel on a side, and it is hard to predict how failing resolution will affect the accuracy of box counting as box size gets smaller. Hence, another experiment was under-

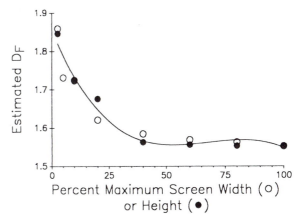

FIG. 7. Relationship between proportion of the computer graphics screen used for plotting and the resulting estimate of D_F.

taken to determine how the estimate of D_F changes as a function of diminishing box size.

A normal woman and a normal man each sustained vowels for ~3 s at comfortable pitch and loudness. In addition, the man produced ~3 s of phonation using pulse register. The fundamental periods of all glottal cycles in each of these productions was determined (using the methods described later). The box-counting method was used to estimate D_F of the first 300 consecutive values of each of these productions. Divisor values varied from 10 to 60 in increments of 5, and the estimated D_F was recalculated as each new divisor (from 15 to 60) was added. The results are plotted in Fig. 8. Clearly, increasing the divisor values affects the D_F estimate for the different files in different ways, but all three series have settled down to a reasonable approximation of a final D_F value by the time the divisor reaches 55. It was concluded that using divisors from 15 to 55, in increments of 5, would provide sufficient accuracy for the present purposes.

For an initial study of fractal dimension, then, it may be assumed that even the relatively low (200×640) resolution of an IBM-PC/XT CGA adapter is adequate and that screen division need be no greater than 55×55 to provide a reliable estimate of D_F.

Does D_F quantify variability or irregularity?

Two methods were used to assess the extent to which D_F simply reflects the variability of the data set rather than its irregularity. In the first, the variance of an actual set of fundamental frequency (F_0) data was manipulated whereas the geometry of the data record was left unchanged. In the second, the same data set was smoothed.

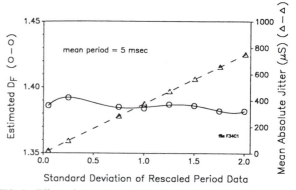

FIG. 9. Effect of changing period SD on D_F and jitter measures when data-set irregularity is held constant.

Effect of data variability: manipulating the standard deviation of periods

The comfortable-pitch male phonation used to derive the data in Fig. 8 was normalized by conversion of its data to z-scores.[2] These were then rescaled to produce fundamental period records with predetermined SDs but with "shapes" or geometries that were identical to that of the original data set. In this way, variability was manipulated while irregularity was preserved. The relative average perturbation (RAP) (6) and the fractal dimension of each of these records was then estimated, with the results shown in Fig. 9. Despite a variation of the SD of the period values from 0.05 to 20.0 ms (a ratio of 1:400) and an associated change of RAP from 0.0022 to 0.090 (a change of more than 40:1), the estimated D_F varied only from 1.382 to 1.392 (~0.7%), a magnitude of change that is probably accounted for by estimate error. The relative immunity of D_F to changes of variability in the face of a constant amount of irregularity seems to be well demonstrated.

Effect of geometric variation: examination of smoothed data files

Linear data smoothing provided a means of documenting that D_F is, in fact, sensitive to the geometric irregularity of the F_0 record, as theory predicts, since the result of smoothing is a decrease in the irregularity of the data record. The first 500 values of the same file that had been rescaled were, therefore, subjected to single-pass linear smoothing, using from 5 to 50 points in the smoothing equa-

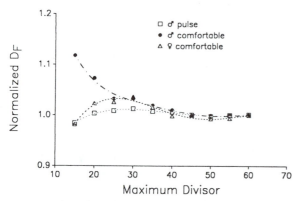

FIG. 8. Effect of maximum plane divisor on the D_F estimate.

---

[2] $z(x) = (x - \text{mean})/\text{SD}$.

tion. (The greater the number of points in the computation, the less irregular the resulting data record.) Figure 10 summarizes the effects of the smoothing process on D_F, period SD, and relative average perturbation. Period SD fell from 0.80 mS to 0.43 mS as smoothing increased from none to 50-point; RAP dropped from 0.02 to 0.0003 across the same smoothing range; and D_F decreased from 1.47 to 1.11.

Summary of preliminary tests of validity

On the basis of preliminary assessment of the behavior of the box-counting algorithm in estimating D_F, the following conclusions were drawn: (a) It is feasible to estimate the D_F of the F_0 record of a sustained vowel using the box-counting algorithm implemented on a microcomputer. (b) The CGA graphics screen resolution of 200×640 pixels is adequate for estimating D_F using a data set 300 periods long. (c) Divisors ranging from 15 to 55, taken in increments of 5, provide a reliable basis for estimating D_F. (d) The D_F of a F_0 record is essentially insensitive to the magnitude of the simple F_0 variability and is, in fact, reflective of the F_0 irregularity. It quantifies a different aspect of the signal from those measured by either SD or a common perturbation measure such as RAP.

FRACTAL DIMENSION OF THE FUNDAMENTAL PERIODS AND AMPLITUDES OF SUSTAINED VOWELS

Having validated the application of D_F estimation in the case of vocal signals, a small study was conducted with the object of providing a first estimate of the likely magnitude of D_F's of the fundamental period and amplitude records of normal voices. In

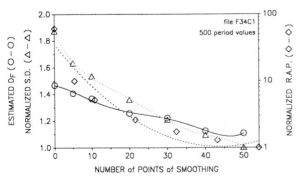

FIG. 10. Effect on D_F and jitter measures of reducing data irregularity by smoothing.

addition, indications were sought about whether D_F seems to vary with vocal F_0, as standard F_0 perturbation measures seem to do (4,43,44), and about whether D_F is influenced by speaker sex. Finally, comparisons were done to validate that D_F does, in fact, quantify something different from the phenomena measured by standard jitter and shimmer indices.

SUBJECTS AND METHOD

The study sample consisted of four men and four women ranging in age from 23 to 59 years (mean = 40.1 years; SD = 11.8 years). All were in good health at the time of testing; none had special training in the use of the speaking voice. No attempt was made to select subjects for uniformity of perceived voice qualities (such as "roughness" or "breathiness"), nor was any formal perceptual scaling of the subjects' voices undertaken.

Each subject sustained the vowel /a/ for as long as possible at a comfortable pitch and loudness, and then at pitches comfortably lower and comfortably higher. The subject's electroglottographic (EGG) (Lx) wave was obtained by a F-J model EG830 ECG having a high-pass cutoff frequency of 30 Hz. The voice signal was transduced by a Knowles model BL1785 electret probe microphone (45) taped to the subject's upper lip. Data signals were captured with 12-bit resolution by a Metrabyte DASH-16 A/D converter at a sampling rate of 20 kilosamples/S/channel and saved to disk.

Interpolated zero-crosses of the increasing-contact phase of the Lx wave demarcated vocal fundamental periods (46), and the peak-to-peak amplitude of each period of the acoustic signal was determined. Software developed for the present study used a box-counting algorithm to estimate D_F of the first 300 periods of each sustained vowel. Mean absolute jitter, relative average perturbation, the SD of the periods, and shimmer in dB were also determined for each 300-period sample.

Table 1 provides the results of the various variability measures,[3] and Table 2 summarizes the D_F findings by test condition. Period D_F ranged from

---

[3] The high-pitch phonation of subject F21 was clearly anomalous, with variability measures falling as far as 36 SDs from the mean of the data for the other female subjects. Summary statistics excluding this trial are provided in the tables, and, where indicated, the outlier data have been eliminated in some analyses.

R. J. BAKEN

TABLE 1. *Fractal dimension of period and amplitude records of sustained vowel phonations*

Subject	Pitch level	SD (ms)	Jitter Absolute (μs)	Jitter RAP (×100)	D_F	Shimmer (dB)	D_F
Male							
M54	COMF	0.067	9.19	0.619	1.396	0.344	1.414
	HIGH	0.035	17.93	0.220	1.557	0.230	1.288
	LOW	0.149	61.51	0.252	1.400	0.578	1.670
M71	COMF	0.082	29.84	0.177	1.430	0.207	1.603
	HIGH	0.075	19.91	0.155	1.258	0.129	1.385
	LOW	0.161	108.17	0.479	1.553	0.407	1.536
M88	COMF	0.049	27.85	0.171	1.494	0.263	1.551
	HIGH	0.063	16.03	0.107	1.416	0.124	1.450
	LOW	0.069	39.59	0.207	1.552	0.289	1.778
M89	COMF	0.074	35.89	0.179	1.475	0.363	1.533
	HIGH	0.023	11.22	0.117	1.475	0.195	1.558
	LOW	0.087	41.01	0.177	1.559	0.383	1.537
Mean		0.077	34.84	0.238	1.464	0.293	1.525
SD		0.041	27.47	0.153	0.090	0.130	0.130
Female							
F21	COMF	0.024	18.04	0.258	1.511	0.130	1.535
	HIGH	0.649	332.13	8.15	1.479	0.125	1.550
	LOW	0.029	12.16	0.138	1.348	0.082	1.542
F34	COMF	0.024	12.39	0.142	1.461	0.115	1.440
	HIGH	0.020	14.39	0.260	1.426	0.106	1.579
	LOW	0.053	28.72	0.245	1.500	0.114	1.542
F58	COMF	0.029	15.62	0.189	1.511	0.171	1.721
	HIGH	0.077	56.27	0.874	1.456	0.481	1.744
	LOW	0.041	9.30	0.108	1.384	0.119	1.392
F59	COMF	0.028	17.17	0.197	1.575	0.236	1.629
	HIGH	0.027	16.21	0.234	1.401	0.162	1.547
	LOW	0.025	16.26	0.198	1.507	0.165	1.525
Mean		0.086	45.72	0.916	1.463	0.167	1.562
SD		0.178	91.06	2.287	0.064	0.107	0.100
(Mean[a]		0.034	19.68	0.258	1.462	0.171	1.563)
(SD[a]		0.017	13.09	0.210	0.067	0.111	0.105)
Grand mean		0.082	40.28	0.577	1.463	0.230	1.544
SD		0.126	66.01	1.622	0.076	0.133	0.115
(Grand mean[a]		0.057	27.59	0.248	1.463	0.234	1.543)
(SD[a]		0.038	22.70	0.179	0.078	0.134	0.118)

[a] Descriptive statistics omit data for subject F21, high-pitch phonation.

1.258 to 1.559 among the men and from 1.348 to 1.575 among the women. The range of amplitude D_F values was larger, from 1.288 to as much as 1.778 among men and from 1.392 to 1.744 among women. A *t* test of the period-amplitude differences (47) yielded $t_{22} = -2.293$, which is significant beyond $\alpha = 0.05$ ($t_{22; 0.05} = 2.074$ [two-tailed]). Analysis of variance (47) failed to demonstrate any significant effect (at $\alpha = 0.05$) of either sex or vocal F_0 on either the amplitude D_F or period D_F. The relationship between the D_F measures of period and amplitude (illustrated in Fig. 11) was a weak one, with a

Pearson correlation coefficient of only 0.28, indicating that the variance of one explains <8% of the variance of the other.

The extent to which the fractal dimension and other measures of variability quantify the same things was explored by evaluating the correlation coefficients among the several variability indices computed from the data samples. None of the correlations (tabulated in Appendix A and illustrated in Fig. 12) was found to be significant at the 0.01 level (48). There is, however, a noticeable tendency for *r* to be higher for correlations with amplitude D_F, sig-

TABLE 2. *Mean period, amplitude D_F and standard deviation (parentheses) by condition*

Pitch level	Mean (SD) of D_F		
	Male	Female	Total
Amplitude			
COMF	1.525	1.581	1.553
	(0.080)	(0.121)	(0.099)
HIGH	1.420	1.605	1.513
	(0.113)	(0.094)	(0.138)
LOW	1.630	1.500	1.565
	(0.117)	(0.073)	(0.114)
Total	1.526	1.562	1.544
	(0.130)	(0.100)	(0.114)
Period			
COMF	1.449	1.514	1.482
	(0.044)	(0.047)	(0.055)
HIGH	1.426	1.441	1.433
	(0.126)	(0.034)	(0.086)
LOW	1.516	1.435	1.475
	(0.077)	(0.081)	(0.085)
Total	1.464	1.463	1.463
	(0.090)	(0.064)	(0.076)

nifying that the distinction between more common measures of variability and D_F is less sharp for the amplitude than for the period record.

Despite its abstractness, D_F does represent something that is visually perceptible in the data record, although it is a quality for which we lack good descriptive terms. Briefly stated, D_F specifies the extent to which a shape (the data set in the present case) tends to occupy empty regions in the metric space that contains it. Figure 13 gives a sense of what this means in the present situation. (The data plots include both period and amplitude records of men and women having four different fractal dimensions that span the range of values observed in the present study.) Note that the data record at the top (for which $D_F = 1.258$) shows an obvious orderliness underlying the variability that is quantified in

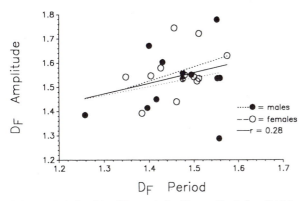

FIG. 11. Relationship of D_F-period to D_F-amplitude for all trials.

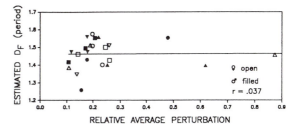

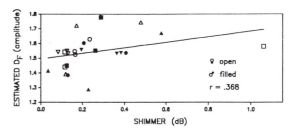

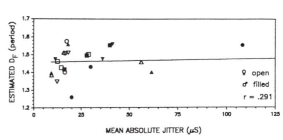

FIG. 12. Relationship of D_F to variability measures for all trials.

its mean absolute jitter of 19.9 μs. Viewed geometrically, this record is like a line that snakes around the plane. There is, however, considerable "openness" within and between the graph's "coils." The data of the second record fill those "inter-coil" spaces more completely, whereas the third graph both wanders over the plane *and* tends to fill in empty spaces. Finally, the bottom record, whose D_F is 1.778, could perhaps be described as a data "smear" that does, in fact, fill up a great deal of the space in which it is located. There is very little evidence of any orderly arrangement of the data points.

DISCUSSION

Determination of the fractal dimension of the period and amplitude records of sustained phonations by application of a box-counting estimation method appears to be a practical procedure of acceptable validity. Even allowing for the small number of normal subjects tested in this pilot study, it is quite clear that D_F quantifies an attribute of the vocal

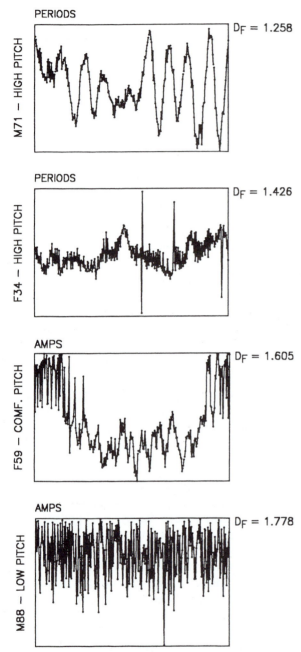

FIG. 13. Sample data sets whose D_F values cover the range found in the present investigation.

signal that is different from that measured by more traditional perturbation measures.

It is also apparent from the summary in Table 3 that the fractal dimension has a much smaller relative variance among normal subjects than the more usual indices of vocal variability. The case of the extreme period perturbational values of the high-pitch phonation of subject F21 is illustrative in this regard: the very high perturbational indices are

nonetheless associated with a period D_F that is very close to the mean for the group. There is thus reason to believe that D_F is fairly robust in the presence of possible defects in the data record.

The fractal dimension of a data set specifies the degree to which it is characterized by "self-similarity" across magnification scales. In theory, a highly self-similar structure could be produced by a generating function that produces a data set that is completely regular but highly complex and space filling. Such structures, exemplified by the Peano curve, Sierpinsky gasket, Hilbert curve, or Koch snowflake have, in fact, been studied extensively by mathematicians (38,40,49). However, such highly regular self-similar structures generally require that the generating function be iterative and recursive, a condition that is improbable in the speech system. Thus, it is fairly safe to conclude that the D_F of the vocal record scales irregularity ("disorderliness").

It is useful to consider, at least in outline, just where vocal irregularity might be produced. Generally, the locus has been most commonly sought at the level of the peripheral physiology. Baer (12), for example, has suggested that F_0 perturbation derives largely from imperfect integration of motor unit contractions in the laryngeal muscles. This kind of explanation is essentially one of additive noise: Random errors are added to an otherwise pure (hypothetical) driving signal, adding a significant "quasi-" to what, in an ideal situation, would be a truly periodic output. There is little doubt of the physiologic validity of such a model, but there is also little reason to believe that it is sufficient.

Recent work in mathematics has brought another possibility to the fore. It has been repeatedly demonstrated that relatively simple nonlinear systems that, at first glance, would be expected to produce completely regular and foreseeable outputs, may behave in unexpected ways, generating products whose characteristics cannot be predicted with any given level of precision in spite of the fact that the output is generated by a function which can be completely specified. The effect has been demonstrated in simple driven oscillators (50). It has also been experimentally observed that when two very simple electronic oscillators, each having a fixed and stable frequency, are coupled together their combined output may be an unpredictable and unstable frequency (51). Physiologic oscillators such as the heart (52,53) and respiratory system (54) show exactly the same effect. An important descriptor of

TABLE 3. *Percent variation[a] of variability measures*

	Period				Amplitude	
	Period SD	Mean absolute jitter	RAP	D_F	dB shimmer	D_F
Male	53.2	78.8	64.2	6.1	44.4	8.5
Female[b]	50.0	66.5	81.4	4.6	64.9	6.7
Total[b]	66.7	82.3	72.2	5.3	57.3	7.6

[a] Defined as (SD/mean) × 100.
[b] Excluding data for subject F21, high-pitch phonation.

the output of any of these systems is its fractal dimension.[4]

Like the heart, the phonatory system (including the supraglottal vocal tract, larynx, and subglottal air supply) is also an oscillator regulated by a very complex set of interconnected control mechanisms. The fractal nature of the phonatory product is likely to reflect not only accidents of peripheral function, but unpredictable irregularity resulting from the nonlinear interactions of the underlying regulatory and driving systems.

To the extent that the noise seen in a system is not simply due to random accidents, but rather results from the very dynamics of the control system, a different view of irregularity emerges. From the perspective of the theories underlying fractal analysis (and the science of chaos, to which they are closely related), the "deterministic noise" of the system represents the system's resources for responding to changing conditions, absorbing functional adversity, and, if necessary, coping with pathology (59). In short, the irregularity that is seen in the output may be a surface indication of the number of degrees of freedom in a system. Irregularity can, therefore, be considered to be adaptive.

In fact, fractal dimensionality provides not only a way of describing a system's irregularity, but also a means of exploring its sources and its relationship to other systems. A number of considerations are important in this regard. First, because D_F is a geometric measure of structure's *shape* rather than a numerical summary of the specific values in a set of data, D_F can be used to compare otherwise dissimilar phenomena. That is, apples can be easily and validly compared to oranges.[5] (In the speech signal,

for example, vocal shimmer could be compared to formant instability.) Next, similar basic phenomena (in the mathematical sense) are characterized by similar fractal dimensions. Finally, the result of joining several systems, each having its own characteristic D_F is a product whose D_F is equal to the highest D_F among the contributing components (40).

Using these facts, it should be possible to trace outward from the glottis seeking relationships and hierarchies. For example, if the D_F of the tension of the vocalis or cricohyoid muscle is very similar to the D_F of the vocal period the former are likely to be the prime basis of the latter. If, however, the tensions have a lower fractal dimension than vocal F_0, the jitter must have a different origin. In a similar way, the D_F of airflow turbulence can be compared to vocal amplitude perturbations.

Thus, fractal analytic methods are likely to have considerable potential for improving understanding of the normal voice. Application to the study of specific pathologies also seems to hold significant promise. There is, for instance, reason to hypothesize that different classes of disorder may well be manifest in different ranges of D_F of one or more parameters of the acoustic or physiologic signal. Consider, for purposes of illustration, that the vocal folds are anatomically divisible into two portions—the cover and the body—that could be modeled as coupled oscillators. The output of such a dual oscillatory system should be characterized by "deterministic noise" that is measurable by a fractal dimension. A change in one of the oscillatory structures (say a tumor of the vocal fold mucosa) will change the system in a way that may result in a

---

[4] The basic concept underlying these phenomena is, of course, that of *chaos* (55), of which D_F is one descriptor. The actual degree of chaos in a system is better specified by the Lyapunov exponent (56–58).
[5] It is, of course, theoretically possible to achieve such comparisons by normalizing the data to obtain a dimensionless parameter. The difficulty, however, is that it is never certain that the correct normalizing function has been selected or that it is sufficient on its own to achieve a true normalization. The use of fractal dimension obviates these concerns.

characteristic shift of an output parameter's fractal dimension. Different underlying pathologies (such as lower motor neuron paresis or CNS disorder) may well cause still different changes in D_F. Perhaps uniquely among available indices of vocal function, fractal dimension can be derived for discontinuous phonation (commonly observed in many dysphonias) in which the vocal signal alternates erratically between quasiperiodic and aperiodic states. This capability should greatly enhance the utility of fractal analysis in the examination of disorder.

Beyond the possibilities of analysis, fractal geometry is likely to be of importance in voice and speech synthesis as well. The use of iterated function systems and the collage theorem (40) have provided powerful tools in the efficient construction of graphic images of enormous complexity and realism. There is no reason to believe that similar methods cannot be applied to the generation of synthetic acoustic signals, perhaps making them much more "natural" and acceptable to listeners.

Fractal geometry shows considerable potential for expanding understanding of the speech signal and for characterizing its essential features. And it promises to be a potent tool in the exploration of speech and voice mechanisms.

APPENDIX A

Correlations Among the Several Variability Measures and the D_F of the Period and Amplitude Records

	Period D_F		Amplitude D_F	
	r	(r^2)	r	(r^2)
Period				
Mean absolute jitter				
Male	0.3561	(0.1268)	0.3736	(0.1396)
Female	0.1685	(0.0284)	0.6260	(0.3919)
Total	0.2906	(0.0844)	0.3407	(0.1161)
RAP				
Male	0.0108	(0.0001)	−0.1429	(0.0204)
Female	0.0688	(0.0047)	−0.5381	(0.2896)
Total	0.0369	(0.0014)	−0.2786	(0.0776)
Amplitude				
dB shimmer				
Male	−0.0649	(0.0042)	0.4138	(0.1712)
Female	0.2314	(0.0536)	0.6831	(0.4666)
Total	−0.0018	(0.0000)	0.3684	(0.1357)

REFERENCES

1. Davis SB. *Computer evaluation of laryngeal pathology based on inverse filtering of speech.* (*SCRL Monograph 13*). Santa Barbara, California: Speech Communications Research Lab, 1976.

2. Deal RE, Emanuel FW. Some waveform and spectral features of vowel roughness. *J Speech Hear Res* 1978;21:250–64.

3. Hecker MHL, Kreul EJ. Descriptions of the speech of patients with cancer of the vocal folds. Part I: Measures of fundamental frequency. *J Acoust Soc Am* 1971;49:1275–82.

4. Horii Y. Fundamental frequency perturbation observed in sustained phonation. *J Speech Hear Res* 1979;22:5–19.

5. Horii Y. Vocal shimmer in sustained phonation. *J Speech Hear Res* 1980;23:202–9.

6. Koike Y. Application of some acoustic measures for the evaluation of laryngeal dysfunction. *Studia Phonologica* 1973;7:17–23.

7. Koike Y, Takahashi H, Calcaterra TC. Acoustic measures for detecting laryngeal pathology. *Acta Otolaryngol* 1977;84:105–17.

8. Lieberman P. Perturbations of vocal pitch. *J Acoust Soc Am* 1961;33:597–603.

9. Lieberman P. Some acoustic measures of the fundamental periodicity of normal and pathologic larynges. *J Acoust Soc Am* 1963;35:344–53.

10. Ludlow C, Coulter D, Gentges F. The differential sensitivity of measures of fundamental frequency perturbation to laryngeal neoplasms and neuropathologies. In: Bless DM, Abbs JH, eds. *Vocal fold physiology: Contemporary research and clinical issues.* San Diego, California: College-Hill Press, 1983:381–92.

11. Takahashi H, Koike Y. Some perceptual dimensions and acoustical correlates of pathologic voices. *Acta Otolaryngol* 1975;suppl 338:1–24.

12. Baer T. Vocal jitter: a neuromuscular explanation. In: Lawrence V, ed. *Transcripts of the eighth symposium: Care of the professional voice.* New York: The Voice Foundation, 1980:19–22.

13. Cavallo S, Baken RJ, Shaiman S. Frequency perturbation characteristics of pulse-register phonation. *J Commun Dis* 1984;17:231–43.

14. Hirano M, Hiki S, Imaizumi S, Kakita Y, Matsushita H. Acoustic analysis of pathological voice. In: Lawrence V, ed. *Transcripts of the seventh symposium: Care of the professional voice. Part III: Medical/surgical therapy.* New York: The Voice Foundation, 1979:50–7.

15. Horii Y. Jitter and shimmer differences among sustained vowel phonations. *J Speech Hear Res* 1982;25:12–4.

16. Ishizaka K, Isshiki N. Computer simulation of pathological vocal-cord vibration. *J Acoust Soc Am* 1976;60:1193–8.

17. Isshiki N, Tanabe M, Ishizaka K, Broad D. Clinical significance of asymmetrical vocal cord tension. *Ann Otol Rhinol Laryngol* 1977;86:58–66.

18. Larson CR, Kempster GB. Voice fundamental frequency changes following discharge of laryngeal motor units. In: Titze IR, Scherer RC, eds. *Vocal fold physiology: Biomechanics, acoustics, and phonatory control.* Denver, Colorado: Denver Center for the Performing Arts, 1983:91–103.

19. Larson CR, Kempster GB, Kistler MK. Changes in voice fundamental frequency following discharge of single motor units in cricothyroid and thyroarytenoid muscles. *J Speech Hear Res* 1987;30:552–8.

20. Sorensen D, Horii Y. Frequency and amplitude perturbation in the voices of female speakers. *J Commun Dis* 1983;16:57–61.

21. Wilcox K, Horii Y. Age and changes in vocal jitter. *J Gerontol* 1980;35:194–8.

22. Beckett RL. Pitch perturbation as a function of subjective vocal constriction. *Folia Phoniatr* 1969;21:416–25.

23. Bowler NW. A fundamental frequency analysis of harsh vocal quality. *Speech Monographs* 1964;31:128–34.

24. Davis SB. Acoustic characteristics of normal and pathologic voices. In: Lass NJ, ed. *Speech and language: Advances in basic research and practice. Vol. I.* New York: Academic Press, 1979:271–335.

25. Davis SB. Acoustic characteristics of normal and pathologic voices. In: Ludlow CL, Hart MO, eds. *Proceedings of the conference on the assessment of vocal pathology. (ASHA Reports no. 11).* Rockville, Maryland: American Speech-Language-Hearing Association, 1981:97–115.

26. Dunker E, Schlosshauer B. Unregelmassige Stimmlippenschwingungen bei functionellen Stimmstorungen. *Zeitschr Laryngol Rhinol* 1961;40:919–34.

27. Isshiki N. Yanagihara N. Morimoto M. Approach to the objective diagnosis of hoarseness. *Folia Phoniatr* 1966;18:393–400.

28. Klingholz F, Martin F. Quantitative spectral evaluation of shimmer and jitter. *J Speech Hear Res* 1985;28:169–74.

29. Koike Y. Application of some acoustic measures for the evaluation of laryngeal dysfunction. *J Acoust Soc Am* 1967;42:1209.

30. Moore P, Thompson CL. Comments on physiology of hoarseness. *Arch Otolaryngol* 1965;81:97–102.

31. von Leden H, Moore P, Timcke R. Laryngeal vibrations: Measurements of the glottic save. Part III: The pathologic larynx. *Arch Otolaryngol* 1960;71:16–35.

32. Wendahl RW. Some parameters of auditory roughness. *Folia Phoniatr* 1966;18:26–32.

33. Zyski BJ, Bull GL, McDonald WE, Johns ME. Perturbation analysis of normal and pathologic larynges. *Folia Phoniatr* 1984;36:190–8.

34. Ludlow CL, Bassich CJ, Connor NP, Coulter DC, Lee YJ. The validity of using phonatory jitter and shimmer to detect laryngeal pathology. In: Baer T, Sasaki C, Harris KS, eds. *Laryngeal function in phonation and respiration.* Boston: Little, Brown, 1987:492–508.

35. Baken RJ. *Clinical measurement of speech and voice.* Boston: Little, Brown, 1987.

36. Pickover CA, Khorasani A. Fractal characterization of speech waveform graphs. *Computer Graphics* 1986;10:51–61.

37. Mandelbrot B. How long is the coast of Britain: Statistical self-similarity and fractional dimension. *Science* 1978;156:636–8.

38. Mandelbrot BB. *The fractal geometry of nature.* New York: WH Freeman, 1983.

39. Greenside HS, Wolf A, Swift J, Pignataro T. Impracticality of a box-counting algorithm for calculating the dimensionality of strange attractors. *Physical Review A* 1982;25:3453–6.

40. Barnsley M. *Fractals everywhere.* Boston: Academic Press, 1988.

41. Framer JD. Dimension, fractal measures, and chaotic dynamics. In: Haken H, ed. *Evolution of order and chaos.* New York: Springer, 1982:228–46.

42. Voss RF. Fractals in nature: From characterization to simulation. In: Peitgen H-O, Saupe D, eds. *The science of fractal images.* New York: Springer, 1988:21–70.

43. Hollien M, Michel J, Doherty ET. A method for analyzing vocal jitter in sustained phonation. *J Phonet* 1973;1:85–91.

44. Orlikoff RF, Baken RJ. Consideration of the relationship between the fundamental frequency of phonation and vocal jitter. *Folia Phoniatr* 1990;42:31–40.

45. Villchur E, Killion MC. Probe-tube microphone assembly. *J Acoust Soc Am* 1975;57:238–40.

46. Titze IR, Horii Y, Scherer RC. Some technical considerations in voice perturbation measurements. *J Speech Hear Res* 1987;30:252–60.

47. Winer BJ. *Statistical principles in experimental design.* New York: McGraw-Hill, 1962.

48. Guenther WC. *Concepts of statistical inference.* New York: McGraw-Hill, 1965.

49. Saupe D. Algorithms for random fractals. In: Peitgen H-O, Saupe D, eds. *The science of fractal images.* New York: Springer, 1988:71–136.

50. Parlitz U., Lauterborn W. Period-doubling cascades and devil's staircases of the driven van der Pol oscillator. *Physical Review A* 1987;36:1428–34.

51. Gollub JP, Brunner TO, Danly BG. Periodicity and chaos in coupled nonlinear oscillators. *Science* 1978;200:48–50.

52. Glass L, Shrier A, Belair J. Chaotic cardiac rhythms. In: Holden AV, ed. *Chaos.* Princeton, NJ: Princeton University Press, 1986:237–56.

53. Goldberger Al, West BJ, Bhargava V. Nonlinear mechanisms in physiology and pathophysiology: Towards a dynamical theory of health and disease. In: Eisenfeld J, Witten M, eds. *Modelling of Biomedical Systems.* The Hague: Elsevier Science Publishers BV, 1986:227–33.

54. Mackey MC, Glass L. Oscillation and chaos in physiological control systems. *Science* 1977;197:287–9.

55. Gleick J. *Chaos: Making a new science.* New York: Viking Press, 1987.

56. Eckmann J-P, Kamphorst SO, Ruelle D, Ciliberto S. Liapunov [*sic*] exponents from time series. *Physical Review A* 1986;34:4971–9.

57. Sano M, Sawada Y. Measurement of the Lyapunov spectrum from a chaotic time series. *Physical Review Letters* 1985;55:1082–5.

58. Wolf A, Swift JB, Swinney HL, Vastano JA. Determining Lyapunov exponents from a time series. *Physica* 1985;16D:285–317.

59. Conrad M. What is the use of chaos? In: Holden AV, ed. *Chaos.* Princeton, New Jersey: Princeton University Press, 1986:3–14.

Journal of Sound and Vibration (1990) **136**(1), 151–156

BIFURCATION PORTRAIT OF THE HUMAN VOCAL CORD OSCILLATIONS

1. INTRODUCTION

Chaotic behaviour in deterministic non-linear oscillators [1–6] shows that our present knowledge cannot explain all the possible complex dynamics of even simple non-linear systems. On the other hand, however, it is well known that the qualitative change in the behaviour of the system with the accompanying change of one or more parameters is due to bifurcations. There are examples where period-doubling bifurcation or bifurcation of the periodic orbits leads to chaos [7, 8]. The standard classical methods based on initial value problems are not efficient enough to give a general structure of the bifurcations in a parameter space. For instance, they do not allow for the accurate calculation of non-visible (unstable) attractors and the bifurcation points.

For these reasons this letter is concerned with a systematic approach for tracing the behaviour of the system by varying one (or more) chosen parameters. The procedure includes the calculation of steady state solutions, Hopf bifurcation points and the branches of periodic orbits which emanate from the Hopf bifurcation points. Then, by tracing the evolution of the characteristic multipliers one can observe the changes of stability of these solutions and possibly further branching to resonance or quasi-periodic motion. This approach is based on solving a boundary value problem by using the shooting method and is a development of earlier work by Brommundt [9], in which Urabe's method [10] was used. A similar strategy of calculation branches and branching points has been presented by Seydel [11].

2. THE METHOD

Non-dimensional non-linear differential equations modelling the vibrations of the human vocal cords were established by Cronjaeger [12]. They can be cast in the following form:

$$\ddot{x} + d\dot{x} + (k_x + k_c((x - X_0)^2 + y^2))(x - X_0) - k_{xy}y + k_s x^{-4}(1 - d_x \dot{x}) = Ep,$$

$$\ddot{y} + d\dot{y} + (k_y + k_c((x - X_0)^2 + y^2))y - k_{xy}(x - X_0) = Ep,$$

$$p = Q - \begin{cases} (x-1)p^{1/2} & \text{for } x > 1 \\ 0 & \text{for } x \leqslant 1 \end{cases}. \tag{1}$$

Here d is the damping coefficient of the vocal cords, $k_x(k_y)$ is a horizontal (vertical) stiffness of the vocal cords, k_{xy} is a stiffness of the couplings between the two directions of motion, k_c is a cubic type stiffness, k_s is a hyperbolic type stiffness, d_s is a damping coefficient, X_0 is the unloaded equilibrium position ($Q = 0$), E is average pressure, and Q is air flow. The co-ordinates x, y are the horizontal and vertical displacements of the vocal cord, while p is the air pressure. Among the ten parameters the following are fixed: $k_x = 1$, $k_y = 0.3$, $k_c = 0.001$, $k_s = 0.001$, $d_s = 0.5$, $k_{xy} = 0.3$, $X_0 = 0.4$, $E = 0.4$, $Q = 7$. For convenience the equations of motion can be concisely expressed as

$$\mathbf{h}(\mathbf{z}', \mathbf{z}, \boldsymbol{\eta}) = 0, \tag{2}$$

where $\mathbf{z} = (x, \dot{x}, y, \dot{y}, p)$ and $\boldsymbol{\eta}$ is the vector of parameters. For the constant solution $\mathbf{z} = \mathbf{z}_0$ one obtains

$$\mathbf{h}(\mathbf{0}, \mathbf{z}_0, \boldsymbol{\eta}_0) = 0. \tag{3}$$

151

0022–460X/90/010151+06 $03.00 0

Equation (3) was solved numerically by Newton's method. From equation (2) one can obtain the linear first order variation equation

$$\Delta z' = H \, \Delta z, \tag{4}$$

where H is a constant matrix and Δz is a vector of small perturbations of the constant solution. The eigenvalue problem of equation (4) yields the five eigenvalues and corresponding eigenvectors.

During the computer calculations these values are found by reduction of the real matrix to Hessenberg form. The eigenvectors are normalized so that the sum of the squares of the moduli of the elements is equal to 1 and the element of largest modulus is real. This ensures that real eigenvalues have real eigenvectors. Cronjaeger [12] has shown using an analytical method that the matrix H possesses only real negative or conjugate complex eigenvalues.

When a pair of complex eigenvalues crosses the imaginary axis with non-zero velocity Hopf bifurcation occurs. A Hopf bifurcation point is the starting point of a branch of periodic solutions of equations (1). The solution $z(z_0, \tau)$, where $z_0 = z(\tau_0)$, is a periodic solution. For the exactly periodic solution the shooting method has been used here:

$$z(z_0, \tau) - z_0 = 0. \tag{5}$$

The vector z_0 has been calculated numerically by using Newton's method. In the k-iteration step

$$(I - J^{(k)}) \, \Delta z^{(k)} = z^{(k)}(z_0, \tau_0 + 2\pi) - z^{(k)}(z_0, \tau_0), \qquad z_0^{(k+1)} = z^{(k)} + \Delta z^{(k)}, \tag{6}$$

where the Jacobian matrix is taken at $z = z^{(k)}$ and the derivatives for its elements are calculated numerically.

Numerical integration yields the fundamental matrix of which the eigenvalues are the characteristic multipliers. If four eigenvalues (because one is always equal to 1) are inside the unit circle in the complex plane, then the periodic orbit considered is stable. If one real eigenvalue, or the pair of complex conjugate eigenvalues, crosses the unit circle, branching of periodic solution occurs. Following Arnold [13] one can expect birth or annihilation of the limit cycle, transcritical or pitchfork bifurcation if one eigenvalue crosses the unit circle at $+1$, period-doubling if one eigenvalue crosses this circle at -1 and finally non-linear resonance or bifurcation into tori if a pair of eigenvalue crosses the unit circle with non-zero imaginary parts. In the last case general topologically versal deformations are not known and may not exist.

During the calculations, the frequency ω and relative time $\tau = \omega t$ are introduced. The frequency ω enters the equations as a parameter to be kept fixed when one looks at a special solution. Periodic solutions $z(t)$ with the period T correspond to periodic solutions $z(\tau, \omega)$ with the period 2π. Because the system (1) is autonomous a phase condition $\dot{x} = 0$ is prescribed in order to fix the unknown frequency ω. If the solution is unfavorably stated (not uniquely solvable for $z(\omega)$), an exchange of the fastest varying z_i removes the numerical difficulties (z_i is chosen, ω calculated). During numerical integration, because of the non-linear term x^{-4}, the standard methods based on the Runge–Kutta algorithm are not sufficiently accurate for integration of the stiff equations system being considered. Hence a variable-order, variable-step Gear method with the small step (for $\dot{x} = 0$) has been used and calculations were made with double precision.

The branching diagram for damping $0 \cdot 01 < d < 0 \cdot 35$ is shown in Figure 1. The previous stable steady state solution becomes unstable for $d = 0 \cdot 35$ and the periodic limit cycle emanates from Hopf bifurcation point H1. At this point a new periodic solution has a frequency $\omega = 1 \cdot 169$ which is equal to the imaginary eigenvalue obtained from equation (4). Then the period of this solution is normalized to 2π and the branch H1PD1 is obtained. As can be seen from the corresponding diagram with multipliers (Figure 2) for

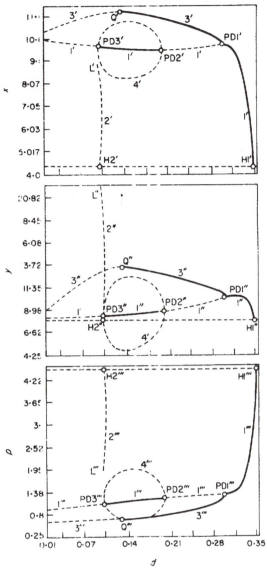

Figure 1. Bifurcation structure of the oscillations of the human vocal cords. At the bifurcation points H1, H2 and PD1 only one branch of the new emanating solutions is marked in order to present the phase shift between the demonstrated variables $y_1 = x$, $y_3 = y$, $y_5 = p$. The solid line indicates stable solutions.

$d = 0.295$ the real eigenvalue crosses the unit circle at -1 and the second subharmonic solution has appeared with $\omega = 1.197$. The previous periodic solution becomes unstable. However, with the further decrease of damping the real eigenvalue turns to the right and for $d = 0.19$ ($\omega = 1.332$) crosses the unit circle at -1 again. After this all eigenvalues are inside the unit circle and the solution considered, marked as 1, is stable. Points PD2 ($d = 0.19$, $\omega = 1.332$) and PD3 ($d = 0.1$, $\omega = 1.402$) belong to the envelope of self-excited oscillations which correspond to the second unstable subharmonic solution (coded as 4). After crossing the point PD3 the 2π periodic solution considered becomes unstable again. Another subharmonic solution branches the point PD1. This solution has period 4π, but during the calculations it is normalized to 2π with $\omega = 0.608$ at the point PD1. With decrease of d, the frequency ω increases and for $d = 0.01$ it reaches the value 0.695.

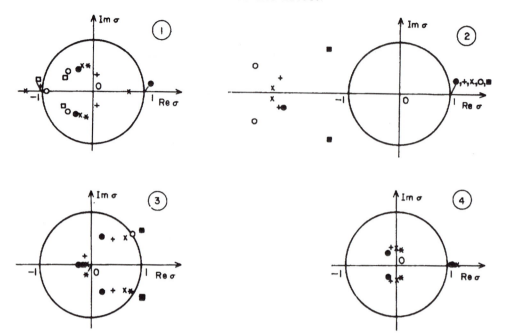

Figure 2. Discrete trajectories of the characteristic multipliers with the changing of damping d on the complex plane with respect to the unit circle. Each of the five examples corresponds to the marked branches in Figure 1. Only three multipliers are presented because one of the multipliers is equal to 1 (autonomous system) whereas another is very small in comparison to the others. d values for ①: •, 0·34; ×, 0·315; +, 0·295; *, 0·25; ○, 0·15; ◐, 0·1. d values for ②: •, 0·10021; +, 0·10052; ×, 0·10184; ○, 0·10202; ■, 0·09578. d values for ③: •, 0·27315; +, 0·20375; ×, 0·16; *, 0·14; ○, 0·13; ■, 0·1. d values for ④: •, 0·18551; +, 0·16; ×, 0·13; *, 0·11.

With the decrease of d (see Figure 3(a)) two complex conjugate eigenvalues approach the unit circle and for $d = 0·13$ cross it. The subharmonic solution marked as 3 becomes unstable and the situation does not change in the considered interval of the parameter d. Another solution branches from the point Q ($d = 0·13$). The question arises if this solution is periodic or quasiperiodic. The two conjugate multipliers σ_μ lie on the unit circle when $\sigma_\mu = e^{2\pi i \omega_\mu}$ and $= (1/2\pi) \arg(\sigma_\mu)$. In this case the eigenvalues lying on the unit circle are $(0·80, \pm0·60)$ and $\omega_\mu \neq l/k$, where l, k are relatively prime integers. This means that at this point a new quasi-periodic solution is born.

The periodic solution 2, which is unstable, branches from the second Hopf bifurcation point H2. For some narrow interval for the fixed d value there exist two unstable periodic solutions. From the last numerically obtained point (L) belonging to the curve 2, further progress of the numerical continuation was impossible. The solution has left the real plane. Calculated stable and unstable limit cycles are shown (see Figure 3) for such values of d which belong to all the separated branches (see Figure 2). Generally, attractors of the system considered possess ten projections of the (y_i, y_j) plane, where $i, j = 1, \ldots, 5$. Corresponding to the trajectory of the vocal cord, only one is presented (y_1, y_3).

3. CONCLUDING REMARKS

To conclude, a calculation method to obtain bifurcation diagrams of a fifth order system of differential non-linear equations has been presented. This system of equations describes the self-excited vibrations of the vocal cords. For the interval of damping considered it has been shown that this system possesses two Hopf bifurcation points, three period-doubling bifurcation points and one Q point. After Q is crossed, a quasi-periodic torus

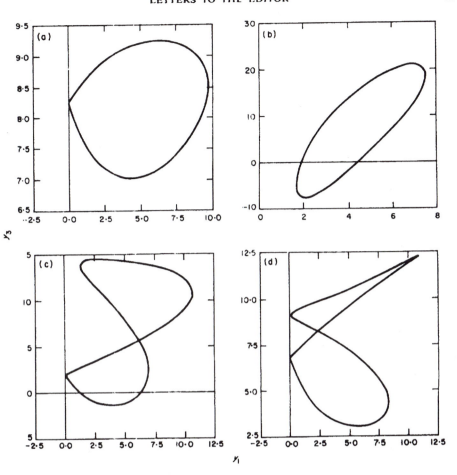

Figure 3. Calculation examples of the stable and unstable limit cycles. The trajectory of the vocal cord corresponds to the branches from Figure 1 as follows: (a) to 1, (b) to 2, (c) to 3 and (d) to 4. The calculations were made for the following values of damping d: (a) $d = 0.13$; (b) $d = 0.10062$; (c) $d = 0.04$; (d) $d = 0.13$.

is born. There is an interval of damping for which two stable 2π periodic and 4π periodic solutions exist. It is possible to jump from one solution to another. Harmonic and subharmonic unstable solutions also exist for this interval of damping.

ACKNOWLEDGMENT

The author would like to thank E. Brommundt for helpful discussion relating to this investigation. Thanks also to H. Staben who assisted in numerical calculations. This work was supported by the Alexander von Humboldt Foundation.

Technical University, Institute of Technical Mechanics,   J. AWREJCEWICZ[†]
Spielmannstrasse 11, 3300 Braunschweig, West Germany

(*Received* 24 April 1989)

[†] On leave from the Technical University, Institute of Applied Mechanics, B. Stefanowskiego 1/15, 90-924 Lodz, Poland.

156   LETTERS TO THE EDITOR

REFERENCES

1. E. N. LORENZ 1963 *Journal of Atmospheric Sciences* **20**, 130–141. Deterministic nonperiodic flow.
2. Y. UEDA 1979 *Journal of Statistical Physics* **20**, 181–186. Randomly transitional phenomena in the system governed by Duffing's equation.
3. R. RATY, H. M. ISOMÄKI and J. VON BOEHM 1984 *Acta Polytechnica Scandinavica Me* **85**, 1–30. Chaotic motion of a classical anharmonic oscillator.
4. R. SEYDEL 1980 *Report TU-München, Institut für Mathematik, TUM-M*8019. The strange attractors of a Duffing equation dependence on the exciting frequency.
5. J. AWREJCEWICZ 1986 *Journal of Sound and Vibration* **109**, 178–180. Chaos in simple mechanical systems with friction.
6. T. KAPITANIAK, J. AWREJCEWICZ and W.-H. STEEB 1987 *Journal of Physics A: Mathematical and General* **20**, L355–L358. Chaotic behaviour of an anharmonic oscillator with almost periodic excitation.
7. M. J. FEIGENBAUM 1978 *Journal of Statistical Physics* **19**, 25–52. Quantitative universality for a class of nonlinear transformations.
8. J. CURRY and J. YORKE 1978 *Lecture Notes in Mathematics* **668**, 48–68. Berlin, Heidelberg, New York: Springer-Verlag. A transition from Hopf bifurcation to chaos; a computer experiments on maps in R^2. The structure of attractors in dynamical systems.
9. E. BROMMUNDT 1977 *Proceedings of the VII International Conference on Nonlinear Vibrations,* 123–134. Berlin: Akademik-Verlag. Bifurcation of self-excited rotor vibrations.
10. M. URABE and A. REITER 1966 *Journal of Applied Mathematical Analysis* **14**, 107–140. Numerical computation of nonlinear forced oscillations by Galerkin's procedure.
11. R. SEYDEL 1988 *From Equilibrium to Chaos: Practical Bifurcation and Stability Analysis.* New York: Elsevier.
12. R. CRONJAEGER 1978 *Ph.D. Thesis, Braunschweig Technical University.* Model of the sound generation in a human larynx.
13. V. I. ARNOLD 1983 *Geometrical Methods in the Theory of Ordinary Differential Equations.* New York, Heidelberg, Berlin: Springer-Verlag.

Observation of perturbations in a lumped-element model of the vocal folds with application to some pathological cases

Darrell Wong, Mabo R. Ito, and Neil B. Cox
Department of Electrical Engineering, University of British Columbia, Vancouver, British Columbia V6T 1W5, Canada

Ingo R. Titze
Voice Acoustics and Biomechanics Laboratory, Department of Speech Pathology and Audiology, University of Iowa, Iowa City, Iowa 52242

(Received 13 June 1989; accepted for publication 7 August 1990)

In this paper a mass–spring model is developed that is a hybrid of the two-mass and the longitudinal string models, proposed by Ishizaka and Flanagan [Bell Sys. Tech. J. **51**, 1233–1268 (1972)] and Titze [Phonetica **28**, 129–170 (1973)], respectively. The model is used to simulate the vibratory motion of both the normal and asymmetric vocal folds. Mouth-output pressure, lateral tissue displacement, phase plots, and energy diagrams are presented to demonstrate the interaction between vocal fold tissue and the aerodynamic flow between the folds. The results of the study suggest that this interaction is necessary for sustained large amplitude oscillation because the flow supplies the energy lost by the tissue damping. Tissue mass and stiffness were varied locally or uniformly. Decreased stress in the longitudinal string tension produced subharmonic and chaotic vibrations in the displacement, velocity and acceleration phase diagrams. Similar vibratory characteristics also appeared in pathological speech data analyzed using time domain jitter and shimmer measures and a harmonics-to-noise ratio metric. The subharmonics create an effect that has been perceptually described as diplophonia.

PACS numbers: 43.70.Bk, 43.70.Aj

INTRODUCTION

Past studies of the self-oscillation mechanism of the vocal fold (Ishizaka and Matsudaira, 1972), (Ishizaka and Flanagan, 1972), (Titze, 1973, 1980, 1985, 1988) have simulated the physics of oscillation to understand the phenomena observed in vowel speech data and high-speed films of laryngeal vibration. These studies have focused on the characteristics of the normal fold.

Isshiki and Ishizaka (1976) used the two-mass model (Ishizaka and Flanagan, 1972) to investigate the effects of asymmetrical biomechanical parameters on tissue vibration, e.g., lateral tissue stiffness and initial area of opening of the glottis. Asymmetric and perturbed tissue vibrations, with significant jitter in the mouth-output pressure, were observed in the model and in canine laryngeal film sequences. Unfortunately, the study did not explain the observations in terms of the driving forces on the tissue or the mechanisms of perturbation. Furthermore, the model did not have longitudinally distributed masses, making it impossible to simulate vocal folds with localized parameter changes.

This paper presents a study of vibrations produced by asymmetrical folds. A multiple mass model, which is a hybrid of the Ishizaka and Flanagan (1972) and Titze (1973) models (hereafter called the IF and T73 models) has been developed and combined with a vocal tract model. In this paper the model's equations will be presented, and its adequacy in representing the normal fold will be demonstrated. Perturbed vibrations resulting from local and nonlocal model parameter changes will then be simulated. Mouth-output

sound pressure perturbations have been characterized using time domain jitter and shimmer measures and a harmonics-to-noise ratio energy metric. A comparison is made between simulation results and voice disorder cases from a pathology data base using these metrics.

I. MODEL STRUCTURE

A. Vocal fold model

The proposed model is similar to the IF two-mass model, but in addition it divides each mass longitudinally in the anterior–posterior direction, as in the T73 model. In this model, however, only lateral motion is permitted (as in the IF model). Vertical motion, which was permitted by the T73 model, is not modeled since the T73 model behavior was similar to the IF model in the vertical plane once steady state was reached. Vertical motion was therefore not expected to contribute critical information for steady-state oscillation but would make the flow calculation much more difficult with asymmetric vocal folds.

Figures 1 and 2 are frontal and perspective views of the vocal folds. Masses m_l and m_u represent the lower and upper portions of the vocal fold (a subscript i, indicating the ith local mass in the longitudinal string, has been excluded from the figure for clarity). The upper and lower elements do not represent specific parts of the fold, but describe the effect of the surface wave that occurs in the mucosal tissue of the fold. The masses are connected to the wall by nonlinear springs with a cubic response, with k_l and k_u representing the linear

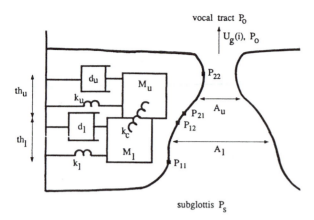

FIG. 1. Side view of proposed model.

stiffness coefficient of the tissue and η_l and η_u the cubic coefficients (see Appendix A). The form of these springs is the same as for the IF model. The upper and lower masses are coupled by a nonlinear cubic spring with coefficients k_c and η_c. Aerodynamic pressures within the glottis (indicated as $P_{11}, P_{12}, P_{21}, P_{22}$, and defined in the IF model) are dependent on time and glottal shape. Here, A_l and A_u are glottal areas and P_s and P_0 are the pressures just below and above the vocal folds, respectively.

The dampers d_l and d_u in Figs. 1 and 2 represent the viscous resistance within the tissue, and T_l and T_u (the lower and upper longitudinal tensions) are coupling tensions between each mass in the string as defined in the T73 model. The tension T_l consists of a strain-dependent function plus a constant component T_{act} representing the muscular contraction during voicing. Only the lateral components of T_u and T_l forces are exerted on the adjacent masses. This is because the model does not permit longitudinal motion of the masses. Large particle displacements are permitted and the end points of the longitudinally tensed "strings" are fixed. Five masses per row have been chosen to minimize the computation effort, while still permitting the localization of

parameters. The number of longitudinal eigenmodes has been reduced from infinity (for a continuum model) to a maximum of five. This is justifiable since the energy in higher modes should be negligible (Titze, 1973). With five masses, it is expected that the first three modes will be identifiable.

The dynamic equations for any mass pair (upper and lower) can be written in terms of the driving forces and all the nearest-neighbor coupling forces:

$$m_l(i)\ddot{x}_l(i) = F_{dl}(i) + F_{tla}(i) + F_{tlp}(i) + F_{kl}(i)$$
$$+ F_{kc}(i) + F_{lcol}(i) + F_{el}(i) = F_l(i),$$
$$m_u(i)\ddot{x}_u(i) = F_{du}(i) + F_{tua}(i) + F_{tup}(i) + F_{ku}(i)$$
$$- F_{kc}(i) + F_{ucol}(i) + F_{eu}(i) = F_u(i). \quad (1)$$

Figure 3 is the free body diagram of the ith upper mass, from which we can see the components of the dynamic equations. Here, $F_{du}(i)$ is the damping force, $F_{ku}(i)$ and $F_{kc}(i)$ are the lateral spring forces attaching the upper portion to the wall and to the lower portion, $F_{ucol}(i)$ is an additional force generated only during collisions, and $F_{tua}(i)$ and $F_{tup}(i)$ (not shown in Fig. 3) are the lateral components of $T_u(i)$ and $T_u(i+1)$, respectively. Also, $F_{eu}(i)$ is the external force generated by the air flow, $\ddot{x}_l(i)$ and $\ddot{x}_u(i)$ are the lateral tissue accelerations of the centers of gravity of the masses, and $F_l(i)$ and $F_u(i)$ are the total forces acting on each element. These forces are fully described in Appendix A.

B. Vocal tract and subglottal models

The vocal tract is modeled as a transmission line, using ten cylindrical hard-walled acoustic tubes of variable cross-sectional areas and lengths. The acoustic impedances are derived from (Flanagan, 1960). In this study the vocal tract shape for the vowel /a/ (Fant, 1960) was used. The glottal constriction is coupled to the lungs via the tracheal subglottal tube. Ishizaka et al. (1976) estimated the lung–trachea subglottal system to be equivalent to an acoustic tube 20 cm long and 2.5 cm² in area, terminated by a constant lung pressure.

C. Network representation

With five vocal fold masses in the longitudinal dimension and two in the vertical (lung to tract) dimension, the

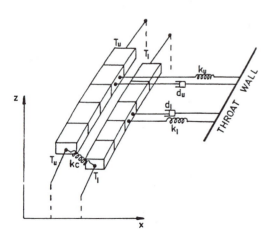

FIG. 2. Perspective view of right fold.

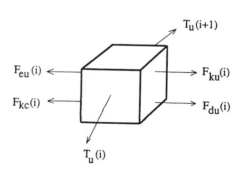

FIG. 3. Free body diagram of the ith upper mass.

glottal flow is the sum of the five parallel flows through each of the upper–lower pairs. The summed flow represents the overall volume velocity. Vocal tract and subglottal tract models for the vowel /a/ are concatenated to the glottal model to complete the speech system (see Fig. 4). Note that the glottal impedances are time-varying nonlinear functions of the constriction areas while the vocal tract and subglottal impedances are fixed. The network in Fig. 4 was solved with loop analysis using the continuous simulation language ACSL on a VAX 11/750. The Adams–Moulton variable step integration algorithm was used with a minimum relative and absolute error tolerance of 10^{-4}. An error size of 10^{-5} was also used with no difference in the results.

For the left and right vocal folds, the equations are duplicated so that the folds are modeled separately, but coupled together through the common air flow. The area through which the flow occurs is then calculated as

$$A_l(i) = w\left(\left(x_{ll}(i) - \frac{th_l}{2}\right) + \left(x_{lr}(i) - \frac{th_l}{2}\right)\right), \tag{2}$$
$$A_u(i) = w\left(\left(x_{ul}(i) - \frac{th_u}{2}\right) + \left(x_{ur}(i) - \frac{th_u}{2}\right)\right),$$

where the left and right lateral displacements x_{ll} and x_{lr} are measured from the glottal midline to the center of gravity of each mass, and th_l is the lateral thickness. Thus $[x_{lr}(i) - th_l/2]$ is the distance to the surface of the mass and w is the distance between the adjacent masses in the longitudinal direction.

II. VOCAL FOLD OSCILLATION MEASUREMENTS

Tissue parameter values used in this model have been taken from works by Kaneko and Ishizaka (1968), Titze

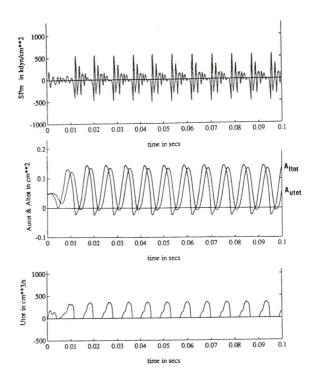

FIG. 5. Mouth-output sound pressure (SP_m), areas (A_{ltot} and A_{utot}), and glottal flow (U_{tot}) for simulated normal vocal folds.

(1973), Hirano (1979), and Ishizaka and Flanagan (1972). The parameters for the hybrid model are generally within the same order of magnitude as the parameters in these works. Values chosen for the normal vocal fold can be found in Appendix B.

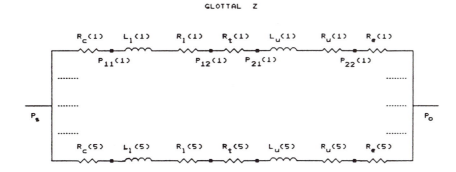

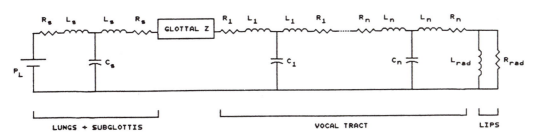

FIG. 4. Model of phonation as an impedance network.

Plots of the mouth-output sound pressure (SP_m in kdyn/cm^2), glottal volume velocity (U_{tot} in cm^3/s), and glottal area are used to illustrate the vibratory characteristics for the normal fold (Fig. 5) and for abnormal parameter values (illustrated later). All values are in cgs units. The SP_m waves have been analyzed using fundamental period (fp) and peak amplitude (pa) versus period number plots (Cox, 1986), and a harmonics-to-noise ratio measure (Yumoto et al., 1982).

Area waves representing the total glottal area open to the flow are measured at the upper (A_{utot}) and lower (A_{ltot}) margins. The area waveforms shown in Fig. 5 have the same shapes as those generated by the IF model. The SP_m and U_{tot} waveforms are also similar. As in the IF model, a negative A_{utot} excursion indicates when the left and right surfaces collide. The negative area occurs when the center of gravities continue to travel after collision, causing the surface edges to pass through one another (in reality the folds would be distorted).

III. SIMULATION OF THE NORMAL FOLDS

A. Phase plane plots

Figure 6 is a phase plane plot of the lower lateral displacement (x_{lr}) versus edge velocity ($\dot{x}_{lr}$) of the right vocal cord (element 3). The system reaches a single stable but asymmetric limit cycle. The asymmetry is the result of the impact during collision. Note that the trajectory crosses over itself. This is not possible unless the system is driven by an external harmonic force, or the system is greater than second order (Minorsky, 1962).

Figure 7 plots the restoring force (F_{lr}) versus displacement (x_{lr}) of the third mass on the lower longitudinal string on the right fold. Figure 7 may also be thought of as an averaged acceleration versus displacement, or an energy exchange plot (the direction of the trajectory indicates the gain or loss of energy by the mass). We can compare our result with Titze (1985), reproduced in Fig. 8. Although the force and displacement was measured midway between the upper

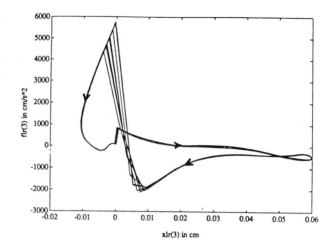

FIG. 7. Equivalent restoring force (F_{lr}) versus displacement $x_{lr}(3)$ for the third lower right mass, showing energy exchange.

and lower lateral edges in Titze's plot, our results are quite similar. Points to note in Fig. 7 are as follows.

(1) The upper left enclosed area, when the displacement is negative, is traversed anticlockwise, indicating energy dissipation. The energy of the mass (the area under the curve) as it enters collision is greater than the energy when it leaves the collision. This implies a net loss of energy by the mass during the negative displacement part of the cycle. Similarly, since the lower right enclosed area is traversed clockwise, energy is absorbed by the mass over the positive part of the cycle. When steady-state oscillation is reached, the sum of the areas enclosed by clockwise areas should be equal to anticlockwise areas indicating a constant energy level.

(2) Figure 7 has characteristics that differ from Fig. 8. The loops of Fig. 8 lie along the $-kx$ axis because Titze (1985) assumed a linear stiffness. In Fig. 7, however, a cubic stiffness characteristic suggesting a $-kx^3$ "spine" is used, which distorts the axis.

(3) The two figures also differ due to the modeling of collisions between the folds. Extra spring forces were intro-

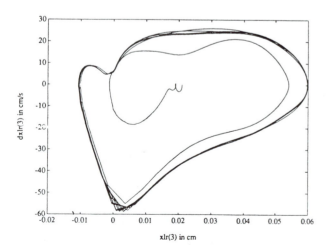

FIG. 6. Velocity-displacement phase plot for the third lower right mass showing a stable limit cycle for the normal fold.

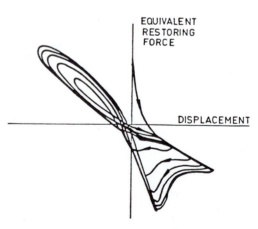

FIG. 8. Equivalent restoring force versus displacement (Titze, 1985).

duced to simulate collision. These forces result in a force of collision much larger than that found by Titze (1985), who did not model the collision. Consequently, the anticlockwise loop is even more upright than the cubic stiffness would dictate.

B. Air flow and tissue interaction

Time plots of $A_{l\text{tot}}$, $A_{u\text{tot}}$, and $F_{lr}(3)$ reveal the changes occurring as the folds oscillate. From Fig. 9 we can observe the following.

(1) Just prior to the lower margin closing (point a), the force due to the Bernoulli effect is large and negative. Negative forces due to vertical phasing and inertial vocal tract loading also help to generate a large, impulsive, negative force (Titze, 1988).

(2) Just after the closure of the lower margin (point b), the lower mass is subjected to a buildup in pressure due to the subglottal pressure. Here, P_s is momentarily very large (Koike, 1980), and as a consequence, the hydrostatic force [proportional to $(P_s + P_0)/2$] increases to a very large value. At this time P_0, the pressure just above the glottis, is negative due to air mass inertia, although its magnitude is relatively small in comparison to P_s. The negative P_o aids in bringing the upper edges together.

(3) At point c the upper edge breaks contact, and the air begins to flow again. At this time, the lower edge is wider than the upper edge, producing glottal convergence and positive pressure in the glottis.

(4) The points discussed above indicate that the direction of the aerodynamic forces near closure are generally in phase with the velocity of the tissue, as described by Titze (1980). Thus energy flows from the air into the folds as the folds part, and energy is dissipated into the air as the folds come together.

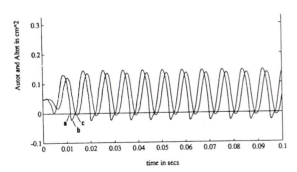

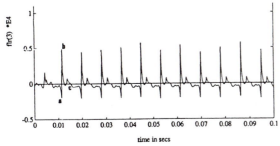

FIG. 9. Areas and $F_{lr}(3)$ as functions of time.

IV. PERTURBATION ANALYSIS

An overall numerical metric of perturbation, the harmonics-to-noise ratio (HNR), and time plots of jitter and shimmer errors were used to measure perturbations in the speech wave.

The HNR is a measure of the cycle to cycle similarity of the waveform, separating the periodic component from the aperiodic component (Yumoto et al., 1982). An average signal for a period is determined by taking the average of a succession of periods. The energy of this average wavelet is the harmonic content of the signal. Then each individual period is compared to the average and the absolute magnitude of the deviations is accumulated as the noise.

HNR is highly sensitive to pitch period estimation, and so a more accurate period estimation scheme has been employed (Cox, 1986). This sensitivity occurs because poor estimation can introduce errors interpreted as jitter. After sampling at 20 kHz a simple visual estimation scheme is used and then a parabolic interpolation of the peak in the autocorrelation wave of the speech signal is employed as a more accurate estimate, using the initial estimate to indicate the region of interest.

The fundamental period length (fp in ms) and peak amplitude (pa) for each period (in kdyn/cm^2), versus period (or wavelet) number are time domain measures used to characterize perturbations. For each period, fp is that period's length. It is a crude instantaneous measure of the jitter. Parameter pa is the magnitude of the largest positive peak value in each period. For the simulated normal case of Fig. 5, both fp and pa plots were smooth, indicating very little jitter and shimmer, and therefore they have not been presented.

For Fig. 5 HNR = 37.7 dB, which is very high when compared to real speech data that were 7 to 25 dB for non-pathological voices (Yumoto et al., 1982). This is not unexpected, since we have not modeled turbulence or neurological jitter that would probably contribute a significant noise component. We have also removed the portion of jitter error due to poor period estimation. As a comparison, a human subject with normal vocal folds measured 22.3 dB using the improved marking scheme.

V. ASYMMETRICAL PARAMETER CHANGES

Modeling pathologies is a difficult task. While some parameters for the normal fold have been published (Kaneko and Ishizaka, 1968), there have been few studies on parameter values for pathologies. Hirano (1979) suggests relative changes from the normal case for some parameters, but specific values are not given. Isshiki and Ishizaka's study (1976) using the IF model has provided some results. Their work, however, used a simulation model rather than real larynges with pathologies.

Although no new mechanical parameter data for pathologies were obtained for this study, comparative examples from a patient database are presented. The approach taken here in simulating pathologies was to vary the masses m_u and m_l, and the lateral stiffnesses (k_l, k_c, and k_u), either locally or by changing an entire fold (unilaterally, right side only). A constant tension parameter, T_{act}, in the T73 model reflecting the longitudinal stress in the vocalis muscle, was also varied, but not locally. The mass or stiffness was increased by a nominal factor of 2.0, and T_{act} (g/cm^2) was reduced from 150 (normal) to 25 (flaccid).

The four asymmetrical cases to be considered—local mass, local stiffness, unilateral mass, and unilateral stiffness (k_u and k_l) changes, were simulated for the normal value of $T_{act} = 150$ g/cm^2 (on both folds). The HNR ratios are listed in Table I ("s" indicates subharmonic modulation of the fundamental, and "r" indicates random perturbations). Values greater than 20 dB indicate very little aperiodicity in the speech signal. This is also shown in SP$_m$ and U_{tot} plots, which are stable and periodic. These plots are not presented here since their appearance is much the same as for the normal case. Increasing the mass or stiffness locally or wholly (unilaterally) on one side resulted in a phase difference in lateral displacement for one side [as reported by Ishiki and Ishizaka (1976)] but no significant perturbations were found, probably due to the high value of T_{act}, which is likely to dampen any harmonics.

A. Unilateral stiffness increase

We now describe the effects of unilateral increase of k_u and k_l for all masses on the right fold by a factor of 2. These perturbations did not appear until T_{act} was decreased to a value of 25 (on both folds).

(1) SP$_m$, area, and U_{tot} waves are shown in Fig. 10. Significant changes on alternating cycles can be observed in all three plots. The phenomenon appears in the displacement (or equivalently the area waves), where the amplitudes indicate the possible presence of a 1/2 subharmonic, commonly described as diplophonia or dichrotic motion.

(2) The energy exchange plot (Fig. 11) shows two major trajectories, with the system alternating from one to the other. Unequal clockwise and anticlockwise areas are enclosed, indicating a net gain in energy for the particular mass examined. Since the overall system exhibits stable oscillation, other masses must be net dissipators of energy to maintain equilibrium. The velocity phase plane plot (not shown) also displays two trajectories.

(3) The pa plot presented in Fig. 12(a) shows the sub-

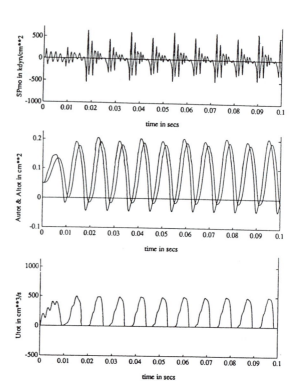

FIG. 10. The SP$_m$, areas and flow (U_{tot}, T) plots for a unilateral stiffness increase in the right fold, $T_{act} = 25$.

harmonic variation in peak amplitude. The subharmonic appears as an up-down motion in the pa curve. The fp plot (not shown) shows a similar trend.

(4) HNR $= 16.8$ dB, indicating significant perturbation in comparison to a normal simulation value of greater than 30 dB.

B. Local stiffness increase

The lateral stiffnesses, k_l, k_c, and k_u for the second and third masses of the right fold were increased by a factor of 2, while $T_{act} = 25$ for both folds.

TABLE I. HNR values (in dB) for simulations and patient data.

Simulation	HNR (dB) ($T_{act} = 150$ g/cm^2)	HNR (dB) ($T_{act} = 25$ g/cm^2)
no changes	37.7	17.5 (*s*)
unilateral stiffness	35.9	16.8 (*s*)
local stiffness	36.1	18.6 (*s,r*)
unilateral mass	40.3	40.8
local mass	35.7	7.9 (*r*)
bilateral local mass		0.38 (*r*)
Patient data		HNR
normal		22.3
chronic laryngitis		4.5 (*s,r*)
T1 glottic cancer (1)		5.5 (*s,r*)
T1 glottic cancer (2)		12.0 (*r*)

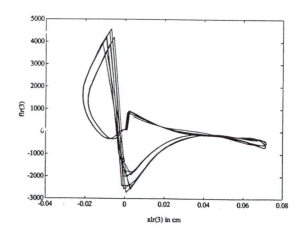

FIG. 11. Energy exchange plot for a unilateral stiffness increase $T_{act} = 25$.

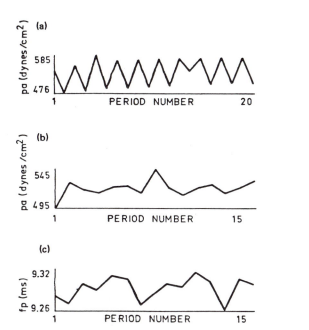

FIG. 12. (a) pa for unilateral stiffness change; (b) pa for local stiffness change; (c) fp for local stiffness change; (in all cases $T_{act} = 25$).

(1) The pa and fp plots [Fig. 12(b) and (c)] have slightly smaller shimmer (pa) and jitter (fp) components than for the unilateral stiffness increase. There is also an irregularity in the plots.

(2) The velocity-displacement phase plot (Fig. 13) shows a system that takes longer to settle into the subharmonic trajectory. Eventually it settles into a trajectory with two major paths, but with an irregular peak amplitude.

(3) HNR = 18.6 dB, indicating that the irregular components produce significant noise. Note that the combination of the subharmonic and the irregular motions produce a higher HNR than for the unilateral stiffness case.

C. Discussion of stiffness changes

Perturbations did not occur until T_{act} was decreased to a value of 25 (both folds). Large amplitude oscillation occurred, causing the lateral springs to enter the nonlinear stiffness region and possibly excite subharmonics.

To determine whether the stiffness asymmetry or the low value of T_{act} is more important, the lateral stiffness of the right side was returned to normal, so that the model was symmetric, with a decreased value of T_{act} for both folds. The subharmonic still appeared, showing that a small value of T_{act} is more important than asymmetry in the lateral stiffness.

Stiffness changes for a complete fold did not affect the presence of the subharmonic (Sec. V A) but local stiffness changes tended to dampen the subharmonic slightly. The perturbation became more irregular, perhaps a combination of other subharmonics and harmonics.

The 1/2 subharmonic manifested itself by modulating the lateral tissue displacement, causing the amplitude of vibration to be reduced on alternate cycles. As a result, the glottal flow pulse, which is proportional to the displacement, also alternates in magnitude and duration. The closing slope of the flow wave is steeper for the large amplitude cycles, and consequently the sound pressure at the mouth (SP_m) receives more energy, since it is proportional to dU_{tot}/dt. This energy appears as alternately large and small peak amplitudes. It also changes the period duration, since the the time of flow closure will vary with the closing slope.

A further simulation (Fig. 14) was carried out in which the right fold T_{act} was set to 25 while the left fold was set to 150. The lateral stiffnesses of the right and left folds were set to their normal values. Neither of the folds were able to produce a subharmonic. By increasing the T_{act} for the left fold, one would expect a smaller amplitude and increased frequency just for this fold. However, in Fig. 14, while the amplitude (d_{ll}) of the stiffer fold (left) has decreased, both the left and right cords have synchronized at the same frequency. This result agrees with experiments performed by Tanabe (1972) who used canine larynges and found the same phenomenon. Frequency synchronization occurs because

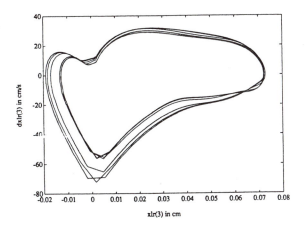

FIG. 13. Velocity-displacement phase plot for $T_{act} = 25$, local stiffness changes.

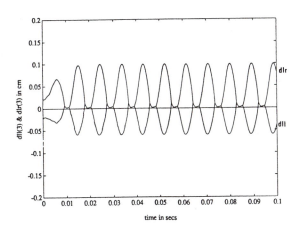

FIG. 14. Left and right displacements, unilateral stiffness change, $T_{actl} = 150$ and $T_{actr} = 25$, show mutual frequency entrainment.

the folds are coupled across the glottal gap by the common air flow, resulting in a mutually synchronized fundamental frequency approximately midway between the expected left and right frequencies. Thus the synchronization between the upper and lower margins within a fold (vertical phasing), due to the explicit spring coupling k_c (Ishizaka, 1980), also occurs between the left and right folds due to aerodynamic coupling.

The pathology that a low T_{act} might represent is superior laryngeal nerve paralysis, a flaccid dysphonia in which the paralyzed fold is characterized by a decrease in longitudinal tension. This may be bilateral or unilateral in its effect, depending on where the lesion occurs. Gerratt and Hanson (1985) produced photoglottograms of patients with this paralysis and a regular perturbation was observed. They described the perturbation as possessing a regular component in which the third pulse was consistently larger, indicating a 1/3 subharmonic.

The effect of local and unilateral mass changes, again with $T_{\text{act}} = 25$ on both folds, was then examined.

D. Unilateral mass increase

For the unilateral case all masses on the right fold (both the upper and lower strings) were increased by a factor of 2. Points to note are: (1) the SP_m, $A_{u\text{tot}}$, $A_{l\text{tot}}$, and U_{tot} waves (not presented) did not reveal any observable perturbations; (2) the phase plot (also not presented), after an initial build-up, settled into a stable trajectory similar to that for the normal case; (3) HNR = 40.8 dB.

E. Localized mass increase

The second and third masses of the right lower and upper strings were increased by a factor of 2. Points to note are:

(1) The SP_m and glottal flow waves appear in Fig. 15. There is an unstable irregular component, causing the closure point to vary. This produces large variations in the SP_m wave.

(2) Figure 16 shows an energy exchange diagram for the right fold. Both the right and left fold (not presented) showed an iregular trajectory. Since only the right fold had local mass changes, the iregular motion of the left fold is excited due to the air flow that couples the left fold with the irregular motion of the right fold. The velocity-displacement phase plot (not shown) of the third mass on the right fold also showed a highly unstable trajectory, although the subharmonic seemed to be present but dominated by the irregular effects.

(3) Plots of pa and fp in Fig. 17(a) and (b) show significant random jitter and shimmer, with about 10-Hz variation about a fundamental of 94 Hz.

(4) HNR = 7.9 dB, a value that is much less than normal and likely to be pathological (Yumoto et al., 1982).

F. Discussion of mass changes

With $T_{\text{act}} = 25$, perturbations appeared for localized mass changes but not for changes in an entire fold. Unilateral mass increases appear to inhibit the subharmonic whereas unilateral stiffness increases enhance the effect.

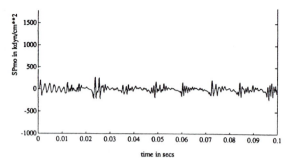
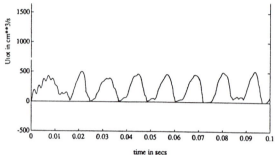

FIG. 15. The SP_m and U_{tot} for local mass changes (elements 2 and 3), $T_{\text{act}} = 25$.

Local mass changes result in a phase plot trajectory with a significant irregular component that seems to dominate any subharmonic. The combined irregular and subharmonic effects decrease the HNR. Local mass changes affected the SP_m wave more than local stiffness changes (which randomized the trajectory to a small extent but dampened the 1/2 subharmonic).

To determine whether the random components were due to the asymmetry of the model, local mass changes were made to both folds. The resulting SP_m and flow waves (not presented, but similar to Fig. 15) showed the irregular behavior was still present again indicating that asymmetry is unimportant. The irregular jitter was even more apparent than in Fig. 15. HNR was 0.38 dB, indicating a very poor harmonic structure. This simulation of symmetrical mass

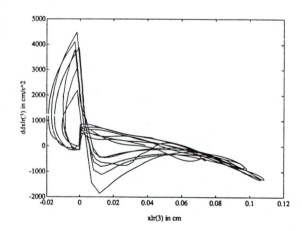

FIG. 16. Energy exchange plot for right fold, local mass changes (elements 2 and 3), $T_{\text{act}} = 25$.

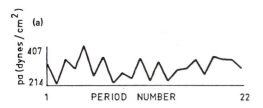

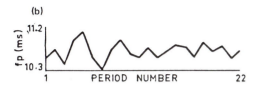

FIG. 17. Plots of (a) pa for local mass change; (b) fp for local mass change; $T_{act} = 25$.

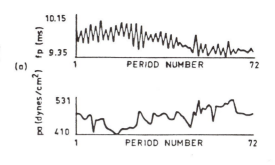

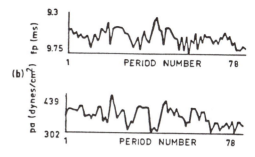

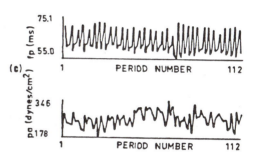

FIG. 18. Plots of pa and fp for: (a) a 63-y-old male with chronic laryngitis (b) a 62-y-old male with T1 glottic cancer (c) a 65-y-old male with T1 glottic cancer.

changes might be analogous to vocal nodules, polyps, or bilateral cancer, in which both folds are affected at the same location.

The asymmetric mass changes were an attempt to model cancer, which can be local and can invade both the surface and the muscle layers.

VI. COMPARISONS WITH OTHER DATA

The model has demonstrated interesting perturbation phenomena, but the appearance of this phenomena in real pathological speech is necessary to validate the model. In this section we present patient data showing subharmonics and random perturbations. Three cases from a database of pathologies at Vancouver General Hospital were analyzed using the HNR, pa, and fp plots. The pa and fp plots are presented in Fig. 18, and the HNR values can be found in Table I.

The first case is a 63-y-old male suffering from chronic laryngitis. The vocal folds were described as weak and flaccid. Figure 18(a) shows the fp and pa plots for this case. The fp plot shows a 1/2 subharmonic with a frequency range of 98 to 107 Hz, and HNR = 4.5 dB, indicating severe hoarseness.

The second case, a 62-y-old male, has T1 glottic cancer. The fp and pa plots [Fig. 18(b)] are almost completely random, with a frequency range from 107 to 114 Hz. HNR = 12.0 dB, again within the range for pathologies.

The third case is a 65-yr-old male also with T1 glottic cancer. The fp plot [Fig. 18(c)] reveals a strong 1/3 subharmonic structure, ranging from 132 to 181 Hz. The pa plot shows a random shimmer effect. HNR = 5.5 dB, also indicating severe hoarseness.

Each patient illustrates one of the phenonena observed in the simulations, although the effects appear to be even more pronounced in this data set than in the simulations.

Frequency versus period number plots produced by Monsen (1981), in a study of the vocal function of hoarse voices, also demonstrated these phemomena. For dry hoarse voice a 1/2 subharmonic appeared, while for harsh hoarse voice a random component modulated the subharmonic, paralleling the phenomena observed in our simulations.

VII. SUMMARY

A hybrid lumped element model based upon the Ishizaka and Flanagan (1972) and Titze (1973) models has been established and used to investigate perturbed oscillations resulting from changes in biomechanical parameters.

Phase and energy exchange plots have been presented to demonstrate oscillatory stability. Displacement and time dependence of the interchange of energy between the glottal flow and the tissue was demonstrated. The plots relate driving forces such as the Bernoulli effect and vocal fold convergence and divergence to the displacement of the tissue.

Fundamental period (fp) and peak amplitude (pa) plots, which are time-dependent end point jitter and shimmer measures, and the harmonics-to-noise ratio metric (an energy measurement) were used to quantify the perturbation in the speech signal. The fp and pa plots only measure the changes that occur at the end of each period, while the HNR is a cumulative measure for the entire signal.

Stiffness and mass were altered separately in order to isolate their effects. The results have been compared to pathologies such as laryngeal paralysis, vocal nodules, and cancer. Isolated parameter changes have been made for two reasons. First, very little is known about the biomechanical parameters to be used in simulating pathologies. Second, more information may be gained by separating the effects of mass and stiffness than by simulating a combination of changes that are poorly understood. In interpreting the results of this study, one should not assume, for example, that cancer can be modeled by local mass changes alone. Our results merely indicate that mass changes such as these are contributing factors.

Significant features shown in these simulations are:

(1) A low value of constant longitudinal tension is necessary for any perturbations to occur, indicating that large values inhibit or dampen the perturbation. Decreasing longitudinal tension causes the damping factor calculated in Appendix A to decrease, probably permitting harmonics other than the fundamental to arise.

(2) Subharmonics of order 1/2 occur for a small value of longitudinal tension in both folds even when the lateral stiffnesses and masses are normal, indicating that asymmetry is not necessary.

(3) Unilateral stiffness increases enhanced the subharmonic.

(4) Unilateral mass increases inhibited the subharmonic.

(5) Local stiffness increases introduced an irregular component but dampened the subharmonic.

(6) Local mass increases produced a large irregular component. The observed randomness may be indicative of chaos.

(7) Bilateral localized mass increases also resulted in a large irregular component.

(8) HNR values are higher than those obtained by Kojima et al. (1980) and Yumoto et al. (1982) because turbulent flow and neurological jitter were not modeled in these simulations, and, most importantly, the period estimation process has been refined to reduce erroneous jitter.

(9) HNR values are much lower for local mass changes than for all other cases due to the random modulation.

A patient database of pathologies demonstrated regular subharmonics and irregular random perturbations (which appear to be a combination of subharmonic and random effects). The model was able to reproduce the effects observed in the patient data, but it is not known if the magnitude of the parameter changes are closely related to physiology. The parameter changes chosen in these experiments (and the resulting phenomena) may not be the only factors affecting perturbed oscillation, but these results indicate that they are possibly significant contributors.

APPENDIX A: TISSUE FORCES

The lateral spring forces are described by the IF model as

$$F_{kl}(i) = k_l(i)\{[x_l(i) - x_{l0}(i)] + \eta_l [x_l(i) - x_{l0}(i)]^3\}. \quad (A1)$$

The l subscript can be replaced by u or c to represent the lateral upper force or the coupling force between the upper and lower masses. The initial displacements are x_{l0} and x_{u0}.

Additional forces during a collision are:

$$F_{lcol}(i) = h_l(i)\{[x_l(i) - x_{lcol}(i)] + \eta_{lcol}[x_l(i) - x_{lcol}(i)]^3\}, \quad (A2)$$

where (1) $x_{lcol}(i)$ and $x_{ucol}(i)$ are the displacements from the midpoint at the instant the surfaces enter a collision; (2) h_l, h_u, η_{lcol}, and η_{ucol} are the stiffness coefficients during collisions.

Only the lateral components of the longitudinal tensor forces are used. These forces depend on the relative positions of adjacent masses. The equations presented here are derived from the T73 model.

Given local tension values $T_l(i)$ and $T_l(i + 1)$ on either side of the ith lower mass, the lateral components of the restoring forces are proportional to the sine of the angle created between adjacent masses. Thus

$$F_{tla}(i) = T_l(i)\{[x_l(i-1) - x_l(i)]/r_l(i)\}, \quad (A3)$$
$$F_{tlp}(i) = T_l(i)\{[x_l(i+1) - x_l(i)]/r_l(i+1)\},$$

where $r_l(i)$ is the distance between the centroids of the masses. Subscripts a and p indicate anterior (front of the throat) and posterior (back of the throat) positions.

The longitudinal tensors T_u and T_l are due to nonlinear local strain, and $T_u(i)$ is a nonlinear function of the relative strain between adjacent upper masses. From the T73 model:

$$T_u(i) = \pm g\tau_u \, \text{th}_u(i)\text{dep}_u(i)\cdot\ln[1 - |S_u(i)|/S_{umax}], \quad (A4)$$

where $T_u(i)$ is the tension in dyn, S_{umax} is the maximum permissible strain, τ_u is a stress constant in g/cm^2, $S_u(i)$ is the local strain, g is the acceleration due to gravity in cm/s^2 and $\text{th}_u(i)\cdot\text{dep}_u(i)$ is the cross-sectional area in cm^2 through which the tensile force acts. The $\pm$ sign indicates expansion or compression. When S_u is positive, the negative sign is used to make T positive since the logarithm will always be negative. Conversely, when S_u is negative, the positive sign is used.

Here, $T_l(i)$ includes the passive elastic effects of the ligament lig, and the vocalis muscle, combined with an active tension T_{act}. The tension T_{act} can be thought of as the stress due to vocalis muscle contraction, varying from 0 to 1000 g/cm^2. For steady phonation, T_{act} is constant. T_l is then

$$T_l(i) = \pm g\tau_{lig}\text{th}_{lig}(i)\text{dep}_{lig}(i)$$
$$\cdot\ln(1 - |S_l(i)|/S_{ligmax}) + g\,\text{th}_l(i)\text{dep}_l(i)T_{act}$$
$$\pm g\tau_l\,\text{th}_l(i)\text{dep}_l(i)\cdot\ln(1 - |S_l(i)|/S_{lmax}).$$

The strains are calculated in the following manner from $r(i)$:

$$r_l(i) = \sqrt{[x_l(i-1) - x_l(i)]^2 + w^2}, \quad (A5)$$
$$S_l(i) = [r_l(i) - r_{l0}(i)]/r_{l0}(i),$$

$r_{l0}(i)$ is the pre-phonatory nearest-neighbor distance.

The damping coefficients are calculated from the T73 model in terms of a dimensionless ratio ρ such that $d = 2\rho\sqrt{km}$. With this definition, the localized lower mass damping factor is

$$d_l(i) = 2\rho_l(i)\sqrt{m_l(i)[k_l(i) + k_c(i) + |T_l(i)|]/r_l(i) + |T_l(i+1)|/r_l(i+1)}, \qquad \text{(A6)}$$

where T_l/r_l is the equivalent lateral spring stiffness due to longitudinal tension, k_l and k_c are the linear components of the lateral stiffness constants, and ρ_l is the damping factor for the vocalis muscle. The force due to damping is then

$$F_{dl}(i) = -d_l(i)\dot{x}_l(i), \qquad \text{(A7)}$$

where $\dot{x}_l(i)$ is the lateral tissue velocity.

The external forces arise due to air flow from the lungs. The pressures on the medial surfaces can be estimated using fluid mechanics (Ishizaka and Matsudaira, 1972). These pressures change during contraction and expansion of the glottal constriction and the regions just upstream and downstream. The resulting pressure profile is thus:

$$P_s - P_{11}(i) = R_c(i)U_g(i),$$

$$P_{11}(i) - P_{12}(i) = R_l(i)U_g(i) + L_l(i)\frac{dU_g(i)}{dt},$$

$$P_{12}(i) - P_{21}(i) = R_t(i)U_g(i),$$

$$P_{21}(i) - P_{22}(i) = R_u(i)U_g(i) + L_u(i)\frac{dU_g(i)}{dt},$$

$$P_{22}(i) - P_0 = R_e(i)U_g(i), \qquad \text{(A8)}$$

where the pressure points are shown in Fig. 1. The impedances are as defined by Ishizaka and Matsudaira (1972). Here, R_c is the impedance causing the pressure drop due to the rapid contraction of the glottis, and subsequent formation of a vena contracta; R_l and R_u are impedances representing the viscous friction of the walls; R_t is the impedance representing the pressure discontinuity in moving from the lower to the upper surfaces; and R_e represents the pressure recovery as the flow leaves the glottis and enters the larger vocal tract chamber. Also, R_e, R_t, and R_c are flow-dependent resistances; L_l and L_u are inductive impedances representing the inertia of the air mass; and U_g is the flow.

The external forces can then be calculated (when the glottis is open) as

$$F_{el}(i) = w\{[P_{11}(i) + P_{12}(i)]/2\}\text{th}_l(i),$$

$$F_{eu}(i) = w\{[P_{21}(i) + P_{22}(i)]/2\}\text{th}_u(i), \qquad \text{(A9)}$$

where $\text{th}_l(i)$ and $\text{th}_u(i)$ are the vertical thicknesses of the masses (in the direction of the flow). When closure occurs, there is no flow. There are, however, aerodynamic forces generated during collision in addition to F_{col}. These arise due to the transglottal pressure. The subglottal and post-glottal pressures are present regardless of closure, building up when the glottis is closed and helping to force the masses apart. Thus, for different closure conditions alternative equations for F_{el} and F_{eu} are:

(i) when only the upper medial edge is sealed,

$$F_{eu}(i) = w[(P_s + P_0)/2]\text{th}_u(i),$$

$$F_{el}(i) = wP_s\,\text{th}_l(i); \qquad \text{(A10)}$$

(ii) when only the lower surface is closed,

$$F_{eu}(i) = wP_0\,\text{th}_u(i),$$

$$F_{el}(i) = w[(P_s + P_0)/2]\text{th}_l(i); \qquad \text{(A11)}$$

(iii) when both surfaces are closed,

$$F_{eu}(i) = w\frac{P_s + P_0}{2}\left(\frac{\text{th}_u(i)}{\text{th}_l(i) + \text{th}_u(i)}\right)\text{th}_u(i),$$

$$F_{el}(i) = w\frac{P_s + P_0}{2}\left(\frac{\text{th}_l(i)}{\text{th}_l(i) + \text{th}_u(i)}\right)\text{th}_l(i), \qquad \text{(A12)}$$

where P_0 is the pressure just above the glottis. Note that in most of our simulations we used $(P_s - P_0)/2$ rather than $(P_s + P_0)/2$ as this was used by Titze (1973). Subsequent corrected simulations have indicated little difference in the results.

APPENDIX B: VALUES FOR THE NORMAL VOCAL FOLD

The following parameters represent the normal vocal cord and apply to both left and right cords.

(1) Mass—as in Ishizaka and Flannagan's models, i.e., $m_l(i) = 0.025$ g and $m_u(i) = 0.005$ g for $i = 1$ to 5.

(2) Lung pressure P_L, from Hirano (1977) is 10 kdyn/cm^2.

(3) Dimensions—the longitudinal length, vertical depth, and lateral thickness are taken from Titze (1973) to be

$$w = 0.28 \text{ cm}, \quad \text{dep}_l(i) = 0.25 \text{ cm},$$

$$\text{dep}_u(i) = 0.1 \text{ cm}, \quad \text{dep}_{\text{lig}}(i) = 0.1 \text{ cm},$$

$$\text{th}_l(i) = 0.25 \text{ cm}, \quad \text{th}_u(i) = 0.05 \text{ cm},$$

$$\text{th}_{\text{lig}}(i) = 0.1 \text{ cm}.$$

The dep dimension is the depth of the mass. The ligament is included in the tension equation for the lower portion. The equations can be found in Appendix A.

(4) Lateral stiffness—values have been determined by trial and error to be $k_l(i) = 5$ kdyn/cm and $k_u(i) = 0.5$ kdyn/cm. These parameters permit the maximum lateral excursion of the mucosal and vocalis masses to be approximately ± 0.12 cm without collision, and the glottal flow to be between 300 and 500 cm^3/s, which is typical for healthy folds (Hirano, 1981). $k_c(i) = 3.5$ kdyn/cm gives a phase lage of 60° between the upper and lower masses. This agrees with Baer (1975) who estimates a 1-m/s vertical traveling wave velocity and a 60° lag for a glottis of similar dimensions.

(5) Nonlinear lateral coefficients are

$$\eta_l,\eta_c,\eta_u = 100 \text{ cm}^{-2}, \quad h_l = 3k_l = 15 \text{ kdyn/cm},$$

$$h_u = 3k_u = 1.5 \text{ kdyn/cm}, \quad \eta_{l\text{col}},\eta_{u\text{col}} = 500 \text{ cm}^{-2}.$$

These values are based upon measurements by Ishizaka and Kaneko (1968) of static stress–strain measurements for an excised human larynx.

(6) Longitudinal stiffness—stress constants and maximum strains have been estimated by Hirano using canine tissue, and assumed to be the same for humans. The equations relating these values to the tensions can be found in Appendix A: $\tau_u = \tau_{\text{lig}} = 800$, $\tau_l = 300$, $S_{u\text{max}} = 0.3$, $S_{\text{ligmax}} = 0.4$, $S_{l\text{max}} = 0.8$, $T_{\text{act}} = 150$ g/cm^2. These values differ from Titze's discrete model, but the vibratory patterns

agree with the IF model. Here, T_{act} values between 25 and 200 g/cm^2 rather than the 500 g/cm^2 proposed by Titze were used since collision was not achieved using the greater value.

(7) Damping—ρ_l and ρ_u have been experimentally estimated by Kaneko and Ishizaka (1968) to be of the order of 0.1 and 0.6, respectively, when not in collision, and 1.1 and 1.6 during collision (representing deformation of the tissue).

(8) Initial configuration—the pre-phonatory position of the masses is controlled by muscular adjustment. Typical initial glottal cross sectional areas are 0.05 cm^2 for both the upper and lower margins. An oval constriction shape is used with the following initial displacement values:

$$x_{l0}(1), x_{l0}(5) = 0.012 \text{ cm},$$
$$x_{l0}(2), x_{l0}(3), x_{l0}(4) = 0.021 \text{ cm}. \tag{B13}$$

Baer, T. (**1975**). "Investigation of phonation using excised larynges," unpublished Ph.D. thesis, MIT, Cambridge, MA.

Cox, N., Morrison, M.D., and Ito, M. R. (**1986**). "Optimising pitch period markers prior to extracting features from isolated vowels," ICA12, Toronto, 1986.

Fant, G. (**1960**). *Acoustic Theory of Speech Production* (Mouton, S-Gravehenge, The Netherlands).

Flanagan, J. L. (**1960**). *Speech Analysis, Synthesis, and Perception* (Springer-Verlag, New York).

Gerratt, B. R., and Hanson, D. G. (**1985**). "Glottographic measures of laryngeal function in individuals with abnormal motor control," paper presented at the Fourth International Conference on Vocal Fold Physiology, June 1985.

Hirano, M. (**1977**). "Structure and vibratory behaviour of the vocal folds," in *Dynamic Aspects of Speech Production,* edited by M. Sawashima and F. S. Cooper (University of Tokyo Press, Tokyo), pp. 13–27.

Hirano, M. (**1979**). "Biomechanical parameters of the vocal folds in normal and pathological states," in Proc. Conf. on the Assessment of Vocal Pathology, ASHA Reports 11, American Speech–Language–Hearing Association, Maryland, pp. 11–30.

Hirano, M. (**1981**). *Clinical Examination of the Voice* (Springer-Verlag, Vienna).

Ishizaka, K. (**1980**). "Equivalent lumped mass models of vocal fold vibration," in *Vocal Fold Physiology*, edited by K. N. Stevens and M. Hirano (University of Tokyo Press, Tokyo), pp. 231–244.

Ishizaka, K., and Flanagan, J. L. (**1972**). "Synthesis of voiced sounds from a two mass model of the vocal cords," Bell Sys. Tech. J. **51**, 1233–1268.

Ishizaka, K., and Matsudaira, M. (**1972**). "Fluid Mechanical Consideration of Vocal Cord Vibration," SCRL Monograph 8, Santa Barbara, CA.

Ishizaka K., Matsudaira, M., and Kaneko, T. (**1976**). "Input acoustic-impedance measurement of the subglottal system," J. Acoust. Soc. Am. **60**, 190–197.

Isshiki, N., and Ishizaka, K. (**1976**). "Computer simulation of pathological vocal cord vibration," J. Acoust. Soc. Am. **60**, 1193–1198.

Kaneko, T., and Ishizaka, K. (**1968**). "On equivalent mechanical constants of the vocal cords," J. Acoust. Soc. Jpn. **24**, 312–313.

Kojima, H., Gould, W. J., Lambiase, A., and Isshiki, N. (**1980**). "Computer analysis of hoarseness," Acta Otolaryngolog. **89**, 547–554.

Koike, Y. (**1980**). "Sub and supraglottal pressure variation during phonation," in *Vocal Fold Physiology*, edited by K. N. Stevens and M. Hirano (University of Tokyo Press, Tokyo), pp. 181–188.

Minorsky, N. (**1962**). *Nonlinear Oscillations* (Van Nostrand, Princeton, NJ).

Monsen, R. B. (**1981**). "The use of a reflectionless tube to assess vocal function," Proc. Conf. on the Assessment of Vocal Pathology, ASHA Reports 11, American Speech–Language–Hearing Association, Maryland, pp. 141–150.

Tanabe, M. (**1972**). "Vibratory pattern of the vocal cord in unilateral paralysis of the cricothyroid muscle," Acta Otolaryngolog. (Stockholm) **74**, 339–345.

Titze, I. R. (**1973**). "The human vocal cords: a mathematical model, Part 1," Phonetica **28**, 129–170.

Titze, I. R. (**1980**). "Comments on the myoelastic-aerodynamic theory of phonation," J. Speech Hear. Res. **23**, 495–510.

Titze, I. R. (**1985**). "Mechanisms of sustained oscillation of the vocal folds," in *Vocal Fold Physiology*, edited by I. R. Titze and R. C. Scherer (Denver Center for the Performing Arts, Denver), pp. 349–357.

Titze, I. R. (**1988**). "The physics of small amplitude oscillation of the vocal folds," J. Acoust. Soc. Am. **83**, 1536–1552.

Yumoto, H., Gould, W. J., and Baer, T. (**1982**). "Harmonics to noise ratio as an index of the degree of hoarseness," J. Acoust. Soc. Am. **71**, 1544–1550.

Volume 145, number 8,9   PHYSICS LETTERS A   30 April 1990

418

Bifurcations and Chaos in Newborn Infant Cries

W. Mende

Department of Mathematics and Cybernetics, Academy of Sciences, Berlin, GDR

H. Herzel

Department of Physics, Humboldt University of Berlin, Berlin, GDR

and

K. Wermke

University Hospital, Department of General Biology, Humboldt University of Berlin, Berlin, GDR

Received 4 September 1989; revised manuscript received 22 February 1990; accepted for publication March 1990
Communicated by A.P. Fordy

Several cries of newborn infants are analyzed using computer spectrograms and methods from nonlinear dynamics. A rich variety of bifurcations (e.g. period doubling) and episodes of irregular behavior are observed. Poincaré sections and the analysis of the underlying attractor suggest that these noise-like episodes are low-dimensional deterministic chaos. Possible implications for the very early diagnosis of brain disorders are discussed.

Speech production is a rather complicated process conditioned by nearly periodic oscillations of the vocal cords which excite resonances in the vocal tract. Moreover, there are certain feedback mechanisms to the central nervous system controlling phonation and articulation. In spite of intense investigations [1,2] many questions are still open. From a physical point of view certain features of speech production are related to the problem of turbulence which is one of the most difficult areas of modern science. However, in the last decade much progress has been made in this field which is intimately related to the term "deterministic chaos" [3]. Recently, typical bifurcation scenarios to turbulence were discovered [4] (e.g. period doubling) and powerful new methods of time series analysis are now available [5,6].

In this paper these ideas are applied to newborn cries as a specific kind of phonation. It was pointed out earlier [7,8] that cries are closely connected with regu-

lating mechanisms of the brain and may serve, therefore, as an indicator of certain cerebral dysfunctions.

Up to now cries of 70 infants were analyzed at the age of 1–5 days. In some cases the analyses were extended beyond the first week. About one third of the infants had peri- and post-natal complications. In the framework of cry diagnosis a high-accuracy pitch determination method was implemented. Especially, indicators which measure fine and fast pitch modulation (microvariability) were proven to be suitable for early detection of certain CNS disorders [9].

With the aid of high-resolution spectrograms diverse bifurcation and episode-like noise behaviour have been observed in a great number of cries. In the following we argue that these irregular segments are manifestations of low-dimensional deterministic chaos.

The signals are recorded on tape, filtered with a 4 kHz Butterworth low-pass filter — to avoid aliasing — and then digitized with a sampling rate of 25 kHz and

419   Volume 145, number 8,9   PHYSICS LETTERS A   30 April 1990

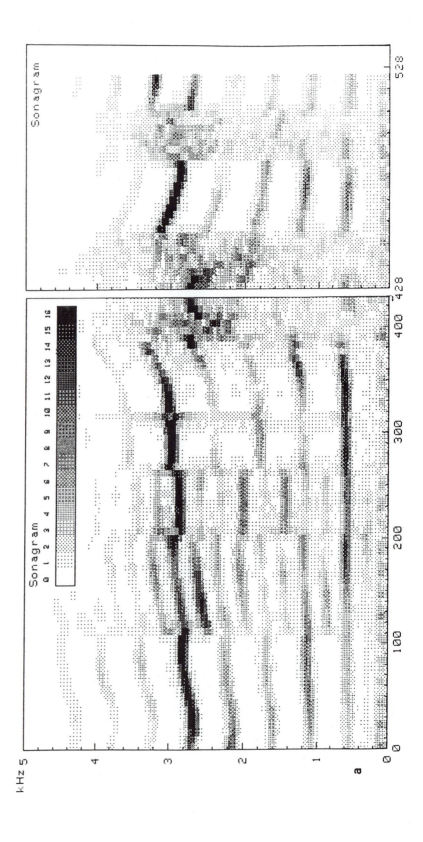

Volume 145, number 8,9   PHYSICS LETTERS A   30 April 1990

420

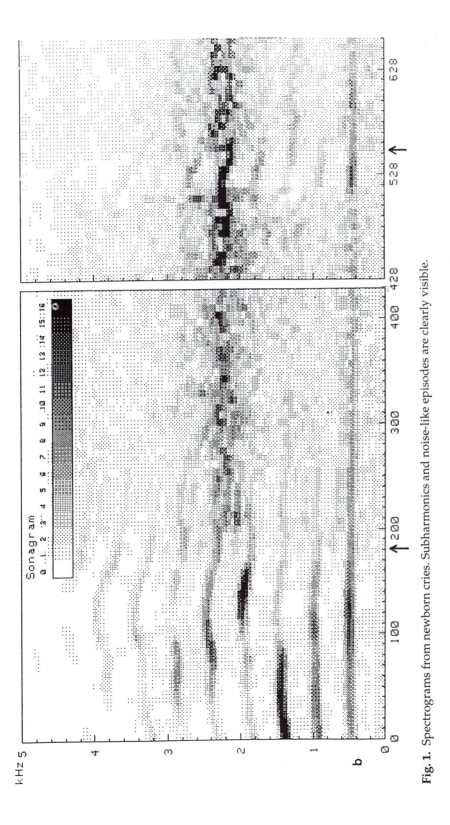

Fig. 1. Spectrograms from newborn cries. Subharmonics and noise-like episodes are clearly visible.

421   Volume 145, number 8,9   PHYSICS LETTERS A   30 April 1990

with 12 bit resolution. In contrast to well controlled hydrodynamic [10] or acoustic [11] experiments, cries are unstationary processes. Therefore, any statistical analysis should be restricted to appropriate segments of 10–20 ms which are assumed to be relatively stationary. However, the instationarity has also an advantage: due to slowly varying parameters many qualitative changes ("bifurcations") become observable during a single cry (see fig. 1). In order to visualize the evolution of the spectral density during a cry, so-called spectrograms (termed also sonagrams) are appropriate. They are based on hundreds of subsequent short-time power spectra of overlapping segments of the whole sample. We have chosen Hamming windowed segments of 512 data points and a shift of 170 points. In this way a good compromise between spectral and time resolution is obtained. The spectral amplitude encoded as a four-bit grey scale is plotted as a function of time and frequency.

Fig. 1 shows two representative spectrograms displaying a rich bifurcation structure. The first one is from a premature infant (28 weeks) with respiratory complications. The cry was recorded two weeks after birth. The second spectrogram is obtained from a term born healthy infant four days after birth.

At the beginning of each spectrogram only the fundamental frequency of about 500 Hz is present together with its pronounced harmonics. Then remarkably sharp transitions to more complicated states are visible. At first subharmonics and later on noise-like broad-band regions appear. A subharmonic at one half of the fundamental frequency corresponds to period-doubling in the time domain. In our spectrograms such subharmonic bifurcations often turn out to be precursors of noisy segments. In another spectrogram which is not shown here three successive period triplings have been identified ahead of a noise-like region [8]. The main features of our spectrograms amazingly resemble bifurcation diagrams from acoustic-cavitation experiments [11]. In that case the complex bifurcations and noise-like regions are well described by a low-dimensional model exhibiting deterministic chaos.

Moreover, we find abrupt transitions which are very reminiscent to alternating sequences of periodic and chaotic states in the Belousov-Zhabotinsky reaction [12]. For example at the end of the first spectrogram a nonperiodic episode is seen which is not accompanied by subharmonics. Around 500 ms we find a noise-like region in between two distinct periodic states. On the left side of the broad band region we have in the time domain five-peak oscillations, i.e. during a fundamental period five maxima occur, and on the right side six-peak oscillations are recorded. Thus we conjecture that the irregular segments of infant cries are manifes-

tations of low-dimensional deterministic chaos. Below, further indications are presented which support this conjecture.

For this purpose the cry in fig. 1b which exhibits long noisy episodes is analyzed in the time domain. Fig. 2 shows characteristics segments of the sound signal. In order to give evidence that the non-periodicity is not random noise but deterministic chaos, we will apply recently developed methods of time-series analysis.

It is instructive to visualize the dynamics in an abstract m-dimensional phase space spanned by delay-coordinates. Thus, instead of a single measurement $x(t)$ the vector

$$x(t) \equiv \{x(t), x(t+\tau), \ldots, x(t+(m-1)\tau)\} \tag{1}$$

is considered. In this way one state of the system becomes a point in the phase space and a time-series defines a curve, the trajectory. As time progresses, trajectories of a dissipative system reach a state of a permanent regime, the attractor. Deterministic chaos is related to "strange attractors" with a non-integer (fractal) dimension. In contrast to this, a random signal corresponds to an unstructured cloud in the phase space. The detection of an attractor is therefore a widely used method to distinguish deterministic chaos from random fluctuations. Rather than analyzing the attractor in the phase space, it is easier to study next-amplitude maps or Poincaré sections. In fig. 3a, a plot of consecutive maxima of the time-series in fig. 2 is presented. The data appear to fall approximately on a curve, indicating that the system is deterministic. Another possibility to derive discrete maps from the data is to use Poincaré sections [3]. Fig. 3b shows a Poincaré map determined by the intersection of trajectories with the plane $x(t) = x(t+\tau)$. Again some nearly one-dimensional structure is evident.

The estimation of the attractor dimension allows chaos to be identified more quantitatively. For this purpose, the numbers $N(r, m)$ of pairs (x_i, x_j) with a distance less than r are investigated. For sufficiently high embedding dimensions m and proper distances r, one can hope to find the scaling law

$$N(r, m) \sim r^{D_2} \tag{2}$$

for attractors. Here D_2 denotes the correlation dimension (for a mathematical justification and technical details see ref. [6]). Along these lines, the dimension D_2 can be determined from log–log plots of $N(r, m)$ versus r. It is convenient to display the slopes of these plots as well (see fig. 4b). If there is a range of r with a reasonable constant slope (a plateau in fig. 4b), this cor-

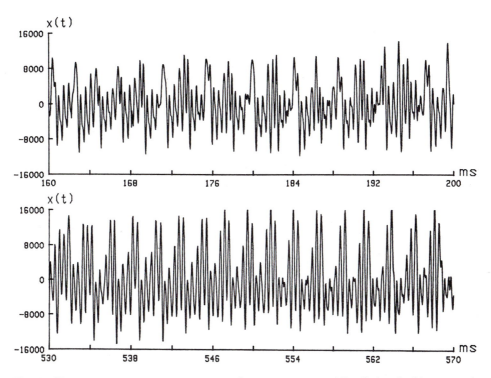

Fig. 2. Characteristic time-series corresponding to segments of fig. 1b (marked by arrows). Below a transition from five-peak oscillations to a non-periodic state is shown.

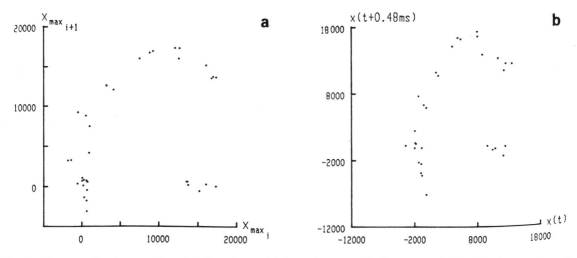

Fig. 3. Next-amplitude map (a) and Poincaré map (b) from the nonperiodic segment behind the five-peak oscillations in fig. 2.

respond to self-similarity. A saturation of the slope with increasing embedding dimension m is a sign of a low-dimensional attractor since random signals lead typically to a permanent increase of the slope.

Fig. 4 displays the results for the first 16 ms of fig. 2. It can be regarded as additional indication of chaos due

to the saturation of the slope with increasing embedding dimension which suggests a correlation dimension around three.

Another approach for the estimation of attractor dimensions is based on nearest neighbour statistics: If $r_k(x_i)$ denotes the distance between point x_i and its kth

423   Volume 145, number 8,9   PHYSICS LETTERS A   30 April 1990

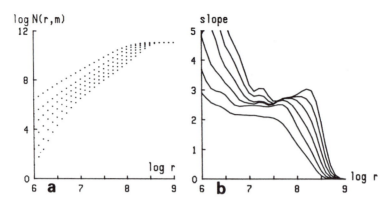

Fig. 4. Number of interpoint distances $N(r, m)$ versus r (a) and the slopes of the log–log plot (b). The curves correspond, from bottom to top, to embedding dimensions $m = 3, 4, ..., 8$.

nearest neighbour, then the average distance depends on k as follows [13]:

$$\langle r_k \rangle \sim G(k, D)k^{1/D}, \qquad (3)$$

with

$$G(k,D) = k^{-1/D} \frac{\Gamma(k+1/D)}{\Gamma(k)}.$$

The prefactor $G(k, D)$ is close to unity and, therefore, a first guess for D is obtained by setting $G(k, D) = 1$, and computing the slope of a log–log plot k versus $\langle r_k \rangle$. The resulting first estimate of D can be improved iteratively [14]. The curves in fig. 5 indicate that for $k > 10$ a power-law holds approximately with $D = 3$ (dashed line). This result is consistent with our previous estimation using interpoint distances (see fig. 4).

At this point some remarks about the validity and accuracy of our analysis are necessary. Due to the limited stationarity, only segments of about 500 data points are studied and, therefore, all quantitative results should be considered with circumspection. However, tests with other chaotic systems support the assumption that such short records could yield reliable results [15].

In conclusion, we emphasize that the spectrograms, the discrete maps and the dimension analysis suggest consistently that the analyzed cries are manifestations of low-dimensional deterministic chaos. This low dimensionality has to be well distinguished from high-dimensional turbulent noise in connection with fricative processes which can be considered as developed turbulence [2]. Our results suggest that in speech production beside limit cycles (vocals are typically periodic signals) and developed turbulence (fricatives)

also low-dimensional chaos plays an essential role. Thus, already several years ago irregularities of voiced speech were reported [16].

Our observations of complex bifurcations and chaos give some hints for modelling certain aspects of the sound production of the vocal system. Most of the described effects have been found also in low-dimensional nonlinear models in other fields (see e.g. ref. [11]). Already a preliminary vocalization model which includes the usually neglected feedback from the vocal tract to the glottis, exhibits indeed certain features of the observed records. Such a model will be the subject matter of a forthcoming paper.

Subharmonics and chaotic episodes have been found in cries of healthy infants as well as in infants with several perinatal complications [8,18]. However, the frequency of occurrence and the duration of chaotic episodes could have diagnostic relevance. In these early stages of development of phonation abnormalities could indicate that the underlying cerebral control mechanisms are disturbed or not yet completely ma-

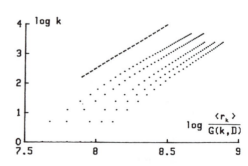

Fig. 5. Nearest neighbour statistics (see eq. (3)) for the same data as in fig. 4. The slopes give estimates of the attractor dimension (dashed line: $D = 3$).

tured. This conjecture is consistent with our experience that chaos appears less frequently with increasing age of children. Perhaps one can even conclude that older speakers learn to control those phenomena. However, vocalizations of adults with certain laryngeal pathologies are again characterized by enhanced frequencies of subharmonic components [19].

Because of the suitability of phonation for the detection of cerebral dysfunctions, further investigations in this field may help to provide diagnostic tools for the early recognition of brain disorders. Moreover, the discovered low-dimensional chaos provides perhaps a new approach to the understanding of some aspects of speech production.

We would like to thank K. Wilzopolski for assistance in signal analysis.

REFERENCES

[1] G. Fant, Acoustic theory of speech production (Mouton, The Hague, 1960).

[2] W.N. Sorokin, The theory of speech production (Radio and Communication, Moscow, 1985) [in Russian].

[3] J.P. Eckmann and D. Ruelle, Rev. Mod. Phys. 57 (1985) 617.

[4] J.P. Eckmann, Rev. Mod. Phys. 53 (1981) 643.

[5] A.V. Holden, ed., Chaos (Manchester Univ. Press, Manchester, 1986);
G. Mayer-Kress, ed., Dimensions and entropies in chaotic systems (Springer, Berlin, 1986);
D.S. Broomhead and R. Jones, Proc. R. Soc. A 423 (1989) 103.

[6] P. Grassberger and I. Procaccia, Physica D 9 (1983) 189.

[7] J. Lind, Newborn infant cry (Almquist and Wiksells Boktrycken, Uppsala, 1965).

[8] K. Wermke, Thesis, Humboldt University of Berlin (1987).

[9] W. Mende, K. Wermke, S. Schindler, K. Wilzopolski and S. Hoeck, submitted to Early Child Dev. Care.

[10] A. Brandstater and H.L. Swinney, Phys. Rev. A 35 (1987) 2207.

[11] W. Lauterborn, in: Frontiers in physical acoustics (Soc. Italiana di Fisica, Bologna, 1986);
W. Lauterborn and J. Holzfuss, Phys. Lett. A 115 (1986) 369.

[12] J.L. Hudson, M. Hart and D. Marinko, J. Chem. Phys. 71 (1979) 1601.

[13] K.W. Pettis, T.A. Bailey, A.K. Jain and R.C. Dubes, IEEE Trans. PAMI-1 (1979) 25.

[14] W. van der Water and P. Schram, Phys. Rev. A 37 (1988) 3118.

[15] N.B. Abraham, A.M. Albano, B. Das, G. de Guzman, S. Yong, R.S. Gioggia, G.P. Puccioni and J.R. Tredicce, Phys. Lett. A 114 (1986) 217;
J. Kurths and H. Herzel, Physica D 25 (1987) 165.

[16] L. Dolansky and P. Terlund, IEEE Trans. AU-16 (1968) 51;
R.B. Monsen and A.M. Engebretson, J. Acoust. Soc. Am. 62 (1977) 981.

[17] H. Herzel, W. Mende and K. Wermke, in preparation.

[18] K. Michelsson and O. Wasz-Hoeckert, in: Infant communication: cry and early speech (College Hill Press, Houston, 1980).

[19] A.W. Kelman, M.T. Gordon, F.M. Morton and T.C. Simpson, Folia Phoniatr. 33 (1981) 51.

CHAPTER 4

*Evidence of Chaos in
Vocal Fold Vibration*

INGO R. TITZE, Ph.D.
R. J. BAKEN, Ph.D.
HANSPETER HERZEL, Ph.D.

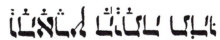

— And the earth was chaos and void.
Genesis I

The classical view of the natural world — which has strongly biased our perceptions of how things are and how they are supposed to behave — inclines us to categorize physical phenomena into two broad classes. Some processes are apparently regular, predictable, and (at least in some metaphorical sense) smooth. Others, however, are described as unstable, erratic, unpredictable, or random. Much of what we understand of nature concerns regular, "lawful" events, simply because they are amenable to relatively easy description and to classical modeling. Many important phenomena fall into the unstable/erratic class, however (fluid turbulence is a prime example). They have proven to be highly refractory, primarily due to the lack of an adequate conceptual base for structuring their investigation. Often they have been regarded simply as "noise." Thus we have had an overly simplistic dichotomy between predictability (determinism) and unpredictability (randomness).

143

Another view of the physical world has its origins in the seminal papers on topology by Poincaré (1881, 1882, 1885). The ability to simulate natural processes (with powerful digital computers) has resulted in the discovery that systems governed by simple mathematical laws can behave in a highly irregular (unpredictable) fashion. Although the response of such systems is *determined* entirely by internal properties and initial conditions, *predictability* over the long range is limited. The behavior can appear chaotic. Analysis of systems of this type has fallen under the rubric of nonlinear dynamics. It uses geometric methods to move beyond simple time-course descriptions of a phenomenon, sketching a portrait of the system's overall dynamic properties. The portrait can in turn be dissected to reveal crucial bases of the system's behavior. We begin with some observations that relate to vocal fold vibration.

CHAOS, FRACTALS, AND VOCAL FOLD VIBRATION

In vocal fold vibration, the displacement of isolated fleshpoints reveals a complex pattern of motion that varies from locus to locus (Baer, 1981a, b). Such motion can be simulated by computer (Titze and Alipour, in review). In Figure 4-1, trajectories of "fleshpoints" of a finite element simulation of vocal fold movement are shown (right side). There is an orderliness in the fleshpoint movements. After a start-up transient, the orbits are primarily elliptical. In Figure 4-2, however, the trajectories are very disorderly, covering virtually every conceivable position. Not much has been changed in the model to go from one condition to the other. Only the Young's modulus of the cover has been reduced.

Tools of analysis of nonlinear dynamics may allow us to summarize many of the dynamic properties of the vocal folds in pictures that are comprehensible at a glance. Before proceeding with further analysis of vocal fold vibration, however, a simpler example is instructive.

A SIMPLE EXAMPLE OF CHAOS

Perhaps the best way of demonstrating what is at issue is to use an example that has become very familiar in the literature of nonlinear dynamics theory. Consider a recursive quadratic function that generates sequences of numbers x_n by the relation

$$x_n = r(x_{n-1})(1 - x_{n-1}) \,, \tag{4-1}$$

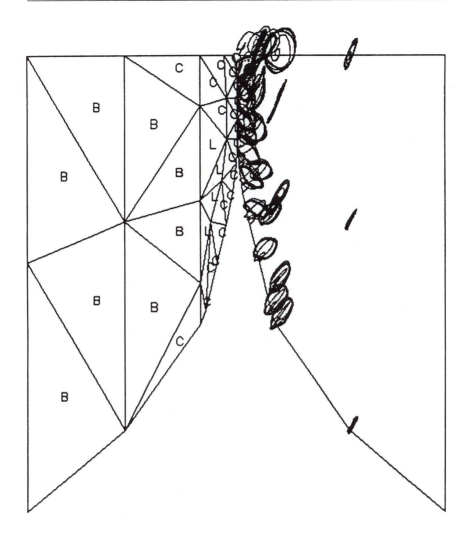

Figure 4-1. Frontal section through vocal folds of a finite element computer simulation model. Left side shows tissue elements for body (B), ligament (L), and cover (C). Right side shows trajectories of nodal points during self-oscillation.

This is known as the *logistic equation*[1]. Let the parameter *r* be set at 2.0. If we choose an arbitrary starting value $x_{n-1} = 0.20$, we find that the

[1] The logistic equation was originally proposed as a model of insect population changes, and has since been extensively analyzed by May (1974, 1976, 1980).

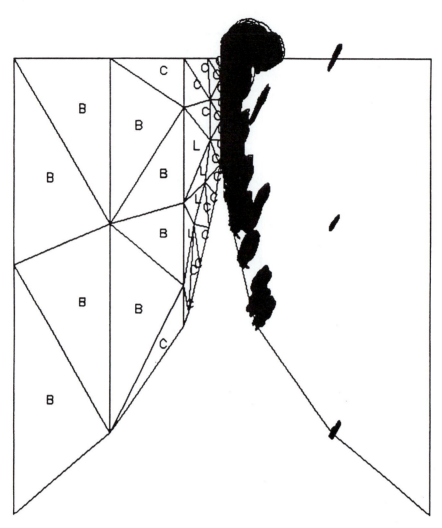

Figure 4-2. Same as Figure 4-1, but the Young's modulus of the cover was reduced from 1.5 KPa to 0.5 KPa.

following series of output values results: 0.320, 0.435, 0.492, 0.499, 0.500, 0.500. . . The recursive series converges relatively quickly on a final value. When the parameter *r* is set to 2.5, starting with x_{n-1} = 0.20 yields the convergent series 0.400, 0.600, 0.600. . . Such convergence suggests that the system modeled by the function could be described as "stable."

Consider, however, what happens when *r* is set at 3.4. The output series becomes 0.544, 0.843, 0.449. . .0.842, 0.452, 0.842, 0.452, 0.842, 0.452,

0.842. . . . The output thus oscillates between two final values. If r = 3.5, the series converges to 0.382, 0.827, 0.501, 0.875, 0.382, 0.827, 0.501, 0.875. . ., an oscillation among 4 final values. Finally, when r = 3.8, the output is 0.789, 0.633, 0.883, 0.392, 0.906. . . without any suggestion of convergence. The very complex behavior of this simple recursive model is plotted as a function of the parameter r in Figure 4-3. Note that for part of the domain over which r varies, the function converges to a single value. As r increases, however, the output alternates between two stable values (for example, at r=3.25), or four (at r=3.5) or 8 or more.

For $r < 3.57$ stability seems to be lost. But the points in this region show a faint patterning, suggesting some underlying order. And an enlargement of part of this domain (Figure 4-4) shows occasional zones where stability is clearly present (as at $r \approx 3.84$). Furthermore, it can

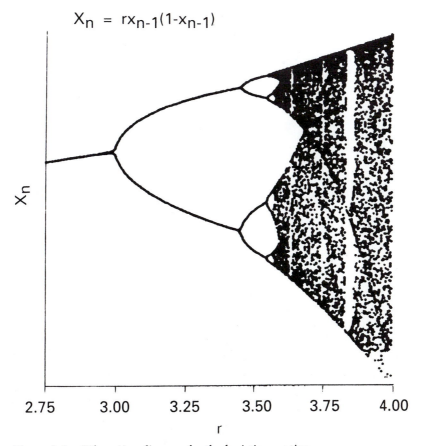

Figure 4-3. Bifurcation diagram for the logistic equation.

$$X_n = rx_{n-1}(1-x_{n-1})$$

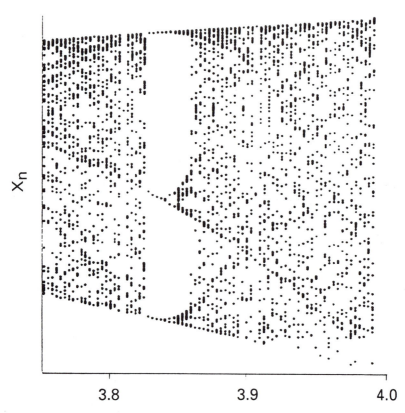

Figure 4-4. Enlargement of a portion of the bifurcation diagram of Figure 4-3.

be shown that an increasing enlargement of any given region in the domain $3.57 < r < 4.0$ will show increasing numbers of such zones of stability. If the logistic equation were a model of vocal fold function, we might say that some adjustments produced stable phonation, some produce diplophonia, some "quadriphonia" or other stable but peculiar F_o trains, and some adjustments produce aperiodicity.

The disorganized regions are themselves quite interesting. It turns out that they are not nearly as unstructured as they seem. If, as shown in Figure 4-5, we plot just a few of the successive outputs of the recursion at a given r in the region of disorganization on the coordinates x_n, x_{n-1} (which define a "pseudo phase space") we find that they fall into a very discernible pattern. (Sequential points do not lie next to each other, however. They are scattered; only in the aggregate

r = 3.97

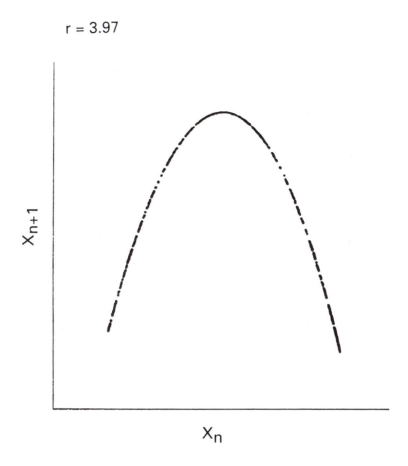

X$_{n+1}$

X$_n$

Figure 4-5. Attractor for the logistic equation.

do they describe a geometric structure. In other words, it is not possible to connect successive points with lines and preserve the pattern shown.) The geometric shape that is formed is an *attractor*. It is, in some sense, a picture of the ordering principle that underlies the seemingly random sequence of outputs of the equation.

The logistic equation represents a purely deterministic system that has unpredictable outputs. But even the erratic outputs are clearly not random, as the attractor shows. The system is said (in the technical sense) to be *chaotic*. Any system is potentially chaotic if:

(a) it is deterministic and nonlinear;
(b) it shows sudden qualitative changes in its output, that is, it demonstrates *bifurcations* such as those shown in Figure 4-3 (the

system may exhibit, at certain parameter values, nonperiodic behavior that appears as intermittent bursts of irregularity [transients], or the output may be exquisitely dependent on initial conditions and tiny parameter changes. For example, infinitesimal differences in r of the logistic equation may result in enormous differences in the regularity of the output);

(c) its representation in phase space shows fractal properties.

The essential properties of chaotic systems are discussed in a large number of texts that have appeared in the last few years. Among the better sources are Berg, Pomeau & Vidal (1984), Moon (1987), Thompson and Stewart (1986) and Rasband (1990).

Criterion (c) above introduces a new concept — *fractal dimension* — that has been shown to be of importance in understanding both structures and processes of the natural world. It will require a bit more explanation.

FRACTAL DIMENSIONS

Classical geometry limits dimensions to integer values. A point has dimension 0, a line 1, a plane 2, and so forth. The problem, however, has been that many geometric structures are not effectively described within those integer values. A classic example explored by Mandelbrot (1967) — who is largely responsible for the creation of the field of fractal geometry — is the natural coastline of a country. Euclidean geometry holds that it is a highly irregular line (and hence its dimension = 1). In classical mathematics, this irregularity is made tractable by assuming that if any segment were sufficiently enlarged, straight line segments would appear. But this is clearly not the case for a coastline (or many other structures). An enlargement of a bay (an irregularity) shows smaller bays along its margins. These in turn have rocks and boulders that stick out to make the bays' edges erratic. The rocks themselves are jagged, and every jagged area is formed by the mineral grains of which the rock is made. The grains, in turn, are composed of aggregated crystals, . . . and so on. At every scale of magnification there is a similar degree of irregularity. A coastline is an example of a geometric structure that is "self similar at all scalings." If one tries to measure such a line, one finds that the length obtained depends on the size of the ruler used. Longer rulers follow fewer irregularities, and hence give a shorter length than do smaller rulers than can follow the line more closely. The result of this, as Mandelbrot demonstrates, is that the dimension of the coastline must be greater than 1. However, its dimension cannot be as much as 2, which is the dimension of a plane. Hence, the dimension of such a line must be *fractional*, and the line itself is said to be *fractal*. Any geometric structure (of any number of Euclidean dimensions) that shows such self-similarity is fractal. An entire geometry of fractality has been developed in the last several years (Barnsley, 1988).

There are a number of ways to estimate the fractal dimension of natural structures (Barnsley, 1988; Farmer, Ott, and Yorke, 1983; Froehling et al., 1981; Farmer, 1982; Grassberger, 1986). What that dimension represents is the degree of the structure's irregularity. Irregularity is different from variability. For example, the completely regular function $F(x) = \sin x$ has a very distinct variability, which could be expressed as the standard deviation of $F(x)$. But a plot of the points $F(x)$ is not at all self-similar and, on measurement, its dimension will be found to be 1, indicating that it really is a line.

The combination of nonlinear dynamics and fractal geometry has considerable potential for explaining many biological phenomena, a number of which are of particular importance in physiology or medicine. It has been found, for example, that strange attractors are associated with electroencephalographic activity and that they change, and their associated dimension is altered, in response to alterations of consciousness level, cognitive activity of the brain, or the presentation of stimuli (Rapp et al., 1990; Samar and Rosenberg, 1990; Freeman, 1990). Chaotic behavior has also been observed in the ventilatory system (Mackey and Glass, 1977) and in the heart rhythm (Glass, Shrier, and Bélair, 1986; Goldberger, West, and Bhargava, 1986; Goldberger and Rigney, 1990).

Where there are fractal dimensions, there is the possibility of chaotic behavior. Glass and Mackey (1988), after a review of potentially or demonstrably chaotic functions in a number of abnormal physiological conditions, have proposed that disorders in which normal organization is disrupted and replaced by abnormal dynamics, such as Cheyne-Stokes breathing, certain cardiac arrhythmias, and epilepsy, may be most appropriately categorized as "dynamical diseases."

RECENT DISCOVERIES IN VOICE SOURCE CHARACTERISTICS

The vocal folds, together with glottal airflow, constitute a nonlinear oscillating system. This system is amenable to nonlinear dynamics analysis, which can provide an entirely different perspective on the underlying basis of phonatory function. This effort has just barely begun. Notable contributions are those of Pickover and Khorsani, (1986); Awrejcewicz, (1991); Wong, Ito, Cox, and Titze, (1990); Mende, Herzel, and Wermke, (1990); and Herzel, Steinecke, Mende, and Wermke, (1991). The objective of these was to certify the applicability of nonlinear systems theory to vocal functioning and to derive initial suggestions about the dynamical nature of the system. Unfortunately, time series data (that is, data that come from a real physical system) are notoriously difficult to deal with. They inevitably include stochastic functions and cannot be made immune to the influences of contaminating variables. Thus, the work goes slowly and definitive answers even to the simple questions concerning applicability are not yet available. The findings already at hand, however, afford veiled glimpses of the value of a nonlinear dynamics approach to the voice. Of specific significance was the early modeling study by Isshiki and Ishizaka (1976), who showed that asymmetry in vocal fold vibration yielded subharmonic structure.

Herzel and his coworkers (Herzel et al. 1991; Mende, Herzel, and Wermke, 1990) have undertaken preliminary examination of the cries of newborn infants and have found numerous bifurcations in the sound pressure signal, including period doublings and sudden transitions to aperiodicity. Their analysis of these phenomena strongly suggest the presence of low-dimensional chaos, and they have established the consistency of these phenomena with two-mass models of the vocal folds. The more intensive modelling experience of Awrejcewicz (1990) has examined the trajectory of the vocal folds and supports the findings of Herzel et al. (1991). It would appear, then, that the vocal folds are, in principle, capable of chaotic behavior.

Baken (1990) has undertaken a preliminary examination of the fractal dimension (D_F) of normal vocal F_o and amplitude. Using a box-counting algorithm for estimation of D_F, he has found that a data record of sequential period values had a D_F of 1.46, which was unaffected by speaker sex or by the mean F_o of phonation. Records of sequential peak intensities of the same phonations had a significantly different mean D_F of 1.54, which also was unaffected by speaker sex or by mean vocal F_o. D_F was at best weakly correlated to measures of vocal variability such as relative average perturbation or shimmer. This work demonstrated that fractal geometry can be useful for measuring irregularity of vocal fold oscillation, independent of oscillatory variability (which, of course, can be the result of organized behavior).

Exploratory, and somewhat informal, examination of vocal F_o and amplitude in cases of several different types of vocal disorder undertaken by Baken (in press) have demonstrated that the fractal dimension is often different from normal, but the differences do not seem related to traditional categories of laryngeal disorder. In fact, this result is not surprising: dynamical theory suggests that a different taxonomy of disorder may be necessary.

But is the vocal fold system potentially chaotic? In principle, it should be. Research now in progress should show whether it is in practice. There are, in the meantime, some suggestions that chaotic behavior does appear in certain circumstances. The baby-cry studies of Herzel and his coworkers certainly point in that direction, although it could be argued that the infant larynx and nervous system do not provide a suitable model for adult vocal production. Perhaps more telling is an investigation by Baken, Watson, and Dembowski, (in preparation) of F_o variation in spasmodic dysphonic patients. It was designed as the proverbial "fishing expedition," based on the intuitive idea that interesting things might be happening to vocal F_o in these patients. Recordings of several male and female spasmodic dysphonic patients were drawn from the extensive collection that has been built up at the University of Texas at Dallas. Fundamental period values for all glottal cycles during sustained vowels were extracted using CSpeech, and a contour of these periods was prepared. Figure 4-6a is typical of one of the records that resulted.

What is interesting about this record is that it demonstrates period doubling bifurcations. Note that, at the start of the trial, successive periods are relatively stable, but after about 50 periods the contour oscillates between two values. This is seen in an expanded plot in Figure 4-6b. Toward the end of the phonation another bifurcation occurs, and the period oscillates between 4 values (Figure 4-6c). These bifurcations are extremely abrupt, the transition from one state to another requiring only a few milliseconds. Another record (Figure 4-7) shows a more complex bifurcation, as the period undergoes a transient change from 2-cycle alternation to a more complicated pattern involving 8-10 periods (see expanded portion in part b).

At this point it is appropriate to reflect on the possible contributors to irregularity in vocal fold vibration. Without attempting to sort out which contributors lead to which kind of pattern, we simply list a number of possible candidates.

1. Unsteadiness in muscle contractions in the laryngeal and respiratory system. In particular, the incomplete summation of muscle twitches in an attempt to form a "smooth tetanus" brings about a fundamental frequency jitter (Baer, 1981b; more recently, the process has been modeled by Titze, 1991).
2. Turbulence in the glottal airstream.
3. Vortex shedding and instability in the jet emerging from the glottis (this differs from the turbulence above). The jet may flip-flop from side to side, even if turbulence does not exist.
4. Asymmetry in the mechanical or geometrical properties of the two vocal folds. Usually, a dominant oscillation mode exists due to synchronization of two similar oscillators by the airflow, but excessive asymmetry may create desynchronization.
5. Nonlinearity in the mechanical properties of vocal fold tissues (the

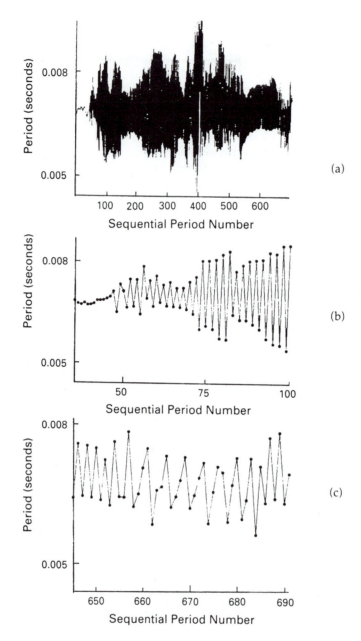

Figure 4-6. Fundamental period of vocal fold oscillation plotted as a function of period number. Spasmodic patient (a) full utterance, (b) expanded segment showing period doubling, (c) expanded segment showing period doubling changing to period quadrupling.

154

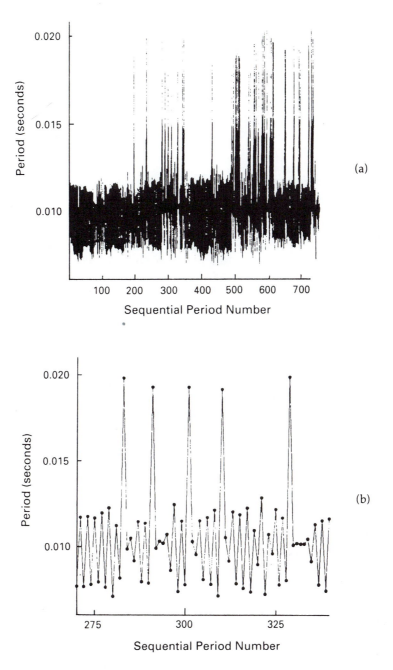

Figure 4-7. Fundamental period of vocal fold oscillation plotted as a function of period number. Spasmodic patient (a) full utterance, (b) expanded segment showing complex patterns involving multiple periods.

constitutive equation) and the pressure-flow relations. Nonlinearities complicate the mode structure of a vibrating system.

6. Coupling between the vocal folds and the vocal tract. Acoustic pressures in the subglottal and supraglottal region may play a part in driving the vocal folds. If these pressures change dynamically, oscillation may be perturbed.

7. Mucus riding on the surface of vocal fold tissue. The mucus could reorient itself from cycle to cycle, causing disturbances in the vibration pattern.

Several of these sources of irregularity can exist in combination with others. Some of them, like mucus and air turbulence, may result in high-dimensionality chaos; others, like left-right asymmetry, may lead to low-dimensionality chaos. It is important to study the sources one at a time to get a better understanding of their effect on vocal fold vibration. Some of this work can be done with physical models and excised larynges, where the effects of neural inputs, the vocal tract, or mucus can be selectively eliminated.

In the following section, some basic principles of nonlinear dynamics will be reviewed that will be helpful in interpretations of data obtained on humans, excised larynges, and computer simulation models.

INTRODUCTION TO NONLINEAR DYNAMICS

A *linear* dynamical system is described by equations of the form

$$\dot{x}_1 = f_1 \, (x_1, x_2 \ldots x_n, \dot{x}_2, \dot{x}_3 \ldots \dot{x}_n, t) \tag{4-2}$$

$$\dot{x}_n = f_n \, (x_1, x_2 \ldots x_n, \dot{x}_1, \dot{x}_2 \ldots \dot{x}_{n-1}, t) \tag{4-3}$$

where $x_1, x_2 \ldots x_n$ are components of displacement or velocity and the dots indicate time differentiation. All of the displacements and all of the velocities are regarded as separate variables in time. Solution of these coupled equations is usually obtained by assuming complex exponential functions for x_i, finding the eigenvalues (which determine the characteristic frequencies of the system), and using the principle of superposition to express the total response as a sum of eigenresponses (transients) and driven responses (steady states).

For example, the dynamical equations for a second order mass-spring-damper system are written as

$$\dot{x}_1 = x_2 \tag{4-4}$$

$$\dot{x}_2 = [-b\dot{x}_1 - kx_1 + F(t)]/m, \qquad (4\text{-}5)$$

where x_1 is displacement from equilibrium, x_2 is velocity, b is the damping coefficient, k is spring stiffness, m is mass, and $F(t)$ is the driving force. Solution of these equations is of the form

$$x_1 = Ae^{\gamma_1 t} + Be^{\gamma_2 t} + G(t), \qquad (4\text{-}6)$$

where A and B are constants (to be evaluated by initial conditions) and γ_1 and γ_2 are eigenvalues of the characteristic equation [found from 4-4 and 4-5 by setting F = 0]. The function $G(t)$ is the steady-state solution.

In *nonlinear* dynamical systems, the variables x_i and $\dot{x}_i$ in equations (4-2) and (4-3) form product terms (e.g., $x_2\dot{x}_3$), or contain higher order terms (e.g., x_1^2). Solutions are much less straightforward and must usually be obtained numerically. More importantly, the nonlinear coupling between displacements and velocities makes the principle of superposition no longer applicable: *a large-signal response is not simply a scaled-up version of a small-signal response.* Different excitations may result in totally different time-courses, described by totally different mathematical functions. The system may be very sensitive to small changes in a parameter (such as a spring constant k or a damping coefficient b), or to an initial condition. Recall that this was demonstrated for the logistic equation (4-1) with the parameter r and with the starting value of x_{n-1}. [Equation 4-1 is nonlinear differential equation written in discrete time steps x_n rather than in continuous form $x(t)$.]

NONLINEARITY IN VOCAL FOLD MECHANICS

Nonlinearity is exhibited in vocal fold mechanics in at least two ways. First, tissue deformation does not follow a simple Hooke's law for elastic springs. The restoring force $-kx_1$ in equation (4-5) is usually augmented by a quadratic or cubic function (involving x_1^2 or x_1^3 terms) in simple vocal fold models, or by an exponential term $e^{\alpha x}$ in more complex models. Second, the pressure-flow relation in the glottis is nonlinear. For steady flow and steady glottal configurations, the flow varies with the square root of the transglottal pressure. For oscillatory flow, the relation may become somewhat "linearized," but only over limited ranges (to be discussed later).

Consider first the mechanical properties of vocal fold tissues in more detail. A universal property of soft biological tissues is that the stress-strain curve is not only nonlinear, but also time-dependent. There is no unique relation between mechanical load and tissue deformation unless a history of the deformation is included. Thus, if one step-elongates a piece of tissue to achieve a specific tension, the tension will not remain constant, but will relax with time. The combined nonlinear and time-dependent characteristics can be observed in a stretch-release experiment. Figure 4-8 shows results of such an experiment for the thyroarytenoid muscle. Three cycles of stretch and release, which occurred at a rate of 1 Hz, are shown. Note that the tissue exhibits less stress during release than during stretch at the same value of strain. This suggests that stress "leaks out" during the cycle. Not all the stored energy is given back. From a Carnot cycle point of view, the area inside the stretch-release loop represents the energy lost per cycle.

Figure 4-9 shows results of the same stretch-release experiment performed on vocal fold cover tissue. The main difference is the degree

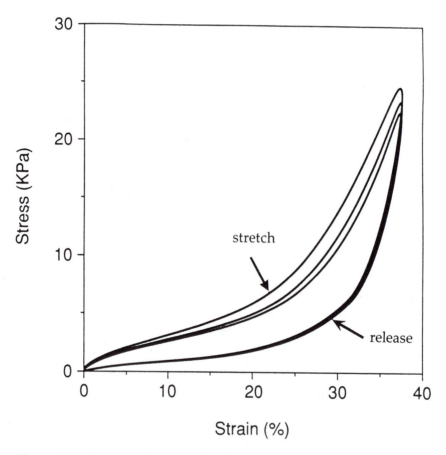

Figure 4-8. Stress-strain curve for three cycles of stretch and release performed on the thyroarytenoid muscle.

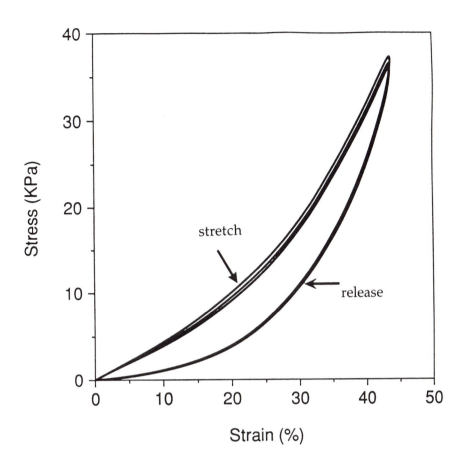

Figure 4-9. Stress-strain curve for three cycles of stretch and release performed on the vocal fold cover.

of nonlinearity. The "banana shape" has a gentler curve above the 30% strain level. But how does this nonlinearity affect phonation? The key parameter is the amplitude-to-length ratio (A/L) of the vocal folds. If the human larynx were to belong to a family of stringed instruments, its major peculiarity would be the shortness of the string in relation to its amplitude of vibration. For the dominant string mode, which is characterized by a half-wavelength between the anterior and posterior boundary attachments, the usual small-amplitude criterion is not met at all. A/L is between 0.1 and 1.0 (amplitudes in excess of 1 mm are observed for vocal fold lengths less than 1 cm). For a piano or violin string, on the other hand, the same ratio is on the order of 0.001. (A 1 mm amplitude of vibration for a 1 m piano string is not atypical).

Many of the simplifying assumptions of elementary vibrating string theory (e.g. small angular deflections and constant tension) do not apply to the vocal folds. Tensions are dynamically varying, which produces mathematical nonlinearities in the effective restoring force (Titze, 1989).

Consider now the relation between transglottal pressure and glottal airflow. For a hard-walled constriction in a pipe,

$$P = \left(\frac{k}{2}\right)\rho U^2 / A_g^2, \qquad (4\text{-}7)$$

where P is the pressure drop across the constriction (the glottis), ρ is the air density, U is the flow, A_g is the minimum cross-sectional area in the constriction, and k is a pressure coefficient. This nonlinear relation between transglottal pressure and glottal airflow, together with a tissue mode that allows for alternating convergent and divergent glottal shapes, provides the necessary instability for flow-induced oscillation (Ishizaka and Matsudaira, 1972; Titze, 1988).

For a yielding wall, the area A_g increases with pressure. Titze (1989) found that under dynamic conditions, the relation

$$A_g = CP^{1/2} \qquad (4\text{-}8)$$

approximated the experimental results obtained in excised canine larynges, where C is a constant that varied with vocal fold length. This nonlinearity is related to the stress-strain nonlinearity of the tissue. The amplitude of vibration, and hence the glottal area, does not increase linearly with driving pressure because the tissue becomes stiffer under greater stretch. This may actually be an advantage from a control standpoint. A simple substitution of (4-8) into (4-7) reveals that

$$P = \frac{1}{C}\sqrt{\frac{k\rho}{2}}\,U, \qquad (4\text{-}9)$$

suggesting a more linear relation between pressure and flow. Recent experiments by Sundberg, Titze, and Scherer (1992) and Titze and Sundberg (1992) on singers have confirmed this relation, at least in some portions of the intensity and fundamental frequency ranges. Although this linearization may simplify the *control* process for phonation, it does not eliminate the nonlinearities. It simply "plays" one nonlinearity against the other. A sophisticated control system may look for regions of operation where complex relations between control variables can be simplified.

ATTRACTORS IN PHASE SPACE

The crucial condition for the applicability of nonlinear dynamics is the dominance of a relatively low number of variables $x_i(t)$ (i = 1, 2, ..., m). Then, time-series can be projected into a *phase space*, which is spanned by these m coordinates. Under the assumption of fixed parameters (i.e. the external conditions are held constant) the m-dimensional vector $\underline{x}(t)$, termed *trajectory*, settles down on an *attractor* after some transient behavior (see Figure 4-10, which represents the lateral motion of one of the finite element nodal points of Figure 4-1. Lateral velocity is plotted as a function of lateral position). Note the transient behavior, indicated by orbits in the middle, followed by asymptotic behavior (nearly periodic) toward the outside. The outside orbits constitute the attractor. They determine the long-term behavior of the system.

A stylized attractor in phase space is shown enlarged in Figure 4-11. In addition to the overall phase portrait, *Poincaré maps* are often enlightening. Such maps are obtained if only the intersections of the orbits with a transversal section are studied. A variety of known attractor-types, together with their Poincaré maps, are illustrated in Figure 4-12:

   i) stable stationary point (i.e. $x_i(t)$ are constant)
   ii) stable limit cycle ($x_i(t)$ are periodic)
   iii) stable n-torus ($x_i(t)$ is governed by n incommensurate frequencies)
   iv) chaotic attractors ($x_i(t)$ nonperiodic).

A limit cycle in phase space corresponds to a fixed point of the Poincaré map, a 2-torus gives a closed curve, and a low-dimensional chaotic attractor may lead to a pattern with a fractal structure.

Several attractors can coexist in phase space. Each attractor then has its own *basin of attraction*. The basin boundaries can be either smooth or fractal. In the latter case, *transient chaos* is possible, i.e. the trajectories change erratically over long periods of time and reach the attractor only after these extended periods. Some phonatory samples will be presented later that demonstrate the various dynamical regimes in phase space.

ATTRACTOR DIMENSIONS AND LYAPUNOV EXPONENTS

We now discuss the quantitative characterization of attractors. The selection of phase space variables x_i is somewhat arbitrary. However, certain quantities, such as attractor dimension, Lyapunov exponents, and the Kolmogorov entropy, are independent of the chosen coordinate system (Eckmann and Ruelle, 1985).

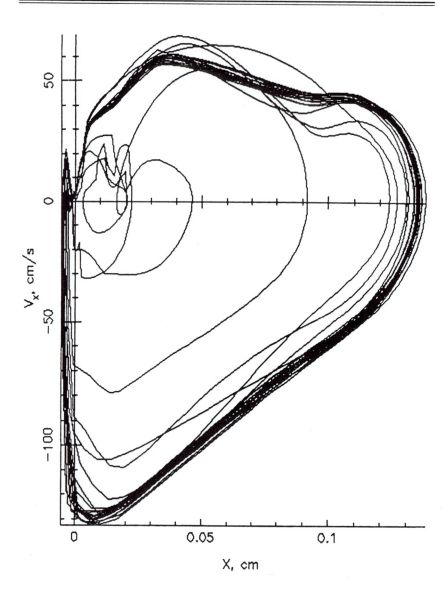

Figure 4-10. Phase plane trajectory for one nodal point of Figure 4-1. Lateral velocity v_x is plotted against lateral displacement x.

We start with some remarks on attractor dimensions. As already discussed earlier, the scaling behavior of various quantities can be exploited to define dimensions. The concept of *pointwise dimensions*

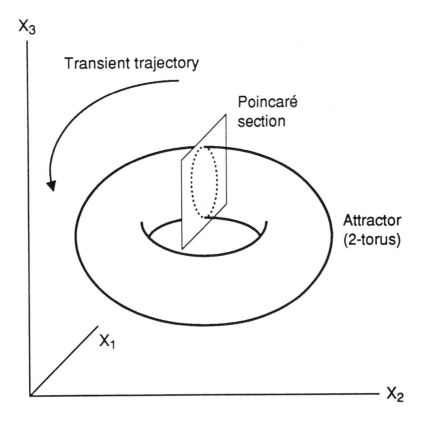

Figure 4-11. Stylized visualization of an attractor in phase space, together with a Poincaré section.

turns out to be useful for the characterization of attractors in phase space: Let us assume that we have a large number of attractor points $\underline{x}(t_i) = \underline{x}_i$ ($i = 1,2,...,N$) (each vector $\underline{x}_i$ corresponds to a point in the m-dimensional phase space). The number of neighbors of an attractor point $\underline{x}_i$ within a distance ε is termed local density $n_i(\varepsilon)$:

$$n_i(\varepsilon) = \sum_{j=1}^{N} \theta\left(\varepsilon - \|\underline{x}_i - \underline{x}_j\|\right), \qquad (4\text{-}10)$$

where $\theta(s)$ is a unit step (Heaviside) function, defined with a dummy variable s as

$$\theta(s) = \begin{cases} 0 & if \ s \leq 0 \\ 1 & s > 0 \end{cases} \qquad (4\text{-}11)$$

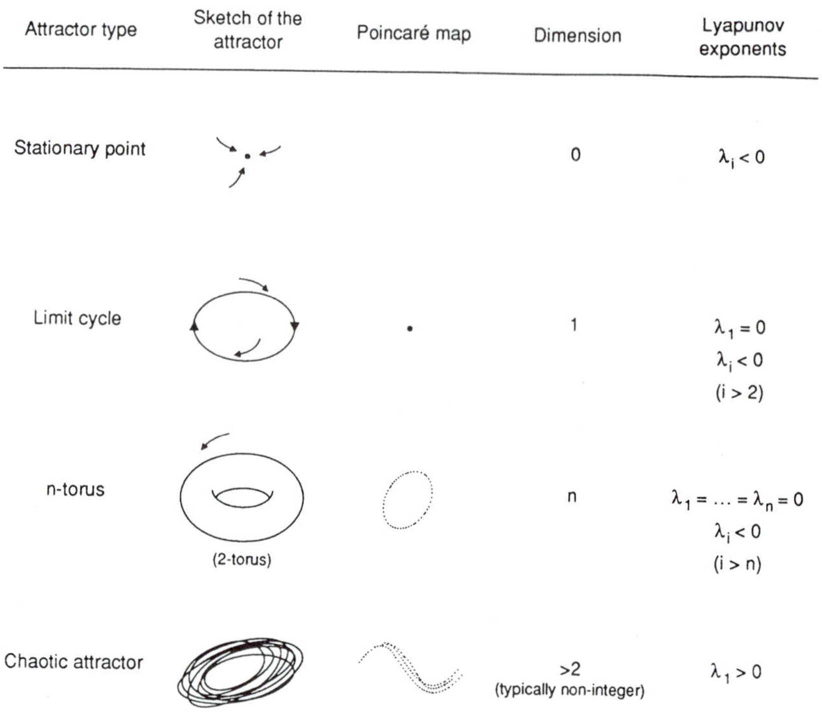

Attractor type	Sketch of the attractor	Poincaré map	Dimension	Lyapunov exponents
Stationary point			0	$\lambda_i < 0$
Limit cycle		.	1	$\lambda_1 = 0$ $\lambda_i < 0$ $(i > 2)$
n-torus	(2-torus)		n	$\lambda_1 = \dots = \lambda_n = 0$ $\lambda_i < 0$ $(i > n)$
Chaotic attractor			>2 (typically non-integer)	$\lambda_1 > 0$

Figure 4-12. Various attractors and their characteristics.

If we find a power-law $n_i(\varepsilon) \sim \varepsilon^{D_p}$ over a certain ε-region, we can take D_p as an estimate of the pointwise dimension. For simple attractors this definition coincides with the familiar notion of a dimension (the "topological dimension"). For example, a line gives $n_i(\varepsilon) \sim \varepsilon^1$ (i.e. $D_p = 1$) and a surface corresponds to $n_i(\varepsilon) \sim \varepsilon^2$. Chaotic attractors typically have noninteger dimensions greater than two.

In order to get reliable dimension estimates, the density $n_i(\varepsilon) \sim \varepsilon^{D_p}$ has to be averaged over many attractor points $\underline{x}_i$, leading to the correlation dimension D_2 (to be discussed later).

Attractors can also be characterized by m Lyapunov exponents $\lambda_1 \geq \lambda_2 \geq \dots \geq \lambda_m$. These quantities describe the stability properties of trajectories in different directions (see Eckmann and Ruelle, 1985 for details). A positive Lyapunov exponent λ_1 is of particular interest since its presence marks a system as chaotic. For $\lambda_1 > 0$ we find that sufficiently small deviations from a trajectory grow, in the mean, according to the function $\exp(\lambda_1 t)$, indicating a strong instability within the attractor. This inherent instability of chaotic systems implies limited predictability of the future if the initial state is known with only finite precision. Chaotic time-series have much in common with stochastic processes (decaying autocorrelations, limited predictability) but the detection of attractors and exponential instability (i.e. $\lambda_1 > 0$) allows chaos to be distinguished from noise.

BIFURCATIONS

Up to now we have assumed fixed parameters; that is, stationary external conditions. In these situations, the essential features of the dynamics are the attractors and their basins of attraction. If parameters of the dynamical system are varied, however, qualitative changes of attractors known as bifurcations are possible. For example, if one decreases the damping of an oscillatory system, one may switch from damped oscillation (fixed point attractor) to self-sustained oscillations (limit cycle). This transition is called a *Hopf bifurcation*. A limit cycle can bifurcate to a 2 torus, with two incommensurate frequencies, via a secondary Hopf bifurcation.

Another prominent kind of bifurcation is period-doubling (see e.g. Feigenbaum, 1983). In this case a limit cycle loses its stability and a periodic orbit of the double period is born. This bifurcation is accompanied by the appearance of subharmonics in the spectrum.

The chart of bifurcation lines in parameter space are termed *bifurcation diagrams*. As an important example we discuss the bifurcation diagram of coupled nonlinear oscillators (see Figure 4-13). The frequency ratio ω_1/ω_2 and the coupling strength K are taken as parameters. The qualitative behavior can be summarized as follows:

K = 0: For almost all ratios ω_1/ω_2 the frequencies are incommensurate and we have a 2-torus.

K small: Each rational value $\omega_1/\omega_2 = p/q$ (with p and q integers) leads to a resonance tongue. Inside these resonance tongues the oscillators are *entrained*, i.e. they oscillate with a fixed phase shift. The attractor is therefore a limit cycle with long periods for large q. The width of these resonance zones shrinks drastically with increasing denominator q, that is, experimentally only the main resonances (1/1, 1/2, 2/3, ...) are visible.

K large: For increasing coupling strength, the tongues overlap. This may lead to coexisting attractors and chaos. Within the resonances, chaos may occur via a cascade of period-doubling bifurcations (Feigenbaum scenario; recall Figure 4-3, which is rotated 90° from Figure 4-13, with the parameter r begun similar to parameter k). Small changes of parameter values may result in drastic changes of the dynamic behavior.

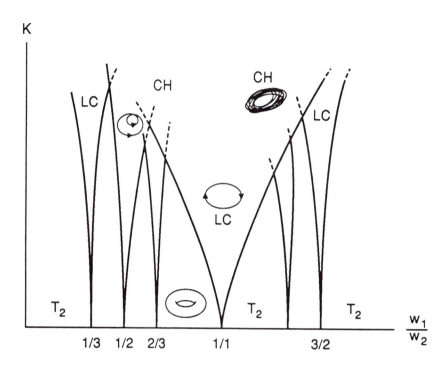

Figure 4-13. Schematic bifurcation diagram of coupled nonlinear oscillators and sketches of the corresponding attractors (LC is a limit cycle inside a resonance zone; T_2 is a 2-torus; CH is a chaotic attractor.

Obviously, the bifurcation diagrams of nonlinear dynamical systems capable of producing deterministic chaos are extremely complicated. As a general result one can say that tori and period-doubling bifurcations are often precursors of chaotic dynamics. Particularly, coupled nonlinear oscillators exhibit complicated limit cycles (entrainment in resonances with $q \geq 2$), 2-tori, and chaotic behavior.

FROM OBSERVATION TO SYSTEM CHARACTERIZATION

It was emphasized in the first section that nonperiodic measurements can be understood either as random processes or as manifestations of chaotic dynamics. In the case of random processes, the classical methods of time-series analysis, such as power spectra and autoregressive models, are appropriate. In the case of chaotic dynamics that can be modeled by relatively few variables, a qualitative theory of dynamical systems should be applied.

PHONATORY SAMPLES

Phenomena that are presumably manifestations of nonlinear dynamics (roughness, creaky voice, octave jumps, voice breaks, diplophonia) are frequently described in the literature (see e.g. Lieberman, 1963; Dolansky and Tjernlund, 1968; Koike, 1969; Monsen, 1979; Kelman, 1981; Imaizumi, 1986; Hirano, 1989). Particularly, newborn cries exhibit frequent voice breaks and irregularities (Lind, 1965). In a recent paper (Mende et al., 1990) these observations are interpreted as bifurcations and low-dimensional chaos.

We now analyze some examples of vocalizations recorded at the university hospital (Charité) of the Humboldt-University (see Wendler et al., 1986 for details). The samples include normal as well as pathological voices. Each record of sustained vowels was classified perceptually according to its degrees of hoarseness (H), roughness (R), and breathiness (B). A four point grading was applied with 0 indicating normality, 1 slight, 2 moderate, and 3 extreme deviations.

The acoustic signals (sustained vowels at comfortable pitch) were digitized with a sampling rate of 20 kHz and 12 bit resolution. Figure 4-14 shows representative samples, labeled according to the diseases and the results of perceptual evaluation. The normal voice in Figure 4-14(a) is taken in the following as a standard of comparison. The pathological voices (parts b-d) exhibit large deviations from periodicity (jitter of more than 10% and shimmer from 15% to 50%). But it is evident that the deviations are by no means random. Therefore, the concept of nonlinear dynamics should be applied in order to detect the "hidden rules" that are related to attractors.

RECONSTRUCTION OF ATTRACTORS FROM TIME-SERIES

In the previous section, the phase space spanned by the relevant dynamical variables x_i (i = 1,2,...m) was introduced. Ideally, these variables are positions and velocities of fleshpoints. In many laboratory situations, however, kinematic variables are not available. Furthermore, often only a single signal $x(t)$ is measured with sufficient accuracy (in our case the acoustic signal). Nevertheless, a pseudo phase space can be constructed easily in the following way (Froehling et al., 1981):

$$\underline{x}(t) = \{ x(t), x(t+\tau), ..., x(t+(m-1)\tau) \} \qquad (4\text{-}12)$$

A vector is reconstructed in "pseudo phase space" by m "delay-co-ordinates." The selection of a delay-time τ and an embedding dimension m is somewhat arbitrary, but attractor dimensions and Lyapunov exponents should not depend on τ and m, provided that m is sufficiently

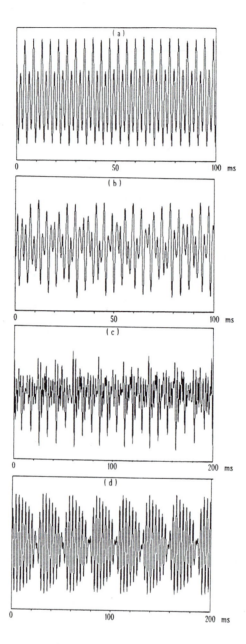

Figure 4-14. Acoustic waveforms from sustained vowels: (a) normal female voice; vowel "i"; (b) female voice, papillomas of the vocal folds; vowel "u"; (c) female voice, polyposis of the vocal folds; vowel "i"; and (d) male voice, papillomas of the vocal folds; vowel "u."

large (Eckmann and Ruelle, 1985). A variation of the embedding parameters can serve, therefore, as a consistency test of the algorithms discussed below.

In Figure 4-15 phase portraits in the pseudo phase space are shown for some of the signals. The periodic signal of the normal voice corresponds to a limit cycle with two loops, whereas the nonperiodic signal leads to a more complicated attractor.

The Poincaré maps in Figure 4-16 indicate a limit cycle with two intersections per period and a 2-torus. In the case of a randomly perturbed signal (e.g. a very breathy voice) an unstructured cloud of points would appear in the Poincaré map. Thus, the appearance of regular structures in phase portraits and Poincaré maps are first indications of low-dimensional dynamics.

QUANTITATIVE CHARACTERIZATIONS OF ATTRACTORS

Several techniques have been developed for the estimation of attractor dimensions (see e.g. Mayer-Kress, 1986). The most popular method is based on averaging the local densities $n_i(\varepsilon)$ introduced in the previous section:

$$< n_i(\varepsilon) > \sim \sum_{i,j} \theta\left(\varepsilon - \| \underline{x}_1 - \underline{x}_j \|\right) \sim C(\varepsilon) \sim \varepsilon^{D_2} \qquad (4\text{-}13)$$

Here the brackets $< \ldots >$ denote averaging over many attractor points $\underline{x}_i$. The double sum is simply the number of distances between attractor points less than ε which is proportional to the so-called correlation integral $C(\varepsilon)$.

If $C(\varepsilon)$ scales as ε^{D_2}, then D_2 can be taken as an estimation of the correlation dimension (Grassberger and Procaccia, 1983). The estimate D_2 can be obtained from the slopes of log-log plots of the correlation integral $C(\varepsilon)$ versus the length scale ε. In the case of a low-dimensional attractor, one expects a scaling region with a constant slope D_2 (see Figure 4-17).

The dotted curves in Figure 4-17 refer to another method for the estimation of dimensions that is related to near-neighbor statistics (van der Water and Schram, 1988). If $r_k(\underline{x}_i)$ denotes the distance between an attractor point $\underline{x}_i$ to its k-th nearest neighbor, then the average distance depends on k as follows:

$$< r_k(\underline{x}_i) > \sim G(k,D)\, k^{1/D} \qquad (4\text{-}14)$$

$$with\; G(k,D) = \frac{\Gamma\left(k = 1/D\right)}{\Gamma(k)} \qquad (4\text{-}15)$$

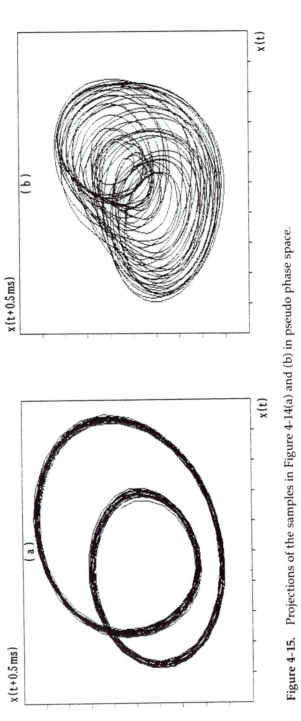

Figure 4-15. Projections of the samples in Figure 4-14(a) and (b) in pseudo phase space.

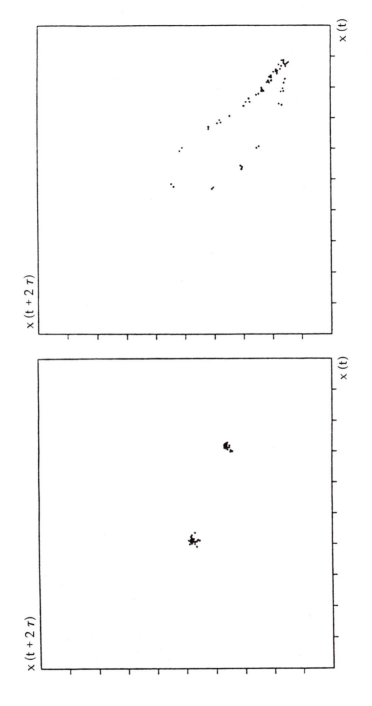

Figure 4-16. Poincaré maps of the samples in Figure 4-14(a) and (d) from intersections with the plane $x(t+\tau) = 0$ for decreasing $x(t+\tau)$ (delay $\tau = 1$ ms and 0.9 ms).

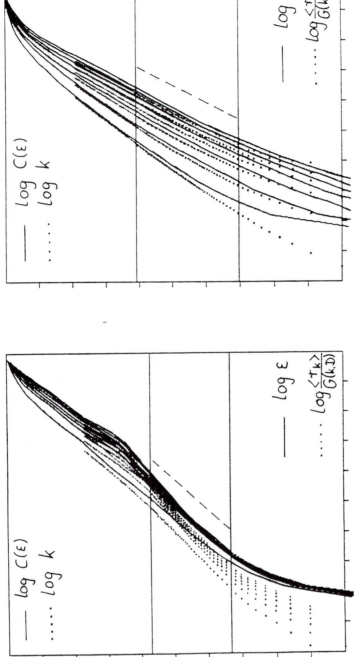

Figure 4-17. Log-log plots for the estimation of attractor dimensions derived from the records in Figure 4-14(a) and (b). Embedding dimensions: M = 2,3,...8 (from above). full lines: correlations integral C(ε) versus length scale ε. dotted lines: near-neighbor statistics (the horizontal lines delimit the approximate scaling region; the dashed lines indicate a slope of 1.0 and 2.6, respectively).

Again, the dimension D can be estimated from the slopes of the corresponding log-log plots. The prefactor $G(k,D)$ is close to unity. Therefore, a first guess of D can be obtained by setting $G(k,D) = 1$. The resulting first estimation can be improved iteratively with the use of the Gamma function Γ.

The application of these techniques is demonstrated in Figure 4-17 for fixed delay-time τ and varying embedding dimensions m (other values of τ give comparable results). It can be seen that both methods give nearly identical slopes. As expected, the periodic signal of Figure 4-14(a) leads to a slope of about $D_2 = D = 1$, whereas the nonperiodic time-series of Figure 4-14(c) corresponds to the estimation $D_2 = D = 2.6$; a chaotic attractor is indicated.

Now we turn to the estimation of the maximum Lyapunov exponent λ_1. Chaotic dynamics (i.e. $\lambda_1 > 0$) implies that nearby trajectories diverge (on the average) exponentially with a rate of λ_1. This property can be exploited to estimate the exponent λ_1. We use an algorithm by Wolf et al. (1985) in a modified version (Herzel et al., 1991). The algorithm contains the following steps:

i) choose nearby points $\underline{x}_1 = \underline{x}(t_i)$ and $\underline{x}(t_j)$ with an initial distance $d(0) = \| \underline{x}(t_i) - \underline{x}(t_j) \|$

ii) compute their distance $d(T) = \| \underline{x}(t_i + T) - \underline{x}(t_j + T) \|$ after an "evolution time" T

iii) find a new close neighbor of the reference point $\underline{x}(t_i + T)$ in such a way that the orientation of the separation vector is most nearly preserved (thus, a new initial distance $d(0)$ results)

iv) average the local growth rate $ln\frac{d(T)}{d(0)}$ over many separations.

The "normalization" in the third step ensures that only small distances are probed for sufficiently small evolution times T and that the separation vector is oriented along the most unstable direction.

An indication of chaos is found if there is a linear growth in $< ln\frac{d(t)}{d(0)} >$ over a range of evolution times T. Moreover, one has to check that different embedding parameters τ and m lead to the same estimation of the exponent λ_1.

Figure 4-18 demonstrates robust estimation results. The analysis of the normal voice is consistent with the expected value $\lambda_1 = 0$ and the presumably chaotic time-series leads to $\lambda_1 \approx 0.1$ ms^{-1}.

Summarizing, we can say that the records of pathological voices in Figure 4-14 are, indeed, manifestations of low-dimensional attractors. Moreover, we have shown that time-series analysis inspired by nonlinear dynamics is applicable to phonatory samples.

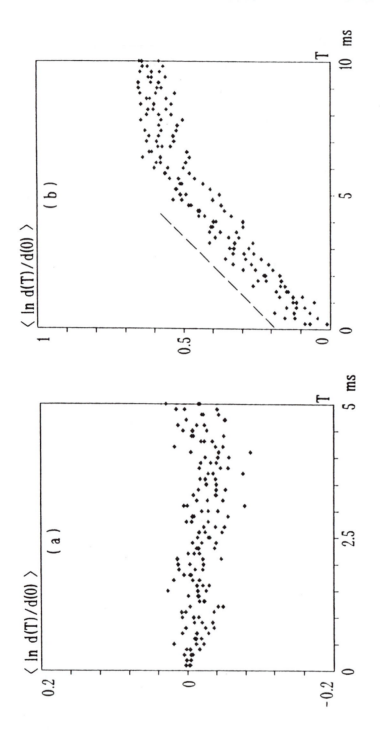

Figure 4-18. Average growth of the distance of initially nearby orbits with evolution time T. Three sets of embedding parameters are superimposed. (a) Record from Figure 4-14(a) $m=6$ and $\tau=0.3$ ms; $m=6$ and $\tau=0.5$ ms; $m=4$ and $\tau=0.5$ ms. (b) Record from Figure 4-14(c) $m=6$ and $\tau=0.6$ ms; $m=6$ and $\tau=1$ ms; $m=5$ and $\tau=1$ ms. The dashed line indicates a slope of $\lambda_1 = 0.1$ ms^{-1}.

BIFURCATIONS IN PHONATORY SIGNALS

The characterization of attractors above was based on the assumption of stationarity. However, even during sustained vowels, changes of pitch and amplitudes are observed due to varying parameters such as muscle tension and subglottal pressure. On one hand such instationarities complicate the attractor analysis. On the other hand, qualitative changes of the signals due to drifting parameters provide additional clues. These transitions can be interpreted as bifurcations of the underlying dynamical system. It was emphasized previously that bifurcation diagrams of potentially chaotic systems are extremely complicated. Consequently, we do not understand the entire collection of observed bifurcations in phonatory records. A few more examples will be given that demonstrate the rich variety of transitions.

Figure 4-19 gives a sense of the multitude of bifurcations possible in newborn cries. At the beginning of the spectrogram, only the fundamental frequency of about 500 Hz is present, together with its pronounced harmonics. Then, in connection with increasing energy and pitch, remarkably sharp transitions to more complicated states are visible. Particularly, the sudden appearances of subharmonics around 100 ms might be related to a jump from a 1:1 to a 1:2 resonance zone in the schematic bifurcation diagram of Figure 4-13. Such transitions to "subharmonic regimes" might be audible as octave jumps and are related to period-doubling bifurcations. Parametrically, the bifurcations may relate to dynamically changing tissue stress. In newborns, the amplitude to length ratio discussed earlier is extremely large, resulting in strong nonlinearities in the restoring forces.

It has been shown with the aid of Poincaré sections and dimension analysis that noisy segments of newborn cries can be interpreted as low-dimensional chaos (Mende et al., 1990). Although the spectrogram in Figure 4-19 is from a premature infant (28 weeks) with respiratory complications, we underscore that complex bifurcations and chaos were found in cries of healthy infants as well as in infants with complications (Lind, 1965; Mende et al., 1990).

The record from a pathological voice in Figure 4-20(a) displays another interesting sequence of transitions. From a nearly periodic state, with a period of about 2.3 ms, a transition to a "low-frequency regime" with large amplitudes is observed. The reverse transition to a high-pitched regime occurs via a segment of nonperiodic oscillation (from 180 to 280 ms), which could be interpreted as a "chaotic transient." The results are in some ways similar to those obtained on a spasmodic patient discussed earlier in Figures 4-6 and 4-7.

The voice of the patient with cancer in Figure 4-20(b) is characterized by a strong instability, showing as multiple transitions during sustained

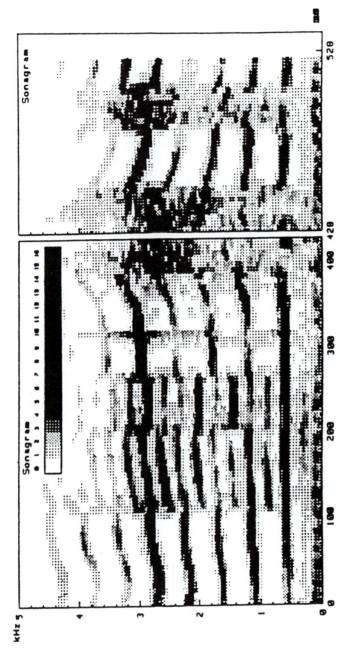

Figure 4-19. Spectrogram from a newborn infant cry. Subharmonics and chaotic episodes are clearly visible.

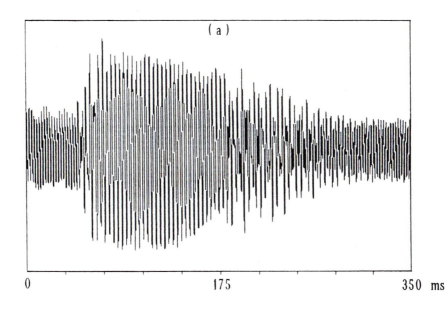

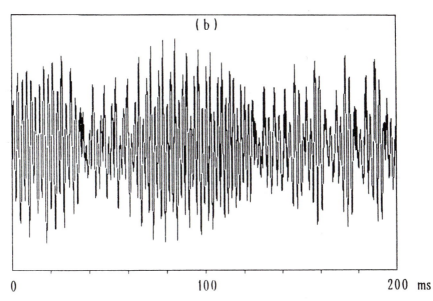

Figure 4-20. Acoustic waveforms from pathological voices displaying bifurcations (see text): (a) female voice, papillomas of the vocal folds (the same as in Figure 4-14(b); vowel "i"; and (b) male voice, with cancer of the vocal folds; vowel "e."

vowels. The displayed signal starts with fast oscillations, then switches to a subharmonic regime, and it ends up in a slowly modulated shape.

Generally, many of the observed transitions remind us of the bifurcations of coupled oscillators. Thus, the relevant problem is to identify the relevant oscillating modes which are desynchronized due to diseases.

CONCLUDING REMARKS

The purpose of this chapter was to demonstrate the existence of low-dimensional chaotic dynamics in phonation. Attractors and bifurcations were identified using methods from nonlinear dynamics and simulation models. Similar phenomena have been seen in earlier models of vocal fold vibrations (Ishizaka and Isshiki, 1976; Herzel et al., 1991).

Exploitation of these findings for clinical diagnosis is still a subject of future work. The estimation of attractor dimensions and Lyapunov exponents may be too complicated for clinical applications, but the presence of low-dimensional dynamics can also be detected by much simpler quantities. In contrast to random perturbations, toroidal and chaotic behavior are characterized by strong correlations over several pitch periods. Thus, previously introduced methods for correlating pitch periods and amplitudes (Koike, 1969; Imaizumi, 1986) might be useful. Fundamental frequency or amplitude contours are intimately related to Poincaré sections introduced in this paper. Such plots are quite easily obtained from voice records and give hints about the underlying attractor. We point out, however, that the widely used perturbation measures jitter, shimmer, or perturbation factor (Liebermann, 1963) are not appropriate for distinguishing chaos from random perturbations. They give only average deviations from a trend and are not sensitive to the salient patterns in the amplitude or F_o contour.

Summarizing, we emphasize that the understanding of pathological voices can benefit from the theory of nonlinear dynamics. Many observed phenomena can be understood as typical occurrences at the borderline of the 1:1 synchronization zone of oscillating modes. However, the precise identification of the essential modes and of the relevant nonlinearities is not yet clear. Specifically, a unification between analysis and synthesis must yet be achieved. A quantitative comparison of observed bifurcations and bifurcation diagrams from sophisticated models of vocal fold vibrations will, hopefully, give answers to the great variety of questions that still exist.

ACKNOWLEDGMENTS

This work was supported, in part, by grant Nos. R01-DC00387-06 and P60-DC00976-01 from the National Institute on Deafness and Other Communication Disorders.

DISCUSSION

Dr. Scherer: What criteria are used to determine when you have an adequate sampling to estimate a fractal dimension?

Dr. Baken: Unfortunately, to the best of my knowledge, there is no pat method for the minimal size of a valid sample of real-world time-series data. The number of points required depends on the nature of the data, and (at least for the variables that are likely to interest us) must be determined empirically. I provide an example in my *Journal of Voice* article (Baken, 1990).

Dr. Scherer: Are the phase plane portraits that you showed adequate for practical use (clinically or otherwise)?   *Dr. Baken:* Except in some trivial senses, not yet. My view is that it is far too early in our exploration of this theoretical framework to be thinking about practical applications.

Dr. Partridge: Regarding the issue of adequate sample and constant parameters, when we study chaos we presume sustained movement on a strange attractor, which in some sense has no information content. In neural function or speech transient conditions, do they carry the information of what these functions are about? Is chaotic behavior really relevant to function?

Dr. Baken: If it is true — as it certainly seems to be — that the phonatory signal is the product of a chaotic system, then we may generate a large number of novel hypotheses that go to the issue of why and how phonation may fail or become aberrant in pathological situations. In at least this sense, chaos theory is eminently relevant.

Dr. Alipour: Regarding partial fractals, can we say that fractal geometry in a complete mathematical sense may not be observed in nature, i.e., there may be repetitious patterns for limited times but not infinite times? Examples are leaves on tree or snowflake.

Dr. Baken: Fractal dimensionality was first extensively explored for mathematical functions—such as the Koch snowflake—whose fractal dimensions are exactly specifiable through analytic methods. It is certainly true that concrete structures or discrete time-series data suffer serious practical limits of scaling. I believe, however, that if our variables are chosen with reasonable care and if our data sets are critically examined before being subjected to the mysteries of our software, we will avoid significantly compromising the validity of our estimates of fractal dimension.

Dr. Fujimura: Nonlinearity is a necessary but not sufficient condition for chaos. A perfectly periodic oscillation is commonly observed in electronic oscillations, which must be nonlinear in order to sustain steady oscillation.

Dr. Titze: This is correct. Nevertheless, we look for nonlinearity and asynchronization of coupled oscillators as primary explanations for *potential* chaos.

Dr. Shadle: In addition to the studies reported of normal and pathological adults uttering vowels, have you observed or considered observing normal adults doing other phonatory tasks, such as shouting, singing (by trained singers), or crying? In which of these tasks would you expect to see chaotic behavior? Finally, I would assume that trained singers learn to avoid chaotic behavior. Is this true, and if so, is it because they stay well away from the "boundaries," or because they extend those boundaries through training?

Dr. Titze: Your comments and observations are very insightful. We should (and will) study vocalizations such as crying, shouting, laughing, etc. I believe that when the system is driven to its boundaries (large intensity, extremely high or low pitch) the nonlinearities become more important and chaos is more likely to occur. This has already been shown by Pabon and Plomp (1988) with a voice range profile. Phonation at the extremes of the intensity and F_o ranges was less stable than phonation near the middle. Singers usually claim that they have a practice range and a performance range, the latter being smaller to avoid breakdowns near the extremes.

Drs. Davies and McGowan: Can you tell us more about the coupling between flow and force. These may be the two "stable" nonlinear components that when coupled create bifurcation.

Dr. Titze: By force you mean vocal fold driving force, I assume, which is related to the mean intraglottal pressure. Indeed, the flow entrains three oscillators: two vocal folds and a vocal tract. The stability of the fluid pressure against the wall, and hence the driving force, depends on how tightly these oscillators are coupled.

Dr. Partridge: Chaos is often described as an effect of a low order system, and statistical theory assumes combination of high dimensionality of elements. At what dimensionality level do we have a transition from chaotic to pseudo random? Is there any true randomness in nature?

Dr. Titze: Chaos can occur in both high-dimensional systems and low-dimensional systems. It's a matter of practicality to apply the detailed phase-plane analysis only to systems with a few degrees of freedom (or at least to those that have a few dominant modes). For example, reducing a three-dimensional phase space to two dimensions (by taking a section) is a significant reduction of complexity. On the contrary, reducing a 10-dimensional space to a 9-dimensional one does not help much. Thus, the transition you mention has less to do with the system, but more with conceptualization and convenience in analysis.

Dr. Partridge: Digital computation (mapping) introduces fine-grained chaos on top of a theoretical limit-cycle oscillation when modeled in a state variable form.

Dr. Titze: Yes, it does. This is why the limit cycles that we showed with the simulation model do have a finite width. It's a challenge to sort out the physical (deterministic) chaos from computational noise.

Dr. Hirano: The term CHAOS is new to us medical people. Physicians have empirically known that human beings are basically "chaotic." There should be some reasons why chaos has been booming up among voice scientists rather recently. Could any of you comment on this?

Dr. Titze: The recent burst of activity stems mainly from the fact that computers are now fast enough to allow us to simulate complex systems over long periods of time, a luxury we did not have before. One has to observe vocal fold vibration over many cycles, and over many parametric conditions, to make sense out of irregularity. Regular vibration can be understood by observing 2 or 3 cycles.

Dr. Baken: There are two other reasons that I believe are important in accounting for the seemingly sudden eruption of chaos theory in our field. The last several years have seen very rapid development of both theory and techniques for identifying and dealing with chaotic phenomena. Our tools are still very far from refined, but they have afforded us a glimpse of enormous possibilities for dealing with some hitherto intractable problems and for clarifying the currently inexplicable.

But perhaps an even more powerful impetus has been the fact that the theory of nonlinear dynamics has been very successful in promoting new points of view and generating novel hypotheses in several other branches of physiology that deal with oscillatory functions. Many of us have been convinced that there is much that this emerging science can offer us, too.

Dr. McGowan: You seem to be confident in your statement that chaos occurs in phonation. Please list the tests you apply.

Dr. Herzel: As we have shown, the time-series and spectrograms exhibit the characteristic features of nonlinear dynamics. Phase portraits and Poincaré sections are used to visualize the attractors. Moreover, dimensions and Lyapunov exponents are estimated. All these techniques indicate consistently the presence of low-dimensional chaos. However, it is impossible to prove the existence of chaos rigorously from experimental time-series.

Dr. McGowan: Do you see an asymptotic approach to a particular dimension as embedding dimension is increased?

Dr. Herzel: Testing the saturation of the estimated attractor dimension with increasing embedding dimension is an essential part of the algorithm. It is just the independence of the estimated value on the embedding parameters that distinguishes chaos from random processes.

Dr. Scherer: What do you think is going to be the physiological predictive power, rather than descriptive power, using chaotic techniques?

Dr. Herzel: A first step might be the selection of appropriate perturbation measures that are able to distinguish the various sources of irregularities. If we know, for example, the acoustic consequences of asymmetric vocal fold vibration, then we can hopefully exploit signal analysis inspired by chaos-theory for diagnostic purposes. However, quite a lot of work has to be done in that direction.

Dr. Titze: We need to solve the forward problem (physiology to acoustics) for isolated sources of irregularity before we can solve the inverse problem (acoustics to physiology) for combined sources in typical speech. By exploiting physical models, together with excised larynx models and human subjects, hopefully the sources of irregularity can be studied individually. We can then "tune" our detectors to look for specific patterns in speech.

Dr. Sataloff: A child's normal cry evokes a strong response regardless of education and culture. Your comments described chaotic signals mixed with non-chaotic segments in a child's cry, and absent in an adult cry. Teleologically, one must wonder why? Do you believe there is a difference in *perception* of chaotic stimuli? Perhaps they carry a code that evokes specific responses, especially if chaotic processes are operative in the brain, as suspected. Are you aware of anyone studying perception of chaotic stimuli?

Dr. Herzel: Chaos in newborn cries can clearly be perceived and evokes natural emotions. However, we interpret the occurrence of chaos mainly from the point of view of biomechanics. If newborns cry, for example, with extreme intensity they can reach the borderline of normal phonation, and therefore chaos might occur. Certainly, older speakers learn to control those phenomena.

EVIDENCE OF CHAOS IN VOCAL FOLD VIBRATION: RESPONSE

OSAMU FUJIMURA, Ph.D.

Voice source characteristics constitute one of the two physical aspects of the nature of speech, according to the standard acoustical theory of speech production. The other aspect involves the articulatory characteristics. With respect to the linguistic functions of speech, voice control, combined with temporal organization and vocalic modulation, constitutes the base function of the speech utterance. Superimposed upon this vocalic base function are consonantal gestures for syllable margins (Fujimura, 1992). Voice control plays a dual role in this picture of speech organization. One is modulation of the base function. In this respect, most phonetic concern traditionally has been limited to voice pitch control. There is an increasing interest, however, in the role of voice quality control. The other role of voice control is consonantal modulation. The primary aspect of this modulation, as far as vocal fold adjustment is concerned, is adduction-abduction.

The discussion of this chapter, from a linguistic/phonemic point of view, is most directly relevant to the first role, *i.e.*, base function control, implementing the so-called prosodic organization of speech. In particular, temporal change of timbre crucially depends on nonlinear dynamics. However, understanding the physical mechanism as discussed in this chapter, is also crucial for explaining how transitional phenomena around voice onset/offset occur in relation to consonantal perturbation. Many specific details of such transient phenomena, which are often considered *ad hoc* choices in individual languages, may well be explained parsimoniously according to basic general principles and a few language-dependent parameters, once the mechanism is correctly understood.

Pathological consideration receives an even more direct impact from this discussion. There, any serious deviation from periodicity of voice is a central issue. However, I would like to point out that this issue is in itself chaotic. Normal voice also is characterized by aperiodicity, and sometimes shows clear bifurcation such as switching to subharmonics. Whether it is considered normal or abnormal depends on the situation in which it occurs. When, for example, switching F_0 to an octave lower occurs toward the weakened end of an utterance in low pitch, it is perfectly normal. I will play a tape to demonstrate that, when it is a matter of discontinuously shifting from a fundamental frequency to its half or double value, the appearance or disappearance of subharmonics is perceived quite differently depending on the direction of the change. What is physically irregular is not necessarily perceptually irregular; as a matter of fact, irregularity may enhance normal voice quality (Fujimura, 1968).

Thus, the diagnostic evaluation of how irregular the vocal fold vibration is must be based also on the correct understanding of the chaotic situation and its phonetic significance. We have to understand why, under certain circumstances, such a phenomenon is disturbing, and is indicative of pathological conditions, while under other circumstances it does not matter perceptually, or even enhances naturalness and is normal. This issue is crucial also for designing, for example, an appropriate speech synthesis system that can handle various expressive features.

Pitch is usually considered a one-dimensional quantity. The concept of F_0 assumes inherently a perfect periodicity, and it is only an approximation to this concept that applies to real voice pitch. When the aperiodicity becomes serious, even the approximate validity of the concept falls apart: this is the situation we are dealing with here. Suppose we have two extreme conditions:

1. perfect periodicity: regular oscillation repeats the same waveform indefinitely. F_0 is well-defined, and the spectrum takes an infinitely sharp comb-like shape (harmonic structure).

2. total randomness: apparently there is no order in the observed phenomenon. Vocal folds flap around randomly, as far as we can interpret. No rules or equations can be found to describe or predict the time function (of *e.g.*, the position of a sample flesh point).

Voicing, normal or abnormal, is always somewhere in between. The question is whether we start with case (1), perfect periodicity, approaching reality by gradually introducing small perturbation of various sorts (call this approach A) or, we start from a general random situation (2), and introduce occasional and intermittent regularity into random phenomena (approach B). The approach of deterministic chaos (approach C) is neither A nor B. It is a generalization of A, not of B. That is, periodicity is described as a special case of C, which is a general deterministic situation. Therefore, C can handle a continuously varying degree of aperiodicity correctly, without "stretching" the theoretical limit of validity. The interesting point is, while the property of the system is continuously modified, the resultant phenomenon at some point shows an abrupt qualitative change. In other words, even though we may observe totally erratic jumps from time to time, in pitch, for example, as determined by a pitch detector, the underlying controlled or uncontrolled variables are only continuously changing.

This is not a new or unusual situation for those who have closely examined the situations of voicing onset/offset control. Laryngeal (or any other) control does not need any abrupt change in the motor control to cause sudden onset or offset of voicing. Such a situation represents some nonlinearity of the system involved. The vocal folds form a system which interacts with air flow and the oscillatory system contains many elements of nonlinearity, with respect to the relation between control variables and vibration parameters. As Ingo Titze suggested, even apparent linearity over a limited range of variable values can be a "coincidental" result of cancellation of two nonlinearities, and therefore the system may be inherently nonlinear and only deceptively linear. Generally, small perturbation of the system, part of which may be random, can cause large qualitative changes in the output.

Finally, I would like to emphasize the danger of blindly applying statistics to the data before we understand the governing principles. Statistics is generally capable of handling data produced by locally linear or nearly-linear systems. If the system is inherently and significantly nonlinear, it is advisable to apply some nonlinear transformation of data variables so that the new variables describe a system that linearly relates them to quantities that represent the underlying factors of interest. Then statistics can be applied effectively to those transformed variables. Often, though not necessarily, this nonlinear variable mapping amounts to inferring a set of underlying control variables. This is one of the reasons effective modeling of physical systems is important for speech research, whether dealing with the vocal folds or the articulatory system (Fujimura, 1990). Particularly when directly observable phenomena are chaotic, it is important to understand the nature of the process that relates the control variables to such observed irregularities. While the study of vocal fold vibration using chaos theory is only in its infancy, I think the serious effort along this direction is critically important for further progress of our research.

REFERENCES

Alipour-Haghighi, F., and Titze, I. (1985). Viscoelastic modeling of canine vocalis muscle in relaxation. *Journal of the Acoustical Society of America, 78(6),* 1939-1943.

Alipour-Haghighi, F., and Titze, I. (1990). Elastic models of vocal fold tissues. *Journal of the Acoustical Society of America* (in review).

Awrejcewicz, J. (1990). Bifurcation portrait of the human vocal cord oscillations. *Journal of Sound and Vibration, 136,* 151-156.

Baer, T. (1981a). Observation of vocal fold vibration: Measurements of excised larynges. In Stevens, K. N. and Hirano, M. (eds.) *Vocal Fold Physiology* (pp 119-133). Tokyo: University of Tokyo Press.

Baer, T. (1981b). Investigation of the phonatory mechanism. *ASHA Reports, 11,* 38-46.

Baken, R.J. (1991). Géométrie fractale et évaluation de la voix: Application préliminaire á la dysphonie. *Bull. d'Audiophonogie. Ann. Sc. Univ. Franche-Comté* 7(5-6), 731-749.

Baken, R.J. (1990). Irregularity of vocal period and amplitude: A first approach to the fractal analysis of voice. *Journal of Voice, 4,* 185-197.

Barnsley, M. (1988). *Fractals everywhere.* New York: Academic Press.

Bergé, P., Pomeau, Y. and Vidal, C. (1984). *Order within chaos. Towards a deterministic approach to turbulence.* John Wiley and Sons, New York.

Dolansky, L., Tjernlund, P. (1968). On certain irregularities of voiced-speech waveforms, *IEEE Trans. AU-16,* 51-56.

Eckmann, J.-P., Ruelle, D. (1985). Ergodic theory of chaotic and strange attractors, *Rev. Mod. Phys. 57,* 617-656.

Farmer, J.D. (1982). Dimension, fractal measures, and chaotic dynamics. In Haken, H. (ed.), *Evolution of Order and Chaos* (228-246). New York: Springer-Verlag.

Farmer, J.D., Ott, E., and Yorke, J.A. (1983). The dimension of chaotic attractors. *Physica, 7D,* 153-180.

Feigenbaum, M. (1983). Universal behavior in nonlinear systems, *Physica 7D,* 16-39.

Freeman, W.J. (1990). Searching for signal and noise in the chaos of brain waves. In Krasner, S. (ed.), *The ubiquity of chaos* (pp 47-55). Washington, D.C.: American Association for the Advancement of Science.

Froehling, H., Crutchfield, J.P., Farmer, J.D., Packard, and N.H., Shaw, S.H. (1981). On determining the dimension of chaotic flows. *Physica 3D,* 605-617.

Fujimura, O. (1968). An approximation to voice aperiodicity. *IEEE Trans. Audio Electroacoustics, AU-16,* 68-72.

Fujimura, O. (1990). Methods and goals of speech production research. *Language and Speech, 3(3),* 195-258.

Fujimura, O. (1992). Phonology and phonetics — a syllable-based model of artic-ulatory organization. *Journal of the Acoustical Society, Japan, (English) 13,* 39-48.

Glass, L. and Mackey, M.C. (1988). *From clocks to chaos.* Princeton, NJ: Princeton University Press.

Glass, L., Shrier, A. and Blair, J. (1986). Chaotic cardiac rhythms. In Holden, A. V. *Chaos* (pp 327-356). Princeton, NJ: Princeton University Press.

Goldberger, A. and Rigney, D.R. (1990). Sudden death is not chaos. In Krasner, S. (ed.), *The ubiquity of chaos.* Washington, D.C.: American Association for the Advancement of Science, 23-34.

Goldberger, A., West, B.J., and Bhargava, V. (1986). Nonlinear mechanisms in physiology and pathophysiology: Towards a dynamical theory of health and disease. In Eisenfeld, J. and Witten, M. (eds.), *Modelling of biomedical systems* (pp 227-233). The Hague: Elsevier.

Grassberger, P. (1986). Estimating the fractal dimensions and entropies of strange attractors. In Holden, A. V. *Chaos* (pp 291-311). Princeton, NJ: Princeton University Press.

Grassberger, P. and Proccaccia, I. (1983). Measuring the strangeness of strange attractors. *Physica 9D,* 189-208.

Herzel, H., Plath, P., Svensson, P. (1991). Experimental evidence of homoclinic chaos and type-II intermittency during the oxidation of methanol. *Physica, 48D,* 340-352.

Herzel, H., Steinecke, I., Mende, W., and Wermke, K. (1991). Chaos and bifurcations during voiced speech. In E. Mosekilde, (ed.), *Complexity, Chaos and Biological Evolution,* New York, NY: Plenum Press, 41-50.

Hirano, M. (1989). Objective evaluation of the human voice: Clinical aspects. *Folia Phoniatr. 41,* 89-144.

Hirano, M., Kurita, S., and Nakashima, T. (1983). Growth, development and aging of human vocal folds. In D. Bless and J. Abbs (eds.), *Vocal Fold Physiology: Contemporary Research and Clinical Issues,* (pp 22-43). San Diego, CA: College Hill Press.

Imaizumi, S. (1986). Acoustic measures of roughness in pathological voice, *Journal of Phonetics 14,* 457-462.

Ishizaka, K., Isshiki, N. (1976). Computer simulation of pathological vocal-cord vibration, *Journal of the Acoustical Society of America, 60,* 1193-1198.

Ishizaka, K. and Matsudaira, M. (1972). Fluid mechanical considerations of vocal cord vibration. *SCRL Monograph 8,* Santa Barbara, CA, Speech Communication Research Laboratory.

Kahane, J.C. (1983). A survey of age-related changes in the connective tissues of the human adult larynx. In D. Bless and J. Abbs (eds.), *Vocal Fold Physiology: Contemporary Research and Clinical Issues,* (pp 44-49). San Diego, CA: College Hill Press.

Kelman, A.W. (1981). Vibratory pattern of the vocal folds, *Folia Phoniatrica, 33,* 73-99.

Koike, Y. (1969). Vowel amplitude modulations in patients with laryngeal diseases, *Journal of the Acoustical Society of America, 45,* 839-844.

Liebermann, P. (1963). Some acoustic measures of the fundamental periodicity of normal and pathological larynges, *Journal of the Acoustical Society of America, 35,* 344-353.

Mackey, M.C. and Glass, L. (1977). Oscillation and chaos in physiological control systems. *Science, 197,* 287-289.

Mandelbrot, B. (1967). How long is the coast of Britain: Statistical self-similarity and fractional dimension. *Science, 156,* 636-638.

May, R.M. (1974). Biological populations with nonoverlapping generations: Stable points, stable cycles, and chaos. *Science, 186,* 645-647.

May, R.M. (1976). Simple mathematical models with very complicated dynamics. *Nature, 261,* 459-467.

May, R.M. (1980). Nonlinear phenomena in ecology and epidemiology. *Annals of the New York Academy of Sciences, 357,* 267-281.

Mayer-Kress, G. (Ed.) (1986). *Dimensions and entropies in chaotic systems,* Berlin: Springer-Verlag.

Mende, W., Herzel, H., Wermke, K. (1990). Bifurcations and chaos in newborn cries. *Phys. Lett. 145 A,* 418-424.

Monsen, R.B. (1979). Acoustic qualities of phonation in young hearing-impaired children. *Journal of Speech and Hearing Research 22,* 270-288.

Moon, F.C. (1987). *Chaotic vibrations: An introduction for applied scientists and engineers.* New York: Wiley.

Pabon, J.P.H. and Plomp, R. (1972). Automatic phonetogram recording supplemented with acoustical voice quality parameters. *Journal of Speech and Hearing Research, 31,* 710-722.

Pickover, C.A. and Khorsani, A. (1986). Fractal characterizations of speech waveform graphs. *Computers and Graphics, 10,* 51-61.

Poincaré, H. (1881). Mémoire sur les courbes définies par une équation différentielle. *Journal de Mathématique, 3e sér., 7,* 375-422.

Poincaré, H. (1882). Mémoire sur les courbes définies par une équation différentielle. *Journal de Mathématique, 3e sér., 8,* 251-296.

Poincaré, H. (1885). Sur les courbes définies par les équations différentielles. *Journal de Mathématiques Pures et Appliquées, 4e sér. 1,* 167-244.

Rapp, P.E., Bashore, T.R., Zimmerman, I.D., Martinerie, J.M., Albano, A.M., and Mees, A.I. (1990). Dynamical characterization of brain electrical activity. In Krasner, S. (ed.), *The ubiquity of chaos* (pp 10-22). Washington, D.C.: American Association for the Advancement of Science.

Rasband, S.N. (1990). *Chaotic dynamics of nonlinear systems.* New York: Wiley.

Samar, V.J. and Rosenberg, S. (1990). A technique for the extraction of chaotic attractors from evoked response data: Toward the discovery of event related chaotic potentials. Presentation at the meeting of TENNET (Theoretical and Experimental Neuropsychology-Neuropsychologie Expérimentale et Théorique).

Sundberg, J., Scherer, R., and Titze, I. (in press). Phonatory control in male singing: A study of the effects of subglottal pressure, fundamental frequency, and mode of phonation on the voice source. *Journal of Voice.*

Thompson, J.M.T. and Stewart, H.B. (1986). *Nonlinear dynamics and chaos.* New York: Wiley.

Titze, I.R. (1988). The physics of small-amplitude oscillation of the vocal folds. *Journal of the Acoustical Society of America, 83(4),* 1536-1552.

Titze, I.R. (1989). On the relation between subglottal pressure and fundamental frequency in phonation. *Journal of the Acoustical Society of America, 85(2),* 901-906.

Titze, I.R. (1991). A model for neurologic sources of aperiodicity in vocal fold vibration. *Journal of Speech and Hearing Research, 34,* 460-472.

Titze, I.R., and Sundberg, J. (1992). Vocal intensity in speakers and singers. *Journal of the Acoustical Society of America, 91(5),* 2936-2946.

Titze, I.R. and Alipour, F. (in review). Three source models for voice synthesis. *Journal of the Acoustical Society of America.*

van de Water, W., Schram, P. (1988). Generalized dimension from near-neighbor information. *Physical Review A, 37,* 3118-3125.

Wendler, J., Rauhut, A., and Krüger, H. (1986). Classification of voice qualities. *Journal of Phonetics, 14,* 485-488.

Wolf, A., Swift, J.B., Swinney, H.L., and Vastano, J.A. (1985). Determining Lyapunov exponents from a time-series. *Physica, 16D,* 285-317.

Wong, D., Ito, M.R., Cox, N.B., and Titze, I.R. (1991). Observation of perturbations in a lumped-element model of the vocal folds with application to some pathological cases. *Journal of the Acoustical Society of America, 89,* 383-394.

AMERICAN
SPEECH-LANGUAGE-
HEARING
ASSOCIATION

Journal of Speech and Hearing Research, Volume 37, 1008–1019, October 1994

Analysis of Vocal Disorders With Methods From Nonlinear Dynamics

Hanspeter Herzel
Technical University
Berlin, Germany

David Berry
Ingo R. Titze
Department of Speech Pathology and
Audiology
National Center for Voice and Speech
The University of Iowa
Iowa City

Marwa Saleh
Ain Shams University, Egypt

Several authors have recently demonstrated the intimate relationship between nonlinear dynamics and observations in vocal fold vibration (Herzel, 1993; Mende, Herzel, & Wermke, 1990; Titze, Baken, & Herzel, 1993). The aim of this paper is to analyze vocal disorders from a nonlinear dynamics point of view. Basic concepts and analysis techniques from nonlinear dynamics are reviewed and related to voice. The voices of several patients with vocal disorders are analyzed using traditional voice analysis techniques and methods from nonlinear dynamics. The two methods are shown to complement each other in many ways. Likely physiological mechanisms of the observed nonlinear phenomena are presented, and it is shown how much of the terminology in the literature describing rough voice can be unified within the framework of nonlinear dynamics.

KEY WORDS: vocal disorders, nonlinear dynamics, voice analysis, bifurcations

Beginning with Lorenz (1963), researchers from many disciplines have observed that complex, unpredictable signals may be generated by low-dimensional, deterministic systems (systems with no random components, e.g., systems whose time-varying history is completely specified by initial conditions and applicable dynamical laws). One might ask, "What can be unpredictable about a completely deterministic system?" The answer is: If the system is nonlinear, errors in measuring the initial state of a system may grow exponentially in time. When this occurs, only a small uncertainty in measuring the initial state of a system may soon result in near total uncertainty about the state of the system. Thus, nothing short of infinite precision in measuring initial conditions (which is not possible) would allow prediction of future events in the long term.

Systems that are both deterministic and unpredictable are said to be "chaotic." To exhibit chaos, a deterministic system must include some type of nonlinearity and must possess several degrees of freedom (i.e., must occupy at least three dimensions in *phase space*, a concept to be introduced shortly). In practice, nonlinear systems are much more common than linear ones, and most systems have at least several degrees of freedom. Consequently, a great variety of systems are potentially chaotic.

In our own field, many studies are beginning to suggest that *some* of the complexities observed in rough, disordered voices are not caused by random external input to the vocal apparatus, but by the intrinsic nonlinear dynamics of vocal fold movement. Given the nonlinearities associated with the laryngeal source (e.g., the nonlinear pressure-flow relation in the glottis, the nonlinear stress-strain curves of vocal fold tissues, or the nonlinearities associated with vocal fold collision), this should not come as a great surprise. Even the simplest models of the vocal folds incorporate nonlinearities (Ishizaka & Flanagan, 1972). Indeed, low-dimensional chaos has been observed in a wide variety of vocal fold models (Awrejcewicz, 1990; Herzel, 1993; Herzel, Steinecke, Mende, & Wermke, 1991; Titze, Baken, & Herzel, 1993; Wong, Ito, Cox, & Titze, 1991). Furthermore, the acoustical analysis of many types of rough voice (e.g., creaky voice, vocal fry, vocal disorders, and newborn infant cries) has

0022-4685/94/3705-1008

been shown to be consistent with output from a low-dimensional dynamical system (Herzel & Wendler, 1991; Mende, Herzel, & Wermke, 1990; Titze et al., 1993).

Such observations are exciting because they lend hope that, eventually, many of the complex and unpredictable vibration patterns associated with laryngeal pathology may be explained and conceptualized in terms of a low-dimensional, nonlinear laryngeal model. Ideally, such a model could be designed to simulate both normal and pathological phonation.

Apart from simulation, insights into vocal dynamics may also be gained by employing a nonlinear dynamics perspective in the *analysis* of voice signals. The primary aim of this paper is to present simple techniques (i.e., techniques accessible to virtually any voice researcher) to identify hints of nonlinear dynamics in voice signals. First, a brief introduction to chaos theory is given to motivate the analysis techniques. Next, the techniques are presented and demonstrated on our own collection of pathological voices. Although the techniques overlap considerably with traditional methods of voice analysis, the key is to use existing techniques, as well as some new ones, cued for the great variety of outputs that are possible from a nonlinear (and potentially chaotic) system. Then, within the context of chaos theory, an attempt is made to clarify and standardize some of the terms that have been used to describe rough, disordered voices in the literature. Finally, possible physiological mechanisms of rough voice are discussed, as well as future directions of research.

Basic Concepts From Nonlinear Dynamics

In this section, we give a brief introduction to a few of the basic concepts prerequisite to an understanding of the results in the next sections. A more detailed introduction to the theory of nonlinear dynamics as applied to phonation can be found in a chapter of a recent book (Titze, 1993). Also, the texts by Bergé, Pomeau, & Vidal (1986), Holden (1986), and Glass & Mackey (1988) are recommended.

In biomechanical modeling of sustained phonation, the elongations of the vocal folds and the glottal airflow are the key variables. Muscle tension and subglottal pressure are often taken as constant parameters. In the space of these variables, nonlinear phenomena have been studied recently (Berry, Herzel, Titze, & Krischer, in press; Herzel et al., 1991; Steinecke & Herzel, 1994). Unfortunately, in human phonations these variables and parameters are not directly measurable. We will illustrate that valuable information can be extracted from a single time series, such as the acoustic signal of a sustained vowel.

Phase Space

Conventional time-series analysis is carried out either in the time domain or the frequency domain. Nonlinear dynamics is based on an embedding of the time series in a "phase space." The most convenient way to embed the series is to introduce delay-coordinates:

$$x(t) = \{x(t), x(t + \tau),\ldots, x[t + (m - 1)\tau]\}. \qquad (1)$$

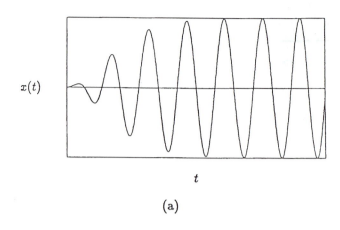

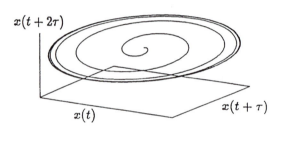

FIGURE 1. An example of the embedding of a time series (a) into phase space (b). In this case, the resultant attractor in (b) is a limit cycle.

With these coordinates, a scalar time series, x(t), generates an orbit in an *m*-dimensional phase space. Obviously, the choice of the delay time τ and of the embedding dimension *m* introduces some arbitrariness. However, several features of the dynamics are essentially independent of the specific embedding parameters. Figure 1 illustrates the embedding of a time series into a three-dimensional phase space ($m = 3$).

Attractors

If the external parameters of a dissipative dynamical system are held constant, the orbit in phase space approaches an asymptotic regime after a transient response. The geometrical object in phase space corresponding to the asymptotic regime is termed an attractor. In Figure 1, for example, the attractor is a closed curve, or a "limit cycle." The spiraling into the limit cycle corresponds to the initial transient. Attractors can be classified as follows: (a) stable stationary states; (b) limit cycles (periodic oscillations as in Figure 1); (c) tori (superposition of two or more oscillations with no rationally dependent frequencies); and (d) chaotic attractors (nonperiodic behavior).

1010 *Journal of Speech and Hearing Research*　　　　　　　37　1008–1019　October 1994

It has been recognized in the last two decades that complicated nonperiodic oscillations ("chaos") can occur in nonlinear systems without any random perturbations. Thus, the discovery of "deterministic chaos" provides a new approach for understanding irregular observations.

Bifurcations

Up to now we have assumed fixed parametric conditions. If parameters of the dynamical system such as muscle tension are varied, qualitative changes of the attractors might appear. Such transitions are termed *bifurcations*. An example is the onset of self-sustained oscillations due to increasing subglottal pressure (see, e.g., Titze, 1988). Such a transition from a steady state (resting fold) to periodic oscillations (phonation) is a manifestation of a "Hopf bifurcation."

For simplicity, we assume here that normal phonation corresponds to a limit cycle and we do not discuss at this point the omnipresent small deviations from periodicity of a normal healthy voice (jitter and shimmer on the order of a percent). Whether or not physiological jitter and shimmer may be regarded as additive noise or as manifestations of an underlying dynamical system, is certainly of interest (Titze, 1991), but we focus in our paper on large deviations from periodicity. Then, the question arises whether or not observed sudden transitions from periodicity to other regimes can be interpreted in terms of bifurcations of a limit cycle.

The most important bifurcations are period-doublings and secondary Hopf bifurcations. In the first case, a new limit cycle with roughly double the original period becomes stable (i.e., in the time domain we may observe an alternation of large and small amplitudes or periods). In the spectral domain one would observe the appearance of subharmonics of the original F_o (fundamental frequency).

A secondary Hopf bifurcation corresponds to a modulation of the signal with another independent frequency (i.e., a torus appears in phase space). It will be shown in this paper that indications of these bifurcations can be found in pathological voices. Another frequently observed bifurcation is the sudden jump from the original limit cycle to another limit cycle with another period and amplitude. Different attractors may coexist in nonlinear systems and, therefore, even extremely tiny changes of parameters (e.g., muscle tension) may lead to abrupt jumps to other regimes.

The theory of nonlinear dynamics predicts that period-doublings, bifurcations, tori, and coexisting limit cycles are often accompanied by "deterministic chaos." Thus, the detection of bifurcations in voice signals supports the idea that some of the irregularities in vocal disorders are manifestations of chaotic dynamics.

Voice Samples

Our study is based on the analysis of 95 dysphonic patients with various pathologies. The patients can be grouped as follows (Saleh, 1991):

1. *Dysphonia with minimal associated pathological lesions*:

Nodules	14 patients
Polyps	8 patients
Cysts	5 patients
Reinke's edema	8 patients

2. *Organic dysphonia*:

Paralysis	16 patients
Neoplastic dysphonia	8 patients

3. *Functional dysphonia*:

Phonasthenia	11 patients
Hypofunctional dysphonia	4 patients
Hyperfunctional dysphonia	11 patients
Hyperfunctional childhood dysphonia	6 patients
Mutational voice disorders	4 patients

For each patient, three utterances of the sustained vowel "a" have been digitally recorded at a sampling rate of 20 kHz and a resolution of 16 bits (Saleh, 1991). The aim of our study was not a detailed and comprehensive analysis of all these cases, but a first estimation of the relevance of the discussed nonlinear phenomena. Moreover, we wanted to test what measures are appropriate for an analysis of bifurcations and chaos.

In about one fourth of the patients, we found indications of attractors and bifurcations. These phenomena were found in patients from all three groups discussed above. In a previous study (Herzel & Wendler, 1991) bifurcations and chaos were detected in about one half of the patients. In that case, all patients had very hoarse voices. In the present analysis, the voice quality ranged from normal to severely hoarse; therefore, the frequency of occurrence of nonlinear phenomena was somewhat less in this data set. We underscore that not all hoarse voices can be interpreted in terms of low-dimensional dynamics. In severely breathy voices, for example, there are manifestations of large amounts of turbulence; many phonations are too unstable to allow for detection of attractors.

Methods

In this section, we briefly describe the techniques used to detect and quantify the nonlinear phenomena. The applicability of the methods is exemplified using characteristic recordings of a few samples of pathological voices.

Perceptual Evaluation

Perceptual evaluation provides the first clues as to whether or not nonlinear phenomena are present in the voice signals. For example, episodes of subharmonic vocalization are perceived as intermittent roughness. If subharmonic components or modulation frequencies are sufficiently low (below about 70 Hz), the acoustic signal is often perceived as vocal fry phonation. Although vocal fry is considered linguistically normal (Hollien & Michel, 1968), fry is often symptomatic in voice pathology (Scherer, 1989; Titze, 1989). Indeed, episodes of low-frequency modulations have been found in several of our recordings.

According to the theory of psychoacoustics (Zwicker & Fastl, 1990), modulations around 70 Hz lead to the perception of roughness. Consequently, our observations of subharmonic vocalizations, low-frequency modulations, and chaos are intimately related to rough voice quality since

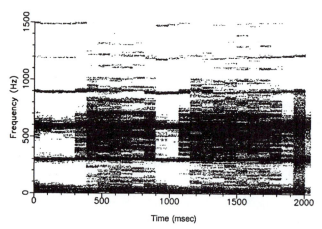

FIGURE 2. Narrow-band computer spectrogram for a patient with a hyperfunctional childhood disorder. Abrupt transitions to subharmonics are visible. Note, especially, the subharmonic corresponding to period-tripling from 300–800 msec and from 1200–1800 msec. In several instances, a low-frequency modulation around 20 Hz also appears.

these phenomena typically lead to an increased amount of low-frequency components.

Spectrographic Displays

Besides listening, inspection of acoustic waveforms, EGG signals, and spectrograms are helpful for the detection of bifurcations and chaos. Subharmonics, biphonation (i.e., two independent frequencies), and chaotic segments have been effectively identified using narrow-band spectrograms (Kel-

man, 1981; Mende et al., 1990; Robb & Saxman, 1988; Sirviö & Michelsson, 1976).

Figure 2 shows abrupt transitions to subharmonic regimes spectrographically, which can be interpreted as bifurcations. The patient (with a hyperfunctional childhood disorder) has a characteristic fundamental frequency around 300 Hz; however, a strong subharmonic appears between 300 and 800 msec, which corresponds to a period-tripling. Although the relative energy of the signal around 100 Hz is so low that it cannot be seen on the spectrogram, the spacing of the harmonics reveals that the subharmonic is, indeed, present. Between 1200 and 1800 msec, the subharmonic appears again. Moreover, low-frequency modulations around 20 Hz are noticeable.

Waveform Displays

An acoustic waveform displaying sudden onsets of deep amplitude modulation is shown in Figure 3. Such transitions resemble secondary Hopf bifurcation, that is, the appearance of a superimposed frequency. The figure displays 1000 msec of an utterance from a patient with unilateral recurrent nerve paralysis. Parts (a)–(e) are serial segments in time. Note that (b) and (d) show amplitude modulations, whereas (a), (c), and (d) look relatively normal. The example illustrates that one may classify instabilities in terms of a bifurcation theory, but no direct conclusions about the underlying mechanisms can be drawn. The modulations may result from either an instability in the biomechanical system or may be introduced by separate motor events.

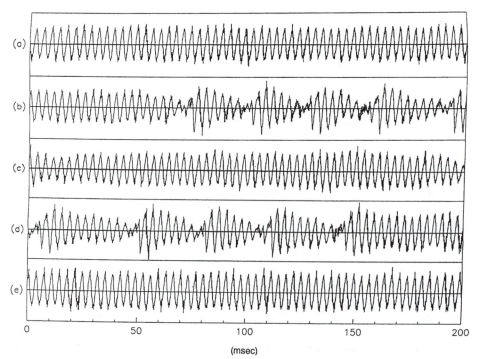

FIGURE 3. A 1000 msec utterance (with 200 msec per line) from a patient with laryngeal paralysis. Bifurcations to low-frequency modulations are shown in lines (b) and (d).

1012 *Journal of Speech and Hearing Research*   37   1008–1019   October 1994

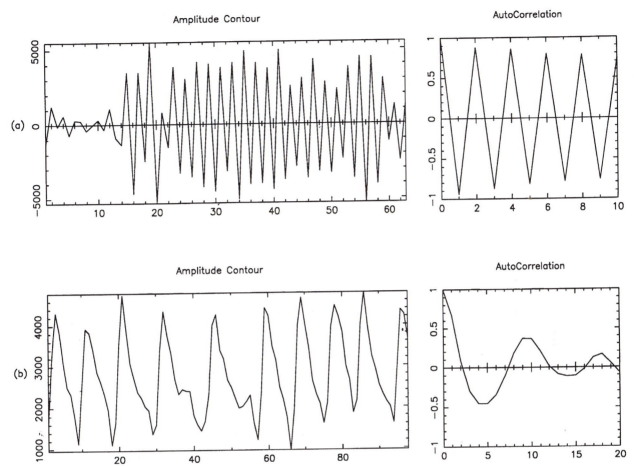

FIGURE 4. Amplitude contours (and corresponding autocorrelation functions) clearly illustrating (a) a period-doubling for a patient with nodules and (b) a low-frequency modulation around 30 Hz for a patient with paralytic dysphonia. The linear trend remover described in the text was applied to the contour in (a). Figure 4b is derived from another utterance of the speaker in Figure 3.

F_o and Amplitude Contours

Traditional perturbation analysis, based on the detection of fundamental frequency and amplitude, can be exploited for the characterization of nonlinear phenomena. In the first step, the acoustic (or EGG) signal is low-pass filtered with a cut-off frequency slightly above F_o (typically at 200 Hz for a male voice). The zero-crossings of the filtered signal are used to locate the approximate period boundaries. Based on these markers, the precise estimates for F_o are found from the unfiltered speech signal using a least mean squares or waveform matching technique (Milenkovic, 1987). Details concerning this algorithm and comparison to other algorithms can be found in Titze & Liang (1993). Since the cutoff frequency of the low-pass filter and the allowed range of the fundamental frequencies can be varied interactively, the algorithm provides the necessary flexibility and user-control for analyzing even severely hoarse voices. After extraction of the periods, the differences between the maximum and minimum value within each cycle are computed and referred to as amplitudes.

Figure 4 shows representative examples of the contours (left panels) and their corresponding autocorrelation functions (right panels) derived from patients with nodules and

paralysis. In Figure 4a, a period-doubling is clearly visible (note the alternating amplitudes starting around the 15th cycle of the contour), whereas Figure 4b shows a low-frequency modulation around 30 Hz, which was audible as vocal fry.

From the F_o and amplitude contours, various perturbation measures can be derived (Pinto & Titze, 1990). However, traditional jitter and shimmer analysis may have limited value for our purposes. In particular, some average perturbation measures cannot distinguish between short-correlated turbulent noise and modulations of the signal over several cycles. In order to detect such modulations, which are characteristic of subharmonic vocalization and biphonation, the autocorrelation function of the F_o (or amplitude) contour has proven useful. Autocorrelation functions of the contours have been used by others (Imaizumi, 1986; Koike, 1969) to describe rough voices.

If the cutoff frequency of the low-pass filter for F_o detection is above the normal fundamental frequency, period markers are set according to this characteristic frequency even if bifurcations do occur. Consequently, period doublings appear as alternating periods (or amplitudes), and modulations are seen as lower F_o and amplitude fluctuations.

Since voice signals exhibit common nonstationarities such as long-term trends and drifts, analysis of the F_o and amplitude contour is mostly based on second-order perturbation functions that measure the deviations from a linear trend (Pinto & Titze, 1990):

$$F_i = \frac{f_{i+1} + f_{i-1}}{2} - f_i \qquad (2)$$

$$A_i = \frac{a_{i+1} + a_{i-1}}{2} - a_i \qquad (3)$$

Here f_i (or a_i) denotes the i-th extracted frequency (or amplitude). Usually, the second order perturbation functions are more stationary than the original contours and contain, nevertheless, information on period-doublings, modulations, and so on.

Phase Portraits

If relatively stationary segments of the signal have been found, a more detailed analysis of the corresponding attractors is possible. A first step is the representation of the signal in a reconstructive phase space. For this purpose, delay-coordinates are useful (Equation 1).

For visualizing the attractor, embedding dimensions of $m = 2$ or $m = 3$ are appropriate. The delay-time τ is chosen as a fraction of the pitch period, which gives a proper representation of the attractor. Figure 5 shows some representative phase portraits. Figure 5a shows a limit cycle resulting from a sample of "normal" phonation. Figure 5b shows a more complicated attractor that takes the shape of a cylindrical surface. This relatively complicated attractor was found in a patient with laryngeal nerve paralysis (see also Figure 7 referring to the same patient).

Attractors can be characterized by discrete maps as well. For example, the intersections of orbits in phase space with a predefined plane (Poincaré plane) can be analyzed. If the attractor is a torus, such a Poincaré section yields a closed curve of intersection points (a torus is a two-dimensional manifold and, hence, its intersection with a Poincaré plane leads to a curve).

Next Amplitude or Next Period Maps

Similar to such Poincaré sections are next amplitude or next period maps. Such maps are easily derived from the F_o (or amplitude) contour. It has been exemplified that such maps give valuable information on the attractor (Lorenz, 1963; Titze et al., 1993). Next, amplitude (or period) maps can reveal additional dependencies in the contours that are not necessarily covered by the autocorrelation function that measures only linear correlations. An example of a next amplitude map, derived from the amplitude contour of Figure 4b (paralytic dysphonia), is shown in Figure 6.

Despite nonstationarities, the points shown in Figure 6 approximate a closed, ellipsoidal curve. This suggests that the corresponding attractor in phase space is a two-dimensional

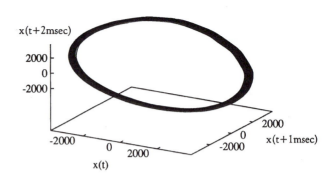

(a)

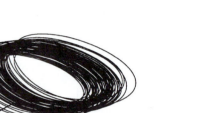

(b)

FIGURE 5. Phase portraits generated from (a) normal phonation and (b) a patient with laryngeal paralysis. The signals have been low-pass filtered slightly above the fundamental frequency.

torus, as might be expected assuming independence of the low-frequency modulation and the fundamental frequency.

Beside these methods to visualize the attractors, methods have been derived to describe the attractors quantitatively with fractal dimensions and Lyapunov exponents (Bergé et al., 1983; Eckmann & Ruelle, 1985; Holden, 1986; Mayer-Kress, 1986). It has been shown (Herzel & Wendler, 1991; Mende et al., 1990; Titze et al., 1993) that these techniques apply to sufficiently stationary phonatory signals. However, these relatively sophisticated methods are beyond the scope of this paper.

Analysis of Characteristic Voice Samples

In this section, sustained vowels of four patients are analyzed in detail in order to (a) provide further evidence of bifurcations and chaos in phonatory signals, and (b) illustrate the application of the techniques described above. First, vocalizations from a male patient with paralytic dysphonia, previously introduced in Figure 5b, are further analyzed. The voice sounded breathy and slightly rough. Figure 7a shows an unfiltered acoustic waveform with pronounced amplitude

1014 *Journal of Speech and Hearing Research*   *37* 1008–1019 October 1994

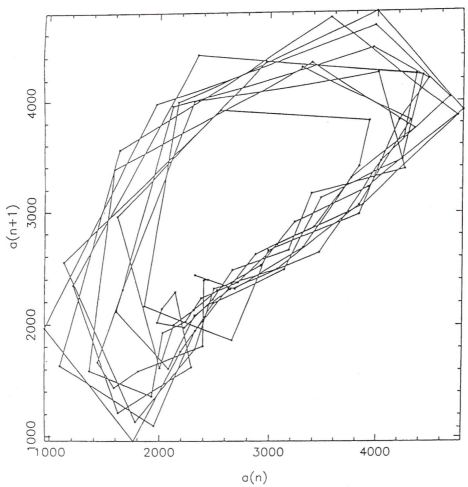

FIGURE 6. A next amplitude map that approximates a closed, ellipsoidal curve, suggesting that the corresponding attractor in phase space is a torus (i.e., there are two independent frequencies in the system).

fluctuations (shimmer around 5%). Subharmonics or bifurcations are not immediately visible. However, the amplitude contour, and especially the corresponding autocorrelation function in Figure 7b, indicate that the amplitude variations are not totally random.

This observation can be substantiated using next amplitude (period) maps (see Figure 7c). Due to noise and nonstationarities, the structure is not as obvious as in Figure 6. However, with enumeration of the points, a rotational motion becomes visible. The rotation angle is about 120°, which indicates that the dynamics is close to period-three motion. Indeed, period-three is also detected by the autocorrelation (Figure 7b, right panel).

Summarizing the above observations, we can conclude that the hoarseness of the patient is not only due to turbulent noise, but also due to complicated vibratory pattern of the folds related to period-tripling. The subharmonics are also clearly visible in the EGG records. This case demonstrates that often several sources of hoarseness superimpose on each other. Indications of period-doubling or tripling and of low-frequency modulations have also been found in the vocalizations of four other patients of paralytic dysphonia (see, e.g., Figures 3, 4b and 6). Moreover, from a total number of eight

cancer patients, we have found three with indications of bifurcations. However, these voices were relatively unstable and, therefore, a detailed quantitative analysis was difficult due to nonstationarity. A characteristic example of a vowel with various transitions is presented in Figure 8. There are low-frequency modulations as well as abrupt transitions to other regimes that might be related to bifurcations.

Even though Aronson, Peterson, and Litin (1964) have already mentioned diplophonia, low-pitched segments, and "intermittent squeaking noises" for functional voice disorders, these vocal disorders have been studied less extensively. Out of 36 speakers, we have found 6 with clear signs of bifurcations. As a first example, we discuss a voice with hyperfunctional childhood dysphonia. A spectrogram of the first utterance of this speaker was already shown in Figure 2. All three recorded utterances exhibit audible low-frequency episodes. Figure 9 displays a time series with various transitions. Again, amplitude and pitch contours are helpful tools for the analysis. Figure 10a is an amplitude contour showing a fairly strong period-tripling. Figure 10b shows the fundamental frequency contour near the end of an utterance, at which point a low-frequency modulation appears that was perceived as vocal fry.

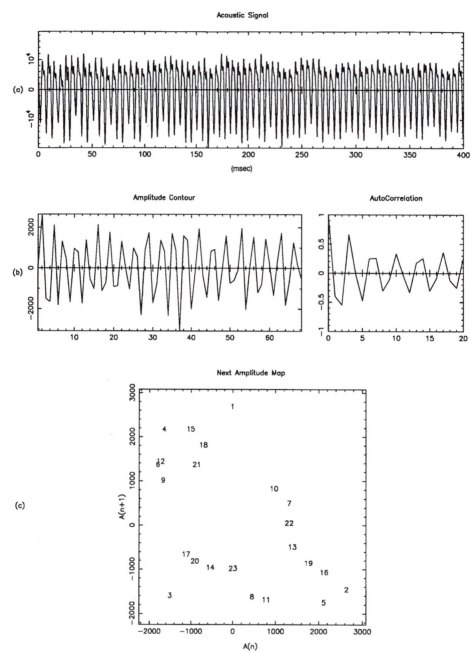

FIGURE 7. Displays of an (a) acoustic waveform, (b) amplitude contour and autocorrelation function, and (c) enumerated next-amplitude plot from a patient with paralytic dysphonia.

Finally, we present the voice of a male speaker with hyperfunctional dysphonia (Figure 11). The signal displays two interesting transitions. First, toward the end of line (c), a period-doubling is visible. Then, on line (d), an amplitude modulation of about 40 Hz is seen. Consequently, vocal fry episodes can be perceived. These bifurcations are also reflected in the corresponding amplitude contour. Similar transitions occur in a second utterance of the same speaker. The example in Figure 11 reflects a general observation that often several bifurcations occur within a single vocalization if the borderline of normal phonation is reached.

The phonatory signals analyzed in this section have illustrated that a variety of bifurcations are found in pathological

voices. Possible mechanisms leading to bifurcations and chaos will now be discussed.

Discussion

Chaos and bifurcations have been reported in many acoustic systems besides the voice. Examples are bubbles in water driven by a sound field (Lauterborn & Parlitz, 1988) and woodwind musical instruments (Keefe & Laden, 1991; Maganza & Caussé, 1986). But the vocal folds are particularly prone to chaotic behavior because of nonlinearities in airflow and tissue dynamics (Titze et al., 1993).

1016 *Journal of Speech and Hearing Research*
37   1008–1019   October 1994

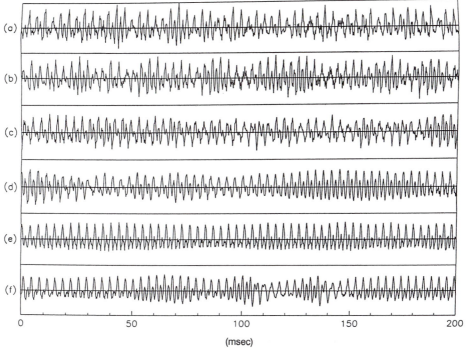

FIGURE 8. A characteristic utterance from a cancer patient showing beating-like segments and sudden jumps to other phonatory regimes.

Mechanisms

Qualitatively, the origin of bifurcations and low-dimensional attractors can be understood as follows: Normal phonation corresponds to an essentially synchronized motion of all vibratory modes. A change of parameters such as muscle tension or localized vocal fold lesions may lead to a desynchronization of certain modes resulting in bifurcations and chaos. The desynchronization of the following modes might be of particular relevance:

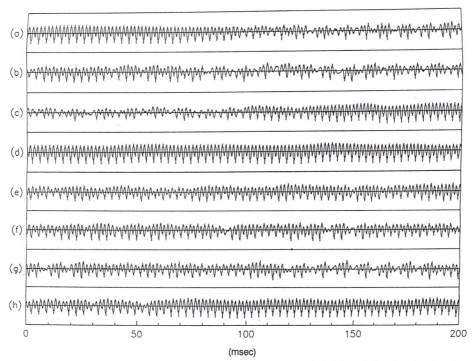

FIGURE 9. An utterance from a patient with hyperfunctional childhood dysphonia showing various transitions.

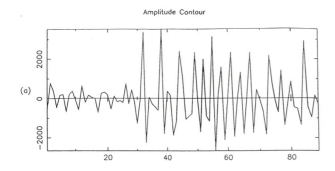

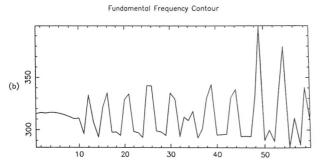

FIGURE 10. (a) A segment of an amplitude contour from a patient with hyperfunctional childhood dysphonia. A transition to a subharmonic regime close to period-tripling appears to be present, (b) a segment of a fundamental frequency contour for the same patient. An onset of a modulation is present that is perceived as vocal fry.

- desynchronized motion of the left and right vocal fold (e.g., for localized vocal fold lesions and unilateral paralysis);

- desynchronization of horizontal and vertical modes (such "symmetric chaos" might be relevant for an understanding of vocal fry phonation);
- interaction of the ventricular and vocal folds (e.g., for pressed voice);
- interaction of vocal fold vibrations with sub- and supraglottal acoustic resonances and vortices generated at the glottis.

Obviously, quite a lot of experimental and theoretical work is necessary to assign the various acoustic observations to these physiological mechanisms. However, nonlinear dynamics provides a framework to understand the underlying mechanisms. If low-dimensional attractors can be identified as the origin of a rough voice, then the phenomena are due to the nonlinear interaction of a few degrees of freedom. It is already known (Glass & Mackey, 1988; Titze et al., 1993) that period-doubling, frequency jumps, beating-like modulations, and chaos can be found in a system of two coupled oscillators. Thus, it makes sense to look for the specific modes that are desynchronized.

Moreover, vocal fry or simulated creaky voice might be a good starting point to understand the physiological mechanisms of complicated vocal fold vibrations. Simulations with a finite element model of the vocal folds (Titze & Alipour-Haghighi, in preparation) and a two-mass model (Herzel et al., 1991) suggest that vocal fry can be generated due to the desynchronization of the horizontal movement of the folds dictated by the body and the vertical motion that is very slow due to a lax cover. The computer simulations show strong correlations with the high-speed film observations of Moore and von Leden (1958). A detailed analysis of the computer

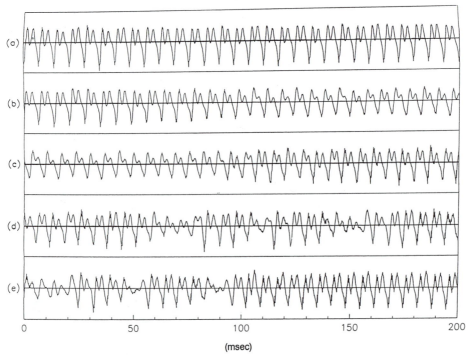

FIGURE 11. An acoustic waveform from a male speaker with hyperfunctional dysphonia showing two interesting transitions: a period-doubling toward the end of line (c), and an amplitude modulation of about 40 Hz on line (d).

1018 *Journal of Speech and Hearing Research*

37 1008–1019 October 1994

simulations in terms of bifurcations and chaos is given in Berry, Herzel, Titze, & Krischer (in press).

Terminology

In the literature, a rich variety of terms is used to describe nonlinear phenomena. Among them are dicrotic dysphonia, diplophonia, creaky voice, subharmonic vocalization, double harmonic break, biphonation, octave jump, and noise concentrations. We review several of the observations in the literature indicating nonlinear phenomena in vocalizations.

"Diplophonia" and "dicrotic patterns of vocal fold vibrations" have been observed for several centuries (see Cooper, 1989). Quite similar findings have been reported for several decades in newborn cry studies based on sound-spectrographic investigations (Sirviö & Michelsson, 1976). In cry analysis, "double harmonic break" refers to the sudden appearance of subharmonics, "biphonation" describes two independent pitches, and "noise concentrations" probably correspond to chaotic episodes (Mende et al., 1990; Sirviö & Michelsson, 1976). Period-doublings and biphonation also appear in noncry vocalizations of young children (Robb & Saxman, 1988).

Occasionally, irregularities are also observed in normal healthy voices (Dolansky & Tjernlund, 1968; Klatt & Klatt, 1990; Moore & von Leden, 1958). In particular, some vocal fry phonation is characterized by glottal pulses of alternating amplitudes or by irregular trains of pulses (Hollien & Michel, 1968; Scherer, 1989).

Several authors report the appearance of subharmonics in cases of unilateral or localized vocal fold lesions. Periodicities of 2–12 pitch periods are found by Koike (1969) for patients with laryngeal neoplasms. For a female speaker with papilloma, period-doubling was termed "zig-zag sections in the fundamental frequency curve" (Askenfelt & Hammarberg, 1986). In a recent paper, subharmonics have been identified for patients with cysts and nodules (Remacle & Trigoux, 1991).

Clear indications of bifurcations and chaos can be found also in studies on unilateral laryngeal nerve paralysis (Fritzell, Gauffin, & Sundberg, 1986; Ishizaka & Isshiki, 1976; Ptok, Sesterhenn, & Arold, 1993; Smith, Berke, Gerratt, & Kreiman, 1992). In these cases, the desynchronization of the right and left vocal fold is presumably the origin of bifurcations.

Most neurobiological disorders of the larynx lead also to phonatory instabilities (Ramig & Scherer, 1991). Diplophonia has been reported for patients with Shy-Drager Syndrome (Ludlow, Coulter, & Gentages, 1983) and spasmodic dysphonia (Titze et al., 1993). In a study by Wieser (1981) octave jumps, two pitches, and noise segments are already considered as characteristics of spastic dysphonia. Sudden drops in fundamental frequency of approximately one octave are found in patients with Huntington's Disease and also for individuals at risk for this disease (Ramig, Scherer, Titze, & Ringel, 1988).

Sometimes, authors assign different meanings to various terms describing rough voices. For example, diplophonia is often used to describe alternating amplitudes of glottal pulses, whereas in other instances it is used to denote the appearance of two fundamental frequencies. Thus, an important contribution of nonlinear systems theory might be a well-defined terminology to classify the observations.

According to nonlinear systems theory, stationary deterministic signals can be assigned to three attractor types: limit cycle (periodic), torus (two or more independent frequencies), or chaotic attractors (nonperiodic). Sudden transitions due to parameter changes can be interpreted as bifurcations. For example, an octave jump is related to a period-doubling bifurcation and the appearance of a modulation might be a manifestation of a secondary Hopf bifurcation.

Summary

Our study was devoted to specific features of voice signals, such as sudden frequency jumps, appearance of a second frequency and noisy episodes. It was discussed that these phenomena can be identified in various kinds of voice disorders, but can also appear in normal healthy voices and in children's vocalizations. Nonlinear dynamics provides an approach to understand these features in a unified manner.

Chaos theory guided our choice of analysis procedures. In addition to conventional time and frequency domain techniques, the embedding of a time series in a reconstructed phase space often yielded new information and insight. Attractors were also visualized with phase portraits and next period (amplitude) maps. For example, modulations (i.e., tori in our terminology) were detected as rotational motion in next-amplitude plots. A more sophisticated attractor analysis would involve the estimation of dimensions and Lyapunov exponents (Titze et al., 1993). However, these techniques would require relatively long, stationary time series, which are often not available.

Much information was obtained from conventional F_o and amplitude contours and their corresponding autocorrelation functions. In these plots, period-doublings appeared as zig-zag sections and low-frequency modulations were easy to visualize. Sometimes it was desirable to remove long-term trends by taking the second derivative of the contours.

We claim that the nonlinear dynamics approach offers new ways of understanding certain features of voice signals. Various observations can be interpreted from a physical perspective. Sources of irregularity can often be traced back to the desynchronization of principal vibratory modes.

Acknowledgments

This work was supported by Grant No. P60 00976 from the National Institute on Deafness and Other Communication Disorders. We gratefully acknowledge Julie Lemke for manuscript preparation.

References

Aronson, A., Peterson, H., Jr., & Litin, E. (1964). Voice symptomatology in functional dysphonia and aphonia. *Journal of Speech and Hearing Disorders, 4,* 367–381.

Askenfelt, A. G., & Hammarberg, B. (1986). Speech waveform perturbation analysis: A perceptual-acoustical comparison of seven measures. *Journal of Speech and Hearing Research, 29,* 50–64.

Awrejcewicz, J. (1990). Bifurcation portrait of human vocal cord oscillations. *Journal of Sound and Vibration, 136,* 151–156.

Bergé, P., Pomeau, Y., & Vidal, C. (1986). *Order within chaos.* New York: Wiley.

Berry, D., Herzel, H., Titze, I., & Krischer, K. (in press). Interpretation of biomechanical simulations of normal and chaotic vocal fold oscillations with empirical eigenfunctions. *Journal of the Acoustical Society of America.*

Cooper, D. S. (1989). Voice: A historical perspective. *Journal of Voice, 3,* 187–203.

Dolansky, L., & Tjernlund, P. (1968). On certain irregularities of voiced speech waveforms. *IEEE Trans. AU-16,* 51–56.

Eckmann, J.-P., & Ruelle, D. (1985). Ergodic theory of chaos and strange attractors. *Reviews of Modern Physics, 57,* 617–656.

Glass, L., & Mackey, M. (1988). *From clocks to chaos.* Princeton: University Press.

Hammarberg, B., Fritzell, B., Gauffin, J., & Sundberg, J. (1986). Acoustic and perceptual analysis of vocal dysfunction. *Journal of Phonetics, 14,* 533–547.

Herzel, H. (1993). Bifurcations and chaos in voice signals. *Applied Mechanics Review, 46,* 399–413.

Herzel, H., & Wendler, J. (1991). Evidence of chaos in phonatory samples. *Proceedings of EUROSPEECH,* Genova.

Herzel, H., Steinecke, I., Mende, W., & Wermke, K. (1991). Chaos and bifurcations during voiced speech. In E. Mosekilde & L. Mosekilde (Eds.), *Complexity, chaos and biological evolution* (pp. 41–50). New York: Plenum Press.

Holden, A. V. (Ed.) (1986). *Chaos.* Manchester: University Press.

Hollien, H., & Michel, J. (1968). Vocal fry as a phonational register. *Journal of Speech and Hearing Research, 11,* 600–604.

Imaizumi, S. (1986). Acoustic measures of roughness in pathological voice. *Journal of Phonetics, 14,* 457–462.

Ishizaka, K., & Flanagan, J. L. (1972). Synthesis of voiced sounds from a two-mass model of the vocal cords. *Bell System Technology Journal, 51,* 1233–1268.

Ishizaka, K., & Isshiki, N. (1976). Computer simulation of pathological vocal-cord vibration. *Journal of the Acoustical Society of America, 60,* 1193–1198.

Keefe, D. H., & Laden, B. (1991). Correlation dimension of woodwind multiphonic tones. *Journal of the Acoustical Society of America, 90,* 1754–1765.

Kelman, A. W. (1981). Vibratory pattern of the vocal folds. *Folia Phoniatrica, 33,* 73–99.

Klatt, D. H., & Klatt, L. C. (1990). Analysis, synthesis, and perception of voice quality vibrations among female and male talkers. *Journal of the Acoustical Society of America, 87,* 820–841.

Koike, Y. (1969). Amplitude modulations in patients with laryngeal diseases. *Journal of the Acoustical Society of America, 45,* 839–844.

Lauterborn, W., & Parlitz, U. (1988). Methods of chaos physics and their application to acoustics. *Journal of the Acoustical Society of America, 84,* 1975–1993.

Lorenz, E. N. (1963). Deterministic nonperiodic flow. *Journal of Atmospherical Sciences, 20,* 130–141.

Ludlow, C., Coulter, D., & Gentages, F. (1983). The differential sensitivity of frequency perturbation to laryngeal neoplasms and neuropathologies. In D. Bless & J. Abbs (Eds.), *Vocal fold physiology: Contemporary research and clinical issues* (pp. 381–392). San Diego: College Hill Press.

Maganza, C., & Caussé, R. (1986). Bifurcations, period doublings and chaos on clarinet-like systems. *Europhysics Letters, 1,* 295–302.

Mayer-Kress, G. (1986). *Dimensions and Entropies in Chaotic Systems.* Berlin: Springer.

Mende, W., Herzel, H., & Wermke, K. (1990). Bifurcations and chaos in newborn infant cries. *Physics Letters A 145,* 418–424.

Milenkovic, P. (1987). Least mean square measures of voice perturbation. *Journal of Speech and Hearing Research, 30,* 529–538.

Moore, G., & van Leden, H. (1958). Dynamic variation of the vibratory pattern in the normal larynx. *Folia Phoniatrica, 10,* 205–238.

Pinto, N. B., & Titze, I. R. (1990). Unification of perturbation measures in speech signals. *Journal of the Acoustical Society of America, 87,* 1278–1289.

Ptok, M., Sesterhenn, G., & Arold, R. (1993). Bewertung der laryngealen Klanggeneration mit der FFT-Analyse der glottischen Impedanz bei Patienten mit Rekurrensparese. *Folia Phoniatrica, 45,* 182–198.

Ramig, L. O., & Scherer, R. C. (1991). Speech therapy for neurological disorders of the larynx. *NCVS Report 1,* 167–190.

Ramig, L. A., Scherer, R. C., Titze, I. R., & Ringel, S. P. (1988). Acoustic analysis of voices of patients with neurologic disease: A rationale and preliminary data. *Annals of Otology, Rhinology and Laryngology, 97,* 164–172.

Remacle, M., & Trigoux, I. (1991). Characteristics of nodules through the high-resolution frequency analyzer. *Folia Phoniatrica, 43,* 53–59.

Robb, L., & Saxman, J. (1988). Acoustic observations in young children's noncry vocalizations. *Journal of the Acoustical Society of America, 83,* 1876–1882.

Saleh, M. M. H. (1991). *Acoustic Analysis of Voice in Certain Types of Dysphonia.* Unpublished doctoral dissertation. Ain Shams University, Egypt.

Scherer, R. (1989). Physiology of creaky voice and vocal fry. *Journal of the Acoustical Society of America, 86* (S1), S25(A).

Sirviö, P., & Michelsson, K. (1976). Sound-spectrographic cry analysis of normal and abnormal newborn infants. *Folia Phoniatrica, 28,* 161–173.

Smith, M. E., Berke, G. S., Gerratt, B. R., & Kreiman, J. (1992). Laryngeal paralysis: Theoretical considerations and effects on laryngeal vibration. *Journal of Speech and Hearing Research, 35,* 545–554.

Steinecke, I., & Herzel, H. (1994). *Bifurcations in an asymmetric vocal fold model.* Manuscript submitted for publication.

Titze, I. (1991). A model of neurologic sources of aperiodicities in vocal fold vibration. *Journal of Speech and Hearing Research, 34,* 460–472.

Titze, I., Baken, R., & Herzel, H. (1993). Evidence of chaos in vocal fold vibration. In I. Titze (Ed.), *Vocal fold physiology: New frontiers in basic science* (pp. 143–188). San Diego: Singular Publishing Group.

Titze, I. R. (1988). The physics of small-amplitude oscillation of the vocal folds. *Journal of the Acoustical Society of America, 83,* 1536–1552.

Titze, I. R. (1989). Acoustics of creaky voice. *Journal of the Acoustical Society of America, 86* (S1), S26(A).

Titze, I. R. (Ed.) (1993). *Vocal fold physiology: New frontiers in basic science.* San Diego: Singular Publishing Group.

Titze, I. R., & Alipour-Haghighi, F. (in preparation). *The Myoelastic-aerodynamic theory of phonation.*

Titze, I. R., & Liang, H. (1993). Comparison of F_o extraction methods for high precision voice perturbation measurements. *Journal of Speech and Hearing Research, 36,* 1120–1133.

Wieser, M. (1981). Periodendaueranalyse bei spastischen Dysphonien. *Folia Phoniatrica, 33,* 314–324.

Wong, D., Ito, M. R., Cox, N. B., & Titze, I. R. (1991). Observation of perturbation in a lumped-element model of the vocal fold with application to some pathological cases. *Journal of the Acoustical Society of America, 89,* 383–394.

Zwicker, E., & Fastl, H. (1990). *Psychoacoustics.* Berlin: Springer.

Received October 25, 1992
Accepted March 30, 1994

Contact author: Ingo Titze, PhD, Department of Speech Pathology and National Center for Voice and Speech, the University of Iowa, 330 SHC, Iowa City 52242-1012, E-mail: ingo-titze@uiowa.edu

Bifurcations and chaos in voice signals

Hanspeter Herzel

Institute of Theoretical Physics, Humboldt University, Invalidenstraße 42,
O-1040 Berlin, Germany

The basic physical mechanisms of speech production is described. A rich variety of bifurcations and episodes of irregular behaviour are observed. Poincaré sections and the analysis of the underlying attractor suggest that these noise-like episodes are low-dimensional deterministic chaos. Possible implications for the very early diagnosis of brain disorder are discussed.

1. INTRODUCTION

Speech research is a wide field finding many important applications. The theory of speech production is, for example, of considerable interest in speech synthesis and recognition, in voice pathology, and the performing arts (see Fant: 1960, Flanagan: 1972, Titze: 1992).

Using parametrized models of voice sources and linear filter theory to model the vocal tract, certain aspects of speech synthesis have been treated relatively succesfully. However, at the borderline of normal speech various observations of complicated nonlinear phenomena are documented, and only very recently bifurcation theory has been applied to those phenomena. The aim of this paper is to give a review over various observations of bifurcations and chaos in cries of newborns, normal speech and, pariculary, voice pathology. Furthermore, bifurcations in biomechanical models of speech production are discussed.

The basic physical mechanisms of speech production are sketched in the next section. Section 3 to 6 are devoted to the analysis of phonatory records using methods from nonlinear dynamics. The biomechanical and aerodynamical modeling of phonation is discussedin section 7. Then, a two-mass model is studied in some detail in sections 8 and 9. Several open questions concerning the physiological mechanisms of bifurcations are formulated in the discussion. Moreover, the clinical relevance of nonlinear dynamics for diagnosis and treatment of voice disorders is discussed.

2. MECHANISMS OF SPEECH PRODUCTION

The generation of speech is characterized by the combined action of respiration, phonation and articulation. The driving force is the air flow, typically from the lungs via the bronchi and trachea. Voiceless signals like, e.g., fricatives are produced if the Reynolds number at a constriction of the vocal apparatus exceeds a critical value of about 1700 (Catford: 1977). The resulting acoustic noise is characterized by a relatively flat power spectrum centered approximately at $\omega = 0.2 \cdot U \cdot A^{-3/2}$ (Sorokin: 1985). Here U denotes the volume velocity of the flow and A is the cross-sectional area of the constriction.

The generated turbulent noise is quite irregular, reflecting the high dimensionality of developed turbulence. By contrast, voiced sound is much more regular. According to the accepted myoelastic theory of voice production, the vocal folds are set in vibration by the combined effects of the subglottal pressure, the elastic properties of the folds, and the Bernoulli effect. The air passing into the vocal tract is usually in the form of discrete puffs (see Fig.1.b). The effective length, mass and tension of the vocal folds are determined by muscle action, and in this way the fundamental frequency F_0 ("pitch") and the glottal waveform can be controlled.

The pitch of an adult voice is typically between 100 Hz and 300 Hz (female voice 200-300 Hz, male voice: 100-150 Hz). A more detailed discussion of the mechanisms of phonation can be found in section 7 in connection with modeling.

The vocal tract acts as a filter which transforms the generated primary signals into meaningful speech (Helmholtz: 1870). The order of magnitude of the resonance frequencies of the tract is easily obtained from the characteristic length of the tract of 17.5 cm and the speed of sound (350 ms^{-1}). The resonance frequencies, termed formants, range from 250 Hz to 3500 Hz. The lower formants F_1 and F_2 determine the vowel, and the higher formants characterize the speaker.

The main sources of dissipation in the vocal tract are viscosity, friction, vibrating walls and radiation, leading to a bandwith of the formants of 50 to 200 Hz.

part of "Chaos and noise in dynamic systems" edited by T Kapitaniak and J Brindley
Appl Mech Rev vol 46, no 7, July 1993

ASME Reprint No AMR130 $59

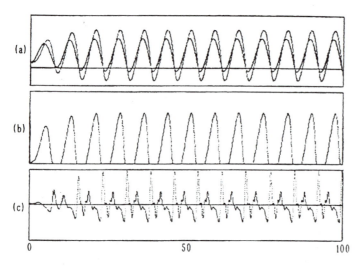

FIG.1 Simulation of voiced sound generation:
(a) Elongation of the lower and upper parts of the vocal folds
(b) Volume velocity at the glottis
(c) Mouth sound pressure

1990) for details. Fig.2 displays a computer spectrogram of the vowel "a" (all vowels are spoken according to German pronunciation rules). The fundamental frequency of about 200 Hz together with its harmonics is clearly visible. The fourth and fifth harmonics are particularly intense since the main formants of the vowel "a" are located around 1 kHz.

It can be seen from Fig.2 that phonatory records might be relatively stationary over about 100 ms. Thus, an attractor analysis during these stationary episodes makes sense. For example, the periodic signal in Fig.2 corresponds to a limit cycle in a corresponding phase space. The attractor analysis of more complicated phonatory records will be given below.

Fig.1 illustrates the production of voiced sound. The data are obtained from the integration of a two-mass model of the vocal folds together with a two-tube approximation of the vocal tract see (Herzel et al.: 1991a) for details.

Since the human auditive system is adapted to resolve many details of the frequency composition of speech (the frequency resolution of the ear is better then one percent) it is appropriate to analyze the generation of sound also in the frequency domain. The discrete puffs of air at the glottis generate a nearly periodic signal with intense harmonic components. This primary signal is modified by the characteristics of the vocal tract and by radiation.

A powerful technique for the analysis of the resulting acoustic signal are sonagrams or computer spectrograms. They are based on many subsequent short-time power spectra of overlapping segments, see (Mende et al.:

3. BIFURCATIONS IN NEWBORN INFANT CRIES

The acoustic properties of newborn cries are comparable to sustained vowels of adults as e.g., shown in Fig.2. Both sustained vowel phonation and neonatal cries serve to minimize the variation in vocal fold state. Therefore, these vocalizations are well suited for comparative studies.

Mainly due to the small size of the vocal apparatus (tract length of about 7 cm), the frequencies are shifted to higher values. The fundamental frequencies are distributed around the "concert pitch" of 440 Hz, and the main resonances of the tract lie typically between 2 kHz and 3 kHz.

A review on early sound-spectrographic investigations of newborn cries is given in the paper by Sirvio and Michelsson (Sirvio and Michelsson: 1976). These authors describe several phenomena which are clearly manifestations of bifurcations and chaos: Their term "double harmonic break" refers to the sudden appearance of subharmonics, and "biphonation" describes two independent fundamental frequencies. "Furcation" denotes in their vocabulary a split in the fundamental frequency. Moreover, "noise concentrations" are mentioned, corres-ponding probably to chaotic episodes. A schematic drawing of such sound-spectrographic observations is given in Fig.3.

It is reported (Sirviö and Michelsson: 1976, Michelsson et al.: 1984) that double harmonic breaks are fairly common in cries of healthy infants. Contrarily, biphonation, furcation and noise concentration are seldom in normal crying, but appear frequently in cries of infants with diseases affecting the central nervous system.

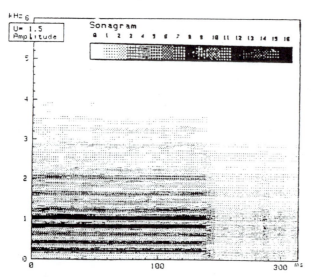

FIG.2 Spectrogram of a sustained vowel "a" (all spectrograms in this paper by courtessy of Werner Mende)

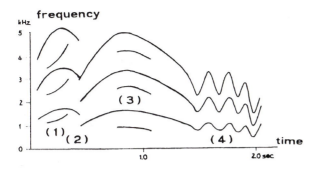

FIG.3 Sketch of a cry-spectrogram with biphonation (1), pitch shift (2), double harmonic break (3), and vibrato (4) (after Sirvio and Michelsson 1976)

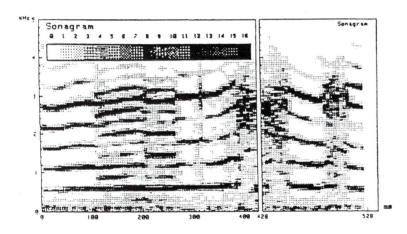

FIG.4 Computer spectrogram of a newborn cry with subharmonic episodes and chaotic segments (after Mende et al. 1990)

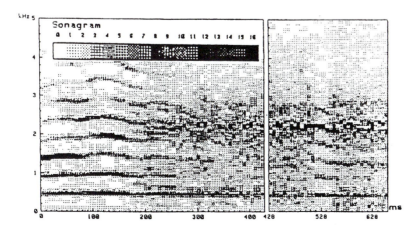

FIG.5 Spectrogram from a healthy newborn (after Mende et al.1990)

It is remarkable that Sirvi and Michelsson were able to relate specific diseases to certain spectrographic features. For instance, furcations occur in newborn cries with jaundice, and noise concentrations have been found in infants with brain infections caused by herpes virus. Biphonation was common in infants with brain damages due to severe oxygen deficiencies, meningitis or hydrocephalus.

It is impressively demonstrated in the book of Hirschberg and Szende (Hirschberg and Szende: 1985) that the majority of infant pathologies lead to characteristic abnormalities of cries.

Thus, an understanding of the various phenomena can provide a helpful noninvasive tool for early diagnosis. Only very recently the observed bifurcations have been interpreted in terms of chaos-theory (Mende et al.: 1990). Fig.4 shows a spectrogram of a premature newborn (28 weeks) with respiratory complications.

At the beginning only the fundamental frequency of about 500 Hz is present together with its pronounced harmonics. Then remarkably sharp transitions to more complicated states are visible. At first subharmonics and later on noise-like regions appear. Often, subharmonic bifurcations turn out to be precursors of noisy segments. In another sonagram (Wermke: 1987) successive period-triplings have been identified ahead of a noise-like region. The newborn cry displayed in Fig.5 exemplifies that also cries of healty full-term newborns may exhibit bifurcations and chaos.

The record in Fig.5 is relatively stationary and, therefore, it was possible to apply various techniques of nonlinear dynamics to this time-series (Mende et al.: 1990). Poincare sections and next-maximum maps from segments near the "window" around 530 ms display the deterministic character of the signal. Moreover, dimension analysis with the Grassberger-Procaccia algorithm and with near-neighbor statistics indicate a low-dimensional attractor (Mende et al.: 1990).

Summarizing this section we emphasize that bifurcations and chaos are quite common in vocalizations of newborn. This was already recognized in 1965 (of course, without refering to chaos-theory): "Perhaps equally as common as the simple 'basic cry' is the markedly complicated phonated egression ...." (from Lind: 1965). It is worth mentioning that also during non-cry vocalization of young children period-doubling and biphonation are normally occuring phonatory events (Robb and Saxmann: 1988). Particularly, speech of hearing-impaired children show often sudden appearance of

Appl Mech Rev vol 46, no 7, July 1993

subharmonics at one-half or one-third of the preceding frequency (Monsen: 1979).

We underline that bifurcations and chaos have been found in vocalization of healthy infants as well as in infant with several complications. However, the frequency of occurence and   specific features of the cries (e.g., biphonation) have diagnostic relevance (Michelsson et al.: 1984, Hirschberg and Szende: 1985). Newborn phonation is based on an already well-developed laryngeal coordination and, therefore, one can hope to detect even mild disturbances of brain functions in cry signals (Mende et al.: 1991, Herzel et al.: 1992).

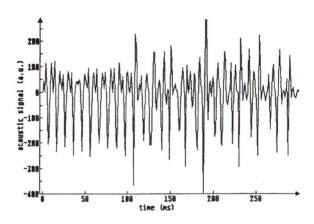

FIG.6 Transition from the sustained vowel "a" to vocal fry phonation

4. BIFURCATIONS DURING VOICED SPEECH

As shown in Figs.1 and 2 acoustic signals of sustained vowels are nearly periodic, although small perturbations are always present. This normal variability is relatively small (in the order of one percent) but it is nevertheless of importance for the naturalness of speech and may even provide diagnostic information for the recognition of brain functions (Mende et al.: 1991).

In the following large deviations from periodicity are discussed, audible for example as hoarseness.

Occasionally, also normal healthy voices exhibit irregularities (Moore and von Leden: 1958, Dolansky and Tjerlund: 1968). However, much more frequent and of immediate clinical   relevance are perturbations of pathological voices.

Various terms are used in the phonetic literature to describe voice perturbations: hoarseness, harshness, raucous voice, husky voice or creaky voice. Of particular interest are the notions of breathiness and roughness since they refer to the main sources of audible noise. Breathiness is intimately related to turbulent noise due to glottal leakage, whereas roughness is related to complicated vibratory pattern of the vocal folds. Thus, especially the understanding of rough voices should benefit from the theory of nonlinear dynamics.

As in the case of infants, the sudden appearance of subharmonics is a common phenomenon in voice records (Kelman: 1981, Klatt and Klatt: 1990). For newborns the term   "double harmonic   break" was designated for this observation. For adult voices terms as "vocal fry", "diplophonia", "dicrotic dysphonia", "creaky voice" or "subharmonic vocalization" describe such transitions to subharmonic regimes. Often, abrupt drops of the fundamental frequency to one-half ("octave jump") or one-third of the preceding frequency are observed (Bowler: 1964, Ramig et al.: 1988, Howard: 1989, Herzel et al.: 1991a).

Vocal fry ("Strohbass" in German) can be produced voluntarily at the lower end of the pitch range (below 100 Hz), and has been termed "vocal fry register" (Hollien and Michel: 1968). A characteristic feature of vocal fry phonation is the alternation of large and small glottal pulses. Fig.6 displays the transition to the vocal fry register for a normal healthy voice.

The observations of vocal fry and simulated creaky voice (Roch et al.: 1990) for healthy voices reveal that complicated pattern of vocal fold vibrations are not restricted to pathological voices. For normal voices they appear typically at the borderline of the voice range ("Stimmfeld").

Very early observations of diplophonia and other nonlinear phenomena are reviewed by Cooper (Cooper: 1989). Thus, Ferrein (Ferrein: 1746) describes "a tone different from the other one". Dicrotic patterns of vocal fold vibrations have also been discussed in the last century by Miller (Miller: 1837) and Rossbach (Rossbach: 1872).

Below, the implications of bifurcations and chaos for the diagnosis of pathological voices are discussed. At first, some few phonatory records are analyzed in detail with methods from nonlinear dynamics. Then, in section 6, the clinical importance of these finding are discussed.

The analysis in this section is based on hundreds of samples of normal and pathological voices recorded at our university hospital (Charit, Phoniatric Department of the ENT-Clinic). In previous studies, the vocalizations were characterized using spectral analysis and perceptual classification (Wendler et al.: 1986).

Acoustic signals of sustained vowels at comfortable pitch are digitized with a sampling rate of 20 kHz and with 12 bit resolution. Each vowel was classified according to the degree of hoarseness (H), roughness (R) and breathiness (B). A four point grading was applied with 0 indicating normality, 1 slight, 2 moderate and 3 extreme deviations.

Up to now signals from 22 patients with strong hoarseness (H3) have been analyzed from the point of view of chaos-theory. In about one half of these phonatory records indications of bifurcations or low-dimensional attractors have been found (subharmonics, toroidal oscillations, ...). Thus, the examples in the following figures are by no means exceptional recordings.

Even during sustained vowels, slightly varying parameters as muscle tension or subglottal pressure may induce qualitative changes of the signal. Transitions as in Fig.7 can be regarded as manifestations of bifurcations of the underlying dynamical system. The record in Fig.7.a displays a transition from a state with a pitch period of about 2.3 ms to a "subharmonic regime" with nearly the double period and

Appl Mech Rev vol 46, no 7, July 1993

large amplitudes. Such "octave jumps" are observed quite commonly and can be interpreted qualitatively as jumps from normal synchronized vibrations of the vocal folds to another limit cycle with the double period.

The backward transition to a high-pitched regime occurs via an episode of nonperiodic oscillations (from 180 to 280 ms) which might be related to a chaotic transient.

The voice of the patient with cancer of the vocal folds (Fig.7.b) is characterized by strong instabilities. The displayed signal starts with fast oscillations, then it switches to a subharmonic regime and it ends up in a slowly modulated shape.

At the moment, we do not understand the whole "zoo" of observed bifurcations. Many of the transitions remind us of the bifurcations of coupled oscillators (jumps to other resonance zones, beating-like behavior at the borderline of Arnold tongues, etc.).

Indeed, in the case of the female voice in Fig.7.a and Fig.8.b the desynchronization of the left and right vocal fold seems to be the underlying mechanism of the bifurcations since large papillomas of the left fold are visible. Such asymmetric vibrations could be verified by videolaryngostroboscopy (Herzel and Wendler: 1991).

The interpretation of the observations in terms of coupled oscillators will be continued in the discussion.

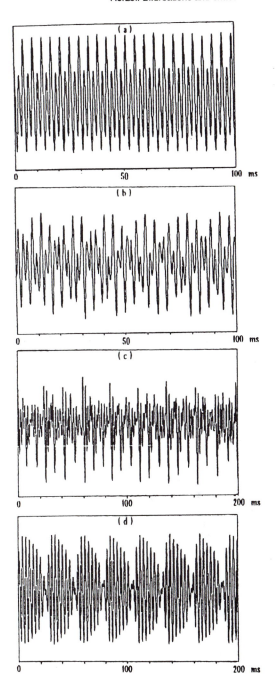

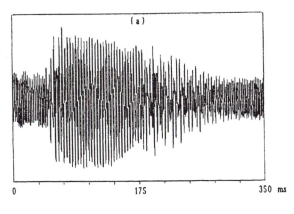

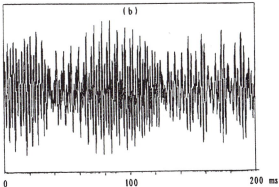

FIG.7 Acoustic waveforms from pathological voices displaying bifurcations:
a) female, papillomas of the vocal folds vowel "i", perceptual evaluation:
H3, R2, B3
b) male, cancer of the vocal folds vowel "e", H3, R2, B2

FIG.8 Acoustic waveforms of sustained vowels
(a) normal female voice,
    vowel "i", H0, R0, B0
(b) female voice, papillomas ofthe vocal folds,
    vowel "u", H3, R2, B3 (same patient in Fig.7.a),
(c) female voice, polyposis of the vocal folds,
    vowel "i", H3, R3, B0
(d) male voice, papillomas of the vocal folds,
    vowel "u", H3, R3, B1

5. ATTRACTOR ANALYSIS OF PHONATORY RECORDS

Vocal fold vibrations are very fast compared to most of the regulatory mechanisms. Consequently, one can find segments of phonatory records with relatively constant parameters as muscle tension and subglottal pressure. Fig.8 shows such relatively stationary signals together with the diseases and the results of perceptual evaluation. The normal voice in Fig.8.a is taken for comparison.

In the following, methods from nonlinear dynamics are applied to the signals in Fig.8.

In order to analyze attractor properties, measured signals have to be projected into a suitable phase space. Even from a single time-series $x(t)$, a phase space can be constructed as follows (Froehling et al.: 1981):

$$\bar{x}(t) = \{x(t), x(t+\tau), x(t+2\tau), ..., x(t+(m-1)\tau)\}. \quad (1)$$

Thus, a point in the reconstructed phase space is given by m "delay-coordinates". The selection of the delay-time τ and the embedding dimension m is somewhat arbitrary, but attractor dimensions and Lyapunov exponents should not depend on τ and m, provided that m is sufficiently large see (Eckmann and Ruelle: 1985) for a review of these problems).

A variation of the embedding parameter can serve, therefore, as consistency test of the algorithms discussed below. Phase portraits from the phonatory signals are shown in Fig.9. The periodic signal of the normal voice corresponds to a limit cycle with two loops, and the nonperiodic signal leads to a more complicated attractor.

Several techniques have been developed for the estimation of attractor dimensions from measured data. The most popular method is based on the correlation integral $C(\epsilon)$:

$$C(\epsilon) \sim \sum_{i,j} \Theta(\epsilon - \|\bar{x}_i - \bar{x}_j\|) \sim \epsilon^{D_2} \quad (2)$$

The double sum counts simply the number of distances between attractor points less then ϵ. The maximum

norm is used in our implementation of the algorithm. Moreover, we take care that the difference $|i-j|$ is sufficiently large such that $\bar{x}$ and $\bar{x}$ can be considered as uncorrelated in the time-domain see (Theiler: 1986) for a discussion of this point.

If the correlation integral $C(\epsilon)$ scales as ϵ^D the value D_2 can be taken as an estimation of the correlation dimension (Grassberger and Procaccia: 1983). An estimate of D_2 can be obtained from the slopes of log-log plots of the correlation integral $C(\epsilon)$ versus the length scale ϵ. In the case of a low-dimensional attractor a scaling region with a constant slope D_2 is expected (see Fig.10).

The dotted curves in Fig.10 refer to another method for the estimation of dimensions which is related to near-neighbor statistics (van de Water and Schram: 1988). If $r_k(\bar{x}_i)$ denotes the distance between an attractor point $\bar{x}_i$ and its k-th nearest neigbor, then the average distance depends on k as follows

$$\langle r_k(\bar{x}_i)\rangle \sim G(k,D) k^{1/D} \quad (3)$$

with

$$G(k,D) = \frac{\Gamma(k+1/D)}{\Gamma(k)}.$$

Again, the dimension D can be estimated from the slopes of the corresponding log-log plots. The prefactor $G(k,D)$ is close to unity and, therefore, a first guess of D can be obtained by setting $G(k,D)=1$. The resulting first estimation is improved iteratively.

The application of these techniques is demonstrated in Fig.10 for fixed delay-time τ and varying embedding dimension (other values of τ give comparable results). It can be seen that both methods give nearly identical slopes, leading to an estimation $D_2 \approx D \approx 2.6$, i.e., a chaotic attractor is indicated.

Now we turn to the estimation of the maximum Lyapunov exponent λ_1. Chaotic dynamics ($\lambda_1 > 0$) implies that adjacent trajectories in phase space diverge on the average exponentially with a rate λ_1. For the estimation of the exponent λ_1 an algorithm by Wolf et al. (Wolf et al.: 1985) is used in a modified version (Herzel et al.: 1991b).

The essence of the method is the analysis of the mean separation rate λ_1 of initially nearby points over an "evolution time" T, i.e., one looks whether or not the following linear growth can be found:

$$\left\langle \ln\frac{d(T)}{d(0)}\right\rangle \sim \lambda_1 T. \quad (4)$$

Here d(0) denotes the initial distance of attractor points. The averaging procedure ensures that only small distances are probed and that the separation along the most unstable direction is analyzed (see Wolf et al. 1985).

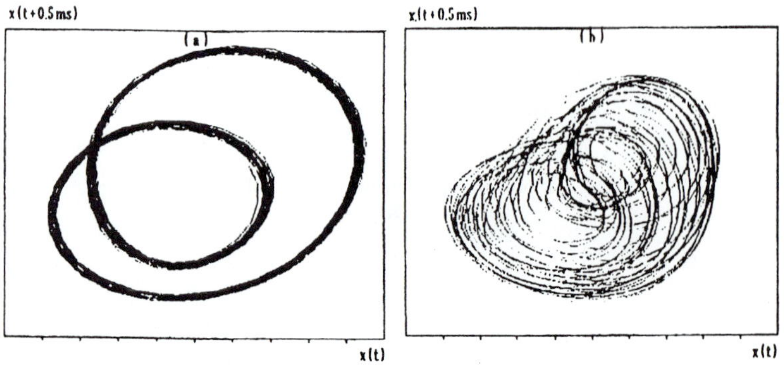

FIG.9 Projections of the records in Fig.8a and 8b in phase space

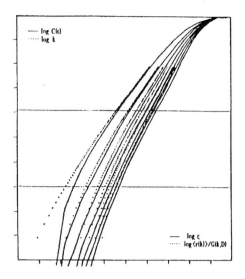

FIG.10 Log-log plot for the estimation of the attractor dimension of the record in Fig.8.b;
embedding dimension: $m = 2,3,...,8$ (from above)
delay-time: $\tau = 0.3$ ms;
full lines: correlation integral $C(\epsilon)$ versus lenght scale ϵ;
dotted: near-neighbor statistics (see eq(3)); the horizontal lines delimit the approximate scaling region leading to $D \approx 2.6$

An indication of chaos is found if there is a linear growth of $\langle \ln(d(T)/d(0) \rangle$ over a range of evolution times T. Moreover, one has to check that different embedding parameters τ and m lead to the same estimation of the exponent λ_I.

Fig.11 shows results of the produce explained above. The analysis of the normal voice is consistent with the expected value $\lambda_I = 0$, and the presumably chaotic time series of Fig.8.c leads to an estimation $\lambda I = 0.1$ ms^{-1}.

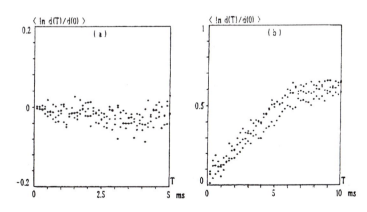

FIG.11 Average growth of the distance of initially nearby orbits with evolution time T. Three sets of embedding parameters are superimposed.
  (a) record from Fig.8a;
    $m = 6$ and $\tau = 0.3$ ms, $m = 6$ and $\tau = 0.5$ ms; $m = 4$ and $\tau = 0.5$ ms
  (b) record from Fig.8c; $m = 6$ and $\tau = 0.6$ ms,
    $m = 6$ and $\tau = 1$ ms; $m = 5$ and $\tau = 1$ ms

Summarizing this section, one can say that the records of pathological voices in Fig.8 are indeed manifestations of low-dimensional attractors.

However, keeping in mind the limited length and stationarity of the signals, the estimation of dimensions and Lyapunov exponents cannot be regarded as proofs of deterministic chaos. Nevertheless, the results of this section are consistent with our emphasized idea that low-dimensional dynamics plays an essential role in voice pathology. Moreover, it was demonstrated that the various techniques are applicable to phonatory signals.

6. IMPLICATIONS FOR THE DIAGNOSIS OF VOICE DISORDERS

There are many techniques to diagnose the various voice disorders as for example perceptual evaluation of the voice, laryngeal mirror examination, stroboscopy, electroglottography and electromyography (Hirano: 1989). During the last decades, the statistical analysis of the acoustic signals became a widely used method. Many acoustic characteristics of the voice have been exploited for diagnosis like, for instance, sound pressure level, pitch range, spectrum envelope, harmonics-to-noise ratio, long-time average spectra and pitch- or amplitude perturbations see (Eskenazi et al.: 1990, Pinto and Titze: 1990, Karnell et al.: 1991) for recent reviews).

Since the pioneering work of Liebermann (Liebermann: 1963), it is believed that appropriate perturbation measures provide significant information on pathologies. However, despite of an enormous effort on such studies, the discrimination of pathologies by acoustic parameters is still unsatisfactory. Even the correlation between the perceptual evaluation of experienced listeners to the acoustic quantities is still a subject of discussion (Arends et al.: 1990, Kreiman et al.: 1990).

One reason of the limited success of acoustic analysis is the inadequate understanding of the physiological sources of voice perturbations. Several sources of irregularities are mentioned in a recent paper (Titze et al.: 1992):
  - turbulence in the airstream
  - instability in the jet emerging from the glottis
  - unsteadiness in muscle contraction
  - mucus riding on the surface of vocal fold tissue
  - complicated vibratory pattern of the vocal folds (perhaps due to asymmetry in the folds, due to nonlinear tissue properties or due to coupling to the subglottal and supraglottal resonances).

Thus, the problem arises to find out the appropriate measures which are adapted to the specific mechanisms of voice perturbations.

Obviously, such widely used measures as the cycle-to-cycle fluctuations of period and amplitude (termed "jitter" and "shimmer") or the signal-to-noise ratio are of limited value since they are not able to discriminate the sources of irregularities. As suggested in the preceding

Appl Mech Rev vol 46, no 7, July 1993

sections bifurcations and chaos of vocal fold vibrations are quite common mechanisms of voice perturbations.

The estimation of attractor dimensions or Lyapunov exponents seems to be too complicated a tool for clinical practice.

However, hints of low-dimensional attractors can be detected by much simpler means. Nowadays, many standard programs for voice analysis compute pitch periods and maxima (or minima) within each glottal cycle. Consequently, plots of subsequent periods or amplitudes are easily obtained. Such next-period-maps or next-maximum-maps are topologically conjugate to Poincaré sections and, therefore, attractor structures can be identified in this way. Fig.12 exemplifies the applicability of these techniques.

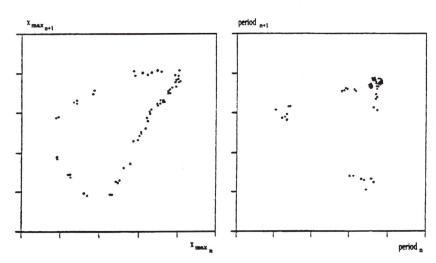

FIG.12 Autocorrelation functions from the sample in Fig.8.b
left: correlogram of the maxima
right: correlogram from the pitch periods (computed via parabolic interpolation of the maxima)

A related measure is the autocorrelation function of pitch periods or amplitudes. Turbulent noise is mainly characterized by short-correlated fluctuations, whereas low-dimensional attractors exhibit often correlations over several pitch periods. Fig.13 demonstrates the applicability of correlation functions.

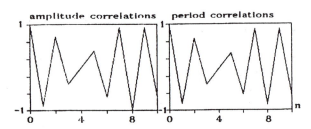

FIG.13 Plots of consecutive maxima (left) and periods (right) from the record in Fig.8.d

It is worth mentioning that such correlation functions have been used already successfully to detect laryngeal diseases (Koike: 1968), to measure roughness in pathological voices (Imazumi: 1986) and in synthetic speech (Hillenbrand: 1988).

A related measure in the spectral domain would be the intensity of subharmonics. It is well known that low-dimensional attractors exhibit often low-frequency components originating for example from period-doubling bifurcations or toroidal oscillations.

In the remainder of this section observations of bifurcations and chaos for specific voice disorders are reviewed.

In the case of bilateral diffuse lesions such as laryngitis, abnormalities of vocal fold vibrations are not very evident. Contrarily, unilateral or localized vocal fold lesions such as polyp, cyst, papilloma or glottic carcinoma are often associated with asymmetric and irregular vibrations (Isshiki et al.: 1966, Hirano: 1989). Several authors clearly demonstrate the appearance of subharmonics for these pathologies: (Koike: 1969) reports long periodicities of 2-12 fundamental periods for patients with laryngeal neoplasms. For a female speaker with papilloma period-doubling is termed "zig-zag sections in the fundamental frequency curve" by Askenfelt and Hammarberg (Askenfelt and Hammarberg: 1986).

In a recent paper, subharmonics have been identified for patients with cysts and nodules (Remacle and Trigoux: 1991).

Distinguishing laryngeal cancer from other laryngeal lesions would allow an earlier detection of cancer. It is known that the tissue in laryngeal cancer is harder, less elastic and more rough-surfaced than for example in polyps (Isshiki et al.: 1969, Hirano et al.: 1986). However, despite of several investigations no sufficient criteria have been developed to reliably discriminate different vocal fold lesions by means of acoustic measures (Hecker and Kreul: 1970, Iwata and von Leden: 1970, Murry and Doherty: 1980). Clear indications of bifurcations and chaos are described also in papers on unilateral laryngeal nerve paralysis (Ishizaka and Isshiki: 1976, Hammarberg et al.: 1986, Smith et al.: 1991). In these cases, the desynchronization of the right and left vocal fold is presumably the origin of bifurcations.

Diplophonia, low-pitched segments and "intermittent squeaking noises" have been reported also for functional voice disorders which result from improper use of the vocal organ or from psychoneurotic mental states (Aronson et al.: 1964).

As in the case of newborn cries (see section 3) voice characteristics may provide diagnostic tools for the diagnosis and management of neurological disorders (Griffiths and Bough: 1989). Even though most neurobiological disorders of the larynx lead to phonatory instabilities (Ramig and Scherer: 1991), a differential diagnosis seems to be possible (Ramig et al.: 1988). Diplophonia (i.e. period-doubling) has

Appl Mech Rev vol 46, no 7, July 1993

been reported for patients with Shy-Drager Syndrome (Ludlow et al.: 1983) and spasmodic dysphonia (Titze et al.: 1992). In a paper by Wieser (Wieser: 1981) octave jumps, two fundamental frequencies and noise segments are considered as characteristics of spastic dysphonia.

The most promising observations in connection with neurological diseases are found in patients with Huntington's disease (Ramig et al.: 1988). During sustained vowel phonation abrupt drops in fundamental frequency of approximately one octave occur. After some few hundred milliseconds reverse transitions to normal phonation take place. Such low-frequency segments occur also sometimes for individuals at risk for Huntington's disease and, therefore, these period-doubling bifurcations can be exploited for early diagnosis and for monitoring of disease progression.

Despite some progress, we have to emphasize that the discrimination of the various diseases is an extremely complicated task. Observed bifurcations reflect primarily the biomechanical conditions of the vocal fold oscillations and only in an indirect way the specific disease. For example, chaos due to asymmetry of the folds can be caused by several pathologies (cysts, cancer, paralysis etc.).

However, an improved understanding of the sources of dyshonias will be surely helpful for diagnosis, treatment and perhaps screening (Laver et al.: 1986, Kasuya et al.: 1986) of diseases and may, additionally, contribute considerably to clinical classification and quantification of different types of hoarseness.

- nonlinear stress-strain characteristics of vocal fold tissue (Titze: 1992)
- strong restoring forces at collision of the folds
- highly nonlinear dependence of the airflow on glottal area

Thus, it is not surprising that complex bifurcations and low-dimensional chaos are observed in phonation. It can be seen with high-speed films or stroboscopy that many degrees of freedom are excited during phonation (left and right fold, vertical movement, surface waves, anterior-posterior oscillations etc.). Low-order models have to be designed which describe the most essential vibratory modes. It was pointed out by several authors that it is mainly the phase difference of the lower and upper margins of the folds which is of central importance for the generation of self-sustained oscillations (Ishizaka and Flanagan: 1972, Stevens: 1977, Broad: 1979). Such a phase shift of about 60 is a crucial mechanism to transfer energy from the airflow to the folds. If the lower part of the folds opens first, the subglottal pressure causes a peeling apart of the vocal folds. During

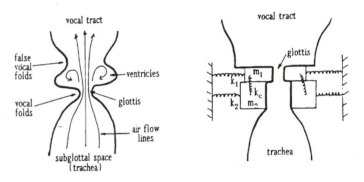

FIG.14 Schematic cross-section through the vocal folds (left) and correspoding two-mass model (right)

7. MODELING VOCAL FOLD VIBRATIONS

Conceptionally, modeling the generation of voiced speech can be separated into a biomechanical part and an aerodynamic part. In principle, partial differential equations should be solved for a comprehensive description. There are indeed sophisticated biomechanical models treating the folds as an layered elastic material capable of propagating compressional, shear, and surface waves (Titze and Talkin: 1979, Titze: 1992). Very recently, also the Navier-Stokes equations within a time-varying glottis have been solved numerically (Liljencrants: 1991).

During these simulations some irregularities have been found, but it is not possible at the moment to understand the underlying bifurcations and attractors in such extensive studies with hundreds of mesh-points.

Consequently, the bifurcation structure of low-order models should be analyzed first (see the next section). Bifurcation theory was only very recently applied to phonation models (Herzel et al.: 1991a, Awrejcewicz: 1991, Wong et al.: 1991, Smith et al.: 1991). However, there is still a large gap between observations and modeling of pathological voices.

Several nonlinearities are involved in the process of vocal fold vibration:

closure, a substantial airflow reduces the static pressure (Bernoulli effect). In this way, the energy supplied from the aerodynamic flow makes up for the losses in the mechanical system.

In order to model the described phase shift two-mass models are appropriate. Fig.14 demonstrates the representation of the vocal folds by such a two-mass model.

The celebrated two-mass model of Ishizaka and Flanagan (Ishizaka and Flanagan: 1972) was shown to exhibit bifurcations and chaos (Herzel et al.: 1991a). However, it contains more than 10 first order equations, and, therefore, a comprehensive analysis is difficult. Consequently, a simplified version has been derived which describes nevertheless many features of phonation (Herzel and Knudsen: 1992). The derivation of this two-mass model and some of the bifurcations are discussed in the next sections.

8. DERIVATION OF A TWO-MASS MODEL

The model is essentially a simplified version of the celebrated Ishizaka-Flanagan (Ishizaka and Flanagan: 1972) model. Their model is capable of reproducing many features

Appl Mech Rev vol 46, no 7, July 1993

of phonation and has been successfully used for speech sythesis. The full model describes beside the mechanical oscillations the volume flow through the glottis and through the vocal tract.

The interaction of the glottal flow with sub- and supraglottal cavities being neglected, a fourth-order model can be derived as follows.

Firstly, constant subglottal pressure P_s and vanishing vocal tract input pressure $P_i = 0$ are assumed. At glottal entry and through the glottis, the flow is presumably nonturbulent and describable by a modified Bernoulli equation. The abrupt contraction at the inlet to the glottis leads to a pressure drop, greater than for an ideal flow. The corresponding entry coefficient is assumed to be 1.37, according to measurements on plaster cast models of the larynx (van den Berg et al.: 1957). U denoting the volume flow through the glottis and A_l the entry area, we obtain:

$$\Delta P_{\text{contraction}} = 1.37 \frac{\rho}{2} \left[\frac{U}{A_1} \right]^2 \qquad (5)$$

A second term, describing the pressure change at the junction between the first and second mass pair, is easily derived from energy conservation (Bernoulli equation):

$$\Delta P_{\text{intra-glotties}} = \frac{\rho}{2} U^2 \left[\frac{1}{A_2^2} - \frac{1}{A_1^2} \right] . \qquad (6)$$

In principle, there is also a pressure difference at the exit, but the exit recovery coefficient is very small and, therefore, this effect can be neglected in a first-order approximation (Cranen and Boves: 1987). Moreover, we have omitted viscous losses and the inertia of the glottal air plug.

Then, the overall equation for the pressure drop across the glottis is given by

$$P_s = \frac{\rho}{2} U^2 \left[0.\frac{37}{A_1^2} + \frac{1}{A_2^2} \right] . \qquad (7)$$

Keeping in mind that airflow is possible only for positive areas we obtain

$$U^2 = \frac{2}{\rho} P_s \left[\frac{A_1^2 A_2^2}{A_1^2 + 0.37 A_2^2} \right] \theta(A_1) \theta(A_2)$$

$$\text{with } \theta(A) = \begin{cases} 1 & \text{for } A > 0 \\ 0 & \text{for } A \le 0 \end{cases} \qquad (8)$$

Combining Eqs.(5) and (8) we find the following pressure P acting on the lower mass pair:

$$P_1 = P_s - 1.37 P_s \frac{1}{0.37 + A_1^2/A_2^2} \theta(A_1) \theta(A_2) \qquad (9)$$

According to our assumptions, no pressure is acting on the upper masses. It is worth mentioning that Eq.(9) just reflects the well known fact that the pressure is high for a convergent glottis (i.e., $A_1 > A_2$) and reduced for a diverging glottis. Consequently, the energy transfer from the flow to the folds is achieved if the glottis is more convergent during opening than during closing. This is observed indeed for chest voice (Stevens: 1977, Hirano: 1977).

Thus, the interplay between glottal geometry and aerodynamic forces is somehow described by our model.

The mechanical restoring forces in the paper of Ishizaka and Flanagan contain besides linear terms also relatively small cubic nonlinearities. In order to keep our model as simple as possible we consider only linear terms.

During collison, Ishizaka and Flanagan applied additional strong restoring forces. To avoid nonanalytic behaviour, we have chosen a hyperbolic contact force according to Awrejcewicz (Awrejcewicz: 1991). The constants were fitted in such a way that the deviations from the original mechanical forces in the Ishizaka-Flanagan model are only a few percent under physiological relevant conditions.

Summarizing, the model equations read as follows:

$$m_1 \ddot{x}_1 + r_1 \dot{x}_1 + k_1 x_1 - c_1 (x_1 + 0.1)^{-3} + \kappa (x_1 - x_2) = P_1 (x_1, x_2)$$
$$m_2 \ddot{x}_2 + r_2 \dot{x}_2 + k_2 x_2 - c_2 (x_2 + 0.1)^{-3} + \kappa (x_2 - x_1) = 0$$

$$P_1(x_1, x_2) = P_s - 1.37 P_s \left[\frac{1}{0.37 + A_1^2/A_2^2} \right] \theta(A_1) \theta(A_2) \qquad (10)$$

$$\text{with} \quad A_i = 0.05 + 2.8 x_i \quad (i = 1, 2).$$

The area-term above implies a rest area of 0.05 and a rectangular slit with a length of 1.4. It is assumed that the pressure P_1 has an effect on an area equal to one. Thus, the numerical value of the force in Eq.(10) is just $P_1(x_1, x_2)$. For numerical simulations the function $\theta(A)$ is approximated by

$$\theta(A) = \frac{1}{\pi} \arctan \ (10000 A) + \frac{1}{2} \qquad (11)$$

The parameters of the model were chosen along the lines of the paper of Ishizaka-Flanagan (Ishizaka-Flanagan: 1972). The following "typical" parameter values serve as starting point to our analysis (Fig.15 displays the corresponding simulations):

$$m_1 = 0.125, \quad m_2 = 0.025, \quad r_1 = 0.1, \quad r_2 = 0.02,$$
$$k_1 = 0.08, \quad k_2 = 0.008, \quad \kappa = 0.025,$$
$$c_1 = 10^{-6}, \quad c_2 = 10^{-7}, \quad P_s = 0.00785 \ (8 \ \text{cm} H_2 O).$$

All parameters are given in units of cm, g and ms and their corresponding combinations.

The above model is of a remarkable simplicity compared to other models. It will be argued below that the equations have, nevertheless, physiological relevance. In

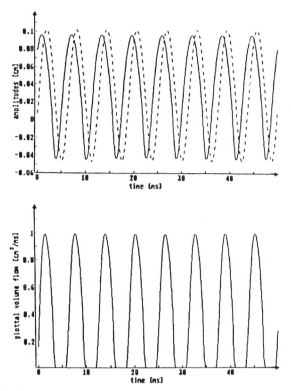

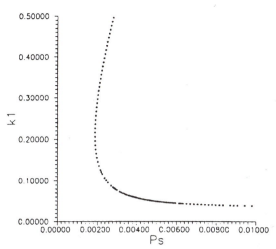

FIG.16 Onset of self-sustained oscillations via a supercritical Hopf-bifurcation. The cross marks the 'typical' parameter values of Fig.15

FIG.15 Simulation of the model (10) for typical parameter values. The dashed line corresponds to the uper part of the folds (i.e., $x_2(t)$)

order to check the relevance of our model we compare the simulation results with several well known physiological facts of normal phonation:
- elongations are in the order of millimeter
- volume flow is in the order of a cm³ per ms
- phase shift of the upper and lower edge is about 60°
- duty factor (i.e., open time divided by period) is about 0.6
- the pulses of the volume flow are asymmetric
- a minimum subglottal pressure of a few cm H_2O is necessary for oscillations
- self-sustained oscillations occur in a wide range of elastic parameters k_1, k_2, κ (modelling muscle tension).

Fig.15 shows the oscillations of the masses and the corresponding volume flow for the parameter values above. It is obvious that many characteristics of normal phonationare reproduced. Moreover, there is a striking similarity to the corresponding figures in the paper of Ishizaka and Flanagan (Ishizaka and Flanagan: 1972).

Using continuation technique (see Knudsen et al.: 1991 for details) the onset of oscillations in the P_s-k_1 parameter plane is analyzed. Fig.16 demonstrates that phonation sets in at realistic pressure values and can be found in a wide range of k_1-values.

It will be shown in the next section that also the other stiffness values k_2 and κ can be varied within a certain range. Despite the convincing explanation of some physiological facts we want to stress that several effects of human vocal fold vibrations are a priori excluded in our simplified approach:
- right-left asymmetry of the folds

- vertical movements
- anterior-posterior degrees of freedom
- source-tract interaction
- viscous losses and vorticity of the flow

Neglecting all these complications has the advantage that we can primarily study the effect of the Bernoulli term in Eqs.(10) and the nonlinear contact forces.

9. BIFURCATIONS OF THE TWO-MASS MODEL

The effective length, mass and tension of the vocal folds are determined by muscle action. Usually, the control of these quantities is much more slower then the vibrations of the folds and, therefore, these quantities can be treated as external parameters. It was demonstrated in the sections 3 and 4 that a drift of parameters can induce qualitative changes of the dynamics. These sudden changes are related to bifurcations of the underlying dynamical systems.

In this section various bifurcations at the borderline of the parameter region of "normal" phonation, as depicted in Fig.15, are studied. We analyze mainly the k_2-κ plane since these elastic parameters can be widely varied by muscle action. Moreover, some limit cases in this plane are of particular interest:
- for $\kappa=0$ the x_2 motion is damped out and, consequently, no self-sustained oscillations are possible
- for $\kappa\to\infty$ no self-oscillations are possible since $x_1=x_2$ leads to $P_1=0$
- for $k_2=0$ the upper mass is coupled only to the lower part like in other approaches (Titze: 1973, Smith et al.: 1991).

Varying the stiffness values k_2 and κ an exceedingly rich variety of bifurcations was found. For example, a large limit cycle with glottal closure (as in Fig.15) coexists with a small limit cycle without collision of the masses. The small limit cycle is "born" via a supercritical Hopf bifurcation from a steady state of an open glottis with $x_1\approx P_s/k_1$. Thus, the full line in Fig.17 corresponds to a soft onset of phonation from folds at rest.

Appl Mech Rev vol 46, no 7, July 1993

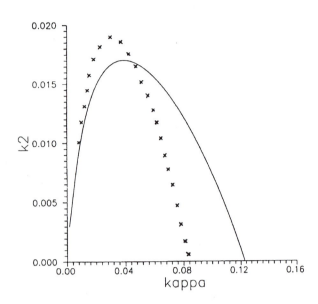

FIG.17 Gross features of the bifurcations in the k_2-κ parameter plane:
___ supercritical Hopf bifurcation of the steady state with $x_1 \approx P_s/k_1$;
× approximate location of bifurcations of the large limit cycle starting parameter variation inside the phonation region

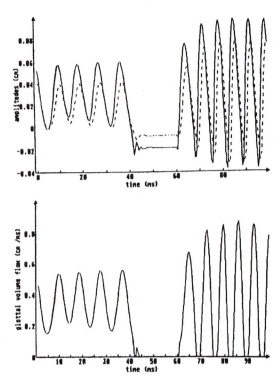

FIG.19 Coexistence of a chaotic attractor, a steady state and a large limit cycle for k_2=0.015 and κ=0.0212.

Starting from the large limit cycle a loss of stability is indicated at the crosses in Fig.17. At these points the large limit cycle either vanishes via a saddle node bifurcation or it "merges" with the small limit cycle in a complicated manner.

A detailed study along the line k_2=0.015 is shown in Fig.18.

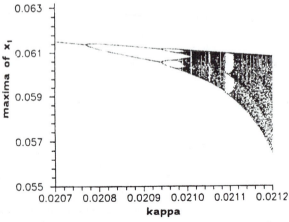

FIG.18 Bifurcation diagram along the line k_2=0.015. The maxima of x_1 are plotted versus the coupling constant κ

Fig.18 displays the well-known transition to chaos via period-doubling bifurcations. Chaotic oscillations for κ=0.0212 are shown during the first 40 ms of Fig.19. The transition from chaos to aphonia at 40 ms is induced by a shift of x_1 of -0.002 and the jump to normal phonation was

achieved by a shift of x_1 of -0.012.

It is worth mentioning that a third attractor coexists which corresponds to a weakly opened lower part ($A \geq 0$; i.e., $x_1 \geq -0.05/2.8$). In this case a negative pressure due to the Bernoulli effect balances the restoring force of the springs.

Summarizing the results above, one can conclude that even in the strongly simplified phonation model complex vibratory pattern are observed at the borderline of the parameter region of normal phonation.

For an understanding of the bifurcation structure it appears to be useful to study the eigenfrequencies of the system (10). For vanishing damping, contact force and aerodynamic forcing one easily obtains the following eigenfrequencies:

$$\omega_{1,2} = \sqrt{\frac{k_1+\kappa}{2m_1} + \frac{k_2+\kappa}{2m_2} \pm \sqrt{\left(\frac{k_1+\kappa}{2m_1} - \frac{k_2+\kappa}{2m_2}\right)^2 + \frac{\kappa^2}{m_1 m_2}}} \qquad (12)$$

For example, the standard parameters in Fig.15 give the eigenfrequencies of 120 and 201 Hz. Generally, phonation occurs if these frequencies are comparable, and if the coupling is sufficiently strong.

It is known from observations and from modeling that complicated vibrations often occur if the vocal folds are slack and thick, i.e., at the lower range of the fundamental frequency range (corresponding to low Q-values in the Ishizaka-Flanagan model). Particularly, at very low

Appl Mech Rev vol 46, no 7, July 1993

frequencies a transition to the "vocal fry register" can occur which is often characterized by an octave-jump (i.e., period-doubling) and irregular fold vibrations. These findings motivated us to analyze also the following set of parameters (corresponding roughly to $Q=0.6$ in the notation of Ishizaka and Flanagan (Ishizaka and Flanagan: 1972)):

$$m_1=0.2, \quad m_2=0.04, \quad r_1=0.02, \quad r_2=0.01,$$
$$k_1=0.05, \quad k_2=0.005, \quad \kappa=0.015,$$
$$c_1=10^{-6}, \quad c_2=10^{-7}, \quad P_s=0.005.$$

The gross features of the bifurcation diagram are similar to the previous analysis. However, at small values of k_2 and κ remarkable phenomena occur.

The two modes are not always in 1:1 resonance, but may oscillate with another frequency ratio (see Fig.20). Consequently, the period is enlarged drastically and low-frequency components appear in the spectrum. Such transitions to low-frequency regimes have been discussed in sections 3 and 4 for newborn cries, vocal fry and pathological voices.

As demonstrated in the Figs.19 and 20 tiny changes of amplitudes or paramters may induce sudden jumps to other regimes comparable to the observations in the sections 3 and 4.

However, despite a certain qualitative agreement of the simulations and observations several remarks are necessary. First of all, no quantitative correspondence between pathological voices and modeling have been achieved so far. Moreover, the parameter regions of the phenomena shown in the Figs.18-20 are rather small. In a forthcoming paper various refinements of the model (10) will

be studied. Particularly, a larger number of biomechanical degrees of freedom and the incorporation of sub- and supraglottal resonances will certainly lead to a rich variety of bifurcations - see e.g. the preliminary results of Wong et al. (Wong et al.: 1991), Smith et al. (Smith et al.: 1991). It should be pointed out finally that particularly two-parameter continuation as in Figs.16 and 17 is an appropriate tool for the understanding of nonlinear dynamics.

10. DISCUSSION

It was emphasized in this paper that nonlinear dynamics plays an essential role in speech research, particularly for an understanding of pathological voices. There are convincing observations of various bifurcations (sections 3 and 4), clear indications of low-dimensional attractors (section 5), and physiologically relevant models showing bifurcations and chaos. An improved theoretical framework will certainly help to understand complicated phonatory processes. The identification of bifurcations and chaos is only the first step. In many cases the underlying physiological mechanisms are not well understood. Careful interpretation of high-speed films and stroboscopic observations might be helpful to identify the relevant modes and the desynchronization mechanisms. The qualitative similarity of many observations to the bifurcations of coupled oscillators gives some hints to possible physiological mechanisms. In normal phonation, all vibratory modes are essentially synchronized. Bifurcations occur consequently at the borderline of 1:1 entrainement zones. The desynchronization of the following modes might be relevant:

- desynchronization of the left and right vocal fold (of particular relevance for localized vocal fold lesions and unilateral paralysis)
- desynchronization of horizontal, vertical and anterior-posterior modes (such "symmetric chaos" might be related, for example, to vocal fry phonation)
- interaction of true and false vocal folds (see Fig.14; many stroboscopic observations of creaky or pressed voice reveal vibrating false vocal folds)
- interaction of the fold vibrations with sub- or supraglottal resonances (this origin of bifurcations should not be overestimated since the resonances of the cavities are significantly damped (Cranen and Boves: 1987)).

Obviously, quite a lot of experimental and theoretical work is necessary in order to understand irregularities in phonation. Signal analysis inspired by nonlinear dynamics and bifurcation diagrams of low-order models are certainly appropriate tools to solve the puzzle.

ACKNOWLEDGEMENT

Thanks are extended to Kathleen Wermke and Werner Mende for introducing me to the field and to Jurgen Wendler for providing me the voice signals. Special thanks also to Ina Steinecke and Carsten Knudsen for assistance in modeling and to Dagmar Rosengarten for manuscript preparation.

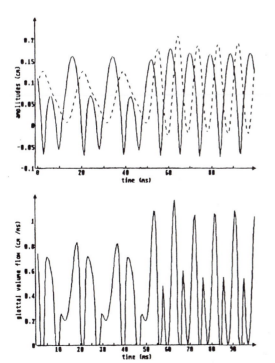

FIG.20 Complex vibrations (2:1 entrainement) for slack vocal folds ($k_2=0$, $\kappa=0.003$, first 50 ms). At 50 ms coupling was increased to $\kappa=0.01$ leading to normal phonation.

Appl Mech Rev vol 46, no 7, July 1993

REFERENCES

Arends N, Povel DJ, van Os E, Speth L (1990), Predicting Voice Quality of Deaf Speakers on the Basis of Glottal Characteristics, *J. Speech Hear. Research* 33 116-122.

Aronson AE, Peterson jr. HW and Litin EM (1964), Voice Symptomatology in Functional Dysphonia and Aphonia, *J. Speech Hear. Disorders* 4 367-381.

Askenfelt AG, Hammarberg B (1986), Speech Waveform Perturbation Analysis: Perceptual-Acoustical Comparison of Seven Measures, *J. Speech Hear. Research* 29 50-64.

Awrejcewicz J (1991), Numerical Analysis of the Oscillations of Human Vocal Cords, *Nonlinear Dynamics* 2 35-52.

Bowler NW (1964), A Fundamental Frequency Analysis of Harsh Voice Quality", *Speech Monogr.* 31 128.

Broad D(1979), The New Theories of Vocal Fold Vibration, in: *Speech and Language: Advances in Basic Research and Practice* (Lass N, ed.), Academic Press, New York.

Catford JC (1977), *Fundamental Problems in Phonetics*, Edinburgh University Press.

Cooper DS Voice (1989), A Historical Perspective", *J. of Voice* 3 187-203.

Cranen B and Boves L (1987), On Subglottal Formant Analysis, *J. Acoust. Soc. Am.* 81 734-746.

Dolansky L and Tjernlund P (1968), On Certain Irregularities of Voiced-Speech Waveforms, *IEEE Trans.* AU-16 51-56.

Eckmann JP and Ruelle D (1985), Ergodic Theory of Chaos and Strange Attractors, *Rev. Mod. Phys.* 57 617-656.

Eskenazi L, Childers DG and Hicks DM (1990), Acoustic Correlates of Vocal Quality, *J. Speech Hear. Research* 33 298-306.

Fant G (1960), *Acoustic Theory of Speech Production*, s'Gravenhage, Mouton.

Flanagan JL (1972) *Speech Analysis, Synthesis and Perception*, Springer, New York.

Froehling H, Crutchfield JP, Farmer JD, Packard NH, and Shaw SH (1981), On Determining the Dimension of Chaotic Flows", *Physica* 3D 605-617.

Grassberger P and Procaccia I (1983), Measuring the Strangeness of Strange Attractors, *Physica* 9D 189-208.

Griffiths C and Bough jr. ID (1989), Neurologic Diseases and Their Effect on Voice, *J. of Voice* 3 148-156.

Hammarberg B, Fritzell B, Gauffin J and Sundberg J (1986), Acoustic and Perceptual Analysis of Vocal Dysfunction, *J. of Phonetics* 14 533-547.

Hecker MHL and Kreul EJ (1971), Descriptions of the Speech of Patients with Cancer of the Vocal Folds. Part I: Measures of Fundamental Frequency, *J. Acoust. Soc. Am.* 49 4.

Helmholtz H (1870), *Die Lehre von den Tonempfindungen als physiologische Grundlage für die Theorie der Musik*, Vieweg und Sohn, Braunschweig.

Herzel H, Steinecke I, Mende W and Wermke K (1991a), Chaos and Bifurcations during Voiced Speech in: *Complexity, Chaos and Biological Evolution* (Mosekilde E, ed.), Plenum Press, New York.

Herzel H, Plath P and Svensson P (1991b), Experimental Evidence of Homoclinic Chaos and Type-II Intermittency during the Oxidation of Methanol, *Physica* 48D 340-352.

Herzel H and Wendler J (1991), Evidence of Chaos in Phonatory Samples, in: *Proc. EUROSPEECH*, Genova.

Herzel H, Mende W and Wermke K (1992), Speech Production - a Dynamical System with Subharmonic Bifurcations and Chaos, in: *Measurement and Selfsimilarity* (Plath P, ed.), Springer, Berlin.

Herzel H and Knudsen C (1993), Bifurcations in a Vocal Fold Model, (in preparation).

Hillenbrand J (1988), Perception of Aperiodicities in Synthetically Generated Voices, *J. Acoust. Soc. Am.* 83 2361-2371.

Hirano M (1977), Structure and Vibratory Behaviour of the Vocal Folds, in: *Dynamic Aspects of Speech Production* (Sawashima M and Cooper FS, eds.), Univ. of Tokyo Press, Tokyo.

Hirano M, Hibi S, Terasawa S and Fujiu M (1986), Relationship Between Aerodynamic, Vibratory, Acoustic and Psychoacoustic Correlates in Dysphonia, *J. of Phonetics* 14 445-456.

Hirano M (1989), Objective Evaluation of the Human Voice: Clinical Aspects, *Folia phoniat.* 41 89-144.

Hirschberg J and Szende T (1985), *Pathologische Schreistimme, Stridor und Hustenton im Säuglingsalter*, Gustav Fischer Verlag, Stuttgart.

Hollien H and Michel JF (1968), Vocal Fry as a Phonational Register, *J. Speech Hear. Research* 11 600-604.

Howard DM (1989), Peak-Picking Fundamental Period Estimation for Hearing Prostheses, *J. Acoust. Soc. Am.* 86 902-910.

Imaizumi S (1986), Acoustic Measures of Roughness in Pathological Voice, *J. of Phonetics* 14 457-462.

Ishizaka K and Flanagan JL (1972), Synthesis of Voiced Sounds from a Two-Mass Model of the Vocal Cords, *Bell Syst. Techn. J.* 51 1233-1268.

Ishizaka K and Isshiki N (1976), Computer Simulation of Pathological Vocal-Cord Vibration, *J. Acoust. Soc. Am.* 60 1193-1198.

Isshiki N, Yanagihara N and Morimoto M (1966), Approach to the Objective Diagnosis of Hoarseness, *Folia phoniat.* 18 393-400.

Isshiki N, Okamura H, Tanabe M and Morimoto M (1969), Differential Diagnosis of Hoarseness, *Folia phoniat.* 21 9-19.

Iwata S and von Leden H (1970), Pitch Perturbations in Normal and Pathologic Voices, *Folia phoniat.* 22 413-424.

Karnell MP, Scherer RS and Fischer LB (1991), Comparison of Acoustic Voice Perturbation Measures Among Three Independent Voice Laboratories, *J. Speech Hear. Research* 34 781-790.

Kasuya H, Masubuchi K, Ebihara S and Yoshida H (1986), Preliminary Experiments on Voice Screening, *J. of Phonetics* 14 463-468.

Kelman AW (1981), Vibratory Pattern of the Vocal Folds, *Folia phoniat.* 33 73-99.

Klatt DH and Klatt LC (1990), Analysis, Synthesis, and Perception of Voice Quality Variations Among Female and Male Talkers, *J. Acoust. Soc. Am.* 87 820-841.

Knudsen C, Sturis J and Thomsen JS (1991), Generic Bifurcation Structures of Arnold Tongues in Forced Oscillators, *Phys. Rev.* A44 3503-3510.

Koike Y (1969), Vowel Amplitude Modulations in Patients with Laryngeal Diseases, *J. Acoust. Soc. Am.* 45 839-844.

Kreiman J, Gerratt BR and Precoda K (1990), Listener Experience and Perception of Voice Quality, *J. Speech Hear. Research* 33 103-115.

Laver J, Hiller S, Mackenzie J and Rooney E (1986), An Acoustic Screening System for the Detection of Laryngeal Pathology, *J. of Phonetics* 14 517-524.

Liebermann P (1963), Some Acoustic Measures of the Fundamental Periodicity of Normal and Pathologic Larynges, *J. Acoust. Soc. Am.* 35 3.

Liljencrants J (1991), Numerical Simulations of Glottal Flow, in: *Proc. EUROSPEECH*, Genova.

Lind J, ed. (1965), Newborn Infant Cry, *Acta paediat. Suppl.* 163.

Ludlow C, Coulter D and Gentages F (1983), The Diffential Sensitivity of Frequency Perturbation to Laryngeal Neoplasms and Neuropathologies, in: *Vocal Fold Physiology - Contemporary Research and Clinical Issues* (Bless D and Abbs J, eds.), College Hill Press, San Diego.

Mende W, Herzel H and Wermke K (1990), Bifurcations and Chaos in Newborn Infant Cries, *Phys. Lett.* A 145 418-424.

Mende W, Wermke K, Schindler S, Wilzopolski K and Huck S (1991), *Variability of the Cry Melody and the Melody Spectrum as Indicators for Certain CNS Disorder*, Early Child Development.

Michelsson K, Raes J and Rinne A (1984), Cry Score - an Aid in Infant Diagnosis, *Folia phoniat.* 36 219-224.

Monsen RB (1979), Acoustic Qualities of Phonation in Young Hearing-Impaired Children, *J. Speech Hear. Res.* 22 270-288.

Moore G and von Leden H (1958), Dynamic Variation of the Vibratory Pattern in the Normal Larynx, *Folia phoniat.* 10 205-238.

Muller J (1837), Handbuch der Physiologie des Menschen, Verlag von J. Holscher, Coblenz.

Murry T and Doherty ET (1980), Selected Acoustic Characteristics of Pathologic and Normal Speakers, *J. Speech Hear. Research* 23 361-369.

Pinto NB and Titze IR (1990), Unification of Perturbation Measures in Speech Signals, *J. Acoust. Soc. Am.* 87 1278-1289.

Ramig LA, Scherer RC, Titze IR and Ringel SP (1988), Acoustic Analysis of Voices of Patients with Neurologic Disease Rational and Preliminary Data, *Ann. Otol. Rhinol. Laryngol.* 97 164-172.

Ramig LO and Scherer RC (1991), Speech Therapy for Neurological Disorders of the Larynx, *NCVS Report* 1 167-190.

Remacle M and Trigaux I (1991), Characteristics of Nodules through the High-Resolution Frequency Analyzer, *Folia phoniat.* 43 53-59.

Robb MP and Saxman JH (1988), Acoustic Observations in Young Children's Non-Cry Vocalizations, *J. Acoust. Soc. Am.* 83 1876-1882.

Roch JB, Comte F, Eyraud A and Dubreuil C (1990), Synchronization of Glottography and Laryngeal Stroboscopy, *Folia phoniat.* 42 289-295.

Rossbach MJ (1872), Doppelt nigkeit der Stimme (Diphthongie) bei ungleicher Spannung der Stimmbunder, *Virchows Arch.* [A]45 571-574.

Sirvi P and Michelsson K (1976), Sound-Spectrographic Cry Analysis of Normal and Abnormal Newborn Infants, *Folia phoniat.* 28 161-173.

Smith ME, Berke GS, Gerratt BR and Kreiman J, Laryngeal Paralyses Theoretical Considerations and Effects on Laryngeal Vibration, *J. Speech Hear. Res.*, (in press).

Sorokin WN (1985), *Theory of Speech Production*, Moscow.

Stevens KN (1977), Physics of Laryngeal Behaviour and Larynx Modes, *Phonetica* 34 264-279.

Theiler J (1986), Spurious Dimension from Correlation Algorithms Applied to Limited Time-Series Data, *Phys. Rev.* **A34** 2427-2432.

Titze IR (1973), The Human Vocal Cords a Mathematical Model, *Phonetica* **28** 129-170.

Titze IR and Talkin DT (1979), A Theoretical Study of the Effects of Various Laryngeal Configurations on the Acoustics of Phonation, *J. Acoust. Soc. Am.* **6** 60-74.

Titze IR ed. (1992), *Vocal Fold Physiology: New Frontiers in Basic Science*, Singular Publ. Group, San Diego.

Titze IR, Baken R and Herzel H (1992), Evidence of Chaos in Vocal Fold Vibration, in: Titze IR ed.

van den Berg J, Zantema JT and Doornenbal P (1987), On the Air Resistence and the Bernoulli Effect of the Human Larynx, *J. Acoust. Soc. Am.* **29** 626-631.

van de Water W and Schram P (1988), Generalized Dimensions from Near-Neighbor Information, *Physical Review* **A37** 3118-3125.

Wendler J, Rauhut A and Kruger H (1986), Classification of Voice Qualities, *J. of Phonetics* **14** 485-488.

Wermke K (1987), *Thesis*, Humboldt-University of Berlin.

Wieser M (1981), Periodendaueranalyse bei spastischen Dysphonien, *Folia phoniat.* **33** 314-324.

Wolf A, Swift JB, Swinney HL and Vastano JA (1985), Determining Lyapunov Exponents from a Time-Series, *Physica* **16D** 285-317.

Wong D, Ito MR, Cox NB and Titze IR (1991), Observation of Perturbation in a Lumped-Element Model of the Vocal Folds with Application to Some Pathological Cases, *J. Acoust. Soc. Am.* **89** 383-394.

Zwicker E and Fastl H (1990), *Psychoacoustics*, Springer, Berlin.

Bifurcations in an asymmetric vocal-fold model

Ina Steinecke
Humboldt-Universität zu Berlin, Institut für Theoretische Physik, Invalidenstrasse 110, D-10099 Berlin, Germany

Hanspeter Herzel
Technische Universität Berlin, Institut für Theoretische Physik, Hardenbergstrasse 36, D-10623 Berlin, Germany

(Received 10 April 1994; accepted for publication 19 October 1994)

A two-mass model of vocal-fold vibrations is analyzed with methods from nonlinear dynamics. Bifurcations are located in parameter planes of physiological interest (subglottal pressure, stiffness of the folds). It is shown that a sufficiently large tension imbalance of the left and right vocal fold induces bifurcations to subharmonic regimes, toroidal oscillations, and chaos. The corresponding attractors are characterized by phase portraits, spectra, and next-maximum maps. The relevance of these simulations for voice disorders such as laryngeal paralysis is discussed.

PACS numbers: 43.70.Aj, 43.70.Dn, 43.70.Gr, 05.45.+b

INTRODUCTION

The development of the theory of nonlinear dynamics in the past years provided the scientific world with a rich variety of methods for investigating dynamical systems. The principal understanding of the mechanisms in such systems was associated with the creation of diverse means for the description and analysis of nonlinear processes. Furthermore, many characteristic phenomena, such as bifurcations and chaos, and their origins could be classified. The new view of the world attracted more and more interest from various sciences [see, e.g., the review (Lauterborn and Parlitz, 1988) on nonlinear dynamics in acoustics and recommendable textbooks (Berge *et al.*, 1984; Glass and Mackey, 1988)]. In this way, the theory of nonlinear dynamics found an application in the analysis of voice signals, too.

Standard methods of voice analysis, such as the estimation of jitter and shimmer and the harmonics-to-noise ratio, are valuable for the characterization of regular phonation. However, in the case of newborn infant cries and voice disorders abrupt changes to other regimes, for example, subharmonic, diplophonic, or irregular ones, occur (Kelman, 1981; Robb and Saxman, 1988; Sirviö and Michelsson, 1976), and these measurements are of limited relevance. The transitions to qualitatively new oscillatory behavior indicate the suitability of the methods from nonlinear dynamics (Herzel and Wendler, 1991; Herzel *et al.*, 1994; Mende *et al.*, 1990; Titze *et al.*, 1993). The theory predicts that in nonlinear systems, such as the voice source, for certain parameter variations periodic oscillations change to subharmonic regimes, oscillations with two frequencies and chaotic dynamics.

The application of nonlinear dynamics to sampled acoustic signals has been demonstrated to be useful. The reconstruction of attractors and the estimation of their properties indicate low dimensionality of the attractors generating the signals (Herzel and Wendler, 1991; Mende *et al.*, 1990; Titze *et al.*, 1993). The investigation of high-dimensional models of vocal-fold vibration supports this assumption. It was shown by means of the empirical orthogonal functions

that normal phonation is well represented by only two eigenmodes. The simulation of disordered voice has shown that the three strongest modes contain 90% of the variance (Berry *et al.*, 1994).

Thus it should be suitable to continue a more detailed analysis of the voice producing system in models representing only a few of the possible modes in vocal-fold vibration. In fact, already the symmetric two-mass model, approximating each vocal fold by two coupled oscillators, shows bifurcations of various types and deterministic chaos (Herzel *et al.*, 1991; Herzel, 1993; Herzel and Knudsen, 1994). Comparable phenomena are found in a high-dimensional model, representing the vocal folds as a nearly real shaped continuum and solving the partial differential equations by the finite element method (Berry *et al.*, 1994; Titze *et al.*, 1993). However, comprehensive bifurcation diagrams in such extensive simulations are not available yet.

Here we study a simplified two-mass model to get detailed bifurcation diagrams. The reduction of the system dimension and of the number of parameters allows us to interpret the effect of the most important parameters quantitatively. We are aware that our study has to be supplemented by a bifurcation analysis of more sophisticated models.

It has been shown that several mechanisms exist which lead to qualitatively different sounds being produced in the larynx. Our attention is directed to the effect of a tension imbalance between the two sides, this is, like in earlier studies, an approach to unilateral laryngeal paralyses (Ishizaka and Isshiki, 1976; Smith *et al.*, 1992; Wong *et al.*, 1991). However, the investigations in these papers were limited to specific simulations of a few representative parameter values.

Moreover, our analysis is supported by improved numerical tools. The available workstation Sparc 2 enabled extensive simulations. Furthermore, the continuation program AUTO has been used for the calculation of phonation onset under various conditions (Doedel, 1986). Continuation techniques allow the location of bifurcation lines in parameter planes with moderate effort (Kubíček and Marek, 1983).

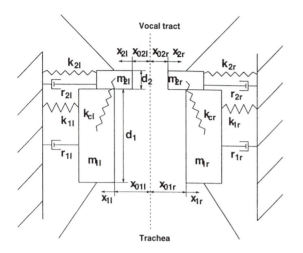

FIG. 1. Schematic representation of the two-mass model of the vocal folds. Each vocal fold is approximated by two coupled oscillators of masses $m_{1\alpha}$ and $m_{2\alpha}$, respectively, arranged one upon the other. Springs $k_{1\alpha}$, $k_{2\alpha}$, and $k_{c\alpha}$ and dampers $r_{1\alpha}$ and $r_{2\alpha}$ represent the viscoelastic properties of vocal-fold tissue. The elongations $x_{1\alpha}$ and $x_{2\alpha}$ are the time-varying variables of our model.

In the next two sections the symmetric version of our model is studied. Then, the effects of asymmetries related to different paralyses are analyzed. In both cases, the relevant bifurcations are located in parameter planes spanned by parameters of physiological meaning. In the symmetric case, the onset of phonation is discussed which corresponds to a Hopf bifurcation from a stable steady state to a limit cycle. In the asymmetric case, instabilities of the limit cycle due to a tension imbalance are described by modeling the transition from normal to disturbed phonation.

I. THE SIMPLIFIED TWO-MASS MODEL

The two-mass model, developed and analyzed by Ishizaka and Flanagan (1972), evolved to a standard for exploring the voice producing system through the years. The main goal of the model was to synthesize voice by a self-oscillating mechanism. The basic principle is intimately related to the observed phase difference between the lower and the upper edge of the vocal fold. This effect can be modeled by representing each fold by two coupled oscillators (Fig. 1). The oscillations are driven by the lung pressure. The induced phase difference of the upper and the lower mass enables the energy transfer from the airstream to the vocal folds. For a sufficiently large subglottal pressure the dissipative losses can be compensated, and phonation sets in.

In comparison with more realistic models, such as those based on partial differential equations simulations (Titze and Talkin, 1979; Titze and Alipour-Haghighi, in press) or systems of more than two coupled oscillators (Story and Titze, 1994; Titze, 1973; Wong et al., 1991), the two-mass model appears to be quite simple. Nevertheless, more than ten coupled ordinary differential equations with many parameters are necessary to solve the mechanical and the aerodynamical problem (Ishizaka and Flanagan, 1972).

That is why we reduced the model to its basic principle, the phase delay between the lower and the upper edge of the

vocal folds. It is emphasized that the interaction of the vocal-fold geometry with the airflow according to the Bernoulli equation is the prerequisite to the self-oscillating motion (van den Berg et al. 1957; Broad, 1979; Stevens, 1977).

Our aim is to analyze instabilities due to the dynamics of the coupled oscillators. Thus we neglect all parts of the description except the basic mechanical equations. Particularly, we neglect the cubic nonlinearities of the oscillators which have been introduced by Ishizaka and Flanagan to describe the nonlinear properties of the tissue. Furthermore, we separate the vocal-fold vibration from the vocal tract dynamics. We are aware that neglecting the influence of vocal tract and subglottal resonances is a strong simplification of the voice source. However, the bifurcations that we expect to occur are also observed in the vibratory patterns of excised larynges (Herzel et al., 1995). This fact supports our approach of analyzing extremely reduced equations, describing solely the vocal-fold dynamics.

In Herzel (1993), Herzel and Knudsen (1994), and Lucero (1993) similar simplifications have been studied and it turned out that the waveforms were quite realistic and similar to simulations of the complete two-mass model (Ishizaka and Flanagan, 1972). Moreover, the phonation onset in such models is found at realistic parameter values (Herzel, 1993; Herzel and Knudsen, 1994; Lucero, 1993).

Another change regards the description of the aerodynamical problem. We neglect the additional pressure drop at the inlet due to the formation of a vena contracta [see Pelorson et al. (1994) for a discussion of this point]. Moreover, we neglect viscous losses inside the glottis and suppose, contrarily to Ishizaka and Flanagan, Bernoulli flow only below the narrowest part of the glottis. Above this constriction, the airstream is considered to be a jet (Story and Titze, 1994; Titze and Alipour-Haghighi, in press). The formation of a free jet downstream for a divergent glottis is studied extensively in Pelorson et al. (1994).

According to the idea of the two-mass model and the modifications mentioned above, we obtain the following equations. The motion of the masses is described by equations of coupled oscillators (see also Fig. 1):

$$m_{i\alpha}\ddot{x}_{i\alpha} + r_{i\alpha}\dot{x}_{i\alpha} + k_{i\alpha}x_{i\alpha} + \Theta(-a_i)c_{i\alpha}(a_i/2l)$$
$$+ k_{c\alpha}(x_{i\alpha} - x_{j\alpha})$$
$$= F_i(x_{1l}, x_{1r}, x_{2l}, x_{2r}) \tag{1}$$

with

$$\Theta(x) = \begin{cases} 1, & x > 0, \\ 0, & x \leq 0. \end{cases} \tag{2}$$

Besides the usual oscillator terms, the Θ function models another restoring force which acts only during the collision of both sides. The forces F_i describe the action of the pressure in the glottis.

The four variables $x_{i\alpha}$ are the displacements of masses $m_{i\alpha}$. The indices mean

$$i, j = \begin{cases} 1\text{—lower mass,} \\ 2\text{—upper mass,} \end{cases} \quad \alpha = \begin{cases} l\text{—left side,} \\ r\text{—right side.} \end{cases}$$

The other variables and parameters are defined as follows:

$a_i = a_{il} + a_{ir}$ lower and upper glottal areas,

$a_{i\alpha} = l(x_{0i\alpha} + x_{i\alpha})$ part of the glottal area formed by the rest position and displacement of mass $m_{i\alpha}$,

$a_{0i} = l(x_{0il} + x_{0ir})$ lower and upper rest areas,

$m_{i\alpha}$ masses,

$k_{i\alpha}$ spring constants,

$k_{c\alpha}$ coupling constants,

$c_{i\alpha}$ additional spring constants during collision,

$r_{i\alpha}$ damping constants,

$x_{0i\alpha}$ distance of the vocal cords from midline in rest position,

l length of the glottis,

d_i thickness of part i,

P_i pressure inside the glottis acting on part i.

The forces F_i acting on the masses $m_{i\alpha}$ are given by

$$F_i = l d_i P_i. \tag{3}$$

The Bernoulli equation, including the assumption of the buildup of the jet, reads as follows:

$$P_s = P_1 + \frac{\varrho}{2}\left(\frac{U}{a_1}\right)^2 = P_0 + \frac{\varrho}{2}\left(\frac{U}{a_{\min}}\right)^2, \tag{4}$$

$$a_{\min} = \min(a_{1l}, a_{2l}) + \min(a_{1r}, a_{2r}). \tag{5}$$

This formula includes the case that $a_{\min}$ is found at the junction of upper and lower masses:

P_s subglottal pressure,

P_0 supraglottal pressure,

U volume flow velocity,

ϱ air density.

Setting $P_0 = 0$ and taking into account that the Bernoulli equation is only relevant when the glottis is open, we can derive the equations

$$P_1 = P_s\left[1 - \Theta(a_{\min})\left(\frac{a_{\min}}{a_1}\right)^2\right]\Theta(a_1), \tag{6}$$

$$P_2 = 0, \tag{7}$$

$$U = \sqrt{2P_s/\varrho}\, a_{\min}\Theta(a_{\min}). \tag{8}$$

For numerical simulations the function $\Theta(x)$ was approximated by

$$\Theta(x) = \begin{cases} \tanh[50(x/x_0)], & x > 0, \\ 0, & x \leq 0. \end{cases} \tag{9}$$

x_0 is a value to measure the gradation of the function $\Theta(x)$. For computation of $\Theta(a_1)$ we used $x_0 = a_{01}$.

In the case of $\Theta(a_{\min})$ we define an implicit Θ function by a new definition of $a_{\min}$,

$$a_{\min} = \max(0, a_{\min}), \tag{10}$$

after calculation of Eq. (5).

This procedure results in a continuous dependence of P_1 from its arguments (Fig. 2). We note that no negative pressure values occur due to our assumption of a jet regime

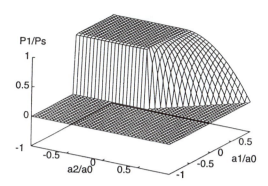

FIG. 2. The normalized pressure profile $P_1(a_1, a_2)$ in the symmetric case shows the effects of the Bernoulli term and the Θ functions which represent closure.

above the narrowest part. Thus the asymmetric model is given by the four mechanical equations (1) and the algebraic pressure equation (6).

II. BIFURCATION ANALYSIS OF THE SYMMETRIC MODEL

The simplified symmetric model shows quite realistic behavior under similar parameters like the original model. The following parameters constitute our standard parameter configuration:

$$m_{1l} = m_{1r} = m_1 = 0.125, \quad r_{1l} = r_{1r} = r_1 = 0.02,$$

$$m_{2l} = m_{2r} = m_2 = 0.025, \quad r_{2l} = r_{2r} = r_2 = 0.02,$$

$$k_{1l} = k_{1r} = k_1 = 0.08, \quad c_{1l} = c_{1r} = c_1 = 3k_1,$$

$$k_{2l} = k_{2r} = k_2 = 0.008, \quad c_{2l} = c_{2r} = c_2 = 3k_2,$$

$$k_{cl} = k_{cr} = k_c = 0.025,$$

$$d_1 = 0.25, \quad a_{01} = a_{01l} + a_{01r} = 0.05,$$

$$d_2 = 0.05, \quad a_{02} = a_{02l} + a_{02r} = 0.05,$$

$$P_s = 0.008 \quad (\approx 8 \text{ cm H}_2\text{O}),$$

$$\varrho = 0.00113.$$

All units are given in centimeters, grams, and milliseconds and their corresponding combinations. The equations of motion can be written as

$$\dot{x}_1 = v_1, \tag{11}$$

$$\dot{v}_1 = \frac{1}{m_1}\left(P_1 l d_1 - r_1 v_1 - k_1 x_1 - \Theta(-a_1)c_1\frac{a_1}{2l}\right.$$

$$\left. - k_c(x_1 - x_2)\right), \tag{12}$$

$$\dot{x}_2 = v_2, \tag{13}$$

$$\dot{v}_2 = \frac{1}{m_2}\left(-r_2 v_2 - k_2 x_2 - \Theta(-a_2)c_2\frac{a_2}{2l} - k_c(x_2 - x_1)\right), \tag{14}$$

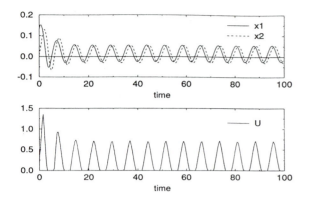

FIG. 3. Simulation for the standard parameter set showing oscillations of the lower and upper masses x_1 and x_2, respectively, and glottal volume flow velocity U of "normal phonation." Note the phase delay between the upper and the lower mass.

$$P_1 = P_s \left[1 - \Theta(a_{min}) \left(\frac{a_{min}}{a_1} \right)^2 \right] \Theta(a_1), \qquad (15)$$

$$a_1 = a_{01} + 2lx_1, \qquad (16)$$

$$a_2 = a_{02} + 2lx_2, \qquad (17)$$

$$a_{min} = \begin{cases} a_1, & \text{if } 0 < x_1 < x_2, \\ a_2, & \text{if } 0 < x_2 \le x_1, \\ 0, & \text{otherwise,} \end{cases} \qquad (18)$$

using the variables x_1, $v_1 = \dot{x}_1$, x_2, and $v_2 = \dot{x}_2$.

Figure 3 shows the oscillations of the lower and the upper mass and the glottal volume flow for the standard parameters. The upper masses are only driven by the lower ones and oscillate with some delay, which refers to the phase difference discussed above.

To describe the voice, one point of interest is the so-called voice range profile or phonetogram. It is defined as the

part of the frequency–intensity plane in which phonation is possible. The phonation onset is associated with a Hopf bifurcation, i.e., a stationary point loses its stability and a stable limit cycle arises. In analogy to the voice range profile, we discuss the phonation onset in the $P_s - k_1$ plane. P_s is intimately related to the intensity and the stiffness k_1 is the principal parameter governing the frequency of the output.

Before we consider bifurcation diagrams, we want to discuss the existence and the stability of the fixed points, or equilibrium positions, of the system. For this simplified model an analytical treatment is possible. To get the equilibrium positions, we set the derivatives of the variables in Eqs. (11)–(14) to zero. From (11) and (13) we obtain

$$v_1 = 0, \qquad (19)$$

$$v_2 = 0. \qquad (20)$$

Equation (14) is solved by

$$x_2 = \frac{k_c}{k_2 + k_c} x_1. \qquad (21)$$

Replacing x_2 by Eq. (21) in Eq. (12) we get a cubic equation for x_1. In the case of a rectangular shaped glottis, we find the trivial solution

$$x_1 = 0, \quad x_2 = 0. \qquad (22)$$

This result is independent of the elastic properties of both sides because the entire pressure is dropped at the glottal inlet in this case. Thus the resulting force F_1 is equal to zero. Due to our assumption of a jet above the smallest area, (22) is a solution for a divergent rest position of the glottis, i.e., $a_{10} < a_{20}$, too, since $P_1 = 0$ follows from $a_{min} = a_1$.

Knowing one solution of the cubic equation for the estimation of the equilibrium position of x_1, the equation can be reduced to a quadratic one, the solutions of which are

$$x_1 = -\frac{a_0}{2l} + \frac{ld_1 P_s}{2} \frac{k_2(k_2 + 2k_c)}{(k_2 + k_c)(k_1 k_2 + k_c(k_1 + k_2))}$$

$$\pm \sqrt{ \left(\frac{ld_1 P_s}{2} \frac{k_2(k_2 + 2k_c)}{(k_2 + k_c)(k_1 k_2 + k_c(k_1 + k_2))} \right)^2 + \frac{a_0 d_1 P_s}{2} \frac{k_2}{k_1 k_2 + k_c(k_1 + k_2)} }. \qquad (23)$$

Ignoring our restriction $x_1 \ge x_2$ (Bernoulli equation applies in our model only to the convergent glottis), this result is comparable to expressions in Lucero (1993). However, due to our assumption of a jet, no negative pressure values occur and hence no steady state with $x_1 < 0$, leading to $a_1 < a_2$, exists. Below a critical value of P_s,

$$P_{crit} = \frac{a_0}{4l^2 d_1} \frac{k_1 k_2 + k_c(k_1 + k_2)}{k_2}, \qquad (24)$$

both solutions of (23) are negative, i.e., only the trivial solution $x_i = 0$ remains.

Note that the solution of (23) corresponding to the minus sign is always less than $-a_0/2l$, indicating a closed glottis. Thus this fixed point does not exist in our model independent of assuming a Bernoulli flow or a jet. Lucero (1993) got a third (stable) equilibrium position for a small pressure interval. The existence of this fixed point is associated with the additional pressure drop due to a vena contracta at the glottal entry. For our assumed idealized Bernoulli flow at this point, this equilibrium position does not occur.

Thus in contrast to Herzel (1993), Herzel and Knudsen (1994), and Lucero (1993), the assumption of the buildup of a jet at the smallest glottal gap leads to only one equilibrium

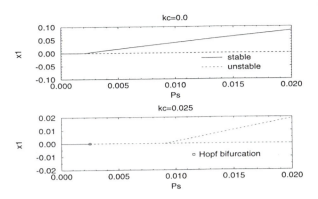

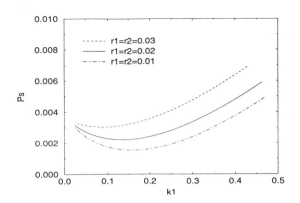

FIG. 4. Stability of the equilibrium positions. Under nonoscillatory conditions ($k_c=0$) the stable fixed point ($x_1=0$, $x_2=0$) becomes unstable at $P_s=0.002$ via a transcritical bifurcation. Another stable fixed point occurs at this parameter value. The bifurcation is associated with a transition from a rectangular glottal shape to a convergent one. Under oscillatory conditions ($k_c=0.025$) the fixed point loses its stability via a Hopf bifurcation and oscillations set in.

FIG. 5. Oscillation threshold pressure as a function of k_1 for different damping parameters. For increasing subglottal pressure P_s the fixed point $x_1=x_2=0$ becomes unstable via a Hopf bifurcation. Consequently, the lines separate parameter regions with a stable equilibrium from regions with self-sustained oscillations. The solid line refers to our standard parameter configuration.

position for $P_s<P_{crit}$ (Steinecke, 1993). P_{crit} is the value at which the positive root of (23) becomes greater than zero, i.e., this branch crosses the trivial solution and becomes relevant.

Now we want to consider briefly the stability properties of the steady states. For this purpose, our system of $n=4$ equations

$$\dot{\mathbf{x}}=\mathbf{f}(\mathbf{x}) \tag{25}$$

is linearized at its fixed points $\mathbf{x}^0$ with $\mathbf{f}(\mathbf{x}^0)=\mathbf{0}$. The evolution of a small deviation $\mathbf{y}=\mathbf{x}-\mathbf{x}^0$ is described by the linearized equations

$$\dot{\mathbf{y}}=\mathbf{A}\mathbf{y}, \quad \mathbf{A}=\left(\frac{\partial\mathbf{f}_i}{\partial\mathbf{x}_k}(\mathbf{x}^0)\right)^n_{i,k=1}. \tag{26}$$

$\mathbf{A}$ is termed a Jacobian matrix. If the real part of at least one eigenvalue is greater than zero, the steady state is unstable. Instead of calculating all the eigenvalues, it is possible to use the Ruth–Hurwitz criterion to get conditions for the signs of all real parts (Jetschke, 1989).

In the case of $k_c=0$, i.e., if both masses are uncoupled, it is possible to calculate the critical values for an instability (bifurcation). Considering the equilibrium position $x_1=0$, $x_2=0$, we get as the result that it becomes unstable for

$$\frac{\partial F_1}{\partial x_1}>k_1. \tag{27}$$

This is equivalent to the requirement (Steinecke, 1993)

$$P_s>P_{crit}. \tag{28}$$

The branch from Eq. (23) which crosses the trivial solution at this point becomes stable, i.e., an exchange of stability, termed transcritical bifurcation, occurs (see also Lucero, 1993).

All in all, there is in contrast to the analysis of Lucero (1993) below P_{crit} only one stable fixed point and for $P_s>P_{crit}$ one stable and one unstable fixed point exist (see Fig. 4). The transcritical bifurcation corresponds to a change

of the glottal shape from a rectangular to a convergent one.

For $k_c>0$ the bifurcations were determined by using the continuation program AUTO (Doedel, 1986). Continuation techniques are a powerful tool to find bifurcations in parameter space (Kubíček and Marek, 1983). At $k_c=0.025$ (Fig. 4) the trivial equilibrium position loses its stability via a Hopf bifurcation and oscillations set in.

For convergent and divergent rest positions analytical calculations are more complicated and beyond the scope of this paper. However, a consequence of our jet assumption for a divergent glottis can be seen immediately: for small displacements the shape remains divergent and according to Eq. (6) the resulting pressure P_1 is equal to zero. Therefore, (22) refers to a stable equilibrium position, and even for large P_s a finite perturbation is necessary for starting oscillations. Moreover, because of (21) a nontrivial fixed point appears only for an overcritical subglottal pressure (a convergent shape has to be reached).

In Figs. 5 and 6 the phonation onset for the rectangular case is drawn as a function of damping parameters and glottal rest area, respectively. Below the lines a stable fixed point exists and oscillations are damped out. For increasing pres-

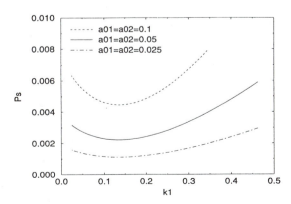

FIG. 6. Oscillation threshold pressure as in Fig. 5 with glottal rest area as the parameter. Note that the phonation threshold pressure is proportional to the glottal rest area as predicted by Titze (1988).

sure phonation sets in. As expected, the threshold increases with the damping constants.

The application of the Ruth–Hurwitz criterion to the trivial equilibrium position (22) in the rectangular case indicates a linear dependence of the phonation threshold pressure on glottal rest area as in Titze (1988). Moreover, oscillations cease to exist for higher values of k_1. These results should be kept in mind insofar that a paralysis of the nervus laryngeus inferior is associated with a fixing of the affected vocal fold in the paramedian or the intermedian position (Wendler and Seidner, 1987) leading to an enlarged glottal rest area.

III. MODELING UNILATERAL PARALYSES

Unilateral laryngeal paralyses lead to changed glottal configurations and tension imbalance between the two sides. It has been shown in experiments with excised canine larynges that such an imbalance results in diverse oscillatory patterns of the vocal folds (Isshiki *et al.*, 1977). Depending on the glottal rest area three patterns could be distinguished. In the case of extremely narrow or wide glottal gaps the oscillations are quite regular with the more tense side preceding the flaccid one. In the case of moderate rest areas the oscillations show alternating amplitudes, and for a very high imbalance the vibrations become irregular (Isshiki *et al.*, 1977).

The degree of the disturbance of the voice quality depends on the localization of the nerve injury (Pahn *et al.*, 1984; Wendler and Seidner, 1987). The laryngeal muscles are essentially innervated by the nervus laryngeus superior and the nervus laryngeus inferior. The superior laryngeal nerve paralysis results in the deficiency of the cricothyroid muscle. This muscle is responsible for the principal tension of the vocal fold. That is why the voice is often limited in the phonation of higher tones. Furthermore, such patients sometimes have difficulties in intonation (Wendler and Seidner, 1987).

In the case of an inferior laryngeal nerve paralysis (recurrent paralysis) all intralaryngeal muscles except the cricothyroid are involved. Therefore the vocalis muscle cannot contract, and because of the absence of adductors the vocal fold cannot be brought into phonatory position. The active cricothyroid muscle partially compensates for this effect by imposing passive stress on the vocal fold which is mostly fixed in the paramedian position or just off midline. The voice quality is highly influenced by this fixing position and the actual position of the arytenoid cartilage (Wendler and Seidner, 1987).

Under conditions of a combined paralysis of both nerves, mostly caused by an injury of the vagus nerve, the vocal fold is often fixed in the intermedian position and the voice is highly disturbed (Pahn *et al.*, 1984; Wendler and Seidner, 1987).

For a very large glottal gap breathiness due to turbulence is the dominant deviation from normal phonation. However, in several cases subharmonics, modulations, and irregularities have been reported for patients with paralytic dysphonia (Hammarberg *et al.*, 1986; Herzel *et al.*, 1994).

Now we want to investigate the simplified two-mass model in unilateral paralysis to examine the relationship be-

tween changes in glottal parameters and the type of vibrations.

For this purpose we define two tension parameters Q and $\tilde{Q}$ as an attempt to describe the activity of the cricothyroid and the vocalis muscle, respectively. The cricothyroid muscle stresses the whole vocal fold. That means that the elastic properties of all parts of the vocal fold are affected. The corresponding parameters Q_α are defined in a similar way as in Ishizaka and Flanagan (1972):

$$k_{i\alpha} = Q_\alpha k_{i\alpha 0}, \qquad (29)$$

$$k_{c\alpha} = Q_\alpha k_{c\alpha 0}, \qquad (30)$$

$$c_{i\alpha} = Q_\alpha c_{i\alpha 0}, \qquad (31)$$

$$m_{i\alpha} = m_{i\alpha 0}/Q_\alpha. \qquad (32)$$

The index 0 denotes the standard parameter set. The tension parameters Q_α describe the change of the eigenfrequencies as follows:

$$\omega_{i\alpha} = Q_\alpha \omega_{i\alpha 0}, \qquad (33)$$

$$\omega_{i\alpha}^2 = k_{i\alpha}/m_{i\alpha}. \qquad (34)$$

The contraction of the vocalis muscle only affects its own tension. Supposing that the properties of the vocalis muscles are represented by the masses $m_{1\alpha}$, $\tilde{Q}_\alpha$ may describe their tensions in the following way (Hirano, 1981; Smith *et al.*, 1992):

$$k_{1\alpha} = \tilde{Q}_\alpha k_{1\alpha 0}, \qquad (35)$$

$$c_{1\alpha} = \tilde{Q}_\alpha c_{1\alpha 0}, \qquad (36)$$

$$m_{1\alpha} = m_{1\alpha 0}/\tilde{Q}_\alpha. \qquad (37)$$

In the next sections we discuss bifurcations due to varying parameters Q and $\tilde{Q}$.

IV. BIFURCATION DIAGRAMS OF ASYMMETRIC VOCAL-FOLD VIBRATION

A. Modeling superior nerve paralysis

Unilateral superior nerve paralysis is modeled by tension imbalance $Q_l \neq Q_r$. Inspections of Eqs. (1) reveal that the transformation of the time $t \to Q_l t$ and of the subglottal pressure $P_s \to P_s/Q_l$ reduces the problem in such a way that the left side remains uninvolved. Hence the asymmetric properties are described solely by $Q = Q_r/Q_l$ as the ratio of the eigenfrequencies of both sides:

$$m_{il} = m_{i0}, \quad k_{il} = k_{i0}, \quad k_{cl} = k_{c0}, \quad c_{il} = c_{i0},$$
$$\qquad (38)$$
$$m_{ir} = m_{i0}/Q, \quad k_{ir} = Qk_{i0}, \quad k_{cr} = Qk_{c0}, \quad c_{ir} = Qc_{i0}.$$

The scaling of the time corresponds to higher frequencies at higher tension; the scaling of the subglottal pressure refers to the necessity of an increased pressure to displace the stressed vocal folds. The transformation implies that we can restrict our analysis to $Q \leq 1$ since any situation with $Q_l > Q_r$ can be rescaled to a case with $Q < 1$.

In addition to Q as a measure of asymmetry, the subglottal pressure P_s takes an important part. P_s is a measure of the energy that is pumped into the system. Furthermore,

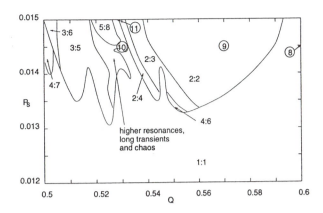

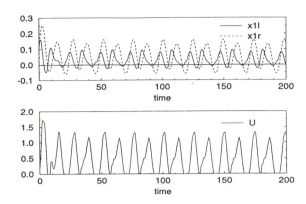

FIG. 7. Two-parameter bifurcation diagram in the Q-P_s plane. The different types of attractors are labeled by the ratio of maxima of x_{1r} and x_{1l} during one total oscillatory cycle. The points labeled by circled numbers indicate the parameter configurations for which time series are presented in Figs. 8–11. The numbers give the corresponding figure numbers.

FIG. 9. Simulations for $P_s = 0.0145$ and $Q = 0.57$ showing 2:2 locking of both folds. The period doubling is indicated by alternating amplitudes of vocal-fold motion and volume flow U, respectively.

the higher P_s, the stronger both sides are coupled by the induced airflow. For $P_s \to 0$ both sides are separated and cannot oscillate.

Along this line, we want to investigate the vibratory behavior in the Q-P_s-parameter plane. According to the transformation and physiological relevance, it is sufficient to consider only values with $0.4 < Q < 1$.

Because bifurcations primarily occur in the case of a significant asymmetry, in Fig. 7 only a part of the Q-P_s plane is shown. The bifurcation diagram is based on 400-ms simulations of the equations of motion on a grid in the plane ($\Delta Q = 0.001$, $\Delta P_s = 0.0002$). Initial conditions are the same for each simulation [$x_{1l}(0) = x_{1r}(0) = 0.1$, $\dot{x}_{1l}(0) = \dot{x}_{1r}(0) = 0.1$, $x_{2l}(0) = x_{2r}(0) = 0$, and $\dot{x}_{2l}(0) = \dot{x}_{2r}(0) = 0$].

In the shown region, $0.5 < Q < 0.6$, a variety of bifurcations can be detected. Regions of different attractors are labeled with the ratio of the number of the maxima of x_{1r} and x_{1l} during one total cycle. For normal phonation one cycle includes just one glottal closure. Thus it corresponds to one maximum of the elongations $x_{i\alpha}$ labeled by 1:1. More complex regimes ("folded limit cycles") correspond to limit

cycles which may contain several closure events. For example, period doubling leads to a limit cycle which includes two closure phases during one total period. It is associated with alternating amplitudes (see Fig. 9). In our notation it means a 2:2 ratio.

The circled numbers in Fig. 7 refer to the parameter values studied in the following Figs. 8–11. In each figure the oscillations of the lower masses and the glottal volume flow velocity are represented. In Fig. 12 the Fourier spectra of the corresponding time series $x_{1r}(t)$ are shown and Figs. 13 and 14 display phase portraits and next-maximum maps of these simulations.

The frequency of the motion is governed by the frequency of the flaccid side, i.e., the lower the Q, the lower the fundamental frequency. This result is related to the inability of patients to phonate higher tones and the difficulty to hit the intended tone.

Figure 8 shows the locking of both sides in a 1:1 ratio. The healthy vocal fold, x_{1l}, precedes the affected side, which oscillates with a greater amplitude. In Fig. 9 we can find period-doubling behavior, leading to alternating pulses in the airflow. Such a subharmonic regime has been often observed in voice pathology and is associated with such terms as "oc-

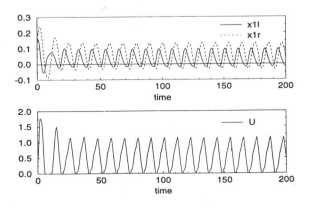

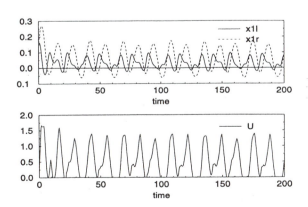

FIG. 8. Simulations for $P_s = 0.0145$ and $Q = 0.6$ showing 1:1 locking of both folds. The more flaccid properties of the "affected side" x_{1r} result in a greater amplitude of x_{1r} and a lower fundamental frequency of the whole system.

FIG. 10. Simulations for $P_s = 0.0145$ and $Q = 0.53$ showing 5:8 locking of both folds. The oscillatory behavior of x_{1r} with a limit cycle of period 5 determines the period of the acoustical signal. The unaffected side x_{1l} is locked with a pattern showing eight maxima during the total cycle.

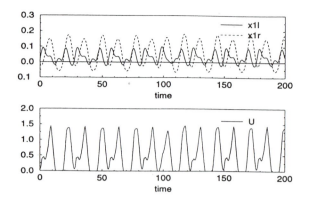

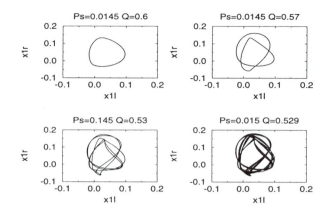

FIG. 11. Simulations for $P_s=0.015$ and $Q=0.529$. The oscillatory patterns show aperiodic behavior.

FIG. 13. The graphs show the attractors from simulations shown in Figs. 8–11 in the x_{1l}-x_{1r} plane. The upper left diagram shows the limit cycle of regular oscillations. The period doubling leads to a folded limit cycle (upper right). Oscillations with period 5 correspond to a folded limit cycle with five loops (lower left). The lower left diagram shows the complicated attractor in the case of chaotic oscillations.

tave jump" or "dicrotic dysphonia." In Fig. 10 the right vocal fold oscillates with "period 5," i.e. the period length is approximately equal to 5× the time between consecutive glottal closure events, which would govern the period in the case of regular phonation. The left side with its higher eigenfrequency is locked in such a way that its motion has eight maxima during one total period of the folded limit cycle. This behavior leads to an increased intensity of subharmonic components (see Fig. 12). For the parameters in Fig. 11 the vibrations become irregular. The corresponding Fourier spectrum in Fig. 12 shows, besides the peaks of the basic frequency and the first subharmonic, a quite unstructured contour.

Another tool for the analysis of complex motion are phase portraits and next-maximum maps. Figure 13 displays the projection of the attractors into the x_{1l}-x_{1r} plane. The plot of consecutive maxima of x_{1r} is shown in Fig. 14. These figures support our claim that the observed complex oscillations corresponds to subharmonic regimes and chaos, respectively.

It is emphasized that qualitative changes in the voice

signal which result from the flow U are governed mainly by the multiple period of the behavior of x_{1r}, i.e., a period doubling, tripling, etc. in the motion of $x_{1r}(t)$ leads to the bifurcation in $U(t)$, whereas the period of x_{1l} influences the sound, i.e., the intensity of harmonics in the spectrum, by forming the shapes of the glottal flow pulses.

All in all, transitions to oscillations with a multiple period dominate in the Q-P_s plane, while chaos seldom occurs. Furthermore, these bifurcations are located at low Q values and relatively high P_s. Note that for tensed vocal folds the subglottal pressure has to be increased even more to obtain the same bifurcations according to the transformation mentioned above. Therefore according to the present model instabilities of the voice are to be expected mostly at high voice effort and low fundamental frequency.

In Fig. 15 the maxima of x_{1r} are plotted versus asymmetry Q. At $P_s=0.010$ a small parameter region shows period doubling and chaos. The plot for higher pressure $P_s=0.015$ is characterized by abrupt transitions to other regimes, indicating hysteresis, i.e., the bifurcations are asso-

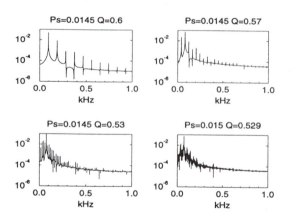

FIG. 12. The graphs show the Fourier spectra of $x_{1r}(t)$ from the simulations shown in Figs. 8–11. The upper left diagram represents the regular spectrum of 1:1 locking. The period doubling is indicated by the occurrence of the first subharmonic (upper right). In the case of 5:8 locking (lower left) we find a spectral peak (and its multiples) at approximately one fifth of the pitch in the 1:1 case. In the lower right diagram the unstructured spectrum of the chaotic oscillations is seen.

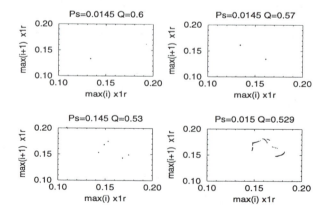

FIG. 14. Plot of consecutive maxima of x_{1r} from simulations shown in Figs. 8–11. These diagrams support the analysis of the attractors. Periodic oscillations of period n result in n points (upper left, upper right, and lower left). The lower right diagram represents the plot for chaotic oscillations.

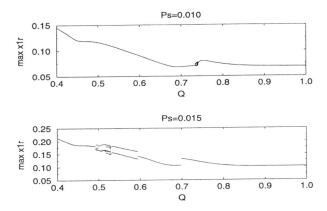

FIG. 15. One-parameter bifurcation diagrams showing maxima of x_{1r} for two values of P_s. The diagrams show the evolution of the attractor as function of the asymmetry Q. For $P_s = 0.01$ the attractor changes smoothly, except for a small parameter interval. In the case of $P_s = 0.015$ abrupt transitions to limit cycles with multiple periods occur.

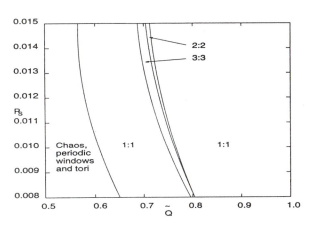

FIG. 17. Two-parameter bifurcation diagram in the $\tilde{Q}$-P_s plane. The different types of attractors are labeled by the ratio of maxima of x_{1r} and x_{1l} during one total oscillatory cycle. The area in the left region of the diagram contains toroidal and chaotic behavior and "periodic windows" (small parameter regions with folded limit cycles).

ciated with the coexistence of two different attractors.

In such a case it is worth studying the basins of attraction of both attractors. Figure 16 shows the basins of the 1:1 and the 2:2 attractor at parameters $Q = 0.585$ and $P_s = 0.0145$ for varying initial displacements of the masses. The structure of the regions is relatively complicated. To see if there is a more differentiated structure, a small parameter region has been tested with a higher precision. In Fig. 16 it is marked by a dark area of the basin of the 1:1 attractor (due to the higher density of points) surrounding a mittenlike area of the 2:2 basin. However, the borderline between the basins seems to be smooth. Intertwined basins of attraction imply that rather weak perturbations may induce abrupt jumps to the other regime as observed in acoustic signals (Herzel *et al.*, 1991; Herzel *et al.*, 1994; Kelman, 1981; Mende *et al.*, 1990; Ramig *et al.*, 1988; Sirviö and Michelsson, 1976).

B. Modeling recurrent nerve paralysis

Recurrent nerve paralysis is associated with a change of the phonation posture. Considering the rectangular shaped glottis, a fixed rest position of only one side does not show any asymmetric effect. The glottal gap affects mainly the phonation onset as discussed in Sec. II.

In this section we want to investigate bifurcations in the $\tilde{Q}$-P_s plane. Despite the absence of a transformation as in preceding section, we restrict the analysis of the $\tilde{Q}$ dependence to the same interval as for Q to underscore the different effects of these parameters.

The bifurcation diagram in the $\tilde{Q}$-P_s plane ($\Delta\tilde{Q} = 0.01$, $\Delta P_S = 0.0002$) in Fig. 17 shows another structure than Fig. 7. There are significant differences to be seen.

The small $\tilde{Q}$ interval with period doubling or tripling at $\tilde{Q} \approx 0.7$ exists over the whole P_s scale. Bifurcations already occur at relatively large values of $\tilde{Q}$, i.e., less asymmetry. The region at $\tilde{Q} \approx 0.5,...,0.6$ shows a variety of different regimes, containing tori and chaos. The one-parameter bifurcation diagram in Fig. 18 displays the occurrence of large regions of irregular motion with interspersed periodic windows. Contrarily to the behavior in the Q-P_s plane, standard subglottal pressure 8 cm H_2O is sufficient to reach these bifurcations.

Figures 19 and 20 show toroidal and chaotic oscillations, respectively. In Figs. 21 and 22 the corresponding spectra,

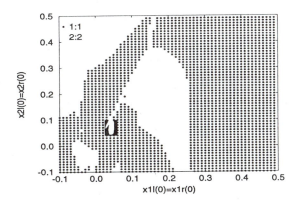

FIG. 16. Basins of attraction of the 1:1 and 2:2 limit cycle, respectively. In the case of coexistence of different attractors (here for $Q = 0.585$ and $P_s = 0.0145$) it depends on the initial conditions which limit cycle is approached. In the diagram the dependence on initial symmetric displacement is shown. Simulations are carried out on a grid in the considered plane [$\Delta x_i(0) = 0.01$]. If the motion finished in the 1:1 attractor, a star was plotted. White areas correspond to the basin of the 2:2 attractor. The borderlines of the basins seem to be smooth.

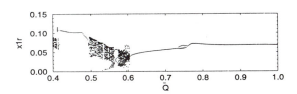

FIG. 18. One-parameter bifurcation diagram for $P_s = 0.010$ showing maxima of x_{1r} of the attractors. The evolution of the attractor as function of $\tilde{Q}$ shows abrupt transitions to other regimes. We can find regions with attractors of multiple period and aperiodic motion. Representative toroidal and chaotic oscillations are shown in the following pictures.

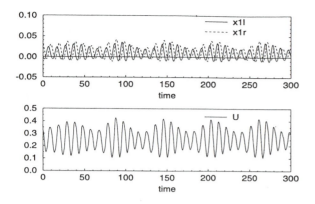

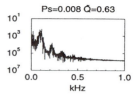

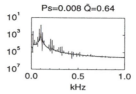

FIG. 21. The graphs show the Fourier spectra of x_{1r} from the simulations shown in Figs. 19 and 20. The spectrum of the toroidal oscillations (left) is characterized by two independent frequencies and their linear combinations. The right diagram shows the unstructured spectrum of chaotic behavior.

FIG. 19. Simulations for $P_s = 0.008$ and $\bar{Q} = 0.64$ showing toroidal oscillations. This type of motion results in a modulated acoustical signal U.

attractors, and consecutive maxima are plotted.

In addition to the occurrence of other types of attractors, bifurcations of the voice signal are not to be seen in the behavior of the affected side. In the case of frequency locking the period of $x_{1r}(t)$ does not necessarily agree with that of the glottal volume flow velocity as in the case of simulations due to the Q asymmetry.

V. SUMMARY AND DISCUSSION

The aim of the paper was to analyze bifurcations which are closely related to observations in voice pathology. For example, in Herzel et al. (1994) period tripling and low-frequency modulation have been analyzed for patients with laryngeal paralysis which are qualitatively comparable to the simulations above. In order to get comprehensive bifurcation diagrams in appropriate parameter planes we had to simplify the classic Ishizaka–Flanagan model. However, inspection of the time series and the study of the phonation onset revealed that the simplified model retained some physiological relevance.

The main focus of the paper was the location of instabilities due to different stiffness values of the left and right vocal fold that are characteristic for laryngeal paralysis. It was found that an overcritical tension imbalance leads to subharmonic regimes, two frequency oscillations, and chaos.

In many cases, the transitions are associated with hysteresis, i.e., in certain parameter regions different attractors coexist. For such a case the basins of attraction of two coexisting limit cycles have been analyzed. It turned out that these basins are intertwined, which implies an additional source of unpredictability. For slightly different initial conditions rather distinct asymptotic dynamics result.

Our paper is embedded in continuing studies on implications of nonlinear dynamics for voice research. In papers devoted to signal analysis three different kinds of attractors have been discussed (Herzel et al., 1994; Titze et al., 1993): subharmonic regimes, toroidal oscillations, and chaotic attractors. These regimes are often observed in newborn cries and voice disorders. They have been termed, for example, "octave jumps," "double harmonic break," "diplophonia," "dicrotic dysphonia," or "creaky voice."

In our model these three attractor types have been identified with the aid of phase portraits, next-maximum maps, and power spectra. The origin of the instabilities in our simplified model can be traced back to the desynchronization of two oscillators, the left and right fold. For sufficiently large effects of nonlinearities (related to large subglottal pressure) and overcritical detuning of the eigenfrequencies, complex oscillation patterns are found. Hence the hypothesis is substantiated that many observed voice instabilities are due to the desynchronization of a few principal modes of vocal-fold vibrations (Berry et al., 1994).

Earlier studies devoted to asymmetric vocal fold models

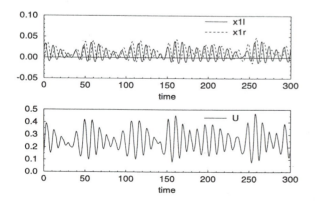

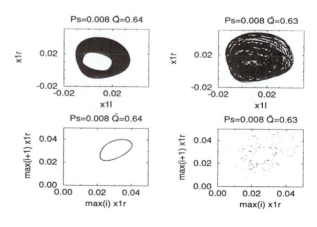

FIG. 22. The diagrams show the attractors in the x_{1l}-x_{1r} plane (upper) and plots of consecutive maxima of x_{1r} (lower), respectively, for simulations shown in Figs. 19 and 20. The difference between a torus (left) and a strange attractor corresponding to chaotic dynamics (right) is seen.

FIG. 20. Simulations for $P_s = 0.008$ and $\bar{Q} = 0.63$ showing chaotic oscillations. This type of motion results in an aperiodic acoustical signal U.

(Ishizaka and Isshiki, 1976; Smith *et al.*, 1992; Wong *et al.*, 1991) were restricted to simulations at a few parameter values or, at most, one-parameter variations. As a major methodical result of our study we claim that the complex bifurcation scenarios require the analysis of (at least) two-parameter variations. Continuation techniques such as AUTO may support direct simulations of the model equations. An already widely used two-parameter "bifurcation diagram" is the phonetogram. The location and characterization of instabilities in such planes of accessible parameters may be the appropriate strategy to compare experimental observations with models quantitatively.

Future studies will be devoted to a quantitative comparison of voice disorders and simulations along this direction. As a first step, bifurcation diagrams, such as Fig. 7 in this paper, based on more sophisticated models and excised larynx studies are desirable.

ACKNOWLEDGMENTS

We gratefully acknowledge the colleagues from the National Center for Voice and Speech for illuminating and stimulating discussions and Katharina Krischer for advice regarding continuation techniques. This work was supported by the Deutsche Forschungsgemeinschaft and by Grant No. P6000976 from the National Institute on Deafness and Other Communication Disorders.

Bergé, P., Pomeau, Y., and Vidal, C. (**1984**). *Order Within Chaos* (Wiley, New York).

Berry, D. A., Titze, I. R., Herzel, H., and Krischer, K. (**1994**). "Interpretation of biomechanical simulations of normal and chaotic vocal fold oscillations with empirical eigenfunctions," J. Acoust. Soc. Am. **95**, 3595–3604.

Broad, D. J. (**1979**). "The new theories of vocal fold vibration," in *Speech and Language: Advances in Basic Research and Practice*, edited by N. J. Lass (Academic, New York), Vol. 2.

Doedel, E. (**1986**). "AUTO: Software for Continuation and Bifurcation Problems in Ordinary Differential Equations," AUTO 86 User Manual.

Glass, L., and Mackey, M. C. (**1988**). *From Clocks to Chaos* (Princeton U.P., Princeton, NJ).

Hammarberg, B., Fritzell, B., Gauffin, J., and Sundberg, J. (**1986**). "Acoustic and perceptual analysis of vocal dysfunction," J. Phon. **14**, 533–547.

Herzel, H., Steinecke, I., Mende, W., and Wermke, K. (**1991**). "Chaos and bifurcations during voiced speech," in *Complexity, Chaos and Biological Evolution* (Plenum, New York), pp. 41–50.

Herzel, H., and Wendler, J. (**1991**). "Evidence of chaos in phonatory signals," in *Proceedings of EUROSPEECH* (European Speech Communication Association, Genova, Italy), pp. 263–266.

Herzel, H. (**1993**). "Bifurcations and chaos in voice signals," Appl. Mech. Rev. **46**, 399–413.

Herzel, H., Berry, D., Titze, I., and Saleh, M. (**1994**). "Analysis of vocal disorders with methods from nonlinear dynamics," J. Speech Hear. Res. **37**, 1008–1019.

Herzel, H., Berry, D., Titze, I., and Steinecke, I. (**1995**). "Nonlinear dynamics of the voice: Signal analysis and biomechanical modeling," Chaos **5** (January 1995).

Herzel, H., and Knudsen, C. (**1994**). "Bifurcations in a vocal fold model," Nonlinear Dyn. (in press).

Hirano, M. (**1981**). "Structure of the vocal fold in normal and disease states

anatomical and physical studies," ASHA, Tech. Rep. No. 11 (unpublished), pp. 11–30.

Ishizaka, K., and Flanagan, J. L. (**1972**). "Synthesis of voiced sounds from a two-mass model of the vocal cords," Bell. Syst. Tech. J. **51**, 1233–1268.

Ishizaka, K., and Isshiki, N. (**1976**). "Computer simulation of pathological vocal-cord vibration," J. Acoust. Soc. Am. **60**, 1193–1198.

Isshiki, N., Tanabe, M., Ishizaka, K., and Broad, D. (**1977**). "Clinical significance of asymmetrical vocal cord tension," Am. Otol. **86**, 58–66.

Jetschke, G. (**1989**). *Mathematik der Selbstorganisation* (Deutscher Verlag der Wissenschaften, Berlin).

Kelman, A. W. (**1981**). "Vibratory pattern of the vocal folds," Folia Phoniatr. **33**, 73–991.

Kubíček, M., and Marek, M. (**1983**). *Computational Methods in Bifurcation Theory and Dissipative Structures* (Springer-Verlag, New York).

Lauterborn, W., and Parlitz, U. (**1988**). "Methods of chaos physics and their application to acoustics," J. Acoust. Soc. Am. **84**, 1975–1993.

Lucero, J. C. (**1993**). "Dynamics of the two-mass model of the vocal folds: Equilibria, bifurcations, and oscillation region," J. Acoust. Soc. Am. **94**, 3104–3111.

Mende, W., Herzel, H., and Wermke, K. (**1990**). "Bifurcations and chaos in newborn infant cries," Phys. Lett. A **145**, 418–424.

Pahn, J., Dettmann, R., and Šram, F. (**1984**). "Zur Verteilung und funktionellen Auswirkung von Paresen der Stimmlippenbewegungs- und -spannungsmuskulatur anhand elektromyographischer Untersuchungen," Folia Phoniatr. **36**, 273–283.

Pelorson, X., Hirschberg, A., van Hassel, R. R., Wijnands, A. P. J., and Auregan, Y. (**1994**). "Theoretical and experimental study of quasi-steady flow separation within the glottis during phonation. Application to a modified two-mass model," J. Acoust. Soc. Am. **96**, 3416–3431.

Ramig, L. A., Scherer, R. C., Titze, I. R., and Ringel, S. P. (**1988**). "Acoustic analysis of voices of patients with neurologic disease: Rationale and preliminary data," Ann. Otol. Rhinol. Laryngol. **97**, 164–172.

Robb, M. P., and Saxman, J. H. (**1988**). "Acoustic observations in young children's non-cry vocalizations," J. Acoust. Am. **83**, 1876–1882.

Sirviö, P., and Michelsson, K. (**1976**). "Sound-spectrographic cry analysis of normal and abnormal newborn infants," Folia Phoniatr. **28**, 161–173.

Smith, M. E., Berke, G. S., Gerratt, B. R., and Kreiman, J. (**1992**). "Laryngeal paralyses: Theoretical considerations and effects on laryngeal vibration," J. Speech. Hear. Res. **35**, 545–554.

Steinecke, I. (**1993**). "Untersuchungen an einem vereinfachten Stimmlippenmodell," Diplomarbeit, Humboldt-Universität zu Berlin.

Stevens, K. N. (**1977**). "Physics of laryngeal behavior and larynx modes," Phonetica **34**, 264–279.

Story, B., and Titze, I. R. (**1995**). "Voice simulation with a body-cover model of the vocal folds," J. Acoust. Soc. Am. **97**, 1249–1260.

Titze, I. R. (**1973**). "The human vocal cords: A mathematical model. Part I," Phonetica **28**, 129–170.

Titze, I. R., and Talkin, D. T. (**1979**). "A theoretical study of the effects of various laryngeal configurations on the acoustics of phonation," J. Acoust. Soc. Am. **66**, 60–74.

Titze, I. R. (**1988**). "The physics of small amplitude oscillation of the vocal folds," J. Acoust. Soc. Am. **83**, 1536–1552.

Titze, I. R., Baken, R., and Herzel, H. (**1993**). "Evidence of chaos in vocal fold vibration," in *Vocal Fold Physiology: New Frontiers in Basic Science*, edited by I. R. Titze (Singular, San Diego), pp. 143–188.

Titze, I. R., and Alipour-Haghighi, F. (**1994**). *Myoelastic Aerodynamic Theory of Phonation* (in press).

van den Berg, J., Zantewa, J. T., and Doornenbal, R. Jr. (**1957**). "On the air resistance and the Bernoulli effect of the human larynx," J. Acoust. Soc. Am. **29**, 626–631.

Wendler, J., and Seidner, W. (**1987**). *Lehrbuch der Phoniatrie* (Georg Thieme Verlag, Leipzig).

Wong, D., Ito, M. R., Cox, N. B., and Titze, I. R. (**1991**). "Observation of perturbation in a lumped-element model of the vocal folds with application to some pathological cases," J. Acoust. Soc. Am. **89**, 383–394.

C H A P T E R
1

Nonlinearity, Complexity, and Control in Vocal Systems

Neville H. Fletcher

Our emphasis in this book is on the complexity of the behavior of the human vocal system. It is trite but true to say that all biological systems are complex and nonlinear in their response—greater stimulus does not simply increase the magnitude of the response but may bring about a qualitative change in its nature. Here we focus on just a small part of that nonlinearity by considering the physical behavior of the vocal folds and the mechanisms and strategies by which their complex behavior can be controlled.

In the case of the human vocal system, we encounter nonlinearity in the vocal fold vibrations themselves, in the aerodynamics of the flow through the vocal fold opening, and in the interaction between these two quantities. This highly nonlinear active part of the vocal system is coupled to passive and very nearly linear multimode vocal tract resonators both downstream and upstream from the glottis, and these interact with the motion and flow mechanics of the vocal folds. While it would seem that the nonlinearity and physical complexity of such a system might make its control a matter of great difficulty, it turns out, paradoxically, that the nonlinearity itself tends to lock the system into stable regimes of oscillation that can be brought under coordinated neural control.

Human speech or song is a combination of phase-locked, harmonic, voiced vowel sounds, and near-chaotic unvoiced stops and consonants, produced in rapid time-sequence. The same is true of the sounds produced by many other animals, although there are cases in which the vocal sound is both voiced and chaotic at the same time. The complexity of this behavior presents a rich field for study.

VOCAL FOLD OSCILLATIONS

The human glottis contains two approximately symmetrical vocal folds which can move to control the air flow through the larynx. Together they form a pressure-controlled valve that can be set into autonomous oscillation through interaction with the acoustic pressures in the respiratory tract above and below the larynx. Simple single-mass models [1,2] exhibit most of the characteristics of such systems for various possible directions of motion of the valve flaps, but realistic models for the human vocal folds must contain many more configurational parameters because of the flexible nature of biological tissue. The two-mass model of Ishizaki and Flanagan [3] is a well-known example of an extension in this direction, though much more complex models have also been developed. Because of the nonlinearities we discuss in the following, it is always necessary to resort to numerical methods to calculate the acoustic behavior of these system models [2,3].

The exact geometry of flow separation at the vocal folds is important to details of the valve operation and has usually been treated simply by assumption. The acoustic impedance of the air passages below the larynx, terminating in the lungs, has surprisingly also been neglected in many models, but it can have a quite significant influence on behavior. Indeed the conditions for autonomous oscillation of the vocal valve involve not only the properties of flow through the valve itself, but also the acoustic impedances of the ducts leading to and from it [1]—the bronchi and lungs upstream and the trachea and mouth downstream of the glottis. Valve oscillation is maintained by a combination of the influences of fluctuating pressure in the regions above and, more importantly, below the glottis, together with pressure differentials caused by Bernoulli effects in the flow through the valve aperture. Which driving mechanism is more important depends upon details of the valve geometry and of the separation of flow though it, and indeed we might expect these details to change progressively throughout the vocal range in the case of singers.

Note that, although there is some similarity between the operation of the vocal folds and that of the lips when playing a brass instrument such as the trumpet, there is also a very significant difference. In the vocal fold case, the frequency of vibration, which is controlled by the mass and muscular tension of the vocal cords, is much less than that of the first resonance of the vocal tract, except for high notes of a soprano voice. When playing a brass instrument, on the other hand, the natural frequency of the lip vibration is adjusted so as to nearly coincide with the frequency of one of the resonances of the instrument horn. This difference has important consequences for the exact physics of the oscillation.

One important point, usually ignored, is that the two vocal folds will generally differ in mass and tension and thus in natural resonance frequency. The motion of the folds can, however, be separated into two normal modes with slightly different frequencies: one in which the two folds move cophase relative to the symmetry plane and therefore close at one extremity of their motion, and one in which they are antiphase, as shown in Figure 1–1. The antiphase motion does not change the flow

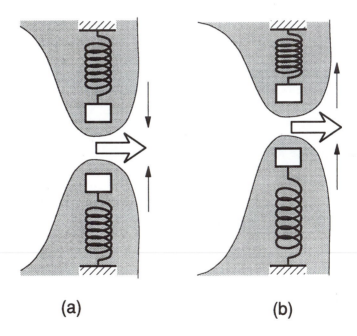

(a)   (b)

Figure 1–1. (a) Symmetric or cophase oscillation; and **(b)** antisymmetric or antiphase oscillation of vocal folds. The underlying model indicated is a "single-mass" model.

through the glottis, so that it cannot be maintained by feedback effects. The cophase motion, however, couples directly to the flow and can be maintained by appropriate feedback from flow-generated pressures. In a real vocal system with appreciable damping, we can therefore usually ignore the antiphase motion and treat the symmetrical cophase motion as the only mode of significance. This is a completely linear effect.

In a more realistic model, and particularly as we approach the reality of a model with a continuous distribution of mass and elastic properties, there are of course many other vibrational modes that should be considered. In the simple two-mass model [3], the larynx is considered to be two-dimensional, with each vocal fold consisting of a pair of masses, one on the leading and one on the trailing edge of the fold, appropriately coupled together by springs as shown in Figure 1–2(a). As is well known, numerical calculations with this model show that the mode of vocal interest is one in which there is a phase difference between the leading and trailing masses or, expressed in another way, a standing

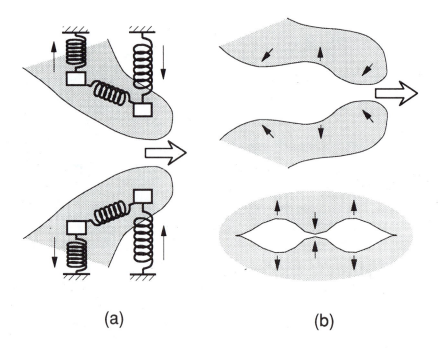

(a)   (b)

Figure 1–2. (a) Phase differences in a simple two-mass model; **(b)** some possible higher vibration modes in a more realistic continuum model. In (b) the upper drawing is a cross section and the lower drawing a face-on view of the glottis.

wave along each vocal fold, in the air flow direction, synchronized with the basic opening and closing mode for the fold pair as shown in Figure 1–2(a). The nonlinearity of the system, which we discuss in a moment, is important in synchronizing these two vibration modes to give a well organized and apparently simple vocal fold oscillation.

In a fully three-dimensional model, which comes closer to physical reality, we must allow for the possibility of phase differences in the motion of the folds, not only parallel to the air flow but also in directions normal to it, as shown in Figure 1–2(b). Each fold, indeed, is able to behave to some extent like a thick elastic plate, though this analogy is of little assistance because of the complex shape of the folds. The various possible vibrational modes of the folds have frequencies that are completely unrelated. Some of these vibrations can be ruled out of consideration in a perfect larynx because their symmetry is such that they do not affect the glottal flow, although the asymmetries of a deformed or damaged vocal fold may reintroduce this coupling.

The principal sources of nonlinearity in the vocal fold oscillation are illustrated in Figure 1–3. In a linear system, the effective vibrating mass, the spring constant, and the damping coefficient are all constant over the oscillation cycle, and the resulting differential equation describing the

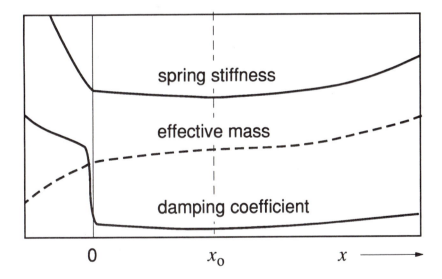

Figure 1–3. Qualitative behavior of the spring constant and the damping coefficient for vocal fold oscillation. The coordinate x measures the opening between the folds, with x_0 being the equilibrium opening distance.

motion is linear, in a mathematical sense. For vocal fold oscillations this is true for very small motions about the equilibrium position x_0 but the approximation breaks down for larger oscillations. As the vocal folds open more widely, the spring stiffness of the biological tissues increases and so does the effective mass recruited into the vibration. As the vocal folds close together, however, the departure of these parameters from constancy becomes extreme—the spring stiffness increases greatly and so does the damping coefficient, because the tissues of the two folds are being distorted by their contact. These nonlinearities are enhanced if the equilibrium opening distance x_0 is small and if the amplitude of the vocal fold oscillations is large.

The effects of nonlinearity upon oscillatory behavior are many and varied. If we consider just a single mode of vibration, for example in a single-mass model, then the effect is simply to distort the normal sinusoidal time variation of the opening dimension x so that the waveform is clipped softly at extreme openings and sharply when the folds close together. This introduces phase-locked harmonics of the fundamental in the motion and hence in the air flow through the glottis. The strength of these harmonic partials increases with the amplitude of the vocal fold vibration; initially the amplitude of the nth harmonic increases as the nth power of the amplitude of the fundamental. This is reflected in the air flow through the glottis and in the sound quality of the voice, which progresses from dull to strident as the subglottal air pressure, which controls vocal fold vibration amplitude, is increased.

In the case of a multimass model of the vocal folds, and in particular for the realistic case in which the mass distribution is continuous, there are many possible vibration modes with frequencies that have no simple numerical relation between them. In is a characteristic of such multimode systems that a sufficient degree of nonlinearity can lock all these vibrations into exact harmonic frequency relationship, so that the resulting motion is simple and periodic [4]. This almost always happens in vocal fold oscillations, because the closing nonlinearity is extreme, and to it we owe the fact that human vowel sounds, and indeed most voiced animal sounds, have strictly harmonic upper partials, as can be seen from the fact that the waveform of the steady sound repeats exactly in each cycle.

As well as the mode-locking behavior that can be induced by strong nonlinearity, nonlinear systems are also capable of a variety of complex behavior, depending upon details of their excitation. If the system is sufficiently simple, such as a single-mass model, then we can find the normal progression from a period-doubling bifurcation, giving a subharmonic an octave below the normal frequency, through further successive bifurcations to chaotic behavior [5]. This chaotic behavior is called deterministic chaos, because it is governed by simple underlying laws, and the tools that have been developed for its study are many. In particular, we can derive much of the detail from a consideration of the time series representing the oscillation [6] and from that a strange attractor with fractal geometry. Needless to say, if the vocal fold oscillation is bifurcated or chaotic, so too will be the flow through the glottis and hence the vocal sound. We return to this later.

Any realistic model of the human vocal folds necessarily involves a description of its configuration involving more than a single displacement parameter—the dimensionality of the system is greater than unity. Such complex systems can again show two sorts of behavior: Either they can become locked into a stable oscillation regime or they can exhibit bifurcations and chaos. The stable regime is simple to treat, since the variations of all coordinates are harmonically related, but the chaotic regime can be very complicated. It is not possible, in general, to derive simple attractor mappings from the time series representing the oscillation, because its description may involve a phase space of many dimensions. Any projection onto a space of lower dimensionality then results in a featureless cloud from which nothing can be deduced.

While examples of chaotic vocal fold oscillation are happily rare in the case of humans, the same is not necessarily true of other animals. An excellent example is provided by the Australian sulfur-crested cockatoo (Cacatua galerita). The syrinx of a bird is in many ways analogous to the larynx of a human, but there are several distinct differences. In the first place, the valve in the syrinx is not a single structure lying in the trachea above the junction of the two bronchi but rather a pair of independent valves, one in each bronchus, lying just below the junction with the trachea. In the second place, each valve consists of a membrane forced into the airway by pressure in a surrounding air sac, rather than a flap of tissue tensed by cartilage. Nevertheless, the operation of the syrinx can be described by a simple nonlinear model that is quite similar to a single-mass model for the human vocal folds [7]. While mostly exhibiting a simple phase-locked oscillation regime similar to that of the human vocal folds, this model can be induced to display complex and chaotic behavior. It is to be expected that a more realistic model, with the syrinx membranes described by several geometric parameters, would behave similarly. The cockatoo Cacatua galerita is one of those birds that can be trained to imitate human speech, but its natural call is an extremely loud and raucous screech with a wide-band spectrum peaking around 7 kHz. Analysis of the resulting time series suggests that the dimensionality of the oscillation is high, reflecting a multiparameter oscillating system, so that it is difficult to treat. We should perhaps be grateful that the normal speech of humans is more disciplined!

FLOW NONLINEARITY

Oscillation of the vocal folds, as we have seen, is nonlinear, with the folds spending an appreciable part of each cycle in the closed state and with the extent of peak opening limited by elastic nonlinearities. The extent of this oscillation nonlinearity will increase as the energy of the oscillation increases, an effect that can be achieved by increasing the pressure below the glottis. Muscular control of the static separation of the vocal folds can also influence the fraction of each period spent in the closed state, although under nearly all assumptions the vocal folds do close once in each cycle.

The source spectrum for the voice is determined by the flow of air through the glottis, and therefore by the product of the area of the glottal opening and the velocity of air flow. The open cross section of the glottis does not behave in a simple sinusoidal fashion, as we have seen, because of elastic nonlinearities and collision of the vocal folds upon closure. The extent of this departure from sinusoidal behavior is at least partially under muscular control. Flow through the vocal fold aperture is itself nonlinear and governed to a good approximation by the Bernoulli equation, which shows that flow velocity is proportional to the square root of the pressure drop across the aperture. This Bernoulli flow nonlinearity is convolved with the nonsinusoidal variation of the aperture area and with the variation of pressure below and above the vocal folds and further distorts the flow waveform. Both the acoustic power in the glottal source and the fraction of energy in high harmonics are increased if the subglottal pressure is high, though the conversion efficiency from pneumatic energy in flow from the lungs to acoustic energy in the vocal tract is typically less than 10%.

As is well known, the flow spectrum is then multiplied by the resonant response of the vocal tract to impress upon it the formants that are a vital part of speech. In principle, there are also formants that include the part of the vocal tract below the glottis during the part of each cycle in which the vocal folds are open. The prominence of these formants depends upon the damping of the complete vocal tract, including its lower termination in the lungs. It seems that this termination is sufficiently resistive in humans that these full-length formants are not observed, though the opposite appears to be true of at least some birds [7]. We should also, in principle, take into account the interaction of the high-frequency pressure fluctuations in the trachea upon the motion of the vocal folds. In practice, however, since these formant oscillations are at frequencies that are a high multiple of the vocal fold vibration frequency, they have little effect. They are important, however, in influencing the instantaneous flow through the open glottis.

Because of flow losses in the glottis and viscous and thermal losses in the vocal tract, the total conversion efficiency from pneumatic energy supplied by the lungs to acoustic energy radiated from the mouth rarely exceeds 1%, and is often much lower [7]. Similar figures apply to sound-producing systems of other types, including musical instruments and electromagnetic loudspeakers.

COMPLEX FLOW BEHAVIOR

Complexity of flow behavior, apart from that introduced by complex behavior of the vocal folds, can arise in two ways. The first, which can occur even in laminar flow, is a variation of the point of detachment of the flow from the trailing edge of the valve aperture, as shown in Figure 1–4. Such a variation can clearly have a large effect on the Bernoulli pres-

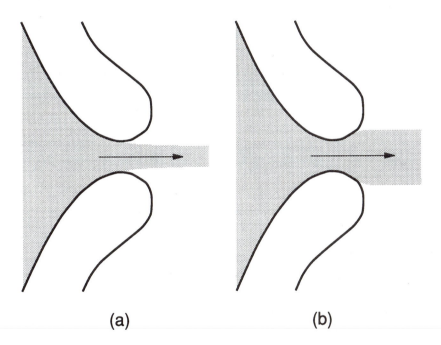

(a)   (b)

Figure 1–4. Variation in flow detachment points. **(a)** Early flow detachment with a vena contracta effect that further reduces the jet cross section; **(b)** late detachment with partial expansion of the jet after the constriction.

sures acting on various parts of the vocal folds and thus upon their motion. If this variation is periodic then it simply adds to the harmonic development, but more complex behavior is possible. Because the process is nonlinear it can exhibit period bifurcation and thus the generation of subharmonics. In the limit this can lead to chaotic behavior and turbulence. Since flow behavior is responsible for acoustic output and also reacts back upon the motion of the vocal folds, these complexities of flow are important for understanding voice quality.

The second effect, which is largely responsible for the wide-band noise associated with fricatives and sibilants, derives from turbulent flow either at the larynx or in the mouth. This turbulence generally has so many possible degrees of freedom that it is truly chaotic rather than deterministically chaotic, as we find with systems of lower dimensionality. There may, however, be deterministic elements embedded in the flow and associated with quasiregular vortex shedding from parts of the bounding structure. It is difficult to do much with turbulence except to describe its fluctuation spectrum and associated radiated acoustic power.

CONTROL

When controlling a linear system, one has simply to set the values of controlling parameters, such as muscular tensions and blowing pressures, and then allow sufficient time for the system to settle into equilibrium. This time is controlled by the system Q value and is typically a few tens of cycles of the fundamental oscillation. In the control of a nonlinear system, on the other hand, we must pay attention not just to the final state but also to the trajectory in parameter space by which that state is approached, since the final oscillation regime can be a function of system history.

This complexity might at first sight appear quite daunting, but in fact it can have some advantages from the point of view of control, particularly when we wish to produce several different kinds of output. A deterministically chaotic system has two important properties. The first is that its trajectory in phase space goes close to every possible point on the attractor and thus to every possible regime of oscillation, usually within rather few cycles of the basic oscillation. The second is that the future behavior of the trajectory, and thus the form of the future oscillation, can be influenced to an extremely large extent by a very small change in the parameters of the system. Together these two facts mean that any desired mode can be stabilized, at least in principle, by repeated application of very small corrections to the system parameters. They also mean that, if we wish to change the regime of oscillation, then we just need to let the system run autonomously for a short time until its trajectory brings it close to a point on the orbit we wish to choose, when a small correction can stabilize this new regime.

When such a control operation is considered ab initio, its possible complexity is daunting. It is quite another thing, however, when the control is exercised by a human neural system. Such a neural system behaves as an elaboration of the simple neural networks that are now exciting increasing attention as intelligent decision and control systems. A simplified example is shown in Figure 1–5. Each element of the system mimics a neuron, in that it has several input connections and a single output, and

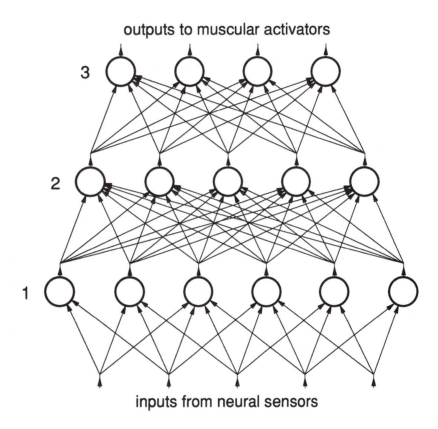

Figure 1–5. A simple neural network. Layer 1 of the network accepts stimuli from neural sensors in various parts of the body, while layer 3 produces control signals for the vocal muscles. Layer 2 is a hidden layer with no external connections. The arrows indicate signal-path connections between the three layers, each connection having an assigned weight that can be changed during the training process.

has only two output states, "on" and "off." Whether a neuron is in the on or the off state is determined by a weighted average of the on or off signals applied to its inputs, the weighting factors for the input links being important parameters of the network. The elements are arranged in at least three layers and there is a great deal of interconnectivity between them. The neurons of the lowest layer sense the physical state of the system at some instant and each turns on or off depending upon the stimulus it receives. The outputs of this layer feed to the second "hidden" layer and turn its elements on or off depending upon the weightings assigned to the network links. The outputs of the elements of the second layer now pass on to the third layer and similarly determine its pattern of on and off states. There is thus a wave of "neural" activity that passes through the system from its first to its third layer, and we can suppose the process to be repeated many times each second as the state of the system changes. The third layer is the output layer of the network, and its pattern of on/off states directly controls muscular actuators that influence the state of the system. Note that the elements of the neural network are highly nonlinear in their response—a small change in the input states can flip a neuron from its off state to its on state. The network as a whole is nonlinear in a very much more subtle and complex way, and its outputs are not simple functions of its inputs.

We can represent this more formally by supposing that O_i is the output signal, either 0 for "off" or +1 for "on," from the ith neuron. The input signal I_j to the jth neuron is then

$$I_j = \sum_i w_{ij} O_j$$

where the w_{ij} are the synaptic weighting factors, either positive or negative, for the links between neurons i and j. Neuron j will now fire and produce an output signal of +1 if $I_j > T$ where T is a threshold value built into the neuron. Each neuron of the network has a similar behavior, but the weighting factors w_{ij} are different for each link of the network.

Neural networks "learn" by modifying the weights assigned to their internal synaptic connections so as to reinforce desired outputs and inhibit those that are undesired. In this way they can maintain a system in a desired state, which may be either constant or else varying in time in a regular manner. The same approach can be applied to system trajectories. The time-varying weighting parameters corresponding to the desired trajectory are stored somewhere outside the network and then passed to it in sequence. This is quite clearly closely related to the way in which humans learn complex tasks—first we learn to maintain steady states such as vowel sounds and then to combine them to produce desired outputs such as phonemes and then words. One might speculate that the problems associated with a "breaking" voice in adolescent male humans are not so much due to physical changes in the larynx, although these are certainly present, but rather to a time lag in adjusting the synaptic weights in the associated neural control system.

With simple neural networks, and even more strikingly with real neural control systems, it is difficult or even impossible to analyze the behavior at a component level—the system is not a conventional von Neumann machine, like an ordinary computer, but something altogether more complex.

CONCLUSIONS

While the physiology and physics of voice production are both interesting subjects in their own right, the importance of studying these matters comes from the fact that vocal communication is a vital part of our everyday life and cultural heritage. The more we can understand about the complexities of the vocal system and its control mechanisms, the better we will be able to repair its defects and to learn or teach about its exploitation.

This book focuses on nonlinearity and complexity in both the vocal system and its neural control. As we have explained above, the nonlinearity of the system is responsible for the richness of vocal sounds, and it is also responsible for the fact that these sounds generally have regularly repeating waveforms and thus harmonic spectra. The nonlinearity locks the behavior of the system into one of a number of regimes of autonomous oscillation, which can then be controlled as stable entities. At the same time, nonlinearity allows the possibility of more complex and even chaotic behavior, and it is generally the objective of the neural control system to avoid these.

A recognition of the nature of the neural control system, and its simplified modeling as a neural network, shows us the role of both imitative practice and conscious thought in achieving both routine vocal utterances and special vocal effects. Certainly this approach has been exploited by evolutionary processes in natural childhood development, and recognized by teachers for millenia. A more thorough understanding of the science upon which these methods are based should make them even more effective.

REFERENCES

1. N.H. Fletcher, "Autonomous vibration of simple pressure-controlled valves in gas flows," *J. Acoust. Soc. Am.* **93**, 2172–2180 (1993).
2. S. Adachi and M. Sato, "Time-domain simulation of sound production in the brass instrument," *J. Acoust. Soc. Am.* **97**, 3850–3861 (1995).
3. K. Ishizaka and J.L. Flanagan, "Synthesis of voiced sounds from a two-mass model of the vocal cords," *Bell Syst. Tech. J.* **51**, 1233–1268 (1972).
4. N.H. Fletcher, "Mode locking in nonlinearly excited inharmonic musical oscillators," *J. Acoust. Soc. Am.* **64**, 1566–1569 (1978).
5. P. Cvitanovic (Ed.), *Universality in Chaos*, (Adam Hilger, Bristol 1984).
6. N.H. Packard, J.P Crutchfield, J.P Farmer and R.S. Shaw, "Geometry from a time series," *Phys. Rev. Lett.* **45**, 712–716 (1980).
7. N.H. Fletcher, *Acoustic Systems in Biology*, (Oxford University Press, New York 1992) Ch. 14.

C H A P T E R
5

Possible Mechanisms of
Vocal Instabilities

Hanspeter Herzel

Much evidence of bifurcations and chaos in voice signals has been given during the past years. Several techniques such as spectrograms, pitch and amplitude contours, phase portraits, Poincaré sections, and dimension calculations have been applied to characterize voice signals from a nonlinear dynamics point of view [1,2]. The analyzed signals include newborn cries [3], fry-like phonation [4,5], and, particularly, vocalizations from voice patients [6].

Furthermore, bifurcation scenarios have been analyzed in a hierarchy of biomechanical vocal fold models [7,8]. For example in a recent paper, asymmetric vocal fold properties have been modeled [9]. The results have relevance for unilateral vocal fold paralyses.

However, there is still a gap between theoretical models of instabilities and clinical observations. For a quantitative comparison of models and experimental data, high-speed video techniques [10] and excised larynx experiments [11] are promising tools. Moreover, the concept of "modes" seems to be a valuable tool to relate computer simulations to observed vibratory patterns.

This chapter is organized as: First the terminus "rough voice" is discussed from different perspectives and it will be concluded that roughness is intimately related to the concept of nonlinear dynamics. Then, various possible mechanisms of voice instabilities are listed and some results from signal analysis, modeling, and excised larynx experiments

63

are presented. The observed instabilities are visualized with the aid of fundamental frequency contours.

CHARACTERISTICS OF ROUGH VOICES

Clinical Observations

Despite some ongoing discussions about the proper terminology, one needs to classify abnormal voices. "Hoarseness" serves as an overall measure for the deviation from a normal voice. The term "breathiness" is related to turbulent noise generated in the vocal apparatus and can be quantified by the amount of high-frequency noise and/or the relative weakness of harmonics of the pitch. Even though turbulence is a manifestation of high-dimensional chaos [12], most tools of nonlinear dynamics apply only to low-dimensional chaos. Consequently, breathiness is out of the scope of this chapter.

"Roughness" is assumed to result from irregular vibrations of the vocal folds. These can be analyzed in the framework of bifurcation theory and chaotic dynamics. Stroboscopy reveals that irregular patterns often appear in various diseases [13,14] such as laryngitis, polyps, Reinke's edema, cysts, carcinoma, and vocal fold paralysis. It is the aim of this chapter to discuss possible methods for an understanding and quantification of these irregularities.

Perception and Acoustic Analyses

There are numerous attempts to relate perceptual categories such as roughness to perturbation measures from acoustic analyses (see e.g. [15,16]). However, results are less than successful. A few authors found a strong correlation between roughness scores and correlated fluctuations of periods and amplitudes [17–19]. These findings suggest that widely used jitter and shimmer calculations that measure only the amount of perturbations (but not its correlations) are not sufficient to quantify roughness.

Hopefully, the understanding of the underlying mechanisms of irregularities will provide hints for a quantification of roughness from acoustic signals.

Psychoacoustic Roughness Measures

Relatively independent of the voice research community, a quantitative characterization of perceived roughness has been developed [20–22].

Actually the unit asper has been introduced to measure roughness. One asper is to the roughness of a 70 Hz amplitude-modulation of a 1 kHz tone (100% modulation). It is found in psychoacoustic experiments that such 70 Hz modulations give the highest roughness scores. For tone frequencies lower than 1 kHz, there is a decrease of modulation frequency that gives maximum roughness. For a carrier frequency of 200 Hz roughness is mostly perceived for modulation frequencies around 30 Hz. Similar results are found for frequency modulation and band-filtered noise. In summary, frequencies between 20 and 70 Hz are sources of perceived roughness.

Bifurcations and Roughness

In the literature, phenomena such as "octave jumps," "biphonation" (two independent pitches), and "noise concentrations" have been reported for decades [23,24]. However, only within the past few years it has been emphasized that these observations can be related to period-doubling bifurcations, tori, and chaos, respectively [2,3].

The theory of coupled nonlinear oscillators predicts that the following phenomena should appear at the borderline of parameter regions corresponding to normal phonation: Subharmonic vocalization (appearance of spectral peaks at F0/2, F0/3, and its multiples), beating-like low-frequency modulations, and low-dimensional chaos with a continuum of spectral components. Acoustic signals from voice patients indeed show often sudden jumps to subharmonic regimes (period doubling or tripling) and low-frequency modulations (tori) [1,6].

At this point the connection of nonlinear phenomena to results of psychoacoustic and perturbation analysis becomes obvious. Subharmonics and modulations induce correlated fluctuations of pitch and amplitudes that were found to correlate to roughness scores. Subharmonics F0/2, F0/3, and so on, plus modulation frequencies often occur in the frequency range below 70 Hz, which gives the impression of roughness according to the psychoacoustic theory [22].

In this way, a consistent unification of different approaches to "roughness" is possible: Nonlinear phenomena of the voice generating system generate low-frequency components that are perceived as a rough voice and can be characterized quantitatively using pitch and amplitude contours. However, the central problem of finding the underlying physiological mechanisms remains to be discussed.

POSSIBLE MECHANISMS OF INSTABILITIES

At the current state of the art, the following list of sources of irregularities has a somewhat speculative character. It is the aim of intense research at the National Center for Voice and Speech of the USA and in other groups to substantiate the ideas below. Some preliminary results are presented in the following sections.

Without making claims about their relative importance, possible candidates are listed:

- **Neurological sources:** Unsteadiness of muscle contraction due to variations in motor unit firing is a possible source of physiological jitter and shimmer [25,26]. Moreover, vibrato and vocal tremor in the frequency range of 3–12 Hz seem to be related to a neural feedback loop [27]. Modulations of higher frequencies (say, e.g., 40 Hz) and subharmonic vocalization have preliminary biomechanical origin, for example, the muscle tension can be regarded as approximately constant. This point of view is supported by computer simulations and excised larynx experiments, which exhibit these phenomena without any variations in neuromuscular control.

- **Aerodynamic instabilities:** Even if the flow is not predominantly turbulent (as for a breathy voice) vortex shedding and instabilities of the jet emerging from the glottis may cause perturbations [28,29]. The interaction of vortex shedding with acoustic resonances may generate whistle-like sound. Moreover, by means of transverse "lift forces" periodically generated vortices can induce self-sustained oscillations of vibrating structures ("vortex-induced vibrations"). Such a vibratory regime was observed recently in excised larynx experiments and might be associated with the so-called whistle-register of the soprano voice [4]. Moreover, the interaction of vortices with vocal resonances might induce secondary frequencies. Two frequencies are observed occasionally in newborn cries [24], excised larynx experiments [4], and vocalizations of voice patients [1].

- **Coupling between vocal folds and sub- and supraglottal resonances:** This coupling might play a role in extreme situations such as pressed voice where supraglottal pressure changes play an essential part in driving the vocal folds.

- **Mucus:** It is a frequent observation in clinical practice that inappropriate management of mucus riding on vocal fold tissue leads to a perturbed voice.

- **Asymmetry of left and right fold:** For certain disorders such as unilateral vocal fold paralyses or highly asymmetric vocal fold lesions the desynchronization of both folds might be the dominant mechanism (see below).

- **Anterior–posterior modes:** Such horizontal motion can frequently be seen in stroboscopy and high-speed movies [10]. However, in many cases these modes are entrained by the main vibratory modes, and hence, they do not induce much irregularity.
- **Desynchronization of horizontal motion ("10-mode" related to opening and closing) and vertical modes ("11-mode" related to the well-known phase shift of upper and lower edge of the folds):** These two vibratory modes are dominating for normal chest voice. Their desynchronization might play a prominent role in voice disorders. For example, vocal fry, which is often symptomatic in voice pathology, seems to be related to this mechanism. Computer simulations have shown [7] that a lax cover that slows down the 11-mode gives rise to vibratory pattern known from high-speed films of vocal fry [30].

In the following sections, some results of earlier and ongoing studies are reported that give some first hints on the underlying physiological mechanisms of vocal instabilities. More detailed information can be gained from the citations.

BIOMECHANICAL INSTABILITIES OF SYMMETRIC VOCAL FOLDS

Vocal fold vibrations are characterized by a huge number of degrees of freedom. In the case of normal phonation, all vibratory modes are essentially synchronized. In this section we consider instabilities that maintain symmetry between both folds. Vocal fry is a well-known example of apparently symmetric complex vibrations. Moreover, period-doubling bifurcations have been also reported for nodules [6,31] that usually appear symmetrically.

Figure 5–1 shows bifurcations for apparently symmetric folds in an excised larynx experiment. Details of the experimental apparatus are given elsewhere [4]. The pitch contour displays alternating cycle lengths as a manifestation of a period-doubling bifurcation. Around cycle 405 a jump to another subharmonic regime with a strong period-three component can be seen.

Comparable bifurcations for symmetric vocal folds have also been analyzed in biomechanical-aerodynamic models of the vocal folds. In Herzel et al. [8], the well-known two-mass model introduced by Ishizaka and Flanagan [32] was analyzed. The model exhibits just two vibratory modes: in-phase and out-of-phase motion of the two masses.

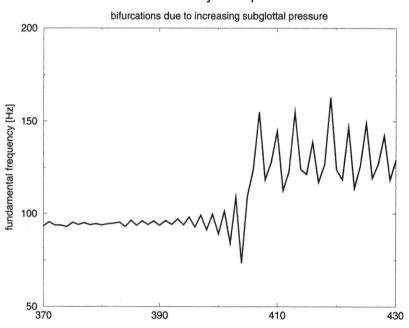

Figure 5–1. Pitch contour for slowly increasing subglottal pressure. The bifurcations are observed around a pressure of 19 cm water gauge. All contours in this chapter are calculated using the voice analysis package GLIMPSES from the National Center for Voice and Speech [39].

It was found that detuning of the two eigenfrequencies by lowering the stiffness of the upper mass gives rise to subharmonics, modulations, and chaos [8]. Similar bifurcations have been found in the symmetric continuum model developed at The University of Iowa [33]. For a decreased transverse Youngs modulus of the cover subharmonics and chaos appear [2,7]. These findings suggest that instabilities do not require asymmetry. Symmetric folds already exhibit many degrees of freedom that can be desynchronized under certain conditions.

Analyzing the output of the finite element model, the concept of modes turned out to be very fruitful. This idea was already introduced by Titze and Strong [34] and is extensively discussed in Berry et al. [7]. Considering vocal folds as a three-dimensional continuum, many possible vibratory modes exist. However, in the case of normal phonation, these different modes are all synchronized to a high degree, and the resulting dynamics appears to be nearly periodic. Due to vocal fold lesions or under extreme conditions (pressed voice, vocal fry, inspiratory phonation, etc.), highly irregular vibrations can appear due to the desynchronization of modes. At least qualitatively, different modes can be detected by high-speed movies [10] and to some extent also by stroboscopy. Consequently, the mode concept provides a unifying framework to interpret computer simulations, excised larynx studies, and clinical observations.

INSTABILITIES DUE TO ASYMMETRY

If the biomechanical properties of the left and right fold are very different, desynchronization of both folds can occur. Hirano et al. [15] compare, for example, vocal fold movement in case of paralysis with "a flag flapping in the wind." Clear indications of bifurcations have been reported in many patients with unilateral laryngeal nerve paralysis [6,35,36]. Figure 5–2 displays three pitch contours from very rough sounding voices from patients with paralysis. The vocalizations have been recorded at the university hospital (Charite) of the Humboldt University [1]. To remove trends, we plot the second derivative of the contour termed second-order perturbation function in Pinto and Titze [37].

The contours display a strong period three (upper graph), period two with superimposed modulations (middle graph), and transitions from period four via irregular perturbations to alternating periods (lower graph).

The role of asymmetry was the focus of recent excised larynx experiments [4]. Elastic asymmetry was imposed by systematic lengthening and shortening of one of the folds. Several instabilities were induced by asymmetry, including fry-like phonation and single fold vibrations. Many of the bifurcations were noted in parameter regions where different phonatory regimes coexist. For instance, the pitch contour in Figure 5–3 was found close to a transition from falsetto-like phonation to chest-like phonation. The contour in Figure 5–3 is characterized by a modulation of about 20 Hz with varying degree of modulation. The corresponding spectrogram shows side-bands around F0, 2 F0, and so on (Figure 3 in [11]).

In computer simulations, asymmetries are studied by assigning different masses and elastic properties to the folds. Alternating amplitudes in an asymmetric two-mass model have been already found by Ishizaka and Isshiki [38]. Recent extensive simulations of an asymmetric two-mass model have shown that a variety of bifurcations occurs for over-critical detuning of the left and right eigenfrequencies and relatively

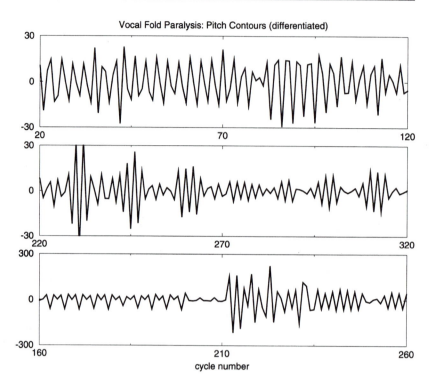

Figure 5–2. Pitch perturbations from patients with recurrent nerve paralyses. Upper graph: male patient, vowel "o," strong subharmonics at multiples of F0/3. middle graph: male patient, vowel "a," spectral peaks at multiples of F0/2. Lower graph: male patient, vowel "e", side bands around F0, 2 F0, etc.

large subglottal pressure [9]. Most frequently one finds sudden jumps to subharmonic regimes at the borderline of normal phonation. Using spectrograms, the qualitative similarity of these simulations to voice disorders have been visualized in [11]. In Figure 5–4 we present bifurcations due to increasing asymmetry with the aid of a pitch contour. The ratio of the eigenfrequencies was reduced in steps of 0.005 from 0.555 to 0.52 for a subglottal pressure of 15 cm H_2O. The low pitch results from the reduction of the stiffness of the affected fold.

Figure 5–4 shows a transition to alternating periods, followed by a subharmonic regime with period five and a final state with period three. Note the qualitative similarity to contours from patients and excised larynx experiments.

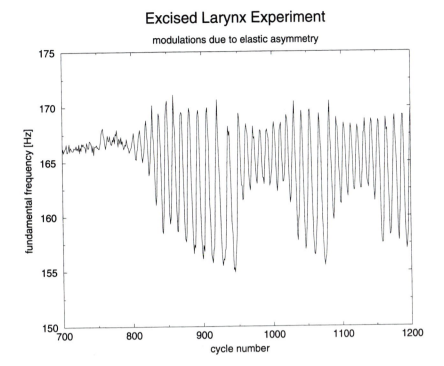

Figure 5–3. Pitch contour with pronounced modulations induced by elastic asymmetry.

Summarizing, asymmetry of mechanical properties of the folds seems to be a relevant source of instabilities. Consequently, a treatment of unilateral paralyses should not only restore the geometric symmetry, but should also equalize the vibratory properties to support synchronization.

SUMMARY AND DISCUSSION

There is now convincing evidence that a rough voice is intimately related to nonlinear phenomena such as period-doubling, toroidal oscillations, and chaos. These regimes can be effectively detected by looking for alternating amplitudes or modulations in pitch or amplitude contours. In frequency domain, these phenomena are often associated with peaks at subharmonics of the fundamental frequencies or with indepen-

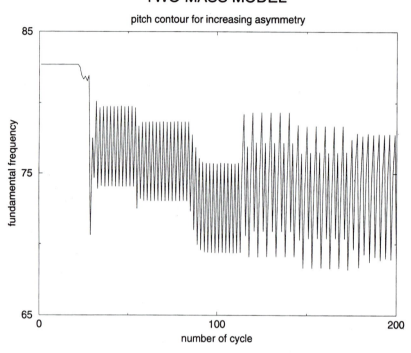

Figure 5–4. Subharmonic bifurcations in an asymmetric two-mass model.

dent frequencies. Since these additional spectral components are often in the range of 20 to 70 Hz (frequently as side-bands of the peaks at F0, 2 F0, etc.), they are perceived as roughness according to the concept of psychoacoustics [21].

However, the interpretation of instabilities as bifurcations is only the very first step. The aim of current research is to detect the physiological mechanisms and to achieve quantitative agreement between observations and computer simulations. Several possible mechanisms have been listed in this chapter, and a few of them (desynchronization of vibratory modes, asymmetry) have been discussed in some detail. Neurological and aerodynamic sources are not explored in this chapter.

The following tools seem to be essential for further progress:

- **Two-parameter-bifurcation diagrams:** This means that the instabilities are located in planes of parameters of physiological interest (subglottal pressure, muscle tension, . . .). For example, voice range profiles (phonetograms) can be regarded as such a diagram where regions of sustained oscillations are separated from regions of no phonation. Bifurcation diagrams have been calculated for the asymmetric two-mass model [9] and measured in excised larynx studies [4].

- **Mode concept:** The characterization of instabilities as desynchronization of vibratory modes provides a framework for the classification of biomechanically induced irregularities in models and observations.
- **Excised larynx studies:** Experiments with human or animal larynges serve as a link between the human voice source in vivo and computer models [25]. They allow controlled and systematic parameter variations and easy observation of vibratory patterns.
- **High speed digital imaging:** A visualization of irregular patterns is of central importance for detecting the physiological mechanisms of instabilities.

These techniques and broad interdisciplinary cooperation will hopefully lead to a better understanding and treatment of voice disorders in the future.

ACKNOWLEDGMENTS

This work is a result of a fruitful cooperation with Juergen Wendler, Ina Steinecke, Ingo Titze, and David Berry. It was supported by the Deutsche Forschungsgemeinschaft and Grant No. P60 00976 from the National Institute on Deafness and Other Communication Disorders.

REFERENCES

1. H. Herzel and J. Wendler, "Evidence of chaos in phonatory samples", in *Proceedings EUROSPEECH* (ESCA, Genova 1991) pp. 263–266
2. I.R. Titze, R. Baken, and H. Herzel, "Evidence of chaos in mbvocal fold vibration", in *Vocal Fold Physiology: Frontiers in Basic Science*, Ed. I.R. Titze (Singular Publishing Group, San Diego 1993) pp. 143–188
3. W. Mende, H. Herzel, and K. Wermke, "Bifurcations and chaos in newborn cries", *Phys. Lett.* A **145**, 418–424 (1990)
4. D. Berry, H. Herzel, I.R. Titze, and B. Story, "Bifurcations in excised larynx experiments", *J. Voice* (submitted 1995)

5. H. Herzel, "Bifurcations and chaos in voice signals", *Appl. Mech. Rev.* **46**, 399–413 (1993)

6. H. Herzel, D. Berry, I.R. Titze, and M. Saleh, "Analysis of vocal disorders with methods from nonlinear dynamics", *J. Speech and Hearing Res.* **37**, 1008–1019 (1994)

7. D.A. Berry, H. Herzel, I.R. Titze, and K. Krischer, "Interpretation of biomechanical simulations of normal and chaotic vocal fold oscillations with empirical eigenfunctions", *J. Acoust. Soc. Am* **95**, 3595–3604 (1994)

8. H. Herzel, I. Steinecke, W. Mende, and K. Wermke, "Chaos and bifurcations during voiced speech", in *Complexity, Chaos and Biological Evolution*, Eds. E. Mosekilde and L. Mosekilde (Plenum Press, New York 1991) pp. 41–50

9. I. Steinecke and H. Herzel, "Bifurcations in an asymmetric vocal fold model", *J. Acoust. Soc. Am.* **97**, 1874–1884 (1995)

10. M.M. Hess, M. Gross, and H. Herzel, "Hochgeschwindigkeitsaufnahmen von Schwingungsmoden der Stimmlippen", *Otorhinolaryngologia NOVA* **4**, 307–312 (1994)

11. Herzel, D. Berry, I.R. Titze, and I. Steinecke, "Nonlinear Dynamics of the voice: Signal analysis and biomechanical modeling", *CHAOS* **5**, 30–34 (1995)

12. S.S. Narayanan and A.A. Alwan, "A nonlinear dynamical systems analysis of fricative consonants", *J. Acoust. Soc. Am.* **97**, 2511–2524 (1995)

13. M. Hirano, "Objective evaluation of the human voice: Clinical aspects", *Folia Phoniatrica 41*, 89–144 (1989)

14. J. Wendler and W. Seidner, *Lehrbuch der Phoniatrie*, (Georg Thieme Verlag, Leipzig 1987)

15. M. Hirano, S. Hibi, R. Terasawa, and M. Fujiu, "Relationship between aerodynamic, vibratory, acoustic and psychoacoustic correlates in dysphonia", *J. Phonetics* **14**, 445–456 (1986)

16. J. Kreiman, B.R. Gerrat, and K. Precoda, "Listener experience and perception of voice quality", *J. Speech and Hearing Res.* **33**, 103–115 (1990)

17. J. Hillenbrand, "Perception of aperiodicities in synthetically generated voices", *J. Acoust. Soc. Am.* **83**, 2361–2371 (1988)

18. S. Imaizumi, "Acoustic measures of roughness in pathological voice", *J. Phonetics* **14**, 475–462 (1986)

19. Y. Koike, "Vowel amplitude modulations in patients with laryngeal diseases", *J. Acoust. Soc. Am.* **45**, 839–844 (1969)

20. W. Aures, "Ein Berechnungsverfahren der Rauhigkeit", *Acustica* **58**, 268–281 (1985)

21. E. Terhardt, "On the perception of periodic sound fluctuation (roughness)", *Acustica* **30**, 201–213 (1974)

22. E. Zwicker and H. Fastl, *Psychoacoustics*, (Springer-Verlag, Berlin 1990)

23. A.W. Kelman, "Vibratory pattern of the vocal folds", *Folia Phoniatrica* **33**, 73–99 (1981)

24. J. Lind (Ed.), *Newborn Infant Cry* (Almquist and Wiksells Boktrycken, Uppsala 1965)

25. T. Baer, "Investigation of the phonatory mechanism", *ASHA Reports* **11**, 38–47 (1981)

26. I.R. Titze, "A model for neurologic sources of aperiodicities in vocal folds", *J. Speech and Hearing Res.* **34**, 460–472 (1991)

27. M. Smith and L.O. Ramig, "Neurological disorders and the voice", *National Center for Voice and Speech Progress and Status Report* **7**, 207–227 (1995)

28. A. Hirschberg, X. Pelorson, G. Hofmans, R.R. van Hassel, and A.P.J. Wijnands, "Starting transient of the flow through an in-vitro model of the vocal folds", (this volume, Ch. 3)

29. X. Pelorson, A. Hirschberg, R.R. van Hassel, and A.P.J. Wijnands, "Theoretical and experimental study of quasisteady-flow separation within the glottis during phonation. Application to a modified two-mass model", *J. Acoust. Soc. Am.* **96**, 3416–3431 (1994)

30. G. Moore and H. von Leden, "Dynamic variation of the vibratory pattern in the normal larynx", *Folia Phoniatrica* **10**, 205–238 (1958)

31. M. Remacle and I. Trigoux, "Characteristics of nodules through the high-resolution frequency analyser", *Folia Phoniatrica* **43**, 53–59 (1991)

32. K. Ishizaka and J.L. Flanagan, "Synthesis of voiced sounds from a two-mass model of the vocal cords", *Bell Syst. Tech. J.* **51**, 1233–1268 (1972)

33. F. Alipour-Haghighi and I.R. Titze, "Elastic models of vocal fold tissues", *J. Acoust. Soc. Am.* **90**, 1326–1331 (1991)

34. I.R. Titze and W. Strong, "Normal modes in vocal fold tissue", *J. Speech and Hearing Res.* **57**, 736–744 (1975)

35. B. Hammarberg, B. Fritzell, J. Gauffin, and J. Sundberg, "Acoustic and perceptual analysis of vocal dysfunction", *J. Phonetics* **14**, 533–547 (1986)

36. M.E. Smith, G.S. Berke, B.R. Gerratt, and J. Kreiman, "Laryngeal paralyses: Theoretical considerations and effects on laryngeal vibrations", *J. Speech and Hearing Res.* **35**, 545–554 (1992)

37. N.B. Pinto and I.R. Titze, "Unification of perturbation measures in speech signals", *J. Acoust. Soc. Am.* **87**, 1278–1289 (1990)

38. K. Ishizaka and N. Isshiki, "Computer simulation of pathological vocal-cord vibration", *J. Acoust. Soc. Am.* **60**, 1193–1198 (1976)

39. I.R. Titze and H. Liang, "Comparison of F0 extraction methods for high precision voice perturbation measurements", *J. Speech and Hearing Res.* **36**, 1120–1133 (1993)

1233

The Bell System Technical Journal
Vol. 51, No. 6, July–August, 1972
Printed in U.S.A.

Synthesis of Voiced Sounds From a Two-Mass Model of the Vocal Cords

By K. Ishizaka and J. L. Flanagan

(Manuscript received January 13, 1972)

A model of voiced-sound generation is derived in which the detailed acoustic behavior of the human vocal cords and the vocal tract is computed. The vocal cords are approximated by a self-oscillating source composed of two stiffness-coupled masses. The vocal tract is represented as a bilateral transmission line. One-dimensional Bernoulli flow through the vocal cords and plane-wave propagation in the tract are used to establish acoustic factors dominant in the generation of voiced speech. A difference-equation description of the continuous system is derived, and the cord-tract system is programmed for interactive study on a DDP-516 computer. Sampled waveforms are calculated for: acoustic volume velocity through the cord opening (glottis); glottal area; and mouth-output sound pressure. Functional relations between fundamental voice frequency, subglottal (lung) pressure, cord tension, glottal area, and duty ratio of cord vibration are also determined.

Results show that the two-mass model duplicates principal features of cord behavior in the human. The variation of fundamental frequency with subglottal pressure is found to be 2 to 3 Hz/cm H_2O, and is essentially independent of vowel configuration in the programmed tract. Acoustic interaction between tract eigenfrequencies and glottal volume flow is strong. Phase difference in motion of the cord edges is in the range of 0 to 60 degrees, and control of cord tension leads to behavior analogous to chest/falsetto conditions in the human. Phonation-neutral, or rest area of cord opening, is shown to be a critical factor in establishing self-oscillation. Finally, the complete synthesis system suggests an efficient, physiological description of the speech signal, namely, in terms of subglottal pressure, cord tension, rest area of cord opening, and vocal-tract shape.

I. GENERATION OF VOICED SOUNDS IN SPEECH

The vocal cords constitute the sound source for all voiced sounds in speech. The cords consist of opposing ligaments which form a constriction at the top of the trachea where it joins to the lower vocal tract. When air is expelled at sufficient velocity through this orifice (the glottis), the cords vibrate and act as an oscillating valve which interrupts the air flow into a series of pulses. These pulses of volume flow serve as the excitation source for the vocal tract in all voiced sounds, and the passive resonances of the vocal tract are excited by the glottal pulses. Voice quality and prosodic features of speech are therefore strongly dependent upon the properties of cord vibration.

In the synthesis of speech by machines (for automatic voice response from computers, for example) it is desirable to make the synthetic voice as natural sounding as possible. Toward this end, it is necessary to understand the fundamental acoustic principles of voiced-sound generation and how these factors might be incorporated into a machine voice. Further, in a rather different area, the successful medical diagnosis (and correction) of voice disorders depends upon an understanding of the critical parameters of vocal-cord behavior. As in the case of computer synthesis, medical diagnosis can be facilitated through an accurate and viable model of the human vocal cords. Applications such as these, together with fundamental interests in the acoustics of speech, provide a motivation for modeling the acoustic behavior of the vocal cords.

The Bell System Technical Journal, July–August 1972

II. SELF-OSCILLATING MODELS OF THE VOCAL CORDS

The first quantitative self-oscillating model of the vocal cords was devised by one of the authors and implemented with a vocal-tract synthesizer on a digital computer.[1,2] This model was subsequently elaborated to include the mechanism of voiceless sound generation as well,[3] and was used for the synthesis of simple speech samples.

In this early work, the vocal cords were approximated as a simple mechanical oscillator, composed of single opposing masses, springs, and nonlinear damping—that is, a so-called one-mass approximation of each vibrating cord. The oscillating masses were permitted only lateral displacement and were driven by a function of the subglottal pressure and the Bernoulli pressure in the glottal orifice. The heretofore much-used assumption of linear separability of sound source and vocal tract was not made, and acoustic factors such as voice pitch, waveform of glottal flow, and glottal duty factor were derived as self-determined functions of physiological parameters, namely, subglottal (lung) pressure, vocal-cord tension (or natural frequency), "neutral" glottal area, and vocal-tract shape.

The waveforms of glottal area and volume velocity obtained in this first study were similar to those observed in high-speed motion pictures of the human vocal cords and in inverse filtering of natural speech. Further, the results revealed how the acoustic interaction between the vocal cords and the vocal-tract shape (through its driving-point impedance) could influence the waveform and period of the glottal flow. Control of the physiological parameters, subglottal pressure, cord tension, neutral area, and vocal-tract shape, were shown to be sufficient for the synthesis of voiced and voiceless sounds.[3]

Although the one-mass model could produce acceptable voiced-sound synthesis and simulate many of the properties of glottal flow, it was inadequate to produce other physiological detail in vocal cord behavior. For example, the amount of acoustic interaction displayed between source and tract was greater than observed in human speech.* The one-mass model was congenitally incapable of sustained oscillation for a capacitive input load of the vocal tract—corresponding to oscillation at a frequency just above a formant (or eigen) frequency of the tract. Also, a physiologically-natural correlate of chest and falsetto registers and phase-difference in the motion of the cord edges were lacking.

To incorporate more physiological properties, multiple-mass representations of the cords were therefore considered.[4-6] The cord ligaments can be mechanically represented with as distributed a system as desired, i.e., periodic structures of masses, springs, and losses. However, theoretical work has shown that a two-mass approximation[6,7] can account for most of the relevant glottal detail, including phase differences of upper and lower edges and oscillation for a capacitive input impedance of the vocal tract. An initial effort at computer simulation of these factors[4] produced realistic phase differences and chest-falsetto dichotomy, but nonrealistic dependence on acoustic load. The difficulty lay in the equivalent circuit of the glottal orifice, the manner of its control, and the physiological data available for the simulation.

The present work seeks a comprehensive and definitive treatment of the relevant acoustic theory and the existing physiological data. As in the earlier study,[2] simulation on an interactive DDP-516 laboratory computer is the tool by which the model is assessed and the unknown constants are estimated. In the sequel, the level of understanding and the realism attained by the two-mass model will be discussed.

III. MECHANICAL RELATIONS FOR THE TWO-MASS MODEL

The vocal cords are assumed to be bilaterally symmetric. The properties of only one cord are therefore discussed, the same being implied for the opposing cord. A schematic diagram of the glottal system is shown in Fig. 1. The trachea, leading to the lungs, is represented by the pipe to the left. The larynx tube, leading to the vocal tract, is to the right. These tubes are assumed to be cylindrical in shape and are fixed in size. The glottis constitutes a constriction between these tubes, and the size of the constriction depends upon the cord displacement. The inlet to the glottal constriction occurs over the contraction distance l_c. Expansion back to the vocal-tract cross section occurs over the distance l_e. Aerodynamic pressures relevant to the following discussion are indicated in Fig. 1.

---

*The amount of interaction is critically dependent upon the trans-glottal pressure distribution. In the first work, van den Berg's measurements of glottal pressure were used.

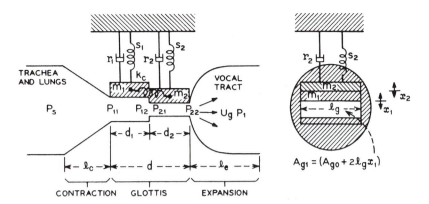

Fig. 1—Schematic diagram of the two-mass approximation of the vocal cords.

In the two-mass model, the vocal cord is divided in depth (thickness) into an upper and a lower part. Each part consists of a simple mechanical oscillator having a mass, spring, and damping (m, s, and r). The two masses of a cord, m_1 and m_2 are permitted only lateral motion, x_1 and x_2, and the masses are coupled by a linear spring, of stiffness k_c, as shown in Fig. 1. Other factors shown in Fig. 1 are:

l_g	the effective length of the vocal cords (or of the glottal slit),
d_1 and d_2	the thickness of m_1 and m_2, respectively,
s_1 and s_2	the equivalent springs,
r_1 and r_2	the equivalent viscous resistances,
A_{g01} and A_{g02}	the cross-sectional areas of the glottal, slit when m_1 and m_2 are at rest (i.e., the "phonation neutral" areas),
U_g	the average volume velocity across the glottal area.

Owing to the assumption of bilateral symmetry, variations in cross-sectional areas due to the lateral displacements x_1 and x_2 are doubled to give the total area variation; that is, the cross-sectional areas at the two masses are:

$$A_{g1} = A_{g01} + 2l_g x_1$$
$$A_{g2} = A_{g02} + 2l_g x_2.$$

3.1 Nature of the Vocal-Cord Springs

The function of the linear coupling spring, k_c, is to represent an effect of flexural stiffness in the lateral direction of the vocal cords. This variable flexural stiffness results from varying the thickness and stiffness of the cords by action of the thyroarytenoid muscle (vocalis).

The springs, s_1 and s_2, are an equivalent representation of the tension of the vocal cords, which becomes firmer due to contraction of the anteriol cricothyroid muscle and other muscles. The springs, s_1 and s_2, are given a nonlinear characteristic to conform to the stiffness as measured on fresh, excised human vocal cords.[8] The nonlinear relation between the deflection from the equilibrium position and the force required to produce this deflection is given by

$$f_{sj} = k_j x_j (1 + \eta_{kj} x_j^2), \qquad j = 1, 2, \tag{1}$$

where f_{sj} is the force required to produce x_j, k_j is the linear stiffness, and η_{kj} is the coefficient describing the nonlinearity of the spring, s_j, being positive in this case.

During closure of the glottis, the model should satisfy realistic conditions at the colliding surfaces of the vibrating masses, m_1 and m_2 with their opposing counterparts. A contact force at collision will cause some deformation in the flesh of the vocal cords. The restoring force at this deformation can be represented by an equivalent spring s_{hj} ($j = 1, 2$). For simplicity, a nonlinear characteristic, similar to eq. (1), is assumed for the spring s_{hj}, that is,

$$f_{hj} = h_j\left(x_j + \frac{A_{g0j}}{2l_g}\right)\left\{1 + \eta_{hj}\left(x_j + \frac{A_{g0j}}{2l_g}\right)^2\right\} \qquad (2)$$

for

$$x_j + A_{g0j}/2l_g \leqq 0 \qquad j = 1, 2,$$

where f_{hj} is the force required to produce the deformation to mass, m_j, during collision, h_j is the linear stiffness, and η_{hj} is a positive coefficient representing the nonlinearity of the contacting vocal cords. The resultant restoring force acting on m_j during closure is, therefore, the sum of f_{sj} and f_{hj}, that is, eq. (1) and eq. (2). This change in spring stiffness at closure is schematically illustrated in Fig. 2.

3.2 Nature of the Vocal-Cord Losses

As in the earlier formulation,[1] the viscous loss of the vibrating cords is assumed piece-wise linear. The loss is caused to increase step-wise on closure of the cords to represent the "stickiness" of the soft, moist contacting surfaces as they form together.

It is convenient to express the equivalent viscous resistances in terms of damping ratios, ζ_1 and ζ_2, for the uncoupled oscillators, where

$$r_1 = 2\zeta_1\sqrt{m_1 k_1} \quad \text{and} \quad r_2 = 2\zeta_2\sqrt{m_2 k_2}, \qquad (3)$$

and where, as shown in eq. (1), k_1 and k_2 are the linear components of stiffness for the springs s_1 and s_2. During the open-glottis condition, the loss is taken as $\zeta_1 = 0.1$ and $\zeta_2 = 0.6$ for a typical condition of the cord model. As in the

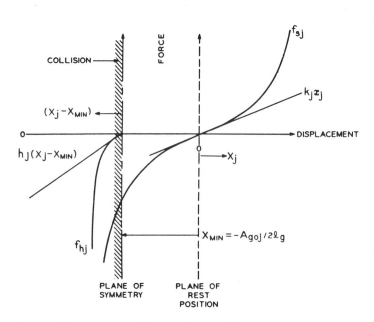

Fig. 2—Characteristics of the nonlinear stiffnesses.

earlier work, the loss during the closed-glottis condition is taken essentially as critical damping, namely

$$\zeta_1 = (1.0 + 0.1) \quad \text{and} \quad \zeta_2 = (1.0 + 0.6). \tag{4}$$

IV. PRESSURE DISTRIBUTION ALONG THE GLOTTIS

Because of the small dimensions of the glottis (compared to a wavelength at the frequencies of interest), and because of the high velocity of the glottal flow (compared to the vocal-cord velocity), we can assume the glottal flow to be quasi-steady.[7] We shall use the Bernoulli equation for one-dimensional flow to obtain the pressure distribution along the glottal flow.

The abrupt contraction in cross-sectional area at the inlet to the glottis produces a *vena contracta* surrounded by stagnant air. The *vena contracta* makes the inlet area A_{g1} appear smaller than it actually is and the pressure drop greater than that dictated by an ideal area change. The loss factor for such a contraction has been studied in fluid flow experiments[9] and found to be on the order of 0.4 to 0.5. Flow measurements by van den Berg, et al.,[10] on plaster cast models of the larynx set the loss figure at 0.37. This latter figure is therefore taken to estimate the pressure drop at the inlet, and we fix this drop at

$$P_{B1}(1.00 + 0.37), \quad \text{or} \quad 0.69\rho(U_g^2 / A_{g1}^2),$$

where $P_{B1} = \frac{1}{2}\rho u_{g1}^2$ is the Bernoulli pressure, ρ the air density, and u_{g1} the particle velocity at the lower cord-edge.

Within the constriction formed by the lower part of the cord, the pressure drop is assumed to be governed by viscous loss, which is also consistent with van den Berg's measurements. In this region the pressure falls linearly with distance according to a resistance to the volume flow equal to $12\mu d_1 l_g^2 / A_{g1}^3$, where μ is the shear viscosity coefficient.

At the junction between the masses m_1 and m_2, the volume flow U_g is continuous, but the particle velocity changes. There is a corresponding abrupt change in pressure equal to the change in kinetic energy per unit volume of the fluid. This pressure change at the junction is

$$\Delta p = 1/2\rho(u_{g1}^2 - u_{g2}^2) \tag{5}$$
$$= 1/2\rho U_g^2(1/A_{g2}^2 - 1/A_{g1}^2).$$

Throughout the constriction formed by the upper cord-edge, m_2, viscous loss is assumed to govern the pressure drop and, like the lower cord portion, the resistance is taken as $(12\mu d_2 l_g^2 / A_{g2}^3)$.

At the abrupt expansion of the glottal outlet, the pressure recovers toward the atmospheric value (assuming no constrictions in the relatively large vocal tract). Van den Berg, in his model flow measurements, found the pressure recovery to be about $0.5\,P_B$. However, for small constrictions this measurement is difficult and uncertain. It seems preferable to base an estimate of the pressure recovery on momentum considerations, which hold in the theory of fluid flow.

Consider at the sudden expansion the relations for Newton's law, $f = (d/dt)(mv)$. Then, because U_g is continuous,

$$\rho U_g(u_1 - u_{g2}) = A_1(P_{22} - P_1)$$

or

$$(P_1 - P_{22}) = 1/2\rho u_{g2}^2 [2N(1-N)]$$
$$= 1/2\rho \frac{U_g^2}{A_{g2}^2}[2N(1-N)]$$
$$= P_{B2}[2N(1-N)], \tag{6}$$

where $N = A_{g2}/A_1$, $P_{B2} = 1/2\rho u_{g2}^2$, and A_1 is the input area to the vocal tract. The value of $2N(1-N)$ is typically in the order of 0.05 to 0.40, which is somewhat smaller than van den Berg's value. This difference is significant to the

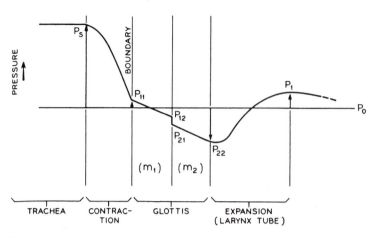

Fig. 3—Pressure distribution along the glottal flow.

acoustic interaction between the vocal tract and the cord source.[1] The pressure distribution along the steady flow through the glottis is indicated in Fig. 3.

In the time-varying condition of the cords, the inertance of the air masses involved should also be taken into account. When combined with the loss terms just discussed, the pressure distribution along the glottis is described by

$$P_8 - P_{11} = 1.37 \frac{\rho}{2}\left(\frac{U_g}{A_{g1}}\right)^2 + \int_0^{lc} \frac{\rho}{A_c(x)}dx \cdot \frac{dU_g}{dt} \quad *$$

$$P_{11} - P_{12} = 12\frac{\mu l_g^2 d_1}{A_{g1}^3} \cdot U_g + \frac{\rho d_1}{A_{g1}} \cdot \frac{dU_g}{dt}$$

$$P_{12} - P_{21} = \frac{\rho}{2}U_g^2\left(\frac{1}{A_{g2}^2} - \frac{1}{A_{g1}^2}\right)$$

$$P_{21} - P_{22} = 12\frac{\mu l_g^2 d_2}{A_{g2}^3}U_g + \frac{\rho d_2}{A_{g2}} \cdot \frac{dU_g}{dt}$$

$$P_{22} - P_1 = -\frac{\rho}{2}\left(\frac{U_g}{A_{g2}}\right)^2 \cdot 2\frac{A_{g2}}{A_1}\left(1 - \frac{A_{g2}}{A_1}\right). \tag{7}$$

V. EQUIVALENT CIRCUIT FOR THE GLOTTIS

On the basis of the pressure difference relations of eq. (7), the acoustic impedance elements of the glottal orifice constitute the equivalent circuit shown in Fig. 4, where the U_g current is continuous. The elements of the acoustic circuit are given by

---

* The $(U_g(dL/dt))$ term in $(d/dt)(LU_g)$ is negligible, where $L = (\rho d/A)$.

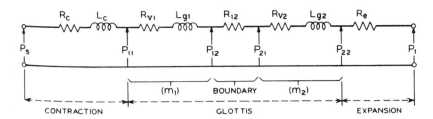

Fig. 4—Equivalent circuit for the glottis.

$$R_c = 1.37 \frac{\rho}{2} \frac{|U_g|}{A_{g1}^2}, \qquad L_c = \int_0^{lc} \frac{dx}{A_c(x)}$$

$$R_{v1} = 12 \frac{\mu l_g^2 d_1}{A_{g1}^3}, \qquad L_{g1} = \frac{\rho d_1}{A_{g1}}$$

$$R_{12} = \frac{\rho}{2}\left(\frac{1}{A_{g2}^2} - \frac{1}{A_{g1}^2}\right)|U_g|$$

$$R_{v2} = 12 \frac{\mu l_g^2 d_2}{A_{g2}^3}, \qquad L_{g2} = \frac{\rho d_2}{A_{g2}}$$

$$R_e = -\frac{\rho}{2} \cdot \frac{2}{A_{g2} A_1}\left(1 - \frac{A_{g2}}{A_1}\right)|U_g|. \tag{8}$$

The total acoustic impedance of the glottis, Z_g, is therefore

$$Z_g = \frac{\rho}{2}|U_g|\left\{\frac{0.37}{A_{g1}^2} + \frac{1 - 2\frac{A_{g2}}{A_1}\left(1 - \frac{A_{g2}}{A_1}\right)}{A_{g1}^2}\right\} + (R_{v1} + R_{v2}) + j\omega(L_{g1} + L_{g2} + L_c) \tag{9}$$

or

$$Z_g = (R_{k1} + R_{k2}) \mid U_g \mid (R_{v1} + R_{v2}) + j\omega(L_{g1} + K_{g2} + L_c),$$
$$Z_g = (R_{k1} + R_{k2}) \mid U_g \mid + (R_{v1} + R_{v2}) + j\omega(L_{g1} + L_{g2} + L_c), \tag{10}$$

where

$$R_{k1} = \frac{0.19\rho}{A_{g1}^2}, \qquad R_{k2} = \frac{\rho\left[0.5 - \frac{A_{g2}}{A_1}\left(1 - \frac{A_{g2}}{A_1}\right)\right]}{A_{g2}^2}.$$

In general, L_c can be neglected in comparison to $(L_{g1} + L_{g2})$.

The glottal impedance relation of eq. (10) can be linked to that obtained in flow measurements by van den Berg et al.[10] Using the pressure recovery found by van den Berg for the glottal outlet, namely $1/2\, P_{B2}$, [instead of the momentum relations in eq. (6) gives a value $R_e = -(\rho/4) \mid U_g \mid / A_{g2}^2$. For the case of $A_{g1} = A_{g2} = A_g$, the total glottal impedance becomes

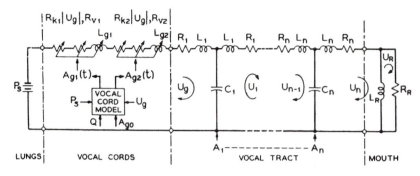

Fig. 5—Network model for the synthesis of voiced sounds.

$$z_g = -0.87 \frac{\rho}{2} \frac{|U_g|}{A_g^2} + 12 \frac{\mu l_g^2 d}{A_g^3} + j\omega L_g.$$

(11)

The real part of this impedance is identical with that given by van den Berg.

VI. MODEL SYSTEM FOR VOICED SOUNDS

A network representation of the vocal system for voiced sounds is shown in Fig. 5. Beginning at the left, the sub-glottal system—comprised of the trachea, bronchi, and lungs—is neglected and, as in the earlier study,[1] the sub-glottal pressure is approximated by a constant excess pressure in the lungs. Neglecting the subglottal system is also based on the finding that its first resonance is relatively high, with a mean value of 650 Hz and a bandwidth of 250 Hz. These values were determined from direct measurements of the subglottal driving-point impedance made on five laryngectomized subjects.[11] The 650 Hz figure is considerably higher than the value of 300 Hz reported by van den Berg.

The vocal tract is represented in Fig. 5 as a transmission line of n cylindrical, hard-walled sections, the element values of which are determined by the cross-sectional areas $A_1 \dots A_n$, and the cylinder lengths $l_1 \dots l_n$.[12] The inductances are $L_n = \rho l_n / 2A_n$ and the capacitances are $C_n = (l_n \cdot A_n / \rho c^2)$, where c is the sound velocity. In the present work $n = 4$.

To account in part for tract losses, serial resistances R_n are taken to have the form of a viscous loss at the pipe wall, namely $R_n = (S_n / A_n^2)\sqrt{\rho\mu\omega/2}$, where S_n is the circumference of the nth section and ω is the radian frequency. The frequency for evaluation of this loss is fixed at the natural frequency of the lower oscillator, $f = (1/2\pi)\sqrt{k_1/m_1}$, and a multiplicative coefficient (ATT) is applied to increase the loss beyond that contributed by viscous loss at the walls and to produce formant bandwidths appropriate to a closed-glottis condition.* (The typical range for ATT is 20 to 25.)

The transmission line is terminated in a radiation load equal to that for a circular piston in an infinite baffle, namely $L_R = 8\rho/3\pi\sqrt{\pi A_n}$ and $R_R = (128\rho c/9\pi^2 A_n)$, where A_n is the final (mouth) area.[12]

From Fig. 5, the differential equations which relate the volume velocities of the system are:

$$(g-\text{loop}) \quad (R_{k1}+R_{k2})|U_g|U_g + (R_{v1}+R_{v2})U_g + (L_{g1}+L_{g2})\frac{dU_g}{dt} + L_1\frac{dU_g}{dt} + R_1 U_g + \frac{1}{C_1}\int_0^t (U_g - U_1)dt - P_8 = 0$$

$$(1-\text{loop}) \quad (L_1+L_2)\frac{dU_1}{dt} + (R_1+R_2)U_1 + \frac{1}{C_2}\int_0^t (U_1-U_2)dt + \frac{1}{C_1}\int_0^t (U_1-U_g)dt = 0$$

---

* Other vocal tract losses not included *per se* are those arising from non-rigid walls and from heat conduction losses at the wall. The former is quite significant in lower-formant damping. The latter is essentially negligible. See Ref. 12.

$$(2-\text{loop}) \quad (L_2+L_3)\frac{dU_2}{dt}+(R_2+R_3)U_2+\frac{1}{C_3}\int_0^t(U_2-U_3)dt+\frac{1}{C_2}\int_0^t(U_2-U_1)dt=0$$

$$(3-\text{loop}) \quad (L_3+L_4)\frac{dU_3}{dt}+(R_3+R_4)U_3+\frac{1}{C_4}\int_0^t(U_3-U_L)dt+\frac{1}{C_3}\int_0^t(U_3-U_2)dt=0$$

$$(4-\text{loop}) \quad (L_4+L_R)\frac{d(U_L)}{dt}+R_4U_L-L_R\frac{d(U_R)}{dt}+\frac{1}{C_4}\int_0^t(U_L-U_3)dt=0$$

$$(5-\text{loop}) \quad L_R\frac{d}{dt}(U_R-U_L)+R_R\cdot U_R=0. \tag{12}$$

VII. FORCING RELATIONS FOR THE VOCAL-CORD OSCILLATOR

The masses of the cord oscillator are driven by mean pressures acting on their exposed faces, namely,

$$P_{m1}=\frac{1}{2}(P_{11}+P_{12})=P_3-1.37\frac{\rho}{2}\left(\frac{U_g}{A_{g1}}\right)^2-\frac{1}{2}\left(R_{v1}U_g+L_{g1}\frac{dU_g}{dt}\right)$$

and

$$P_{m2}=\frac{1}{2}(P_{21}+P_{22})=P_{m1}-\frac{1}{2}\left\{(R_{v1}+R_{v2})U_g+(L_{g1}+L_{g2})\frac{dU_g}{dt}\right\}-\frac{\rho}{2}U_g^2\left(\frac{1}{A_{g2}^2}-\frac{1}{A_{g1}^2}\right). \tag{13}$$

The exposed areas are l_gd_1 and l_gd_2, respectively. A shape of the cords is assumed such that the forces F_1 and F_2 acting on m_1 and m_2 over their displacements x_1 and x_2 are:

x_1	x_2	F_1/l_gd_1	F_2/l_gd_2
$x_1>x_{1\min}$	$x_2>x_{2\min}$	P_{m1}	P_{m2}
$x_1\leqq x_{1\min}$	$x_2>x_{2\min}$	P_8	0
$x_1>x_{1\min}$	$x_2\geqq x_{2\min}$	P_8	P_8
$x_1\leqq x_{1\min}$	$x_2\leqq x_{2\min}$	P_8	$0,$

$$\tag{14}$$

where $x_{1\min}=(A_{g01}/2l_g)$, $x_{2\min}=-(A_{g02}/2l_g)$, and A_{g01}, A_{g02} are the "phonation neutral" values of the glottal area. The equations of motion for the two masses are therefore:

$$m_1\frac{d^2x_1}{dt^2}+r_1\frac{dx_1}{dt}+s_1(x_1)+k_c(x_1-x_2)=F_1$$

$$m_2\frac{d^2x_2}{dt^2}+r_2\frac{dx_2}{dt}+s_2(x_2)+k_c(x_2-x_1)=F_2,$$

where

$$A_{g1}=(A_{g01}+2l_gx_1), \qquad A_{g2}=(A_{g02}+2l_gx_2),$$

$$s_j(x_j)=k_j(x_j+\eta_{kj}\cdot x_j^3), \qquad j=1,2, \text{ for } x_j>-\frac{A_{g0j}}{2l_g},$$

and

$$s_j(x_j)=k_j(x_j+\eta_{kj}\cdot x_j^3)+h_j\left\{\left(x_j+\frac{A_{g0j}}{2l_g}\right)+\eta_{hj}\left(x_j+\frac{A_{g0j}}{2l_g}\right)^3\right\}, \text{ for } x_j\leqq-\frac{A_{g0j}}{2l_g}, \tag{15}$$

and F_1 and F_2 are given by the force table of eq. (14). These equations are coupled to the flow equations through the fact that x_1 and x_2 determine A_{g1} and A_{g2}. Also note that the coupling between the masses, which are permitted only lateral motion, has been linearized to be proportional to $(x_2 - x_1)$. [A more detailed consideration of the elongation produced in the coupling spring by a displacement difference $(x_2 - x_1)$, and of the lateral component of restoring force, leads to modifying the coupling term to $2k_c(x_2 - x_1)^3/(d_1 + d_2)^2$.]

VIII. DIGITAL SIMULATION

The differential equations are approximated by difference equations in which

$$\frac{df(t)}{dt} \cong \frac{f(t_i) - f(t_{i-1})}{(t_i - t_{i-1})} = \frac{f_i - f_{i-1}}{T}$$

$$\int_0^t f(t)dt \cong (t_i - t_{i-1})\sum_{j=0}^{i-1} f(t_j) = T\sum_{j=0}^{i-1} f_j. \tag{16}$$

These discrete approximations applied to eqs. (12) and (15) yield:

$$(g-\text{loop}) \quad (R_{k1i} + R_{k2i})|U_{gi}|U_{gi} + (R_{v1i} + R_{v2i})U_{gi} + (L_{g1i} + L_{g2i})\frac{U_{gi} - U_{gi-1}}{T} + L_1\frac{U_{gi} - U_{gi-1}}{T}$$

$$+R_1 \cdot U_{gi} + \frac{T}{C_1}\sum_{j=0}^{i-1}(U_{gj} - U_{1j}) - P_g = 0$$

$$(1-\text{loop}) \quad \left\{\frac{L_1 + L_2}{T} + (R_1 + R_2)\right\}U_{1i} - \frac{L_1 + L_2}{T}U_{1i-1} + \frac{T}{C_2}\sum_{j=0}^{i-1}(U_{1j} - U_{2j}) + \frac{T}{C_1}\sum_{j=0}^{i-1}(U_{1j} - U_{gj}) = 0$$

$$(2-\text{loop}) \quad \left\{\frac{L_2 + L_3}{T} + (R_2 + R_3)\right\}U_{2i} - \frac{L_2 + L_3}{T}U_{2i-1} + \frac{T}{C_3}\sum_{j=0}^{i-1}(U_{2j} - U_{3j}) + \frac{T}{C_2}\sum_{j=0}^{i-1}(U_{2j} - U_{1j}) = 0$$

$$(3-\text{loop}) \quad \left\{\frac{L_3 + L_4}{T} + (R_3 + R_4)\right\}U_{3i} - \frac{L_3 + L_4}{T}U_{3i-1} + \frac{T}{C_4}\sum_{j=0}^{i-1}(U_{3j} - U_{Lj}) + \frac{T}{C_3}\sum_{j=0}^{i-1}(U_{3j} - U_{2j}) = 0$$

$$(4-\text{loop}) \quad \left\{\frac{L_4 + L_R}{T} + R_4\right\}U_{Li} - \frac{L_4 + L_R}{T}U_{Li-1} - \frac{L_R}{T}(U_{Ri} - U_{Ri-1}) + \frac{T}{C_4}\sum_{j=0}^{i-1}(U_{Lj} - U_{3j}) = 0$$

$$(5-\text{loop}) \quad \frac{L_R}{T}\left\{(U_{Ri} - U_{Li}) - (U_{Ri-1} - U_{Li-1})\right\} + R_R U_{Ri} = 0,$$

where

$$R_{k1i} = \frac{0.19\rho}{A_{g1i-1}^2}, R_{k2i} = \left[\frac{0.5 - \dfrac{A_{g2i-1}}{A(1)}\left(1 - \dfrac{A_{g2i-1}}{A(1)}\right)}{A_{g2i-1}^2}\right]\rho,$$

$$L_{g1i} = \frac{\rho d_1}{A_{g1i-1}}, L_{g2i} = \frac{\rho d_2}{A_{g2i-1}}, R_{v1i} = 12\mu l_g^2 \frac{d_1}{A_{g1i-1}^3},$$

$$R_{v2i} = 12 l_g^2 \frac{d_2}{A_{g2i-1}^3}, \tag{17}$$

and

$$\frac{m_1}{T^2}(x_{1i} - 2x_{1i-1} + x_{1i-2}) + \frac{r_1}{T}(x_{1i} - x_{1i-1}) + s_1(x_{1i}) + k_c(x_{1i-1} - x_{2i-1}) = F_{1i}$$

$$\frac{m_2}{T^2}(x_{2i} - 2x_{2i-1} + x_{2i-2}) + \frac{r_2}{T}(x_{2i} - x_{2i-1}) + s_2(x_{2i}) + k_c(x_{2i-1} - x_{1i-1}) = F_{2i},$$

where

$$A_{g1i} = A_{g01} + 2l_g \cdot x_{1i},$$

$$A_{g2i} = A_{g02} + 2l_g \cdot x_{2i},$$

$$s_1(x_{1i}) = k_1 \cdot \left(x_{1i} + \eta_{k1} \cdot x_{1i-1}^3 \right), \text{ for } x_{1i} > -\frac{A_{g01}}{2l_g},$$

$$s_1(x_{1i}) = k_1 \cdot \left(x_{1i} + \eta_{k1} \cdot x_{1i-1}^3 \right) + h_1 \cdot \left\{ \left(x_{1i} + \frac{A_{g01}}{2l_g} \right) + \eta_{h1} \cdot \left(x_{1i-1} + \frac{A_{g01}}{2l_g} \right)^3 \right\}, \text{ for } x_{1i} \leqq -\frac{A_{g01}}{2l_g},$$

$$s_2(x_{2i}) = k_2 \cdot \left(x_{2i} + \eta_{k2} \cdot x_{2i-1}^3 \right), \text{ for } x_{2i} > -\frac{A_{g02}}{2l_g},$$

$$s_2(x_{2i}) = k_2 \cdot \left(x_{2i} + \eta_{k2} \cdot x_{2i-1}^3 \right) + h_2 \cdot \left\{ \left(x_{2i} + \frac{A_{g02}}{2l_g} \right) + \eta_{h2} \cdot \left(x_{2i-1} + \frac{A_{g02}}{2l_g} \right)^3 \right\}, \text{ for } x_{2i} \leqq -\frac{A_{g02}}{2l_g},$$

$$F_{1i}/d_1 l_g = P_{m1i} = P_s - 1.37 \frac{\rho}{2} \left(\frac{U_{gi}}{A_{g1i-1}} \right)^2 - \frac{1}{2} \left\{ R_{v1i} U_{gi} + \frac{L_{g1i}}{T} (U_{gi} - U_{gi-1}) \right\},$$

$$F_{2i}/d_2 l_g = P_{m2i} = P_{m1i} - \left\{ \frac{1}{2} (R_{v1i} + R_{v2i}) U_{gi} + (L_{g1i} + L_{g2i}) \frac{U_{gi} - U_{gi-1}}{T} \right\} - \frac{\rho}{2} U_{gi}^2 \left(\frac{1}{A_{g2i-1}^2} - \frac{1}{A_{g1i-1}^2} \right). \tag{18}$$

These difference equations were programmed in Fortran IV and compiled for experiment on one of the DDP-516 laboratory computers of the Acoustics Research Department at Bell Laboratories.[13] Simultaneous solution of eqs. (17) and (18) yields all relevant volume velocities, glottal areas, and displacement. The time derivative of the mouth volume velocity (i.e., through the radiation load) is a good approximation to the radiated sound pressure.[12] Time samples of all dependent variables are obtained by iterating the solution for as many samples as are desired.

The sampling interval T is chosen as the longest interval that yields a stable solution to the difference equations. This interval is determined primarily by the time required for sound to transit the shortest length of the vocal tube. Because the distributed vocal tract is approximated as lumped constant T-sections, and because the behavior of these elements is further approximated by finite differences, the sampling interval T must be considerably shorter than the sound transit time through the shortest tube element. In the absence of appropriate sampling theory for this situation, the broad range of stable solutions was determined interactively on the DDP-516 computer and the longest stable interval used. In the present work, sampling rates in the range of 10 kHz to 30 kHz were used.

The iteration "loop" of the equations can be closed owing to the manner in which the glottal impedance elements and the forcing functions are taken to involve samples of glottal area; for example, current values of impedance and forcing function involve only past values of glottal areas. The iteration, therefore, proceeds as follows.

The cords and tract are initially assumed at rest, and initial currents are zero. The first sample of U_{gi} is calculated from loop-g using $A_{gi-1} = A_{g0}$ (i.e., $x_{i-1} = 0$). The initial samples of all other loop currents are likewise calculated, out to the radiation load. The first sample of U_{gi} is then used to calculate the first samples of the forcing functions and, from the mechanical equations, the first samples of the displacements x_{1i} and x_{2i}. The latter dictate new values of A_{g1} and A_{g2} which are entered back into the glottal impedance elements for the calculation of the next sample of U_g and all other currents. The process is continued until as much of the solution as desired is obtained.

For synthesis of continuous speech, the vocal-tract area values change as do the values of P_s, A_{g0}, and cord constants.* These changes are slow by comparison to the sample variations in volume velocities, displacements, and pressure. The solutions for the continuously changing vocal system can therefore be considered as quasi-steady solutions of eqs. (17) and (18), and the mouth output samples taken as the synthetic speech signal.

---

*As indicated in Fig. 5, a cord-tension parameter, Q, constitutes an input to the vocal-cord model. This parameter determines the mechanical constants of the oscillator.

IX. PHYSIOLOGICAL CONSTANTS FOR THE VOCAL-CORD MODEL

Few numerical values are available for the physiological parameters of the vocal cords. Using the sparse data available, the simulation on the DDP-516 computer was used to establish relevant ranges for the parameters.

First, the range of parameters which allows self-oscillation of the model was studied for a uniform vocal tract, 16 cm long, 5 cm^2 in cross-section, and terminated in the radiation load. The DDP-516 computer was used interactively to establish the self-oscillation region. The allowed oscillation range as a function of k_2 and k_c is shown in Fig. 6. In this plot, the axes are normalized by the factor m_1/m_2k_1. The parameters in the figure are the damping coefficients of the mechanical oscillators, ζ_1 and ζ_2. For these cases, all other glottal parameters are held constant at physiologically realistic values: namely, $P_8 = 8$ cm H$_2$O, $l_g = 1.4$ cm, $A_{g01} = A_{g02} = 0.05$ cm^2, thickness of the vocal cords $d_1 + d_2 = 0.3$ cm, total mass $m_1 + m_2 = 0.15$ g, nonlinear coefficient of the springs $\eta_{k1} = \eta_{k2} = 100$ and $\eta_{h1} = \eta_{h2} = 500$, and $h_1 = 3k_1$, $h_2 = 3k_2$. In particular, values for the spring constants are based upon measurements of static tensile stress versus displacement for an excised human larynx.[8] From these measurements, for example, η_k is deduced to be on the order of 50 to 100.

For Fig. 6a, the vocal cords are divided into equal parts, with thickness and mass 0.15 cm and 0.075 g, respectively, and with $k_1 = 50$ kdyn/cm. For Fig. 6b, the lower part of the vocal-cord model is thicker than the upper part, that is, $d_1 = 0.25$ cm and $d_2 = 0.05$ cm, and the masses, $m_1 = 0.125$ g and $m_2 = 0.025$ g, are chosen proportional to the thicknesses, keeping the same total mass of 0.15 g as in Fig. 6a.

Kaneko[11] has measured the damped oscillations of a fresh excised human larynx when excited by a mechanical impulse and with no air flow through the glottis. From this data, the damping ratio for the excised human cords can be estimated to be of the order of 0.1 to 0.2 (which, incidentally, is the same order as deduced in the earlier simulations[1]). This range of damping seems particularly appropriate for the bulk of the cords, that is, for m_1 of the model.*

An acoustic load of the vocal tract, whose driving-point impedance has an inductive reactance at the fundamental frequency of the vocal-cord vibration, acts to enhance oscillation of the model. An increase in damping (loss) of the vocal tract at lower frequencies, as would be caused by wall vibration in the vocal tract, however, acts to oppose oscillation. Also, the tendency to oscillate is suppressed by an increase in the mechanical damping of m_1 and especially of m_2.

The behavior of the vocal-cord model, calculated for values of k_2 and k_c specified by the small circle in Fig. 6b, will now be considered. This glottal condition is chosen as the "typical" one throughout the present study; namely, $k_1 = 80$ kdyn/cm, $k_2 = 8$ dyn/cm, and $k_c = 25$ kdyn/cm.

X. RESULTS OF THE DIGITAL SIMULATION

The vocal-cord and vocal-tract program, specified by eqs. (17) and (18), was used interactively on the DDP-516 computer to calculate waveforms of glottal flow, glottal area, and mouth sound pressure.

10.1 Waveforms for Typical Glottal Conditions

Measurements made at the typical glottal condition and for a uniform vocal tract are illustrated in Fig. 7. Waveforms of A_{g1}, A_{g2}, U_g, and mouth sound pressure are shown for the initial 30 ms of voicing. The negative values of A_{g1} and A_{g2} indicate glottal closure. (One can imagine the cords forming into one another upon contact, and the negative areas correspond to the continued displacement of the center of mass of the cords.)

---

*An equivalent damping ratio for the bulk of the cords can be estimated as follows:

$$(r_1 + r_2) = 2\zeta_1\sqrt{m_1k_1} + 2\zeta_2\sqrt{m_2k_2}.$$

For $k_c \to \infty$

$$(r_1 + r_2) = 2\zeta_{equi}\sqrt{(m_1 + m_2)(k_1 + k_2)}.$$

Substituting (for the "typical" conditions) $m_2 = m_1/5$, $k_2 = k_1/10$, $\zeta_1 = 0.1$, and $\zeta_2 = 0.6$ gives

$$\zeta_{equi} = \frac{1}{\sqrt{66}}\left(\sqrt{50}\,\zeta_1 + \zeta_2\right) = 0.16,$$

which corresponds favorably with Kaneko's measurements.

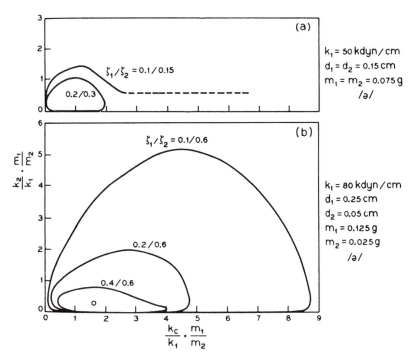

Fig. 6—Allowed regions of oscillation for the two-mass model. The parameter is the open-glottis damping ratio. The vocal-tract shape is for the vowel /ə/.

The results show that the phase difference between m_1 and m_2 is about 55 degrees, and the duty ratio (glottis open time to total period) is about 0.6. These values compare well with observations which have been made on human vocal cords by high-speed motion picture techniques[14] and by inverse filtering.[15] One notices the differences between the glottal area wave and the corresponding glottal flow wave, as pointed out in the earlier work.[1] The glottal flow wave is typically characterized by some temporal detail, asymmetry, and steep falling slope, while the area wave shows little temporal detail, is less steep, and tends to be more symmetrical. Because the cords are massive

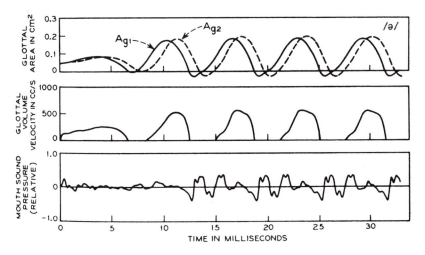

Fig. 7—Vocal-cord and vocal-tract functions computed from the DDP-516 simulation. Glottal areas, A_{g1} and A_{g2}, glottal volume velocity, U_g, and mouth-output sound pressure are shown for the initial 30 ms of voicing for the neutral vowel /ə/.

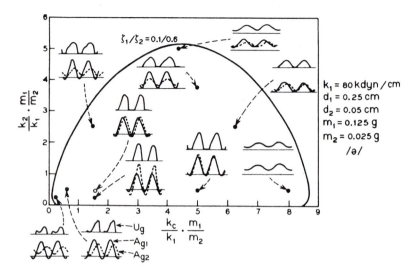

Fig. 8—Sketches of cord-tract functions for points on the k_2–k_c plane. The axes are normalized by the function (m_1/k_1m_2). The vowel is /ə/. Compare with Fig. 6b.

and are generally forced at a frequency above their natural frequency, their mechanical displacement does not reflect the detail of acoustic interaction which the glottal flow displays. The sound output wave reflects the periodicity established by the cord oscillator, and the greatest formant oscillation (or excitation) typically occurs (with about 0.5 ms delay) at the closing phase of the U_g wave. This effect has been observed previously.[2]

10.2 Effect of Cord Stiffnesses

The normalized k_2 versus k_c plane of Fig. 6 is a convenient medium for demonstrating the effects of spring constants. Using this plane, waveforms of U_g, A_{g1}, and A_{g2} are sketched for corresponding stiffnesses in Fig. 8. As before, the vocal tract is a uniform pipe (/ə/ and other glottal conditions are kept at their typical values.

An increase in k_c above the typical value reduces the phase difference between A_{g1} and A_{g2}. It also diminishes the steep falling slope of the flow waveform, and tends to make the wave more symmetrical and triangular. An increase in k_c also produces an increase in the build-up time required for the oscillation to settle to a steady state. For still larger values of k_c, close to the bounds of the oscillation range, both the glottal flow and area waveforms become sinusoidal on a dc component and the glottis does not close.

The range of the sinusoidal behavior is expanded if the damping coefficients are made smaller. This special case is shown in Fig. 6a for the damping coefficients $\eta_{k1} = 0.1$ and $\eta_{k2} = 0.15$. Here, k_c has no limitation for the oscillation when k_2 is less than 20 kdyn/cm. Owing to the large k_c, the two-mass model behaves just as the one-mass model in the extended region in which the oscillation is sustained by the inductive reactance of the vocal tract and glottis. This projecting tail disappears with an increase in the losses, either of the vocal tract or of the vocal cords.

In contrast, an increase in k_2, with other conditions constant, decreases the amplitude of A_{g2} without a change of the phase difference. Further increase of k_2 leads to no closure of A_{g2} while A_{g1} can close completely during the cycle. Owing to the small amplitude of A_{g2} and its dc component, the glottal flow increases in upward roundness and also increases in duty ratio. A small, broad hump appears on the rising slope of the glottal flow wave, at which point the area A_{g1} is equal to A_{g2}.

By comparison, a decrease in k_2 increases the amplitude of A_{g2} and the glottal waves tend to a symmetrical form. This same dependence on k_2 and k_c also occurs for the case of equal thicknesses, $d_1 = d_2 = 0.15$ cm. A change in proportion of the damping coefficients, ζ_1 and ζ_2, also influences the relations between A_{g1} and A_{g2}. For example, the typical condition $\zeta_1 = 0.1$ and $\zeta_2 = 0.6$ produces an amplitude of A_{g1} slightly larger than that of A_{g2} for /ə/, as seen in Fig. 7. A smaller value of ζ_2 for the same values of ζ_1 and other parameters produces an amplitude of A_{g2} larger

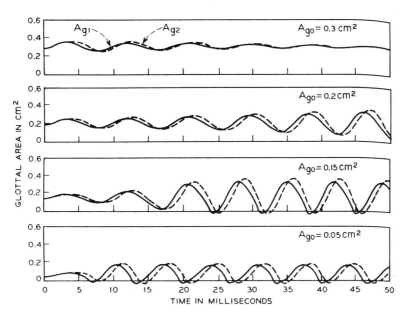

Fig. 9—Effect of the "phonation-neutral" or rest area, A_{g0}, upon the glottal area. The vowel is /i/.

than A_{g1} without a change in phase difference. A steeper rising slope of the glottal area wave also results, but the falling slope remains unchanged.

10.3 Effect of Neutral Area

The behavior of the vocal-cord model with respect to the "phonation-neutral" area, or the equilibrium value A_{g0}, is another case where we can find correspondence between the complex behavior of the human vocal cords and the vibrations of the vocal-cord model. In human phonation the neutral area is maintained by laryngeal adjustment. Typical results from the simulation for different values of A_{g0} are illustrated in Fig. 9. These data were measured for the typical glottal conditions with $\zeta_1 = 0.1$ and $\zeta_2 = 0.6$ and for the vowel /i/. One sees that the build-up time required for the oscillation to reach a steady state increases as A_{g0} gets larger. The value $A_{g0} = 0.30$ cm^2 surpasses a critical limit (about 0.25 cm^2) beyond which the model does not oscillate for these conditions.

During the voicing build-up time the pitch period is much longer than that of the steady-state oscillation. The change in pitch at the onset of voicing is similar to the starting motion of the human cords when they are brought to the phonation position from an open position. In this instance, unestablished low subglottal pressure also contributes to the reduction of the fundamental frequency. The oscillation period before cord closure is a value between the damped natural frequencies of the two mechanical oscillators. This is consistent with the value calculated from the acoustic theory of the two-mass model neglecting the collision and the nonlinearity of the springs.

Although the model, in this case, does not self-oscillate for $A_{g0} > 0.25$ cm^2, the maximum glottal area of phonation depends on the damping of the mechanical oscillators and of the vocal tract and on the subglottal pressure. For $\zeta_1 = 0.2$ and $\zeta_2 = 0.6$, and with $P_s = 8$ cm H$_2$O, the maximum glottal area reduces to about 0.20 cm^2. An increase in the phonation-neutral area also causes an increase in the amplitude of the vibration with no significant change in the period of the steady-state oscillation.

10.4 Effect of Tract Shape

Excitation of the vocal tract by the cord model was studied for several vowels. Area waves, glottal flow, and mouth-output sound pressure are shown for the vowels /i/, /u/, and /a/ in Figs. 10a, b, and c. For all these cases, the typical glottal conditions hold (same as for /ə/ in Fig. 7).

1248   The Bell System Technical Journal, July–August 1972

One notices that the waveforms of glottal area and the fundamental frequency are almost independent of the vocal-tract shape, while the shape can substantially influence the waveform of the glottal flow, similar to the results obtained from the one-mass model in the earlier work.[1] The acoustic interaction between the glottal flow and the acoustic load depends on the resonance characteristics of the vocal tract. Vowels having high resonant Q for the first formant show noticeable interaction in the glottal flow wave, as is seen for /a/. Also a low first formant can affect the glottal flow wave to a considerable extent, for example in /i/. However, the relatively large dissipation of the vocal tract in the frequency range of low first formants (such as for /i/ and /u/) caused primarily by vibration of the vocal-tract walls acts to reduce the interaction, but the glottal flow waveforms still differ markedly from each other. In all these cases, the tract losses are set to give bandwidths for the first formant equal to values measured on the human tract for the closed-glottis condition.[16]

The data of Fig. 10* permit a comparison between the glottal waveform and the speech pressure wave. The comparison is familiar from the results of inverse filtering.[15,17] There is a delay time difference of about 0.5 ms between the waves, corresponding to the time required for the sound to travel from the glottis to the lips. The waveforms for

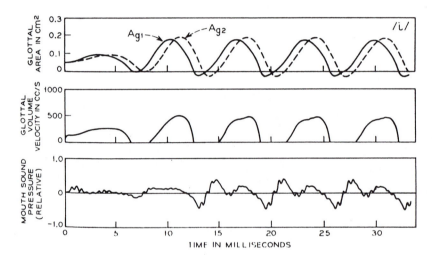

Fig. 10a—Results of the DDP-516 simulation for the vowel /i/ showing area waves, glottal flow, and mouth-output sound pressure.

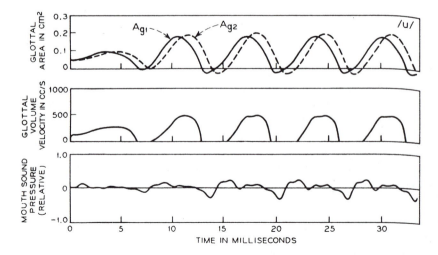

Fig. 10b—Same as Fig. 10a for the vowel /u/.

---

*Sound spectrograms of the computed mouth-output sound pressure are shown for several vowels in Fig. 10d.

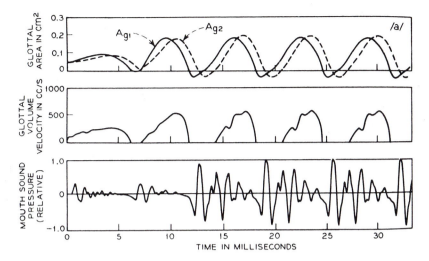

Fig. 10c—Same as Fig. 10a for the vowel /a/.

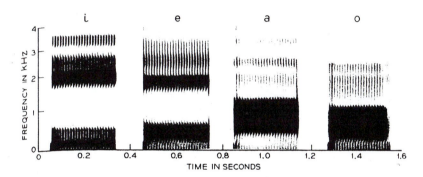

Fig. 10d—Sound spectrograms of the computed mouth-output sound pressure for the vowels /i, e, a, o/.

/a/, /i/, and /u/ show that the formants are excited largely at the closure of the cords. The output pressure waves attenuate rapidly with increasing glottal area during the opening phase of the glottal cycle.

10.5 Effect of Subglottal Pressure

The influence of the subglottal pressure on the fundamental frequency of the vocal-cord vibration is another important aspect of voice production. Typical behavior of the model for these factors is shown in Fig. 11. The nonlinear coefficient of the spring, η_k, is shown as the parameter for the vowel /ə/. The data for the vowels /i/ and /a/ correspond to $\eta_k = 100$ solely. For all these cases, the coefficient describing the nonlinearity in the deformation of the vocal cords at closure is taken as $\eta_k = 5\eta_k$.

The slope of the fundamental frequency as a function of subglottal pressure is seen to be about 2.5 Hz/cm H_2O for $\eta_k = 100$, independent of the vowel configuration. This represents good agreement with measurements which have been made on human speech in the chest register by Hixon, et al.[18] The curve for $\eta_k = 0$, that is, linear springs, shows a saturation characteristic for subglottal pressures greater than 8 cm H_2O. These results suggest that pitch variations with subglottal pressure might be ascribed to two causes. One is the collision of the vocal cords at closure when the amplitude of vibration is not too large and the subglottal pressure is less than several cm H_2O. Another is the nonlinearity of the deflection of the muscles and ligaments at large amplitudes of vibration and at subglottal pressures more than several cm H_2O. In the latter case, the nonlinearity becomes dominant when large displacement amplitude increases the effective stiffness of the springs. This tends to increase fundamental frequency. The minimum subglottal pressure for vowel production is about 2 cm H_2O.

The Bell System Technical Journal, July–August 1972

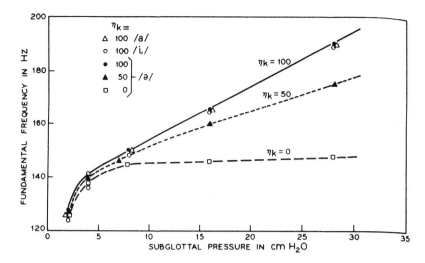

Fig. 11—Variation of fundamental frequency with subglottal pressure. The parameter is the nonlinear coefficient of the stiffnesses, ηk.

In the earlier work with the one-mass model, significant influences were found on fundamental frequency as a function of tract configuration. This influence was due in large part to the pressure recovery assumed at the glottal outlet, namely $1/2\, P_B$ according to van den Berg's data. When the intraglottal pressure distribution derived here is used in the one-mass model, the interaction across vowels and with subglottal pressure is much less.

The two-mass model becomes a one-mass model if k_c is increased to a large value. For this condition, the variation in fundamental frequency with subglottal pressure is shown for several vowels in Fig. 12. The behavior is similar to the two-mass model. Under these conditions, the duty ratio of the former tends to be slightly greater than the latter.

Duty ratio is another aspect of the model that can be compared to human phonation. An increase in subglottal pressure produces an increase in glottal flow and in glottal amplitude. Duty ratio (open time to total period) decreases for this increase in subglottal pressure and is asymptotic to a value around 0.5, as shown in Fig. 13. This value compares well with measurements on natural speech.[12]

10.6 Effect of Cord Tension

As in the previous studies,[1–3] it is convenient to apply a "tension parameter," Q, to control fundamental frequency. This can be achieved by causing the masses and thicknesses to be scaled down and the springs scaled up by the fac-

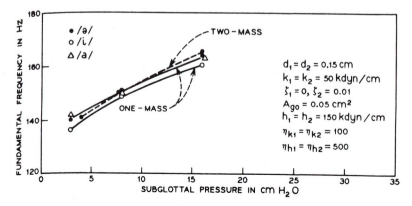

Fig. 12—Variations of fundamental frequency with subglottal pressure for the one-mass and two-mass models. The parameter is vowel configuration.

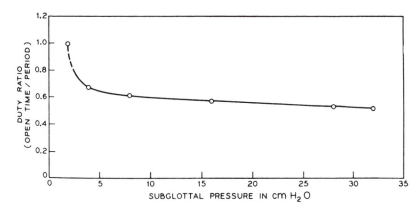

Fig. 13—Variation of duty ratio with subglottal pressure.

tor Q, causing the fundamental frequency to vary proportionally with Q. Phase difference, duty ratio, and glottal area waveforms are essentially uninfluenced by Q, and the amplitudes of glottal area and glottal flow decrease gradually with increasing Q. The glottal flow waveform also varies in detail depending on the fundamental frequency, because the formants contributing to the temporal detail of the glottal flow are unchanged while the period of the glottal flow varies as a function of Q. Changes in flow waveform with pitch variation are greatest in cases where acoustic interaction is especially pronounced (such as for /a/).

In human speech the duty ratio has a tendency to increase with the fundamental frequency.[19] This feature can also be given to the vocal-cord model by modifying the coupling-tension parameter k_c to increase more than in linear proportion to Q. A variation of Q^2 appears more realistic. Physiologically this corresponds to the considerable decrease in compliance and thickness of the vocal cords when they are stretched by contraction of the cricothyroid muscle and other muscles associated with contracting of the vocalis. The increase of k_c more than proportional to Q is equivalent to shifting the glottal operation condition on a line parallel to the abscissa in Fig. 6. As indicated in Fig. 8, a shift to the right reduces the phase difference and increases the duty ratio without changing other features of the cord vibration, except near the boundaries of the oscillation range.

Behavior of the cord model with the Q parameter so defined is shown in Figs. 14 and 15. Variations in waveforms with Q are shown for the vowel /a/ in Fig. 14. The relations between fundamental frequency, duty ratio, and amplitude of glottal area with Q are plotted in Fig. 15. Variation of the duty ratio with frequency falls into the range measured in inverse filtering experiments.[19]

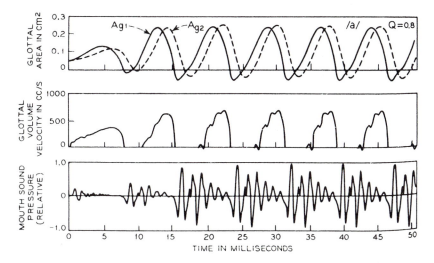

Fig. 14a—Effect of tension parameter, Q, on cord-tract output for the vowel /a/. $Q = 0.8$.

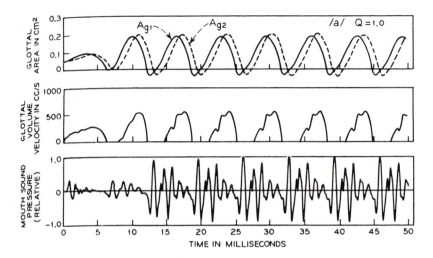

Fig. 14b—Same as Fig. 14a with $Q = 1.0$.

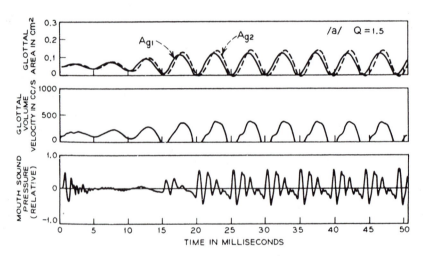

Fig. 14c—Same as Fig. 14a with $Q = 1.5$.

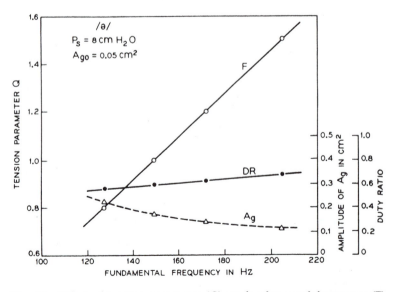

Fig. 15—Effect of tension parameter (Q) on fundamental frequency (F), duty ratio (DR), and glottal area (A_g).

XI. INTERACTION EFFECTS WITH LARGE ACOUSTIC LOADS

11.1 Differences Between Two-Mass and One-Mass Models

The measurements discussed previously show that the fundamental frequency and the area waveforms of the cord model are not strongly influenced by tract geometry. The interaction with glottal flow, however, is marked. We have further investigated the effect of acoustic load by lowering the frequency of the lowest resonance of the acoustic load (the first formant) into the range of the fundamental frequency. This increases the driving-point impedance at the fundamental frequency and strong coupling between source and load is expected.

The formant frequencies are lowered by lengthening the simulated vocal tract. Measurements of the fundamental frequency are shown in Fig. 16 as a function of the length of a uniform vocal-tract tube, 5 cm^2 in cross-section. Data are shown for both the two-mass cord model and an equivalent one-mass model ($k_c \to \infty$). The measurements are for the typical glottal conditions. The shunt impedance of the vocal-tract wall (wall vibration) is not taken into account *per se*, and this effect is only approximated by an increase in damping for the first 16-cm section of the tube (as was used for the /ə/ configuration). The remaining tube is regarded as an ideal hard-wall tube. The first resonance frequency of the vocal-tract tube, F_{01}, is shown by the solid line.

The frequency of the two-mass model decreases more gradually than that of the one-mass model with increasing the tube length. When the oscillation frequency of the former meets the first formant frequency of the vocal-tract tube, a sharp increase of the fundamental frequency occurs for further increase in tube length. The frequency returns to almost the same value as for a short tube. The frequency jump occurs at the resonant frequency of the vocal-tract tube, independent of dissipation and of glottal conditions. For example, an increase in acoustic dissipation of the vocal tract and a decrease in mechanical damping of m_1 and m_2 raises the onset frequency of the jump, but the frequency where the jump occurs is still the first resonant frequency of the tube. The variation of frequency with vocal-tube length is shown for two conditions of damping in Fig. 16.

The curve of F_{01} as a function of tube length marks the boundary between an inductive driving-point impedance (to the left) and a capacitive driving-point impedance (to the right). The frequency jump for the two-mass model, which occurs at F_{01} regardless of the glottal conditions, places its new oscillation in the capacitive region, that is, between the first pole and second zero of the driving-point impedance.

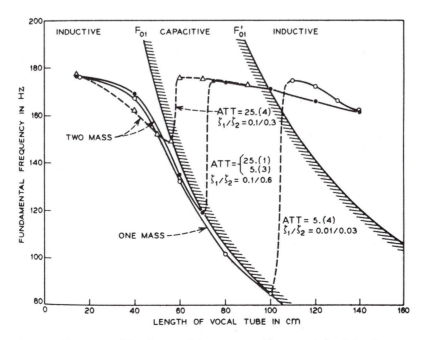

Fig. 16—Variation of fundamental frequency with acoustic load for the two-mass and one-mass models. F_{01} shows the frequency of the first pole of the driving-point impedance, and F_{01}' shows the first zero.

The Bell System Technical Journal, July–August 1972

A frequency jump also occurs in the one-mass model. In this case, however, the jump is to the original frequency for which the driving-point impedance is still an inductive impedance, that is, between the second zero and second pole of the driving-point impedance. This behavior can be predicted by an analysis of the oscillator with a uniform transmission line as a load.

11.2 Effects of Acoustic Load on Human Voicing

For comparison with the model behavior, we have measured similar loading effects in human voicing. To bring a first formant resonance into the range of the voice pitch, subjects phonated into a long metal tube the length of which was periodically changed from 39 cm to 73 cm by a motor (i.e., a bazooka-like sliding pipe). The subjects were instructed to pronounce the sustained vowel /ə/ at medium sound level and with constant glottal adjustment regardless of the change in tube length. Fundamental frequency (pitch) measurements were made at several frequencies in the chest register. Typical results for one subject are shown in Fig. 17.

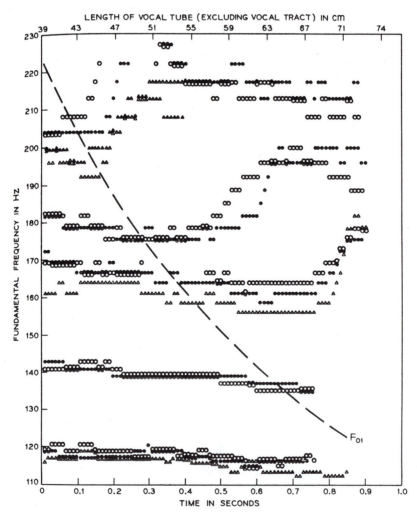

Fig. 17—Fundamental frequency measurements made for a human subject when the acoustic load on his vocal cords is varied. The acoustic load is varied by periodically changing the length of a uniform tube fitted to the subjects' mouth. The broken line show the first resonant (pole) frequency of the uniform tube.

The voice pitch was measured at 10-ms intervals by a pitch-extracting program.[20] The length of the metal tube (exclusive of the subject's vocal tract) is also indicated on the abscissa along with the corresponding time scale for the length change. Adjacent open and closed points (circles or triangles) pertain to different cycles of the pipe in one set of measurements. One sees frequency jumps similar to those in the two-mass model. However, the observed onset frequencies of the jumps are generally higher than the resonant frequency of the compound tube consisting of the metal tube and the subject's vocal tract (neglecting the shunt impedance of the vocal-tract wall). The deviation from the resonant frequency becomes especially noticeable for lower frequencies.

Toward an interpretation, it is known that the shunting impedance caused by vibration of the walls of the vocal tract produces a "cutoff frequency" of the sound transmission and constrains the lowest first formant frequency of the vocal tract.[21] This effect will contribute to raising the resonant frequency of the compound tube in a frequency range near the cutoff frequency. In the present instance, one could conceive of the walls of the cheeks, pharynx, and soft velum to yield to vibration because of the vocal-tract geometry for /ə/ and because of the long wavelength. At the cutoff frequency of the vocal tract, the first resonance frequency of the combined vocal tract and metal pipe is essentially that of the metal pipe alone. The latter is shown in Fig. 17 by the broken line.

From Fig. 17, we can presume the cutoff frequency of the vocal tract for /ə/ to be a little lower than 200 Hz. The effect of the wall vibration could thus account for the rightward shift of the observed pitch jumps. The rightward shift is most noticeable at the lower frequencies as this argument would predict. Even with these uncertainties, we see the close similarity in the dependence of fundamental frequency on acoustic load between the human larynx and the two-mass model.* It is further of interest that the vocal cords can self-oscillate without regenerative feedback from the subglottal and supraglottal system. In addition, the vibration of the soft walls of the vocal tract acts as a buffer to aid stable operation in the presence of coupling between the vocal cords and the vocal tract as the latter takes on a wide variety of shapes.

XII. CONCLUSION

The two-mass formulation of the vocal-cord model is seen to yield physiologically realistic behavior. In particular, the phase differences between upper and lower cord-edges corresponds well with motion observed in high-speed photography. The two-mass formulation also leads to a natural correlate to chest and falsetto register with coupling stiffness (lax in chest and tense in falsetto) being an important factor along with mass and thickness of the cords.

The computer measurements show that the two-mass model is capable of oscillation just above the resonant frequencies of the acoustic load (i.e., the formant frequencies of the vocal tract), duplicating a capability of the human cords. The one-mass model cannot oscillate in this frequency range, where the driving-point reactance is capacitive. Further, the intra-glottal pressure distribution derived for use with the two-mass models yields cord-tract interaction similar to human speech. Fundamental frequency varies with subglottal pressure approximately as 2 to 3 Hz/cm H_2O, and changes in vowel configuration do not markedly influence the fundamental frequency. Closures tighter than those which occur in vowel shapes (for example, at consonant-vowel boundaries) can of course influence the fundamental frequency. The improved intra-glottal pressure distribution is also applicable to a one-mass formulation, and it produces physiologically realistic cord-tract interactions with a one-mass model.

The programmed cord oscillator and the digitally simulated vocal tract constitute a complete synthesizer for voiced sounds. The system so implemented has potential for speech synthesis applications such as computer voice response. Especially for techniques such as text synthesis,[22] the cord model and vocal tract offer means for natural control of tract and larynx parameters, i.e., subglottal pressure, cord tension, neutral area, and tract shape. These parameters appear sufficient for describing both voiced and voiceless sounds in continuous speech.[3] In some synthesis applications, the complexity of the two-mass model may not be needed and a simpler one-mass formulation may serve. In normal voice production, phonation occurs at a fundamental frequency always below the first vocal resonance (formant). Here, the driving-point impedance is inductive and the one-mass oscillator performs acceptably, particularly with the improved intra-glottal pressure distribution.

Note added in proof: After this paper was written, we measured the "cutoff frequency" for the vocal tract and tube combination. We found its value to be 195 Hz.

The two-mass model, because of its physiological detail, also provides a potential tool for medical analyses of voice disorder. Although the present simulation assumes bilateral symmetry of the opposing cords, asymmetric configurations can be implemented. The effects of deficiencies such as unilateral cord paralysis can therefore be investigated and quantified. Biomedical engineering is making increased use of digital simulations of physiological behavior. The simulation technique described here not only permits acoustic analysis of voice functions but of human respiration as well.

XIII. ACKNOWLEDGMENTS

We wish to thank several members of the Acoustics Research Department for their substantial contributions to this study. A. E. Rosenberg collaborated on the design and measurements with the impedance tube, D. E. Dudgeon made early simulations with the two-mass program, D. E. Bock assisted in an interactive implementation of the program on the DDP-516 computer, and K. Shipley programmed the pitch extractor used for the real voice measurements.

REFERENCES

1. Flanagan, J. L., and Landgraf, L. L., "Self-Oscillating Source for Vocal-Tract Synthesizers," Proc. IEEE-AFCRL Symposium on Speech Commun. and Process., Boston, Mass., (Nov. 1967), also published in IEEE Trans. Audio and Electroacoustics, AU-16, (March 1968), pp. 57–64.
2. Flanagan, J. L., "Use of an Interactive Laboratory Computer to Study an Acoustic-Oscillator Model of the Vocal Cords," IEEE Trans. Audio and Electroacoustics, AU-17, (March 1969), pp. 2–6.
3. Flanagan, J. L., and Cherry, L., "Excitation of Vocal-Tract Synthesizers," J. Acoust. Soc. Amer., 45, (March 1969), pp. 2–6.
4. Dudgeon, D. E., "Two-Mass Model of the Vocal Cords," J. Acoust. Soc. Amer., 48, (July 1970), p. 118A.
5. Ishizaka, K., "On Models of the Larynx," J. Acoust. Soc. Japan, 22, 1966, pp. 293–294.
6. Ishizaka, K., and Matsudaira, M., "What Makes the Vocal Cords Vibrate," 6th Int. Congr. Acoust., Tokyo, (Aug. 1968), pp. B1–3.
7. Ishizaka, K., and Matsudaira, M., "Acoustic Theory of a Two-Mass Model of the Vocal Cords," unpublished work.
8. Ishizaka, K., and Kaneko, T., "On Equivalent Mechanical Constants of the Vocal Cords," J. Acoust. Soc. Japan, 24, No. 5, 1968, pp. 312–313.
9. Kaufmann, W., Fluid Mechanics, New York: McGraw-Hill Co., 1963, p. 111.
10. van den Berg, J. W., Zantema, J. T., and Doornenbal, Jr., P., "On the Air Resistance and the Bernoulli Effect of the Human Larynx," J. Acoust. Soc. Amer., 29, 1957, pp. 626–631.
11. Ishizaka, K., Kaneko, T., and Matsudaira, M., unpublished work.
12. Flanagan, J. L., Speech Analysis, Synthesis and Perception, 2nd Edition, New York, Berlin: Springer Verlag, 1972.
13. Flanagan, J. L., "Focal Points in Speech Communication Research," Proc. 7th Int. Cong. Acoust., Budapest, (August 1971). Also, IEEE Trans. Commun. Tech., (December 1971).
14. Farnsworth, D. W., "High-Speed Motion Pictures of the Human Vocal Cords," Bell Labs Record, 18, No. 7 (March 1940), pp. 203–208.
15. Miller, R. L., "Nature of the Vocal Cord Wave," J. Acoust. Soc. Amer,. 31, 1969, pp. 667–677.
16. Fujimura, O., and Lindqvist, J., "Sweep Tone Measurements of Vocal-Tract Characteristics," J. Acoust. Soc. Amer., 49, (Feb. 1971), pp. 554–558.
17. Holmes, J. N., "An Investigation of the Volume Velocity Waveform at the Larynx During Speech by Means of an Inverse Filter," Proc. Speech Commun. Seminar, Stockholm, 1962.
18. Hixon, T. J., Mead, J., and Klatt, D. H., "Influence of Forced Transglottal Pressure Changes on Vocal Fundamental Frequency," J. Acoust. Soc. Amer., 49, (Jan. 1971), p. 105A.
19. Lindqvist, J., "The Voice Source Studied by Means of Inverse Filtering," Quarterly Report, Speech Transmicro Laboratory, Stockholm, Sweden, (Jan. 1970).
20. Gold, B., and Rabiner L., "Parallel Processing Techniques for Estimating Pitch Periods of Speech in the Time Domain," J. Acoust. Soc. Amer., 46, (Aug. 1969), pp. 442–448.
21. Fant, G., "Speech at High Ambient Air-Pressure," STL-QPSR, (Feb. 1964), pp. 9–21.
22. Flanagan, J. L., Coker, C. H., Rabiner, L. R., Schafer, R. W., and Uneda, N., "Synthetic Voices for Computers," IEEE SPECTRUM, 7, (October 1970), pp. 22–45.

APOLONN brings us to the real world
: Learning nonlinear dynamics and fluctuations in nature

Masa-aki SATO, Kazuki Joe, Tatsuya Hirahara

ATR Auditory and Visual Perception Research Laboratories

Sanpeidani Inuidani Seika-cho Soraku-gun Kyoto, 619-02, Japan

ABSTRACT

Recurrent neural networks with arbitrary feedback connections are highly nonlinear dynamical systems and exhibit a variety of complex dynamical behavior. The applications of these temporal behaviors for information processing give us great possibilities. In this article, supervised learning for the recurrent networks are studied with emphasis on learning aperiodic motions. APOLONN (adaptive nonlinear pair oscillators with local connections) is used for a speech synthesis. The naturalness of human's voice seems to come from fluctuations in voice source waveforms. We trained APOLONN to learn the voice source waveforms including fluctuations of amplitudes and periodicities. After the learning, APOLONN was able to generate the waveforms with fluctuations. APOLONN can also generate waveforms with modulated amplitudes and frequencies by a simple scaling of the parameters. Our results encourage further applications of recurrent networks.

1. Introduction

Neural networks can be classified into three categories. The first one is the multilayered feed-forward network. This type of networks is capable of learning complex input-output mapping relations by using error back propagation method [1]. The second one is the asymptotically stable recurrent network. Recurrent networks with symmetric connections have Lyapunov functions [2,3] which monotonically decrease in time. Therefore they are asymptotically stable. This type of networks has been applied to solve optimization problems [4] and used as associative memory [5]. The Bortzmann machine [6] can be considered as this type. Although these networks are dynamical systems and their outputs change in time, only the stable outputs are used for information processing. The last one is the temporal recurrent networks with arbitrary feedback connections. Since these networks are highly nonlinear dynamical systems, they exhibit a variety of complex dynamical behavior. The main purpose of this paper is to apply these dynamical behavior for information processing. There are lots of applications, e.g. , memory of sequence, temporal pattern recognition, oscillating pattern generation, robot control, and system identification of nonlinear dynamical systems. In recent years, supervised learning algorithms for recurrent networks has been derived in various forms by Pineda [7], Williams and Zipper [8], Pearlmutter [9], Gherrity [10], Doya and Yoshizawa [11], and by Sato [12,13]. In this article we will study backpropagation through time method developed by Pearlmutter [9] and one of the authors [13]. In order to learn aperiodic motion, several new techniques are to be introduced. It is shown that the initial values of the hidden units can be considered as

learning parameters. Especially, successive changes of initial conditions are needed to learn aperiodic dynamics. A weak periodic boundary constraint is also introduced to learn periodic motion.

An interesting application of the temporal recurrent networks is a speech synthesis. A lot of effort have made synthetic speech sound quite readable. Its quality, however, still far from human's voice in the viewpoint of naturalness. This problems might be mainly due to the difficulties of obtaining voice sources which have good quality. The voice source of real human speech involves a lot of small waveform and spectral fluctuations, which seems to provide the naturalness, whereas artificial voice source does not have them. If the recurrent networks could learn the voice source waveforms including these fluctuations and if they could reproduce them under some control, a recurrent net driven synthesizer would produce an excellent synthetic speech. We tested this idea in computer simulations. A recurrent network, which composed of locally connected nonlinear pair oscillators, was used. It is called APOLONN. The APOLONN was able to learn the fluctuations of voiced-sources. Although APOLONN can not generate the perfect voiced-source at the moment, the present result is very encouraging. After learning one specific waveform, APOLONN can generate waveforms with modulated amplitudes and frequencies by a simple scale transformation of the parameters.

2. Learning Algorithm

In this section, we will review the backpropagation through time method for recurrent networks [9,13], and develop it so that recurrent networks are able to learn aperiodic motion. Let $X_i(t)$ be the i-th unit output at a time t. Equations of motion for the unit outputs are given as

$$\tau_i \, dX_i/dt = - X_i + G_i(\Sigma W_{ij}X_j) + I_i \, , \qquad (2.1)$$

where τ_i, G_i, I_i and W_{ij} are a time delay constant, a sigmoid function and an external input of the i-th unit, and a connection weight from the j-th unit to the i-th unit, respectively. There is no restriction for the weight values. In the following, (2.1) is written in compact form as

$$\tau_i \, dX_i/dt = F_i(X,W,I) \, , \qquad (2.2)$$

where X, W and I represent sets of all the unit outputs, connection weights and external inputs, respectively.

2.1 Error Measure Function

Some of the units receive time dependent teacher signal, $Q_i(t)$. They are called visible units. The set of visible units is denoted by V. The performance of the networks can be evaluated by a error measure function, E. Usually, E is given by the deviation of the visible outputs from the teacher signal over some

period: $\int_{t1}^{t2} dt \sum_{i \in V} (X_i - Q_i)^2$ or $\int_{t1}^{t2} dt \, e^{\lambda(t-t2)} \sum_{i \in V} (X_i - Q_i)^2$.

In the teacher forcing method [8,9,11], the visible units receive additional external forces, $\xi_i = (\tau_i \, dQ_i/dt - F_i(X,W,I))$, so that the visible unit outputs are clamped to the teacher signal: $X_i(t) = Q_i(t)$ for $i \in V$. In this case, the error can be measured by the magnitude of the external forces: $E = \int_{t1}^{t2} dt \sum_{i \in V} \xi_i^2$. In the following, we will assume a general form for E:

$$E = \int_{t1}^{t2} dt \, L_1(X,Q,dQ/dt,I,W,\tau) + L_2(X(t2),X(t0)) \, , \qquad (2.3)$$

where the initial conditions for the unit outputs are supposed to be given at the time t0.

2.2 Variation of Error Measure Function

In learning process, parameters in the recurrent network are changed so that the error measure function, E, is decreased. Any parameter in the networks considered as an adjustable parameter [9,12]. Here, the weights, W, and the time delay constants, τ, are updated. Learning rules for other parameters can be derived by the same way. The change of E, which is caused by parameter change, can be calculated by a variational method. Since the unit outputs, X, satisfy the equations of motion (2.2), E can be written as

$$E = \int_{t1}^{t0} dt \, L_1 + L_2 - \int_{t0}^{t2} dt \sum_i P_i(\tau_i \, dX_i/dt - F_i) \, , \qquad (2.4)$$

where P_i is the Lagrange multiplier. Note that the time integration for the P_i-term is extended to the time t0 at which the initial condition is imposed. The variation of E can be calculated as

$$\delta E = \int_{t1}^{t2} dt \, [\sum_i (\partial L_1/\partial X_i)\delta X_i + \sum_i (\partial L_1/\partial \tau_i) \, \delta \tau_i$$
$$+ \sum_{i,j} (\partial L_1/\partial W_{ij}) \, \delta W_{ij}]$$

$$+ \int_{t0}^{t2} dt \, [\sum_i (\tau_i \, dP_i/dt + \sum_j P_j \, \partial F_j/\partial X_i) \, \delta X_i$$
$$- \sum_i (P_i \, dX_i/dt) \, \delta \tau_i + \sum_{i,j,k} (P_k \, \partial F_k/\partial W_{ij}) \, \delta W_{ij}]$$

$$+ \sum_i [\partial L_2/\partial X_i(t2) - \tau_i P_i(t2)] \, \delta X_i(t2)$$

$$+ \sum_i [\partial L_2/\partial X_i(t0) + \tau_i P_i(t0)] \, \delta X_i(t0) \, . \qquad (2.5)$$

Assuming the equation of motion for P_i,

$$\tau_i \, dP_i/dt = - \sum_j P_j \, \partial F_j/\partial X_i - \partial L_1/\partial X_i$$
$$\text{for } t1 \leq t < t2, \qquad (2.6a)$$

$$\tau_i \, dP_i/dt = - \sum_j P_j \, \partial F_j/\partial X_i$$
$$\text{for } t0 \leq t < t1, \qquad (2.6b)$$

and the boundary condition,

$$\tau_i P_i(t2) = \partial L_2/\partial X_i(t2) \, , \qquad (2.6c)$$

δE turns out to be

$$\delta E = \int_{t1}^{t2} dt \, [\sum_i (\partial L_1/\partial \tau_i - P_i \, dX_i/dt)\delta \tau_i$$
$$+ \sum_{i,j} (\partial L_1/\partial W_{ij} + \sum_k P_k \, \partial F_k/\partial W_{ij})\delta W_{ij}]$$

$$+ \int_{t0}^{t1} dt \, [- \sum_i (P_i \, dX_i/dt)\delta \tau_i + \sum_{i,j} (\sum_k P_k \, \partial F_k/\partial W_{ij})\delta W_{ij}]$$

$$+ \sum_i [\partial L_2/\partial X_i(t0) + \tau_i P_i(t0)] \, \delta X_i(t0) \, . \qquad (2.7)$$

Form (2.7), the derivatives of E can be derived as

$$\partial E/\partial \tau_i = \int_{t1}^{t2} dt \, (\partial L_1/\partial \tau_i - P_i \, dX_i/dt) - \int_{t0}^{t1} dt \, P_i \, dX_i/dt \, , \qquad (2.8a)$$

$$\partial E/\partial W_{ij} = \int_{t1}^{t2} dt \, (\partial L_1/\partial W_{ij} + \sum_k P_k \, \partial F_k/\partial W_{ij})$$
$$+ \int_{t0}^{t1} dt \sum_k P_k \, \partial F_k/\partial W_{ij} \, , \qquad (2.8b)$$

$$\partial E/\partial X_i(t0) = \tau_i P_i(t0) + \partial L_2/\partial X_i(t0) \, . \qquad (2.8c)$$

These derivatives can be calculated as follows.

(1) The recurrent net is run under fixed parameter values τ and W from t0 to t2 according to (2.2), starting from the initial value X(t0).

(2) The Lagrange multiplier, P_i, is calculated backward in time with the boundary condition (2.6c). From t2 to

t1, the unit error $(\partial L_1/\partial X_i)$ is injected according to (2.6a), while there is no unit error injection from t1 to t0 according to (2.6b).

(3) The derivatives of the error E are obtained according to (2.8).

2.3 Fixed Time Interval Method

Let us first consider periodic motion or a trajectory within a finite time interval. Let [t1,t2] be the basic period or the interval under consideration. The initial condition is given at the time t1 (=t0). The error E is evaluated in the whole interval [t1,t2]. After the network is run for the whole interval, the parameters are updated by the steepest descent method:

$$\Delta\tau_i = -\alpha \ \partial E/\partial\tau_i, \qquad (2.9a)$$
$$\Delta W_{ij} = -\alpha \ \partial E/\partial W_{ij}, \qquad (2.9b)$$

where α is a learning constant. Although the initial condition for the visible units are known, the initial condition for the hidden units are not known. One can impose some fixed initial condition for the hidden units. In this case, an improper choice of the initial condition causes errors of the visible units, even for the desired parameter values. In order to avoid this difficulty, it is possible to change the initial values of the hidden units by the steepest descent method:

$$\Delta X_i(t1) = -\alpha \ \partial E/\partial X_i(t1) \quad \text{for } i \notin V. \qquad (2.10)$$

In the case of periodic motion, one can impose a weak periodic boundary condition for the hidden units by introducing the term, $\Sigma_{i \notin V} (X_i(t2) - X_i(t1))^2$, for the error

function E.

2.4 Learning Aperiodic Motion

A procedure to learn aperiodic motion is given as follows. Let $\underline{t}$ be the current time.

(1) The future error E and its gradients for a time interval [t1,t2] (= $[\underline{t},\underline{t}+T]$) are calculated following the equations (2.2), (2.6) and (2.8). (2) The parameters are changed toward the steepest descent direction according to (2.9). (3) The network with the new parameter value is run for some period T_Δ and the current time is increased by T_Δ. Repeat the above procedures. When the initial condition is imposed at a fixed time t0, it is necessary to propagate P_i back to the initial time t0. It means that the whole past trajectory should be stored. However, if the desired trajectory is stable under small fluctuations, the calculation can be simplified. In this case, the linearlized equations,

$$\tau_i \ dZ_i/dt = \Sigma_j \ (\partial F_i(X,W,I)/\partial X_j) \ Z_j, \qquad (2.11)$$

have negative Lyapunov exponents and the solution dumps exponentially. Since the equations for P_i without the error injection, (2.6b), are the adjoint equations for the linearlized equations (2.11), P_i dumps exponentially backward in time (Note that $d(\Sigma_i\tau_iP_iZ_i)/dt$

= 0) .Therefore, the calculation of P_i and the time integration in (2.8) can be truncated around the time (t1-T_B). The truncation time T_B is estimated by the inverse magnitude of the largest Lyapunov exponent. As pointed out before, it is not necessary to impose a fixed initial condition for the hidden units. Especially, when the desired trajectory is chaotic motion, it is impossible to impose a fixed initial condition because of sensitive dependence on the initial condition [14]. This is reflected by the fact that P_i diverges exponentially backward in time because of positive Lyapunov exponents. The initial condition can be successively changed so that the future error decreases. This can be done by changing the current state according to

$$\Delta X_i(t1) = -\alpha \ \partial E/\partial X_i(t1) = -\alpha \ \tau_iP_i(t1), \qquad (2.12)$$

before proceeding the step (3). Therefore, it is not necessary to backpropagate P_i from t1 to t0.

2.5 Evaluation of Past Error

It is possible to use the past error for the calculation of the parameter change. In this case, the error evaluation interval [t1,t2] is set to $[\underline{t}-T,\underline{t}]$. Since the network parameters have been updated, the parameter values in the interval [t1,t2] are functions of the time in general. Therefore, the derivatives of error, $\partial E/\partial W_{ij}$ and $\partial E/\partial\tau_i$ are ill-defined. However, the variation of the error, (2.7), is well defined. Let us imagine a weight variation for the past weight trajectory:

$$W_{ij}(t) \to W_{ij}(t) + f(\underline{t},t)\delta W_{ij} \qquad \text{for } t \le \underline{t} \quad (2.13)$$

where $f(\underline{t},t)$ is a given function of time t. By using (2.7), one can find δW_{ij}^* which maximally decreases the past error E defined in the interval [t1,t2]:

$$\delta W_{ij}^* = -\alpha \ [\int_{t1}^{t2} dt \ f(\underline{t},t) \ (\partial L_1/\partial W_{ij} + \Sigma_k P_k \ \partial F_k/\partial W_{ij})$$
$$+ \int_{t0}^{t1} dt \ f(\underline{t},t) \ \Sigma_k P_k \ \partial F_k/\partial W_{ij})]. \qquad (2.14)$$

It is reasonable to update the weight value by δW_{ij}^*. The on-line learning algorithms derived by Williams & Zipser [8], Gherrity [10] and Doya & Yoshizawa [11] are equivalent to the choice, $f(\underline{t},t) = 1$. This means that a fixed initial condition is imposed at the time t0 and its effects are incorporated to δW^*. As before one can successively reset the initial condition. This can be done by choosing a $f(\underline{t},t)$ which vanishes for t < t1. This means that the effects before the time t1 are neglected and the initial condition is reset at t1 by the output value at that time. A natural choice is $f(\underline{t},t) = \exp[-2\pi(\underline{t}-t)/T]$. The update rules for the time delay constants can be derived by the same way.

3   Problems in Speech Synthesis

Despite a lot of efforts have been made, the quality and naturalness of a synthesized speech are still insufficient. A speech synthesizer system based on either the LPC and their family or a cascaded Formant consists of a two main functions, sound source generators and filter systems (Fig. 2) [15] . When a proper filter system is exited by a residual signal obtained from a real speech, the quality of the output signal would be good enough. However, it get worse dramatically if the filter system is exited by an artificial voiced-source signal such as a impulse train. In that case, synthesized speech preserve the readability of a language information whereas the quality of a speech sound is quite unnatural. Hence, we could know that the source signal property affects the output qualities.

In order to improve the synthesized speech quality, particularly in the rule-based synthesis system, a number of source waveform and its generation methods have been proposed. One of them is the polynomial approximation of the glottal waveform [16,17]. Another is the combination of the impulse generator and filters which simulate the transfer function of the glottis.[15,16,18]. The third one is a more realistic glottal waveform generator, such as the two-mass model [19]. These source certainly make synthesized speech more natural somehow than the simple impulse train source. However, as far as they generate the same waveform for every pitch period, the output does not sound as that of humans but of machines. Because, small fluctuations of source waveform, amplitude, periodicity, and spectrum affect in giving a naturalness to the output speech.

How can we add these small fluctuations to the source? When the fluctuation is too small, they do not affect the quality improvement since they are masked perceptually. When the excess of the fluctuation is given, the output speech would be a pathologic voice. Moreover, when the fluctuation is given by some simple function, the results would be disappointing even if the statistical characteristics of the fluctuation were preserved within the function. On the other hand, the synthesized speech using the residual signal tell us that the naturalness is preserved if the fluctuations of the original speech waveform are preserved. The experimental result [20] shows at least 32 pitch period is required to make a natural longer duration vowel by concatenating several pitch period waveform. It supports the advantage of using the preserved fluctuations of the original speech. Therefore, we tried to train the recurrent net to generate the source waveform including fluctuations for high quality speech synthesizer.

4. APOLONN

A simple nonlinear oscillator can be composed of a pair of units with asymmetric connections. It exhibits various wave forms depending on its weight values. It can be considered as a basic component of a complex nonlinear oscillation generator. It is called a pair oscillator. Our model is composed of a set of pair oscillators. They are locally connected each other and fully connected with the visible units. [Fig.1]. We call it APOLONN (adaptive nonlinear pair oscillators with local connections). The dynamical degree of freedom is determined by the number of units in the network. It is well known that a simple dynamical system with three degrees of freedom can generate chaotic motion [14]. Therefore, one can expect that APOLONN can generate very complex trajectories by increasing the number of pair oscillators. Since pair oscillators with different time delay constants adjust their weights to different time scale components of the desired trajectory, it is easy for APOLONN to learn complex dynamical behavior. From the computational point of view, APOLONN has advantages over fully connected recurrent networks. A number of connections in APOLONN scales linearly with the number of units, while that of fully connected nets scales like (number of units)^2. APOLONN can be easily implemented in parallel machines than fully connected nets. After learning a specific wave forms, its amplitude and frequency can be modulated by scale transformation of the parameters. For the definiteness, the sigmoid function of the i-th unit, G_i, in (2.1) is supposed to have the following form:

$$G_i(y) = A_i \tanh(B_i \cdot y) + C_i .\qquad (4.1)$$

It can be shown that the equation of motion, (2.1), is invariant under the scale transformation

$$t, \tau_i \rightarrow \beta t, \beta \tau_i \qquad (4.2a)$$
$$X_i, A_i, B_i, C_i \rightarrow r X_i, r A_i, B_i/r, r C_i \qquad (4.2b)$$

It means that the amplitude and frequency can be modulated by the scale transformation of the parameters, A_i, B_i, C_i and τ_i.

5. Computer simulation

We trained APOLONN to generate voiced-source waveforms for the speech synthesizer (Fig. 2). We used several residual signal waveform obtained by 16th order inversefiltering of vowels /a/ and /e/, which are the partials of some Japanese ward. A 20 kHz sampling, 16bits AD was used to digitize these speech. In the simulation we used the discrete time by introducing a sampling time step constant Δt (=0.05msec).

First, learning of one pitch period waveform was examined. Its period length is 8.75 msec. We used APOLONN with 6 pair oscillators. There is only one visible unit and no external input. The fixed time interval method with teacher forcing was used to update weights. The time delay constants was fixed throughout the learning process in this study. These were determined as

$$\tau_i = scale\_factor * i \qquad (5.1)$$

for pair oscillators to introduce several time scales. The time delay constant value of the visible unit greatly affects the learning speed. The best choice was τ_1 (the smallest time delay of the pair oscillators). A typical learning curve is shown in Fig. 3. One can find intermittent increases of the error and the weight change distance. They correspond to the instabilities at the bifurcation points in the weight space. By changing the learning step size adaptively, this behavior can be reduced. After about 3,000 learning cycles, APOLONN generated a periodic trajectory which waveform for one pitch period is shown in Fig. 4. The APOLONN with the same weights can generate trajectories with modulated amplitudes and frequencies by scaling the sigmoid function parameters, the time delay constants and the initial output values according to (4.2). If the time and amplitude scale factors, β and γ in (4.2) are set to 0.5 and 1.25, respectively, APOLONN with the same weights as in Fig.4 generate a modulated trajectory in Fig. 5.

Next, we examined whether the fluctuation of the residual signal of speech sound could be learned by APOLONN with 20 pairs. The teacher signal was composed of 32 pitch periods. The sampling rate in this case was 4kHZ to reduce the number of data. After about 15,000 learning cycles, APOLONN produced the trajectory in Fig. 6. The phase space trajectory in Fig. 7 shows that the trajectory seems to be a chaotic attractor. However, the fluctuations of the amplitude and the periodicity are rather small compared with those of the teacher signal.

6. Conclusion

We proposed a recurrent net called APOLONN to learn complex nonlinear dynamics. It was trained to generate voiced-source waveforms. Complex waveforms in one pitch period was learned by APOLONN fairly well. APOLONN was able to generate fluctuations of the amplitude and the frequency among 32 pitch period, which are crutial to preserve the naturalness of voiced speech. Although APOLONN can not generate the perfect voiced-source for a speech synthesizer at the moment, the above results are encouraging. Much work has to be done to make a recurrent net driven high quality speech synthesizer.

We also proposed new methods to learn aperiodic motion. However, the fixed time interval method proposed in the previous studies [9,13] was used in the current simulation. We expect that the new method may help the learning of the fluctuation. Also, it may help the learning performance to adjust the time delay constants. These methods will be used in our future study. In the simulations, there are free parameters like a learning constant α. The learning performance much more depends on these parameters than in the feedforward backpropagation network. It is necessary to find a systematic way to adjust these parameters. The detailed analysis of the learning behavior near the bifurcation points will be done for future work.

Our results shows the capability of the temporal recurrent net to learn complex nonlinear dynamics and the great possibility of their use for the real world.

References

[1] Hinton GE, Rumelhart DE and Williams RJ, (1986), "Learning internal representation by error propagation", in Parallel Distributed Processing I, edited by Rumelhart DE and McClelland JL, M.I.T.Press, Cambridge, MA, 318-362

[2] Hopfield JJ (1984), "Neurons with graded response have collective computational properties like those of two-state neurons", Proc. Natl. Acad. Sci. USA, 81, 3088-3092

[3] Cohen MA and Grossberg S (1983), "Absolute stability of global pattern formation and parallel memory storage by competitive neural networks", IEEE Trans. on Systems, Man and Cybernetics, 13, 815-825

[4] Hopfield JJ and Tank DW (1985), "Neural computation of decisions in optimization problems", Biol. Cybern., 52, 141-152

[5] Hopfield JJ (1982), "Neural networks and physical systems with emergent collective computational abilities", Proc. Natl. Acad. Sci. USA, 79, 2554-2558

[6] Hinton GE and Sejnowski TJ, (1986), "Learning and relearning in Boltzmann machines", In Parallel Distributed Processing I, eds Rumelhart DE, McClelland JL, Cambridge, MA: M.I.T. Press

[7] Pineda FJ, (1987), "Generalization of back-propagation to recurrent neural networks", Phys. Rev. Lett. 59, 2229-2232

[8] Williams RJ and Zipser D, (1989), "A learning algorithm for continually running fully recurrent neural networks", Neural Computation, 1, 270-280

[9] Pearlmutter BA, (1989), "Learning state space trajectories in recurrent neural network", Neural Computation, 1, 263-269

[10] Gherrity M, (1989), "A learning algorithm for analog, fully recurrent neural networks", in Proceedings of IJCNN, (Washington D.C.), Vol 1, 643-644

[11] Doya K and Yoshizawa S, (1989), "Memorizing oscillatory patterns in the analog neuron network", in Proceeding of IJCNN, (Washington D.C.), Vol 1, 27-32

[12] Sato M, (1989), "A real time learning algorithm for recurrent analog neural networks", Biol. Cybernetics, in press.

[13] Sato M, (1989), "A Learning Algorithm to Teach Spatiotemporal Patterns to Recurrent Neural Networks", Biol. Cybernetics, 62, 259-263.

[14] Berge P, Pomeau Y, Vidal C, (1984), "Order within Chaos", John Wiley & Sons

[15] Klatt DH, (1980), "Software for a cascade/parallel formant synthesizer", J.Acous.Soc.Am.67(3), pp.971-995

[16] Rothenberg M, (1981), "An Interactive Model for the Voice Source", STL-QPSR,KTH,No.4.pp-1-17

[17] Fujisaki H and Lingquist M, (1986), "Proposal and Evaluation of Models for the Glottal Source Waveform", Proc.ICASSP86, pp.1605-1608

[18] Klatt DH, (1987), "Review of text-to-speech conversion for English", J.Acous.Soc.Am.82(3), pp.737-793

[19] Flanagan JL and Ishizaka K, (1978), "Computer Model to Characterize the air displaced by the vibrating vocal cords", J.Acous.Soc.Am.63(5), pp.1559-1565

[20] Hashiba M and Ifukube T,*et.al*, (1988), "A Role of Waveform Fluctuation on Naturality of Vowels", Proc.J.Acous.Soc.Jpn, Fall Meeting, pp.345-346

Fig. 1 APOLONN structure

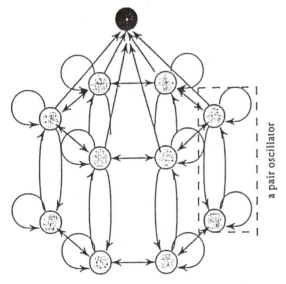

Numbers of pair oscillators are locally connected each other and fully connected with a visible unit.

Fig. 2 Structure of speech synthesizer

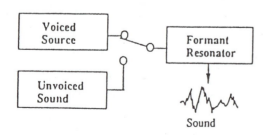

Fig. 3 Learning curve

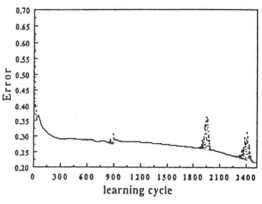

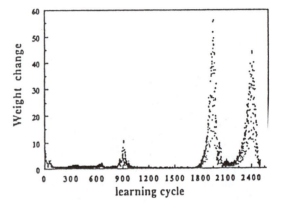

Fig. 5 Modulated trajectory

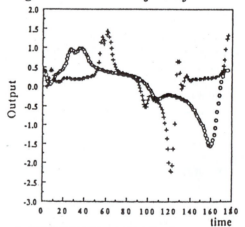

A modulated trajectory (axes) and the original trajectory (circle).
The amplitude and the period length are scaled by factors 1.25 and 0.5, respectively.

Fig. 6 Trajectory in 32 pitch period

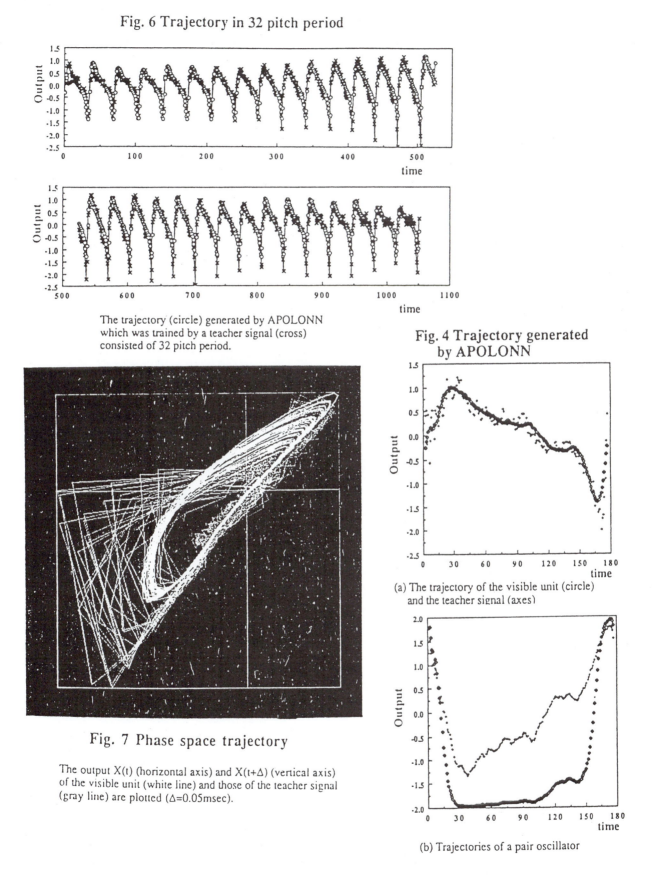

The trajectory (circle) generated by APOLONN
which was trained by a teacher signal (cross)
consisted of 32 pitch period.

Fig. 7 Phase space trajectory

The output X(t) (horizontal axis) and X(t+Δ) (vertical axis)
of the visible unit (white line) and those of the teacher signal
(gray line) are plotted (Δ=0.05msec).

Fig. 4 Trajectory generated
by APOLONN

(a) The trajectory of the visible unit (circle)
and the teacher signal (axes)

(b) Trajectories of a pair oscillator

Nonlinear dynamics of the voice: Signal analysis and biomechanical modeling

Hanspeter Herzel
Institute of Theoretical Physics, Technical University, Hardenbergstrasse 36, D-10623 Berlin, Germany

David Berry and Ingo Titze
National Center for Voice and Speech, The University of Iowa, Iowa City, Iowa 52242

Ina Steinecke
Institute of Theoretical Physics, Humboldt University, Invalidenstrasse 110, D-10115 Berlin, Germany

(Received 17 May 1994; accepted for publication 8 August 1994)

Irregularities in voiced speech are often observed as a consequence of vocal fold lesions, paralyses, and other pathological conditions. Many of these instabilities are related to the intrinsic nonlinearities in the vibrations of the vocal folds. In this paper, bifurcations in voice signals are analyzed using narrow-band spectrograms. We study sustained phonation of patients with laryngeal paralysis and data from an excised larynx experiment. These spectrograms are compared with computer simulations of an asymmetric 2-mass model of the vocal folds. © 1995 American Institute of Physics.

I. INTRODUCTION

The vocal folds, together with glottal airflow, constitute a highly nonlinear self-oscillating system. According to the accepted myoelastic theory of voice production, the vocal folds are set into vibration by the combined effect of subglottal pressure, the viscoelastic properties of the folds, and the Bernoulli effect.[1,2] The effective length, mass, and tension of the vocal folds are determined by muscle action, and in this way the fundamental frequency ("pitch") and the waveform of the glottal pulses can be controlled. The vocal tract acts as a filter which transforms the primary signals into meaningful voiced speech.[3]

Normal sustained voiced sound appears to be nearly periodic, although small perturbations (on the order of a percent) are important for the naturalness of speech. Under certain circumstances, however, much larger irregularities are observed in vocalizations which are often associated with the term "roughness." In the phonetic literature phenomena such as "octave jumps," "biphonation" (two independent pitches), and "noise concentrations" have been reported for decades.[4,5] However, only within the past few years has it been suggested that these observations might be interpreted as period-doubling bifurcations, tori, and chaos, respectively,[6-10] It has been shown using Poincaré sections and estimations of attractor dimension and Lyapunov exponents that newborn cries[6] and vocal disorders[7-10] are intimately related to bifurcations and low-dimensional attractors. On the one hand, subharmonics and irregularities appear occasionally in normal vocalizations (newborn cries,[6] "vocal fry" phonation,[9] and speech[11]). On the other hand, vocal instabilities due to bifurcations are often symptomatic in voice pathology.[7-10] Laryngeal stroboscopy reveals that various voice disorders lead to irregular vibratory patterns of the vocal folds resulting in a rough voice quality.[12] The corresponding acoustic signals often show sudden jumps to subharmonic regimes (period-doubling or -tripling) and low-frequency modulations (tori).[7,8,10] It is the aim of current research to understand the underlying physiological mechanisms of these bifurcations with the aid of high-speed films, excised larynx experiments,[13] and biomechanical modeling.[14,15]

In this paper we analyze voice signals with the aid of narrow-band spectrograms, allowing the detection of bifurcations in systems with slowly varying parameters.[4-6,16,17] Spectrograms are based on many subsequent short-time power spectra of overlapping segments. The spectral amplitude is encoded as a grey scale and, in this way, the (dis)appearance of spectral peaks due to bifurcations of the underlying dynamical system can be monitored. For example, period-doubling is reflected in additional peaks in the middle of the harmonics of the original pitch. Low-frequency modulations lead to sidebands of the main spectral peaks. An amplitude modulation with frequency f induces, e.g., peaks at $F_0 \pm f, 2F_0 \pm f, \ldots$.

While normal phonation is characterized by synchronized motion of all vibratory modes of the vocal folds, various physiological mechanisms lead to the desynchronization of certain modes.[10] One source of instabilities is the tension imbalance of the left and right vocal fold which is relevant for unilateral laryngeal nerve paralyses. In these cases the rest position, the stiffness, and the effective mass of the affected fold may deviate drastically from normality. Often paralysis leads to turbulent fricative noise due to incomplete closure of the folds corresponding to a "breathy voice."[12] Frequently, subharmonics and low-frequency modulations have also been observed.[10,18-20] Here, the left–right asymmetry is presumably the origin of the instabilities.[15,18,21]

In the following sections we present left–right asymmetry from three perspectives. Spectrograms are presented from patients with unilateral paralyses, from excised larynx experiments with artificially induced asymmetry, and from

 1054-1500/95/5(1)/30/5/$6.00

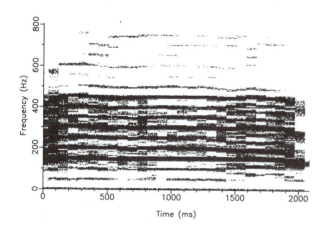

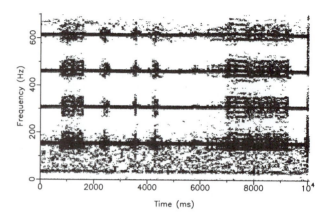

FIG. 1. Computer spectrogram of the vowel [i:] from a male patient with paralysis showing subharmonics. In order to get sufficient spectral resolution to resolve subharmonics and sidebands, segments of 4096 points (about 200 ms) have been used in all spectrograms. Higher frequencies have been boosted for a better visualization of harmonics.

FIG. 3. Spectrogram from an excised larynx experiment with asymmetric elongation of the folds. Around 1000 and 8000 ms episodes with low-frequency modulations of about 20 Hz can be seen.

simulations of an asymmetric 2-mass model of the vocal folds.

II. UNILATERAL LARYNGEAL NERVE PARALYSES

Figure 1 shows a spectrogram of a sustained vowel from a male patient with unilateral recurrent nerve paralysis. The fundamental frequency F_0 of about 150 Hz and its harmonics of 300 Hz and 450 Hz appear as dark horizontal lines. The audible rough voice quality results from the strong subharmonic components. Particularly, period-tripling, i.e. subharmonics at $\frac{1}{3}F_0, \frac{2}{3}F_0,...$ occur between 0 and 1500 ms. Moreover, around 1700 ms another subharmonic regime is found: there are subharmonics at one-fourth of the pitch F_0. Comparable transitions between subharmonic regimes will be discussed later in connection with our 2-mass model.

In Fig. 2 a sustained vowel of another male patient with recurrent nerve paralysis is shown. His voice is characterized by low-frequency modulations typically between 20 and 30 Hz. The modulations appear in the spectrogram as sidebands of the fundamental frequency ($\approx$ 120 Hz) and its harmonics. These toroidal oscillations result in a very rough voice quality. Moreover, the voice sounds breathy due to turbulent air flow. In this case, two sources of hoarseness—complicated vibratory patterns of the folds and turbulence—superimpose on each other.

III. EXCISED LARYNX EXPERIMENTS

Experiments with human or animal larynges serve as a link between the human voice source *in vivo* and computer models.[1,18,22] They allow controlled and systematic parameter variations and easy observation of vibratory patterns.

We have examined three larynges from large (about 25 kg) mongrel dogs coming from coronary research units at The University of Iowa. The dissected larynges were mounted on an apparatus described in detail elsewhere.[13,22] Heated and humified air was supplied from below as the driving force of the oscillations. The device was attached to several micrometers to control the adduction and the elongation of the vocal folds. To facilitate observation of vocal fold movement, a strobe light with adjustable frequency was placed above the glottis. The data were recorded on a color video system and afterwards digitized with 16-bit resolution and a sampling rate of 20 kHz.

In our experiments instabilities have been studied for varying subglottal pressure and for asymmetric adduction and elongation of the vocal folds. 2-parameter bifurcation diagrams can be found elsewhere.[13] Here we only summarize briefly the various dynamic regimes which have been observed for overcritical asymmetry and pressure:

- Symmetric periodic phonation in head-like and chest-like registers;
- periodic vibrations of the lax fold only;
- subharmonics, modulations, and irregular vibrations with both folds involved;

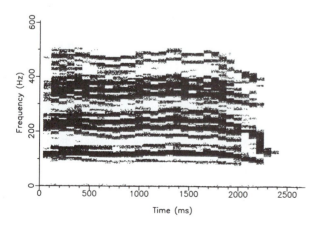

FIG. 2. Spectrogram (vowel [e:], recurrent nerve paralysis) displaying low-frequency modulations visible as sidebands.

- whistle-like sound;
- aphonia, i.e., vibrations ceased for very strong asymmetric tension.

Typically, the parameter ranges of these regimes overlap, i.e., hysteresis is observed. Sometimes spontaneous transitions between different dynamical regimes appeared without external parameter changes. The spectrogram in Fig. 3 shows such transitions from normal phonation to intermittent regimes with a low-frequency modulation of about 20 Hz, as evidenced by the spacing of the sidebands about the harmonics. The longest duration of low-frequency modulations occurs between 7000 and 9000 ms. An example of normal phonation is found between 5000 and 7000 ms. These modulations have been found due to lengthening of one of the folds. Note, that qualitatively comparable modulations appeared in the sustained vowel shown in Fig. 2.

IV. TWO-MASS MODEL

Computer models of speech production are valuable to understand the basic mechanisms of normal and pathological phonation. There are conceptionally simple 2-mass models[9,15,18,21,23] and sophisticated continuum models simulating the viscoelastic equations.[2,8,14,24] In this section we discuss a simplified version of the intensively studied Ishizaka–Flanagan model.[23] For such relatively simple models extensive bifurcation analysis can be carried out.[9,15,25]

In our model, each fold is represented by two oscillators (defined by mass m, stiffness k, damping constant r) which are coupled by a spring with stiffness k_c (see Fig. 4). This realization enables the "vocal folds" to oscillate with a phase difference between the lower and the upper part. Another restoring force with stiffness c acts during collision of the left and the right vocal fold, i.e., if areas a_i become negative. We can describe the elongation of each of the four masses by Newton's law:

$$m_{i\alpha}\ddot{x}_{i\alpha} + r_{i\alpha}\dot{x}_{i\alpha} + k_{i\alpha}x_{i\alpha} + \Theta(-a_i)c_{i\alpha}\left(\frac{a_i}{2l}\right) + k_{c\alpha}(x_{i\alpha} - x_{j\alpha})$$

$$= F_i(x_{1l}, x_{1r}, x_{2l}, x_{2r}), \tag{1}$$

$$a_{i\alpha} = a_{i0\alpha} + l x_{i\alpha},$$

$$a_i = a_{il} + a_{ir}, \tag{2}$$

with $a_{i0\alpha}$ the glottal rest area and l the length of the glottis

$$i, j = \begin{cases} 1 \text{—lower mass,} \\ 2 \text{—upper mass;} \end{cases}$$

$$\alpha = \begin{cases} l \text{—left side,} \\ r \text{—right side,} \end{cases}$$

where $F_i(x_{1l}, x_{1r}, x_{2l}, x_{2r})$ is the force exerted by the pressure P_i on the corresponding part of the glottis,

$$F_i = l d_i P_i, \tag{3}$$

where d_i is the thickness of part i.

The air flow is considered to be laminar and is described by the Bernoulli equation (4). After passing the smallest gap

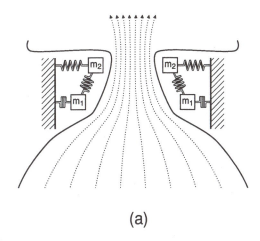

(a)

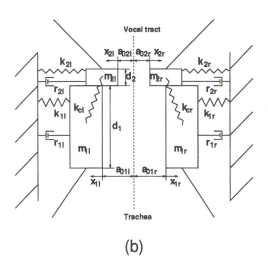

(b)

FIG. 4. (a) A cross section of the vocal folds with the airflow and 2-mass model superimposed. (b) A schematic of the asymmetric 2-mass model of vocal folds.

in the vertical direction with area $a_{\min}$, a jet is built up and the static pressure equals that of the supraglottal system which is set to zero.[2,15]

$$P_s = P_1 + \frac{\rho}{2}\left(\frac{U}{a_1}\right)^2 = \frac{\rho}{2}\left(\frac{U}{a_{\min}}\right)^2,$$

$$a_{\min} = \min(a_{1l}, a_{2l}) + \min(a_{1r}, a_{2r}), \tag{4}$$

where P_s is the subglottal pressure, U the volume flow velocity, and ρ the density of air.

According to these assumptions we get the following pressure equations:

$$P_1 = P_s\left[1 - \Theta(a_{\min})\left(\frac{a_{\min}}{a_1}\right)^2\right]\Theta(a_1), \tag{5}$$

$$P_2 = 0, \tag{6}$$

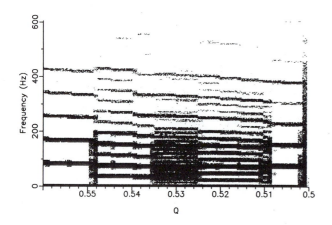

FIG. 5. Spectrogram from the asymmetric 2-mass model (calculated from the flow velocity U). The asymmetry parameter Q was reduced every 400 ms by 0.005 from 0.56 to 0.50. In this way jumps between different subharmonic regimes including period-doubling and -tripling are induced.

$$U = \sqrt{\frac{2P_s}{\rho}}\, a_{\min}. \tag{7}$$

It is emphasized that in this manner the upper masses are only driven by the lower ones. Our default parameter values representing a normal voice are given in the Appendix.

In the above model several aspects have been neglected: vertical motion, incompressibility, and nonlinear tissue properties of the folds. Moreover, the vocal fold vibrations were separated from the vocal tract by assuming constant pressures below and above the glottis. Nevertheless, several features of the human voice source such as the waveforms of glottal pulses and the phonation onset can be captured quite realistically.[9,15] However, we are aware that details such as localized lesions of the vocal folds cannot be treated by 2-mass models.

V. MODELING ASYMMETRY

In this section the effect of asymmetric mechanical properties of the folds is studied as a first approach to unilateral paralysis. Following earlier studies [15,18,21] we introduce an asymmetry parameter Q:

$$k_{ir} = Q k_{il},$$
$$m_{ir} = m_{il}/Q, \tag{8}$$
$$0 < Q < 1.$$

In this way the eigenfrequency of the affected fold is reduced by the factor Q. Instabilities have been found for $Q < 0.6$ and subglottal pressure above $P_s = 0.013$.[15] Typically, at the borderline of normal phonation abrupt jumps to subharmonic regimes are observed.[15] Figure 5 shows a "spectral bifurcation diagram" for slowly decreasing Q. It can be seen that the pitch decreases with the ratio of the eigenfrequencies Q. Around $Q = 0.55$ subharmonics suddenly appear at one-half of the pitch. At $Q = 0.536$ another complicated subharmonic regime is reached. Inspection of the peaks of the elongations x_{1r} and x_{1l} [see Eq. (1)] reveals that during one cycle (about

5 times the original pitch period) five maxima of x_{1r} and eight maxima of x_{1l} occur, i.e., we can interpret this regime as a 5:8 resonance. From $Q = 0.525$ to 0.51 subharmonics of one-third of the original pitch ("period-tripling") dominate corresponding to a 3:5 resonance in the above sense. The sequence of decreasing ratios from 2:3 to 5:8 to 3:5 is reminiscent of "Arnold tongues" in bifurcation diagrams of coupled oscillators.

Our simulations show that for sufficiently large pressures, which couple the left and right folds, the detuning of the eigenfrequencies induces transitions to subharmonic regimes comparable to observations as in Fig. 1. Comprehensive bifurcation diagrams in the $P_s - Q$ parameter plane also reveal the appearance of toroidal and chaotic oscillations.[15]

Despite the qualitative resemblance of our simulations to observations, we have to keep in mind that a 2-mass model is only a crude approximation of the real vocal folds. However, in simulations of a three-dimensional model based on partial differential equations, similar bifurcations to subharmonic regimes and chaos have been found.[8,14] Moreover, the calculation of empirical orthogonal functions from the continuum model reveal that the dynamics is often governed by only a few dominant modes. This can be regarded as a justification to study specific aspects of vocal fold vibrations such as left–right asymmetry with appropriate low-order models.

VI. SUMMARY AND DISCUSSION

Analysis of acoustic signals from newborn cries,[6] voice disorders, and excised larynx studies reveals clear evidence of bifurcations and low-dimensional attractors.[6-10] Since vocal folds are vibrating rather fast compared to slowly varying parameters such as muscle tension and subglottal pressure, different dynamic regimes (normal phonation, subharmonics, modulations) can be characterized. Although the limited stationarity of such data allows no definite proof of chaos, nonlinear phenomena are plausible since the human voice source exhibits several essential nonlinearities:

- Nonlinear stress-strain characteristics of vocal fold tissue;[8,2]
- highly nonlinear relation between pressure and glottal area [cf. Eq. (5)];
- collision of the vocal folds;
- vortices and jet instabilities.

Simulations of the 2-mass model have shown that various bifurcations appear due to the desynchronization of the right and left fold for overcritical asymmetry. The corresponding instabilities are similar to observations of vocalizations of patients with unilateral paralysis. However, a more quantitative comparison would require the use of more sophisticated models and more detailed measurements of the biomechanical properties of vocal fold tissues, especially in the case of pathologies.

In forthcoming studies we plan to analyze the physiological mechanisms of vocal instabilities in detail using the continuum model,[8,14,2] excised larynx experiments, and high-speed films of vocal fold vibrations.

ACKNOWLEDGMENTS

Partial funding for this research was provided by the Deutsche Forschungsgemeinschaft and Grant No. P60 DC00976 from the National Institute of Deafness and Other Communication Disorders. We thank J. Wendler and M. Cebulla for providing data from patients with paralyses.

APPENDIX: PARAMETERS OF THE TWO-MASS MODEL

Following mostly Ishizaka and Flanagan we choose the following parameters to model a normal voice:

$$m_{1l} = m_{1r} = 0.125,$$

$$m_{2l} = m_{2r} = 0.025,$$

$$k_{1l} = k_{1r} = 0.08,$$

$$k_{2l} = k_{2r} = 0.008,$$

$$k_{cl} = k_{cr} = 0.025,$$

$$c_{1l} = c_{1r} = 3k_1,$$

$$c_{2l} = c_{2r} = 3k_2,$$

$$r_{1l} = r_{1r} = 0.02,$$

$$r_{2l} = r_{2r} = 0.02,$$

$$d_1 = 0.25, \qquad a_{01} = a_{01l} + a_{01r} = 0.05,$$

$$d_2 = 0.05, \qquad a_{02} = a_{02l} + a_{02r} = 0.05,$$

$$P_s = 0.008 \qquad (\approx 8\text{cm } H_2O),$$

$$\rho = 0.00113.$$

All units are given in cm, g, ms, and their corresponding combinations.

[1] J. van den Berg, "Myoelastic-aerodynamic theory of voice production," J. Speech Hearing Res. **1**, 227–244 (1958).

[2] I. R. Titze and F. Alipour-Haghighi, "Myoelastic aerodynamic theory of phonation" (in preparation).

[3] G. Fant, *Acoustic Theory of Speech Production* (Mouton, The Hague, 1960).

[4] J. Lind (editor), *Newborn Infant Cry* (Almquist and Wiksells Boktrycken, Uppsala, 1965).

[5] A. W. Kelman, "Vibratory pattern of the vocal folds," Folia Phoniat. **33**, 73–99 (1981).

[6] W. Mende, H. Herzel, and K. Wermke, "Bifurcations and chaos in newborn cries," Phys. Lett. A **145**, 418–424 (1990).

[7] H. Herzel and J. Wendler, "Evidence of chaos in phonatory samples," in *EUROSPEECH* (ESCA, Genova, 1991), pp.263–266.

[8] I. R. Titze, R. Baken, and H. Herzel, "Evidence of chaos in vocal fold vibration," in *Vocal Fold Physiology: Frontiers in Basic Science*, edited by I. R. Titze (Singular Publishing Group, San Diego, 1993), pp.143–188.

[9] H. Herzel, "Bifurcations and chaos in voice signals," Appl. Mech. Rev. **46**, 399–413 (1993).

[10] H. Herzel, D. A. Berry, I. R. Titze, and M. Saleh, "Analysis of vocal disorders with methods from nonlinear dynamics," J. Speech Hearing Res. **37**, 1008–1019 (1994).

[11] L. Dolansky and P. Tjernlund, "On certain irregularities of voiced-speech waveforms," IEEE Trans. Audio **AU-16**, 51–56 (1968).

[12] M. Hirano, "Objective evaluation of the human voice: clinical aspects," Folia Phoniat. **41**, 89–144 (1989).

[13] D. Berry, H. Herzel, and I. R. Titze, "Bifurcations in excised larynx experiments due to asymmetric vocal folds" (in preparation).

[14] B. A. Berry, H. Herzel, I. R. Titze, and K. Krischer, "Interpretation of biomechanical simulations of normal and chaotic vocal fold oscillations with empirical eigenfunctions," J. Acoust. Soc. Am. **95**, 3595–3604 (1994).

[15] I. Steinecke and H. Herzel, "Bifurcations in an asymmetric vocal fold model," J. Acoust. Soc. Am. (in press).

[16] W. Lauterborn and E. Cramer, "Subharmonic routes to chaos observed in acoustics," Phys. Rev. Lett. **47**, 1445–1448 (1981).

[17] M. A. Liauw, K. Koblitz, N. I. Jaeger, and P. Plath, "Periodic perturbation of a drifting heterogeneous catalytic system," J. Phys. Chem. **97**, 11724–11730 (1993).

[18] K. Ishizaka and N. Isshiki, "Computer simulation of pathological vocal-cord vibrations," J. Acoust. Soc. Am. **60**, 1194–1198 (1976).

[19] B. Hammarberg, B. Fritzell, J. Gauffin, and J. Sundberg, "Acoustic and perceptual analysis of vocal dysfunction," J. Phonetics **14**, 533–547 (1986).

[20] M. Ptok, G. Sesterhenn, and R. Arold, "Bewertung der laryngealen Klanggeneration mit der FFT-Analyse der glottischen Impedanz bei Patienten mit Rekurrensparese," Folia Phoniat. **45**, 182–197 (1993).

[21] M. E. Smith, G. S. Berke, B. R. Gerrat, and J. Kreimann, " Laryngeal paralysis: theoretical considerations and effects on laryngeal vibration," J. Speech Hearing Res. **35**, 545–554 (1992).

[22] T. Baer, "Investigation of the phonatory mechanism, " ASHA Rep. **11**, 38–47 (1981).

[23] K. Ishizaka and J. L. Flanagan, "Synthesis of voiced sounds from a two-mass model of the vocal cords," Bell Syst. Technol. J. **51**, 1233–1268 (1972).

[24] I. R. Titze and D. T. Talkin, "A theoretical study of the effects of various laryngeal configurations on the acoustics of phonation," J. Acoust. Soc. Am. **66**, 60–74 (1979).

[25] H. Herzel, I. Steinecke, W. Mende, and K. Wermke, "Chaos and bifurcations during voiced speech," in *Complexity, Chaos and Biological Evolution*, edited by E. Mosekilde and L. Mosekilde (Plenum, New York, 1991), pp. 41–50.

Suggested Readings

Biology

Albano AM, Mees AS, Deguzman GC, Rapp TE. Data requirements for reliable estimation of correlation dimensions. In: Degn, Holden, Olsen, eds. *Chaos in Biological Systems.* New York, NY: Plenum; 1987:207–219.

Avnir D, Farin D, Pfeifer P. Molecular fractal surfaces. *Nature (Lond).* 1984;308:261–263.

Barnsley MF, Massopust P, Strickland H, Sloan AD. Fractal modeling of biological structures. *Ann NY Acad Sci.* 1987;504:179–194.

Bassingthwaighte J, King R, Sambrook JE, van Steenwyk B. Fractal analysis of blood-tissue exchange kinetics. In: Mochizuki, Honig, Koyama, Goldstick, Bruely, eds. *Advances in Experimental Medicine and Biology.* 1988;15–23.

Davidoff F. A touch of cancer: teaching uncertainty, ambiguity in medicine. *ACP Observer.* October 1994;10.

Decroly O, Goldbeter AA. Selection between multiple periodic regimes in a biochemical system: complex dynamic behavior resolved by use of one-dimensional maps. *J Theor Biol.* 1985;113:649–671.

Eberhart RC. Chaos theory for the biomechanical engineer. *IEEE Eng Med Biol Mag.* 1989;8(3):41–45.

Jurgensen H, Lindenmayer A. Inference algorithms for development systems with cell lineages. *Bull Math Biol.* 1987;49:93–123.

Katz NJ. Fractals in the analysis of wave forms. *Comput Biol Med.* 1988;18:145–156.

Korolev SV, Solovyev VV, Tumanyan VG. A new global method for searching functional region of DNA based on fractal geometry representation of nucleotide sequences. *Comput Appl Biosci.* 1992; in press.

Lewis M, Rees DC. Fractal surfaces of proteins. *Science (Wash, DC).* 1985;230:1163–1165.

Liebovitch LS. Analysis of fractal ion channel gating kinetics: kinetic rates, energy levels, and activation energies. *Math Biosci.* 1989;93:97–115.

Liebovitch LS, Fischbarg J, Koniarek JP, Todorova I, Wang M. Fractal model of ion-channel kinetics. *Biochim Biophys Acta.* 1987;896:173–180.

Liebovitch LS, Fischbarg J, Koniarek JP. Ion channel kinetics: a model based on fractal scaling rather than multistate Markov processes. *Math Biosci.* 1987;84:37–68.

Manly BF. *Randomization and Monte-Carlo Methods in Biology.* New York, NY: Chapman and Hall; 1991.

May RM. *Stability and Complexity in Model Ecosystems.* Princeton, NJ: Princeton University Press; 1973.

Meakin P. A new model for biological pattern formation. *J Theor Biol.* 1986;118:101–113.

Meinhardt H. The random character of bifurcations and the reproducible processes of embryonic development. *Ann NY Acad Sci.* 1979;316:188–202.

Ng Y-K, Iannaccone PM. Fractal geometry of mosaic pattern demonstrates liver regeneration is a self-similar process. *Dev Biol.* 1992;151:419–430.

Olsen LF, Degn H. Chaos in biological systems. *Q Rev Biophys.* 1985;18:165–225.

Pecora LM. Fractal growth processes. *Nature (Lond).* 1986;322:789–793.

Smith TG, Marks WB, Lange GD, Sheriff WH, Neale EA. A fractal analysis of cell images. *J Neurosci Methods.* 1989;27:173–180.

Solovyev VV, Korolev SV, Lim HA. A new approach for the classification of functional regions of DNA sequences based on fractal representation. *Int J Genomic Res.* 1992;1:108–127.

Solovyev VV, Korolev SV, Tumanyan VG, Lim HA. A new approach to classification of DNA regions based on fractal representation of functionally similar sequences. *Dokl Biochem,* 1991;319:1496–1500.

Sporns O, Roth S, Seelig F. Chaotic dynamics of two coupled biochemical oscillators. *Physica D.* 1987;26:215–224.

Tsonis AA, Tsonis PA. Fractals: a new look at biological shape and patterning. *Perspect Biol Med.* 1987;30:355–361.

Cardiology

Abboud S, Berenfeld O, Sadeh D. Simulation of high-resolution QRS complex using a ventricular model with a fractal conduction system: effects of ischemia on high-frequency QRS potentials. *Circ Res.* 1991;68(6):1751–1760.

Abboud S, Sadeh D. Power spectrum analysis of foetal heart rate variability using the abdominal maternal electrocardiogram. *J Biomed Eng.* 1990;12:161–164.

Adam DR, Smith JM, Akselrod S, Nyberg S, Powell AO, Cohen RJ. Fluctuations in T-wave morphology and susceptibility to ventricular fibrillation. *J Electrocardiol.* 1984;17:209–218.

Albert DE. Chaos and the ECG: fact and fiction. *J Electrocardiol.* 1991;24(suppl):102–106.

Aoki M, Okamoto Y, Musha T, Harumi KI. Three-dimensional simulation of the ventricular depolarization and repolarization process and body surface potentials; normal heart and bundle branch block. *IEEE Trans Biomed Eng.* 1987;BME34(6):454–462.

Arnsdorf MF (Chairman, postgraduate seminar). *Is Cardiac Chaos Normal or Abnormal?* American Heart Association, 62nd Scientific Sessions, November, 1989.

Babloyant A, Destexhe A. Is the normal heart a periodic oscillator? *Biol Cybern.* 1988;58:203–211.

Bassingthwaighte JB, King RB, Roger SA. Fractal nature of regional myocardial blood flow heterogeneity. *Circ Res.* 1989;65:578–590.

Bassingthwaighte JB, van Beek JB. Lightning and the heart: fractal behavior in cardiac function. *Proc IEEE.* 1988;76:693–699.

Beamish RE. The new science of chaos—implications for cardiology [editorial]. *Can J Cardiol.* 1993;9:607–608.

Berenfeld O. *Simulation of the Ventricular Depolarization Thresses, Using a 3-Dimensional Heart Model with a Self-Similar Conduction System* [masters thesis]. Tel Aviv, Israel: Tel Aviv University; 1989.

Breborowicz G, Moczko J, Gadzinowski J. Quantification of the fetal heart rate variability by spectral analysis in growth-retarded fetuses. *Gynecol Obstet Invest.* 1988;25:186–191.

Burrows ME, Johnson PC. Diameter, wall tension, and flow in mesenteric arterioles during autoregulation. *Am J Physiol.* 1981;241:H829–H837.

Cargill EB, Donohoe K, Kolodny G, Parker JA, Zimmerman RE. Analysis of lung scans using fractals. Proc. SPIE. 1989;1092:2–9.

Chialvo DR, Jalife J. Nonlinear dynamics of cardiac excitation and impulse propagation. *Nature.* 1987;330:749–752.

Chialvo DR, Michaels D, Jalife J. Supernormal excitability as a mechanism of chaotic dynamics of activation in cardiac Purkinje fibres. *Circ Res.* 1990;66:525–545.

Coumel P, Maison-Blanche P. Complex dynamics of cardiac arrythmias. *Chaos.* 1991;1:335–342.

DeBoer RW, Karemaker JM, Strackee J. Comparing spectra of a series of point events particularly for heart rate variability data. *IEEE Trans Biomed Eng.* 1984;31:384–387.

Destexhe A, Babloyantz A. Is the normal heart a periodic ossilator? *J Biol Cybern.* 1988;58:203–211.

Diamond GA. Future imperfect: the limitations of clinical prediction models and the limits of clinical prediction. *J Am Coll Cardiol.* 1989;14:12A–22A.

Evans SJ, Khan SS, Garfinkle A, Kass RM, Albano A, Diamond GA. Is ventricular fibrillation random or chaotic? [abstract]. *Circulation.* 1989;80:II–134.

Frame LH, Rhee EK. Chaotic cycle length oscillation and bifurcation during rentry [abstract]. *Circulation.* 1989;80:II–96.

Garfinkel A, Karagueuzian H, Khan S, Diamond G. Is the proarrhythmic effect of quinidine a chaotic phenomenon? [abstract]. *J Am Coll Cardiol.* 1989;13:186A.

Garfinkel ML, Spano ML, Ditto WL, Weiss JN. Controlling cardiac chaos. *Science.* 1992;257:1230–1235.

Glass L. Complex cardiac rhythms. *Nature.* 1987;330:695–696.

Glass L. Mathematics and cardiac arrhythmias. *Rhythmology.* 1989;85–88.

Glass L. Is cardiac chaos normal or abnormal? *J Cardiovasc Electrophysiol.* 1990;F:481–482.

Glass L, Goldberger AL, Courtemanche M, Shrier A. Nonlinear dynamics, chaos and complex cardiac arryhthmias. *Proc R Soc Lond A,* 1987;413:9–26.

Glass L, Hunter P, McCulloch A. *Theory of Heart Biomechanics, Biophysics, and Nonlinear Dynamics of Cardiac Function.* New York, NY: Springer-Verlag; 1991.

Glass L, Guevara MR, Shrier A. Bifurcation and chaos in a periodically stimulated cardiac oscillator. *Physica D.* 1983;7:89–101.

Glass L, Guevara MR, Shrier A. Universal bifurcations and the classification of cardiac arrhythmias. *Ann NY Acad Sci.* 1987;504:168–178.

Glass L, Shrier A. Bélair J. Chaotic cardiac rhythms. In: Holden AV, ed. *Chaos.* Princeton, NJ: Princeton University Press; 1986:327–356.

Goldberger AL. Nonlinear dynamics, fractals, cardiac physiology and sudden death. In: Rensing L, an der Heiden U, Mackey MC, eds. *Temporal Disorders in Human Oscillatory Systems.* New York, NY: Springer-Verlag; 1987:118–125.

Goldberger AL. Is the normal heartbeat chaotic or homeostatic? *News Physiol Sci.* 1991;6:87–91.

Goldberger AL, Bhargava V, West BJ, Mandell AJ. On a mechanism of cardiac electrical stability. The fractal hypothesis. *Biophys J.* 1985;48:525–528.

Goldberger AL, Bhargava V, West BJ, Mandell AJ. Nonlinear dynamics of the heartbeat II. Subharmonic bifurcations of the cardiac interbeat interval in sinus node disease. *Physica D.* 1985;17:207–214.

Goldberger AL, Bhargava V, West BJ, Mandell AJ. Some observations on the question: Is ventricular fibrillation chaos? *Physica D.* 1986;19:282–289.

Goldberger AL, Findley LJ, Blackburn MR, Mandell AJ. Nonlinear dynamics in heart failure: implications of long-wavelength cardiopulmonary oscillations. *Am Heart J.* 1984;107:612–615.

Goldberger AL, Rigney DR. Sudden death is not chaos. In: Krasner S, ed. *The Ubiquity of Chaos.* Washington, DC: American Association for the Advancement of Science; 1990:23–34.

Goldberger AL, Rigney DR. Nonlinear dynamics at the bedside. In: Glass L, Hunter P, McCulloch A, eds. *Theory of Heart.* New York, NY: Springer-Verlag; 1990.

Goldberger AL, Rigney DR, Mietus J, Antman EM, Greenwald S. Nonlinear dynamics in sudden cardiac death syndrome: heart rate, oscillations and bifurcations. *Experientia.* 1988;44:983–987.

Goldberger AL, Shabetai R, Bhargava V, West BJ, Mandell AJ. Nonlinear dynamics electrical alternans and pericardial tamponade. *Am Heart J.* 1984;107:1297–1299.

Goldberger AL, West BJ. Applications of nonlinear dynamics to clinical cardiology. *Ann NY Acad Sci.* 1987;504:195–213.

Goldberger A, West BJ, Bhargava V. Nonlinear mechanisms in physiology and pathophysiology: towards a dynamic theory of health and disease. In: Eisenfeld J, Witten M, eds. *Modelling of Biomedical Systems.* The Hague, Holland: Elsevier Press; 1986:227–233.

Griffith TM, Edwards DH. EDRF suppresses chaotic pressure oscillations in an isolated resistance artery but does not influence their intrinsic complexity. *Am J Physiol.* 1994;266 (Heart Circ Physiol 35):H1786–H1800.

Griffith TM, Edwards DH. Fractal analysis of role of smooth muscle Ca^{2+} fluxes in genesis of chaotic arterial pressure oscillations. *Am J Physiol.* 1994;267:H1801–H1811.

Guevara MR, Jongsma HJ. Three ways of abolishing automaticity in sinoatrial node: ionic modeling and nonlinear dynamics. *Am J Physiol.* 1992;262:H1268–H1286.

Guevara MR, Glass L, Shrier A. Phase locking, period-doubling bifurcations, and irregular dynamics in periodically stimulated cardiac cells. *Science.* 1981;214:1350–1354.

Guevara MR, Shrier A, Glass L. Phase-locked rhythms in periodically stimulated heart cell aggregates. *Am J Physiol.* 1988;254:H1–H10.

Guevara MR, Shrier A, Glass L. *Chaotic and Complex Cardiac Rhythms in Cardiac Electrophysiology*, Zipes D. Jalife. Philadelphia, Pa: W.B. Saunders Co.; 1990:192–201.

Hudley WG, Renaldo GJ, Levasseur JE, Kontos HA. Vasomotion in cerebral microcirculation of awake rabbits. *Am J Physiol.* 1988;254:H67–H71.

Intaglietta M. Wave-like characteristics of vasomotion. *Prog Appl Microcirc.* 1983;3:83–94.

Jalife J. Chaos theory and the study of arrhythmogenesis: part 1. *Am Coll Cardiol Current Journal Review.* 1993;5.

Johansson B, Bohr DF. Rhythmic activity in smooth muscle from small subcutaneous arteries. *Am J Physiol.* 1966;210:801–806.

Johnson PC. The myogenic response. In: Bohr DF, Somlyo AP, Sparis HV, eds. *Handbook of Physiology: The Cardiovascular System II.* Bethesda, Md: American Physiological Society; 1980.

Kaplan DT. *The Dynamics of Cardiac Electrical Instability* [PhD thesis]. Cambridge, Mass: Harvard University; 1989.

Kaplan DT, Talajic M. Dynamics of heartrate. *Chaos.* 1991;1:251–256.

Kryger MH, Millar T. Cheyne-Stokes respiration: stability of interactive systems in heart failure. *Chaos.* 1991;1:265–269.

Lewis PJ, Guevara MR. A 1/T power law spectrum of the QRS complex does not imply fractal activation of ventricles (letter). *Biophys J.* 1991;60:1297–1300.

Lundahl T, Ohley WJ, Kuklinski WS, Williams DO, Gerwitz H, Most AS. Analysis and interpolation of angiographic images by use of fractals. *Comput Cardiol,* 1985;24:355–358.

Mayer-Cress G, Yates FE, Benton L, et al. Dimensional analysis of nonlinear ossications in brain, heart and muscle. *Math Biosci.* 1988;90:155–182.

Michaels D, Chialvo DR, Matyas EP, Jalife J. Chaotic activity in a mathematical model of the vagally driven sinoatrial node. *Circ Res.* 1989;65:1350–1360.

Myers GA, Martin GJ, Magid NM, Barnett PS, Schaad JW, Weiss JS, Lesch M, Singer DH. Power spectral analysis of heart rate variability in sudden cardiac death: comparison to other methods. *IEEE Trans Biomed Eng.* 1986;33:1149–1156.

Oude Vrielink HHE, Slaaf DW, Tangelder GJ, et al. Analysis of vasomotion waveform changes during pressure reduction and adenosine application. *Am J Physiol.* 1990; 258 (Heart Circ Physiol 27): H29–H37.

Pyeritz RE, Murphy EA. Genetics and congenital heart disease: perspectives and prospects. *J Am Coll Cardiol.* 1989;13:1458–1468.

Rambihar VS. *Chaos. From Cos to Cosmos.* Toronto, Canada: Vashna Publications; 1996.

Rambihar VS. *Chaos: A New Science for Heart Disease and its Prevention.* Toronto, Canada: Vashna Publications; 1996.

Ritzenberg AL, Adam DR, Cohen RJ. Period multiplyng—evidence for nonlinear behavior of the canine heart. *Nature.* 1984;307:159–161.

Sheldon R, Riff K. Changes in heart rate variability during fainting. *Chaos.* 1991;1:257–264.

Skinner JE, Carpeggiani C, Landisman CE, Fulton KW. The chaotic correlation dimension of the heartbeat is reduced in conscious pigs by myocardial ischemia. *Circ Res.* 1991;68:966–976.

Skinner JE, Goldberger AL, Mayer-Kress G, Ideker RE. Chaos in the heart: implications for clinical cardiology. *Biotechnology.* 1990;8:1018–1024.

Stein KM, Kligfield P. Fractal clustering of ventricular ectopy in dilated cardiomyopathy. *Am J Cardiol.* 1990;65:1512.

Vinet A, Chialvo DR, Jalife J. Irregular dynamics of excitation in biologic and mathematical models of cardiac cells. *Ann NY Acad Sci.* 1990;601:281–298.

Weinberg S. The prevention paradox. *J Am Coll Cardiol.* 1993;21(6).

Winfree AT. *When Time Breaks Down: The Three-Dimensional Dynamics of Electrochemical Waves and Cardiac Arrhythmias.* Princeton, NJ: Princeton University Press; 1987.

Yamashiro SM, Slaaf DW, Reneman RS, Tangelder GJ, Bassingthwaighte JB. Fractal analysis of vasomotion. *Ann NY Acad Sci.* 1990;591:410–416.

General

Abraham RH, *Chaos Gaia Eros.* New York, NY: Harper Collins Publishers; 1994.

Adler RJ. *The Geometry of Random Fields.* New York, NY: Wiley Press; 1981.

Albana AM, Mees AI, deGuzman GS, Rapp PE. Data requirements for reliable estimation of correlation dimensions. In: Holden AV, ed. *Chaotic Biological Systems.* New York, NY: Pergamon Press; 1987.

Albert DZ. Bohn's alternative to quantum mechanics. *Aci Am.* May, 1994;270(5):58–67.

Armbruster D, Heiland R, Kostelich EJ, Nicomlaenko B. Phase-space analysis of bursting behavior in Kolmogorov flow. *Physica.* 1992;58D:392–401.

Arneodo A, Coulleet P, Peyraud J, Tresser C. Strange attractors in Volterra equations for species in competition. *J Math Biol.* 1982;14:153–157.

Bak P, Chen K. Self-organized criticality. *Sci Am.* 1991;264(1):46–53.

Barcellos A. The fractal geometry of Mandelbrot. *Coll Math J.* 1984;15:98–114.

Barnsley MF. Fractal functions and interpolation. *Construct Approx.* 1986;2:303–329.

Barnsley MF. *Fractals Everywhere.* San Diego, CA: Academic Press; 1988.

Bassingthwaighte JB. Physiological heterogeneity: fractals link determinism and randomness in structures and functions. *News Physiol Sci.* 1988;3:5–10.

Behar T, McMorris FA, Novotny EA, Barker JL, Dubois-Dalcq M. Growth and differentiation properties of O-2A progenitors purified from rat cerebral hemispheres. *J Neurosci Res.* 1988;21:168–180.

Beloshapkin VV, Chernikov AA, Natenzon MY, Petrovichev BA, Sagdeev RZ, Zaslavsky GM. Chaotic streamlines in preturbulent states. *Nature.* 1989;337:133–137.

Berge P, Pomeau Y, Vidal C. *Order Within Chaos.* New York, NY: John Wiley & Sons; 1984.

Berry MV, Lewis ZV. On the Weierstress-Mandelbrot fractal function. *Proc R Soc Lond.* 1980;370:459–484.

Bevington PR. *Data Reduction and Error Analysis for the Physical Sciences.* New York, NY: McGraw-Hill; 1969.

Blaisdell BE. A measure of the similarity of sets of sequences not requiring sequence alignment. *Proc Natl Acad Sci U S A,* 1986;53:5155–5159.

Blaisdell BE. Effectiveness of measures requiring and not requiring prior sequence alignment for estimating the dissimilarity of natural sequences. *J Mol Evol.* 1989;29:526–537.

Boorstin DJ. *Cleopatra's Nose. Essays on the Unexpected.* New York, NY: Random House; 1994.

Breuer KS, Sirovich L. The use of the Karhunen-Loève procedure for calculation of linear eigenfunctions. *J Comput Phys.* 1991;96:277–296.

Briggs J. Fractals. *The Patterns of Chaos. Discovering a New Aesthetic of Art, Science and Nature.* New York, NY: Touchstone, Simon & Schuster; 1992.

Briggs J, Peat FD. *Turbulent Mirror. An Illustrated Guide to Chaos Theory and the Science of Wholeness.* New York, NY: Harper and Row; 1989.

Buzan T, Buzan B. *The Mind Map Book.* London, England: BBC Enterprise Ltd.; 1992.

Ceccatto HA, Huberman BA. The complexity of hierarchical systems. *Phys Scripta.* 1988;37:145–150.

Chan HP, Doi K, Vyborny CJ, Schmidt RA, Metz CE, Lam KL, Ogura T, Wu Y, MacMahon H. Improvements in radiologists' detection of clustered microcalcifications on mammograms. *Invest Radiol.* 1990;25:1102–1110.

Chen CC, Daponte JS, Fox MD. Fractal features analysis and classification in medical imaging. *IEEE Trans Med Imaging.* 1989;8:133–142.

Chesters S, Wen HY, Lundin M, Kasper G. Fractal-based characteristics of surface texture. *Appl Surf Sci.* 1989;40:185–192.

Claverie JM, Bougueleret L. Heuristic information analysis of sequences. *Nucl Acids Res.* 1986;14:179–196.

Cohen J, Stewart I. *The Collapse of Chaos. Discovering Simplicity in a Complex World.* New York, NY: Penguin Books, USA Inc.; 1994.

Cohen MA, Grossberg S. Absolute stability of global pattern formation and parallel memory storage by competitive neural networks. *IEEE Trans Syst Man Cybern.* 1983;13:815–825.

Conrad M. What is the use of chaos? In: Holden AV, ed. *Chaos.* Princeton, NJ: Princeton University Press; 1986:3–14.

Crutchfield JP, Farmer JD, Packard NJ, Shaw RS. Chaos. *Sci Am.* 1986;255:46–57.

Cutting JE, Garvin JJ. Fractal curves and complexity. *Percept Psychophys.* 1987;42:365–370.

Cvitanovic P, ed. *Universality in chaos.* New York, NY: Adam-Filger; 1989.

Damme HV, Obrecht F, Levitz P, Gatineau L, Laroche C. Fractal viscous fingering in clay slurries. *Nature (Lond),* 1986;320:731–733.

Dauskardt RH, Hanbensak F, Ritche RO. On the interpretation of the fractal character of fracture surfaces. *Acta Metall.* 1986;38:143–159.

Davies P, Gribbin J. *The Matter Myth. Dramatic Discoveries that Challenge Our Understanding of Physical Reality.* New York, NY: Touchstone Books, Simon & Schuster; 1992.

Davis P. *The Mind of God. The Scientific Basis for a Rational World.* New York, NY: Touchstone, Simon & Schuster; 1992.

Davis PJ, Park D. *No Way. The Nature of the Impossible.* New York, NY: Freeman and Company; 1987.

Decroly O, Goldbeter A. Birhythmicity, chaos and other patterns of temporal self-organization in a multiply regulated biochemical system. *Proc Natl Acad Sci.* 1982;79:6917–6921.

Destexhe A, Sepulchre JA, Babloyantz A. A comparative study of the experimental quantification of deterministic chaos. *Phys Lett.* 1988;132:101–106.

Devaney RL. Chaotic bursts in nonlinear dynamical systems. *Science.* 1987;235:342–344.

Ditto WL, Pecora LM. Mastering chaos. *Sci Am.* 1993;269(2):78–84.

Ditto WL, Rauseo SN, Spaino ML. Experimental control of chaos. *Phys Rev Lett.* 1990;65:3211–3214.

Dubuc B, Rogues-Carmes C, Tricot C, Zucker SW. The variation method: a technique to estimate the fractal dimension of surfaces. *Proc SPIE.* 1987;845:241–248.

Eckmann JP, Ruelle D. Ergodic theory of chaos and strange attactors. *Rev Mod Phys.* 1985;57:617–656.

Edgar GA. *Measure, Topology, and Fractal Geometry.* New York, NY: Springer-Verlag; 1990.

Englert BG, Scully MO, Walther H, et al. The duality in matter and light. *Sci Am.* 1994;271:86–92.

Epstein IR. Oscillations and chaos in chemical systems. *Physica D.* 1983;7:47–56.

Eubank S, Farmer D. An introduction to chaos and randomness. In: Jen E, ed. *1989 Lecture in Complex Systems (SFI studies in the sciences of complexity)* Vol 2. Reading, MA: Addison-Wesley; 1990:75.

Farmer D, Crutchfield J, Froehling H, Packard N, Shaw R. Power spectra and mixing properties of strange attractors. *Ann NY Acad Sci.* 1980;357:453–472.

Farmer D, Crutchfield J, Froehling H, Packard N, Shaw R. Power spectra and mixing properties of strange attractors. *Ann NY Acad Sci.* 1989;357:453–472.

Feder J. Fractals. New York, NY: Plenum; 1988.

Feigenbaum MJ. Quantitative universality for a class of nonlinear transformations. *J Stat Phys.* 1978;19:25–52.

Feigenbaum MJ. Universal behavior in nonlinear systems. *Science.* 1980;1:4–27.

Feigenbaum MJ. Universal behavior in nonlinear systems. *Physica D.* 1983;7:16–39.

Feinstein AR. Clinical judgement revisited: the distraction of quantitative models. *Ann Intern Med.* 1994;120(9):799–805.

Ferris T. *The Universe and Eye. Making Sense of the New Science.* San Francisco, CA: Chronicles Books; 1992.

Flook AG. The use of dilation logic on the quantimet to achieve fractal dimension characterization of textured and structured profiles. *Powder Technol.* 1978;21:295–298.

Flook AG. Fractal dimensions: their evaluation and significance in stereological measurements. *Acta Stereol.* 1982;1:79.

Fournier A, Fussel D, Carpenter L. Computer rendering of stochastic models. *Commun ACM.* 1982;25:371–84.

Fractals and Medicine [editorial]. *Lancet.* 1991;338:1425–1426.

Framer JD. Dimension, fractal measures, and chaotic dynamics. In: Haken H, ed. *Evolution of Order and Chaos.* New York, NY: Springer; 1982;228–46.

Freedman DH. Quantum consciousness. *Discover.* 1994;6:89–98.

Galloway MM. Texture analysis using gray level run lengths. *Comput Graphic Image Proc.* 1975;4:172–179.

Gårding J. Properties of fractal intensity surfaces. *Pattern Recognition Lett.* 1988;8:319–324.

Gardner M. White and brown music, fractal curves and one-over-f fluctuations. *Sci Am.* April, 1978;16–32.

Gell-Mann, M. *The Quark and the Jaguar. Adventures in the Simple and the Complex.* New York, NY: Freeman and Company; 1994.

Glass L, Mackey MC. *From Clocks to Chaos: The Rhythms of Life.* Princeton, NJ: Princeton University Press; 1988.

Gleick J. The man who reshaped geometry. *New York Times Magazine.* December 5, 1985;Sect 6:64.

Gleick J. *Chaos: Making a New Science.* New York, NY: Penguin Press; 1987.

Gollub JP, Brunner TO, Danly BG. Periodicity and chaos in coupled nonlinear oscillators. *Science.* 1978; 200:48–50.

Gomes MAF. Fractal geometry in crumpled paper balls. *Am J Phys.* 1989;55:649–690.

Grassberger P, Procaccia I. Characterization of strange attractors. *Phys Rev Lett.* 1983;50:346–349.

Grassberger P, Procaccia I. Estimation of the Kolmogorov entropy from a chaotic signal. *Phys Rev A.* 1983;28:2591–2593.

Grassberger P. Estimating the fractal dimensions and entropies of strange attractors. In: Holden AV, ed. *Chaos.* Princeton, NJ: Princeton University Press; 1986; 291–311.

Grassberger P, Procaccia I. Dimensions and entropies of strange attractors from a fluctuating dynamics approach. *Physica D,* 1984;13:34–54.

Grebogi C, Ott E, Pelikan S, Yorke JA. Strange attractors that are not chaotic. *Physica D.* 1984;13:261–268.

Grebogi C, Ott E, Yorke JA. Chaos, strange attractors, and fractal basin boundaries in nonlinear dynamics. *Science.* 1987;238;632–638.

Gutzwiller MC. Quantum chaos. *Sci Am.* 1992;266(1):79–84.

Haken H: *Advanced Synergetics.* New York, NY: Springer-Verlag; 1983.

Haralick RM, Shanmugan K, Dinstein I. Textural features for image classification. *IEEE Trans Syst Man Cybern.* 1973;SMC—3:610–621.

Harris SL. *Agents of Chaos. Earthquakes, Volcanoes and Other Natural Disasters.* Missoula, MT: Mountain Press Publishing Co.; 1990.

Havstad JW, Ehlers CL. Attractor dimension of nonstationary dynamical systems from small data sets. *Phys Rev A.* 1989;39:845–853.

Hawking S. *A Brief History of Time. From the Big Bang to Black Holes.* New York, NY: Bantam Books; 1988.

Hawking S. *Black Holes and Baby Universes and Other Essays.* New York, NY: Bantam Books; 1993.

Hazlett RD. Fractal application: wettability and contact angle. *J Colloid Interface Sci.* 1990;137:527–533.

Heppenheimer TA. Routes to chaos. *Mosaic.* 1986;17:3–13.

Herzel H, Plath P, Svensson P. Experimental Evidence of Homoclinic Chaos and Type-II Intermittency during the Oxidation of Methanol. *Physica.* 1991;48D:340–352.

Holden AV. Chaos in complicated systems. *Nature.* 1983;305:183.

Holden AV, ed. *Chaos.* Princeton, NJ: Princeton University Press; 1986.

Hollander M, Wolfe DA. *Nonparametric statistical methods.* New York, NY: John Wiley & Sons; 1973;67–70.

Hopfield JJ. Neural networks and physical systems with emergent collective computational abilities. *Proc Natl Acad Sci USA.* 1982;79:2554–2558.

Horgan J. Quantum philosophy. *Sci Am.* 1992;266(1):94–104.

Horgan J. Can science explain consciousness? *Sci Am.* 1994;271(1):88–94.

Hornbogen E. Fractal analysis of grain boundaries in hot-worked poly-crystals. *Zeit Matllk.* 1987;78:622–625.

Hornbogen E. Fractals in microstructure of metals. *Int Mater Rev.* 1989;34:277–296.

Hunt GA. Random Fourier transforms. *Trans Am Math Soc.* 1951;71:38–69.

Jeffrey HJ. Chaos game representation of gene structure. *Nucl Acids Res.* 1990;18:2163–2170.

Jensen RV. Classical chaos. *Am Sci.* 1987;75:168–181.

Jurgens H, Peitgen HO, Saupe D. The language of fractals. *Sci Am.* 1990;263(2):60–67.

Kaplan JL, Yorke JA. The onset of chaos in a fluid flow model of Lorenz. *Ann NY Acad Sci.* 1979;316:400–407.

Katz AJ, Thompson AH. Fractal sandstone pores: implications for conductivity and pore formation. *Phys Rev Lett.* 1985;54:1325–1328.

Kauffman SA. Antichaos and Adaptation. *Sci Am.* 1991;265(2):78–84.

Kauffman SA. *At Home in the Universe.* New York, NY: Oxford University Press; 1995.

Kaye BH. Fractal geometry and the characterization of rock fragments. *Isr Phys Soc.* 1978;21:1.

Kaye BH. Specification of the ruggedness and/or texture of a fine-particle profile by its fractal dimension. *Powder Technol.* 1978;21:1–16.

Kaye BH. Multifractal description of a rugged fine-particle profile. *Part Charact.* 1984;1:14–21.

Kaye BH. Fractal dimension and signature waveform characterization of fine-particle shape. *Am Lab.* 1987;19:55–63.

Kearney RE, Hunter IW. Nonlinear identification of stretch reflex dynamics. *Ann Biomed Eng.* 1988;16:79–94.

Keller JM, Chen S. Crownower: texture description and segmentation through fractal geometry. *Comput Vis Graph Image Proc.* 1989;45:150–166.

Kellert SH. *In the Wake of Chaos.* Chicago: Unviersity of Chicago Press; 1993.

Kloeden PE, Mees AI. Chaotic phenomena. *Bull Math Biol.* 1985;47:697–738.

Kronenberg F. Menopausal hot flashes: randomness or rhythmicity. *Chaos.* 1991;1:271–278.

Kube P, Pentland A. On the imaging of fractal surfaces. *IEEE Trans Pattern Anal Mach Intell.* 1988;10:704–707.

Kubicek M, Marek M. *Computational Methods in Bifurcation Theory and Dissipative Structures.* New York, NY: Springer-Verlag; 1983.

Lafaille R, Fulder S, eds. *Towards a New Science of Health.* London, England: Routledge; 1993.

Lauwerier H. *Fractals: Images of Chaos.* New York, NY: Penguin Books; 1991.

Laws KI. Rapid texture identification: image processing for missle guidance. *Proc SPIE.* 1980;238:376–380.

Lederman L, Teresi D. *The God Particle. If the Universe is the Answer, What is the Question?* New York, NY: Dell Publishing; 1993.

Lewin R. *Complexity: Life at the Edge of Chaos.* New York, NY: Macmillan Publishing Company; 1992.

Lewis PJ, Guevara MR. A $1/f^d$ power law spectrum of the QRS complex does not imply fractal activation of the ventricles (letter). *Biophys J.* 1991;60:1297–1300.

Liauw MA, Koblitz K, Jaeger NI, Plath P. Periodic perturbation of a drifting heterogeneous catalytic system. *J Phys Chem.* 1993;97:11724–11730.

Liebovitch LS, Fischbarg J, Koniarek JP. Ion channel kinetics: a model based on fractal scaling rather than multistate Markov processes. *Math Biosci.* 1987;84:37–68.

Ling, FF. The possible role of fractal geometry in tribology. *Tribology Trans.* 1989;32:497–505.

Lorenz EN. Deterministic nonperiodic flow. *J Atmospheric Sci.* 1963;20:130–141.

Lovejoy S, Mandelbrot BB. Fractal properties of rain, and a fractal model. *Tellus.* 1985;37a:209–232.

Lundahl T, Ohley WJ, Kay SM, Siffert R. Fractional Brownian motion: a maximum likelihood estimator and its application to image texture. *IEEE Trans Med Imaging.* 1986;MI-5:152–161.

Magnin IE, Cluzeau F, Odet CL, Bremond A. Mammographic texture analysis: an evaluation of risk for developing breast cancer. *Opt Eng.* 1986;25:780–784.

Majumdar A, Bhushan B. Role of fractal geometry in roughness characteristics and contact mechanics of surfaces. *J Tribology.* 1990;112:205–216.

Majumdar A, Tien CL. Fractal characterization and simulation of rough surfaces. *Wear.* 1990;136:313–327.

Mandelbrot BB. How long is the coast of Britain? Statistical self-similarity and fractal dimension. *Science.* 1967;156:636–638.

Mandelbrot BB, Passoja DE, Paullay AJ. Fractal character of fracture surfaces of metals. *Nature.* 1987;308:721–722.

Mandelbrot BB, Van Ness JW. Fractional Brownian motions: fractional noises and applications. *SIAM Rev.* 1968;10:422–437.

Marr D, Hildreth E. Theory of edge detection. *Proc R Soc Lond B.* 1980;207:187–217.

Matsushita M. Experimental Observations of Aggregates. In: Avnir D, ed. *The Fractal Approach to Heterogeneous Chemistry. Surfaces, Colloids, Polymers.* New York, NY: J. Wiley Press; 1989;161–179.

Mayer-Kress G. Introductory remarks. In: Mayer-Kress G, ed. *Dimension and Entropies in Chaotic Systems.* New York, NY: Springer-Verlag; 1985.

Mayer-Kress G, Yates FE, Benton L, et al. Dimensional analysis of nonlinear oscillations in brain, heart and muscle. *Math Biosci.* 1988;90:155–182.

Mecholsky JJ, Passoja DE, Fenberg-Ringel KS. Quantitative analysis of brittle fracture surfaces using fractal geometry. *J Am Ceram Soc.* 1989;72:60–65.

Miller A, Knoll W, Möhwald H. Fractal and non-fractal crystalline phospholipid domains in monomolecular layers [abstract]. *Biophys J.* 1986;49:317a.

Miller P, Astley S. Classification of breast tissue by texture analysis. *Image Vision Comput.* 1992;10:277–282.

Moon FC. *Chaotic Vibrations: An Introduction for Applied Scientists and Engineers.* New York, NY: Wiley Press; 1987.

Mussigman U. Texture analysis, fractals and scale space filtering. In: *Proceedings of the 6th Scandinavian Conference on Image Analysis;* 1989; Oula, Finland: 987–994.

Mussigman U. Homogeneous fractals and their application in texture analysis. In: Peitgen HO, Henriques JM, Penedo LF, eds. *Proceedings of the 1st IFIP Conference on Fractals.* Amsterdam, Netherlands: Elsevier Publishing; 1990.

Nayak PR. Random process model of rough surfaces. *J Lubr Tech.* 1971;93:398–407.

Nishihara T. Characterization of metals using fractal theory. *Heat Treat.* 1989;29:99–102.

Orbach R. Dynamics of fractal networks. *Science.* 1986;231:814–819.

Pande CS, Richards LE, Louat N, Dempsey BD, Schwoeble AJ. Fractal characterization of fracture surfaces. *Acta Metall.* 1987;35:1633–1637.

Pappas T. *Fractals, Googols and other Mathematical Tales.* San Carlos, Calif: Wide World Publishing/Tetra; 1993.

Paulus MP, Geyer MA, Gold HL, Mandell AJ. Application of entropy measures derived from the ergodic theory of dynamic systems to rat locomotor behavior. *Proc Natl Acad Sci U S A.* 1990;87:723–727.

Paumgartner D, Losa G, Weibel ER. Resolution effect on the sterological estimation of surface and volume and its interpretation in terms of fractal dimensions. *J Microsc.* 1981;121:51–63.

Peak D, Frame M. *Chaos Under Control. The Art and Science of Complexity.* New York, NY: WH Freeman and Company; 1994.

Pecora LM, Carroll TL. Synchronization in chaotic systems. *Phys Lett.* 1990;64:821–824.

Peitgen HO, Richter PH. *The Beauty of Fractals.* New York, NY: Springer-Verlag; 1986.

Penrose R. *Shadows of the Mind. A Search for the Missing Science of Consciousness.* New York, NY: Oxford University Press; 1994.

Pentland AP. Fractal-based descriptions of natural scenes. *IEEE Trans Pattern Anal Mach Intell.* 1984;PAMI-6:661–674.

Pentland AP. Fractal surface models for communication about terrain. *Proc SPIE.* 1987;845:301–306.

Peters T. *The Pursuit of WOW! Every Person's Guide to Topsy-Turvy Times.* New York, NY: Vintage Books; 1994.

Peters T. *The Tom Peters Seminar. Crazy Times Call for Crazy Organizations.* New York, NY: Vintage Books; 1994.

Pfeifer P, Anvir D. Chemistry in noninteger dimensions between two and three. I. Fractal theory of heterogeneous surfaces. *Surf Sci.* 1983;79:3558–3565.

Pfeifer P, Obert M. Fractals: basic concepts and terminology. In: Avnir D, ed. *The Fractal Approach to Heterogeneous Chemistry. Surfaces, Colloids, Polymers.* New York, NY: J. Wiley Press; 1989;11–14.

Pickover CA. *Computers, Pattern, Chaos and Beauty.* Straub, United Kingdom: Allan Sutton; 1990.

Pincus SM. Approximate entropy as a measure of system complexity. *Proc Natl Acad Sci U S A.* 1991;88:2297–2301.

Pinsker HM, Bell J. Phase plane description of endogenous neuronal oscillators in aplysia. *Biol Cybern.* 1981;39:211–221.

Pool R. Seeing chaos in a simple system. *Science.* 1988; 241:787–788.

Pool R. Is it chaos, or is it just noise? *Science.* 1989; 243:25–28.

Pool R. Ecologists flirt with chaos. *Science.* 1989; 243:310–313.

Pool R. Is it healthy to be chaotic? *Science.* 1989; 243:604–607.

Pressman NJ. Markovian analysis of cervical cell images. *J Histochem Cytochem.* 1976;24:138–144.

Procaccia I. Universal properties of dynamically complex systems: the organization of chaos. *Nature.* 1988;333:618–623.

Rambihar VS. *Chaos. A New Science of Health.* Toronto, Canada: Vashna Publications; 1996.

Rambihar VS. *Chaos: A New Organizating and Management Science.* Toronto, Canada: Vashna Publications; 1996.

Ramon ME. An attempt at classifying nerve cells on the basis of their dendritic patterns. *J Comput Neurol.* 1962; 119:211–227.

Reichenbach A, Siegel A, Senitz D, Smith TG. A comparative fractal analysis of various mammalian astroglial cell types. *Neuroimage.* 1992;1:66–77.

Rigaut JP. An empirical formulation relating boundary lengths to resolution in specimens showing non-ideally fractal dimensions. *J Microsc.* 1984;133:41–54.

Rogers TD, Yang XC, Yip LW. Complete chaos in a simple epidemiological model. *J Math Biol.* 1986;23:263–268.

Roux JC. Experimental studies of bifucations leading to chaos in the Belousof-Zhabotinsky reaction. *Physica D.* 1983;7:57–68.

Rueff M. Scale space filtering and the scaling regions of fractals. In: Simon JC, ed. *From Pixels to Features.* Amsterdam, Netherlands: Elsevier Publishing; 1989:49–60.

Ruelle D. Strange attractors. *Math Intelligence.* 1980;2: 126–137.

Russ JC. *Practical Stereology.* New York, NY: Plenum Press; 1986.

Ruthen R. Adapting to complexity. *Sci. Am.* 1993;268(1): 130–140.

Saaty TL, Bram J. *Nonlinear Mathematics.* New York, NY: Dover Publications; 1964.

Saftlas AF, Szklo M. Mammographic parenchymal patterns and breast cancer risk. *Epidemiol Rev.* 1987;9: 146–174.

Sander LM. Fractal growth. *Sci Am.* 1987;256:94–100.

Saperstein AM. Chaos—a model for the outbreak of war. *Nature.* 1984;309:303–305.

Saupe D. Algorithms for random fractals. In: Peitgen HO, Saupe D, eds. *The Science of Fractal Images.* New York, NY: Springer-Verlag Press; 1988.

Saupe D, ed. *The science of fractal images.* New York, NY: Springer; 1988.

Sayles RS, Thomas TR. Surface topography as a nonstationary random process. *Nature.* 1978;271:431–434.

Schroeder M. Fractals, chaos, power laws: minutes from an incident paradise. New York, NY: WH Freeman; 1991.

Stanley HE, Ostrowksy N, eds. *On Growth and Form, Fractal and Non-Fractal Patterns in Physics.* Boston, Mass: Martinus Nihoff Publishers; 1986.

Stauffer D, Stanley HE. *From Newton to Mandelbrot. The primer in theoretic physics.* New York, NY: Springer-Verlag; 1990.

Stewart I. *Does God Play Dice? The Nathematics of Chaos.* New York, NY: Basil Blackwell, Ltd.; 1989.

Stupak PR, Donovan JA. Fractal analysis of rubber wear surfaces and debris. *J Mater Sci.* 1988;23:2230–2242.

Swinney HL. Observations of order and chaos in nonlinear systems. *Physica D.* 1983;7:3–15.

Takens F. Detecting strange attractors in turbulence. In: Rand DA, Yound LS, eds. *Dynamical Systems and Turbulence,* New York, NY: Springer-Verlag; 1980.

Thibault GE. Appropriate degree of diagnostic certainty. *Engl J Med.* 1994;331(18):1216–1220.

Thompson JMT, Steward HB. *Nonlinear Dynamics and Chaos.* New York, NY: John Wiley & Sons; 1986.

Underwood EE, Banerji K. Fractal analysis of fracture surfaces. *Fractography.* 1987;12:193–198.

Vicenzi AE. Chaos theory and some nursing considerations. *Nurs Sci Q.* 1992;7(1):36–42.

Voss RF. Random fractal forgeries. In: Earnshaw RA, ed. *Fundamental Algorithms for Computer Graphics.* New York, NY: Springer Press; 1985:805–835.

Voss RF. Characterization and measurement of random fractals. *Phys Scripta,* 1986;T13:27–32.

Voss RF. Fractals in nature: from characterization to simulation. In: Peitgen H, Saupe D, eds. *The Science of Fractal Images.* New York, NY, Springer; 1988:21–70.

Waldrop MM. *Complexity: The Emerging Science at the Edge of Order and Chaos.* New York, NY: Simon and Schuster; 1992.

Weinberg S. Life in the universe. *Sci. Am.* 1994;271(4): 44–49.

West BJ, Goldberger AL. Physiology in fractal dimensions. *Am Sci.* 1987;75:354–365.

West BJ. *Fractal Physiology and Chaos in Medicine.* Teaneck, NJ: World Scientific; 1990.

Wolf A. Simplicity and universality in the transition to chaos. *Nature.* 1983;305:182–183.

Wujec T. Pumping Ions. *Games and Exercises to Flex your Mind.* Toronto, Canada: Doubleday Canada Ltd.; 1988.

Zähle U. Sets and measures of fractional dimension. *Inform Process Cybern.* 1984;20:261–269.

Imaging and Radiology

Caldwell CB, Stapleton SJ, Holdsworth DW, Jong RA, Weiser WJ, Cooke G, Yaffe MJ. Characterization of mammographic parenchymal pattern by fractal dimension. *Phys Med Biol.* 1990;35:235–247.

Cargill EB, Barrett HH, Fiete RD, Ker M, Patton DD. Fractal physiology and nuclear medicine scans. *Med Imaging II.* 1988;914:355–361.

Cargill EB, Donohoe KJ, Kolodny G, Parker AJ. Estimation of fractal dimension of parenchymal organs based on power spectrum analysis of nuclear medicine scans. *Information Processing Med Imaging.* 1991;363: 557–570.

Chan HP, Doi K, Vyborny CJ, Schmidt FA, Metz CE, Lam KL, Ogura T, Wu Y, MacMahon H. Improvements in radiologists' detection of clustered microcalcifications on mammograms. *Invest Radiol.* 1990;25:1102–1110.

Chen CC, Daponte JS, Fox MD. Fractal feature analysis and classification in medical imaging. *IEEE Trans Med Imaging.* 1989;MI-8:133–142.

Coggins JM, Jain AK. A spatial filtering approach to texture analysis. *Pattern Recognition Lett.* 1985;3:195–203.

Delleplane S, Serpico SB, Vernazza G, Viviani R. Fractal-based image analysis in radiological applications. *Proc SPIE.* 1987;845:396–403.

Dubuc B, Roques-Carmes C, Tricot C, Zucker SW. The variation method: a technique to estimate the fractal dimension of surfaces. *Proc SPIE.* 1987;845:241–248.

Javanaud C. The application of a fractal model to the scattering of ultrasound in biological media. *J Acoust Soc Am.* 1989;86:493–496.

Katsuragawa S, Doi K, MacMahon H. Image feature analysis and computer-aided diagnosis in digital radiography: classification of normal and abnormal lungs with interstitial disease in chest images. *Med Phys.* 1989;16:38–34.

Kuklinski WS, Chandra K, Ruttimann UE, Webber RL. Application of fractal texture analysis to segmentation of dental radiographs. *Proc SPIE.* 1989;1092: 111–117.

Lee JKT, Sagel SS, Stanle RJ. *Computed body tomography with MRI correlation.* New York, NY: Raven Press; 1989.

Lundahl T, Ohley WJ, Kay SM, Siffert R. Fractional Brownian motion: a maximum likelihood estimator and its application to image texture. *IEEE Trans Med Imaging.* 1986:MI-5;152–161.

Lundahl T, Ohley WJ, Kuklinski WS, Williams DO, Gerwitz H, Most AS. Analysis and interpolation of angiographic images by use of fractals. *Comput Cardiol.* 1985;24:355–8.

Nelson TR. Morphological modeling using fractal geometries. In: *Medical Imaging II: Image Formation Detection, Processing, and Interpretation/Image Data Management and Display.* Bellingham, WA: SPIE–Int Soc Opt. Eng.; 1988;326–333.

Nelson TR. Fractals. Physiologic complexity, scaling, and opporunities for imaging. *Invest Radiol.* 1990;25: 1140–1148.

Neurology/Psychology

Arle JE, Simon RH. An application of fractal dimension to the detection of transients in the electroencephalogram. Electroencephalography, *Clin Neurophysiol.* 1990;75:296–305.

Babloyantz A. Strange attractors in the dynamics of brain activity. In: Haken H, ed. *Complex systems—Operational approaches in neurobiology, physics, and computers.* Berlin, Germany: Springer-Verlag; 1985:116–122.

Babloyantz A. Chaotic dynamics in brain activity. In: Basar E, ed. *Chaos in Brain Function.* Berlin, Germany: Springer-Verlag; 1990:42–48.

Babloyantz A, Destexhe A. Low dimensional chaos in an instance of epilepsy. *Proc Natl Acad Sci U S A.* 1986;83:3513–3517.

Babloyantz A, Nicholis C, Salazar JM. Evidence for chaotic dynamics of brain activity during the sleep cycle. *Phys Lett.* 1985;111:152–156.

Basar E. *Chaos in Brain Function.* New York, NY: Springer-Verlag; 1990.

Behar T, McMorris FA, Novotny EA, Barker JL, Dubois-Dalcq M. Growth and differentiation properties of O-2A progenitors purified from rat cerebral hemispheres. *J Neurosci Res.* 1988;21:168–180.

Beuter A, Labrie C, Vasilakos K. Transient dynamics in motor control of patients with Parkinson's disease. *Chaos.* 1991;1:279–286.

Bullmore ET, Brammer NJ, Alarcon G, Binnie CD. A new technique for fractal analysis applied to human, intracerebrally recorded, ictal and electroencephalographic signals. *Neurosci Lett.* 1992;146:227–230.

Bullmore ET, Brammer NJ, Binnie CD, Alarcon G. Fractal electroencephalography. *Lancet.* 1992;339:618–619.

Bullmore ET, Brammer NJ, Alarcon G, Binnie CD. Synaptic visualization of brain electrical activity during a cluster of eleven epileptic seizures. In: Novak M, ed. *Fractals in the Natural Unapplied Sciences.* Amsterdam, Netherlands: Elsevier Science; 1994:69–80.

Bullmore ET, Brammer NJ, Bourlon P, Alarcon G, Polkey CE, Elwes R, Binnie CD. Fractal analysis of electroencephalographic signals intracerebrally recorded during 35 epileptic seizures: evaluation of a new method for synaptic visualization of ictal events. *Electroencephalogr Clin Neurophysiol.* 1994;91:337–345

Cutting JE, Garvin JJ. Fractal curves and complexity. *Percep Psychophys.* 1987;42:365–370.

Freeman W, Skarda CA. Spatial EEG-patterns, non-linear dynamics and perception: the neo-Sherringtonian view. *Brain Res Rev.* 1985;10:147–175.

Freeman WJ. Searching for signal and noise in the chaos of brain waves. In: Krasner S ed. *The Ubiquity of Chaos.* Washington, DC: American Association for the Advancement of Science; 1990:47–55.

Freeman WJ. Nonlinear neural dynamics in olfaction as a model for cognition. In: Basar E, ed. *Dynamics of Sensory and Cognitive Processing by the Brain.* New York, NY: Springer; 1991:19–29.

Gallez D, Babloyantz A. Predictability of human EGG: a dynamic approach. *Biol Cybern.* 1991;64:381–391.

Graf KE, Elbert T. Dimensional analysis of the waking EEG. In: Basar E, ed. *Chaos in Brain Function.* Berlin, Germany: Springer-Verlag; 1990:135–152.

Gray CN, Freeman WJ, Skinner JE. Changes in the spacial amplitude patterns of rabbits of olfactory EEGR neurepinephrined dependent. *Neurosci Abstracts.* 1984;10:121.

Iasmedis LD, Sackellares JC, Zaveri HP, Williams WJ. Phase space topography and the Lyapunov exponent of electrocorticograms in partial seizures. *Brain Topogr.* 1990;2:187–201.

Janssen BH. Quantitative analysis of electroencephalograms: is there chaos in the future? *Intern J Biomed Comp.* 1991;27:95–123.

King CC. Fractal and chaotic dynamics in nervous systems. *Prog Neurobiol.* 1991;36:279–308.

Lancet D, Greer CA, Kauer JS, Sheppard GM. Mapping of oto-related neuronal activity in the olfactory bulb by high resolution 2-deoxyglucose autoradiography. *Proc Natl Acad Sci U S A.* 1982;79:670–674.

Lashley KS. In search of the engram. *Symp Soc Exp Biol.* 1950;4:454–482.

Mayer-Cress G, Layne SP. Dimensionality of the human electroencephalogram. *Ann NY Acad Sci.* 1986; 504:3513–3517.

Mayer-Cress G, Layne SP. Dimensionality of the human electroencephalogram. *Ann NY Acad Sci.* 1987; 504:62–87.

Moulton DG. Spacial patterning of response to odors in the peripheral olfactory system. *Physiol Rev.* 1976;56:578–593.

Mpitsos GJ, Burton MR, Creech HC, Soinila SO. Evidence for chaos in spike trains of neurons that generate rhythmic motor patterns. *Brain Res Bull.* 1988;21:529–538.

Neale EA, Bowers LM, Smith TG. Early dendrite development described by fractal dimension [abstract]. *Soc Neurosci.* 1991;17:36.

Nicoll RA. Recurrent excitation of secondary olfactory neurons: a possible mechanism for signal amplification. *Science.* 1971;171:824–825.

Pellionisz AJ. Neural geometry: towards a fractal model of neurons. In Cotterill RMJ, ed. *Models of Brain Function.* Cambridge, MA: Cambridge University Press; 1991;453–464.

Pinsker HM, Bell J. Phase plane description of endogenous neuronal oscillators in aplysia. *Biol Cybern.* 1981;39:211–221.

Pradhan N, Narayana Dutt D. *Use of Running Fractal Dimension for the Analysis of Changing Patterns in Electroencephalograms.* 1993.

Rall W, Sheppard GM. Theoretical reconstruction of field potentials and dendrodentritic synaptic interactions in olfactory bulb. *J Neurophys.* 1968;31:884–915.

Rapp PE, Bashore TR, Zimmerman ID, Marinerie JM, Albano AM, Mees AI. Dynamical characterization of brain electrical activity. *Brain Topogr.* 1989;2:99–118.

Rapp PE, Bashore TR, Zimmerman ID, Marinerie JM, Albano AM, Mees AI. Dynamical characterization of brain electrical activity. In: Krasner S, ed. *The Ubiquity of Chaos.* Washington, DC: American Association for the Advancement of Science; 1990:10–22.

Smith TG, Brauer K, Reichenbach A. Quantitative phylogenetic constancy of cerebellar Purkinje morphological complexity. *J Comput Neurol.* 1993;331:402–406.

Smith, TG Jr, Marks WB, Lange GD, Sheriff, WH Jr, Neale EA. Edge detection in images using Marr-Hildreth filtering techniques. *J Neurosci Methods.* 1988;26:75–82.

Soong ACK, Stewart CIJM. Evidence of chaotic dynamics underline the human alpha-rhythm electroencephalogram. *Biol Cybern.* 1989;62:55–62.

Teich MC, Keilson SE, Khanna SM, Brundin L, Ulfendahl M, Flock A. Chaos in the cochlea. In: Lim DJ, ed. *Abstracts of the Fourteenth Midwinter Meeting of the Association for Research in Otolaryngology;* 1991; Des Moine, Iowa. 50.

Viana di Prisco G, Freeman WJ. Otorelated bulbar EEG spacial pattern analysis during appetitive conditioning in rabbits. *Behav Neurosci.* 1985;99:964–978.

Watt RC, Hameroff SR. Phase space analysis of human EEG during general anesthesia. *Ann NY Acad Sci.* 1987;504:286–288.

Watt RC, Hameroff SR. Phase space electroencephalography (EEG): a new mode of intraoperative EEG analysis. *Int J Clin Monit Comput.* 1988;5:3–13.

Xu N, Xu J. The fractal dimension of EEG as a physical measure of conscious human brain activities. *Bull Math Biol.* 1988;50:559–565.

Ophthalmology

Amthor FR. Quantitative fractal analysis of dendritic trees of identified rabbit retinal ganglion cells. *Soc Neurosci Abstr.* 1988;14:603.

Daxer A. Fractals and retinal vessels. *Lancet.* 1992;339:618.

Family F, Masters BR, Platt DE. Fractal pattern formation in human retinal vessels. *Physica D.* 1989;38:98–103.

Kinoshita M, Honda Y. The fractal property of retinal vascular pattern. *Invest Ophthalmol Vis Sci.* 1991;32(suppl):1082.

Mainster MA. The fractal properties of retinal vessels: embryological and clinical applications. *Eye.* 1990;4:235–241.

Masters BR. Fractal analysis of human retinal blood vessel patterns: developmental and diagnostic aspects. In: Master BR, ed. *Noninvasive Diagnostic Techniques in Ophthalmology.* New York, NY: Springer-Verlag; 1990.

Masters BR, Family F, Platt DE. Fractal analysis of human retinal vessels. *Biophys J.* 1989;55(suppl):575a.

Schmeisser ET. Fractal analysis of steady-state-flicker visual evoked potentials: feasibility. *J Opt Soc Am A.* July, 1993;10(7):1637–1640.

Smith, TG Jr, Behar TN. Comparative fractal analysis of cultured glia derived from optic nerve and brain demonstrate different rate of morphological differentiation. *Brain Res.* 1994;634:181–190.

Otology

Goldstein MH. Auditory periphery as speech signal processor. *IEEE Eng Med Biol.* 1994;186–196.

Kelly OE, Johnson DH, Delgutte B, Cariani P. Factors affecting the fractal character of auditory nerve activity. In: Lin DJ, ed. *Abstracts of the Sixteenth Midwinter Research Meeting of the Association for Research in Otolaryngology;* 1993; Des Moine, Iowa. Abstract 369;93.

Koumar AH, Johnson DH. Analyzing and modeling fractal intensity point processes. *J Acoust Soc Am.* 1993:3365–3373.

Lowen SB, Teich MC. Doubly stochastic plauson point process driven by fractal shot noise. *Phy Rev.* 1991;A43:4192–4215.

Lowen SB, Teich MC. Fractal renewal processes generate I/F noise. *Phys Rev.* 1993;E4:992–1001.

Lowen SB, Teich MC. Fractal renewal processes. *IEEE Transinformed Theory.* 1993;39:1669–1671.

Lowen SB, Teich MC. Fractal auditory nerve firing patterns may derive from fractal switching in sensory hair cell ion channels. In: Handel PH, Chung AL, eds. *Noise in Physical Systems and I/F Fluctuations. AIP Conference Proceedings.* New York, NY: American Institute of Physics; 1993;745–748.

Lowen SB, Teich MC. Estimating the dimension of fractal point processes. *Proc SPIE.* 1993;2036:64–76.

Teich MC. Fractal character of the auditory neural spike train. *IEEE Transbiomed Inc.* 1989;36:150–160.

Teich MC. Fractal neuronal firing patterns. In: McKenna, Davis, Zornetzer, eds. *Single Neuron Computation.* Boston, Mass: Academic; 1992:589–625.

Teich MC, Johnson DH, Koumar AH, Tergot RT. Rate fluctuations and fractional power law noise recorded from cells in the lower auditory pathway of the cat. *Hear Res.* 1990;46:41–52.

Teich MC, Keilson SE, Khanna FN, Brundin L, Ulfendahl M, Flach A. Chaos in the cochlea. In: Lin DJ, ed. *Abstracts of Fourteenth Midwinter Meeting of the Association for Research in Otolaryngology.* Des Moine, Iowa 1991;50.

Teich MC, Lowen SB. Fractal patterns in auditory nerve spike trains. *IEEE Eng Med Biol.* 1994;197–202.

Teich MC, Lowen SB, Tergot RT. On possible peripheral origins of the fractal auditory neural spike train. In: Lin DJ, ed. *Abstracts of the Fourteenth Midwinter Research Meeting of the Association for Research in Otolaryngology;* 1991; Des Moine, Iowa. Abstract 154; 50.

Teich MC, Turcott JG, Lowen SB. The fractal doubly stochastic poisson point process as a model for the cochlear neural spike train. In: Dallos P, M Geisler, S Ruggero, eds. *The Mechanics and Biophysics of Hearing.* Springer-Verlag; 1990:387–394.

Physiology

Bassingthwaighte JB. Physiological heterogeneity: fractals link determinism and randomness in structures and functions. *News Physiol Sci.* 1988;3:5–10.

Cederbaum LS, Haller E, Pfeifer P. Fractal dimension function for energy levels. *Phys Rev.* 1985;A31:1869–1871.

Elber R, Karplus M. Low-frequency modes in proteins: use of the effective-medium approximation to interpret the fractal dimension observed in electron-spin relaxation measurements. *Phys Rev Lett.* 1986;56:394–397.

Farmer JD, Ott E, Yorke JA. The dimension of chaotic attractors. *Physica.* 1983;7D:153–180.

Freeman WJ. The physiology of perception. *Sci. Am.* 1991;264(2):78–85.

Froehling H, Crutchfield JP, Framer D, Packard NH, Shaw R. On determining the dimension of chaotic flows. *Physica.* 1981;3:605–617.

Gerstein GL, Mandelbrot BB. Random walk models for the spike activity of a single neuron. *Biophys.* 1964; J4:41–68.

Glass L. Nonlinear dynamics of physiological function and control. *Chaos.* 1991;1:247–250.

Glass L, Mackey MC. Pathological conditions resulting from instabilities in physiological control systems. *Ann NY Acad Sci.* 1979;316:214–235.

Goldberger AL, Rigney D, West B. Chaos and fractals in human physiology. *Sci. Am.* 1990;43–49.

Goldberger AL, West BJ. Fractals in physiology and medicine. *Yale J Biol Med.* 1987;60:421–436.

Goldberger AL, West BJ. Chaos in physiology: health or disease? In: Degn H, Holden AV, Olsen LF, eds. *Chaos in Biological Systems.* New York, NY: Plenum Publishing Corp.; 1987:1–4.

Goldberger AA, West BJ, Bhargava V. Nonlinear mechanisms in physiology and pathophysiology: towards a dynamical theory of health and disease. In: Eisenfeld J, Witten M, eds. *Modeling of Biomedical Systems.* The Hague, Holland: Elsevier Science Publishers BV; 1986:227–233.

Greenside HS, Wolf A, Swift J, Pignataro T. Impracticality of box-counting algorithm for calculating the dimensionality of strange attractors. *Phys Rev A.* 1982;25:3453–3456.

Haken H, Kolpchen HP, eds. *Rhythms in Physiological Systems.* Berlin, Germany: Springer-Verlag; 1991.

Knudsen C, Sturis J, Thomsen JS. Generic bifurcation structures of Arnold tongues in forced oscillators. *Phys Rev A.* 1991;44:3503–3510.

Krumhansl JA. Vibrational anomalies are not generally due to fractal geometry: comments on proteins. *Phys Rev Lett.* 1986;56:2696–2699.

Layton HE, Pitman BE, Moore LC. Bifurcation analysis of TGF-mediated oscillations in SNGFR. *Am J Physiol.* 1991;261(30):F904–F919.

Liebovitch LS. Introduction to the properties and analysis of fractal objects, processes, and data. In: Marmarelis VZ, ed. *Advanced Methods of Physiological System Modeling.* Vol 2. New York, NY: Plenum Press; 1989:225–239.

Liebovitch LS, Fischbarg J, Koniarek JP. Fractal model of ion channel kinetics [abstract]. *J Gen Physiol.* 1986; 88:34a-35a.

Liebovitch LS, Fischbarg JP, Koniarek JP, Todorova I, Wang M. Fractal model of ion channel kinetics. *Biochim Biophys Acta.* 1987;896:173–180.

Lipsitz LA, Goldberger AL. Loss of "complexity" and aging: potential applications of fractals and chaos theory to senescence. *JAMA.* April 1, 1992;267(13):1806–1809.

Mackey MC, Glass L. Oscillation and chaos in physiological control systems. *Science.* 1977;197:287–289.

Oude Vrielink HHE, Slaff DW, Tangelder GJ, Weijmer-Van Velzen S, Reneman RS. Analysis of vasomotion waveform changes during pressure reduction and adenosine application. *Am J Physiol* (Heart Circ Physiol 27). 1990;258:H29–H37.

Pietronero L, Tosatti E, eds. *Fractals in Physics.* Amsterdam, Netherlands: North-Holland Physics; 1986.

Smith LA, Fournier JD, Spiegel EA. Lacunarity and intermittency in fluid turbulence. *Phys Lett A.* 1986;114A: 465–468.

Stapleton HJ, Allen JP, Flynn CP, Stinson DG, Kurtz SR. Fractal form of proteins, *Phys Rev Lett.* 1980; 45:1456–1459.

West BJ. An essay on the importance of being nonlinear. In: Levine S, ed. *Lecture Notes. Biomathematics-62.* New York, NY: Springer-Verlag; 1985.

West BJ. Physiology in fractal dimensions: error tolerance. *Ann Biomed Eng.* 1990;8:135–149.

West BJ. *Fractal Physiology and Chaos in Medicine.* Teaneck, NJ: World Scientific Press; 1990.

West BJ, Bhargava V, Goldberger AL. Beyond the principle of similitude, renormalization in the bronchial tree. *J Appl Physiol.* 1986;60:1089–1097.

West BJ, Goldberger AL. Physiology in fractal dimensions. *Am Sci.* 1987;75:354–365.

Pulmonology

Cargill EB, Donohoe K, Kolodny G, Parker JA, Zimmerman RE. Analysis of lung scans using fractals. *Proc SPIE.* 1989;1092:2–9.

Glenny RW, Robertson HT. Fractal properties of pulmonary blood flow: characterization of spatial heterogeneity. *J Appl Physiol.* 1990;69:532–545.

Glenny RW, Robertson HT. Fractal modeling of pulmonary blood flow hetergeneity. *J Appl Physiol.* 1991;70:1024–1030.

Jagoe JR, Patton KA. Reading chest radiographs for pneumoconiosis by computer. *Br J Int Med.* 1975;32: 267–272.

Katsuragawa S, Doi K, MacMahon H. Image feature analysis and computer-aided diagnosis in digital radiography: classification of normal and abnormal lungs with interstitial disease in chest images. *Med Phys.* 1989;16:38–44.

Kitaok H, Itoh H. Spatial distribution of the peripheral airways: application of fractal geometry. *Forma.* 1991; 6:181–191.

Macefield G, Gandevia SC. The cortical drive to human respiratory muscles in the awake state assessed by premotor cerebral potentials. *J Physiol.* 1991;439:545–558.

Nelson TR, Manchester DK. Modeling of lung morphogenesis using fractal geometries, *IEEE Trans Med Imaging.* 1988;7:321–327.

Nelson TR, West BJ, Goldberger AL. The fractal lung: universal and species related scaling patterns. *Experientia.* 1990;46:251–254.

West BJ, Bhargava V, Goldberger AL. Beyond similitude: renormalization in the bronchial tree. *J Appl Phys.* 1986;60:1089–1097.

Voice

Awrejcewicz J. Numerical analysis of the oscillations of human vocal cords. *Nonlinear Dynamics.* 1991;2:35–52.

Baken RJ. Irregularity of vocal period and amplitude: a first approach to the fractal analysis of voice. *J Voice.* 1990;4:185–197.

Berry D, Herzel H, Titze IR, Krischer K. Interpretation of biomechanical simulations of normal and chaotic vocal fold oscillations with empirical eigenfunctions. *J Acoust Soc Am.* 1994;95:3595–3604.

Berry DA, Herzel H, Titze I, Storey BH. Bifurcations and excised larynx experiments. *J Voice.* 1996;10(2): 129–138.

Borst C, Karemaker JM. Time delays in the human baroreceptor reflex. *J Auton Nerv Syst.* 1983;9:399.

Broad DJ. The new theories of vocal fold vibration. In: Lass NJ, ed. *Speech and Language Advances in Basic Research and Practice.* Vol 2. New York, NY: Academic Press; 1979.

Dolansky L, Tjerlund P. On certain irregularities of voice speech wave forms. *IEEE Trans.* 1968;AU-16: 51–66.

Herzel H. Bifurcations and chaos in voice signals. *Appl Mech Rev.* 1993;46:399–413.

Herzel H, Berry DA, Titze IR. Nonlinear dynamics of the voice: signal analysis and biomedical modeling. *Am Institute Phys.* 1995;5(1):30–34.

Herzel H, Mende W, Wermke K. Speech production— a dynamical system with subharmonic bifurcations and chaos. In: Plath P, ed. *Measurement and Self-Similarity,* Berlin, Germany: Springer Press; 1992.

Herzel H, Plath P, Vensson P. Experimental evidence of homoclinic chaos and type-2 intermittency during the oxidation of methanol. *Physica.* 1991;48D:340–352.

Herzel H, Steincke I, Mende W, Wermke K. Chaos and bifurcations during voiced speech. In: Mosekilde E, ed. *Complexity, Chaos and Biological Evolution.* New York, NY: Plenum; 1991:41.

Herzel H, Wendler J. Evidence of chaos in phonatory samples. In: *Proceedings of EUROSPEECH;* Geneva, Switzerland: ESCA; 1991:263–266.

Ishizaka K, Isshiki N. Computer simulation of pathological vocal cord vibration. *J Acoust Soc Am.* 1976;60:1193–1198.

Ishizaka K, Matsudaira N. Fluid mechanical considerations of vocal fold vibration. *Speech Commun Res Lab.* 1972;8.

Lauterborn W, Cramer E. Subharmonic routes to chaos observed in acoustics. *Phys Rev Lett.* 1981;47:1445–1448.

Lauterborn W, Parlitz U. Methods of chaos physics and their application to acoustics. *J Acoust Soc Am.* 1988;84:1975–1993.

Lucero JC. Dynamics of the two-mass model of the vocal folds: equilibria, bifurcations, and oscillation region. *J Acoust Soc Am.* 1993;94:3104–3111.

Moore G, von Leden H. Dynamic variation of the vibratory pattern in the normal larynx. *Folia Phoniatrica.* 1958;10:205–238.

Pickover CA, Khorsani A. Fractal characterizations of speech waveform graphs. *Comput Graphics.* 1986;10:51–61.

Tenney S. Art and science: where numerology and mathematics touch the lung. *Can Respir J.* 1994;1(4):241–247.

Titze IR. The human vocal cords: A mathematical model, part I. *Phonetica.* 1973;28:129–170.

Titze IR. The physics of small amplitude oscillations of the vocal folds. *J Acoust Soc Am.* 1988;83:1536–1552.

Titze IR. A model of neurologic sources of aperiodicities in vocal fold vibration. *J Speech Hear Res.* 1991;34:460–472.

Titze IR, ed. *Vocal Fold Physiology: New Frontiers in Basic Science.* San Diego, Calif: Singular Publishing Group, Inc.; 1993:143–188.

Voss RF, Clark J. "1/f noise" in music and speech. *Nature (Lond).* 1975;258:317–318.